The Essential Physics of Medical Imaging

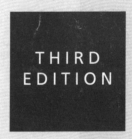

THIRD EDITION

JERROLD T. BUSHBERG, PhD
Clinical Professor of Radiology and Radiation Oncology
University of California, Davis
Sacramento, California

J. ANTHONY SEIBERT, PhD
Professor of Radiology
University of California, Davis
Sacramento, California

EDWIN M. LEIDHOLDT JR, PhD
Clinical Associate Professor of Radiology
University of California, Davis
Sacramento, California

JOHN M. BOONE, PhD
Professor of Radiology and Biomedical Engineering
University of California, Davis
Sacramento, California

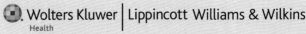 Wolters Kluwer | Lippincott Williams & Wilkins
Health
Philadelphia · Baltimore · New York · London
Buenos Aires · Hong Kong · Sydney · Tokyo

Executive Editor: Charles W. Mitchell
Product Manager: Ryan Shaw
Vendor Manager: Alicia Jackson
Senior Manufacturing Manager: Benjamin Rivera
Senior Marketing Manager: Angela Panetta
Design Coordinator: Stephen Druding
Production Service: SPi Global

Library of Congress Cataloging-in-Publication Data
Bushberg, Jerrold T.
 The essential physics of medical imaging / Jerrold T. Bushberg. — 3rd ed.
   p. ; cm.
 Includes bibliographical references and index.
 ISBN 978-1-4511-1810-0
 1. Diagnostic imaging. 2. Medical physics. I. Title.
 [DNLM: 1. Diagnostic Imaging—methods. WN 200]
 RC78.7.D53E87 2011
 616.07'54—dc22

                                                                    2011004310

Care has been taken to confirm the accuracy of the information presented and to describe generally accepted practices. However, the authors, editors, and publisher are not responsible for errors or omissions or for any consequences from application of the information in this book and make no warranty, expressed or implied, with respect to the currency, completeness, or accuracy of the contents of the publication. Application of the information in a particular situation remains the professional responsibility of the practitioner.

The authors, editors, and publisher have exerted every effort to ensure that drug selection and dosage set forth in this text are in accordance with current recommendations and practice at the time of publication. However, in view of ongoing research, changes in government regulations, and the constant flow of information relating to drug therapy and drug reactions, the reader is urged to check the package insert for each drug for any change in indications and dosage and for added warnings and precautions. This is particularly important when the recommended agent is a new or infrequently employed drug.

Some drugs and medical devices presented in the publication have Food and Drug Administration (FDA) clearance for limited use in restricted research settings. It is the responsibility of the health care provider to ascertain the FDA status of each drug or device planned for use in their clinical practice.

To purchase additional copies of this book, call our customer service department at (800) 638-3030 or fax orders to (301) 223-2320. International customers should call (301) 223-2300.

Visit Lippincott Williams & Wilkins on the Internet: at LWW.com. Lippincott Williams & Wilkins customer service representatives are available from 8:30 am to 6 pm, EST.

10 9 8 7 6 5 4 3 2 1

First and foremost, I offer my most heartfelt love, appreciation and apology to my wife Lori and our children, Alex and Jennifer, who endured my many absences to focus on completing this text with "almost" infinite patience (especially during the last 4 months, when I was typically gone before they woke and got home long after they had gone to sleep). I look forward to spending much more time with my family and even to starting to make a dent in the list of "chores" my wife has been amassing in my absence. I have also had the good fortune to be supported by my extended family and my Oakshore neighbors who never missed an opportunity to offer an encouraging word after my response to their question "Is the book done yet?"

Second, I would like to express my profound gratitude to my coauthors, colleagues, and friends Tony, Ed, and John for their herculean efforts to bring this 3rd edition into existence. Not only would this text not exist without them, but the synergy of their combined skills, expertise, and insights was an invaluable resource at every stage of development of this edition. We all have many more professional obligations now than during the writing of the previous editions. The willingness and ability of my coauthors to add another substantial commitment of time to their already compressed professional lives were truly remarkable and greatly appreciated.

While all of my staff and colleagues have been very helpful and supportive during this effort (for which I am very grateful), two individuals deserve special recognition. Linda Kroger's willingness to proof read several chapters for clarity along with the countless other ways she provided her support and assistance during this effort with her typical intelligent efficiency was invaluable and greatly appreciated. Lorraine Smith has been the coordinator of our annual radiology resident physics review course for as long as I can remember. This course would not be possible without her considerable contribution to its success. Lorraine is one of the most helpful, resourceful, patient, and pleasant individuals I have ever had the pleasure to work with. Her invaluable assistance with this course, from which this book was developed, is gratefully acknowledged and deeply appreciated.

I would also like to thank our publisher Lippincott Williams and Wilkins, Charley Mitchell, Lisa McAllister, and in particular Ryan Shaw (our editor) for the opportunity to develop the 3rd edition. Your patience, support, and firm "encouragement" to complete this effort are truly appreciated.

I dedicate this edition to my parents. My mother, Annette Lorraine Bushberg (1929–1981), had a gift for bringing out the best in me. She cheered my successes, reassured me after my failures, and was an unwavering source of love and support. My father, Norman Talmadge Bushberg, brightens everyone's world with his effortless wit and sense of humor. In addition to his ever present love and encouragement, which have meant more to me than I can find the words to fully express, he continues to inspire me with his belief in each person's ability and responsibility to make a unique contribution. To that end, and at the age of 83, he recently published his first literary contribution, a children's story entitled "Once Upon a Time in Kansas." It is slightly lighter reading than our text and I highly recommend it. However, if getting your child to fall asleep is the problem, then any chapter in our book should do the trick.

J.T.B.

Thanks, TSPOON, for your perseverance, patience, and understanding in regard to your often AWOL dad during these past several years—it's very gratifying to see you prosper in college, and maybe someday you will be involved in writing a book as well! And to you, Julie Rainwater, for adding more than you know to my well-being and happiness.

J.A.S.

To my family, especially my parents and my grandmother Mrs. Pearl Ellett Crowgey, and my teachers, especially my high school mathematics teacher Mrs. Neola Waller, and Drs. James L. Kelly, Roger Rydin, W. Reed Johnson, and Denny D. Watson of the University of Virginia. To two nuclear medicine physicists, Drs. Mark W. Groch and L. Stephen Graham, who contributed to earlier editions of this book, but did not live to see this edition. And to Jacalyn Killeen, who has shown considerable patience during the last year.

E.M.L.

Susan Fris Boone, my wife, makes life on this planet possible and her companionship and support have made my contribution to this book possible. Emily and Julian, children extraordinaire and both wild travelers of the world, have grown up using earlier editions of this book as paperweights, lampstands, and coasters. I appreciate the perspective. Marion (Mom) and Jerry (Dad) passed in the last few years, but the support and love they bestowed on me over their long lives will never be forgotten. Sister Patt demonstrated infinite compassion while nurturing our parents during their final years and is an angel for all but the wings. Brother Bob is a constant reminder of dedication to patient care, and I hope that someday he and I will both win our long-standing bet. Friends Steve and Susan have elevated the fun in life. My recent students, Nathan, Clare, Shonket, Orlando, Lin, Sarah, Nicolas, Anita, and Peymon have helped keep the flag of research flying in the laboratory, and I am especially in debt to Dr. Kai Yang and Mr. George Burkett who have helped hold it all together during my too frequent travel. There are many more to thank, but not enough ink. This book was first published in 1994, and over the many years since, I have had the privilege of sharing the cover credits with my coauthors and good friends Tony, Jerry, and Ed. This has been a wild ride and it would have been far less interesting if not shared with these tres amigos.

J.M.B.

There has been an
Alarming Increase
? in the Number
of Things
I Know
Nothing About

Preface to the Third Edition

The first edition of this text was written in 1993, and the second edition followed in 2002. This third edition, coming almost 10 years after the second edition, reflects the considerable changes that have occurred in medical imaging over the past decade. While the "digitization" of medical images outside of nuclear medicine began in earnest between the publication of the first and second editions, the transformation of medical imaging to an all-digital environment is largely complete at the time of this writing. Recognizing this, we have substantially reduced the treatment of analog modalities in this edition, including only a short discussion on screen-film radiography and mammography, for example. Because the picture archiving and communication system (PACS) is now a concrete reality for virtually all radiological image interpretation, and because of the increasing integration between the radiology information systems (RISs), the PACS, and the electronic medical record (EMR), the informatics section has been expanded considerably.

There is more to know now than 10 years ago, so we reduced some of the detail that existed in previous editions that may be considered *nonessential* today. Detailed discussions of x-ray tube heating and cooling charts, three-phase x-ray generator circuits, and CT generations have been shortened or eliminated.

The cumulative radiation dose to the population of the United States from medical imaging has increased about sixfold since 1980, and the use of unacceptably large radiation doses for imaging patients, including children, has been reported. In recent years, radiation dose from medical imaging and radiation therapy has become the focus of much media attention, with a number of radiologists, radiobiologists, and medical physicists testifying before the FDA and the U.S. Congress regarding the use of radiation in imaging and radiation therapy. The media attention has given rise to heightened interest of patients and regulatory agencies in the topics of reporting and optimizing radiation dose as well as limiting its potentially harmful biological effects. In this edition, we have added an additional chapter devoted to the topic of x-ray dose and substantially expanded the chapters on radiation biology and radiation protection. The current International Commission on Radiological Protection system of estimating the potential detriment (harm) to an irradiated population; the calculation of effective dose and its appropriate use; as well as the most recent National Academy of Sciences *Biological Effects of Ionizing Radiation* (BEIR VII) report recommended approach of computing radiation risk to a specific individual are discussed in several chapters.

Our publisher has indicated that the second edition was used by increasing numbers of graduate students in medical imaging programs. While the target audience of this text is still radiologists-in-training, we have added appendices and other sections with more mathematical rigor than in past editions to increase relevance to scientists-in-training. The goal of providing physicians a text that describes image science and the radiological modalities in plain English remains, but this third edition contains an appendix on Fourier transforms and convolution, and Chapter 4 covers basic image science with some optional mathematics for graduate student readers and for radiologists with calculus-based undergraduate degrees.

A number of new technologies that were research projects 10 years ago have entered clinical use, and this edition discusses the more important of these: tomosynthesis in mammography, cone beam CT, changes in mammography anode composition, the exposure index in radiography, flat panel fluoroscopy, rotational CT on fluoroscopy systems, iterative reconstruction in CT, and dual modality imaging systems such as PET/CT and SPECT/CT. Some new technologies offer the possibility of substantially reducing the radiation dose per imaging procedure.

All of the authors of this book are involved in some way or another with national or international advisory organizations, and we have added some perspectives from published documents from the American Association of Physicists in Medicine, the National Council on Radiation Protection and Measurements, the International Commission on Radiation Units and Measurement, and others.

Lastly, with the third edition we transition to color figures, tables, text headings, and photographs. Most of the figures are newly designed; some are colorized versions of figures from previous editions of the text. This edition has been completely rewritten and a small percentage of the text remains as it was in previous editions. We hope that our efforts on this third edition bring this text to a completely up-to-date status and that we have captured the most important developments in the field of radiology so that the text remains current for several years to come.

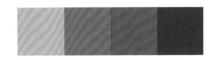

Foreword

Dr. Bushberg and his coauthors have kept the title *The Essential Physics of Medical Imaging* for this third edition. While the first edition in 1994 contained the "essentials," by the time the second edition appeared in 2002, the book had expanded significantly and included not only physics but also a more in depth discussion of radiation protection, dosimetry, and radiation biology. The second edition became the "go to" reference book for medical imaging physics. While not light weekend reading, the book is probably the only one in the field that you will need on your shelf. Residents will be happy to know that the third edition contains the topics recommended by the AAPM and thus likely to appear on future examinations.

Although there are shorter books for board review, those typically are in outline form and may not be sufficient for the necessary understanding of the topics. This book is the one most used by residents, medical imaging faculty, and physicists. On more than one occasion I have heard our university biomedical physicists ask, "What does Bushberg's book say?"

The attractive aspects of the book include its completeness, clarity, and ability to answer questions that I have. This is likely a consequence of the authors having run a resident review course for almost 30 years, during which they have undoubtedly heard every question and point of confusion that a nonphysicist could possibly raise. I must say that on the door to my office I keep displayed a quote from the second edition: "Every day there is an alarming increase in the number of things I know nothing about." Unfortunately, I find this true regarding many things besides medical physics.

My only suggestion to the authors is that in subsequent editions they delete the word "Essentials" from the title, for that word does not do justice to the staggering amount of work they have done in preparing this edition's remarkably clear text or to the 750+ illustrations that will continue to set the standard for books in this field.

Fred A. Mettler Jr, MD, MPH
Clinical and Emeritus Professor
University of New Mexico School of Medicine

Acknowledgments

During the production of this work, several individuals generously gave their time and expertise. Without their help, this new edition would not have been possible. The authors would like to express their gratitude for the invaluable contributions of the following individuals:

Craig Abbey, PhD
University of California, Santa Barbara

Ramsey Badawi, PhD
University of California, Davis

John D. Boice Jr, ScD
Vanderbilt University
Vanderbilt-Ingram Cancer Center

Michael Buonocore, MD, PhD
University of California, Davis

Dianna Cody, PhD
MD Anderson Cancer Center

Michael Cronan, RDMS
University of California, Davis

Brian Dahlin, MD
University of California, Davis

Robert Dixon, PhD
Wake Forest University

Raymond Dougherty, MD
University of California, Davis

Ken Eldridge, RT(R)(N)

William Erwin, MS
UT MD Anderson Cancer Center Houston, TX

Kathryn Held, PhD
Massachusetts General Hospital Harvard Medical School

Jiang Hsieh, PhD
General Electric Medical Systems

Kiran Jain, MD
University of California, Davis

Willi Kalender, PhD
Institute of Medical Physics, Erlangen, Germany

Frederick W. Kremkau, PhD
Wake Forest University School of Medicine

Linda Kroger, MS
University of California, Davis Health System

Ramit Lamba, MD
University of California, Davis

Karen Lindfors, MD
University of California, Davis

Mahadevappa Mahesh, PhD
Johns Hopkins University

Cynthia McCollough, PhD
Mayo Clinic, Rochester

John McGahan, MD
University of California, Davis

Sarah McKenney
University of California, Davis

Michael McNitt-Gray, PhD
University of California. Los Angeles

Fred A. Mettler Jr, MD, MPH
University of New Mexico School of Medicine

Stuart Mirell, PhD
University of California at Los Angeles

Norbert Pelc, ScD
Stanford University

Otto G. Raabe, PhD
University of California, Davis

Werner Roeck, Dipl Eng
University of California, Irvine

John Sabol, PhD
General Electric Medical Systems

D.K. Shelton, MD
University fo California, Davis

Jeffrey Siewerdsen, PhD
Johns Hopkins University

Michael G. Stabin, PhD
Vanderbilt University

Steve Wilkendorf, RDMS
University of California, Davis

Sandra Wootton-Gorges, MD
University of California, Davis

Kai Yang, PhD
University of California, Davis

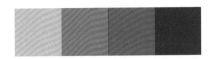

Contents

Basic Concepts

CHAPTER 1

Introduction to Medical Imaging

Medical imaging of the human body requires some form of energy. In the medical imaging techniques used in radiology, the energy used to produce the image must be capable of penetrating tissues. Visible light, which has limited ability to penetrate tissues at depth, is used mostly outside of the radiology department for medical imaging. Visible light images are used in dermatology (skin photography), gastroenterology and obstetrics (endoscopy), and pathology (light microscopy). Of course, all disciplines in medicine use direct visual observation, which also utilizes visible light. In diagnostic radiology, the electromagnetic spectrum outside the visible light region is used for medical imaging, including x-rays in mammography and computed tomography (CT); radiofrequency (RF) in magnetic resonance imaging (MRI), and gamma rays in nuclear medicine. Mechanical energy, in the form of high-frequency sound waves, is used in ultrasound imaging.

With the exception of nuclear medicine, all medical imaging requires that the energy used to penetrate the body's tissues also interacts with those tissues. If energy were to pass through the body and not experience some type of interaction (e.g., absorption or scattering), then the detected energy would not contain any useful information regarding the internal anatomy, and thus it would not be possible to construct an image of the anatomy using that information. In nuclear medicine imaging, radioactive substances are injected or ingested, and it is the physiological *interactions* of the agent that give rise to the information in the images.

While medical images can have an aesthetic appearance, the diagnostic utility of a medical image relates both to the technical quality of the image and the conditions of its acquisition. Consequently, the assessment of image quality in medical imaging involves very little artistic appraisal and a great deal of technical evaluation. In most cases, the image quality that is obtained from medical imaging devices involves compromise—better x-ray images can be made when the radiation dose to the patient is high, better magnetic resonance images can be made when the image acquisition time is long, and better ultrasound images result when the ultrasound power levels are large. Of course, patient safety and comfort must be considered when acquiring medical images; thus, excessive patient dose in the pursuit of a perfect image is not acceptable. Rather, the power and energy used to make medical images require a balance between patient safety and image quality.

1.1 The Modalities

Different types of medical images can be made by varying the types of energies and the acquisition technology used. The different modes of making images are referred to as *modalities*. Each modality has its own applications in medicine.

Radiography

Radiography was the first medical imaging technology, made possible when the physicist Wilhelm Roentgen discovered x-rays on November 8, 1895. Roentgen also made the first radiographic images of human anatomy (Fig. 1-1). Radiography (also called roentgenography) defined the field of radiology and gave rise to radiologists, physicians who specialize in the interpretation of medical images. Radiography is performed with an x-ray source on one side of the patient and a (typically flat) x-ray detector on the other side. A short-duration (typically less than ½ second) pulse of x-rays is emitted by the x-ray tube, a large fraction of the x-rays interact in the patient, and some of the x-rays pass through the patient and reach the detector, where a radiographic image is formed. The homogeneous distribution of x-rays that enters the patient is modified by the degree to which the x-rays are removed from the beam (i.e., attenuated) by scattering and absorption within the tissues. The attenuation properties of tissues such as bone, soft tissue, and air inside the patient are very different, resulting in a heterogeneous distribution of x-rays that emerges from the patient. The radiographic image is a picture of this x-ray distribution. The detector used in radiography can be photographic film (e.g., screen-film radiography) or an electronic detector system (i.e., digital radiography).

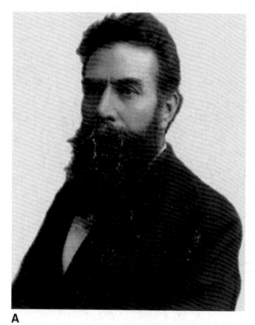 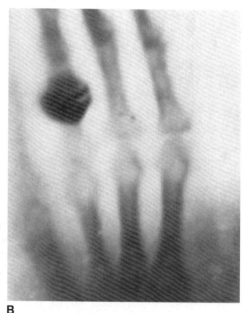

A   **B**

■ **FIGURE 1-1** Wilhelm Conrad Roentgen (1845–1923) in 1896 (**A**). Roentgen received the first Nobel Prize in Physics in 1901 for his discovery of x-rays on November 8, 1895. The beginning of diagnostic radiology is represented by this famous radiographic image, made by Roentgen on December 22, 1895 of his wife's hand (**B**). The bones of her hand as well as two rings on her finger are clearly visible. Within a few months, Roentgen had determined the basic physical properties of x-rays. Roentgen published his findings in a preliminary report entitled "On a New Kind of Rays" on December 28, 1895 in the Proceedings of the Physico-Medical Society of Wurzburg. An English translation was published in the journal Nature on January 23, 1896. Almost simultaneously, as word of the discovery spread around the world, medical applications of this "new kind of ray" rapidly made radiological imaging an essential component of medical care. In keeping with mathematical conventions, Roentgen assigned the letter "x" to represent the unknown nature of the ray and thus the term "x-rays" was born.

Transmission imaging refers to imaging in which the energy source is outside the body on one side, and the energy passes through the body and is detected on the other side of the body. Radiography is a transmission imaging modality. *Projection imaging* refers to the case when each point on the image corresponds to information along a straight-line trajectory through the patient. Radiography is also a projection imaging modality. Radiographic images are useful for a very wide range of medical indications, including the diagnosis of broken bones, lung cancer, cardiovascular disorders, etc. (Fig. 1-2).

Fluoroscopy

Fluoroscopy refers to the continuous acquisition of a sequence of x-ray images over time, essentially a real-time x-ray movie of the patient. It is a transmission projection imaging modality, and is, in essence, just real-time radiography. Fluoroscopic systems use x-ray detector systems capable of producing images in rapid temporal sequence. Fluoroscopy is used for positioning catheters in arteries, visualizing contrast agents in the GI tract, and for other medical applications such as invasive therapeutic procedures where real-time image feedback is necessary. It is also used to make x-ray movies of anatomic motion, such as of the heart or the esophagus.

Mammography

Mammography is radiography of the breast, and is thus a transmission projection type of imaging. To accentuate contrast in the breast, mammography makes use of

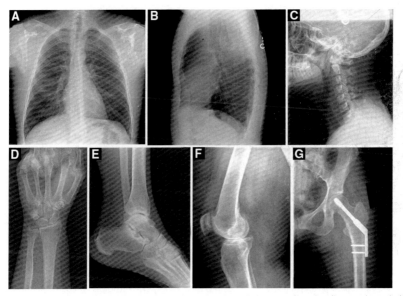

■ FIGURE 1-2 Chest radiography is the most common imaging procedure in diagnostic radiology, often acquired as orthogonal posterior-anterior (**A**) and lateral (**B**) projections to provide information regarding depth and position of the anatomy. High-energy x-rays are used to reduce the conspicuity of the ribs and other bones to permit better visualization of air spaces and soft tissue structures in the thorax. The image is a map of the attenuation of the x-rays: dark areas (high film optical density) correspond to low attenuation, and bright areas (low film optical density) correspond to high attenuation. **C.** Lateral cervical spine radiographs are commonly performed to assess suspected neck injury after trauma, and extremity images of the (**D**) wrist, (**E**) ankle, and (**F**) knee provide low-dose, cost-effective diagnostic information. **G.** Metal objects, such as this orthopedic implant designed for fixation of certain types of femoral fractures, are well seen on radiographs.

much lower x-ray energies than general purpose radiography, and consequently the x-ray and detector systems are designed specifically for breast imaging. Mammography is used to screen asymptomatic women for breast cancer (screening mammography) and is also used to aid in the diagnosis of women with breast symptoms such as the presence of a lump (diagnostic mammography) (Fig. 1-3A). Digital mammography has eclipsed the use of screen-film mammography in the United States, and the use of computer-aided detection is widespread in digital mammography. Some digital mammography systems are now capable of tomosynthesis, whereby the x-ray tube (and in some cases the detector) moves in an arc from approximately 7 to 40 degrees around the breast. This limited angle tomographic method leads to the reconstruction of tomosynthesis images (Fig. 1-3B), which are parallel to the plane of the detector, and can reduce the superimposition of anatomy above and below the in-focus plane.

Computed Tomography

Computed tomography (CT) became clinically available in the early 1970s, and is the first medical imaging modality made possible by the computer. CT images are produced by passing x-rays through the body at a large number of angles, by rotating the x-ray tube around the body. A detector array, opposite the x-ray source, collects the transmission projection data. The numerous data points collected in this manner

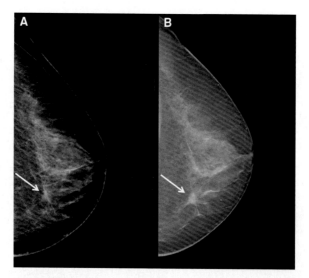

■ **FIGURE 1-3** Mammography is a specialized x-ray projection imaging technique useful for detecting breast anomalies such as masses and calcifications. Dedicated mammography equipment uses low x-ray energies, K-edge filters, compression, screen/film or digital detectors, antiscatter grids and automatic exposure control to produce breast images of high quality and low x-ray dose. The digital mammogram in (**A**) shows glandular and fatty tissues, the skin line of the breast, and a possibly cancerous mass (*arrow*). In projection mammography, superposition of tissues at different depths can mask the features of malignancy or cause artifacts that mimic tumors. The digital tomosynthesis image in (**B**) shows a mid-depth synthesized tomogram. By reducing overlying and underlying anatomy with the tomosynthesis, the suspected mass in the breast is clearly depicted with a spiculated appearance, indicative of cancer. X-ray mammography currently is the procedure of choice for screening and early detection of breast cancer because of high sensitivity, excellent benefit-to-risk ratio, and low cost.

are synthesized by a computer into *tomographic* images of the patient. The term tomography refers to a picture (*graph*) of a slice (*tomo*). CT is a transmission technique that results in images of individual slabs of tissue in the patient. The advantage of CT over radiography is its ability to display three-dimensional (3D) slices of the anatomy of interest, eliminating the superposition of anatomical structures and thereby presenting an unobstructed view of detailed anatomy to the physician.

CT changed the practice of medicine by substantially reducing the need for exploratory surgery. Modern CT scanners can acquire 0.50- to 0.62-mm-thick tomographic images along a 50-cm length of the patient (i.e., 800 images) in 5 seconds, and reveal the presence of cancer, ruptured disks, subdural hematomas, aneurysms, and many other pathologies (Fig. 1-4). The CT volume data set is essentially isotropic, which has led to the increased use of coronal and sagittal CT images, in addition to traditional axial images in CT. There are a number of different acquisition modes available on modern CT scanners, including dual-energy imaging, organ perfusion imaging, and prospectively gated cardiac CT. While CT is usually used for anatomic imaging, the use of iodinated contrast injected intravenously allows the functional assessment of various organs as well.

Because of the speed of acquisition, the high-quality diagnostic images, and the widespread availability of CT in the United States, CT has replaced a number of imaging procedures that were previously performed radiographically. This trend continues. However, the wide-scale incorporation of CT into diagnostic medicine has led to more than 60 million CT scans being performed annually in the United States. This large number has led to an increase in the radiation burden in the United States, such that now about half of medical radiation is due to CT. Radiation levels from medical imaging are now equivalent to background radiation levels in the United States, (NCRP 2009).

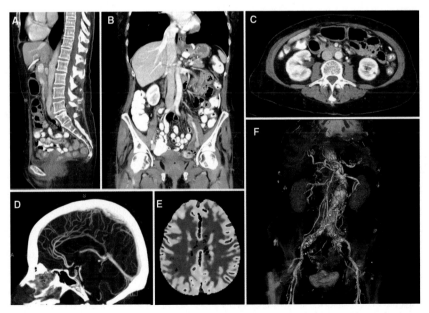

■ **FIGURE 1-4** CT reveals superb anatomical detail, as seen in (**A**) sagittal, (**B**) coronal, and (**C**) axial images from an abdomen-pelvis CT scan. With the injection of iodinated contrast material, CT angiography (CTA) can be performed, here (**D**) showing CTA of the head. Analysis of a sequence of temporal images allows assessment of perfusion; (**E**) demonstrates a color coded map corresponding to blood volume in this patient undergoing evaluation for a suspected cerebrovascular accident ("stroke"). **F.** Image processing can produce pseudocolored 3D representations of the anatomy from the CT data.

Magnetic Resonance Imaging

Magnetic resonance imaging (MRI) scanners use magnetic fields that are about 10,000 to 60,000 times stronger than the earth's magnetic field. Most MRI utilizes the nuclear magnetic resonance properties of the proton—that is, the nucleus of the hydrogen atom, which is very abundant in biological tissues (each cubic millimeter of tissue contains about 10^{18} protons). The proton has a magnetic moment and, when placed in a 1.5 T magnetic field, the proton precesses (wobbles) about its axis and preferentially absorbs radio wave energy at the resonance frequency of about 64 million cycles per second (megahertz—MHz).

In MRI, the patient is placed in the magnetic field, and a pulse of radio waves is generated by antennas ("coils") positioned around the patient. The protons in the patient absorb the radio waves, and subsequently reemit this radio wave energy after a period of time that depends upon the spatially dependent magnetic properties of the tissue. The radio waves emitted by the protons in the patient are detected by the antennas that surround the patient. By slightly changing the strength of the magnetic field as a function of position in the patient using magnetic field *gradients*, the proton resonance frequency varies as a function of position, since frequency is proportional to magnetic field strength. The MRI system uses the frequency and phase of the returning radio waves to determine the position of each signal from the patient. One frequently used mode of operation of MRI systems is referred to as *spin echo* imaging.

MRI produces a set of tomographic images depicting slices through the patient, in which each point in an image depends on the micromagnetic properties of the tissue corresponding to that point. Because different types of tissue such as fat, white and gray matter in the brain, cerebral spinal fluid, and cancer all have different local magnetic properties, images made using MRI demonstrate high sensitivity to anatomical variations and therefore are high in contrast. MRI has demonstrated exceptional utility in neurological imaging (head and spine) and for musculoskeletal applications such as imaging the knee after athletic injury (Fig. 1-5A–D).

MRI is a tomographic imaging modality, and competes with x-ray CT in many clinical applications. The acquisition of the highest quality images using MRI requires tens of minutes, whereas a CT scan of the entire head requires seconds. Thus, for patients where motion cannot be controlled (pediatric patients) or in anatomical areas where involuntary patient motion occurs (the beating heart and churning intestines), CT is often used instead of MRI. Also, because of the large magnetic field used in MRI, only specialized electronic monitoring equipment can be used while the patient is being scanned. Thus, for most trauma, CT is preferred. MRI should not be performed on patients who have cardiac pacemakers or internal ferromagnetic objects such as surgical aneurysm clips, metal plate or rod implants, or metal shards near critical anatomy such as the eye.

Despite some indications for which MRI should not be used, fast image acquisition techniques using special coils have made it possible to produce images in much shorter periods of time, and this has opened up the potential of using MRI for imaging of the motion-prone thorax and abdomen (Fig. 1-5E). MRI scanners can also detect the presence of motion, which is useful for monitoring blood flow through arteries (MR *angiography*—Figure 1-5F), as well as blood flow in the brain (*functional* MR), which leads to the ability to measure brain function correlated to a task (e.g., finger tapping, response to various stimuli, etc.).

An area of MR data collection that allows for analysis of metabolic products in the tissue is MR *spectroscopy*, whereby a single voxel or multiple voxels may be analyzed

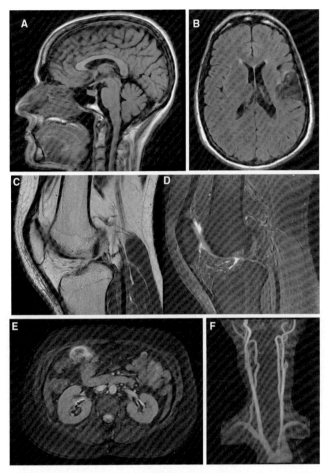

■ **FIGURE 1-5** MRI provides excellent and selectable tissue contrast, determined by acquisition pulse sequences and data acquisition methods. Tomographic images can be acquired and displayed in any plane including conventional axial, sagittal and coronal planes. (**A**) Sagittal T1-weighted contrast image of the brain; (**B**) axial fluid-attenuated inversion recovery (FLAIR) image showing an area of brain infarct; sagittal image of the knee, with (**C**) T1-weighted contrast and (**D**) T1-weighted contrast with "fat saturation" (fat signal is selectively reduced) to visualize structures and signals otherwise overwhelmed by the large fat signal; (**E**) maximum intensity projection generated from the axial tomographic images of a time-of-flight MR angiogram; (**F**) gadolinium contrast-enhanced abdominal image, acquired with a fast imaging employing steady-state acquisition sequence, which allows very short acquisition times to provide high signal-to-noise ratio of fluid-filled structures and reduce the effects of patient motion.

using specialized MRI sequences to evaluate the biochemical composition of tissues in a precisely defined volume. The spectroscopic signal can act as a signature for tumors and other maladies.

Ultrasound Imaging

When a book is dropped on a table, the impact causes pressure waves (called sound) to propagate through the air such that they can be heard at a distance. Mechanical energy in the form of high-frequency ("ultra") sound can be used to generate images of the anatomy of a patient. A short-duration pulse of sound is generated by an ultrasound *transducer* that is in direct physical contact with the tissues being imaged. The sound waves travel into the tissue, and are reflected by internal structures in the body, creating echoes. The reflected sound waves then reach the transducer, which records the returning sound. This mode of operation of an ultrasound device is called *pulse echo* imaging. The sound beam is swept over a slice of the patient line by line using a linear array multielement transducer to produce a rectangular scanned area, or through incremental angles with a phased array multielement transducer to produce a sector scanned area. The echo amplitudes from each line of ultrasound are recorded and used to compute a brightness mode image with grayscale-encoded acoustic signals representing a tomographic slice of the tissues of interest.

Ultrasound is reflected strongly by interfaces, such as the surfaces and internal structures of abdominal organs. Because ultrasound is thought to be less harmful than ionizing radiation to a growing fetus, ultrasound imaging is preferred in obstetrical patients (Fig. 1-6A,B). An interface between tissue and air is highly echoic, and thus, very little sound can penetrate from tissue into an air-filled cavity. Therefore, ultrasound imaging has less utility in the thorax where the air in the lungs presents a

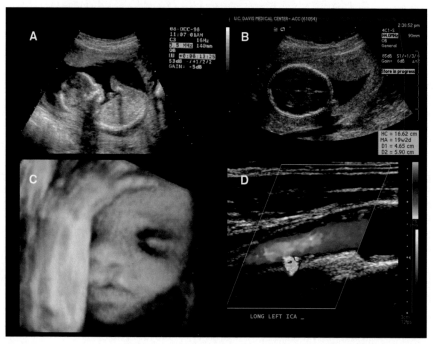

■ **FIGURE 1-6** The ultrasound image is a map of the echoes from tissue boundaries of high-frequency sound wave pulses. **A.** A phased-array transducer operating at 3.5 MHz produced the normal obstetrical ultrasound image (sagittal profile) of Jennifer Lauren Bushberg at 5½ months before her "first birthday." Variations in the image brightness are due to acoustic characteristics of the tissues; for example, the fluid in the placenta is echo free, whereas most fetal tissues are echogenic and produce larger returned signals. Acoustic shadowing is caused by highly attenuating or scattering tissues, such as bone or air, producing the corresponding low intensity streaks distal to the transducer. **B.** Distance measurements (e.g., fetal head diameter assessment for age estimation) are part of the diagnostic evaluation of a cross-sectional brain ultrasound image of a fetus. **C.** From a stack of tomographic images acquired with known geometry and image locations, 3D image rendering of the acoustic image data can show anatomic findings, such as a cleft palate of the fetus. **D.** Vascular assessment using Doppler color-flow imaging can be performed by many ultrasound systems. A color-flow image of the internal carotid artery superimposed on the grayscale image demonstrates an aneurysm in the left internal carotid artery of this patient.

barrier that the sound beam cannot penetrate. Similarly, an interface between tissue and bone is also highly echoic, thus making brain imaging, for example, impractical in most cases. Because each ultrasound image represents a tomographic slice, multiple images spaced a known distance apart represent a volume of tissue, and with specialized algorithms, anatomy can be reconstructed with volume rendering methods as shown in Figure 1-6C.

Doppler Ultrasound

Doppler ultrasound makes use of a phenomenon familiar to train enthusiasts. For the observer standing beside railroad tracks as a rapidly moving train goes by blowing its whistle, the pitch of the whistle is higher as the train approaches and becomes lower as the train passes by the observer and speeds off into the distance. The change in the pitch of the whistle, which is an apparent change in the frequency of the sound, is a result of the Doppler effect. The same phenomenon occurs at ultrasound frequencies, and the change in frequency (the Doppler shift) is used to measure the motion of blood. Both the speed and direction of blood flow can be measured, and within a subarea of the grayscale image, a color flow display typically shows blood flow in one direction as red, and in the other direction as blue. In Figure 1-6D, a color-flow map reveals arterial flow of the left internal carotid artery superimposed upon the grayscale image; the small, multicolored nub on the vessel demonstrates complex flow patterns of an ulcerated aneurysm.

Nuclear Medicine Imaging

Nuclear medicine is the branch of radiology in which a chemical or other substance containing a radioactive isotope is given to the patient orally, by injection or by inhalation. Once the material has distributed itself according to the physiological status of the patient, a radiation detector is used to make projection images from the x- and/or gamma rays emitted during radioactive decay of the agent. Nuclear medicine produces emission images (as opposed to transmission images), because the radioisotopes emit their energy from inside the patient.

Nuclear medicine imaging is a form of functional imaging. Rather than yielding information about just the anatomy of the patient, nuclear medicine images provide information regarding the physiological conditions in the patient. For example, thallium tends to concentrate in normal heart muscle, but in areas that are infarcted or are ischemic, thallium does not concentrate as well. These areas appear as "cold spots" on a nuclear medicine image, and are indicative of the functional status of the heart. Thyroid tissue has a great affinity for iodine, and by administering radioactive iodine (or its analogues), the thyroid can be imaged. If thyroid cancer has metastasized in the patient, then "hot spots" indicating their location may be present on the nuclear medicine images. Thus functional imaging is the forte of nuclear medicine.

Nuclear Medicine Planar Imaging

Nuclear medicine planar images are projection images, since each point on the image is representative of the radioisotope activity along a line projected through the patient. Planar nuclear images are essentially 2D maps of the 3D radioisotope distribution, and are helpful in the evaluation of a large number of disorders (Fig. 1-7).

■ **FIGURE 1-7** Anterior and posterior whole-body bone scan images of a 64-year-old male with prostate cancer. This patient was injected with 925 MBq (25 mCi) of ^{99m}Tc methylenediphosphonate (MDP) and was imaged 3 hours later with a dual-head scintillation camera. The images demonstrate multiple metastatic lesions. Lesions are readily seen in ribs, sternum, spine, pelvis, femurs and left tibia. Planar imaging is still the standard for many nuclear medicine examinations (e.g., whole-body bone scans and hepatobiliary thyroid, renal and pulmonary studies). (Image courtesy of DK Shelton.)

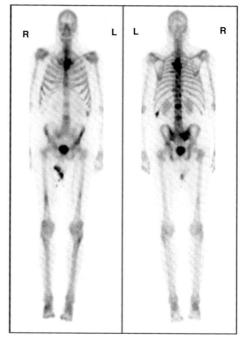

Single Photon Emission Computed Tomography

Single photon emission computed tomography (SPECT) is the tomographic counterpart of nuclear medicine planar imaging, just like CT is the tomographic counterpart of radiography. In SPECT, a nuclear camera records x- or gamma-ray emissions from the patient from a series of different angles around the patient. These projection data are used to reconstruct a series of tomographic emission images. SPECT images provide diagnostic functional information similar to nuclear planar examinations; however, their tomographic nature allows physicians to better understand the precise distribution of the radioactive agent, and to make a better assessment of the function of specific organs or tissues within the body (Fig. 1-8). The same radioactive isotopes are used in both planar nuclear imaging and SPECT.

Positron Emission Tomography

Positrons are positively charged electrons, and are emitted by some radioactive isotopes such as fluorine-18 and oxygen-15. These radioisotopes are incorporated into metabolically relevant compounds, such as ^{18}F-fluorodeoxyglucose (^{18}FDG), which localize in the body after administration. The decay of the isotope produces a positron, which rapidly undergoes a very unique interaction: the positron (e$^+$) combines with an electron (e$^-$) from the surrounding tissue, and the mass of both the e$^+$ and the e$^-$ is converted by annihilation into pure energy, following Einstein's famous equation $E = mc^2$. The energy that is emitted is called *annihilation radiation*. Annihilation radiation production is similar to gamma ray emission, except that two photons are produced, and they are emitted simultaneously in almost exactly opposite directions, that is, 180 degrees from each other. A positron emission tomography (PET) scanner utilizes rings of detectors that surround the patient, and has special circuitry that is capable of identifying the photon pairs produced during

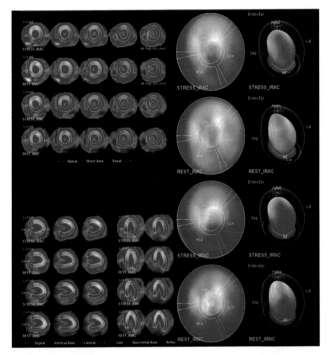

■ **FIGURE 1-8** Two-day stress-rest myocardial perfusion imaging with SPECT/CT was performed on an 89-year-old, obese male with a history of prior CABG, bradycardia, and syncope. This patient had pharmacological stress with regadenoson and was injected with 1.11 GBq (30 mCi) of ^{99m}Tc-tetrofosmin at peak stress. Stress imaging followed 30 minutes later, on a variable-angle two-headed SPECT camera. Image data were acquired over 180 degrees at 20 seconds per stop. The rest imaging was done 24 hours later with a 1.11 GBq (30 mCi) injection of ^{99m}Tc-tetrofosmin. Stress and rest perfusion tomographic images are shown on the left side in the short axis, horizontal long axis, and vertical long axis views. "Bullseye" and 3D tomographic images are shown in the right panel. Stress and rest images on the bottom (IRNC) demonstrate count reduction in the inferior wall due to diaphragmatic attenuation. The same images corrected for attenuation by CT (IRAC) on the top better demonstrate the inferior wall perfusion reduction on stress, which is normal on rest. This is referred to as a "reversible perfusion defect" which is due to coronary disease or ischemia in the distribution of the posterior descending artery. SPECT/CT is becoming the standard for a number of nuclear medicine examinations, including myocardial perfusion imaging. (Image courtesy of DK Shelton.)

annihilation. When a photon pair is detected by two detectors on the scanner, it is assumed that the annihilation event took place somewhere along a straight line between those two detectors. This information is used to mathematically compute the 3D distribution of the PET agent, resulting in a set of tomographic emission images.

Although more expensive than SPECT, PET has clinical advantages in certain diagnostic areas. The PET detector system is more sensitive to the presence of radioisotopes than SPECT cameras, and thus can detect very subtle pathologies. Furthermore, many of the elements that emit positrons (carbon, oxygen, fluorine) are quite physiologically relevant (fluorine is a good substitute for a hydroxyl group), and can be incorporated into a large number of biochemicals. The most important of these is ^{18}FDG, which is concentrated in tissues of high glucose metabolism such as primary tumors and their metastases. PET scans of cancer patients have the ability in many cases to assess the extent of disease, which may be underestimated by CT alone, and to serve as a baseline against which the effectiveness of chemotherapy can be evaluated. PET studies are often combined with CT images acquired immediately before or after the PET scan.

PET/CT combined imaging has applications in oncology, cardiology, neurology, and infection and has become a routine diagnostic tool for cancer staging. Its role in the early assessment of the effectiveness of cancer treatment reduces the time, expense, and morbidity from failed therapy (Fig. 1-9).

Combined Imaging Modalities

Each of the imaging modalities has strengths (e.g., very high spatial resolution in radiography) and limitations (e.g., anatomical superposition in radiography). In particular, nuclear medicine imaging, whether with a scintillation camera or PET, often shows abnormalities with high contrast, but with insufficient anatomic detail to permit identification of the organ or tissue with the lesion. Furthermore, in nuclear medicine, attenuation by the patient of emitted radiation degrades the information in the images. Combining a nuclear medicine imaging system (SPECT or PET) with another imaging system providing good definition of anatomy (CT or MRI) permits the creation of fused images, enabling anatomic localization of abnormalities, and correction of the emission images for attenuation (Fig. 1-10).

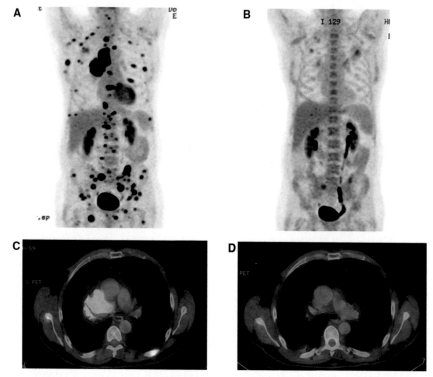

■ FIGURE 1-9 Two whole-body PET/CT studies of a 68-year-old male undergoing treatment for small cell lung cancer. Maximal intensity projection images are shown before (**A**) and after (**B**) chemotherapy. For each study, the patient was injected intravenously with 740 MBq (20 mCi) of ^{18}FDG. The CT acquisition was immediately followed by the PET study, which was acquired for 30 minutes, beginning 60 minutes after injection of the FDG. The bottom panel shows the colorized PET/CT fusion axial images before (**C**) and after (**D**) chemotherapy. The primary tumor in the right hilum (**C**) is very FDG avid (i.e., hypermetabolic). The corresponding axial slice (**D**) was acquired 3 months later, showing dramatic metabolic response to the chemotherapy. The metastatic foci in the right scapula and left posterior rib have also resolved. The unique abilities of the PET/CT scan in this case were to assess the extent of disease, which was underestimated by CT alone, and to assess the effectiveness of chemotherapy. (Images courtesy of DK Shelton.)

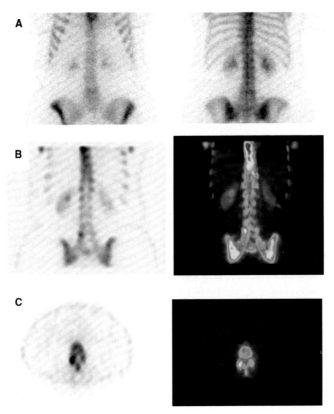

■ **FIGURE 1-10** A planar and SPECT/CT bone scan done 3 hours after injection of 925 MBq (25 mCi) Tc-MDP. **A.** Anterior (**left**) and posterior (**right**) spot views of the spine in this 54-year-old female with back pain. The posterior view shows a faintly seen focus over a lower, right facet of the lumbar spine. **B.** Coronal views of the subsequent SPECT bone scan (**left**) better demonstrate the focus on the right lumbar spine at L4. The colorized image of the SPECT bone scan with CT fusion is shown on right. **C.** The axial views of the SPECT bone scan (**left**) and the colorized SPECT/CT fusion image (**right**) best localizes the abnormality in the right L4 facet, consistent with active facet arthropathy. (Images courtesy of DK Shelton.)

1.2 ## Image Properties

Contrast

Contrast in an image manifests as differences in the grayscale values in the image. A uniformly gray image has no contrast, whereas an image with sharp transitions between dark gray and light gray demonstrates high contrast. The various imaging modalities introduced above generate contrast using a number of different forms of energy, which interact within the patient's tissues based upon different physical properties.

The contrast in x-ray transmission imaging (radiography, fluoroscopy, mammography, and CT) is produced by differences in tissue composition, which determine the local x-ray absorption coefficient, which in turn is dependent upon the density (g/cm^3) and the effective atomic number. The energies of the x-ray photons in the beam (adjusted by the operator) also affect contrast in x-ray images. Because bone has a markedly different effective atomic number ($Z_{eff} \approx 13$) than soft tissue ($Z_{eff} \approx 7$), due to its high concentration of calcium (Z = 20) and phosphorus (Z = 15), bones produce high contrast on x-ray image modalities. The chest radiograph, which demonstrates the lung parenchyma with high tissue and airway contrast, is the most common radiographic procedure performed in the world (Fig. 1-2).

CT's contrast is enhanced over other x-ray imaging modalities due to its tomographic nature. The absence of out-of-slice structures in the CT image greatly improves its image contrast.

Nuclear medicine images (planar images, SPECT, and PET) are maps of the spatial distribution of radioisotopes in the patient. Thus, contrast in nuclear images depends upon the tissue's ability to concentrate the radioactive material. The uptake of a radiopharmaceutical administered to the patient is dependent upon the pharmacological interaction of the agent with the body. PET and SPECT have much better contrast than planar nuclear imaging because, like CT, the images are not obscured by out-of-slice structures.

Contrast in MR imaging is related primarily to the proton density and to relaxation phenomena (i.e., how fast a group of protons gives up its absorbed energy). Proton density is influenced by the mass density (g/cm^3), so MRI can produce images that look somewhat like CT images. Proton density differs among tissue types, and in particular adipose tissues have a higher proportion of protons than other tissues, due to the high concentration of hydrogen in fat ($CH_3(CH_2)_nCOOH$). Two different relaxation mechanisms (spin/lattice and spin/spin) are present in tissue, and the dominance of one over the other can be manipulated by the timing of the RF pulse sequence and magnetic field variations in the MRI system. Through the clever application of different pulse sequences, blood flow can be detected using MRI techniques, giving rise to the field of MR angiography. Contrast mechanisms in MRI are complex, and thus provide for the flexibility and utility of MR as a diagnostic tool.

Contrast in ultrasound imaging is largely determined by the acoustic properties of the tissues being imaged. The difference between the *acoustic impedances* (tissue density × speed of sound in tissue) of two adjacent tissues or other substances affects the amplitude of the returning ultrasound signal. Hence, contrast is quite apparent at tissue interfaces where the differences in acoustic impedance are large. Thus, ultrasound images display unique information about patient anatomy not provided by other imaging modalities. Doppler ultrasound imaging shows the amplitude and direction of blood flow by analyzing the frequency shift in the reflected signal, and thus, motion is the source of contrast.

Spatial Resolution

Just as each modality has different mechanisms for providing contrast, each modality also has different abilities to resolve fine detail in the patient. *Spatial resolution* refers to the ability to see small detail, and an imaging system has *higher* spatial resolution if it can demonstrate the presence of *smaller* objects in the image. The *limiting spatial resolution* is the size of the smallest object that an imaging system can resolve.

Table 1-1 lists the limiting spatial resolution of each of the imaging modalities used in medical imaging. The wavelength of the energy used to probe the object is a fundamental limitation of the spatial resolution of an imaging modality. For example, optical microscopes cannot resolve objects smaller than the wavelengths of visible light, about 400 to 700 nm. The wavelength of x-rays depends on the x-ray energy, but even the longest x-ray wavelengths are tiny—about 1 nm. This is far from the actual resolution in x-ray imaging, but it does represent the theoretical limit on the spatial resolution using x-rays. In ultrasound imaging, the wavelength of sound is the fundamental limit of spatial resolution. At 3.5 MHz, the wavelength of sound in soft tissue is about 500 μm. At 10 MHz, the wavelength is 150 μm.

TABLE 1-1   THE LIMITING SPATIAL RESOLUTIONS OF VARIOUS MEDICAL IMAGING MODALITIES. THE RESOLUTION LEVELS ACHIEVED IN *TYPICAL* CLINICAL USAGE OF THE MODALITY ARE LISTED

MODALITY	SPATIAL RESOLUTION (mm)	COMMENTS
Screen film radiography	0.08	Limited by focal spot size and detector resolution
Digital radiography	0.17	Limited by size of detector elements and focal spot size
Fluoroscopy	0.125	Limited by detector resolution and focal spot size
Screen film mammography	0.03	Highest resolution modality in radiology, limited by same factors as in screen film radiography
Digital mammography	0.05–0.10	Limited by same factors as digital radiography
Computed tomography	0.3	About ½ mm pixels
Nuclear medicine planar imaging	2.5 (detector face), 5 (10 cm from detector)	Spatial resolution degrades substantially with distance from detector
Single photon emission computed tomography	7	Spatial resolution worst towards the center of cross-sectional image slice
Positron emission tomography	5	Better spatial resolution than the other nuclear imaging modalities
Magnetic resonance imaging	1.0	Resolution can improve at higher magnetic fields
Ultrasound imaging (5 MHz)	0.3	Limited by wavelength of sound

MRI poses a paradox to the wavelength-imposed resolution rule—the wavelength of the radiofrequency waves used (at 1.5 T, 64 MHz) is 470 cm, but the spatial resolution of MRI is better than a millimeter. This is because the spatial distribution of the paths of RF energy is not used to form the actual image (contrary to ultrasound, light microscopy, and x-ray images). The radiofrequency energy is collected by a large antenna, and it carries the spatial information of a group of protons encoded in its frequency spectrum.

Medical imaging makes use of a variety of physical parameters as the source of image information. The mechanisms for generating contrast and the spatial resolution properties differ amongst the modalities, thus providing a wide range of diagnostic tools for referring physicians. The optimal detection or assessment of a specific clinical condition depends upon its anatomical location and tissue characteristics. The selection of the best modality for a particular clinical situation requires an understanding of the physical principles of each of the imaging modalities. The following chapters of this book are aimed at giving the medical practitioner just that knowledge.

SELECTED REFERENCE

NCRP 2009: National Council on Radiation Protection and Measurements. Ionizing radiation exposure of the population of the United States (NCRP Report No 160). Bethesda, Md: National Council on Radiation Protection and Measurements; 2009.

CHAPTER 2

Radiation and the Atom

2.1 Radiation

Radiation is energy that travels through space or matter. Two catogories of radiation of importance in medical imaging are electromagnetic (EM) and particulate.

Electromagnetic Radiation

Radio waves, visible light, x-rays, and gamma rays are different types of EM radiation. EM radiation has no mass, is unaffected by either electric or magnetic fields, and has a constant speed in a given medium. Although EM radiation propagates through matter, it does not require matter for its propagation. Its maximal speed (2.998×10^8 m/s) occurs in a vacuum. In matter such as air, water, or glass, its speed is a function of the transport characteristics of the medium. EM radiation travels in straight lines; however, its trajectory can be altered by interaction with matter. The interaction of EM radiation can occur by *scattering* (change in trajectory), *absorption* (removal of the radiation), or, at very higher energies, *transformation* into particulate radiation (energy to mass conversion).

EM radiation is commonly characterized by wavelength (λ), frequency (v), and energy per photon (E). EM radiation over a wide range of wavelengths, frequencies, and energy per photon comprises the EM spectrum. For convenient reference, the EM spectrum is divided into categories including the radio spectrum (that includes transmissions from familiar technologies such as AM, FM, and TV broadcasting; cellular and cordless telephone systems; as well as other wireless communications technologies); infrared radiation (i.e., radiant heat); visible, ultraviolet (UV); and x-ray and gamma-ray regions (Fig. 2-1).

Several forms of EM radiation are used in diagnostic imaging. Gamma rays, emitted by the nuclei of radioactive atoms, are used to image the distributions of radiopharmaceuticals. X-rays, produced outside the nuclei of atoms, are used in radiography, fluoroscopy, and computed tomography. Visible light is produced when x-rays or gamma rays interact with various scintillators in the detectors used in several imaging modalities and is also used to display images. Radiofrequency EM radiation, near the FM frequency region, is used as the excitation and reception signals for magnetic resonance imaging.

Wave-Particle Duality

There are two equally correct ways of describing EM radiation—as waves and as discrete particle-like packets or *quanta* of energy called *photons*. A central tenet of quantum mechanics is that all particles exhibit wave-like properties and all waves exhibit particle-like properties. *Wave—particle duality* addresses the inadequacy of classical Newtonian mechanics in fully describing the behavior of atomic and sub-atomic-scale objects.

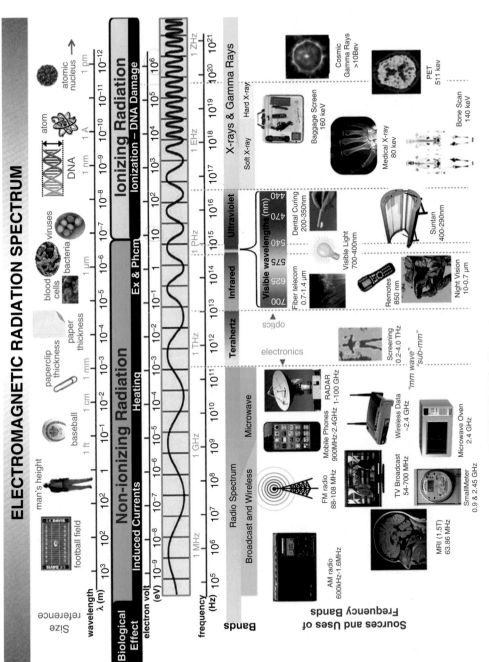

■ FIGURE 2-1 The EM spectrum.

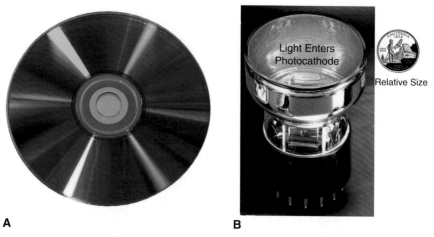

A   **B**

■ **FIGURE 2-2** Wave- and particle-like properties of light. **A.** Colors on the CD are produced as light waves interact with the periodic structure of the tracks on a CD. This diffraction grating effect of the CD tracks splits and diffracts light into several beams of different frequencies (color) traveling in different directions. **B.** The imaging chain in nuclear medicine begins when gamma rays, which are not intercepted by the lead collimator, interact with the NaI crystal of a gamma camera (not shown) producing light photons. The NaI crystal is optically coupled to the surface of a number of PMTs like the one shown above. Just below the glass surface of the PMT, light photons strike the photocathode, ejecting electrons in a classical billiard ball (particle-like) fashion. The ejected electrons are subsequently accelerated and amplified in the PMT, thus increasing gain of the signals used to localize the gamma ray interactions. Further details of nuclear medicine imaging systems are provided in Chapters 18 and 19.

Wave characteristics are more apparent when EM radiation interacts with objects of similar dimensions as the photon's wavelength. For example, light is separated into colors by the diffraction grating effect of the tracks on a compact disc (CD) where the track separation distance is of the same order of magnitude as the wavelength of the visible light, Figure 2-2A.

Particle characteristics of EM radiation, on the other hand, are more evident when an object's dimensions are much smaller than the photon's wavelength. For example, UV and visible light photons exhibit particle-like behavior during the detection and localization of gamma rays in a nuclear medicine gamma camera. Light photons, produced by the interaction of gamma rays with the NaI crystal of a gamma camera, interact with and eject electrons from atoms in the photocathode of a photomultiplier tubes (PMTs) (Fig. 2-2B). The PMTs are optically coupled to the crystal, thereby producing electrical signals for image formation (discussed in greater detail in Chapter 18). The particle-like behavior of x-rays is exemplified by the classical "billiard-ball" type of collision between an x-ray photon and an orbital electron during a *Compton scattering* event. Similarly the x-ray photon's energy is completely absorbed by, and results in the ejection of, an orbital electron (a *photoelectron*), in the *photoelectric effect*. Each of these interactions is important to medical imaging and will be discussed in greater detail in Chapter 3. Prior to the development of quantum mechanics, the classical wave description of EM radiation could not explain the observation that the kinetic energies of the photoelectrons were dependent on the energy (or wavelength) of the incident radiation, rather than the intensity or quantity of incident photons. Albert Einstein received the Nobel Prize in 1921 for his explanation of the photoelectric effect.

Wave Characteristics

Any wave (EM or mechanical, such as sound) can be characterized by their *amplitude* (maximal height), *wavelength* (λ), *frequency* (ν), and *period* (τ). The amplitude is the intensity of the wave. The wavelength is the distance between any two identical points on adjacent cycles. The time required to complete one cycle of a wave (i.e., one λ) is the period. The number of periods that occur per second is the frequency (1/τ). Phase is the temporal shift of one wave with respect to the other. Some of these quantities are depicted in Figure 2-3. The speed (*c*), wavelength, and frequency of any wave are related by

$$c = \lambda \nu \qquad\qquad\qquad [2\text{-}1]$$

Because the speed of EM radiation is constant in a given medium, its frequency and wavelength are inversely proportional. Wavelengths of x-rays and gamma rays are typically measured in fractions of *nanometers* (nm), where 1 nm = 10^{-9} m. Frequency is expressed in *hertz* (Hz), where 1 Hz = 1 cycle/s = 1 s^{-1}.

EM radiation propagates as a pair of oscillating and mutually reinforcing electric and magnetic fields that are orthogonal (perpendicular) to one another and to the direction of propagation, as shown in Figure 2-4.

Problem: Find the frequency of blue light with a wavelength of 400 nm in a vacuum.

Solution: From Equation 2-1,

$$\nu = \frac{c}{\lambda} = \frac{(3 \times 10^{8}\, m\, s^{-1})(10^{9}\, nm\, m^{-1})}{400\, nm} = 7.5 \times 10^{14}\, s^{-1} = 7.5 \times 10^{14}\, Hz$$

Particle Characteristics

The discrete (particle-like) packets (or *quanta*) of EM energy are called *photons*. The energy of a photon is given by

$$E = h\nu = \frac{hc}{\lambda} \qquad\qquad\qquad [2\text{-}2]$$

where *h* (Planck's constant) = 6.626×10^{-34} J-s = 4.136×10^{-18} keV-s. When *E* is expressed in keV and λ in nanometers (nm),

$$E\ (\text{keV}) = \frac{1.24}{\lambda\ (\text{nm})} \qquad\qquad\qquad [2\text{-}3]$$

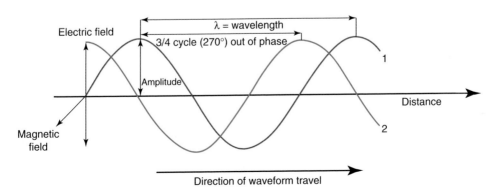

■ FIGURE 2-3 Characterization of waves.

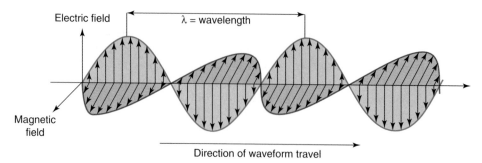

Electric field

λ = wavelength

Magnetic
field

Direction of waveform travel

■ **FIGURE 2-4** Electric and magnetic field components of EM radiation.

The energies of photons are commonly expressed in electron volts (eV). One electron volt is defined as the energy acquired by an electron as it traverses an electrical potential difference (voltage) of one volt in a vacuum. Multiples of the eV common to medical imaging are the keV (1,000 eV) and the MeV (1,000,000 eV).

Ionizing Radiation

An atom or molecule that has lost or gained one or more electrons has a net electrical charge and is called an ion (e.g., sodium ion or Na$^+$). Some but not all electromagnetic and particulate radiations can cause ionization. In general, photons of higher frequency than the far UV region of the spectrum (i.e., wavelengths greater than 200 nm) have sufficient energy per photon to remove bound electrons from atomic shells, thereby producing ionized atoms and molecules. Radiation in this portion of the spectrum (e.g., x-rays and gamma rays) is called *ionizing radiation*. EM radiation with photon energies in and below the UV region (e.g., visible, infrared, terahertz, microwave and radio waves) is called *nonionizing radiation*.

The threshold energy for ionization depends on the type and state of matter. The minimum energies necessary to remove an electron (referred to as the *ionization energy*) from calcium (Ca), glucose ($C_6H_{12}O_6$), and liquid water (H_2O) are 6.1, 8.8, and 11.2 eV respectively. As water is the most abundant (thus most likely) molecular target for radiation interaction in the body, a practical radiobiological demarcation between ionizing and nonionizing EM radiation is approximately 11 eV. While 11 eV is the lowest photon energy capable of producing ionization in water, in a random set of ionization events evoked in a medium by ionization radiation, the average energy expended per ion pair (W) is larger than the minimum ionization energy. For water and tissue equivalent gas, W is about 30 eV. Particulate radiations such high speed electrons and alpha particles (discussed below) can also cause ionization. Particulate and EM ionizing radiation interactions are discussed in more detail in Chapter 3.

Particulate Radiation

The physical properties of the most important particulate radiations associated with medical imaging are listed in Table 2-1. Protons are found in the nuclei of all atoms. A proton has a positive electrical charge and is identical to the nucleus of a hydrogen-1 atom. An atomic orbital electron has a negative electrical charge, equal in magnitude to that of a proton, and is approximately 1/1,800 the mass of a proton. Electrons emitted by the nuclei of radioactive atoms are referred to as *beta particles*. Except for their nuclear origin, negatively charged beta-minus particles (β^-), or *negatrons*, are indistinguishable from ordinary orbital electrons. However, there are also positively charged electrons, referred to as beta-plus particles (β^+), or *positrons*; they are a form of antimatter that ultimately combines with matter in a unique transformation in which all of their mass is instantaneously

TABLE 2-1 PROPERTIES OF PARTICULATE RADIATION

PARTICLE	SYMBOL	ELEMENTARY CHARGE	REST MASS (amu)	ENERGY EQUIVALENT (MeV)
Alpha	α, $^4He^{2-}$	+2	4.00154	3,727
Proton	p, $^1H^+$	+1	1.007276	938
Electron	e^-	−1	0.000549	0.511
Negatron (beta minus)	β^-	−1	0.000549	0.511
Positron (beta plus)	β^+	+1	0.000549	0.511
Neutron	n^0	0	1.008665	940

amu, atomic mass unit , defined as 1/12th the mass of a carbon-12 atom. Elementary charge is a unit of electric charge where 1 is equal in magnitude to the charge of an electron.

converted to an equivalent amount of energy in the form of high-energy gamma rays. This mass-energy conversion and its relevance to medical imaging are discussed briefly below and in more detail in Chapters 3 and 15. Unless otherwise specified, common usage of the term beta particle refers to β^-, whereas β^+ particles are usually referred to as positrons. A neutron is an uncharged nuclear particle that has a mass slightly greater than that of a proton. Neutrons are released by nuclear fission and are used for radionuclide production (Chapter 16). An alpha particle (α) consists of two protons and two neutrons; it thus has a +2 charge and is identical to the nucleus of a helium atom ($^4He^{2+}$). Alpha particles are emitted by many high atomic number radioactive elements, such as uranium, thorium, and radium. Following emission, the α particle eventually acquires two electrons from the surrounding medium and becomes an uncharged helium atom (^4He). Whereas alpha particles emitted outside the body are harmless, alpha particles emitted inside the body cause more extensive cellular damage per unit energy deposited in tissue than any type of radiation used in medical imaging. The emission of alpha particles during radioactive decay is discussed in Chapter 15, and the radiobiological aspects of internally deposited alpha particles are discussed in Chapter 20.

Mass-Energy Equivalence

Within months of Einstein's ground breaking work uniting the concepts of space and time in his special theory of relativity, he theorized that mass and energy were also two aspects of the same entity and in fact were interchangeable. In any reaction, the sum of mass and energy must be conserved. In classical physics, there are two separate conservation laws, one for mass and one for energy. While these separate conservation laws provided satisfactory explanations of the behavior of objects moving at relatively low speeds, they fail to explain some nuclear processes in which particles approach the speed of light. For example, the production of the pairs of 511 keV annihilation photons used in position emission tomography (PET) could not be explained if not for Einstein's insight that neither mass nor energy is necessarily conserved separately, but can be transformed, one into the other, and it is only the total *mass-energy* that is always conserved. The relationship between the mass and the energy is expressed in one of the most famous equations in science:

$$E = mc^2 \qquad\qquad [2\text{-}4]$$

where E (in joules -symbol "J" where $1\ kg\ m^2\ s^{-2} = 1\ J$) represents the energy equivalent to mass m at rest and c is the speed of light in a vacuum (2.998×10^8 m/s). For example, the energy equivalent of an electron with a rest mass (m) of 9.109×10^{-31} kg is

$$E = mc^2$$

$$E = (9.109 \times 10^{-31} \text{ kg}) (2.998 \times 10^8 \text{ m/s})^2$$

$$E = 8.187 \times 10^{-14} \text{ J} = (8.187 \times 10^{-14} \text{ J}) (1 \text{ MeV}/1.602 \times 10^{-13} \text{ J})$$
$$= 0.511 \text{ Mev} = 511 \text{ keV}$$

The conversion between mass and energy occurs in other phenomena discussed later in this book including pair production, radioactive decay and annihilation radiation (used in positron emission tomography), (Chapters 3, 15 and 19 respectively).

A common unit of mass used in atomic and nuclear physics is the atomic mass unit (amu), defined as $\frac{1}{12}$th of the mass of an atom of ^{12}C. One amu is equivalent to 931.5 MeV of energy.

2.2   Structure of the Atom

The atom is the smallest division of an element in which the chemical identity of the element is maintained. The atom is composed of an extremely dense positively charged nucleus, containing protons and neutrons, and an extranuclear cloud of light negatively charged electrons. In its nonionized state, an atom is electrically neutral because the number of protons equals the number of electrons. The radius of an atom is approximately 10^{-10} m, whereas that of the nucleus is only about 10^{-14} m. Thus, the atom is largely unoccupied space, in which the volume of the nucleus is only 10^{-12} (a millionth of a millionth) the volume of the atom. If the empty space in an atom could be removed, a cubic centimeter of protons would have a mass of approximately 4 million metric tons!

Electron Orbits and Electron Binding Energy

In the Bohr model of the atom (Niels Bohr 1913), electrons orbit around a dense, positively charged nucleus at fixed distances (Bohr radii). Bohr combined the classical Newtonian laws of motion and Coulomb's law of electrostatic attraction with quantum theory. In this model of the atom, each electron occupies a discrete energy state in a given electron shell. These electron shells are assigned the letters K L, M, N,..., with K denoting the innermost shell, in which the electrons have the lowest energies. The shells are also assigned the *quantum numbers* 1, 2, 3, 4,..., with the quantum number 1 designating the K shell. Each shell can contain a maximum number of electrons given by ($2n^2$), where n is the quantum number of the shell. Thus, the K shell ($n = 1$) can only hold 2 electrons, the L shell ($n = 2$) can hold $2(2)^2$ or 8 electrons, and so on, as shown in Figure 2-5. The outer electron shell of an atom, the *valence shell*, determines the chemical properties of the element. Advances in atomic physics and quantum mechanics led to refinements of the Bohr model. According to contemporary views on atomic structure, the location of an orbital electron is more properly described in terms of the probability of its occupying a given location within the atom with both wave and particle properties. At any given moment, there is even a probability, albeit very low, that an electron can be within the atom's nucleus. However, the highest probabilities are associated with Bohr's original atomic radii.

The energy required to remove an orbital electron completely from the atom is called its *orbital binding energy*. Thus, for radiation to be ionizing, the energy transferred

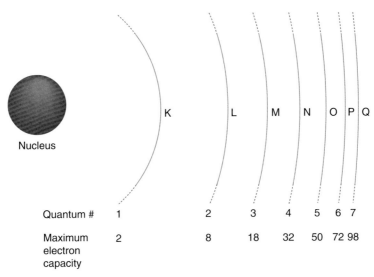

Quantum #   1   2   3   4   5   6   7

Maximum   2   8   18   32   50 72 98
electron
capacity

■ **FIGURE 2-5** Electron shell designations and orbital filling rules.

to the electron must equal or exceed its binding energy. Due to the closer proximity of the electrons to the positively charged nucleus, the binding energy of the K-shell is greater than that of outer shells. For a particular electron shell, binding energy also increases with the number of protons in the nucleus (i.e., atomic number). In Figure 2-6, electron binding energies are compared for hydrogen (Z = 1) and tungsten (Z = 74). A K shell electron of tungsten with 74 protons in the nucleus is much more

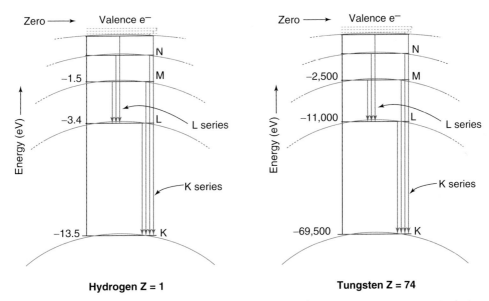

■ **FIGURE 2-6** Energy-level diagrams for hydrogen and tungsten. The energy necessary to separate electrons in particular orbits from the atom (not drawn to scale) increases with Z and decreases with distance from the nucleus. Note that zero energy represents the point at which the electron is experiencing essentially no Coulomb attractive force from the protons in the nucleus (often referred to as a "free" electron). For a bound electron to reach that state, energy has to be absorbed. Thus, the energy states of the electrons within the atom must be below zero and are thus represented as negative numbers. The vertical lines represent various transitions (e.g., K and L series) of the electrons from one energy level to another.

tightly bound (~69,500 eV) than the *K* shell electron of hydrogen orbiting a nucleus with a single proton (~13.5 eV). The energy required to move an electron from the innermost electron orbit (*K* shell) to the next orbit (*L* shell) is the difference between the binding energies of the two orbits (i.e., $E_{bK} - E_{bL}$ equals the transition energy).

Hydrogen:

$$13.5 \text{ eV} - 3.4 \text{ eV} = 10.1 \text{ eV}$$

Tungsten:

$$69,500 \text{ eV} - 11,000 \text{ eV} = 58,500 \text{ eV} (58.5 \text{ keV})$$

Radiation from Electron Transitions

When an electron is removed from its shell by an x-ray or gamma ray photon or a charged particle interaction, a vacancy is created in that shell. This vacancy is usually filled by an electron from an outer shell, leaving a vacancy in the outer shell that in turn may be filled by an electron transition from a more distant shell. This series of transitions is called an *electron cascade*. The energy released by each transition is equal to the difference in binding energy between the original and final shells of the electron. This energy may be released by the atom as characteristic x-rays or Auger electrons.

Characteristic X-rays

Electron transitions between atomic shells can result in the emission of radiation in the visible, UV, and x-ray portions of the EM spectrum. The energy of this radiation is characteristic of each atom, since the electron binding energies depend on Z. Emissions from transitions exceeding 100 eV are called *characteristic* or *fluorescent* x-rays. Characteristic x-rays are named according to the orbital in which the vacancy occurred. For example, the radiation resulting from a vacancy in the *K* shell is called a *K*-characteristic x-ray, and the radiation resulting from a vacancy in the *L* shell is called an *L* characteristic x-ray. If the vacancy in one shell is filled by the adjacent shell, it is identified by a subscript alpha (e.g., $L \rightarrow K$ transition $= K_\alpha$, $M \rightarrow L$ transition $= L_\alpha$). If the electron vacancy is filled from a nonadjacent shell, the subscript beta is used (e.g., $M \rightarrow K$ transition $= K_\beta$). The energy of the characteristic x-ray ($E_{\text{x-ray}}$) is the difference between the electron binding energies (E_b) of the respective shells:

$$E_{\text{x-ray}} = E_{b \text{ vacant shell}} - E_{b \text{ transition shell}} \qquad [2\text{-}5]$$

Thus, as illustrated in Figure 2-7A, an *M* to *K* shell transition in tungsten would produce a K_β characteristic x-ray of

$$E(K_\beta) = E_{bK} - E_{bM}$$
$$E(K_\beta) = 69.5 \text{ keV} - 2.5 \text{ keV} = 67 \text{ keV}$$

Auger Electrons and Fluorescent Yield

An electron cascade does not always result in the production of a characteristic x–ray or x-rays. A competing process that predominates in low Z elements is *Auger electron emission*. In this case, the energy released is transferred to an orbital electron, typically in the same shell as the cascading electron (Fig. 2-7B). The ejected Auger electron possesses kinetic energy equal to the difference between the transition energy and the binding energy of the ejected electron.

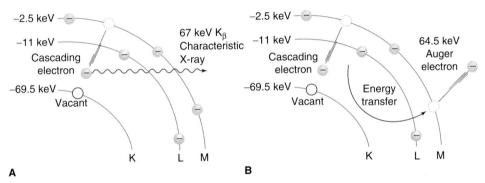

A

B

■ FIGURE 2-7 De-excitation of a tungsten atom. An electron transition filling a vacancy in an orbit closer to the nucleus will be accompanied by either the emission of characteristic radiation (**A**) or the emission of an Auger electron (**B**).

The probability that the electron transition will result in the emission of a characteristic x-ray is called the *fluorescent yield* (ω). Thus, $1 - \omega$ is the probability that the transition will result in the ejection of an Auger electron. Auger emission predominates in low Z elements and in electron transitions of the outer shells of heavy elements. The K-shell fluorescent yield is essentially zero ($\leq 1\%$) for elements $Z < 10$ (i.e., the elements comprising the majority of soft tissue), about 15% for calcium ($Z = 20$), about 65% for iodine ($Z = 53$), and approaches 80% for $Z > 60$.

The Atomic Nucleus

Composition of the Nucleus

The nucleus is composed of protons and neutrons, known collectively as *nucleons*. The number of protons in the nucleus is the *atomic number* (Z), and the total number of protons and neutrons within the nucleus is the *mass number* (A). It is important not to confuse the mass number with the atomic mass, which is the actual mass of the atom. For example, the mass number of oxygen-16 is 16 (8 protons and 8 neutrons), whereas its atomic mass is 15.9994 amu. The notation specifying an atom with the chemical symbol X is $_{Z}^{A}X_{N}$, where N is the number of neutrons in the nucleus. In this notation, Z and X are redundant because the chemical symbol identifies the element and thus the number of protons. For example, the symbols H, He, and Li refer to atoms with $Z = 1$, 2, and 3, respectively. The number of neutrons is calculated as $N = A - Z$. For example, $_{53}^{131}I_{78}$ is usually written as ^{131}I or as I-131. The charge on an atom is indicated by a superscript to the right of the chemical symbol. For example, Ca^{2+} indicates that the calcium atom has lost two electrons and thus has a net charge of $+2$.

Nuclear Forces and Energy Levels

There are two main forces that act in opposite directions on particles in the nucleus. The coulombic force between the protons is repulsive and is countered by the attractive force resulting from the exchange of gluons (subnuclear particles) among all nucleons. The exchange forces, also called the *strong force*, hold the nucleus together but operate only over very short (nuclear) distances ($<10^{-14}$ m).

The nucleus has energy levels that are analogous to orbital electron shells, although often much higher in energy. The lowest energy state is called the *ground*

TABLE 2-2   NUCLEAR FAMILIES: ISOTOPES, ISOBARS, ISOTONES, AND ISOMERS

FAMILY	NUCLIDES WITH SAME	EXAMPLE
Isotopes	Atomic number (Z)	I-131 and I-125: Z = 53
Isobars	Mass number (A)	Mo-99 and Tc-99: A = 99
Isotones	Number of neutrons (A–Z)	$_{53}$I-131: 131 – 53 = 78 $_{54}$Xe-132: 132 – 54 = 78
Isomers	Atomic and mass numbers but different energy states in the nucleus	Tc-99m and Tc-99: Z = 43 A = 99 Energy of Tc-99m > Tc-99: ΔE = 142 keV

Note: See text for description of the italicized letters in the nuclear family terms.

state of an atomic nucleus. Nuclei with energy in excess of the ground state are said to be in an *excited state*. The average lifetimes of excited states range from 10^{-16} s to more than 100 y. Excited states that exist longer than 10^{-12} s are referred to as *metastable* or *isomeric states*. Metastable states with longer lifetimes are denoted by the letter m after the mass number of the atom (e.g., Tc-99m).

Classification of Nuclides

Species of atoms characterized by the number of protons and neutrons and the energy content of the atomic nuclei are called *nuclides*. Isotopes, isobars, isotones, and isomers are families of nuclides that share specific properties (Table 2-2). An easy way to remember these relationships is to associate the *p* in isoto*p*es with the same number of protons, the *a* in isob*a*rs with the same atomic mass number, the *n* in isoto*n*es with the same number of neutrons, and the *e* in isom*e*r with the different nuclear energy states.

Nuclear Stability and Radioactivity

Only certain combinations of neutrons and protons in the nucleus are stable; the others are radioactive. On a plot of Z versus N, these stable nuclides fall along a "line of stability" for which the N/Z ratio is approximately 1 for low Z nuclides and approximately 1.5 for high Z nuclides, as shown in Figure 2-8. A higher neutron-to-proton ratio is required in heavy elements to offset the Coulomb repulsive forces between protons. Only four nuclides with odd numbers of neutrons and odd numbers of protons are stable, whereas many more nuclides with even numbers of neutrons and even numbers of protons are stable. The number of stable nuclides identified for different combinations of neutrons and protons is shown in Table 2-3. Nuclides with an odd number of nucleons are capable of producing a nuclear magnetic resonance signal, as described in Chapter 12.

While atoms with unstable combinations of neutrons and protons exist, over time they will transform to nuclei that are stable. Two kinds of instability are neutron excess and neutron deficiency (i.e., proton excess). Such nuclei have excess internal energy compared with a stable arrangement of neutrons and protons. They achieve stability by the conversion of a neutron to a proton or vice versa, and these events are accompanied by the emission of energy. The energy emissions include particulate

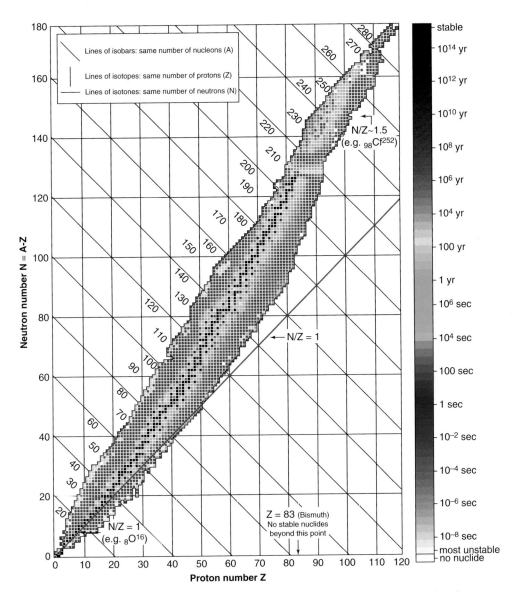

■ **FIGURE 2-8** A plot of the nuclides where the number of protons (i.e., atomic number or Z) and neutrons of each nuclide is shown on the x- and y-axes, respectively. The outlined area containing all the black and colored squares represents the range of known nuclides. The stable nuclides are indicated by small black squares, whereas the colored squares represent radioactive (i.e., unstable) nuclides or *radionuclides*. The stable nuclides form the so-called *line of stability* in which the neutron-to-proton ratio is approximately 1 for low Z nuclides and increases to approximately 1.5 for high Z nuclides. The color code indicates the physical half-life of each of the radionuclides. Note that all nuclides with Z > 83 (bismuth) are radioactive and that, in general, the further the radionuclide is from the line of stability, the more unstable it is and the shorter the half-life it has. Radionuclides to the left of the line of stability are neutron rich and are likely to undergo beta-minus decay, while radionuclides to the right of the line of stability are neutron poor and thus often decay by positron emission or electron capture. Extremely unstable radionuclides and those with high Z often decay by alpha particle emission.

TABLE 2-3 DISTRIBUTION OF STABLE NUCLIDES AS A FUNCTION OF NEUTRON AND PROTON NUMBER

NUMBER OF PROTONS (Z)	NUMBER OF NEUTRONS (N)	NUMBER OF STABLE NUCLIDES
Even	Even	165
Even	Odd	57 (NMR signal)
Odd	Even	53 (NMR signal)
Odd	Odd	4 (NMR signal)
	Total	279

NMR, nuclear magnetic resonance.

and EM radiations. Nuclides that decay (i.e., transform) to more stable nuclei are said to be *radioactive*, and the transformation process itself is called *radioactive decay* (radioactive disintegration). There are several types of radioactive decay, and these are discussed in detail in Chapter 15. A nucleus may undergo several decays before a stable configuration is achieved. These "decay chains" are often found in nature. For example, the decay of uranium 238 (U-238) is followed by 13 successive decays before the stable nuclide, lead 206 (Pb-206), is formed. The radionuclide at the beginning of a particular decay sequence is referred to as the *parent*, and the nuclide produced by the decay of the parent is referred to as the *daughter*. The daughter may be either stable or radioactive.

Gamma Rays

Radioactive decay often results in the formation of a daughter nucleus in an excited state. The EM radiation emitted from the nucleus as the excited state transitions to a lower (more stable) energy state is called a *gamma ray*. This energy transition is analogous to the emission of characteristic x-rays following electron transition. However, gamma rays (by definition), emanate from the nucleus. Because the spacing of the energy states within the nucleus is usually considerably larger than those of atomic orbital electron energy states, electron transitions, gamma rays are often much more energetic than characteristic x-rays. When this nuclear de-excitation process takes place in an isomer (e.g., Tc-99m), it is called *isomeric transition* (discussed in Chapter 15). In isomeric transition, the nuclear energy state is reduced with no change in A or Z.

Internal Conversion Electrons

Nuclear de-excitation does not always result in the emission of a gamma ray. An alternative form of de-excitation is *internal conversion*, in which the de-excitation energy is completely transferred to an orbital (typically *K, L,* or *M shell*) electron. The conversion electron is ejected from the atom, with a kinetic energy equal to that of the gamma ray less the electron binding energy. The vacancy produced by the ejection of the conversion electron will be filled by an electron cascade and associated characteristic x-rays and Auger electrons as described previously. The internal conversion energy transfer process is analogous to the emission of an auger electron in lieu of characteristic x-ray energy emission. However, the kinetic energy of the internal conversion electron is often much greater than that of Auger electrons due to the greater energy associated with most gamma ray emissions compared to characteristic x-ray energies.

Nuclear Binding Energy and Mass Defect

The energy required to separate an atom into its constituent parts is the *atomic binding energy*. It is the sum of the orbital electron binding energy and the nuclear binding energy. The *nuclear binding energy* is the energy necessary to disassociate a nucleus into its constituent parts and is the result of the strong forces acting between nucleons. Compared with the nuclear binding energy, the orbital electron binding energy is negligible. When two subatomic particles approach each other under the influence of this strong nuclear force, their total energy decreases and the lost energy is emitted in the form of radiation. Thus, the total energy of the bound particles is less than that of the separated free particles.

The binding energy can be calculated by subtracting the mass of the atom from the total mass of its constituent protons, neutrons, and electrons; this mass difference is called the *mass defect*. For example, the mass of an N-14 atom, which is composed of 7 electrons, 7 protons, and 7 neutrons, is 14.00307 amu. The total mass of its constituent particles in the unbound state is

$$
\begin{aligned}
\text{mass of 7 protons} &= 7(1.007276 \text{ amu}) = 7.050932 \text{ amu} \\
\text{mass of 7 neutrons} &= 7(1.008665 \text{ amu}) = 7.060655 \text{ amu} \\
\text{mass of 7 electrons} &= 7(0.000549 \text{ amu}) = \underline{0.003843 \text{ amu}} \\
\text{mass of component particles of N-14} &= 14.11543 \text{ amu}
\end{aligned}
$$

Thus, the mass defect of the N-14 atom, the difference between the mass of its constituent particles and its atomic mass, is 14.11543 amu − 14.003074 amu = 0.112356 amu. According to the formula for mass energy equivalence (Equation 2-4), this mass defect is equal to (0.112356 amu) (931.5 MeV/amu) = 104.7 MeV.

An extremely important observation is made by carrying the binding energy calculation a bit further. The total binding energy of the nucleus may be divided by the mass number A to obtain the average binding energy per nucleon. Figure 2-9 shows the average binding energy per nucleon for stable nuclides as a function of mass number. The fact that this curve reaches its maximum near the middle elements and decreases at either end predicts that large quantities of energy can be released from a small amount of matter. The two processes by which this can occur are called *nuclear fission* and *nuclear fusion*.

Nuclear Fission and Fusion

During nuclear fission, a nucleus with a large atomic mass splits into two usually unequal parts called *fission fragments*, each with an average binding energy per nucleon greater than that of the original nucleus. In this reaction, the total nuclear binding energy increases. The change in the nuclear binding energy is released as EM and particulate radiation and as kinetic energy of the fission fragments. Fission is typically accompanied by the release of several neutrons. For example, the absorption of a single neutron by the nucleus of a U-235 atom can result in the instantaneous fission of U-236 into two fission fragments (e.g., Sn-131 and Mo-102), and two or three energetic neutrons. This reaction results in a mass defect equivalent to approximately 200 MeV, which is released as kinetic energy of the fission fragments (~165 MeV); neutrons (~5 MeV); *prompt* (instantaneous) gamma radiation (~7 MeV) and radiation from the decay of the fission products (~23 MeV). The probability of fission increases with the neutron flux, which is the number of neutrons per cm^2/s. Fission is used in nuclear powered electrical generating plants and in the design of "atom" bombs. The use of nuclear fission for radionuclide production is discussed in Chapter 16.

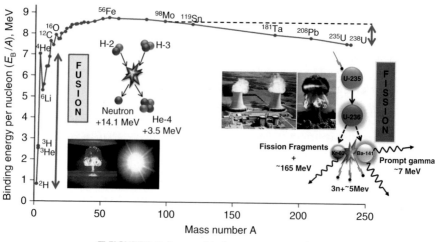

■ **FIGURE 2-9** Average binding energy per nucleon.

Energy is also released from the fusion (combining) of light atomic nuclei. For example, the fusion of deuterium (H-2) and tritium (He-3) nuclei results in the production of helium-4 and a neutron. As can be seen in Figure 2-9, the helium-4 atom has a much higher average binding energy per nucleon than either tritium (H-3) or deuterium (H-2). The energy associated with the mass defect of this reaction is about 17.6 MeV. The nuclei involved in fusion reactions require exceptionally high kinetic energies in order to overcome Coulomb repulsive forces. Fusion of hydrogen nuclei in stars, where extreme gravitational forces result in extraordinarily high temperatures, is the first step in subsequent self-sustaining fusion reactions that produce helium-4. The *H-bomb* is a fusion device that uses the detonation of an atom bomb (a fission device) to generate the temperature and pressure necessary for fusion. H-bombs are also referred to as "thermonuclear" weapons.

SUGGESTED READING

Cherry, R., Simon et.al. Physics in Nuclear Medicine. 4th ed., Philadelphia: Saunders, 2011.

Evans RD. *The atomic nucleus*. Malabar, FL: Robert E. Krieger, 1982.

Turner, J. E. *Atoms, radiation, and radiation protection*, 3rd ed. Weinheim, Germany: Wiley-VCH Verlag GmbH & Co. KGaA 2007.

CHAPTER 3

Interaction of Radiation with Matter

 ## 3.1 Particle Interactions

Particles of ionizing radiation include charged particles, such as alpha particles (α^{+2}), protons (p^+), beta particles (β^-), positrons (β^+), energetic extranuclear electrons (e^-) and uncharged particles, such as neutrons. The behavior of heavy charged particles (e.g., alpha particles and protons) is different from that of lighter charged particles such as electrons and positrons.

Excitation, Ionization, and Radiative Losses

Energetic charged particles interact with matter by electrical (i.e., coulombic) forces and lose kinetic energy via *excitation, ionization,* and *radiative losses.* Excitation and ionization occur when charged particles lose energy by interacting with orbital electrons in the medium. These interactional, or *collisional,* losses refer to the coulombic forces exerted on charged particles when they pass in proximity to the electric field generated by the atom's electrons and protons. Excitation is the transfer of some of the incident particles' energy to electrons in the absorbing material, promoting them to electron orbits farther from the nucleus (i.e., higher energy level). In excitation, the energy transferred to an electron does not exceed its binding energy. Following excitation, the electron will return to a lower energy level, with the emission of the excitation energy in the form of electromagnetic radiation or Auger electrons. This process is referred to as *de-excitation* (Fig. 3-1A). If the transferred energy exceeds the binding energy of the electron, ionization occurs, whereby the electron is ejected from the atom (Fig. 3-1B). The result of ionization is an *ion pair* consisting of the ejected electron and the positively charged atom. Sometimes, the ejected electrons possess sufficient energy to produce further ionizations called *secondary ionization*. These electrons are called *delta rays*.

Approximately 70% of the energy deposition of energetic electrons in soft tissue occurs via ionization. However, as electron energy decreases the probability of energy loss via excitation increases. For very low energy electron (~40 eV) the probabilities of excitation and ionization are equal and with further reductions in electron energy the probability of ionization rapidly diminishes becoming zero (in tissue) below the first ionization state of liquid water at approximately 11.2 eV. So, while the smallest binding energies for electrons in carbon, nitrogen, and oxygen are less than 10 eV, the average energy deposited per ion pair produced in air (mostly nitrogen and oxygen) and soft tissue (mostly hydrogen, carbon, and oxygen) are approximately 34 eV and 22 eV, respectively. The energy difference is the result of the excitation process. Medical imaging with x-rays and gamma rays results in the production of energetic electrons by mechanisms discussed later in this chapter. It should be appreciated that, owing to the relatively modest amount of energy necessary to produce a secondary electron, each of these energetic electrons will result in a abundance of secondary electrons as they deposit

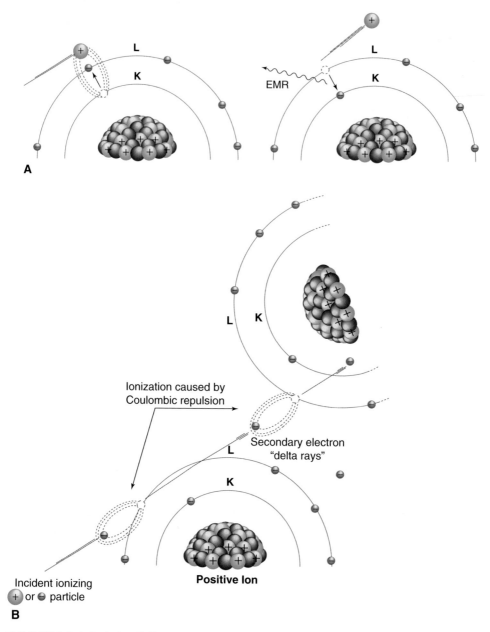

A

B

Ionization caused by
Coulombic repulsion

Secondary electron
"delta rays"

Positive Ion

Incident ionizing
+ or ⊖ particle

■ **FIGURE 3-1 A.** Excitation (**left**) and de-excitation (**right**) with the subsequent release of electromagnetic radiation. **B.** Ionization and the production of delta rays.

their energy in tissue. For example, a 10 keV electron will result in the production of over 450 secondary electrons, most with energies between 10– and 70 eV.

Specific Ionization

The average number of primary and secondary ion pairs produced per unit length of the charged particle's path is called the *specific ionization,* expressed in ion pairs (IP)/mm. Specific ionization increases with the square of the electrical charge (Q) of the particle and decreases with the square of the incident particle velocity (v); thus,

$SI \propto \dfrac{Q^2}{v^2}$. A larger charge produces a greater coulombic field; as the particle loses

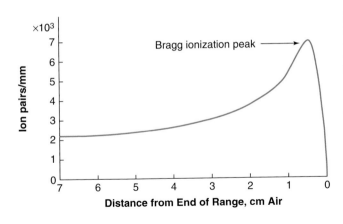

■ **FIGURE 3-2** Specific ionization (ion pairs/mm) as a function of distance from the end of range in air for a 7.69-MeV alpha particle from ^{214}Po. Rapid increase in specific ionization reaches a maximum (Bragg peak) and then drops off sharply as the particle kinetic energy is exhausted and the charged particle is neutralized.

kinetic energy, it slows down, allowing the coulombic field to interact at a given location for a longer period of time. The kinetic energies of alpha particles emitted by naturally occurring radionuclides extend from a minimum of about 4.05 MeV (Th-232) to a maximum of about 10.53 MeV (Po-212). The ranges of alpha particles in matter are quite limited and, for the alpha particle energies mentioned above, their ranges in air are 2.49 and 11.6 cm respectively. In tissue the alpha particle range is reduced to less than the diameter of a dozen or so cells, (~30 to 130 μm). The specific ionization of an alpha particle can be as high as approximately 7,000 IP/mm in air and about 10 million IP/mm in soft tissue. The specific ionization as a function of the particle's path is shown for a 7.69-MeV alpha particle from ^{214}Po in air (Fig. 3-2). As the alpha particle slows, the specific ionization increases to a maximum (called the *Bragg peak*), beyond which it decreases rapidly as the alpha particle acquires electrons and becomes electrically neutral, thus losing its capacity for further ionization. The large Bragg peak associated with heavy charged particles has applications in radiation therapy. For example, several proton therapy centers have been built over the past decade. By adjusting the kinetic energy of heavy charged particles, a large radiation dose can be delivered at a particular depth and over a fairly narrow range of tissue containing a lesion. On either side of the Bragg peak, the dose to tissue is substantially lower. Heavy particle accelerators are used at some medical facilities to provide this treatment in lieu of surgical excision or conventional radiation therapy. Compared to heavy charged particles, the specific ionization of electrons is much lower (in the range of 5 to 10 IP/mm of air).

Charged Particle Tracks

Another important distinction between heavy charged particles and electrons is their paths in matter. Electrons follow tortuous paths in matter as the result of multiple scattering events caused by coulombic deflections (repulsion and/or attraction). The sparse tortuous ionization track of an electron is illustrated in Figure 3-3A. On the other hand, the larger mass of a heavy charged particle results in a dense and usually linear ionization track (Fig. 3-3B). The *path length* of a particle is defined as the distance the particle travels. The *range* of a particle is defined as the depth of penetration of the particle in matter. As illustrated in Figure 3-3, the path length of the electron almost always exceeds its range, whereas the typically straight ionization track of a heavy charged particle results in the path length and range being nearly equal. Additional information on the pattern of energy deposition of charged particles at the cellular level and their radiobiological significance is presented in Chapter 20.

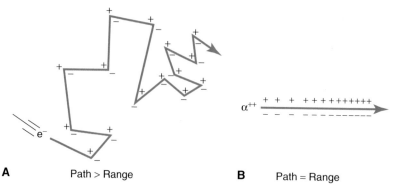

A   Path > Range   **B**   Path = Range

■ **FIGURE 3-3** **A.** Electron scattering results in the path length of the electron being greater than its range. **B.** Heavily charged particles, like alpha particles, produce a dense, nearly linear ionization track, resulting in the path and range being essentially equal.

Linear Energy Transfer

While specific ionization reflects all energy losses that occur before an ion pair is produced, the linear energy transfer (LET) is a measure of the average amount of energy deposited locally (near the incident particle track) in the absorber per unit path length. LET is often expressed in units of keV or eV per μm. The LET of a charged particle is proportional to the square of the charge and inversely proportional to the particle's kinetic energy (i.e., LET $\propto Q^2/E_k$). The LET of a particular type of radiation describes the local energy deposition density, which can have a substantial impact on the biologic consequences of radiation exposure. In general, for a given absorbed dose, the dense ionization tracks of "high LET" radiations (alpha particles, protons, etc.) deposit their energy over a much shorter range and are much more damaging to cells than the spare ionization pattern associated with "low LET" radiations. Low LET radiation includes energetic electrons (e.g., β^- and β^+) and ionizing electromagnetic radiation (gamma and x-rays, whose interactions set electrons into motion). By way of perspective the exposure of patients to diagnostic x-rays results in the production of energetic electrons with an average LET of approximately 3 keV/μm in soft tissue, whereas the average LET of 5-MeV alpha particles in soft tissue is approximately 100 keV/μm. Despite their typically much higher initial kinetic energy, the range of high LET radiation is much less than that of low LET radiation. For example at the point where an alpha particle and electron traversing tissue have the same kinetic energy, say 100 keV, their range from that point will be 1.4 and 200 μm respectively.

Scattering

Scattering refers to an interaction that deflects a particle or photon from its original trajectory. A scattering event in which the total kinetic energy of the colliding particles is unchanged is called *elastic*. Billiard ball collisions, for example, are elastic (disregarding frictional losses). When scattering occurs with a loss of kinetic energy (i.e., the total kinetic energy of the scattered particles is less than that of the particles before the interaction), the interaction is said to be *inelastic*. For example, the process of ionization can be considered an elastic interaction if the binding energy of the electron is negligible compared to the kinetic energy of the incident electron (i.e., the kinetic energy of the ejected electron is equal to the kinetic energy lost by the incident electron). If the binding energy that must be overcome to ionize the atom is not insignificant compared to the kinetic energy of the incident electron (i.e., the kinetic energy of the ejected electron is less than the kinetic energy lost by the incident electron), the process is said to be inelastic.

Radiative Interactions—Bremsstrahlung

While most electron interactions with the atomic nuclei are elastic, electrons can undergo inelastic interactions in which the path of the electron is deflected by the positively charged nucleus, with a loss of kinetic energy. This energy is instantaneously emitted as electromagnetic radiation (i.e., x-rays). Energy is conserved, as the energy of the radiation is equal to the kinetic energy lost by the electron.

The radiation emission accompanying electron deceleration is called *bremsstrahlung*, a German word meaning "braking radiation" (Fig. 3-4). The deceleration of the high-speed electrons in an x-ray tube produces the bremsstrahlung x-rays used in diagnostic imaging.

Total bremsstrahlung emission per atom is proportional to Z^2, where Z is the atomic number of the absorber, and inversely proportional to the square of the mass of the incident particle, that is, Z^2/m^2. Due to the strong influence of the particle's mass, bremsstrahlung production by heavier charged particles such as protons and alpha particles will be less than one millionth of that produced by electrons.

The energy of a bremsstrahlung x-ray photon can be any value up to and including the entire kinetic energy of the deflected electron. Thus, when many electrons undergo bremsstrahlung interactions, the result is a continuous spectrum of x-ray energies. This radiative energy loss is responsible for the majority of the x-rays produced by x-ray tubes and is discussed in greater detail in Chapter 6.

Positron Annihilation

The fate of positrons (β^+) is unlike that of negatively charged electrons (e$^-$ and β^-) that ultimately become bound to atoms. As mentioned above, all energetic electrons (positively and negatively charged) lose their kinetic energy by excitation, ionization, and radiative interactions. When a positron (a form of antimatter) reaches the end of its range, it interacts with a negatively charged electron, resulting in the annihilation of the electron-positron pair and the complete conversion of their rest mass to energy in the form of two oppositely directed 0.511-MeV *annihilation photons*. This process occurs following radionuclide decay by positron emission (see Chapter 15). Imaging of the distribution of positron-emitting radiopharmaceuticals in patients is accomplished by the detection of the annihilation photon pairs during positron emission tomography (PET) (see Chapter 19). The annihilation photons are not often emitted at exactly 180 degrees apart because there is often a small amount of residual momentum in the positron when it interacts with the oppositely charged electron. This *noncolinearity* is not severe (~0.5 degree), and its blurring effect in the typical PET imaging system is not clinically significant.

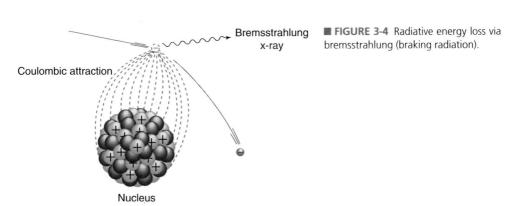

Bremsstrahlung
x-ray

Coulombic attraction

Nucleus

■ **FIGURE 3-4** Radiative energy loss via bremsstrahlung (braking radiation).

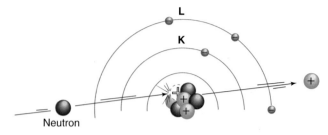

■ **FIGURE 3-5** Schematic example of collisional energy loss. An uncharged particle (neutron) interacts with the atomic nucleus of an atom resulting in the ejection of a proton. This interaction results in transformation of the atom into a new element with an atomic number (Z) reduced by 1.

Neutron Interactions

Unlike protons and electrons, neutrons, being uncharged particles, cannot cause excitation and ionization via coulombic interactions with orbital electrons. They can, however, interact with atomic nuclei, sometimes liberating charged particles or nuclear fragments that can directly cause excitation and ionization (Fig. 3-5). Neutrons often interact with atomic nuclei of light elements (e.g., H, C, O) by scattering in "billiard ball"–like collisions, producing recoil nuclei that lose their energy via excitation and ionization. In tissue, energetic neutrons interact primarily with the hydrogen in water, producing recoil protons (hydrogen nuclei). Neutrons may also be captured by atomic nuclei. Neutron capture results in a large energy release (typically 2 to 7 MeV) due to the large binding energy of the neutron. In some cases, one or more neutrons are reemitted; in other cases, the neutron is retained, converting the atom into a different isotope. For example, the capture of a neutron by a hydrogen atom (^{1}H) results in deuterium (^{2}H) and the emission of a 2.22-MeV gamma ray, reflecting the increase in the binding energy of the nucleus:

$$^1H + {}^1n \rightarrow {}^2H + \gamma \quad \text{Gamma ray energy } (E_\gamma) = 2.22 \text{ MeV}$$

Some nuclides produced by neutron absorption are stable, and others are radioactive (i.e., unstable). As discussed in Chapter 2, neutron absorption in some very heavy nuclides such as ^{235}U can cause nuclear fission, producing very energetic fission fragments, neutrons, and gamma rays. Neutron interactions important to the production of radiopharmaceuticals are described in greater detail in Chapter 16.

3.2 X-ray and Gamma-Ray Interactions

When traversing matter, photons will penetrate without interaction, scatter, or be absorbed. There are four major types of interactions of x-ray and gamma-ray photons with matter, the first three of which play a role in diagnostic radiology and nuclear medicine: (a) Rayleigh scattering, (b) Compton scattering, (c) photoelectric absorption, and (d) pair production.

Rayleigh Scattering

In Rayleigh scattering, the incident photon interacts with and excites the *total atom,* as opposed to individual electrons as in Compton scattering or the photoelectric effect (discussed later). This interaction occurs mainly with very low energy x-rays, such as those used in mammography (15 to 30 keV). During the Rayleigh scattering event, the electric field of the incident photon's electromagnetic wave expends energy, causing all of the electrons in the scattering atom to oscillate in phase. The atom's electron cloud immediately radiates this energy, emitting a photon of the same

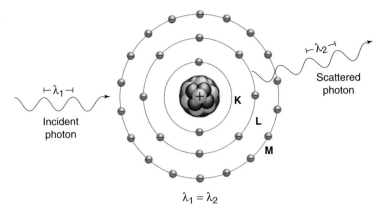

■ FIGURE 3-6 Rayleigh scattering. The diagram shows that the incident photon λ_1 interacts with an atom and the scattered photon λ_2 is being emitted with the same wavelength and energy. Rayleigh scattered photons are typically emitted in the forward direction fairly close to the trajectory of the incident photon. *K, L,* and *M* are electron shells.

energy but in a slightly different direction (Fig. 3-6). In this interaction, electrons are not ejected, and thus, ionization does not occur. In general, the average scattering angle decreases as the x-ray energy increases. In medical imaging, detection of the scattered x-ray will have a deleterious effect on image quality. However, this type of interaction has a low probability of occurrence in the diagnostic energy range. In soft tissue, Rayleigh scattering accounts for less than 5% of x-ray interactions above 70 keV and at most only accounts for about 10% of interactions at 30 keV. Rayleigh interactions are also referred to as "coherent" or "classical" scattering.

Compton Scattering

Compton scattering (also called inelastic or nonclassical scattering) is the predominant interaction of x-ray and gamma-ray photons in the diagnostic energy range with soft tissue. In fact, Compton scattering not only predominates in the diagnostic energy range above 26 keV in soft tissue but also continues to predominate well beyond diagnostic energies to approximately 30 MeV. This interaction is most likely to occur between photons and outer ("valence")-shell electrons (Fig. 3-7). The electron is ejected from the atom, and the scattered photon is emitted with some reduction in energy relative to the incident photon. As with all types of interactions, both energy and momentum must be conserved. Thus, the energy of the incident photon (E_0) is equal to the sum of the energy of the scattered photon (E_{sc}) and the kinetic energy of the ejected electron (E_{e-}), as shown in Equation 3-1. The binding energy of the electron that was ejected is comparatively small and can be ignored.

$$E_o = E_{sc} + E_{e-} \qquad [3\text{-}1]$$

Compton scattering results in the ionization of the atom and a division of the incident photon's energy between the scattered photon and the ejected electron. The ejected electron will lose its kinetic energy via excitation and ionization of atoms in the surrounding material. The Compton scattered photon may traverse the medium without interaction or may undergo subsequent interactions such as Compton scattering, photoelectric absorption (to be discussed shortly), or Rayleigh scattering.

The energy of the scattered photon can be calculated from the energy of the incident photon and the angle (with respect to the incident trajectory) of the scattered photon:

■ **FIGURE** 3-7 Compton scattering. The diagram shows the incident photon with energy E_o, interacting with a valence-shell electron that results in the ejection of the Compton electron (E_{e-}) and the simultaneous emission of a Compton scattered photon E_{sc} emerging at an angle θ relative to the trajectory of the incident photon. *K, L,* and *M* are electron shells.

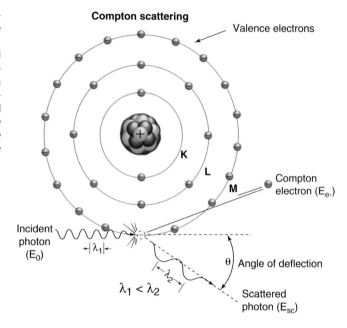

$$E_{sc} = \frac{E_o}{1 + \dfrac{E_o}{511 \text{ keV}}(1 - \cos \theta)} \qquad [3\text{-}2]$$

where E_{sc} = the energy of the scattered photon, E_o = the incident photon energy, and θ = the angle of the scattered photon.

As the incident photon energy increases, both scattered photons and electrons are scattered more toward the forward direction (Fig. 3-8). In x-ray transmission imaging, these photons are much more likely to be detected by the image receptor. In addition, for a given scattering angle, the fraction of energy transferred to the scattered photon decreases with increasing incident photon energy. Thus, for higher energy incident photons, the majority of the energy is transferred to the scattered electron. For example, for a 60-degree scattering angle, the scattered photon energy (E_{sc}) is 90% of the incident photon energy (E_o) at 100 keV but only 17% at 5 MeV.

■ **FIGURE 3-8** Graph illustrates relative Compton scatter probability as a function of scattering angle for 20-, 80-, and 140-keV photons in tissue. Each curve is normalized to 100%. (From Bushberg JT. The AAPM/RSNA physics tutorial for residents. X-ray interactions. *RadioGraphics* 1998;18:457–468, with permission.)

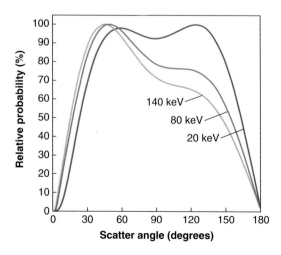

When Compton scattering occurs at the lower x-ray energies used in diagnostic imaging (15 to 150 keV), the majority of the incident photon energy is transferred to the scattered photon. For example, following the Compton interaction of an 80-keV photon, the minimum energy of the scattered photon is 61 keV. Thus, even with maximal energy loss, the scattered photons have relatively high energies and tissue penetrability. In x-ray transmission imaging and nuclear emission imaging, the detection of scattered photons by the image receptors results in a degradation of image contrast and an increase in random noise. These concepts, and many others related to image quality, will be discussed in Chapter 4.

The laws of conservation of energy and momentum place limits on both scattering angle and energy transfer. For example, the maximal energy transfer to the Compton electron (and thus, the maximum reduction in incident photon energy) occurs with a 180-degree photon scatter (backscatter). In fact, the maximal energy of the scattered photon is limited to 511 keV at 90 degrees scattering and to 255 keV for a 180-degree scattering event. These limits on scattered photon energy hold even for extremely high-energy photons (e.g., therapeutic energy range). The scattering angle of the ejected electron cannot exceed 90 degrees, whereas that of the scattered photon can be any value including a 180-degree backscatter. In contrast to the scattered photon, the energy of the ejected electron is usually absorbed near the scattering site.

The incident photon energy must be substantially greater than the electron's binding energy before a Compton interaction is likely to take place. Thus, the relative probability of a Compton interaction increases, compared to Rayleigh scattering or photoelectric absorption, as the incident photon energy increases. The probability of Compton interaction also depends on the electron density (number of electrons/g × density). With the exception of hydrogen, the total number of electrons/g is fairly constant in tissue; thus, the probability of Compton scattering per unit mass is nearly independent of Z, and the probability of Compton scattering per unit volume is approximately proportional to the density of the material. Compared to other elements, the absence of neutrons in the hydrogen atom results in an approximate doubling of electron density. Thus, hydrogenous materials have a higher probability of Compton scattering than anhydrogenous material of equal mass.

The Photoelectric Effect

In the photoelectric effect, all of the incident photon energy is transferred to an electron, which is ejected from the atom. The kinetic energy of the ejected *photoelectron* (E_{pe}) is equal to the incident photon energy (E_0) minus the binding energy of the orbital electron (E_b) (Fig. 3-9 left).

$$E_{pe} = E_0 - E_b \qquad [3\text{-}3]$$

In order for photoelectric absorption to occur, the incident photon energy must be greater than or equal to the binding energy of the electron that is ejected. The ejected electron is most likely one whose binding energy is closest to, but less than, the incident photon energy. For example, for photons whose energies exceed the *K*-shell binding energy, photoelectric interactions with *K*-shell electrons are most probable. Following a photoelectric interaction, the atom is ionized, with an inner-shell electron vacancy. This vacancy will be filled by an electron from a shell with a lower binding energy. This creates another vacancy, which, in turn, is filled by an electron from an even lower binding energy shell. Thus, an electron cascade from outer to inner shells occurs. The difference in binding energy is released as either characteristic x-rays or Auger electrons (see Chapter 2). The probability of characteristic x-ray emission decreases as the atomic number of the absorber decreases, and

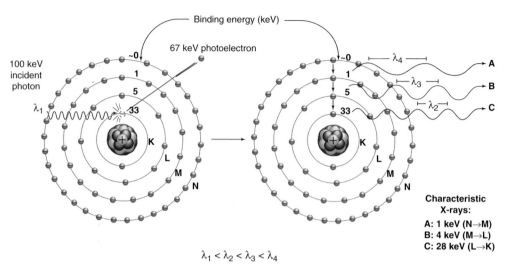

$$\lambda_1 < \lambda_2 < \lambda_3 < \lambda_4$$

■ **FIGURE 3-9** Photoelectric absorption. **Left**. The diagram shows that a 100-keV photon is undergoing photoelectric absorption with an iodine atom. In this case, the *K*-shell electron is ejected with a kinetic energy equal to the difference (67 keV) between the incident photon energy (100 keV) and the *K*-shell binding energy (33 keV). **Right**. The vacancy created in the *K* shell results in the transition of an electron from the *L* shell to the *K* shell. The difference in their binding energies (i.e., 33 and 5 keV) results in a 28-keV K_α characteristic x-ray. This electron cascade will continue, resulting in the production of other characteristic x-rays of lower energies. Note that the sum of the characteristic x-ray energies equals the binding energy of the ejected photoelectron (33 keV). Although not shown on this diagram, Auger electrons of various energies could be emitted in lieu of the characteristic x-ray emissions.

thus, characteristic x-ray emission does not occur frequently for diagnostic energy photon interactions in soft tissue. The photoelectric effect can and does occur with valence shell electrons such as when light photons strike the high Z materials that comprise the photocathode (e.g., cesium, rubidium and antimony) of a photomultiplier tube. These materials are specially selected to provide weakly bound electrons (i.e., electrons with a low work function), so when illuminated the photocathode readily releases electrons (see Chapter 17). In this case, no inner shell electron cascade occurs and thus no characteristic x-rays are produced.

EXAMPLE: The *K*- and *L*-shell electron binding energies of iodine are 33 and 5 keV, respectively. If a 100-keV photon is absorbed by a *K*-shell electron in a photoelectric interaction, the photoelectron is ejected with a kinetic energy equal to $E_o - E_b = 100 - 33 = 67$ keV. A characteristic x-ray or Auger electron is emitted as an outer-shell electron fills the *K*-shell vacancy (e.g., *L* to *K* transition is $33 - 5 = 28$ keV). The remaining energy is released by subsequent cascading events in the outer shells of the atom (i.e., *M* to *L* and *N* to *M* transitions). Note that the total of all the characteristic x-ray emissions in this example equals the binding energy of the *K*-shell photoelectron (Fig. 3-9, right).

Thus, photoelectric absorption results in the production of

1. A photoelectron
2. A positive ion (ionized atom)
3. Characteristic x-rays or Auger electrons

The probability of photoelectric absorption per unit mass is approximately proportional to Z^3/E^3, where Z is the atomic number and E is the energy of the incident photon. For example, the photoelectric interaction probability in iodine (Z = 53) is $(53/20)^3$ or 18.6 times greater than in calcium (Z = 20) for a photon of a particular energy.

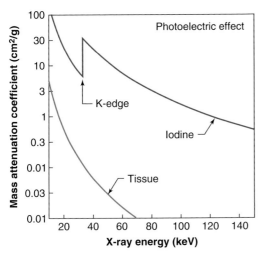

■ **FIGURE 3-10** Photoelectric mass attenuation coefficients for tissue ($Z_{effective}$ = 7), and iodine (Z = 53) as a function of energy. Abrupt increase in the attenuation coefficients called "absorption edges" occur due to increased probability of photoelectric absorption when the photon energy just exceeds the binding energy of inner-shell electrons (e.g., K, L, M,...), thus increasing the number of electrons available for interaction. This process is very significant in high-Z elements, such as iodine and barium, for x-rays in the diagnostic energy range.

The benefit of photoelectric absorption in x-ray transmission imaging is that there are no scattered photons to degrade the image. The fact that the probability of photoelectric interaction is proportional to $1/E^3$ explains, in part, why image contrast decreases when higher x-ray energies are used in the imaging process (see Chapters 4 and 7). If the photon energies are doubled, the probability of photoelectric interaction is decreased eightfold: $(½)^3 = 1/8$.

Although the probability of the photoelectric effect decreases, in general, with increasing photon energy, there is an exception. For every element, the probability of the photoelectric effect, as a function of photon energy, exhibits sharp discontinuities called *absorption edges* (see Fig. 3-10). The probability of interaction for photons of energy just above an absorption edge is much greater than that of photons of energy slightly below the edge. For example, a 33.2-keV x-ray photon is about six times as likely to have a photoelectric interaction with an iodine atom as a 33.1-keV photon.

As mentioned above, a photon cannot undergo a photoelectric interaction with an electron in a particular atomic shell or subshell if the photon's energy is less than the binding energy of that shell or subshell. This causes the dramatic decrease in the probability of photoelectric absorption for photons whose energies are just below the binding energy of a shell. Thus, the photon energy corresponding to an absorption edge is the binding energy of the electrons in that particular shell or subshell. An absorption edge is designated by a letter, representing the atomic shell of the electrons, followed by a roman numeral subscript denoting the subshell (e.g., K, L_1, L_{II}, L_{III}). The photon energy corresponding to a particular absorption edge increases with the atomic number (Z) of the element. For example, the primary elements comprising soft tissue (H, C, N, and O) have absorption edges below 1 keV. The element iodine (Z = 53) commonly used in radiographic contrast agents to provide enhanced x-ray attenuation, has a K-absorption edge of 33.2 keV (Fig. 3-10). The K-edge energy of the target material in most x-ray tubes (tungsten, Z = 74) is 69.5 keV. The K- and L-shell binding energies for elements with atomic numbers 1 to 100 are provided in Appendix C, Table C-3.

The photoelectric process predominates when lower energy photons interact with high Z materials (Fig. 3-11). In fact, photoelectric absorption is the primary mode of interaction of diagnostic x-rays with image receptors, radiographic contrast materials, and radiation shielding, all of which have much higher atomic numbers than soft tissue. Conversely, Compton scattering predominates at most diagnostic and therapeutic photon energies in materials of lower atomic number such as tissue and air. At photon energies below 50 keV, photoelectric interactions in soft tissue

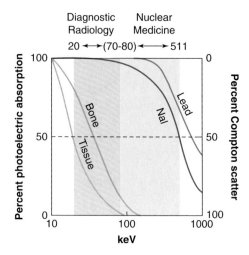

■ **FIGURE 3-11** Graph of the percentage of contribution of photoelectric (**left scale**) and Compton (**right scale**) attenuation processes for various materials as a function of energy. When diagnostic energy photons (i.e., diagnostic x-ray effective energy of 20 to 80 keV; nuclear medicine imaging photons of 70 to 511 keV) interact with materials of low atomic number (e.g., soft tissue), the Compton process dominates.

play an important role in medical imaging. The photoelectric absorption process can be used to amplify differences in attenuation between tissues with slightly different atomic numbers, thereby improving image contrast. This differential absorption is exploited to improve image contrast through the selection of x-ray tube target material and filters in mammography (see Chapter 8).

Pair Production

Pair production can only occur when the energies of x-rays and gamma rays exceed 1.02 MeV. In pair production, an x-ray or gamma ray interacts with the electric field of the nucleus of an atom. The photon's energy is transformed into an electron-positron pair (Fig. 3-12A). The rest mass energy equivalent of each electron is 0.511 MeV, and this is why the energy threshold for this reaction is 1.02 MeV. Photon energy in excess of this threshold is imparted to the electron (also referred to as a negatron or beta minus particle) and positron as kinetic energy. The electron and positron lose their kinetic energy via excitation and ionization. As discussed previously, when the positron comes to rest, it interacts with a negatively charged electron, resulting in the formation of two oppositely directed 0.511-MeV annihilation photons (Fig. 3-12B).

Pair production does not occur in diagnostic x-ray imaging because the threshold photon energy is well beyond even the highest energies used in medical imaging. In fact, pair production does not become significant until the photon energies greatly exceed the 1.02-MeV energy threshold.

3.3 Attenuation of X-rays and Gamma Rays

Attenuation is the removal of photons from a beam of x-rays or gamma rays as it passes through matter. Attenuation is caused by both absorption and scattering of the primary photons. The interaction mechanisms discussed in the previous section, in varying degrees, cause the attenuation. At low photon energies (less than 26 keV), the photoelectric effect dominates the attenuation processes in soft tissue. However, as previously discussed, the probability of photoelectric absorption is highly dependent on photon energy and the atomic number of the absorber. When higher energy photons interact with low Z materials (e.g., soft tissue), Compton scattering dominates (Fig. 3-13). Rayleigh scattering occurs in medical imaging with low probability,

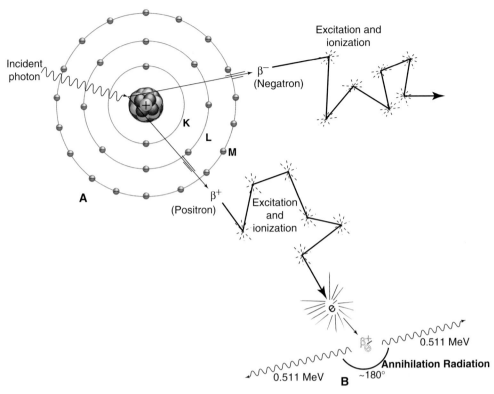

■ FIGURE 3-12 Pair production. **A.** The diagram illustrates the pair production process in which a high-energy incident photon, under the influence of the atomic nucleus, is converted to an electron-positron pair. Both electrons (positron and negatron) expend their kinetic energy by excitation and ionization in the matter they traverse. **B.** However, when the positron comes to rest, it combines with an electron producing the two 511-keV annihilation radiation photons. *K, L,* and *M* are electron shells.

comprising about 10% of the interactions in mammography and 5% in chest radiography. Only at very high photon energies (greater than 1.02 MeV), well beyond the range of diagnostic and nuclear radiology, does pair production contribute to attenuation.

Linear Attenuation Coefficient

The fraction of photons removed from a monoenergetic beam of x-rays or gamma rays per unit thickness of material is called the *linear attenuation coefficient* (μ), typically expressed in units of inverse centimeters (cm^{-1}). The number of photons removed from the beam traversing a very small thickness Δx can be expressed as

$$n = \mu \, N \, \Delta x \qquad\qquad [3\text{-}4]$$

where n = the number of photons removed from the beam, and N = the number of photons incident on the material.

For example, for 100-keV photons traversing soft tissue, the linear attenuation coefficient is 0.016 mm^{-1}. This signifies that for every 1,000 monoenergetic photons incident upon a 1-mm thickness of tissue, approximately 16 will be removed from the beam, by either absorption or scattering.

As the thickness increases, however, the relationship is not linear. For example, it would not be correct to conclude from Equation 3-4 that 6 cm of tissue would attenuate 960 (96%) of the incident photons. To accurately calculate the number of

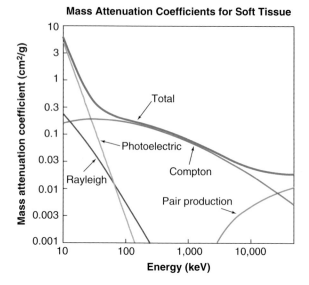

■ FIGURE 3-13 Graph of the Rayleigh, photoelectric, Compton, pair production, and total mass attenuation coefficients for soft tissue (Z ≈ 7) as a function of photon energy.

photons removed from the beam using Equation 3-4, multiple calculations utilizing very small thicknesses of material (Δx) would be required. Alternatively, calculus can be employed to simplify this otherwise tedious process. For a monoenergetic beam of photons incident upon either thick or thin slabs of material, an exponential relationship exists between the number of incident photons (N_0) and those that are transmitted (N) through a thickness x without interaction:

$$N = N_0 e^{-\mu x} \qquad [3\text{-}5]$$

Thus, using the example above, the fraction of 100-keV photons transmitted through 6 cm of tissue is

$$N/N_0 = e^{-(0.16\ \text{cm}^{-1})(6\ \text{cm})} = 0.38$$

This result indicates that, on average, 380 of the 1,000 incident photons (i.e., 38%) would be transmitted through the 6-cm slab of tissue without interacting. Thus, the actual attenuation (1 − 0.38 or 62%) is much lower than would have been predicted from Equation 3-4.

The linear attenuation coefficient is the sum of the individual linear attenuation coefficients for each type of interaction:

$$\mu = \mu_{\text{Rayleigh}} + \mu_{\text{photoelectric effect}} + \mu_{\text{Compton scatter}} + \mu_{\text{pair production}} \qquad [3\text{-}6]$$

In the diagnostic energy range, the linear attenuation coefficient decreases with increasing energy except at absorption edges (e.g., K-edge). The linear attenuation coefficient for soft tissue ranges from approximately 0.35 to 0.16 cm^{-1} for photon energies ranging from 30 to 100 keV.

For a given thickness of material, the probability of interaction depends on the number of atoms the x-rays or gamma rays encounter per unit distance. The density (ρ, in g/cm^3) of the material affects this number. For example, if the density is doubled, the photons will encounter twice as many atoms per unit distance through the material. Thus, the linear attenuation coefficient is proportional to the density of the material, for instance:

$$\mu_{\text{water}} > \mu_{\text{ice}} > \mu_{\text{water vapor}}$$

The relationship among material density, electron density, electrons per mass, and the linear attenuation coefficient (at 50 keV) for several materials is shown in Table 3-1.

TABLE 3-1 MATERIAL DENSITY, ELECTRONS PER MASS, ELECTRON DENSITY, AND THE LINEAR ATTENUATION COEFFICIENT (AT 50 keV) FOR SEVERAL MATERIALS

MATERIAL	DENSITY (g/cm³)	ELECTRONS PER MASS (e/g) × 10²³	ELECTRON DENSITY (e/cm³) × 10²³	μ @ 50 keV (cm⁻¹)
Hydrogen gas	0.000084	5.97	0.0005	0.000028
Water vapor	0.000598	3.34	0.002	0.000128
Air	0.00129	3.006	0.0038	0.000290
Fat	0.91	3.34	3.04	0.193
Ice	0.917	3.34	3.06	0.196
Water	1	3.34	3.34	0.214
Compact bone	1.85	3.192	5.91	0.573

Mass Attenuation Coefficient

For a given material and thickness, the probability of interaction is proportional to the number of atoms per volume. This dependency can be overcome by normalizing the linear attenuation coefficient for the density of the material. The linear attenuation coefficient, normalized to unit density, is called the *mass attenuation coefficient*.

$$\text{Mass Attenuation Coefficient } (\mu/\rho)\left[\text{cm}^2/\text{g}\right]$$

$$= \frac{\text{Linear Attenuation Coefficient } (\mu)\text{cm}^{-1}]}{\text{Density of Material } (\rho) \, [\text{g/cm}^3]} \qquad [3\text{-}7]$$

The linear attenuation coefficient is usually expressed in units of cm⁻¹, whereas the units of the mass attenuation coefficient are usually cm²/g.

The mass attenuation coefficient is *independent* of density. Therefore, for a given photon energy,

$$\mu_{\text{water}}/\rho_{\text{water}} = \mu_{\text{ice}}/\rho_{\text{ice}} = \mu_{\text{water vapor}}/\rho_{\text{water vapor}}$$

However, in radiology, we do not usually compare equal masses. Instead, we usually compare regions of an image that correspond to irradiation of adjacent volumes of tissue. Therefore, density, the mass contained within a given volume, plays an important role. Thus, one can radiographically visualize ice in a cup of water due to the density difference between the ice and the surrounding water (Fig. 3-14).

To calculate the linear attenuation coefficient for a density other than 1 g/cm³, the density ρ of the material is multiplied by the mass attenuation coefficient to yield the linear attenuation coefficient. For example, the mass attenuation coefficient of air, for 60-keV photons, is 0.186 cm²/g. At typical room conditions, the density of air is 0.00129 g/cm³. Therefore, the linear attenuation coefficient of air under these conditions is

$$\mu = (\mu/\rho_o)\rho = (0.186 \text{ cm}^2/\text{g}) (0.00129 \text{ g/cm}^3) = 0.000240 \text{ cm}^{-1}$$

To use the mass attenuation coefficient to compute attenuation, Equation 3-5 can be rewritten as

$$N = N_o e^{-\left(\frac{\mu}{\rho}\right)\rho x} \qquad [3\text{-}8]$$

Because the use of the mass attenuation coefficient is so common, scientists in this field tend to think of thickness not as a linear distance *x* (in cm) but rather in

■ **FIGURE 3-14** Radiograph (acquired at 125 kV with an antiscatter grid) of two ice cubes in a plastic container of water. The ice cubes can be visualized because of their lower electron density relative to that of liquid water. The small radiolucent objects seen at several locations are the result of air bubbles in the water. (From Bushberg JT. The AAPM/RSNA physics tutorial for residents. X-ray interactions. *RadioGraphics* 1998;18:457–468, with permission.)

terms of mass per unit area ρx (in g/cm^2). The product ρx is called the *mass thickness* or *areal thickness*.

Half-Value Layer

The half-value layer (HVL) is defined as the thickness of material required to reduce the intensity (e.g., air kerma rate) of an x-ray or gamma-ray beam to one half of its initial value. The HVL of a beam is an indirect measure of the photon energies (also referred to as the *quality*) of a beam, when measured under conditions of *narrow-beam geometry*. Narrow-beam geometry refers to an experimental configuration that is designed to exclude scattered photons from being measured by the detector (Fig. 3-15A). In *broad-beam geometry*, the beam is sufficiently wide that a substantial fraction of scattered photons remain in the beam. These scattered photons reaching the detector (Fig. 3-15B) result in an underestimation of the attenuation coefficient

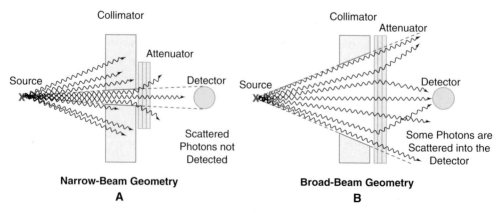

■ **FIGURE 3-15 A.** Narrow-beam geometry means that the relationship between the source shield and the detector is such that almost no scattered photons interact with the detector. **B.** In broad-beam geometry, scattered photons may reach the detector; thus, the measured attenuation is less compared with narrow-beam conditions.

(i.e., an overestimated HVL). Most practical applications of attenuation (e.g., patient imaging) occur under broad-beam conditions. The tenth-value layer (TVL) is analogous to the HVL, except that it is the thickness of material that is necessary to reduce the intensity of the beam to a tenth of its initial value. The TVL is often used in x-ray room shielding design calculations (see Chapter 21).

For monoenergetic photons under narrow-beam geometry conditions, the probability of attenuation remains the same for each additional HVL thickness placed in the beam. Reduction in beam intensity can be expressed as $(1/2)^n$, where n equals the number of HVLs. For example, the fraction of monoenergetic photons transmitted through 5 HVLs of material is

$$\frac{1}{2} \times \frac{1}{2} \times \frac{1}{2} \times \frac{1}{2} \times \frac{1}{2} = (1/2)^5 = 1/32 = 0.031 \text{ or } 3.1\%$$

Therefore, 97% of the photons are attenuated (removed from the beam). The HVL of a diagnostic x-ray beam, measured in millimeters of aluminum under narrow-beam conditions, is a surrogate measure of the penetrability of an x-ray spectrum.

It is important to understand the relationship between μ and HVL. In Equation 3-5, N is equal to $N_o/2$ when the thickness of the absorber is 1 HVL. Thus, for a monoenergetic beam,

$$N_o/2 = N_o e^{-\mu(\text{HVL})}$$
$$1/2 = e^{-\mu(\text{HVL})}$$
$$\ln(1/2) = \ln e^{-\mu(\text{HVL})}$$
$$-0.693 = -\mu(\text{HVL})$$
$$\text{HVL} = 0.693/\mu \qquad [3\text{-}9]$$

For a monoenergetic incident photon beam, the HVL can be easily calculated from the linear attenuation coefficient, and vice versa. For example, given
1. $\mu = 0.35 \text{ cm}^{-1}$

$$\text{HVL} = 0.693/0.35 \text{ cm}^{-1} = 1.98 \text{ cm}$$

2. $\text{HVL} = 2.5 \text{ mm} = 0.25 \text{ cm}$

$$\mu = 0.693/0.25 \text{ cm} = 2.8 \text{ cm}^{-1}$$

The HVL and μ can also be calculated if the percent transmission is measured under narrow-beam geometry.

EXAMPLE: If a 0.2-cm thickness of material transmits 25% of a monoenergetic beam of photons, calculate the HVL of the beam for that material.

STEP 1. $0.25 = e^{-\mu(0.2 \text{ cm})}$

STEP 2. $\ln 0.25 = -\mu(0.2 \text{ cm})$

STEP 3. $\mu = (-\ln 0.25)/(0.2 \text{ cm}) = 6.93 \text{ cm}^{-1}$

STEP 4. $\text{HVL} = 0.693/\mu = 0.693/6.93 \text{ cm}^{-1} = 0.1 \text{ cm}$

HVLs for photons from three commonly used diagnostic radionuclides (^{201}Tl, ^{99m}Tc, and ^{18}F) are listed for tissue and lead in Table 3-2. Thus, the HVL is a function of (a) photon energy, (b) geometry, and (c) attenuating material.

Effective Energy

X-ray beams in radiology are *polyenergetic*, meaning that they are composed of a spectrum of x-ray energies. The determination of the HVL in diagnostic radiology is a way of characterizing the penetrability of the x-ray beam. The HVL, usually measured

TABLE 3-2   HVLs OF TISSUE, ALUMINUM, AND LEAD FOR X-RAYS AND GAMMA RAYS COMMONLY USED IN NUCLEAR MEDICINE

	HALF VALUE LAYER (mm)	
PHOTON SOURCE	TISSUE	LEAD
70 keV x-rays (^{201}Tl)	37	0.2
140 keV γ-rays (^{99m}Tc)	44	0.3
511 keV γ-rays (^{18}F)	75	4.1

Tc, technetium; Tl, thallium; Fl, fluorine.
Note: These values are based on the narrow-beam geometry attenuation and neglecting the effect of scatter. Shielding calculations (discussed in Chapter 21) are typically for broad-beam conditions.

in millimeters of aluminum (mm Al) in diagnostic radiology, can be converted to a quantity called the *effective energy*. The effective energy of a polyenergetic x-ray beam is an estimate of the penetration power of the x-ray beam, expressed as the energy of a monoenergetic beam that would exhibit the same "effective" penetrability. The relationship between HVL (in mm Al) and effective energy is given in Table 3-3. The effective energy of an x-ray beam from a typical diagnostic x-ray tube is one third to one half the maximal value.

Mean Free Path

One cannot predict the range of a single photon in matter. In fact, the range can vary from zero to infinity. However, the average distance traveled before interaction can

TABLE 3-3   HVL AS A FUNCTION OF THE EFFECTIVE ENERGY OF AN X-RAY BEAM

HVL (mm Al)	EFFECTIVE ENERGY (keV)
0.26	14
0.75	20
1.25	24
1.90	28
3.34	35
4.52	40
5.76	45
6.97	50
9.24	60
11.15	70
12.73	80
14.01	90
15.06	100

Al, aluminum.

Average Photon Energy and HVL Increases

Photon Intensity (i.e. quantity) decreases

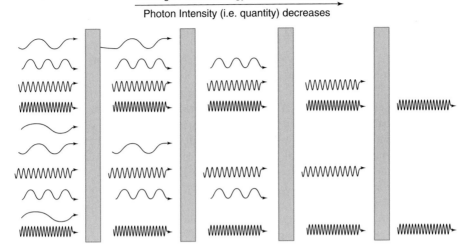

■ **FIGURE 3-16** Beam hardening results from preferential absorption of lower energy photons as the x-rays traverse matter.

be calculated from the linear attenuation coefficient or the HVL of the beam. This length, called the *mean free path* (MFP) of the photon beam, is

$$\text{MFP} = \frac{1}{\mu} = \frac{1}{0.693 \, / \, \text{HVL}} = 1.44 \, \text{HVL} \qquad [3\text{-}10]$$

Beam Hardening

The lower energy photons of the polyenergetic x-ray beam will preferentially be removed from the beam while passing through matter. The shift of the x-ray spectrum to higher effective energies as the beam transverses matter is called *beam hardening* (Fig. 3-16). Low-energy (soft) x-rays will not penetrate the entire thickness of the body; thus, their removal reduces patient dose without affecting the diagnostic quality of the exam. X-ray machines remove most of this soft radiation with filters, thin plates of aluminum, copper, or other materials placed in the beam. This added filtration will result in an x-ray beam with a higher effective energy and thus a greater HVL.

The homogeneity coefficient is the ratio of the first to the second HVL and describes the polyenergetic character of the beam. The first HVL is the thickness that reduces the incident intensity to 50%, and the second HVL reduces it to 25% of its original intensity (i.e., $0.5 \times 0.5 = 0.25$). For most of diagnostic x-ray imaging the homogeneity coefficient of the x-ray spectrum is between 0.5–0.7. However for special applications such as conventional projection mammography with factors optimized to enhance the spectral uniformity of the x-ray beam the homogeneity coefficient can be as high as 0.97. A monoenergetic source of gamma rays has a homogeneity coefficient equal to 1.

The maximal x-ray energy of a polyenergetic spectrum can be estimated by monitoring the homogeneity coefficient of two heavily filtered beams (e.g., 15th and 16th HVLs). As the coefficient approaches 1, the beam is essentially monoenergetic. Measuring μ for the material in question under heavy filtration conditions and matching it to known values of μ for monoenergetic beams provides an approximation of the maximal energy.

3.4 Absorption of Energy from X-rays and Gamma Rays

Radiation Units and Measurements

The International System of units (SI) provides a common system of units for science and technology. The system consists of seven base units: meter (m) for length, kilogram (kg) for mass, second (s) for time, ampere (A) for electric current, kelvin (K) for temperature, candela (cd) for luminous intensity, and mole (mol) for the amount of substance. In addition to the seven base units, there are *derived units* defined as combinations of the base units. Examples of derived units are speed (m/s) and density (kg/m³). Details regarding derived units used in the measurement and calculation of radiation dose for specific applications can be found in the documents of the International Commission on Radiation Units and Measurements (ICRU) and the International Commission on Radiological Protection (ICRP). Several of these units are described below, whereas others related to specific imaging modalities or those having specific regulatory significance are described in the relevant chapters.

Fluence, Flux, and Energy Fluence

The number of photons or particles passing through a unit cross-sectional area is referred to as the *fluence* and is typically expressed in units of cm^{-2}. The fluence is given the symbol Φ.

$$\Phi = \frac{Photons}{Area} \qquad [3\text{-}11]$$

The fluence rate (e.g., the rate at which photons or particles pass through a unit area per unit time) is called the *flux*. The flux, given the symbol $\dot{\Phi}$, is simply the fluence per unit time.

$$\dot{\Phi} = \frac{Photons}{Area \cdot Time} \qquad [3\text{-}12]$$

The flux is useful in situations in which the photon beam is on for extended periods of time, such as in fluoroscopy. Flux has the units of cm^{-2} s^{-1}.

The amount of energy passing through a unit cross-sectional area is referred to as the *energy fluence*. For a monoenergetic beam of photons, the energy fluence (Ψ) is simply the product of the fluence (Φ) and the energy per photon (E).

$$\Psi = \Phi \left(\frac{Photons}{Area} \right) \times E \left(\frac{Energy}{Photon} \right) \qquad [3\text{-}13]$$

The units of Ψ are energy per unit area, J m^{-2}, or joules per m². For a polyenergetic spectrum, the total energy in the beam is tabulated by multiplying the number of photons at each energy by that energy and adding these products. The energy fluence rate or energy flux is the energy fluence per unit time.

Kerma

As a beam of indirectly (uncharged) ionizing radiation (e.g., x-rays or gamma rays or neutrons) passes through a medium, it deposits energy in the medium in a two-step process:
Step 1. Energy carried by the photons (or other indirectly ionizing radiation) is transformed into kinetic energy of charged particles (such as electrons). In the case of x-rays and gamma rays, the energy is transferred by photoelectric absorption, Compton scattering, and, for very high energy photons, pair production.

Step 2. The directly ionizing (charged) particles deposit their energy in the medium by excitation and ionization. In some cases, the range of the charged particles is sufficiently large that energy deposition is some distance away from the initial interactions.

Kerma (K) is an acronym for *kinetic energy released in matter*. Kerma is defined at the kinetic energy transferred to charged particles by indirectly ionizing radiation per unit mass, as described in Step 1 above. The SI unit of Kerma is the joule per kilogram with the special name of the *gray* (Gy) or milligray (mGy), where $1 \text{ Gy} = 1 \text{ J kg}^{-1}$. For x-rays and gamma rays, kerma can be calculated from the mass energy transfer coefficient of the material and the energy fluence.

Mass Energy Transfer Coefficient

The mass energy transfer coefficient is given the symbol:

$$\left(\frac{\mu_{tr}}{\rho_o} \right)$$

The mass energy transfer coefficient is the mass attenuation coefficient multiplied by the fraction of the energy of the interacting photons that is transferred to charged particles as kinetic energy. As was mentioned above, energy deposition in matter by photons is largely delivered by the energetic charged particles produced by photon interactions. The energy in scattered photons that escape the interaction site is not transferred to charged particles in the volume of interest. Furthermore, when pair production occurs, 1.02 MeV of the incident photon's energy is required to produce the electron-positron pair and only the remaining energy (E_{photon} − 1.02 MeV) is given to the electron and positron as kinetic energy. Therefore, the mass energy transfer coefficient will always be less than the mass attenuation coefficient.

For 20-keV photons in tissue, for example, the ratio of the energy transfer coefficient to the attenuation coefficient (μ_{tr}/μ) is 0.68, but this reduces to 0.18 for 50-keV photons, as the amount of Compton scattering increases relative to photoelectric absorption.

Calculation of Kerma

For a monoenergetic photon beam with an energy fluence Ψ and energy E, the kerma K is given by

$$K = \Psi \left(\frac{\mu_{tr}}{\rho_o} \right)_E \tag{3-14}$$

where $\left(\dfrac{\mu_{tr}}{\rho_o} \right)_E$ is the mass energy transfer coefficient of the absorber at energy E. The SI units of energy fluence are J m^{-2}, and the SI units of the mass energy transfer coefficient are $\text{m}^2 \text{ kg}^{-1}$, and thus their product, kerma, has units of J kg^{-1} ($1 \text{ J kg}^{-1} = 1 \text{ Gy}$).

Absorbed Dose

The quantity *absorbed dose* (D) is defined as the energy (E) imparted by ionizing radiation per unit mass of irradiated material (m):

$$D = \frac{E}{m} \tag{3-15}$$

Unlike Kerma, absorbed dose is defined for all types of ionizing radiation (i.e., directly and indirectly ionizing). However, the SI unit of absorbed dose and kerma, is the same (gray), where $1 \text{ Gy} = 1 \text{ J kg}^{-1}$. The older unit of absorbed dose is the *rad* (an acronym for *radiation absorbed dose*). One rad is equal to 0.01 J kg^{-1}. Thus, there are 100 rads in a gray, and 1 rad $= 10$ mGy.

If the energy imparted to charged particles is deposited locally and the bremsstrahlung produced by the energetic electrons is negligible, the absorbed dose will be equal to the kerma. For x-rays and gamma rays, the absorbed dose can be calculated from the mass energy absorption coefficient and the energy fluence of the beam.

Mass Energy Absorption Coefficient

The mass energy transfer coefficient discussed above describes the fraction of the mass attenuation coefficient that gives rise to the initial kinetic energy of electrons in a small volume of absorber. The mass energy absorption coefficient will be the same as the mass energy transfer coefficient when all transferred energy is locally absorbed. However, energetic electrons may subsequently produce bremsstrahlung radiation (x-rays), which can escape the small volume of interest. Thus, the mass energy absorption coefficient may be slightly smaller than the mass energy transfer coefficient. For the energies used in diagnostic radiology and for low-Z absorbers (air, water, tissue), the amount of radiative losses (bremsstrahlung) is very small. Thus, for diagnostic radiology,

$$\left(\frac{\mu_{en}}{\rho_{0}}\right) \cong \left(\frac{\mu_{tr}}{\rho_{0}}\right)$$

The mass energy absorption coefficient is useful when energy deposition calculations are to be made.

Calculation of Dose

The distinction between kerma and dose is slight for the relatively low x-ray energies used in diagnostic radiology. The dose in any material is given by

$$D = \Psi \left(\frac{\mu_{en}}{\rho_{0}}\right)_{E}$$
[3-16]

The difference between the calculation of kerma and dose for air is that kerma is defined using the mass energy transfer coefficient, whereas dose is defined using the mass energy absorption coefficient. The mass energy transfer coefficient defines the energy transferred to charged particles, but these energetic charged particles (mostly electrons) in the absorber may experience radiative losses, which can exit the small volume of interest. The coefficient

$$\left(\frac{\mu_{en}}{\rho_{0}}\right)_{E}$$

takes into account the radiative losses, and thus

$$\left(\frac{\mu_{tr}}{\rho_{0}}\right)_{E} \geq \left(\frac{\mu_{en}}{\rho_{0}}\right)_{E}$$

Exposure

The amount of electrical charge (Q) produced by ionizing electromagnetic radiation per mass (*m*) of air is called *exposure* (*X*):

$$X = \frac{Q}{m}$$
[3-17]

Exposure is expressed in the units of charge per mass, that is, coulombs per kg ($C \, kg^{-1}$). The historical unit of exposure is the roentgen (abbreviated R), which is defined as

$$1 \, R = 2.58 \times 10^{-4} \, C \, kg^{-1} \, \text{(exactly)}$$

Radiation beams are often expressed as an exposure rate (R/h or mR/min). The output intensity of an x-ray machine can be measured and expressed as an exposure (R) per unit of current times exposure duration (milliampere second or mAs) under specified operating conditions (e.g., 5 mR/mAs at 70 kV for a source-image distance of 100 cm, and with an x-ray beam filtration equivalent to 2 mm Al).

Exposure is a useful quantity because ionization can be directly measured with air-filled radiation detectors, and the effective atomic numbers of air and soft tissue are approximately the same. Thus, exposure is nearly proportional to dose in soft tissue over the range of photon energies commonly used in radiology. However, the quantity of exposure is limited in that it applies only to the interaction of ionizing photons (not charged particle radiation) in air (not any other substance).

The exposure can be calculated from the dose to air. Let the ratio of the dose (D) to the exposure (X) in air be W and substituting in the above expressions for D and X yields

$$W = \frac{D}{X} = \frac{E}{Q} \qquad [3\text{-}18]$$

W, the average energy deposited per ion pair in air, is approximately constant as a function of energy. The value of W is 33.85 eV/ion pair or 33.85 J/C.

In terms of the traditional unit of exposure, the roentgen, the dose to air is

$$K_{air} = W \times X \left(\frac{2.58 \times 10^{-4} \, C}{kg \cdot R} \right)$$

or

$$K_{air} \, (Gy) = 0.00873 \left(\frac{Gy}{R} \right) \times X \qquad [3\text{-}19]$$

Thus, one R of exposure results in 8.73 mGy of air dose. The quantity exposure is still in common use in the United States, but the equivalent SI quantities of air dose or air kerma are used exclusively in most other countries. These conversions can be simplified to

$$K_{air} \, (mGy) = \frac{X \, (mR)}{114.5 (mR / mGy)} \qquad [3\text{-}20]$$

$$K_{air} (\mu Gy) = \frac{X (\mu R)}{114.5 (\mu R / \mu Gy)} \qquad [3\text{-}21]$$

3.5 Imparted Energy, Equivalent Dose, and Effective Dose

Imparted Energy

The total amount of energy deposited in matter, called the *imparted energy* (ε), is the product of the dose and the mass over which the energy is imparted. The unit of imparted energy is the joule.

$$\varepsilon = (J/kg) \times kg = J \qquad [3\text{-}22]$$

For example, assume a head computed tomography (CT) scan delivers a 30 mGy dose to the tissue in each 5-mm slice. If the scan covers 15 cm, the dose to the irradiated volume is 30 mGy; however, the imparted (absorbed) energy is approximately 15 times that in a single scan slice.

Other modality-specific dosimetric quantities such as the CT dose index (CTDI), the dose-length product (DLP), multiple scan average dose (MSAD) used in computed tomography, and the entrance skin dose (ESD) and kerma-area-product (KAP) used in fluoroscopy will be introduced in context with their imaging modalities and discussed again in greater detail in Chapter 11. Mammography-specific dosimetric quantities such as the average glandular dose (AGD) are presented in Chapter 8. The methods for calculating doses from radiopharmaceuticals used in nuclear imaging utilizing the Medical Internal Radionuclide Dosimetry (MIRD) scheme are discussed in Chapter 16. Dose quantities that are defined by regulatory agencies, such as the total effective dose equivalent (TEDE) used by the Nuclear Regulatory Commission (NRC), are presented in Chapter 21.

Equivalent Dose

Not all types of ionizing radiation cause the same biological damage per unit absorbed dose. To modify the dose to reflect the relative effectiveness of the type of radiation in producing biologic damage, a *radiation weighting factor* (w_R) was established by the ICRP as part of an overall system for radiation protection (see Chapter 21), High LET radiations that produce dense ionization tracks cause more biologic damage per unit dose than low LET radiations. This type of biological damage (discussed in greater detail in chapter 20) can increase the probability of stochastic effects like cancer and thus are assigned higher radiation weighting factors. The product of the absorbed dose (D) and the radiation weighing factor is the *equivalent dose* (H).

$$H = D \, w_R \qquad\qquad [3\text{-}23]$$

The SI unit for equivalent dose is joule per kilogram with the special name of the *sievert* (Sv), where $1 \, Sv = 1 \, J \, kg^{-1}$. Radiations used in diagnostic imaging (x-rays and gamma rays) as well as the energetic electrons set into motion when these photons interact with tissue or when electrons are emitted during radioactive decay, have a w_R

TABLE 3-4   RADIATION WEIGHTING FACTORS (w_R) FOR VARIOUS TYPES OF RADIATION

TYPE OF RADIATION	RADIATION WEIGHTING FACTOR (W_R)
X-rays, gamma rays, beta particles, and electrons	1
Protons	2
Neutrons (energy dependent)[a]	2.5–20
Alpha particles and other multiple-charged particles	20

Note: For radiations principally used in medical imaging (x-rays and gamma rays) and beta particles, $w_R = 1$; thus, the absorbed dose and equivalent dose are equal (i.e., 1 Gy = 1 Sv).
[a]w_R values are a continuous function of energy with a maximum of 20 at approximately 1 Mev, minimum of 2.5 at 1 keV and 5 at 1 BeV). Adapted from ICRP Publication 103, *The 2007 Recommendations of the International Commission on Radiological Protection. Ann. ICRP 37 (2–4), Elsevier, 2008.*

of 1: thus, 1 mGy $\times$ 1 (w_R) = 1 mSv. For heavy charged particles such as alpha particles, the LET is much higher, and thus, the biologic damage and the associated w_R are much greater (Table 3-4). For example, 10 mGy from alpha radiation may have the same biologic effectiveness as 200 mGy of x-rays.

The quantity H replaces an earlier but similar quantity, the *dose equivalent*, which is the product of the absorbed dose and the *quality factor* (Q) (Equation 3-24). The quality factor is similar to w_R.

$$H = DQ \qquad\qquad [3\text{-}24]$$

The need to present these out-of-date dose quantities arise because regulatory agencies in the United States have not kept pace with current recommendations of national and international organizations for radiation protection and measurement. The traditional unit for both the dose equivalent and the equivalent dose is the rem. A sievert is equal to 100 rem, and 1 rem is equal to 10 mSv.

Effective Dose

Biological tissues vary in sensitivity to the effects of ionizing radiation. Tissue weighting factors (w_T) were also established by the ICRP as part of their radiation protection

TABLE 3-5 TISSUE WEIGHTING FACTORS ASSIGNED BY THE INTERNATIONAL COMMISSION ON RADIOLOGICAL PROTECTION (ICRP REPORT 103)

ORGAN/TISSUE	w_T	% OF TOTAL DETRIMENT
Breast	0.12	
Bone marrow	0.12	
Colon[a]	0.12	
Lung	0.12	72
Stomach	0.12	
Remainder[b]	0.12	
Gonads[c]	0.08	8
Bladder	0.04	
Esophagus	0.04	16
Liver	0.04	
Thyroid	0.04	
Bone surface	0.01	
Brain	0.01	4
Salivary gland	0.01	
Skin	0.01	
Total	**1.0**	**100**

[a]The dose to the colon is taken to be the mass-weighted mean of upper and lower large intestine doses.
[b]Shared by remainder tissues (14 in total, 13 in each sex) are adrenals, extrathoracic tissue, gallbladder, heart, kidneys, lymphatic nodes, muscle, oral mucosa, pancreas, prostate (male), small intestine, spleen, thymus, uterus/cervix (female).
[c]The w_T for gonads is applied to the mean of the doses to testes and ovaries.
Adapted from ICRP Publication 103, *The 2007 Recommendations of the International Commission on Radiological Protection. Ann. ICRP 37 (2–4),* Elsevier, 2008.

TABLE 3-6 RADIOLOGICAL QUANTITIES, SYSTEM INTERNATIONAL (SI) UNITS, AND TRADITIONAL UNITS

QUANTITY	DESCRIPTION OF QUANTITY	SI UNITS (ABBREVIATIONS) AND DEFINITIONS	TRADITIONAL UNITS (ABBREVIATIONS) AND DEFINITIONS	SYMBOL	DEFINITIONS AND CONVERSION FACTORS
Exposure	Amount of ionization per mass of air due to x-rays and gamma rays	C kg^{-1}	Roentgen (R)	X	1R = 2.58×10^{-4} C kg^{-1} 1R = 8.708 mGy air kerma @ 30 kV 1R = 8.767 mGy air kerma @ 60 kV 1R = 8.883 mGy air kerma @ 100 kV
Absorbed dose	Amount of energy imparted by radiation per mass	Gray (Gy) 1 Gy = J kg^{-1}	rad 1 rad = 0.01 J kg^{-1}	D	1 rad = 10 mGy 100 rad = 1 Gy
Kerma	Kinetic energy transferred to charged particles per unit mass	Gray (Gy) 1 Gy = J kg^{-1}	—	K	—
Air kerma	Kinetic energy transferred to charged particles per unit mass of air	Gray (Gy) 1 Gy = J kg^{-1}	—	K_{air}	1 mGy = 0.115 R @ 30 kV 1 mGy = 0.114 R @ 60 kV 1 mGy = 0.113 R @ 100 kV 1 mGy ≅ 0.140 rad (dose to skin)[a] 1 mGy ≅ 1.4 mGy (dose to skin)[a]
Imparted energy	Total radiation energy imparted to matter	Joule (J)	—	ε	Dose (J kg^{-1}) × mass (kg) = J
Dose equivalent (defined by ICRP in 1977)	A measure of absorbed dose weighted for the biological effectiveness of the type(s) of radiation (relative to low LET photons and electrons) to produce stochastic health effects in humans	Sievert (Sv)	rem	H	$H = Q\,D$ 1 rem = 10 mSv 100 rem = 1 Sv
Equivalent dose (defined by ICRP in 1990 to replace dose equivalent)	A measure of absorbed dose weighted for the biological effectiveness of the type(s) of radiation (relative to low LET photons and electrons) to produce stochastic health effects in humans	Sievert (Sv)	rem	H	$H = w_R\,D$ 1 rem = 10 mSv 100 rem = 1 Sv
Effective dose equivalent (defined by ICRP in 1977)	A measure of dose equivalent, weighted for the biological sensitivity of the exposed tissues and organs (relative to whole body exposure) to stochastic health effects in humans	Sievert (Sv)	rem	H_E	$H_E = \sum_T w_T H_T$
Effective dose (defined by ICRP in 1990 to replace effective dose equivalent and modified in 2007 with different w_T values)	A measure of equivalent dose, weighted for the biological sensitivity of the exposed tissues and organs (relative to whole body exposure) to stochastic health effects in humans	Sievert (Sv)	rem	E	$E = \sum_T w_T H_T$

[a]Includes backscatter (discussed in Chapters 9 and 11).
ICRP, International Commission on Radiological Protection.

system to assign a particular organ or tissue (T) the proportion of the detriment[1] from stochastic effects (e.g., cancer and hereditary effects, discussed further in Chapter 20) resulting from irradiation of that tissue compared to uniform whole-body irradiation (ICRP Publication 103, 2007). These tissue weighting factors are shown in Table 3-5. The sum of the products of the equivalent dose to each organ or tissue irradiated (H_T) and the corresponding weighting factor (w_T) for that organ or tissue is called the *effective dose (E)*.

$$E(Sv) = \sum_T [w_T \times H_T(Sv)] \qquad [3\text{-}25]$$

The effective dose is expressed in the same units as the equivalent dose (sievert or rem).

The w_T values were developed for a reference population of equal numbers of both genders and a wide range of ages. Thus effective dose applies to a population, not to a specific individual and should not be used as the patient's dose for the purpose of assigning risk. This all too common misuse of effective dose, for a purpose for which it was never intended and does not apply, is discussed in further detail in Chapters 11 and 16. ICRP's initial recommendations for w_T values (ICRP Publication 26, 1977) were applied as shown in Equation 3-25, the product of which was referred to as the *effective dose equivalent (H_E)*. Many regulatory agencies in the United States, including the NRC, have not as yet adopted the current ICRP Publication 103 w_T values. While there is a current effort to update these regulations, they are, at present, still using the old (1977) ICRP Publication 26 dosimetric quantities.

Summary

Most other countries and all the scientific literature use SI units exclusively. While some legacy (traditional) radiation units and terms are still being used for regulatory compliance purposes and some radiation detection instruments are still calibrated in these units, students are encouraged to use the current SI units discussed above. A summary of the SI units and their equivalents in traditional units is given in Table 3-6. A discussion of these radiation dose terms in the context of x-ray dosimetry in projection imaging and CT is presented in Chapter 11.

SUGGESTED READING

Bushberg JT. The AAPM/RSNA physics tutorial for residents. X-ray interactions. *RadioGraphics* 1998;18:457–468.

International Commission on Radiation Units and Measurements. *Fundamental quantities and units for ionizing radiation.* Journal of the ICRU Vol 11 No 1 (2011) Report 85.

International Commission on Radiological Protection, *Recommendations of the ICRP.* Annals of the ICRP 37(2–4), Publication 103, 2007.

Johns HE, Cunningham JR. *The physics of radiology*, 4th ed. Springfield, IL: Charles C Thomas, 1983.

McKetty MH. The AAPM/ RSNA physics tutorial for residents. X-ray attenuation. *RadioGraphics* 1998; 18:151–163.

---

[1]The total harm to health experienced by an exposed group and its descendants as a result of the group's exposure to a radiation source. Detriment is a multimentional concept. Its principal components are the stochastic quantities: probability of attributable fatal cancer, weighted probability of attributable non-fatal cancer, weighted probability of severe heritable effects, and length of life lost if the harm occurs.

CHAPTER 4

Image Quality

Unlike snapshots taken on the ubiquitous digital camera, medical images are acquired not for aesthetic purposes but out of medical necessity. The image quality on a medical image is related not to how pretty it looks but rather to how well it conveys anatomical or functional information to the interpreting physician such that an accurate diagnosis can be made. Indeed, radiological images acquired with ionizing radiation can almost always be made much prettier simply by turning up the radiation levels used, but the radiation dose to the patient then becomes an important concern. Diagnostic medical images therefore require a number of important trade-offs in which image quality is not necessarily *maximized* but rather is *optimized* to perform the specific diagnostic task for which the exam was ordered.

The following discussion of image quality is also meant to familiarize the reader with the terms that describe it, and thus the vernacular introduced here is important as well. This chapter, more than most in this book, includes some mathematical discussion that is relevant to the topic of image science. To physicians in training, the details of the mathematics should not be considered an impediment to understanding but rather as a general illustration of the methods. To image scientists in training, the mathematics in this chapter are a necessary basic look at the essentials of imaging system analysis.

4.1 Spatial Resolution

Spatial resolution describes the level of detail that can be seen on an image. In simple terms, the spatial resolution relates to how small an object can be seen on a particular imaging system—and this would be the limiting spatial resolution. However, robust methods used to describe the spatial resolution for an imaging system provide a measure of how well the imaging system performs over a continuous range of object dimensions. Spatial resolution measurements are generally performed at high dose levels in x-ray and γ-ray imaging systems, so that a precise (low noise) assessment can be made. The vast majority of imaging systems in radiology are digital, and clearly the size of the picture element (pixel) in an image sets a limit on what can theoretically be resolved in that image. While it is true that one cannot *resolve* an object that is smaller than the pixel size, it is also true that one may be able to detect a high-contrast object that is smaller than the pixel size if its signal amplitude is large enough to significantly affect the gray scale value of that pixel. It is also true that while images with small pixels have the *potential* to deliver high spatial resolution, many other factors also affect spatial resolution, and in many cases, it is not the pixel size that is the limiting factor in spatial resolution.

The Spatial Domain

In radiology, images vary in size from small spot images acquired in mammography ($\sim$50 mm $\times$ 50 mm) to the chest radiograph, which is 350 mm $\times$ 430 mm. These images

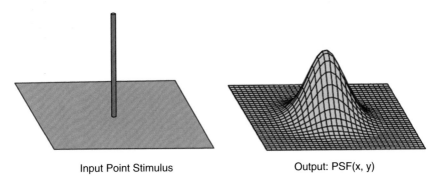

Input Point Stimulus   Output: PSF(x, y)

■ **FIGURE 4-1** A point stimulus to an imaging system is illustrated (**left**), and the response of the imaging system, the point spread function (PSF) is shown (**right**). This PSF is rotationally symmetric.

are acquired and viewed in the spatial domain. The spatial domain refers to the two dimensions of a single image, or to the three dimensions of a set of tomographic images such as computed tomography (CT) or magnetic resonance imaging (MRI). A number of metrics that are measured in the spatial domain and that describe the spatial resolution of an imaging system are discussed below.

The Point Spread Function, PSF

The point spread function (PSF) is the most basic measure of the resolution properties of an imaging system, and it is perhaps the most intuitive as well. A point source is input to the imaging system, and the PSF is (by definition) the response of the imaging system to that point input (Fig. 4-1). The PSF is also called the impulse response function. The PSF is a two-dimensional (2D) function, typically described in the x and y dimensions of a 2D image, *PSF(x,y)*. Note that the PSF can be rotationally symmetric, or not, and an asymmetrical PSF is illustrated in Figure 4-2. The diameter of the "point" input should theoretically be infinitely small, but practically speaking, the diameter of the point input should be five to ten times smaller than the width of the detector element in the imaging system being evaluated.

To produce a point input on a planar imaging system such as in digital radiography or fluoroscopy, a sheet of attenuating metal such as lead, with a very small hole in it*, is placed covering the detector, and x-rays are produced. High exposure levels need to be used to deliver a measurable signal, given the tiny hole. For a tomographic

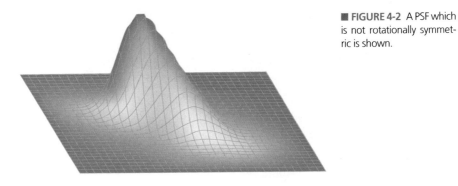

■ **FIGURE 4-2** A PSF which is not rotationally symmetric is shown.

---

*In reality, PSF and other resolution test objects are precision-machined tools and can cost over a thousand dollars.

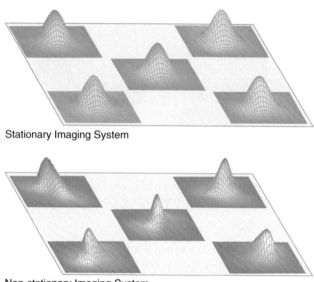

Stationary Imaging System

Non-stationary Imaging System

■ **FIGURE 4-3** A stationary or shift-invariant imaging system is one in which the PSF remains constant over the field of view of the imaging system. A nonstationary system has a different PSF, depending on the location in the field of view.

system, a small-diameter wire or fiber can be imaged with the wire placed normal to the tomographic plane to be acquired.

An imaging system with the same PSF at all locations in the field of view is called *stationary* or *shift invariant*, while a system that has PSFs that vary depending on the position in the field of view is called *nonstationary* (Fig. 4-3). In general, medical imaging systems are considered stationary—even if some small nonstationary effects are present. Pixelated digital imaging systems have finite detector elements (dexels), commonly square in shape (but not always), and in some cases, the detector element is uniformly sensitive to the signal energy across its surface. This implies that if there are no other factors that degrade spatial resolution, the digital sampling matrix will impose a PSF, which is square in shape (Fig. 4-4) and where the dimensions of the square are the dimensions of the dexels.

The PSF describes the extent of *blurring* that is introduced by an imaging system, and this blurring is the manifestation of physical events during the image acquisition

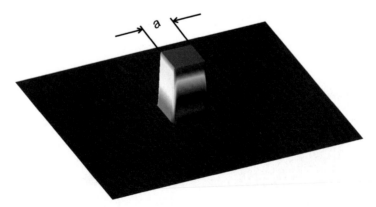

■ **FIGURE 4-4** A 2D RECT function is shown, illustrating the PSF of a digital imaging system with square detector elements of width a, in the absence of any other blurring phenomenon. This PSF is the best possible for a digital imaging system.

or reconstruction process. Mathematically, for a linear stationary system, the input image is *convolved* with the PSF and that results in the output image. Convolution is a mathematical operation discussed later in this chapter.

The Line Spread Function, LSF

When an imaging system is stimulated with a signal in the form of a line, the line spread function (LSF) can be evaluated. For a planar imaging system, a slit in some attenuating material can be imaged and would result in a line on the image. For a tomographic imaging system, a thin plane of material can be imaged normal to the tomographic plane, and that also would result in a line being produced in the image (Fig. 4-5). Once the line is produced on the image (e.g., parallel to the y-axis), a profile through that line is then measured perpendicular to the line (i.e., along the x-axis). The profile is a measure of gray scale as a function of position. Once this profile is normalized such that the area is unity, it becomes the *LSF(x)*. As will be discussed later, the LSF has an important role in the practical assessment of spatial resolution.

For an analog imaging system such as radiographic film, a device called a scanning microdensitometer is required to measure the optical density as a function of position. The optical density trace would then have to be corrected for its nonlinear relationship with incident exposure, before the LSF can be computed. For digital x-ray imaging systems that have a linear response to x-rays such as digital radiography or CT, the profile can be easily determined from the digital image using appropriate software. Profiles from ultrasound and MR images can also be used to compute the LSF, as long as the signal is converted in a linear fashion into gray scale on the images.

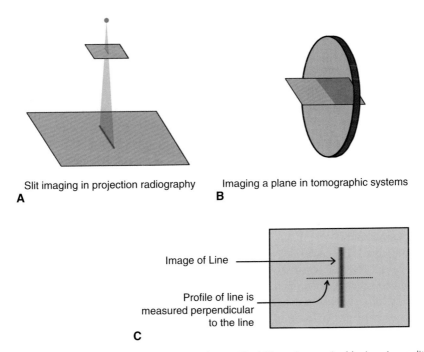

Slit imaging in projection radiography   Imaging a plane in tomographic systems
A   **B**

Image of Line ⟶

Profile of line is
measured perpendicular
to the line

C

■ **FIGURE 4-5** Methods for acquiring the LSF are shown. The LSF can be acquired by imaging a slit image (**A**), or by imaging a thin plane of material in a tomographic imaging system such as CT, MRI, or ultrasound (**B**). **C**. The LSF is computed by taking an orthogonal profile across the measured slit image.

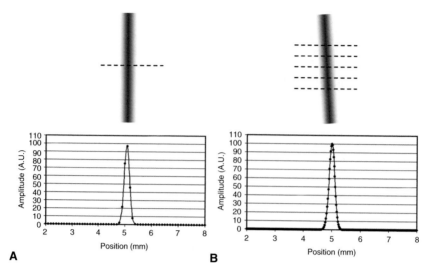

■ **FIGURE 4-6 A.** The conventional approach to measuring the LSF involves the acquisition of a slit image along the y-axis, and a profile (gray scale versus position) across it (in the x-axis) is evaluated. This approach is legitimate but is limited by the sampling pitch of the detector. **B.** An alternative approach to computing the LSF was proposed by Fujita. Here, the slit image is acquired at a slight angle (~5 degrees) relative to the y-axis. At any row along the vertical slit, a single LSF can be measured. However, because of the angle, a composite LSF can be synthesized by combining the LSFs from a number of rows in the image. The angle of the slit creates a small differential phase shift of the LSF from row to row—this can be exploited to synthesize an LSF with much better sampling than the pixel pitch. This oversampled LSF is called the presampled LSF.

For a system with good spatial resolution, the LSF will be quite thin, and thus on the measured profile, the LSF will only be few pixels wide, and the LSF measurement will consequently suffer from coarse pixel sampling in the image. One way to get around this is to place the slit at a small angle (e.g., 2 to 8 degrees) to the detector element columns during the physical measurement procedure. Then, instead of taking one profile through the slit image, a number of profiles are taken at different locations vertically (Fig. 4-6) and the data are synthesized into a *presampled LSF*. Due to the angulation of the slit, the profiles taken at different vertical positions (Fig. 4-6) intersect the slit image at different phases (horizontally) through the pixel width—this allows the LSF to be synthesized with sub-pixel spacing intervals, and a better sampled LSF measurement results.

The Edge Spread Function, ESF

In some situations, PSF and LSF measurements are not ideally suited for a specific imaging application, where the edge spread function (ESF) can be measured. Instead of stimulating the imaging system with a slit image as with the LSF, a sharp edge is presented. The *edge gradient* that results in the image can then be used to measure the *ESF(x)*. The ESF is particularly useful when the spatial distribution characteristics of glare or scatter phenomenon are the subject of interest—since a large fraction of the field of view is stimulated, low-amplitude effects such as glare or scatter (or both) become appreciable enough in amplitude to be measurable. By comparison, the tiny area of the detector receiving signal in the PSF or LSF measurements would not be sufficient to cause enough optical glare or x-ray scatter to be measured. A sharp, straight edge is also less expensive to manufacture than a point or slit phantom.

An example of spatial domain spread functions is shown in Figure 4-7.

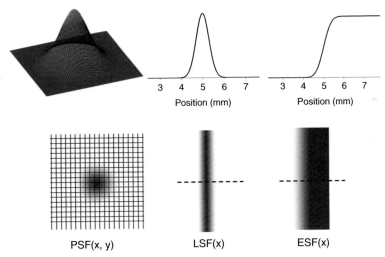

PSF(x, y)   LSF(x)   ESF(x)

■ **FIGURE 4-7** The three basic spread functions in the spatial domain are shown—the PSF(x,y) is a 2D spread function. The LSF and ESF are both 1D spread functions. There is mathematical relationship between the three spread functions, as discussed in the text.

4.2 Convolution

Convolution is an integral calculus procedure that accurately describes mathematically what the blurring process does physically. The convolution process is also an important mathematical component of image reconstruction, and understanding the basics of convolution is essential to a complete understanding of imaging systems. Below, a basic description of the convolution process is provided. Convolution in 1D is given by

$$G(x) = \int_{-\infty}^{\infty} H(x')\, k(x - x')\, dx' = H(x) \otimes k(x) \qquad [4\text{-}1]$$

where $\otimes$ is the mathematical symbol for convolution. Convolution can occur in two or three dimensions as well, and the extension to multidimensional convolution is straightforward. Referring to Figure 4-8, a column of numbers H is to be convolved with the *convolution kernel*, resulting in column G. The function H can also be thought

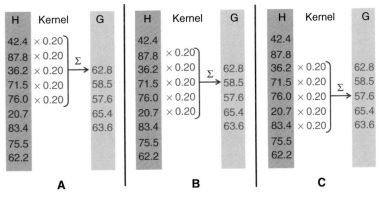

■ **FIGURE 4-8** The basic operation of discrete convolution is illustrated in this figure. In the three panes (**A–C**), the function H is convolved with the convolution kernel, resulting in the function G. The process proceeds by indexing one data element in the array, and this is shown in the three different panes. The entire convolution is performed over the entire length of the input array H.

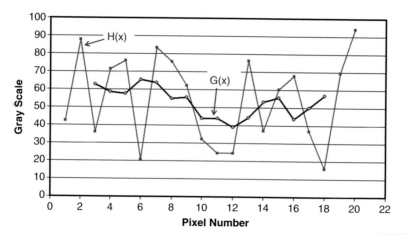

■ **FIGURE 4-9** A plot of the noisy input data H(x), and of the smoothed function G(x), is shown. The first elements in the data shown on this plot correspond to the data illustrated in Figure 4-8. The input function H(x) is simply random noise. The convolution process with the RECT function results in substantial smoothing, and this is evident by the much smoother G(x) function in comparison to H(x).

of as a row of pixel data on a 1D image. The kernel in this example is five elements long, and its value sums to unity. In pane A, the first five numbers of H are multiplied by the corresponding elements in the kernel (here, each element of the kernel has a numerical value of 0.20); these five products are summed, resulting in the first entry in column G. In pane B, the convolution algorithm proceeds by shifting down one element in column H, and the same operation is computed, resulting in the second entry in column G. In pane C, the kernel shifts down another element in the array of numbers, and the same process is followed. This shift, multiply, and add procedure is the discrete implementation of convolution—it is the way this operation is performed in a computer. A plot of the values in columns H and G is shown in Figure 4-9, and H in this case is randomly generated noise. The values of G are smoothed relative to H, and that is because the elements of the convolution kernel in this case are designed to perform data smoothing—essentially by averaging five adjacent values in Column H. A plot of various five-element kernels is shown in Figure 4-10. The

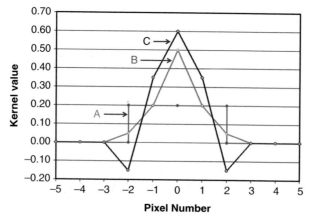

■ **FIGURE 4-10** Three convolution kernels are illustrated. A is a RECT function defined by [0.2, 0.2, 0.2, 0.2, 0.2], and the convolution process with this function is illustrated in Figures 4-8. Kernel B illustrates another possible smoothing kernel, with values [0.05, 0.20, 0.50, 0.20, 0.05]. Kernel C has the values [−0.15, 0.35, 0.50, 0.35, −0.15]. The negative sidebands of this kernel cause edge enhancement during a convolution procedure, but this can also increase the noise in the resulting function.

kernel illustrated in Figure 4-8 is kernel A in Figure 4-10, and the shape is that of a rectangle (a RECT function), because all of the values in the kernel are the same. Use of such a kernel in data analysis is also called a *boxcar average* or *running average*, with applications in economics and elsewhere. Kernel B in Figure 4-10 has an appearance a bit similar to a bell-shaped curve, to the extent that only five values can describe such a shape. Both kernels A and B have all positive values, and therefore, they will always result in data smoothing. Kernel C has some negative edges on it, and when negative values are found in a kernel, some edge enhancement will result. In Equation 4-1 or Figure 4-8, it can be seen that negative values in the kernel will result in weighted subtraction of adjacent elements of the input function, and this brings out edges or discontinuities in the input function, and it tends to exacerbate noise in the data as well. It is worth noting that if the kernel was [0, 0, 1, 0, 0], G would be equal to H. This kernel is called a *delta* function.

Convolution can use kernels of any length, and for image processing, kernels from 3 elements to 511 or more elements are used. Although not required, most kernels that are smaller in length are odd, so that there is a center element. For a kernel of length N_k (odd), convolution is ill defined at the edges of the image for $(N_k - 1)/2$ pixels (Fig. 4-8); however, assuming that the image has zero-valued pixels adjacent to its edges is a common method for dealing with this. Above, only 1D convolution using 1D kernels was discussed, but convolution is routinely performed in two dimensions using 2D kernels. In such case, 3×3, 5×5, and other odd kernel dimensions are routinely used. Examples of 2D convolution kernels are illustrated in Figure 4-11. Three-dimensional convolution techniques are also used in medical imaging processing. Convolution is a mathematical process that describes physical blurring phenomena, but convolution techniques can be used to restore (improve) spatial resolution as well—in such cases the process is called *deconvolution*. While deconvolution can improve spatial resolution in some cases, it also amplifies the noise levels in the image.

Relationships Between Spread Functions

There are mathematical relationships between the spatial domain spread functions PSF, LSF, and ESF. The specific mathematical relationships are described here, but the take-home message is that under most circumstances, given a

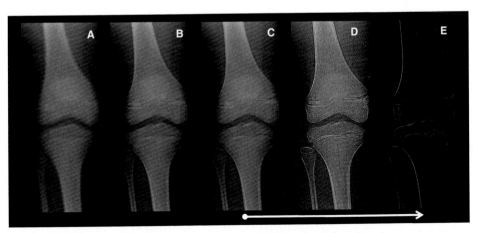

gaussian blur   original   increasing edge enhancement

■ **FIGURE 4-11** This figure illustrates the results of 2D image processing using a variety of different convolution kernels. The original image is shown as image **B**. Image **A** is a smoothed version, while images **C–E** show the effect of edge enhancement kernels with increasing edge enhancement from images **C** to **E**.

measurement of one of the spread functions, the others can be computed. This feature adds to the flexibility of using the most appropriate measurement method for characterizing an imaging system. These statements presume a rotationally symmetric PSF, but in general, that is the case in many (but not all) medical imaging systems.

The LSF and ESF are related to the PSF by the convolution equation. The LSF can be computed by convolving the PSF with a line[†]:

$$LSF(x) = PSF(x, y) \otimes LINE(y) \qquad [4\text{-}2]$$

Because a line is purely a 1D function, the convolution shown in Equation 4-2 reduces to a simple integral

$$LSF(x) = \int_{y=-\infty}^{\infty} PSF(x, y)\, dy \qquad [4\text{-}3]$$

Convolution of the PSF with an edge[‡] results in the ESF

$$ESF(x) = PSF(x, y) \otimes EDGE(y) \qquad [4\text{-}4]$$

In addition to the above relationships, the LSF and ESF are related as well. The ESF is the integral of the LSF, and this implies that the LSF is the derivative of the ESF.

$$ESF(x) = \int_{x'=-\infty}^{x} LSF(x')\, dx' \qquad [4\text{-}5]$$

One can also compute the LSF from the ESF, and the PSF can be computed from the LSF; however, the assumption of rotational symmetry with the PSF is necessary in the latter case.

4.3 Physical Mechanisms of Blurring

There are many different mechanisms in medical imaging that cause blurring, and some of these mechanisms will be discussed in length in subsequent chapters. The spatial resolution of an image produced by any optical device (such as in an image intensifier/TV-based fluoroscopy system) can be reduced by accidental defocusing. When an x-ray strikes an intensifying screen or other phosphor, it produces a burst of light photons that propagate by optical diffusion though the screen matrix. For thicker screens, the diffusion path toward the screen's surface is longer and more lateral diffusion occurs, which results in a broader spot of light reaching the surface of the screen and consequently more blurring. Digital sampling usually results in the integration of the 2D signal over the surface of the detector element, and this occurs in digital x-ray, CT, nuclear medicine, ultrasound, and other modalities. Figure 4-4 illustrates the 2D RECT function that represents digital sampling, and the spatial resolution decreases as the width of the RECT function increases. These are just some examples of physical factors that reduce spatial resolution; many other processes can degrade resolution as well.

The measurement of the various spread functions discussed above is used to characterize the impact of physical blurring phenomena in medical imaging systems. Subsequent analyses on spread functions, and in particular on the LSF, are often performed to characterize the frequency dependence of spatial resolution, as described below.

[†]Line(y) = 1, where y = 0,
         = 0, elsewhere
[‡]Edge(y) = 1, where y > 0,
          = 0, elsewhere

4.4 ## The Frequency Domain

The PSF, LSF, and ESF are apt descriptions of the resolution properties of an imaging system in the spatial domain. Another useful way to express the resolution of an imaging system is to make use of the spatial *frequency domain*. By analogy, the amplitude of sound waves vary as a function of time (measured in seconds), and temporal frequency is measured in units of cycles/s (s^{-1}), also known as Hertz. For example, the middle A key on a well-tuned piano corresponds to 440 Hz. If the period of a sound wave occurs within shorter periods of time, the sound wave is of higher frequency. Spatial frequency is similar to temporal frequency except that distance (in mm) is used instead of time. In the spatial frequency domain, smaller objects correspond to higher frequencies, and larger objects correspond to lower frequencies.

There are some technical nuances to the statement, but to a first approximation, spatial frequency can be thought of as just a different way of thinking about object size—low spatial frequencies correspond to larger objects in the image, and higher spatial frequencies correspond to smaller objects. If the size of an object (Δ) is known, it can be converted to spatial frequency ($F = 1/2\Delta$), and if the spatial frequency (F) is known, it can be converted to object size ($\Delta = 1/2F$). Here, the dimensions of Δ are mm, and the dimensions of F are cycles/mm, which is equivalent to mm^{-1} or 1/mm. These statements are true, but a rigorous mathematical description of the relationship between Δ and F would involve the shape, size, and periodicity of the object, but that discussion is not necessary here.

Fourier Series and the Fourier Transform

In Figure 4-12, let the solid black line be a trace of gray scale as a function of position across an image. Nineteenth-century French mathematician Joseph Fourier developed a method for decomposing a function such as this gray scale profile into the sum of a number of sine waves. Each sine wave has three parameters that characterize its shape: amplitude (a), frequency (f), and phase (Ψ), where

$$g(x) = a \sin(2\pi f x + \psi) \qquad [4\text{-}6]$$

Figure 4-12 illustrates the sum of four different sine waves (*solid black line*), which approximates the shape of two rectangular functions (*dashed lines*). Only four

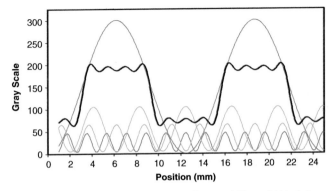

■ **FIGURE 4-12** The basic concept of Fourier Series analysis is illustrated. The *solid black lines* are the sum of the four sets of sine waves, and approximate the two RECT functions (*dashed lines*). Only four sine waves are summed here, but with a more complete set, the RECT functions could be almost perfectly matched. The Fourier transform breaks any arbitrary signal down into the sum of a set of sine waves of different phase, frequency, and amplitude.

sine waves were used in this figure for clarity; however, if more sine waves (a more complete Fourier series) were used, the shape of the two rectangular functions could in principle be matched.

The Fourier transform is an algorithm that decomposes a spatial or time domain signal into a series of sine waves that, when summed, replicate that signal. Once a spatial domain signal is Fourier transformed, the resulting data are considered to be in the *frequency domain*. The Fourier transform is given by

$$G(f) = \int_{x=-\infty}^{\infty} g(x) e^{-2\pi i f x} \, dx \qquad [4\text{-}7]$$

where i is $\sqrt{-1}$. If, for example, the input signal $g(x)$ to the Fourier transform is a sine wave with a frequency v, the function $G(f)$ will be a plot with spikes at frequencies $\pm v$, and it will be zero elsewhere. The function $G(f)$ will in general consist of complex numbers, with real and imaginary components.

The Fourier transform, $FT[]$, converts a temporal or spatial signal into the frequency domain, while the inverse Fourier transform, $FT^{-1}[]$, converts the frequency domain signal back to the temporal or spatial domain. The Fourier transform can be used to perform convolution. Referring back to Equation 4-1, the function $G(x)$ can be alternatively computed as

$$G(x) = FT^{-1} \left\{ FT[H(x)] \times FT[k(x)] \right\} \qquad [4\text{-}8]$$

Equation 4-8 computes the same function $G(x)$ as in Equation 4-1, but compared to the convolution procedure, in most cases the Fourier transform computation runs faster on a computer. Therefore, image processing methods that employ convolution filtration procedures such as in CT are often performed in the frequency domain for computational speed. Indeed, the kernel used in CT is often described in the frequency domain (descriptors such as *ramp, Shepp-Logan, bone kernel, B41*), so it is more common to discuss the shape of the kernel in the frequency domain (e.g., $FT[k(x)]$) rather than in the spatial domain (i.e., $k(x)$), in the parlance of clinical CT.

Fourier computations are a routine part of medical imaging systems. Fourier transforms are used to perform the filtering procedure in filtered back projection, for CT reconstruction. Inverse Fourier transforms are used in MRI to convert the measured time domain signal into a spatial signal. Fourier transforms are also used in ultrasound imaging and Doppler systems.

The Modulation Transfer Function, *MTF(f)*

Conceptual Description

Imagine that it is possible to stimulate an imaging system spatially with a pure sinusoidal wave form, as illustrated in Figure 4-13A. The system will detect the incoming sinusoidal signal at frequency f, and as long as the frequency does not exceed the Nyquist frequency (discussed later) of the imaging system (i.e., $f < F_N$), it will produce an image at that same frequency but in most cases with reduced contrast (Fig. 4-13A, right side). The reduction in contrast transfer is the result of resolution losses in the imaging system. For the input sinusoidal signals with frequencies of 1, 2, and 4 cycles/mm (shown in Fig 4-13A), the recorded contrast levels were 87%, 56%, and 13%, respectively, on the measured images. For any one of these three frequencies measured individually, if the Fourier transform was computed on the recorded signal, the result would be a peak at the corresponding frequency (Fig. 4-13A, right side). Three such peaks are shown in Figure 4-13B, representing three sequentially and individually acquired (and then Fourier transformed) signals. The amplitude of the peak at each frequency reflects the contrast transfer (retained) at that frequency, with contrast losses due to resolution limitations in the system. Interestingly, due to the characteristics of the Fourier transform, the three sinusoidal input waves shown in Figure 4-13A could be acquired simultaneously by the detector system, and the

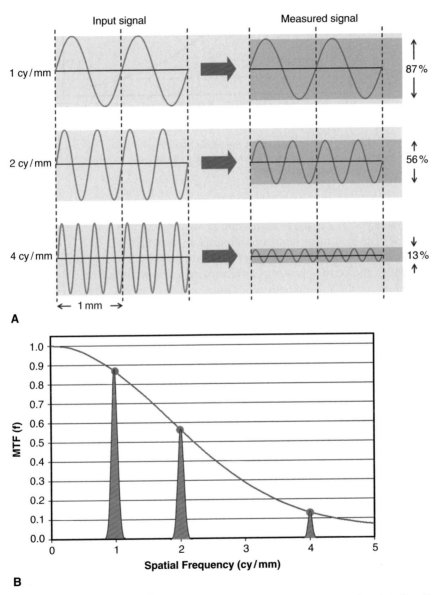

■ **FIGURE 4-13 A**. Sinusoidal input signals are incident on a detector (intensity as a function of position), and three different frequencies are shown as input functions (**left**). The signals measured by the imaging system are shown on the right—the frequency is the same as the inputs in all cases, but the amplitude of the measured signal is reduced compared to that of the input signal. This reduction in amplitude is a result of resolution losses in the imaging system, which are greater with signals of higher frequencies. For the input at 1 cycle/mm, the original 100% amplitude was attenuated to 87%, and with the 2- and 4-cycle/mm input functions, the resulting signal amplitudes were reduced to 56% and 13%, respectively. **B**. This figure shows the amplitude reduction as a function of spatial frequency shown in **A**. At 1 cycle/mm, the system reduced the contrast to 87% of the input. For 2 mm^{-1} and 4 mm^{-1}, the signal was modulated as shown. This plot shows the MTF, which illustrates the spatial resolution of an imaging system as a function of the spatial frequency of the input signal.

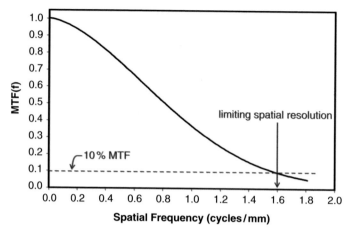

■ FIGURE 4-14 The limiting spatial resolution is the spatial frequency at which the amplitude of the MTF decreases to some agreed-upon level. Here the limiting spatial resolution is shown at 10% modulation, and the limiting spatial resolution is 1.6 cycles/mm.

Fourier Transform could separate the individual frequencies and produce the three peaks at F = 1, 2, and 4 cycles/mm shown in Figure 4-13B. Indeed, if an input signal contained more numerous sinusoidal waves (10, 50, 100,....) than the three shown in Figure 4-13A, the Fourier transform would still be able to separate these frequencies and convey their respective amplitudes from the recorded signal, ultimately resulting in the full, smooth modulation transfer function (MTF) curve shown in Figure 4-13B.

Practical Measurement

It is not possible in general to stimulate a detector system with individual, spatial sinusoidal signals as described in the paragraph above. Rather, the LSF, discussed previously and illustrated in Figures 4-6 and 4-7, is used to determine the MTF in experimental settings. A perfect line source input (called a delta-function), it turns out, is represented in the frequency domain by an infinite number of sinusoidal functions spanning the frequency spectrum. Therefore, the Fourier transform of the $LSF(x)$ computes the full MTF curve as shown in Figure 4-13B. Prior to the computation, the $LSF(x)$ is normalized to have unity area

$$\int_{x=-\infty}^{\infty} LSF(x)dx = 1 \qquad \text{[4-9]}$$

Then the Fourier transform is computed, and the modulus (brackets) is taken, resulting in the $MTF(f)$

$$MTF(f) = \left| \int_{x=-\infty}^{\infty} LSF(x)e^{-2\pi ifx} dx \right| \qquad \text{[4-10]}$$

Limiting Resolution

The MTF gives a rich description of spatial resolution, and is the accepted standard for the rigorous characterization of spatial resolution. However, it is often useful to have a single number value that characterizes the approximate resolution limit of an imaging system. The limiting spatial resolution is often considered to be the frequency at which the MTF crosses the 10% level (see Fig. 4-14), or some other agreed-upon and specified level.

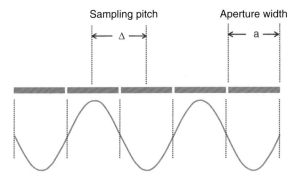

■ FIGURE 4-15 This figure illustrates a side view of detector elements in a hypothetical detector system. Detector systems whose center-to-center spacing (pitch) is about equal to the detector width are very common, and these represent contiguous detector elements. The sampling pitch affects aliasing in the image, while the aperture width of the detector element influences the spatial resolution (the LSF and MTF). A sine wave (shown) where each period just matches the width of two detector elements is the highest frequency sine wave that can be imaged with these detectors due to their sampling pitch.

Nyquist Frequency

Let's look at an example of an imaging system where the center-to-center spacing between each detector element (dexel) is Δ in mm. In the corresponding image, it would take two adjacent pixels to display a full cycle of a sine wave (Fig. 4-15)—one pixel for the upward lobe of the sine wave, and the other for the downward lobe. This sine wave is the highest frequency that can be accurately measured on the imaging system. The period of this sine wave is 2Δ, and the corresponding spatial frequency is $F_N = 1/2\Delta$. This frequency is called the Nyquist frequency (F_N), and it sets the upper bound on the spatial frequency that can be detected for a digital detector system with detector pitch Δ. For example, for $\Delta = 0.05$ mm, $F_N = 10$ cycles/mm, and for $\Delta = 0.25$ mm, $F_N = 2.0$ cycles/mm.

If a sinusoidal signal greater than the Nyquist frequency were to be incident upon the detector system, its true frequency would not be recorded, but rather it would be *aliased*. Aliasing occurs when frequencies higher than the Nyquist frequency are imaged (Fig. 4-16). The frequency that is recorded is lower than the incident frequency, and indeed the recorded frequency *wraps around* the Nyquist frequency. For example, for a system with $\Delta = 0.100$ mm, and thus $F_N = 5.0$ cycles/mm, sinusoidal inputs of 2, 3, and 4 cycles/mm are recorded accurately because they obey the Nyquist Criterion. The Fourier transform of the detected signals would result in a

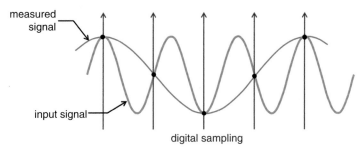

■ FIGURE 4-16 The concept of aliasing is illustrated. The input sine wave is sampled with the sampling comb (*arrows*), but the Nyquist criterion is violated here because the input sine wave is higher than the Nyquist frequency. Thus, the sampled image data will be aliased and the lower frequency sine wave will be seen as the measured signal on the image.

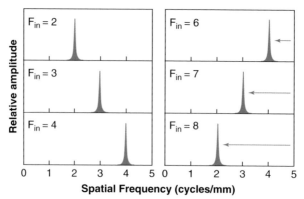

■ FIGURE 4-17 For a single-frequency sinusoidal input function to an imaging system (sinusoidally varying intensity versus position), the Fourier transform of the image results in a spike (delta function) indicating the measured frequency. The Nyquist frequency in this example is 5 cycles/mm. For the three input frequencies in the left panel, all are below the Nyquist frequency and obey the Nyquist criterion, and the measured (recorded) frequencies are exactly what was input into the imaging system. On the right panel, the input frequencies were higher than the Nyquist frequency, and the recorded frequencies in all cases were aliased—they wrapped around the Nyquist frequency—that is, the measured frequencies were lower than the Nyquist frequency by the same amount by which the input frequencies exceeded the Nyquist frequency.

histogram of the frequency distribution of the measured sinusoid frequencies, but since the input functions are single frequencies, the Fourier transform appears as a spike at that frequency (Fig. 4-17). For sinusoidal inputs with frequencies greater than the Nyquist frequency, the signal wraps around the Nyquist frequency—a frequency of 6 cycles/mm ($F_N + 1$) is recorded as 4 cycles/mm ($F_N - 1$), and a frequency of 7 cycles/mm ($F_N + 2$) is recorded as 3 cycles/mm ($F_N - 2$), and so on. This is seen on Figure 4-17 as well. Aliasing is visible when there is a periodic pattern that is imaged, such as an x-ray antiscatter grid, and aliasing appears visually in many cases as a Moiré pattern or wavy lines.

The Presampled MTF

Aliasing can pose limitations on the measurement of the MTF, and the finite size of the pixels in an image can cause sampling problems with the LSF that is measured to compute the MTF (Equation 4-10). Figure 4-6 shows the angled slit method for determining the presampled LSF, and this provides a methodology for computing the so-called presampled MTF. Using a single line perpendicular to the slit image (Fig. 4-6A), the sampling of the LSF measurements is Δ, and the maximum frequency that can be computed for the MTF is then $1/2\Delta$. However, for many medical imaging systems it is both possible and probable that the MTF has nonzero amplitude beyond the Nyquist limit of $F_N = 1/2\Delta$. In order to measure the presampled MTF, the angled-slit method is used to synthesize the presampled LSF. By using a slight angle between the long axis of the slit and the columns of detector elements in the physical measurement of the LSF, different (nearly) normal lines can be sampled (Fig. 4-6B). The LSF computed from each individual line is limited by the Δ sampling pitch, but multiple lines of data can be used to synthesize an LSF, which has much better sampling than Δ. Indeed, oversampling can be by a factor of 5 or 10, depending on the measurement procedure and how long the slit is. The details of how the presampled LSF is computed are beyond the scope of the current discussion; however, by decreasing the sampling pitch from Δ to, for example, $\Delta/5$, the

Nyquist limit goes from F_N to $5F_N$, which is sufficient to accurately measure the presampled MTF.

RECT Functions and SINC

We have seen in the above discussion on aliasing, that the discrete sampling in digital detector systems imposes the Nyquist Criterion (i.e., $F_N = 1/2\Delta$) and if this criterion is not met, then aliasing may occur. Digital detector systems such as flat panel detector systems (as a concrete example) have detector elements that are essentially contiguous (i.e., very little dead space between adjacent detector elements). Thus, for a detector where the detector *pitch* (the center-to-center distance between adjacent detector elements) is Δ, the width of each detector element (a) is about the same (Fig. 4-16), that is, $a \cong \Delta$. This finite width of each detector element means that all of the signal which is incident on each dexel is essentially averaged together, and one number (the gray scale value) is produced for each detector element (in general). This means that on top of any blurring that may occur from other sources, the width of the dexel imposes a fundamental limit on spatial resolution. In a very literal sense, the detector width—idealized as a rectangular (RECT) response function—is the best the LSF can ever get on a digital imaging system. The RECT function is a rectangle-shaped function of width a, usually centered at $x = 0$, such that the RECT function runs from $-a/2$ to $+a/2$. Let the LSF be a RECT function with width a, and the MTF is then computed as the Fourier transform of the LSF. This Fourier transform can be computed analytically, and the resulting MTF will be given by

$$MTF(f) = \int_{x=-\infty}^{\infty} RECT\left(\frac{x}{a}\right)e^{-2\pi i f x}dx = a\ sinc(af) \qquad [4\text{-}11]$$

A plot of this MTF is illustrated in Figure 4-18. The function on the right side of Equation 4-11 is commonly called a **sinc** function. The **sinc** function goes to zero at $F = 1/a$, but aliasing occurs above the Nyquist frequency at $1/2\Delta$. Thus, for a system which has an MTF defined by the **sinc** function, the possibility of aliasing is high

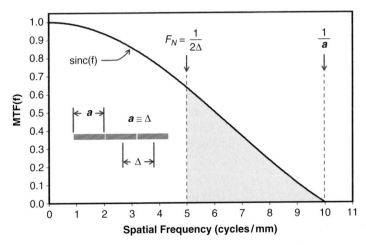

■ **FIGURE 4-18** This figure shows the MTF for a RECT input function of width **a**. Here, **a** = 0.100 mm. This was a contiguous detector; so the sampling pitch, Δ, was equal to **a**. Thus, the Nyquist frequency is 5 cycles/mm and the amplitude of the MTF goes to zero at 1/**a** = 10 cycles/mm. This MTF shows the SINC function—the analytical Fourier transform of the RECT function of width **a**. For an imaging system with a detector aperture of width **a**, this curve represents the best MTF possible for that detector.

■ FIGURE 4-19 Line pair phantoms are used for practical estimates of the spatial resolution in field tests of clinical imaging equipment. An ideal test phantom (**left**) is imaged, and the system blurs the image of the object as shown here (**right**). The observer reads the spatial frequency (not indicated here) corresponding to the smallest set of bars that were visible, and this measurement is considered the *limiting spatial resolution*.

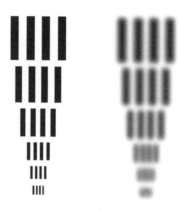

since the MTF still has nonzero amplitude above F_N. An imaging system that has an MTF defined by the **sinc** function is performing at its theoretical maximum in terms of spatial resolution.

Field Measurements of Resolution Using Resolution Templates

Spatial resolution should be monitored on a routine basis for many imaging modalities. However, measuring the LSF or the MTF is more detailed than necessary for routine quality assurance purposes. For most clinical imaging systems, the evaluation of spatial resolution using resolution test phantoms is adequate for routine quality assurance purposes. The test phantoms are usually line pair phantoms or star patterns (Fig. 4-19). The test phantoms are imaged, and the images are viewed to estimate the limiting spatial resolution of the imaging system. There is a degree of subjectivity in such an evaluation, but in general viewers will agree within acceptable limits. These measurements are routinely performed on fluoroscopic equipment, radiographic systems, nuclear cameras, and in CT.

 ## Contrast Resolution

Contrast resolution refers to the ability to detect very subtle changes in gray scale and distinguish them from the noise in the image. Contrast resolution is characterized by measurements that pertain to the signal-to-noise ratio (SNR) in an image. Contrast resolution is not a concept that is focused on physically small objects per se (that is the concept of spatial resolution); rather, contrast resolution relates more to anatomical structures that produce small changes in signal intensity (image gray scale), which make it difficult for the radiologist to pick out (detect) that structure from a noisy background.

Basic Notions of Accuracy and Precision

Accuracy and precision are illustrated using targets in Figure 4-20. Accuracy relates to how close one gets to the "truth" (the bull's-eye, in this case), while precision is a description of the variation, scatter, or reproducibility in a measurement. Measurements (or marksmanship) with low precision have higher levels of noise. Improving precision in a measurement may require new equipment (a better target rifle) or more practice in the case of the marksman, and once the

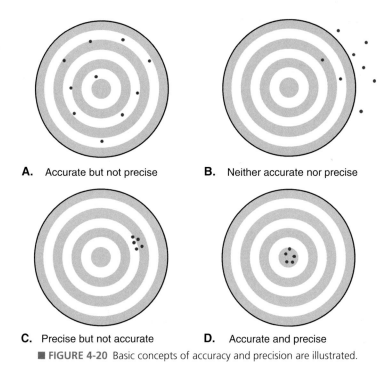

■ **FIGURE 4-20** Basic concepts of accuracy and precision are illustrated.

marksman becomes more reproducible, he or she can make adjustments to correct for *bias* that may affect accuracy. In Figure 4-20C, a tight pattern is achieved (high precision) but there is a bias to the upper right of the bull's-eye. Correction for this bias may require adjustments to the rifle's sites, and after such adjustments (Fig. 4-20D), accuracy with precision is achieved. This is an example where the bias can be corrected for.

In medical images, precision has to do with the amount of noise in the image. In the case of x-ray and gamma ray imaging, which are typically *quantum limited*, precision can almost always be improved by collecting more photons (quanta) to make the image—by increasing the time of the image acquisition, turning up the intensity of the source (or injecting more isotope), or both. In MRI, a number of redundant signal measurements are made and are averaged together to improve precision and reduce noise.

Sources of Image Noise

Grain Noise

When radiographic film is exposed and processed, the increase in observed darkness (optical density) in the film corresponds to an increase in the density of reduced silver grains adhering to the film support. The actual distribution of the silver grains is random and is a function of the manufacturing and development processes. Normally, the individual grains are not resolvable by the unaided human eye, and thus grain noise is not a factor when reading a film radiograph on a view box. However, in screen-film mammography, it is the standard of practice that the breast imager uses a magnifying glass to scan for small microcalcifications on the image. Depending on the magnification factor, it is theoretically possible to observe the silver grains, and thus, they would become a source of image noise in that instance (Fig. 4-21A).

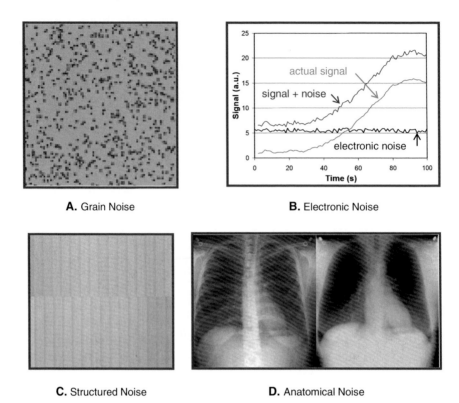

A. Grain Noise

B. Electronic Noise

C. Structured Noise

D. Anatomical Noise

■ **FIGURE 4-21** Various sources of image noise are illustrated. **A.** Grain noise results in screen film radiography, where the image is formed by millions of silver grains attached to the clear film substrate. In general, grain noise is too small to be resolved in general radiography. **B.** Electronic noise is typically additive noise from various sources that does not scale with the signal level. For the "signal + noise" curve in the figure, most of the "measured" information is noise. This plot illustrates that additive noise is worst in areas of low actual signal in the detector. **C.** Structured noise represents a reproducible pattern on the image that reflects differences in the gain of individual detector elements or groups of detector elements. Structured noise can be corrected using a flat field algorithm. **D.** Anatomical noise refers to anatomy in the patient which is not pertinent to the specific imaging examination. For example, ribs are a source of anatomical noise in a chest radiograph, where the lung parenchyma is the anatomy of interest. Ribs can be removed by using dual-energy x-ray imaging techniques.

Electronic Noise

Electronic detector systems can be analog or digital, but the flow of electrons (current) conveys the signal at one or more points in the imaging chain. There are electrons that resulted from actual signal detection events (in CT, MRI, nuclear imaging, etc.), and there are also electrons that are added to the signal that are not the result of signal detection events—this added electronic noise can be from thermal noise, shot noise, and other electronic noise sources. If the electrons associated with noise are added into the signal prior to amplification circuits, then their noise contribution will be amplified as well. In some imaging situations, especially when signal levels are low, the added noise can be substantial and can contribute appreciably to the overall noise levels in the image (Fig. 4-21B). There are several ways to reduce electronic noise, including cooling the detector system to reduce thermal noise, designing in noise reduction circuitry (e.g., double correlated sampling), or shielding electronics to avoid stray electronic signal induction.

Electronic noise is a real problem in some clinical applications, such as the use of thin film transistor panels for fluoroscopy or cone beam CT, or in very low dose CT situations.

Structure Noise

Most pixelated detectors have a number of parallel channels for reading out the array of detector elements, and this reduces readout time. Each channel uses its own amplifier circuits and these circuits cannot be perfectly tuned with respect to each other. As a result, groups of detector elements that are read out may have different offset noise and gain characteristics, and these cause structured or fixed pattern noise in digital detector systems (Fig. 4-21C). The key to correcting for structured noise is that it is spatially constant for a period of time. This allows the offset and gain factors for each individual detector element to be characterized by exposing the detector to radiation in the absence of an object (the so-called *gain* image). The *offset* image is measured with no radiation incident on the detector. These two calibration images can then be used to correct for structured noise using the so-called flat field correction algorithm[8]. In addition to a visible structure on uncorrected images due to amplifier configuration, each individual detector element has its own gain and offset characteristics which are also corrected by the flat field correction algorithm. Because it is probable that the structured noise pattern can change over time, for many imaging systems it is routine to acquire the offset and gain images necessary for calibration frequently—hourly, daily, or monthly, depending on the system.

There are other causes for structured noise—a splash of iodinated contrast agent on the input surface of an image intensifier (II) used in angiography will cause a dark spot that is always at the same location in the image (except when magnification modes are applied). Flat field correction approaches will correct for these blemishes as well, but if the II is cleaned and the flat field images are not recomputed, then the blemish will be overcompensated for—it will be a bright spot.

Anatomical Noise

Anatomical noise is the pattern on the image that is generated by patient anatomy that is always present but not important for the diagnosis. For example, in abdominal angiography, the vascular system is the anatomy of interest, and other sources of image contrast such as bowel gas and spine just get in the way. Using digital subtraction angiography, images are acquired before and after the injection of vascular contrast agents, and these images are subtracted, revealing only the vascular anatomy. Chest radiographs are acquired for the evaluation of the pulmonary anatomy and mediastinum; the ribs are a source of anatomical noise. Using dual-energy subtraction techniques (Fig. 4-21D), the ribs (and other bones) can be subtracted revealing only the soft tissue contrast in the image. Both temporal and dual-energy subtraction methods are performed primarily to reduce anatomical noise.

One of the underappreciated aspects of modern tomographic imaging, such as CT, MRI, and ultrasound, is that these images eliminate overlapping anatomical structures, and this substantially reduces anatomical noise by reducing or eliminating the superposition of normal tissue structures. Much of the *power of tomography*, then, is in its ability to reduce anatomical noise through spatial isolation. Thus, anatomical noise can be reduced using a number of approaches that capitalize on the temporal, energy, or spatial characteristics of the image formation process.

---

[8] $I_{corrected} = g\dfrac{I_{raw} - I_{offset(r)}}{I_{gain} - I_{offset(g)}}$, where g is the mean gray scale of the denominator, and the offsets are

for the raw (r) and gain (g) images, respectively.

Quantum Noise

The term *quanta* refers to any number of particles or objects that can be counted, such as electrons, x-ray photons, optical photons, or even brush strokes on impressionist paintings. The modern human visual experience involves quantum-rich viewing—a sunny day, a well-illuminated room, a bright flat panel monitor. When the number of quanta used to illuminate a scene is large, there is virtually no noise in the visual image. In low-light imaging environments, such as when night vision glasses are used, significant levels of optical quantum noise are seen. In the radiology department, to reduce radiation dose to the patient from x-rays or gamma rays, imaging modalities based upon ionizing radiation use relatively few quanta to form the image—indeed, the numbers of quanta are so low that for most medical images involving x-rays or gamma rays, appreciable noise in the image results, and this noise is called *quantum noise*. Before directly addressing the topic of imaging in a quantum-limited setting, it is useful to review the topic of statistical distributions.

Statistical Distributions

There is a large field devoted to the evaluation of random variation in data, and most readers will likely have more than one book on statistics on their bookshelf. Here, a basic discussion of statistical distributions is presented as a prelim to a more focused discussion on contrast resolution in medical imaging.

Nonparametric Measures of Noise

Nonparametric metrics of a data distribution use measures that assume no underlying statistical distribution to the data distribution. The *median* is the point in the distribution where 50% of the observations are greater, and 50% are less. It is the halfway point in the observed data set. The *mode* is the most frequent observation, the highest point in the histogram (Fig. 4-22). The width of the distribution is characterized by the *range*, and there is flexibility in the fractional range that one uses—the 100% range would be subject to outliers, and so often a smaller fraction of the range is quoted, such as the 50% or 90% range.

Nonparametric characterizations of two distributions can be used to test for differences, for example. Appropriate nonparametric statistical tests (Wilcoxon rank sum, etc.) are used. The use of nonparametric statistical tests is applicable to any distribution; however, there is greater power in tests of statistical inference when an underlying parametric distribution (such as the normal distribution) can be assumed. The normal distribution is discussed in the next section.

■ FIGURE 4-22 An arbitrary distribution is shown, with the nonparametric parameters of *median*, *mode*, and *range* illustrated.

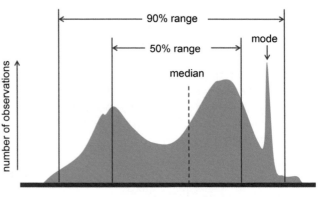

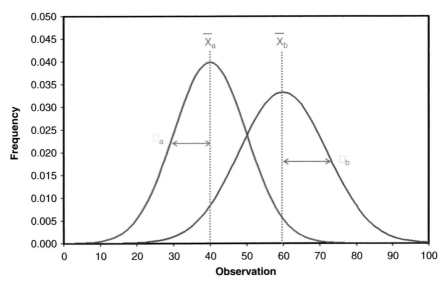

■ **FIGURE 4-23** Two normal distributions are illustrated. The normal distribution has two parameters, which determine its shape, and position the mean $\bar{x}$, and standard deviation σ.

Most textbooks on statistical distributions start with a discussion of the *binomial distribution*, which is a discrete distribution and is useful for discussing coin tosses and the like. The normal distribution and the Poisson distributions are extensions of the binomial distribution, and are the predominant statistical distributions used in medical imaging. For that reason, we refer readers interested in the binomial distribution to any basic text on statistics.

The Normal Distribution

The normal distribution, also called the gaussian distribution, is the most widely used statistical distribution in scientific analysis and other observational settings. The well-known bell-shaped curve (Fig. 4-23) is characterized by two parameters—the mean ($\bar{x}$) and the standard deviation (σ). The square of the standard deviation is the variance, σ^2. On a 2D plot of the distribution, the x-axis parameter typically is called the independent variable, and the y-axis parameter is the dependent variable (y, $G(x)$, etc). The normal distribution is given by the equation

$$G(x) = \frac{1}{\sigma\sqrt{2\pi}}\, e^{-\frac{1}{2}\left(\frac{x-\bar{x}}{\sigma}\right)^2}, \qquad [4\text{-}12]$$

where x is the independent variable, $\bar{x}$ and σ are the parameters of interest, and the first term to the right of the equal sign simply normalizes the area of $G(x)$ to unity. Two normal distributions are illustrated in Figure 4-23, one with a mean of 40 and the other with a mean of 60. It is clear from the graph that the mean describes the center of the bell-shaped curve, and the value of σ determines the width of each distribution. The value of σ is the half width at 61% of full height, and that is useful for estimating the value of σ on generic bell-shaped plots. The mean can be computed from a series of N observations x_i, such as $x_1, x_2, x_3, \ldots\ldots x_N$, where

$$\bar{x} = \frac{1}{N}\sum_{i=1}^{N} x_i. \qquad [4\text{-}13]$$

The variance is computed as

$$\sigma^2 = \frac{\sum_{i=1}^{N}(\bar{x}-x)^2}{N-1} \qquad [4\text{-}14]$$

and the standard deviation is the square root of the variance

$$\sigma = \sqrt{\sigma^2}. \qquad [4\text{-}15]$$

The dependence on two parameters ($\bar{x}$ and σ) means that the normal distribution is flexible and can be used to model a number of physical situations and laboratory measurements. Furthermore, the value of each parameter, $\bar{x}$ and σ, can have a physical interpretation—not just a statistical one. The following simple example will illustrate this:

A large elementary school has a number of classes from kindergarten to the sixth grade. The mean height of the children in the fourth grade (~age 9) is 135 cm, while the mean height of all the sixth graders (~age 11) is 147 cm. It is not surprising that grade-school children grow rapidly in height as they age, and thus the fact that the mean height of sixth graders is greater than that of fourth graders is logical and easy to understand. It has physical meaning. But what about the standard deviation? This school is large and has 3 fourth grades (three classes of 30 students each) to accommodate enrollment. While the average height of all the fourth graders in this particular school is 135.7 cm (simulated data were used in this example), the standard deviation across all 90 students was 6.4 cm. Let us say that the students were assigned *randomly* to each classroom, and then the mean and standard deviation were measured—for Class 4A it was 134.4 cm ($\sigma = 6.4$ cm), Class 4B was 137.7 cm ($\sigma = 6.0$ cm), and Class 4C was 135.3 cm ($\sigma = 7.0$ cm). Instead of randomly assigning children to each class, what if the fourth graders were assigned to each class by height—line all 90 children up by height; the shortest 30 go to Class 4A, the tallest 30 go to Class 4C, and the rest are assigned to Class 4B (Fig. 4-24). In this case, the mean and standard deviation for these classes are 128.2 cm (2.3 cm), 135.5 cm

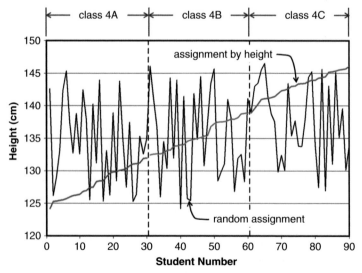

■ **FIGURE 4-24** The *black line* shows the heights of 90 children in fourth grade, and this is simply a random order. The three sections show the heights of children in three different classrooms, where the children were assigned to each classroom by height. The purpose of this illustration is to show the value of the two-parameter normal distribution in describing physical observations.

(2.2 cm), and 143.1 cm (1.9 cm). It is not surprising that, because the students in this latter example were assigned by height, Class 4A is shorter, Class 4B is next, and Class 4C has the largest mean height. Also, because the children were selected by height, there is less variation in height in each class, and that is why the standard deviation for each classroom for this latter assignment approach is substantially less ($\bar{\sigma} = 2.1$) than random assignment ($\bar{\sigma} = 6.5$). There is less variation in height in each classroom, and thus the standard deviation measured in each class is lower—this makes physical sense.

In regard to the first randomization scheme mentioned in the above paragraph, what methods would result in a true random assignment to each of the 3 fourth-grade classrooms? What if alphabetical order based on the last name of the child was used, would this be random? Probably not, since last names can be related to ethnicity, and there is a relationship between ethnicity and height. Such a scheme would probably add *bias* to the assignment scheme that may not be recognized. What if the child's birth date was used for the assignment? Those with birthdays in December and January are bound to be older than those children with birthdays in June and August, and since older children are in general taller (even just a little), this randomization scheme would suffer from bias as well. This example is meant to illustrate how unintentional bias can enter an experiment—or, in radiology, selection criteria for a clinical trial. Perhaps the easiest way to eliminate bias in the above example is to print the numbers 1 through 90 on identical chits, thoroughly mix them up in a hat, and let each child pick from the hat—Numbers 1 to 30 go to Class 4A, 31 to 60 to Class 4B, and 61 to 90 go to Class 4C.

Relative Areas of the Normal Distribution

With the normal distribution, the relative area of the curve as a function of $\pm\sigma$ (in both the negative and positive directions) is useful to know. Measurements that fall within $\bar{x} \pm 1\sigma$ represent 68% of the observations that are being characterized by the normal distribution (Fig. 4-25). Values falling within $\bar{x} \pm 2\sigma$ represent 95% of

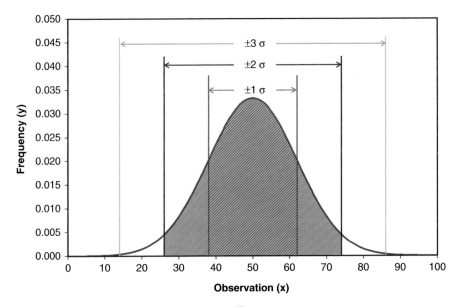

■ **FIGURE 4-25** The areas of the normal distribution for $\bar{x} \pm n\sigma$, for n = 1, 2, and 3 are shown. For $\bar{x} \pm 1\sigma$, the area is 68%, for $\bar{x} \pm 2\sigma$ it is 95%, and for $\bar{x} \pm 3\sigma$ the area is 99% of the total area of the normal distribution.

the observations, and values falling into the range $\bar{x} \pm 3\sigma$ encompass 99% of the observations. In scientific papers, it is common to plot curves with error bars spanning $\pm 2\sigma$, and this demonstrates to the observer that 95% of expected observations for each data point should fall between the ends of the error bars. A p-value of 0.05 is commonly used as the threshold for statistical significance, and this states that there is a 95% probability $(1-0.05)$ that an observation that obeys the normal distribution will fall *inside* the $\bar{x} \pm 2\sigma$ range, and a 5% probability (0.05) that it will fall *outside* that range.

The Poisson Distribution

The normal distribution is a very commonly used statistical distribution; however, it is not the only one. Another important statistical distribution that is relevant in radiological imaging is the Poisson distribution, $P(x)$, which is given by

$$P(x) = \frac{m^x}{x!} e^{-m} \qquad [4\text{-}16]$$

where m is the mean and x is the independent variable. The very important thing about the Poisson distribution is that its shape is governed by only one parameter (m), not two parameters as we saw for the normal distribution. Figure 4-26 illustrates the Poisson distribution with $m = 50$ (*dashed line*), along with the normal distribution with $\bar{x}=50$ and $\sigma = \sqrt{\bar{x}}$. The normal distribution is often used to approximate the Poisson distribution, in part because the factorial ($x!$, i.e., $5! = 1 \times 2 \times 3 \times 4 \times 5$) in Equation 4-16 makes computation difficult for large values of x (e.g., $70!$ $> 10^{100}$). Therefore, we can approximate the Poisson distribution with the normal distribution, but only when we stipulate that $\sigma = \sqrt{\bar{x}}$. This is a very important stipulation, with very important ramifications in imaging.

X ray and γ-ray counting statistics obey the Poisson distribution, and this is quite fortunate for radiology. *Why?* We will use an x-ray imaging example (i.e., radiography, mammography, fluoroscopy, CT), but this pertains to nuclear

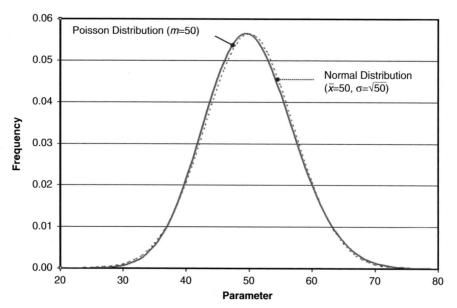

■ **FIGURE 4-26** This figure shows that the normal distribution with $\bar{x} = 50$ and $\sigma = \sqrt{50}$, closely conforms to the Poisson distribution with $m = 50$.

imaging as well. If an x-ray beam with a photon fluence ϕ (photons/mm²) is incident on a digital x-ray detector system with detection efficiency ϵ and with detector elements of area A (in mm²), the average number of x-rays recorded in each detector element will be N, where $\phi A \epsilon = N$. Using the normal distribution assumption for the Poisson distribution, and now using N to represent the mean number of photons (instead of the symbol $\bar{x}$ used previously) in the image, the noise per pixel is given by

$$\sigma = \sqrt{N} \qquad [4\text{-}17]$$

The above equation *is* the stipulation that allows the normal distribution to approximate the Poisson distribution. In other words, we are constraining the two-parameter normal distribution so that it now behaves like a one-parameter distribution. This allows us to adjust the technique parameters (N) in x-ray imaging a priori, to control the noise levels perceived in the image. The relative noise on an image is equal to the coefficient of variation (COV):

$$\text{Relative noise} = \text{COV} = \frac{\sigma}{N} \qquad [4\text{-}18]$$

So, we can adjust N in an x-ray image, as it is proportional to various settings on the x-ray system discussed later in this text. In nuclear imaging, N is determined by the amount of isotope injected and the scan time, amongst other factors. In general (at the same energy), N is also linearly proportional to the radiation dose to the patient. By adjusting N, we are also adjusting σ (Equation 4-17), which in turn means that we are adjusting the relative noise in the image (Equation 4-18). Therefore, we can predict the relative noise in the image and use this knowledge to adjust the value of N (and hence σ and COV) for the clinical imaging task, *before* we acquire that image.

A clinical example will help illustrate the power of Equation 4-18. In fluoroscopy, we only need to see a catheter advance in a vessel for part of the interventional vascular procedure, so we know that we can use a relatively small value of N (per pixel per image) for this task, acknowledging that the fluoroscopic images will be noisy, but experience has shown that this is adequate for providing the radiologist the image quality necessary to advance the catheter. This saves dose to the patient for what can ultimately be a time-consuming, high-dose procedure. By comparison, mammography requires very low relative noise levels in order to determine, from a statistical standpoint, that there are small microcalcifications on the image. This means that we need to use a relatively high value of N per pixel for breast imaging. The fluoroscopic and mammography systems are adjusted to deliver a certain N per pixel in the resulting images, but it is the Poisson Distribution, and its handier normal distribution approximation, that allow us to predict the noise in the image from the mean photon fluence to the detector. The bottom line is that because the noise level in an image (σ/N) is determined by setting N, this allows the compromise between radiation dose to the patient and noise in the image to be determined a priori.

There are very important dose ramifications when working in an environment where the Poisson distribution is in play: Doubling the radiation dose to the patient implies adjusting the photon fluence from N to $2N$, but since $\sigma = \sqrt{N}$, this will reduce the noise by a factor of $\sqrt{2} = 1.41$. Hence, doubling the dose results in a 41% reduction in noise. To reduce the noise by half, a fourfold increase in radiation dose to the patient is needed. Table 4-1 illustrates how noise and SNR change as a function of N.

TABLE 4-1   EXAMPLES OF NOISE VERSUS PHOTONS

PHOTONS/PIXEL (N)	NOISE (σ) ($\sigma = \sqrt{N}$)	RELATIVE NOISE (σ/N) (%)	SNR (N/σ)
10	3.2	32	3.2
100	10	10	10
1,000	31.6	3.2	32
10,000	100	1.0	100
100,000	316.2	0.3	316

SNR, signal-to-noise ratio.

4.6   Noise Texture: The Noise Power Spectrum

The measurement that is characterized by the variance, σ^2 is a simple metric which can quantify the noise in an image using Equation 4-14, but this metric does not quantify the noise *texture*. In Figure 4-27, the two CT images of a test object have the same variance in the background, but there is a perceptible difference in appearance of the way the noise *looks*. Although the noise variance is the same, the frequency dependence of the noise is different. The frequency dependence of the noise variance is characterized by the *noise power spectrum*, NPS(f), where for a 2D image $I(x,y)$

$$NPS(f_x, f_y) = \left| \int_x \int_y \left[I(x,y) - \overline{I} \right] e^{-2\pi i (xf_x + yf_y)} \, dx \, dy \right|^2 \qquad [4\text{-}19]$$

where f_x is the frequency corresponding to the x-dimension and f_y is the frequency corresponding to the y-dimension, and $\overline{I}$ is the mean of image $I(x,y)$. Just as the MTF(f) gives a richer, frequency-dependent measure of how an imaging system operates on an input signal, the NPS(f) yields an informative, frequency-dependent measure of how an imaging system operates on the noise input into the system. The NPS is essentially a frequency-dependent breakdown of the variance, and indeed the integral of the NPS over all frequencies equals the variance σ^2.

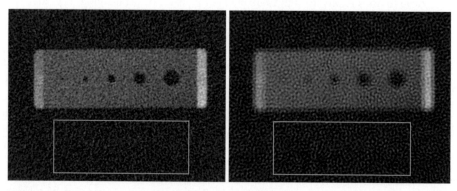

■ **FIGURE 4-27** Two CT images of a test object are shown, and the standard deviation in the highlighted boxes is identical. However, the noise texture—the way the noise looks—is different. These differences in noise texture are characterized using the frequency dependent noise power spectrum, *NPS(f)*.

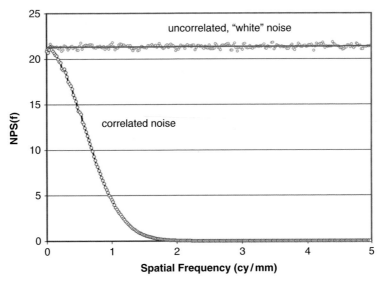

FIGURE 4-28 The noise power spectrum, *NPS(f)*, is shown for uncorrelated noise and for correlated noise.

$$\sigma^2 = \int_{f_x} \int_{f_y} NPS(f_x, f_y)\, df_x\, df_y \qquad \text{[4-20]}$$

If the noise in each pixel of a 2D image is not dependent upon the noise values in any of its surrounding pixels, then there will be no *noise correlation* and the *NPS(f)* will essentially be a flat, horizontal line (Fig. 4-28). This type of uncorrelated noise is called *white noise*. Real imaging systems have some blur phenomenon that results in the finite width of the *PSF(x)* or *LSF(x)*. This blurring means that noise from detector elements can leak into the adjacent detector elements, leading to noise correlation between adjacent pixels in the image. There are many types and causes of noise correlation (including anticorrelation, where positive noise in one pixel will tend to induce a negative noise value in adjacent pixels), including reconstruction algorithms in tomography, but in general, the result of noise correlation is that the NPS is no longer white—and the shape of the *NPS(f)* for a given imaging system then is a technical description of this broader sense of *noise texture* (see Fig. 4-28).

The noise power spectrum is an analytical tool that is used by imaging scientists but is not generally used in the clinical radiology setting. It is an important metric when considering the design of new imaging systems, and in the comprehensive evaluation of research imaging systems. Nevertheless, some familiarity with the concept of the NPS is useful to the clinically focused reader, because reconstructed images such as in CT have a wide array of noise textures that are plainly visible on clinical images, and these textures depend on the reconstruction methodology and kernels used.

We will return to concepts of the NPS later in this chapter.

4.7 Contrast

Subject Contrast

Subject contrast is the fundamental contrast that arises in the signal, after it has interacted with the patient but before it has been detected. The example of projection radiography is illustrated in Figure 4-29. In the case of x-ray projection imaging, an

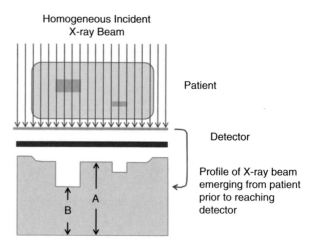

■ FIGURE 4-29 An x-ray beam is incident on a simple "patient," and the incident beam of x-ray photons is modulated by attenuation processes in the patient, resulting in a heterogeneous pattern of x-rays emerging from the patient, which then are incident upon the x-ray detector. Subject contrast is defined as the differences in the x-ray beam fluence across the beam, emmerging from the patient which is incident upon the detector.

approximately homogeneous x-ray beam is incident upon the patient, and the x-rays then interact via various interaction mechanisms, resulting in the majority of x-rays being attenuated, but a small fraction will emerge from the patient unattenuated. Although this beam cannot be measured in reality until it reaches a detector, the concept of subject contrast involves the fundamental interaction between the x-ray beam and the object. The subject contrast is defined as

$$C_s = \frac{(A - B)}{A} \qquad [4\text{-}21]$$

where the photon fluence levels of A and B are shown in Figure 4-29, and for Equation 4-21, A > B. This requirement means that contrast runs from 0 to 1 (i.e., 0% to 100%).

Subject contrast has intrinsic factors and extrinsic factors—the intrinsic component of subject contrast relates to the actual anatomical or functional changes in the patient's tissues, which give rise to contrast. That is, the patient walks into the imaging center with intrinsic, physical or physiological properties that give rise to subject contrast. For a single pulmonary nodule in the lung, for example, the lesion is of greater density than the surrounding lung tissue, and this allows it to be seen on chest radiography or thoracic CT or thoracic MRI. The lesion may also exhibit higher metabolism, and thus, when a sugar molecule labeled with radioisotope is injected into the patient, more of that biomarker will accumulate in the lesion than in the surrounding lung due to its greater metabolism, and the radioisotope emission resulting from this concentration difference results in subject contrast.

Extrinsic factors in subject contrast relate to how the image-acquisition protocol can be optimized to enhance subject contrast. Possible protocol enhancements include changing the x-ray energy, using a different radiopharmaceutical, injecting an iodine (CT) or gadolinium (MR) contrast agent, changing the delay between contrast injection and imaging, changing the pulse sequence in MR, or changing the angle of the ultrasound probe with respect to the vessel in Doppler imaging. These are just a few examples of ways in which subject contrast can be optimized; many more parameters are available for optimization.

Detector Contrast

The incident beam of energy from the imaging system will eventually reach the detector(s), and again radiography is used as an example (Fig. 4-30). The same log

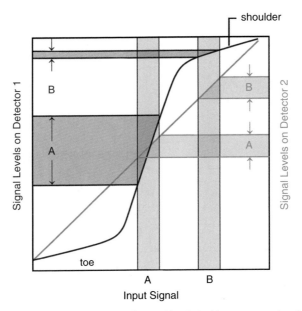

■ **FIGURE 4-30** For a log input signal (x-axis) with two identical objects attenuating the beam at different fluence levels in the beam (inputs A and B), the signal levels on Detector 1 (screen-film system) are dramatically influenced by the nonlinear characteristic curve of the detector. By comparison, the linear detector system (detector 2) produces signals that are proportional to the input signal trends. Detector 1 amplifies the signal contrast in the steep area of the curve, while a reduction in signal contrast is realized in the toe and shoulder of detector 1's characteristic curve.

relative exposure differences are shown on the x-axis, and two different detector responses are shown—a nonlinear response to x-rays (screen-film radiography) is shown on the left vertical axis, and a linear response (typical of many digital x-ray detectors) is shown on the right vertical axis. This figure illustrates that the detector system can have a profound impact on how the subject contrast incident upon it is converted to the final image.

Displayed Contrast

The detector contrast acts to modulate the subject contrast, but the acquisition procedure ultimately results in the capture of digital image data on a computer's hard drive. For modalities where subsequent image processing occurs, such as image processing in many digital radiography systems, or image reconstruction in CT, MRI, SPECT, PET, etc., the raw image information is processed into an image that is finally meant for physician viewing (*for presentation* images, in the parlance of PACS).

The majority of medical images have bit depths ranging from 10, 12, and even 14 bits, which run from 1,024, 4,096, to 16,384 shades of gray, respectively. Modern displays, however, are only capable of displaying 8-bit (256 shades of gray) to 10-bit (1,024 shades of gray) images. The display computer needs to convert the higher bit depth data encoded on the image to the spectrum of gray scale on the monitor, and there is a *look-up table* (LUT) that is used to make this transformation. Various LUTs are illustrated in Figure 4-31. The LUT transforms the gray scale of each pixel of the image stored in memory on the computer, ultimately to be displayed as gray scale on the monitor. The most commonly used LUT in radiological imaging is the so-called window/level, which is depicted in Figure 4-31. This is generally a nonlinear LUT that causes saturation to black below L−W/2 and saturation to white above

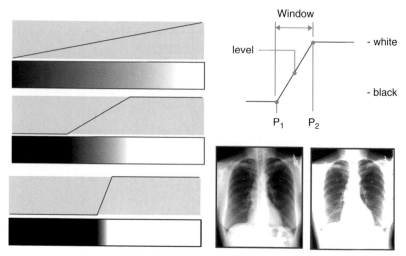

■ **FIGURE 4-31** A digital image is represented as a matrix of gray scale values in the memory of a computer, but the look-up table (LUT) describes how that gray scale is converted to actual densities on the display. Three different "window/level" settings are shown on the left. The diagram shows the window width and level, and the image data is saturated to black at $P_1 = L - W/2$, and is saturated white at $P_2 = L + W/2$. Chest radiographs are shown with different window/level settings.

$L + W/2$. Because the monitor cannot depict the depth of gray scale from the entire image, it is routine for the interpreting physician to routinely change the window/level settings for a given image, so that the entire range of gray scale on the acquired image can be evaluated. While freely changing the window and level setting is possible on most image workstations, several preset window and level settings are generally used to expedite viewing.

There is another approach for medical image display, which reduces the need for the physician to view images using multiple LUT settings. Simple image processing techniques can reduce the dynamic range of the native image for display down to a point where all gray scale in the image can be viewed using one window and level setting—one LUT (Fig. 4-32). While there are many examples of this, the most obvious is that of digital mammography—where the raw 14-bit image is collapsed down to a displayable 10-bit image using image processing methods akin to *blurred mask subtraction*.

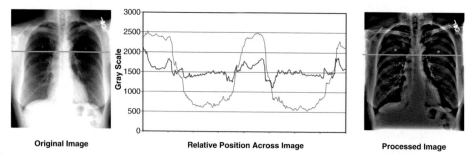

■ **FIGURE 4-32** A standard chest x-ray is shown on the **left**, and the corresponding trace through it is shown in the **graph**. Image processing methods such as blurred mask subtraction or other high pass filtering techniques can be used to compress the gray scale necessary for the display of the image (**right image**). The gray scale versus position trace of the processed image has less dynamic range than in the original image.

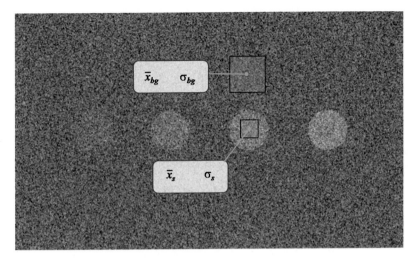

Mean BG = 127.5332
Noise = 10.2949
Steps are 5, 10, 15, 20

■ **FIGURE 4-33** The CNR is illustrated. The CNR is an area-independent measure of the contrast, relative to the noise, in an image. The CNR is useful for optimizing image acquisition parameters for generic objects of variable sizes and shapes. The CNRs in this figure (in the disks running from left to right) are 0.39, 1.03, 1.32, and 1.70.

Contrast-to-Noise Ratio

The contrast-to-noise ratio (CNR) is an object *size-independent* measure of the signal level in the presence of noise. Take the example of a disk as the object (Fig. 4-33). The contrast in this example is the difference between the average gray scale of a region of interest (ROI) in the disk $(\overline{x}_S)$ and that in an ROI in the background $(\overline{x}_{BG})$, and the noise can be calculated from the background ROI as well. Thus, the CNR is given by

$$CNR = \frac{(\overline{x}_S - \overline{x}_{bg})}{\sigma_{bg}} \qquad [4\text{-}22]$$

The CNR is a good metric for describing the signal amplitude relative to the ambient noise in an image, and this is particularly useful for simple objects. Because the CNR is computed using the difference in mean values between the signal region and the background, this metric is most applicable when test objects that generate a homogeneous signal level are used—that is, where the mean gray scale in the signal ROI is representative of the entire object. Example uses of the CNR metric include optimizing the kV of an imaging study to maximize bone contrast at a fixed dose level, computing the dose necessary to achieve a given CNR for a given object, or computing the minimum concentration of contrast agent that could be seen on given test phantom with fixed dose.

4.9 Signal-to-Noise Ratio

The SNR is a metric similar to the CNR, except that the size and shape of the object is explicitly included in the computation. In addition, the SNR does not require the test object that generates the signal to be homogeneous; however, the background

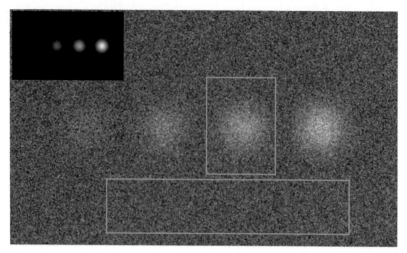

■ **FIGURE 4-34** Signal regions with a gaussian-based intensities are shown. The SNR has a fundamental relationship with detectability, and the Rose Criterion states that if SNR > 5, the signal region will be detectable in most situations.

does need to be homogeneous in principle—a series of gaussian "blobs" is used to illustrate this point (Fig. 4-34). The numerator in the SNR is the signal integrated over the entire dimensions of the object of interest. The signal amplitude of each pixel is the amount in which this patch of the image is elevated relative to the mean background signal—thus, for a mean background of $\bar{x}_{BG}$, the signal at each pixel i in the image is $x_i - \bar{x}_{BG}$. The denominator is the standard deviation in the homogeneous background region of the image (σ_{BG}), and thus the SNR represents the integrated signal over an ROI, which encapsulates the object of interest, divided by the noise

$$SNR = \frac{\sum_i (x_i - \bar{x}_{BG})}{\sigma_{BG}}$$

[4-23]

The SNR can be computed by summing the difference values over a rectangular ROI, which surrounds the signal region. Notice that this definition of the SNR allows the computation to be performed even when the signal region is not homogeneous in gray scale (see Fig. 4-34). The SNR computed in Equation 4-23 does require that the measurement of $\bar{x}_{BG}$ be accurate, and thus it should be computed over as large a region as possible.

The SNR is one of the most meaningful metrics that describes the conspicuity of an object—how well it will be seen by the typical observer. Indeed, Albert Rose recognized this and was able to demonstrate that if SNR ≥ 5, then an object will almost always be recognized (detected), but that detection performance continuously degrades as SNR approaches zero. This is called the *Rose Criterion*.

4.10 Contrast-Detail Diagrams

In this chapter, we have discussed spatial resolution and contrast resolution as if they were separate entities, but of course both of these quantities matter on a given image. In particular, it does not matter if the imaging receptor has excellent spatial resolution if the noise in the detector is high (i.e., the contrast resolution is low) and the

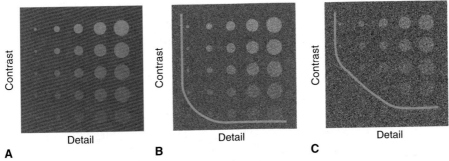

■ FIGURE 4-35 Contrast-detail diagrams are illustrated. **A.** The (noiseless) CD phantom is illustrated, where disks are smaller to the left and have less contrast toward the bottom. **B.** Some resolution loss and added noise is present, and the smallest and lowest in contrast disk can no longer be seen with confidence. The *yellow line* is the line of demarcation between disks that can be seen (upper right) and those that cannot be seen (lower left). **C.** More noise is added, and more of the subtle disks (including the entire, low-contrast bottom row) cannot be reliably seen.

statistical integrity of the image is not sufficient to detect a small object. The contrast detail diagram, or *CD diagram*, is a conceptual, visual method for combining the concepts of spatial resolution and contrast resolution.

A standard CD phantom is illustrated in Figure 4-35A. Here, the disk diameter decreases toward the left, so the greatest detail (smallest disks) is along the left column of the CD diagram. The contrast of each disk decreases from top to bottom, and thus the bottom row of the CD diagram has the lowest contrast—and the disks in the bottom row will therefore be most difficult to see in a noisy image. Figure 4-35B illustrates the CD diagram, but with some resolution loss and with increased noise. It is important to remember that the most difficult disk to see is in the lower left (smallest with lowest contrast), and the easiest disk to see is the upper right (largest with highest contrast) on this CD diagram. The line (see Fig. 4-35B) on a CD diagram is the line of demarcation, separating the disks that you can see from the ones that you cannot see. To the left and below the line are disks that cannot be seen well, and above and to the right of the line are disks that can be seen. Figure 4-35C shows the CD diagram with even more noise, and in this image the line of demarcation (the CD curve) has changed because the increased noise level has reduced our ability to see the disks with the most subtle contrast levels.

Figure 4-35 illustrates CD diagrams with the actual test images superimposed behind the graph; however, Figure 4-36 illustrates an actual CD diagram. The two curves in Figure 4-36A correspond to imaging systems A and B, but how can the differences in these two imaging systems be interpreted? Let curve A in Figure 4-36A be a standard radiographic procedure and curve B represents a low-dose radiograph. The dose does not change the detail in the image, and thus the two curves come together in the upper left (where the contrast is the highest) to describe the same detail level. However, because curve A corresponds to an image that was acquired with higher radiation dose—the noise in the image is less, and the CD diagram shows that curve A has better contrast resolution—because (lower contrast) disks lower down on the CD diagram can be seen (relative to curve B).

Figure 4-36B shows another example of a CD diagram. The two curves A and B on this CD diagram describe two different image processing procedures for the same image. Let curve B be the original acquired data of the CD phantom on some imaging modality, and curve A has been smoothed using image processing techniques (see Fig. 4-11). The smoothing process blurs edges (reduces detail) but reduces image

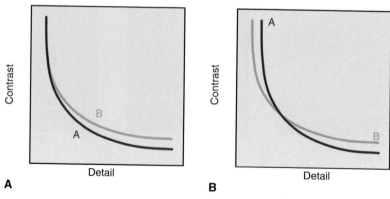

A (left graph) — Contrast vs Detail with curves A and B.
B (right graph) — Contrast vs Detail with curves A and B.

■ **FIGURE 4-36 A**. CD curves are shown. Both curves demonstrate the same detail (in the limit of high-contrast objects), but curve A extends to lower contrast. One explanation is that curve A corresponds to a higher dose version of curve B. **B**. Curve A has less detail but more contrast resolution than Curve B, and one explanation would be that Curve A corresponds to an image that was smoothed, relative to the image corresponding to curve B.

noise as well (increases contrast resolution). Thus, relative to curve B, curve A has less detail (does not go as far left as curve B) due to the blurring procedure, but has better contrast resolution (curve A goes lower on the CD diagram) because blurring smoothes noise.

The use of CD diagrams unites the concepts of spatial resolution (i.e., detail) and contrast resolution (i e., SNR) on the same graph. It is a subjective visual test, and so it is excellent in conveying the relationships visually but it is not quantitative. The detective quantum efficiency (DQE), discussed in the next section, also combines the concepts of spatial resolution and contrast resolution; however, the methods of DQE analysis are less visual and more quantitative.

4.11 Detective Quantum Efficiency

The DQE of an imaging system is a characterization of an x-ray imaging system, used by imaging scientists, which describes the overall frequency-dependent SNR performance of the system. In conceptual terms, the DQE can be defined as the ratio of the SNR^2 output from the system to the SNR^2 of the signal input into the system

$$DQE(f) = \frac{SNR^2_{OUT}}{SNR^2_{IN}}$$ [4-24]

The SNR_{IN} to an x-ray imaging system is simply $SNR_{IN} = N/\sigma = N/\sqrt{N} = \sqrt{N}$ (Equation 4-17), and thus $SNR^2_{IN} = N$, the mean photon fluence incident upon the imaging system.

The SNR^2_{OUT} is a function of the MTF and the NPS. The $MTF(f)$ describes how well an imaging system *processes signal,* and the $NPS(f)$ describes how well an imaging system *processes noise* in the image.

Combining these concepts, the numerator of Equation 4-19 is given by

$$SNR^2_{OUT} = \frac{[MTF(f)]^2}{NPS(f)}$$ [4-25]

The NPS(f) is the noise variance, so it is already squared. Equation 4-25 also describes the Noise Equivalent Quanta (NEQ).

With the above definitions for SNR^2_{IN} and SNR^2_{OUT}, the DQE(f) is given by

$$DQE(f) = \frac{k\,[MTF(f)]^2}{N\,NPS(f)}$$ [4-26]

where k is a constant that converts units, and its value is usually defined as the square of the mean pixel value in the image(s) used to measure NPS(f). Its role is to convert the gray scale units of the imaging system to generic relative noise so as to be comparable with N (the Poisson noise term). The NPS(f) is determined from an image (or images) acquired at a mean photon fluence of N photons/mm². Thus, the units of the DQE(f) are mm^{-2}. The DQE(f) for a given detector system is shown as a function of different exposure levels to the detector in Figure 4-37. The DQE(f) has become the standard by which the performance of x-ray imaging systems is measured in the research environment. The DQE(f) is an excellent description of the dose efficiency of an x-ray detector system—that is how well the imaging system converts SNR² incident on the detector into SNR² in the image. The DQE(f), is a frequency-dependent description, and at zero frequency (f = 0) in the absence of appreciable electronic noise, the DQE(0) essentially converges to the detector's *quantum detection efficiency*, the QDE. The QDE reflects the efficiency of x-ray detection, neglecting other elements in the imaging chain that inject or amplify noise. It can also be estimated using

$$QDE = \frac{\int_E \phi(E)\left[1 - e^{-\mu(E)T}\right]dE}{\int_E \phi(E)\,dE}$$ [4-27]

where $\phi(E)$ is the x-ray spectrum, $\mu(E)$ represents the energy dependent linear attenuation coefficient of the x-ray detector material, and T is the thickness of the detector material. For a monoenergetic x-ray beam, Equation 4-27 collapses to the term in the square brackets.

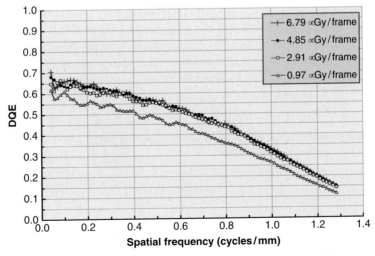

■ FIGURE 4-37 The DQE(f), is shown for a flat panel detector used on a cone beam CT system is shown. Four curves were generated at different exposure levels per image, as indicated. The curve at the lowest exposure level (0.97 μGy/frame) shows reduced DQE(f), likely due to the presence of added electronic noise. The electronic noise is present in the other curves as well, but the higher exposure levels dominate the signal intensity, and thus the electronic noise has less of an influence in degrading performance.

4.12 Receiver Operating Characteristic Curves

Image quality can be quantified using a number of metrics that have been discussed above. Ultimately, however, the quality of an image relates to how well it conveys diagnostic information to the interpreting physician. This can be tested using the concept of the receiver operating characteristic (ROC) curve. ROC performance includes not only the quality of the image data produced by an imaging system for a specific task, but in some cases the skill of the interpreting physician in assessing this data is also included.

The starting point of ROC analysis is the 2 × 2 *decision matrix* (sometimes called the truth table), shown in Figure 4-38. The patient either has the suspected disease (actually abnormal) or not (actually normal), and this gold standard is considered the "truth." The diagnostician has to make a binary decision about whether he or she thinks the patient has the suspected disease or not—based upon one or more diagnostic tests (including imaging examinations), he or she calls the patient either normal (does not have the disease) or abnormal (has the disease). The 2 × 2 decision matrix defines the terms *true positive (TP), true negative (TN), false positive (FP),* and *false negative (FN)* (see Fig. 4-38). Most of the work in performing patient-based ROC studies is the independent confirmation of the "truth," and this may require biopsy confirmation, long-term patient follow-up, or other methods to ascertain the true diagnosis.

In most radiology applications, the decision criterion is not just one feature or number, but is rather an overall impression derived from a number of factors, sometimes referred to as *gestalt*—essentially, the gut feeling of the experienced radiologist. Figure 4-39A illustrates two distributions of cases, those that are normal (left curve) and those that are abnormal (right curve). The generic descriptors *normal* and *abnormal* are used here, but these can be more specific for a given diagnostic task. For example, for mammography, the abnormal patients may have breast cancer and the normal patients do not. Overlap occurs between normal and abnormal findings in imaging, and thus these curves have overlap. Even though there is some ambiguity in the decision due to the overlap of the two curves, the radiologist is often responsible for diagnosing each case one way or another (e.g., to make the decision to biopsy or not). Hence, the patient is either determined to be *normal* or *abnormal*—a binary decision. In this case the diagnostician sets his or her own *decision threshold* (Fig. 4-39A). Patients to the right of the decision threshold are considered abnormal, and patients to the left of the threshold are considered normal. When the threshold is set, the values of TP, TN, FP, and FN can be determined (see Fig. 4-39).

■ FIGURE 4-38 The 2 × 2 decision matrix is illustrated.

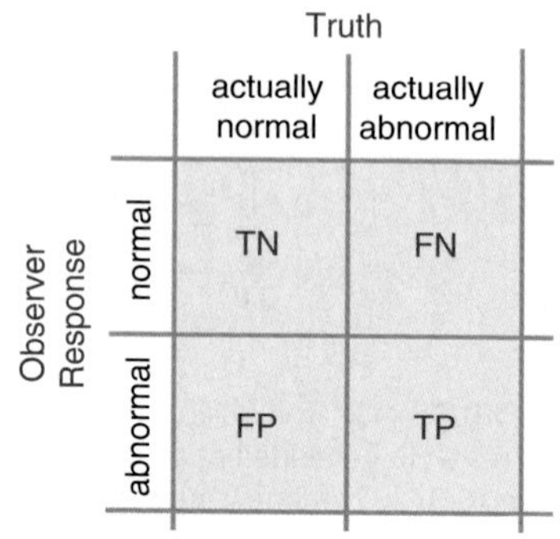

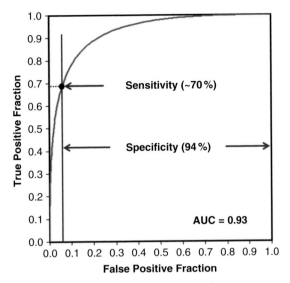

■ **FIGURE 4-40** An ROC curve is shown, and this curve is plausible for breast cancer screening using mammography. The ROC *curve* describes the theoretical performance of a skilled observer, but this observer will generally operate at a given point on the curve, called the *operating point* (*black dot*). This figure demonstrates the trade-offs of decision performance—compared to the operating point shown, the radiologist could increase sensitivity but generally this will come at a reduction in specificity—the operating point will move upward and to the right along the curve. More cancers will be detected (sensitivity will be increased), but far more women will be called back and asked to undergo additional imaging procedures and potentially biopsies (reduced specificity).

positives), and accuracy would be approximately 99.7%. Although the specificity would be 100%, the sensitivity would be 0%—obviously a useless test in such a case. For these reasons, diagnostic accuracy defined in Equation 4-31 is rarely used as a metric for the performance of a diagnostic test.

The *positive predictive value* (PPV) refers to the probability that the patient is actually abnormal (TP), when the diagnostician *says* the patient is abnormal (TP + FP).

$$\text{Positive predictive value} = \frac{\text{TP}}{\text{TP} + \text{FP}} \qquad [4\text{-}32]$$

Conversely, the negative predictive value (NPV) refers to the probability that the patient is actually normal (TN), when the diagnostician *says* the patient is normal (TN + FN).

$$\text{Negative predictive value} = \frac{\text{TN}}{\text{TN} + \text{FN}} \qquad [4\text{-}33]$$

The PPV and NPV of a diagnostic test (such as an imaging examination with radiologist interpretation) are useful metrics for referring physicians as they weigh the information from a number of diagnostic tests (some which may be contradictory) for a given patient, in the process of determining their diagnosis.

SUGGESTED READING

Barrett HH, Swindell W. *Radiological imaging: the theory of image formation, detection, and processing*, vols. 1 and 2. New York, NY: Academic Press, 1981.

Bracewell RN. *The Fourier transform and its applications*. New York, NY: McGraw-Hill, 1978.

Boone JM. Determination of the presampled MTF in computed tomography. *Med Phys* 2001;28:356–360.

Dainty JC, Shaw R. *Image science*. New York, NY: Academic Press, 1974.

Fugita H, Tsai D-Y, Itoh T, et al. A simple method for determing the modulation transfer function in digital radiography, *IEEE Trans Med Imaging* 1992;MI-11:34–39.

Hasegawa BH. *The physics of medical x-ray imaging*, 2nd ed. Madison, WI: Medical Physics, 1991.

Metz CE. Basic principles of ROC analysis. *Semin Nucl Med* 1978;8:283–298.

Rose A. *Vision: human and electronic*. New York, NY: Plenum Press, 1973.

CHAPTER 5

Medical Imaging Informatics

Medical imaging informatics is a multidisciplinary field of science and engineering that addresses the gathering, transfer, storage, processing, display, perception, and use of information in medicine. It overlaps many other disciplines such as electrical engineering, computer and information sciences, medical physics, and perceptual physiology and psychology.

This chapter begins by discussing number systems, the analog and digital representation of information, and the conversion of information between analog and digital representations. It next discusses digital radiological images and briefly describes digital computers and digital information storage technology. After this is a discussion of the display of digital radiological images. This is followed by a description of computer networks, which permit the rapid transfer of information over short and long distances. The next section addresses picture archiving and communications systems (PACS), which store and supply digital medical images for display. The last sections review image processing methods and measures for the security of medical information stored in digital form or transferred using computer networks.

5.1 Analog and Digital Representation of Data

Number Systems

Our culture uses a number system based on ten, probably because humans have five fingers on each hand and number systems having evolved from the simple act of counting on the fingers. Computers use the binary system for the storage and manipulation of numbers.

Decimal Form (Base 10)

In the decimal form, the ten digits 0 through 9 are used to represent numbers. To represent numbers greater than 9, several digits are placed in a row. The value of each digit in a number depends on its position in the row; the value of a digit in any position is *ten* times the value it would represent if it were shifted one place to the right. For example, the decimal number 3,506 actually represents

$$(3\times10^3)+(5\times10^2)+(0\times10^1)+(6\times10^0)$$

where $10^1=10$ and $10^0=1$. The leftmost digit in a number is called the *most significant digit* and the rightmost digit is called the *least significant digit*.

Binary Form (Base 2)

In binary form, the two digits 0 and 1 are used to represent numbers. Each digit, by itself, has the same meaning that it has in the decimal form. To represent numbers greater than 1, several digits are placed in a row. The value of each digit in a number

TABLE 5-1   NUMBERS IN DECIMAL AND BINARY FORMS

DECIMAL	BINARY	DECIMAL	BINARY
0	0	8	1000
1	1	9	1001
2	10	10	1010
3	11	11	1011
4	100	12	1100
5	101	13	1101
6	110	14	1110
7	111	15	1111
		16	10000

depends on its position in the row; the value of a digit in any position is *two* times the value it would represent if it were shifted one place to the right. For example, the binary number 1101 represents

$$(1\times2^3)+(1\times2^2)+(0\times2^1)+(1\times2^0)$$

where $2^3=8$, $2^2=4$, $2^1=2$, and $2^0=1$.

To count in binary form, 1 is added to the least significant digit of a number. If the least significant digit is 1, it is replaced by 0 and 1 is added to the next more significant digit. If several contiguous digits on the right are 1, each is replaced by 0 and 1 is added to the least significant digit that was not 1. Counting in the binary system is illustrated in Table 5-1.

Conversions Between Decimal and Binary Forms

To convert a number from binary to decimal form, the binary number is expressed as a series of powers of two and the terms in the series are added. For example, to convert the binary number 101011 to decimal form

$$101011 \text{ (binary)} = (1 \times 2^5) + (0 \times 2^4) + (1 \times 2^3) + (0 \times 2^2) + (1 \times 2^1) + (1 \times 2^0)$$
$$= (1 \times 32) + (1 \times 8) + (1 \times 2) + (1 \times 1) = 43 \text{ (decimal)}.$$

To convert a number from decimal into binary representation, it is repeatedly divided by two. Each division determines one digit of the binary representation, starting with the least significant. If there is no remainder from the division, the digit is 0; if the remainder is 1, the digit is 1. The conversion of 42 (decimal) into binary form is illustrated in Table 5-2.

Considerations Regarding Number Systems

Whenever it is not clear which form is being used, the form is written in parentheses after the number or denoted by a subscript of 2 for binary form and 10 for decimal form. For example, the number five can be written as 101 (binary), 101_2, 5 (decimal), or 5_{10}. If the form is not specified, it can usually be assumed that a number is in decimal form. It is important not to confuse the binary representation of a number with its more familiar decimal representation. For example, 10 (binary) and 10 (decimal) represent different numbers, although they look alike. On the other hand,

TABLE 5-2   CONVERSION OF 42 (DECIMAL) INTO BINARY FORM

DIVISION	RESULT		REMAINDER
42/2 =	21	0	Least significant digit
21/2 =	10	1	
10/2 =	5	0	
5/2 =	2	1	
2/2 =	1	0	
1/2 =	0	1	Most significant digit

Note: The decimal value is repeatedly divided by 2, with the remainder recorded after each division. The binary equivalent of 42 (decimal) is therefore 101010.

1010 (binary) and 10 (decimal) represent the same number. The only numbers that appear the same in both systems are 0 and 1.

Analog and Digital Representations

The detectors of medical imaging devices inherently produce analog data. Image display devices, discussed later in this chapter, require image information in analog form or must convert it to analog form. For many years, information in medical imaging systems was in analog form from signal detection to image display. For example, during these years, information in fluoroscopes, nuclear medicine scintillation cameras, and ultrasound imaging systems was entirely in analog form. Later, at some stages in these devices, the information was converted into digital form for processing and perhaps storage. Other imaging systems, such as x-ray computed tomography (CT) systems, from inception converted analog information from the detectors into digital form for processing. Today, in nearly all radiological imaging systems, analog information from the detectors is converted to digital form; processed, stored, and transferred in digital form; and converted to analog form only in the last stages of the image display systems.

Analog Representation of Data

In analog form, information is represented by a physical quantity whose allowed values are continuous, that is, the quantity in theory can have an infinite number of possible values between a lower and an upper limit. Most analog signals are also continuous in time; such a signal has a value at every point in time. In electronic circuits, numerical data can be represented in analog form by a voltage or voltage pulse whose amplitude is proportional to the number being represented, as shown in Figure 5-1A. An example of analog representation is a voltage pulse produced by a photomultiplier tube attached to a scintillation detector. The amplitude (peak voltage) of the pulse is proportional to the amount of energy deposited in the detector by an x- or gamma ray. Another example is the signal from the video camera attached to the image intensifier tube of a fluoroscopy system; the voltage at each point in time is proportional to the intensity of the x-rays incident on a portion of the input phosphor of the image intensifier tube (Fig. 5-1B). Numerical data can also be represented in analog form in electronic circuits by the frequency or phase of an alternating sinusoidal voltage, but these will not be discussed in this chapter.

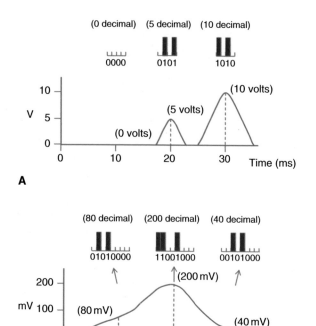

■ FIGURE 5-1 Analog and digital representation of numerical data. **A.** Three analog voltage pulses, similar to those produced by a photomultiplier tube attached to a scintillator, are illustrated. The height of each pulse represents a number, for instance, energy. Data are "sampled" at 10, 20, and 30 ms in time. Above the graph, these same amplitudes are represented in digital form with a sequence of four binary digits as on = 1, off = 0 binary states. Digital sampling occurs over a much shorter time scale than depicted on the x-axis. **B.** A continuously varying analog signal, such as a single video trace from the video camera in a fluoroscopy system, is shown. This analog signal varies in proportion to x-ray induced light intensities falling upon a photoconductive TV target, and produces an output voltage, in millivolts, as a function of time. The amplitude of the signal is sampled and converted to a corresponding digital value; shown are digital samples at 20, 40 and 60 μs. The values are represented in digital form as sequences of 8 binary digits, with binary values that correspond to the signal amplitude in mV.

Digital Representation of Information

Information in digital form is represented by a physical quantity that is allowed to have one of only a limited number of discrete (separated) values at any moment in time. In digital form, a number or other unit of information such as a letter of the alphabet is represented by a sequence of digits, each of which is limited to a defined number of values. Most digital signals are binary, that is, they consist of digits, each of which is limited to only two allowed values, but digital signals that consist of digits with more than two allowed values are possible and used in some situations.

The portion of a binary signal that is limited to one of two values is referred to as a binary digit (*bit*). In an electronic circuit, a bit might be a voltage of either 0 or 5 V, maintained for a defined length of time. (In a practical digital circuit, a range of voltages about each of these two voltages is permitted, but the two ranges are separated by a wide gap.) In microprocessors, computer memory, and mass storage devices, a bit is a physical entity. A bit in a microprocessor may be an electronic switch that has two stable states. In most solid-state computer memory, each bit is a capacitor; charged above a specific voltage is one state and not charged is the other. In magnetic storage media, such as magnetic disks and magnetic tape, a bit is a small portion of the disk or tape that may be magnetized

TABLE 5-3   UNITS TO DESCRIBE COMPUTER MEMORY CAPACITY AND INFORMATION STORAGE CAPACITY

Computer memory capacity
1 kilobyte (kB) = 2^{10} bytes = 1,024 bytes ≈ a thousand bytes
1 megabyte (MB) = 2^{20} bytes = 1,024 kilobytes = 1,048,576 bytes ≈ a million bytes
1 gigabyte (GB) = 2^{30} bytes = 1,024 megabytes = 1,073,741,824 bytes ≈ a billion bytes
Digital storage device or media capacity
1 kilobyte (kB) = 10^3 bytes = 1,000 bytes = a thousand bytes
1 megabyte (MB) = 10^6 bytes = 1,000 kilobytes = 1,000,000 bytes = a million bytes
1 gigabyte (GB) = 10^9 bytes = 1,000 megabytes = 1,000,000,000 bytes = a billion bytes
1 terabyte (TB) = 10^{12} bytes = 1,000 gigabytes = 1,000,000,000,000 bytes = a trillion bytes
1 petabyte (PB) = 10^{15} bytes = 1,000 terabytes = 1,000,000,000,000,000 bytes

Note: Note that the prefixes *kilo-, mega-,* and *giga-* have slightly different meanings when used to describe computer memory capacity than in standard scientific usage, whereas they have the standard scientific meanings when used to describe digital storage device or media capacity. To avoid confusion, some standards organizations have advocated the units kibibyte (kiB, 1 kiB = 2^{10} bytes), mibibyte (MiB, 1 MiB = 2^{20} bytes), and gibibyte (GiB, 1 GiB = 2^{30} bytes) for describing memory capacity.

in a specific direction. Because a bit is limited to one of two values, it can only represent two numbers.

To represent more than two values, several bits must be used. For example, a series of bits can be used to represent a number or another unit of information. The binary number system allows a group of several bits to represent a number.

Bits, Bytes, and Words

As mentioned above, most digital signals and digital memory and storage consist of many elements called bits (for binary digits), each of which can be in one of two states. Bits are grouped into *bytes,* each consisting of eight bits. The capacity of a computer memory, a storage device, or a unit of storage media is usually described in kilobytes, megabytes, gigabytes, or terabytes (Table 5-3). (As noted in that table, the prefixes kilo-, mega-, and giga-, when used to describe computer memory capacity, commonly have slightly different meanings than standard usage, whereas these prefixes have their usual meanings when used to describe digital information storage devices and media.) Bits are also grouped into *words.* The number of bits in a word depends on the computer system; 16-, 32-, and 64-bit words are common.

Digital Representation of Different Types of Information

General-purpose computers must be able to store and process several types of information in digital form. For example, if a computer is to execute a word processing program or a program that stores and retrieves patient data, it must be able to represent alphanumeric information (text), such as a patient's name, in digital form. Computers must also be able to represent numbers in digital form. Most computers have several formats for numbers. For example, one computer system provides formats for 1-, 2-, 4-, and 8-byte positive integers; 1-, 2-, 4-, and 8-byte signed integers ("signed" meaning that they may have positive or negative values); and 4- and 8-byte floating-point numbers (to be discussed shortly).

When numbers can assume very large or very small values or must be represented with great accuracy, formats requiring a large amount of storage per number must be used. However, if numbers are restricted to integers within a limited range of values, considerable savings in storage and processing time may be realized. For instance, the grayscale values in ultrasound images typically range from 0 (black) to 255 (white), a range of 256 numbers. As will be seen in the following section, any grayscale value within this range can be represented by only eight bits. The following sections describe schemes for the digital representation of different types of information.

As discussed above, computer memory and storage consist of many bits. Each bit can be in one of two states and can therefore represent the numbers 0 or 1. Two bits have four possible configurations (00, 01, 10, or 11) that in decimal form are 0, 1, 2, and 3. Three bits have eight possible configurations (000, 001, 010, 011, 100, 101, 110, or 111) that can represent the decimal numbers 0, 1, 2, 3, 4, 5, 6, and 7. In general, N bits have 2^N possible configurations and can represent integers from 0 to $2^N - 1$. One byte can therefore store integers from 0 to 255 and a 16-bit word can store integers from 0 to 65,535 (Table 5-4).

The previous discussion dealt only with positive integers. It is often necessary for computers to manipulate integers that can have positive or negative values. There are many ways to represent signed integers in binary form. The simplest method is to reserve the first bit of a number for the sign of the number. Setting the first bit to 0 can indicate that the number is positive, whereas setting it to 1 indicates that the number is negative. For an 8-bit number, 11111111 (binary) = -127 (decimal) is the most negative number and 01111111 (binary) = 127 (decimal) positive number. Most computers use a different scheme called "twos complement notation" to represent signed integers, which simplifies the circuitry needed to add positive and negative integers.

Computers used for scientific purposes must be able to manipulate very large numbers, such as Avogadro's number (6.022×10^{23} molecules per gram-mole) and very small numbers, such as the mass of a proton (1.673×10^{-27} kg). These numbers are usually represented in floating-point form. Floating-point form is similar to scientific notation, in which a number is expressed as a decimal fraction times ten raised to a power. A number can be also written as a binary fraction times two to a power. For example, Avogadro's number can be written as

$$0.11111111 \text{ (binary)} \times 2^{01001111 \text{ (binary)}}.$$

When a computer stores this number in floating-point form, it stores the pair of signed binary integers, 11111111 and 01001111.

It is often necessary for computers to store and manipulate alphanumeric data, such as a patient's name or the text of this book. A common method for representing alphanumeric data in binary form has been the American Standard Code for Information Inter-

TABLE 5-4   NUMBER OF BITS REQUIRED TO STORE INTEGERS

NUMBER OF BITS	POSSIBLE CONFIGURATIONS	NUMBER OF CONFIGURATIONS	REPRESENT INTEGERS (DECIMAL FORM)
1	0,1	2	0,1
2	00,01,10,11	4	0,1,2,3
3	000,001,010,011,100,101,110,111	8	0,1,2,3,4,5,6,7
8	00000000 to 11111111	256	0 to 255
16	0000000000000000 to 1111111111111111	65,536	0 to 65,535
N		2^N	0 to $2^N - 1$

change (ASCII). Each character is stored in seven bits. The byte values from 00000000 to 01111111 (binary) represent 128 characters, including the upper- and lowercase English letters, the integers 0 through 9, many punctuation marks, and several carriage-control characters such as line feed. For example, the uppercase letter "A" is represented by 01000001, the comma is represented by 00111010, and the digit "2" is represented by 00110010. ASCII is being superseded by text encoding schemes that permit more than 128 characters to be represented in digital form. Unicode is a system for encoding the characters of the world's languages and other symbols. Unicode incorporates ASCII. In Unicode, as many as four bytes may be needed to represent a character.

Transfers of Information in Digital Form

Information is transferred between the various components of a computer, such as the memory and central processing unit, in binary form. A voltage of fixed value (such as 5 V) and fixed duration on a wire can be used to represent the binary number 1 and a voltage of 0 V for the same duration can represent 0. A group of such voltage pulses can be used to represent a number, an alphanumeric character, or other unit of information. (This scheme is called "unipolar" digital encoding. Many other digital encoding schemes exist.)

A group of wires used to transfer data between several devices is called a *data bus*. Each device connected to the bus is identified by an address or a range of addresses. Only one device at a time can transmit information on a bus, and in most cases only one device receives the information. The sending device transmits both the information and the address of the device that is intended to receive the information.

Advantages and Disadvantages of Analog and Digital Forms

There is a major disadvantage to the electronic transmission of information in analog form –the signals become distorted, causing a loss of fidelity of the information. Causes of this distortion include inaccuracies when signals are amplified, attenuation losses, and electronic noise –small stray voltages that exist on circuits and become superimposed on the signal. The more the information is transferred, the more distorted it becomes. On the other hand, information stored or transferred in digital form is remarkably immune to the accumulation of errors because of signal distortion. These distortions are seldom of sufficient amplitude cause a 0 to be mistaken for a 1 or vice versa. Furthermore, most digital circuits do not amplify the incoming information, but make fresh copies of it, thus preventing distortions from accumulating during multiple transfers.

The digital form facilitates other safeguards. Additional redundant information can be sent with each group of bits to permit the receiving device to detect errors or even correct them. A simple error detection method uses parity bits. An additional bit is transmitted with each group of bits, typically with each byte. The bit value designates whether an even or an odd number of bits were in the "1" state. The receiving device determines the parity and compares it with the received parity bit. If the parity of the data and the parity bit do not match, an odd number of bits in the group have errors.

There are advantages to analog form. Information can often be transferred in less time using the analog form. However, digital circuits are likely to be less expensive.

Conversion Between Analog and Digital Forms

Conversion of Data from Analog to Digital Form

The transducers, sensors, or detectors of most electronic measuring equipment, including medical imaging devices, produce analog data. The data must be converted to digital form if they are to be processed by a computer, transferred over a network, or stored on a digital storage device. Devices that perform this function are called *analog-to-digital converters* (ADCs, also A/Ds). ADCs are essential components of all medical imaging systems producing digital images and of multichannel analyzers, discussed in Chapter 17.

The conversion of an analog signal into a digital signal is called *digitization*. There are two steps in digitization—sampling and quantization. Most analog signals are continuous in time, meaning that at every point in time the signal has a value. However, it is not possible to convert the analog signal to a digital signal at every point in time. Instead, certain points in time must be selected at which the conversion is to be performed. This process is called *sampling*. Each analog sample is then converted into a digital signal. This conversion is called *quantization*.

An ADC is characterized by its *sampling rate* and the *number of bits of output* it provides. The sampling rate is the number of times a second that it can sample and digitize an input signal. Most radiologic applications require very high sampling rates. An ADC produces a digital signal of a fixed number of bits. For example, an ADC may produce an 8-bit, a 10-bit, a 12-bit, a 14-bit, or even a 16-bit digital signal. The number of bits of output is just the number of bits in the digital number produced each time the ADC samples and quantizes the input analog signal.

As discussed above, the digital representation of data is superior to analog representation in its resistance to the accumulation of errors. However, there are also disadvantages to digital representation, an important one being that *the conversion of an analog signal to digital form causes a loss of information*. This loss is due to both sampling and quantization. Because an ADC samples the input signal, the values of the analog signal between the moments of sampling are lost. If the sampling rate of the ADC is sufficiently rapid that the analog signal being digitized varies only slightly during the intervals between sampling, the sampling error will be small. There is a minimum sampling rate requirement, the *Nyquist limit* (discussed in Chapter 4) that ensures the accurate representation of a signal.

Quantization also causes a loss of information. As mentioned previously, an analog signal is continuous in magnitude, meaning that it can have any of an infinite number of values between a minimum and a maximum. For example, an analog voltage signal may be 1.0, 2.5, or 1.7893 V. In contrast, a digital signal is limited to a finite number of possible values, determined by the number of bits used for the signal. As was shown earlier in this chapter, a 1-bit digital signal is limited to two values, a 2-bit signal is limited to four values, and an N-bit signal is restricted to 2^N possible values. The quantization error is similar to the error introduced when a number is "rounded off." Table 5-5 lists the maximal percent errors associated with digital signals of various numbers of bits.

There are additional sources of error in analog-to-digital conversion other than the sampling and quantization effects described above. For example, some averaging

TABLE 5-5   MAXIMAL ERRORS WHEN DIFFERENT NUMBERS OF BITS ARE USED TO APPROXIMATE AN ANALOG SIGNAL

NUMBER OF BITS	NUMBER OF VALUES	MAXIMAL QUANTIZATION ERROR (%)
1	2	25
2	4	12.5
3	8	6.2
8	256	0.20
12	4,096	0.012

of the analog signal occurs at the time of sampling, and there are inaccuracies in the quantization process. In summary, a digital signal can only approximate the value of an analog signal, causing a loss of information during analog-to-digital conversion.

No analog signal is a perfect representation of the quantity being measured. Statistical effects in the measurement process and stray electronic voltages ("noise") cause every analog signal to have some uncertainty associated with it. To convert an analog signal to digital form without a significant loss of information content, the ADC must sample at a sufficiently high rate and provide a sufficient number of bits so that the error is less than the uncertainty in the analog signal being digitized. In other words, an analog signal with a large *signal-to-noise ratio* (SNR) requires an ADC providing a large number of bits to avoid reducing the SNR.

Digital-to-Analog Conversion

It is often necessary to convert a digital signal to analog form. For example, to display digital images from a CT scanner on a display monitor, the image information must be converted from digital form to analog voltage signals. This conversion is performed by a *digital-to-analog converter* (DAC). It is important to recognize that the information lost by analog-to-digital conversion is not restored by sending the signal through a DAC (Fig. 5-2).

Digital Radiological Images

A digital image is a rectangular, sometimes square, array of picture elements called *pixels*. In most radiological images, each pixel is represented by a single number and the image can be stored as a matrix of these numbers. For example, in nuclear medicine planar images, a pixel contains the number of counts detected by the corresponding portion of the crystal of a scintillation camera. In tomographic imaging (e.g., x-ray CT and positron emission tomography [PET]), each pixel describes a property of a corresponding volume element (voxel) in the patient. In projection imaging (e.g., radiography), each pixel describes a property regarding the voxels along a line projected through the patient. Figure 5-3 shows a digital image in four different pixel formats. The number in each pixel is converted into a visible light intensity when the image is displayed on a display monitor. Typical image formats used in radiology are listed in Table 5-5.

Imaging modalities with higher spatial resolution and larger fields of view require more pixels per image so the image format does not degrade the resolution. In general, an image format should be selected so that the pixel size is half or less than the size of the smallest object to be seen. In the case of a fluoroscope with a 23-cm field of view, the 512^2 pixel format would be adequate for detecting objects as small as

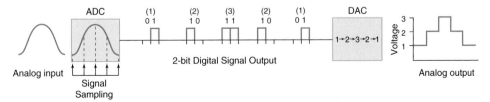

■ **FIGURE 5-2** Analog-to-digital conversion and digital-to-analog conversion. In this figure, a 2-bit ADC samples the input signal five times. Note that the output signal from the DAC is only an approximation of the input signal to the ADC because the five 2-bit digital numbers produced by the ADC can only approximate the continuously varying analog signal. More rapid sampling and digital numbers with more bits would provide a more accurate representation.

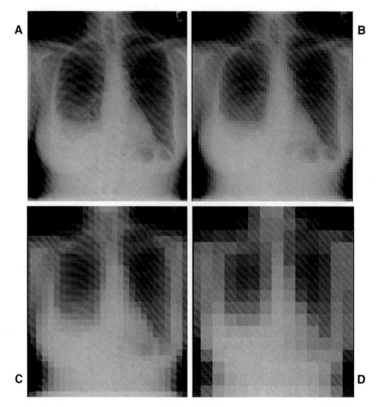

■ **FIGURE 5-3** Effect of pixel size on image quality—digital chest image in formats of $1,024^2$, 64^2, 32^2, and 16^2 pixels (**A, B, C,** and **D,** respectively).

about a millimeter in size close to the image receptor. To detect objects half this size, a larger format, such as 1,024 by 1,024, should be selected. When it is necessary to depict the shape of an object, such as a microcalcification in x-ray mammography, an image pixel matrix much larger than that needed to merely detect the object is required. Figure 5-3 shows the degradation of spatial resolution caused by using too small an image matrix. The penalty for using larger pixel matrices is increased storage and processing requirements and slower transfer of images.

The largest number that can be stored in a single pixel is determined by the number of bits or bytes used for each pixel. If 1 byte (8 bits) is used, the maximal number that can be stored in one pixel is 255 ($2^8 - 1$). If 2 bytes (16 bits) are used, the maximal number that can be stored is 65,535 ($2^{16} - 1$). The contrast resolution provided by an imaging modality determines the number of bits required per pixel. Therefore, imaging modalities with higher contrast resolution require more bits per pixel. For example, the limited contrast resolution of ultrasound usually requires only 6 or 7 bits, and so 8 bits are commonly used for each pixel. On the other hand, x-ray CT provides high contrast resolution and 12 bits are required to represent the full range of CT numbers. Figure 5-4 shows the degradation of contrast resolution caused by using too few bits per pixel.

Pixel size is calculated by dividing the distance between two points in the subject being imaged by the number of pixels between these two points in the image. It is approximately equal to the field of view of the imaging device divided by the number of pixels across the image. For example, if a fluoroscope has a 23-cm (9-inch) field of view and the images are acquired in a 512-by-512 format, then the approximate size of a pixel is 23 cm/512 = 0.045 cm = 0.45 mm for objects at the face of the image receptor.

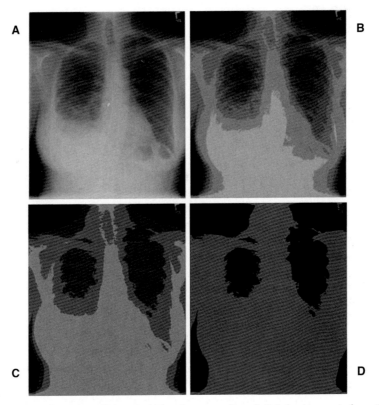

■ FIGURE 5-4 Effect of number of bits per pixel on image quality—digital chest image in formats of 8, 3, 2, and 1 bits per pixel (**A, B, C,** and **D,** respectively). Too few bits per pixel not only causes loss of contrast resolution, but also creates the appearance of false contours.

The total number of bytes required to store an image is the number of pixels in the image multiplied by the number of bytes per pixel. For example, the number of bytes required to store a 512-by-512 pixel image, if one byte is used per pixel, is

$$(512 \times 512 \text{ pixels}) \, (1 \text{ byte/pixel}) \, / \, (1{,}000 \text{ bytes/kB}) = 262 \text{ kB}.$$

Similarly, the number of 512-by-512 images that may be stored on a 60-GB optical disk, if 16 bits (2 bytes) are used per pixel, is

$$(60 \text{ GB/disk}) \, (10^9 \text{ bytes/GB}) \, / \, [(512 \times 512 \text{ pixels/image}) \, (2 \text{ bytes/pixel})]$$
$$\approx 114{,}000 \text{ images/disk,}$$

if no other information is stored on the disk.

If these are CT studies and an average of 500 images per study is stored, this disk would hold about 114,000 images/500 images per study ≈228 studies. In practice, other information stored with the studies would slightly reduce the number of studies that could be stored on the disk.

5.3 Digital Computers

Computers were originally designed to perform mathematical computations and other information processing tasks very quickly. Since then, they have come to be used for many other purposes, including information display, information storage, and, in conjunction with computer networks, information transfer and communications.

Computers were introduced in medical imaging in the early 1970s and have become increasingly important since that time. Today, computers are essential to most imaging modalities, including x-ray CT, magnetic resonance imaging (MRI), single photon emission computed tomography (SPECT), and PET.

Any function that can be performed by a computer can also be performed by a hard-wired electronic circuit. The advantage of the computer over a hard-wired circuit is its flexibility. The function of the computer can be modified merely by changing the program that controls the computer, whereas modifying the function of a hard-wired circuit usually requires replacing the circuit. Although the computer is a very complicated and powerful information processing device, the actual operations performed by a computer are very simple. The power of the computer is mainly due to its speed in performing these operations and its ability to store large volumes of information.

The components and functioning of computers are discussed in Appendix B. The remainder of this section will define several terms regarding computers that will be used in the following parts of this chapter.

The term *hardware* refers to the physical components of a computer or other device, whereas *software* refers to the programs, consisting of sequences of instructions, that are executed by a computer. Software is commonly categorized as applications programs or systems software.

An *applications program*, commonly referred to as an *application*, is a program that performs a specific function or functions for a user. Examples of applications are e-mail programs, word processing programs, web browsers, and image display programs.

A computer's operating system is a fundamental program that is executing even when a computer seems to be idle and awaiting a command. When the user instructs a computer to run a particular program, the operating system copies the program into memory from a disk, transfers control to it, and regains control of the computer when the program has finished. An operating system handles many "housekeeping" tasks, such as details of storage of information on disks and magnetic tapes, apportioning system resources amongst applications and amongst users in a multiuser system, and handling interrupts, for example, when a user activates a pointing device. Examples of operating systems are Microsoft Windows and Linux on IBM compatible PCs; OS X on Apple computers; and Unix, used on a wide variety of computers.

A *workstation* is a computer designed for use by a single person at a time. A workstation is usually equipped with one or more display monitors for the visual display of information, a keyboard for the entry of alphanumeric information, and a pointing device, such as a mouse.

5.4 Information Storage Devices

Mass storage devices permit the nonvolatile (i.e., data are not lost when power is turned off) storage of information. Most mass storage devices have mechanical components, but at least one newer storage modality, flash memory, is entirely electronic. Mass storage devices with mechanical components include magnetic disk drives, magnetic tape drives, and optical (laser) disk units. Each of these devices consists of a mechanical drive; the storage medium, which may be removable; and an electronic controller. Despite the wide variety of storage media, there is not one best medium for all purposes, because they differ in storage capacity, data access time, data transfer rate, cost, and other factors.

When the CPU or another device sends data to memory or a mass storage device, it is said to be *writing* data, and when it requests data stored in memory or on a storage device, it is said to be *reading* data. Data storage devices permit either random access or sequential access to the data. The term *random access* describes a storage medium in which the locations of the data may be read or written in any order, and *sequential access* describes a medium in which data storage locations can only be accessed in a serial manner. Most solid-state memories, magnetic disks, and optical disks are random access, whereas magnetic tape typically permits only sequential access.

Magnetic Disks

Magnetic disks are spinning disks coated with a material that may be readily magnetized. Close to the surface of the spinning disk is a read-write head that, to read data, senses the magnetization of individual locations on the disk and, to write data, changes the direction of the magnetization of individual locations on the disk. Most disk drives have a read-write head on each side of a platter so that both sides can be used for data storage. Information is stored on the disk in concentric rings called *tracks*. The read-write heads move radially over the disk to access data on individual tracks. The *access time* of a disk is the time required for the read-write head to reach the proper track (head seek time) and for the spinning of the disk to bring the information of interest to the head (rotational latency). The *data transfer rate* is the rate at which data are read from or written to the disk once the head and disk are in the proper orientation; it is primarily determined by the rotational speed of the disk and the density of information storage in a track.

A typical hard magnetic disk drive, as shown in Figure 5-5, has several rigid platters stacked above each other on a common spindle, with a read-write head for each side of each platter. Hard disks with nonremovable platters are called fixed disks. The platters continuously rotate at a high speed (typically 5,400 to 15,000 rpm). The read-write heads aerodynamically float at distances less than a micron above and below the disk surfaces on air currents generated by the spinning platters. A spinning hard disk drive should

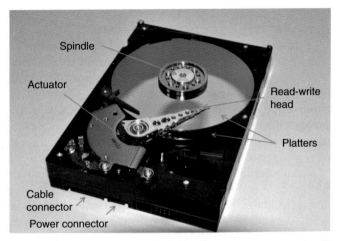

■ **FIGURE 5-5** Hard magnetic disk drive with 500 GB storage capacity. A read-write head is visible at the end of the actuator arm overlying the top disk platter. There is a read-write head for each surface of each platter.

not be jarred because that might cause a "head crash" in which the head strikes the disk, gouging the disk surface and destroying the head, with a concomitant loss of information. The portion of a disk drive containing the disks and read-write heads is sealed to keep dirt from damaging them. Hard disks have very large storage capacities, up to 2 TB each. Although their access times and data transfer rates are very slow compared to solid-state memory, they are much faster than those of most other storage media. For these reasons, hard disks are used on most computers to store frequently used programs and data.

Flash Memory

A type of solid-state memory called *flash memory* stores digital information as small electric charges. Flash memory does not require electrical power to maintain stored information and thus can replace spinning magnetic disks and other storage media. Today, flash memory is much more expensive per unit storage capacity than magnetic disks and other storage media and so is not used commonly for the storage of large amounts of information. However, it is replacing spinning magnetic disks on some portable "laptop" computers. "Flash drives," which connect to the USB ports of workstations and laptops, have mostly replaced "floppy" disk drives and are rapidly replacing optical (CD and DVD) disks because of their portability and relatively large capacities.

Magnetic Tape

Magnetic tape is plastic tape coated with a magnetizable substance. Its average data access times are very long, because the tape must be read serially from the beginning to locate a particular item of information. Magnetic tape was originally stored on reels, but today is obtained in cartridges or cassettes. There are several competing cartridge or cassette formats available today. A single tape cartridge or cassette can store a very large amount of data, up to about 1.5 TB uncompressed. Common uses are to "back up" (make a copy for the purpose of safety) large amounts of important information and archival storage of digital images.

Optical Disks

An optical disk is a removable disk that rotates during data access and from which information is read and written using a laser. There are three categories of optical disks—read-only; write-once, read-many-times (WORM); and rewritable. Read-only disks are encoded with data that cannot be modified. To read data, the laser illuminates a point on the surface of the spinning disk and a photodetector senses the intensity of the reflected light. WORM devices permit any portion of the disk surface to be written upon only once, but to be read many times. This largely limits the use of WORM optical disks to archival storage. To store information, a laser at a high intensity burns small holes in a layer of the disk. To read information, the laser, at a lower intensity, illuminates a point on the spinning disk and a photodetector senses the intensity of the reflected light. Rewritable optical disks permit the stored data to be changed many times. Most rewritable optical disks today use phase-change technology. The recording material of a phase-change disk has the property that, if heated to one temperature and allowed to cool, it becomes crystalline, whereas if heated to another temperature, it cools to an amorphous phase. To write data on a phase-change disk, the laser heats a point on the recording film, changing its phase from crystalline to amorphous or vice versa. The transparency of the amorphous material differs from that in the crystalline phase. Above the layer of recording material is a reflective layer. Information is read as described above for WORM disks.

CDs, which have capacities of about 650 MB, are available as WORM and rewritable optical disks. The CD has been partially displaced by a newer standard for optical disks, the DVD, that provides a much larger storage capacity because the laser beam is focused to a smaller spot on the recording layer. DVDs are also available in WORM and rewritable forms and provide storage capacities of about 4.5 GB. Optical disks using 405 nm wavelength blue-violet lasers are now available. The blue-violet beam can be focused onto a smaller area because of its shorter wavelength, increasing the storage capacity substantially. There are two competing standards for these disks, both available in WORM and rewritable formats, providing up to 50 or 60 GB per disk. Optical disks provide much prompter data access than magnetic tape and better information security than most other media because they are not subject to head crashes, as are magnetic disks; are not as vulnerable to wear and damage as magnetic tape; and are not affected by magnetic fields.

Table 5-6 compares the characteristics of mass storage devices and memory. Because there is no best device or medium for all purposes, most computer systems today have at least a hard magnetic disk drive and a drive capable of reading optical disks.

Technologies for Large Archives

Medical imaging can produce very large amounts of information. For example, a medium size medical center with a radiology department, cardiac catheterization laboratory, and several services performing fluoroscopically guided interventional procedures typically produces several terabytes of image information each year. There are technologies that permit automated storage and retrieval of such massive amounts of information.

TABLE 5-6   COMPARISON OF CHARACTERISTICS OF MASS STORAGE MEDIA AND MEMORY

	REMOVABLE	STORAGE CAPACITY	ACCESS TIME (AVERAGE)	TRANSFER RATE	COST PER DISK/TAPE	MEDIA COST PER GB
Hard magnetic disk	Usually not	20 GB–2 TB	6–15 ms	3–170 MB/s	NA	$0.05
Solid state "disk" (flash memory)	Yes or no	20 GB–2 TB	~0.1 ms	Up to 740 MB/s	NA	$2.00
Optical disk, CD-R, CD-RW	Yes	usually 650 MB	100–150 ms (for 24×)	3.6 MB/s (for 24×)	$0.25, $1.00	$0.40, $1.50
Optical disk, DVD-R, DVD-RAM	Yes	3–6 GB		26 MB/s (for 20×)	$0.20, $2.00	$0.04, $0.40
Optical disk, blue-violet laser	Yes	23–60 GB	25 ms	12 MB/s	$60 (UDO2)	$1.00 (UDO2)
Magnetic tape (cartridge or cassette)	Yes	45 MB–1.5 TB	Seconds to minutes	0.125–140 MB/s	$85 (1.5 TB LTO-5	$0.05 (1.5 TB LTO-5)
DRAM solid-state memory	No	NA	1–80 ns	0.5–3 GB/s	NA	NA

Note: Values are typical for 2011. Cost refers to one disk or tape cartridge or tape cassette. Storage capacities and transfer rates are for uncompressed data; they would be higher for compressed data.

ms, milliseconds; ns, nanoseconds (10^6 ns = 1 ms); MB, megabytes; GB, gigabytes; TB, terabytes; LTO, linear tape open. Prices and capabilities of "enterprise quality" (high reliability and long lifetime) disks are ~10 × higher than commodity grade disks.

A technology called RAID (redundant array of independent disks) can provide a large amount of on-line storage. RAID permits several or many small and inexpensive hard magnetic disk drives to be linked together to function as a single very large drive. There are several implementations of RAID, designated as RAID Levels 0, 1, 2, 3, 4, 5, and 10. In RAID Level 0, portions of each file stored are written simultaneously on several disk drives, with different portions on each disk drive. This produces very fast reads and writes, but with no redundancy, and so the loss of one of these drives results in the loss of the file. In RAID Level 1, called *disk mirroring*, all information is written simultaneously onto two or more drives. Because duplicate copies of each file are stored on each of the mirrored disk drives, Level 1 provides excellent data protection, but without any improvement in data transfer rate and with at least a doubling of required storage capacity. The other RAID levels provide various compromises among fault tolerance, data transfer rate, and storage capacity. Most RAID implementations provide sufficient redundancy that no information is lost by the failure of a single disk drive. Figure 5-6 shows RAID modules.

Another technology permitting the storage of very large amounts of information is automated magnetic tape or optical disk libraries, commonly referred to as *jukeboxes*. In these devices, magnetic tape cartridges or cassettes or optical disks are stored in large racks. Robotic arms load the media into or remove them from drives that read and write information on the media. These automated libraries commonly have two or more drives, permitting simultaneous access to more than one unit of media. The storage capacity of a jukebox is the product of the storage capacity of a unit of media and the number of media units that can be stored on the racks. The access time for a study stored on media in a jukebox includes a few seconds for the disk, cartridge, or cassette to be loaded into a drive as well as the access time for the media.

5.5 Display of Digital Images

As mentioned above, an important function of many computers, particularly workstations, is to display information. In medical imaging, the purpose of the display may be to permit technologists to visually assess the adequacy of acquired images, for physicians to interpret images, or to guide physicians performing interventional procedures. The designs of display systems should take into account the human visual system.

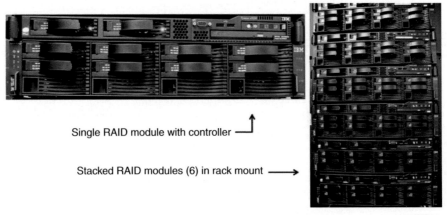

Single RAID module with controller

Stacked RAID modules (6) in rack mount

■ **FIGURE 5-6** Stackable RAID modules. Each module contains a dual CPU processor, two 140 GB disks for the CPU and software, and eight 300 GB disk drives in a RAID-5 configuration, with one hot-swappable drive. Total storage is 2 TB per module, 1.6 of which are usable for data storage (0.8 TB used for redundancy). The 6 stacked modules provide about 10 TB of uncompressed data storage (1/2 rack) with dimensions of approximately 2 × 3 × 4 ft (w × d × h).

The display system of a workstation or other computer typically consists of a display interface, also referred to by terms such as "video interface" and "graphics adapter," in the computer; one or more display monitors connected to the display interface by a cable or cables that carry electrical signals; and software to control the display system. The display interface and display monitor(s) may be consumer-grade commercial products or they may be more expensive devices designed for the high-fidelity display of medical images.

A display system may be designed to display color images or only monochrome (grayscale) images. A system that can display color images can also display grayscale images. Nearly all general-purpose commercial display systems are designed to display images in color. However, images from the radiological modalities, consisting of rectangular arrays of numbers, in general do not benefit from being displayed in color and so are commonly displayed on high-quality grayscale monitors for interpretation. However, some radiological images, such as co-registered dual modality images (e.g., SPECT/CT and PET/CT), false color images (commonly used in nuclear medicine myocardial perfusion imaging), and volume rendered displays (discussed later in this chapter) of three-dimensional image sets, benefit from being displayed partly or entirely in color.

Color is a perception created by some animals' visual systems. In the retina of the human eye, cone cells provide color vision. In most humans, there are three types of cone cells, which differ in spectral sensitivity. One is most sensitive to yellow-green light (although largely responsible for the perception of red), another to green light, and the third to blue light. A mixture of red, green, and blue light, in the proper proportion, can cause the impression of many colors and of white. In a color display monitor, each displayed pixel generates red, green, and blue light, with the intensities of each independently controlled. The construction of display monitors is described below.

In grayscale radiological images, each pixel value is typically represented by a single integer, commonly stored in 16 bits, although fewer than 16 of the bits may be used. For example, the range of CT numbers requires only 12 bits. In color images, each pixel is commonly represented by three integers, commonly 8 or 10 bits each, which are contained in a 32-bit word. The three integers designate the intensities of the red, green, and blue light to be generated for that pixel.

Display Interface and Conversion of a Digital Image into Analog Signals for Display

A computer's display interface converts a digital image into a signal that is displayed by a display monitor. Most display interfaces contain memories to store the images being displayed. For a digital image to be displayed, it is first sent to this display memory by the computer's CPU under the control of an application program. Once it is stored in this memory, the display interface of the computer reads the pixels in the image sequentially and sends these values to the monitor for display. Older display interfaces produce analog signals that are displayed by monitors; such a display interface contains one or more digital-to-analog converters (DACs), which convert each digital number to an analog voltage signal. Newer display interfaces send the image information in digital form to the display monitors; these monitors contain DACs to convert the digital pixel values to analog signals.

Display Monitors

For approximately 80 years, cathode ray tubes (CRTs) were used for the electronic display of images. CRT displays are rapidly being replaced by flat-panel displays and can no longer be obtained on most medical imaging equipment. There are several types of flat-panel displays, including gas plasma, light emitting diode, organic light emitting diode, and field emissive displays. However, most flat-panel monitors used today to display medical images have liquid crystal displays (LCDs) because of their superior performance and longevity.

The term "pixel," when referring to display monitors, has a meaning different from a picture element of an image; it refers to a physical structure in a monitor that displays a single pixel of an image. Most types of monitors have physical pixels, although CRT monitors do not.

Cathode Ray Tube Monitors

A CRT in a display monitor is an evacuated container, usually made of glass, with components that generate, focus, and modulate the intensity of one or more electron beams directed onto a fluorescent screen. When a voltage is applied between a pair of electrodes, the negative electrode is called the *cathode* and the positive electrode is called the *anode*. If electrons are released from the cathode, the electric field accelerates them toward the anode. These electrons are called *cathode rays*. A grayscale CRT monitor (Fig. 5-7) generates a single electron beam. The source of the electrons is a cathode that is heated by an electrical current and the anode is a thin aluminum layer in contact with the fluorescent screen. A large constant voltage, typically 10 to 30 kV, applied between these two electrodes creates an electric field that accelerates the electrons to high kinetic energies and directs them onto the screen. The electron beam is focused, electrically or magnetically, onto a very small area on the screen. Between the cathode and the screen is a grid electrode. A voltage applied to the grid electrode is used to vary the electric current (electrons per second) of the beam. The electrons deposit their energy in the phosphor of the screen, causing the emission of visible light. The intensity of the light from any location on the screen is proportional to the electric current in the beam, which is determined by the analog voltage signal applied to the grid electrode. The electron beam is steered, either electrically or magnetically, in a raster pattern as shown in Figure 5-8.

The CRT of a color monitor is similar to that of a grayscale monitor, but has three electron guns instead of one, producing three electron beams. The three electron beams

■ **FIGURE 5-7** Grayscale CRT display monitor. The electron gun contains a heated cathode, the source of the electrons in the beam, and a grid electrode, which modulates the intensity (electrical current) of the beam. This CRT uses an electromagnet to focus the beam and two pairs of electromagnets to steer the beam. (One pair, not shown, is perpendicular to the pair in the diagram.) Alternatively, electrodes placed inside the CRT can perform these functions.

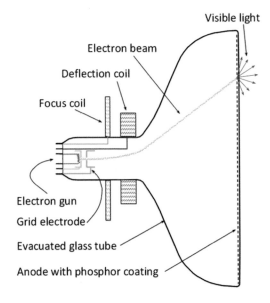

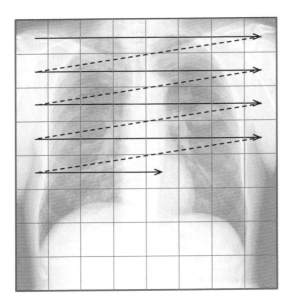

■ **FIGURE 5-8** Order of conversion of pixels in a digital image to analog voltages to form a video signal (*raster scan*). Data is scanned from left to right, with a retrace to the next row (*dashed line*). The actual size of the matrix is much smaller than depicted.

are close to one another and are steered as one, but their intensities are modulated separately. The fluorescent screen consists of triads of tiny dots or stripes of phosphors emitting red, green, and blue light. Just before the screen is a thin metal sheet containing holes or slits so that each electron beam only strikes the phosphor emitting a single color. Thus one electron beam produces red light, another produces green light, and the third produces blue light. As mentioned above, mixtures of red, green, and blue light can create the perception of many colors by the human visual system.

Liquid Crystal Display Monitors

In LCDs, the pixels are physical structures; in many grayscale LCDs and all color LCDs, each pixel consists of three subpixels, whose light intensities are independently controlled. The liquid crystal (LC) material of an LCD does not produce light. Instead, it modulates the intensity of light from another source. All high image quality LCDs are illuminated from behind (backlit). A backlit LCD consists of a uniform light source, typically containing fluorescent tubes or light emitting diodes and a layer of diffusing material; a layer of LC material between two glass plates; and a polarizing filter on each side of the glass holding the LC material (Fig. 5-9).

Visible light, like any electromagnetic radiation, may be considered to consist of oscillating electrical and magnetic fields, as described in Chapter 2. The oscillations are perpendicular to the direction of travel of the light. Unpolarized light consists of light waves whose oscillations are randomly oriented. A polarizing filter is a layer of material that permits components of light waves oscillating in one direction to pass, but absorbs components oscillating in the perpendicular direction. When unpolarized light is incident on a single layer of polarizing material, the intensity of the transmitted light is half that of the incident light. When a second polarizing filter is placed in the beam of polarized light, parallel to the first filter, the intensity of the beam transmitted through the second filter depends on the orientation of the second filter with respect to the first. If both filters have the same orientation, the intensity of the beam transmitted through both filters is almost the same as that transmitted through the first. However, if the second filter is rotated with respect to the first, the intensity of the transmitted light is reduced. When the second filter is oriented so that its polarization is perpendicular to that of the first filter, almost no light is transmitted.

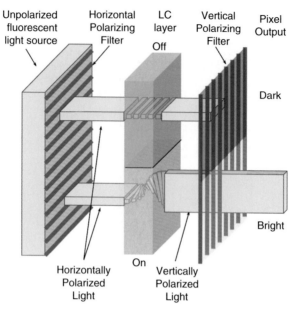

■ FIGURE 5-9 Two subpixels of a grayscale backlit LCD monitor. On each side of the LC layer in each subpixel is a transparent electrode. In the top subpixel, no voltage is applied across the LC layer. The polarization of the light is unchanged as it passes through the LC layer, causing most of the light to be absorbed by the second polarizing filter and thereby producing a dark subpixel. In the bottom subpixel, a voltage is applied across the LC layer. The applied voltage causes the molecules in the LC layer to twist. The twisted molecules change the polarization of the light, enabling it to pass through the second filter with an intensity that increases with the applied voltage; with full voltage on the LC layer, the output light is vertically polarized, causing the subpixel to transmit the brightest luminance. (The *bars* shown in the polarizing filters are merely an artist's rendition to indicate the direction of the polarization, as is depicting the polarized light as a ribbon.) Variations in grayscale are achieved by varying the voltage provided to each LCD subpixel.

An LC material consists of long organic molecules and has properties of both a liquid and a crystalline material. For example, it flows like a liquid. On the other hand, the molecules tend to align parallel to one another. The material has additional properties that are used in LCDs. If a layer of LC material is in contact with a surface with fine grooves, the molecules align with the grooves. If an electric field is present, the molecules will align with the field. If polarized light passes through a layer of LC material, the LC material can change the polarization of the light.

In an LCD display, the light that has passed through the first filter is polarized. Next, the light passes through a thin layer of LC material contained between two glass plates. The sides of the glass plates in contact with the LC material have fine parallel grooves to orient the LC molecules. Each pixel or subpixel of an LCD has a pair of electrodes. When a voltage is applied to the pair of electrodes, an electric field is created, changing the orientation of the LC molecules and the polarization of the light. The amount of change in the orientation of the molecules and the polarization of the light increases with the magnitude of the applied voltage. The light then passes through the second polarizing filter, which can be oriented so that pixels or subpixels are bright when no voltage is applied, or so that they are black when no voltage is applied. Figure 5-9 shows the filters oriented so that the subpixels are dark when no voltage is applied. Thus, when no voltage is applied to a pixel or subpixel, the light is polarized by the first filter, passes through the LC material, and then is absorbed by the second polarizing filter, resulting in a dark pixel or subpixel. As the voltage applied to the pixel or subpixel is increased, the LC molecules twist, changing the polarization of the light and decreasing the fraction absorbed by the second filter, thereby making the pixel or subpixel brighter.

Three major variants of LCD technology are twisted nematic (TN), in-plane switching (IPS), and patterned vertical alignment (PVA). The differences among these designs, discussed in some of the references listed at the end of this chapter, are mainly due to the positions of the two electrodes in each subpixel and in the orientations of the LC molecules without applied voltage and when voltage is applied. The performance of these designs is more important to the user. TN LCDs, commonly used in inexpensive home and office monitors, suffer from very limited viewing angles and thus should be avoided when purchasing medical image displays. More expensive IPS panels have significantly improved viewing angles and excellent color reproduction. PVA was implemented as a compromise between the TN and IPS technologies, with an intermediate price.

A color LCD has an additional layer containing color filters. Each pixel consists of three subpixels, one containing a filter transmitting only red light, the second transmitting only green light, and the third transmitting only blue light. As mentioned previously, mixtures of red, green, and blue light can create the perception of most colors. Because these color filters absorb light, they reduce the luminance of the display, in comparison to an equivalent monochrome LCD, by about a factor of three.

In theory, each pixel or subpixel of a flat-panel display could be controlled by its own electrical conductor. If this were done, a three-megapixel grayscale display would contain at least 3 million electrical conductors and a color display of the same pixel format would have three times as many. In practice, flat-panel displays are matrix controlled, with one conductor serving each row of pixels and one serving each column. For a three-megapixel grayscale display (2,048 by 1,536 pixels), only 2,048 row pathways and 1,536 column pathways (if there are not subpixels) are required. A signal is sent to a specific pixel by simultaneously providing voltages to the row conductor and the column conductor for that pixel.

The intensity of each pixel must be maintained while signals are sent to other pixels. In active matrix LCDs, each pixel or subpixel has a transistor and capacitor. The electrical charge stored on the capacitor maintains the voltage signal for the pixel or subpixel while signals are sent to other pixels. The transistors and capacitors are constructed on a sheet of glass or quartz coated with silicon. This sheet is incorporated as a layer within the LCD. Active matrix LCDs are also called thin film transistor (TFT) displays. TFT technology, without the polarizing filters and LC material, is used in flat-panel x-ray image receptors and is discussed in Chapter 7.

Performance of Display Monitors

Display monitors usually are the final component of the imaging chain and their performance can significantly affect radiological imaging. Monitors are characterized by parameters such as spatial resolution, spatial distortion, contrast resolution, aspect ratio, maximal luminance, black level, dynamic range, uniformity of luminance, noise, lag, and refresh rate.

The photometric quantity* describing the brightness of a monitor (or other light source) is *luminance*. Luminance is the rate of light energy emitted or reflected from a

---

*Photometric quantities and units describe the energy per unit time carried by light, modified to account for the spectral sensitivity of the human eye. A person with normal vision perceives a given radiance of green light as being brighter than, for example, an equal radiance of red or blue light.

surface per unit area, per unit solid angle, corrected for the photopic[†] spectral sensitivity of the human eye. The SI unit of luminance is the candela per square meter (cd/m^2). Perceived brightness is not proportional to luminance; for example, the human visual system will perceive a doubling of luminance as only a small increase in brightness. The contrast resolution of a monitor is mainly determined by its dynamic range, defined as the difference between its maximal and minimal luminance. (Sometimes, the dynamic range is defined as the ratio of the maximal to minimal luminance.)

Studies have been undertaken with light boxes and display monitors on the effect of maximal luminance on diagnostic performance (Goo et al, 2004; Krupinski, 2006). Studies involving light boxes and some of those involving display monitors showed better accuracy with higher luminance. However, other studies using display monitors, particularly those in which contrast adjustment (e.g., windowing and leveling) by the observer was permitted, showed little or no effect of maximal luminance on diagnostic performance. At least one study showed that lower luminance increased the time to reach diagnostic decisions. A likely explanation is that contrast adjustment can, at least partially, compensate for the adverse effect of lower maximal monitor luminance.

Especially bright monitors should be used for the display of radiological images to provide adequate dynamic range. The American College of Radiology has published the ACR *Technical Standard for Electronic Practice of Medical Imaging*; the current standard specifies that grayscale (monochrome) monitors of interpretation workstations should provide maximal luminances of at least 171 cd/m^2, whereas those for mammography should provide at least 250 cd/m^2 and, for optimal contrast, at least 450 cd/m^2. Grayscale monitors for displaying medical images for interpretation can typically provide maximal luminances of about 600 to 900 cd/m^2 when new and are usually calibrated to provide maximal luminances of about 400 to 500 cd/m^2 that can be sustained for several tens of thousands of operating hours. Grayscale LCD monitors provide about three times larger maximal luminances than do color LCD monitors with backlights of equal intensity; this is because the red, green, and blue filters in color LCDs absorb light to create color images. Color LCD monitors providing sustained luminances exceeding 400 cd/m^2 are available; however, they are not able to sustain these luminances as long as comparable grayscale monitors. To provide the same maximal luminance, an LCD with smaller pixels must have a brighter backlight than one with larger pixels. The stability of the luminance of an LCD monitor depends upon the constancy of the luminance of the backlight. Most LCD monitors designed for medical imaging have light sensors that are used to keep the luminance constant; in some cases, the sensor is in the back of the monitor and in other cases, it is in front and measures the luminance seen by the viewer.

The minimal luminance of a monitor, measured in total darkness with the entire screen black, is called the *black level*. LCD monitors have much higher black levels (the luminance is higher) than the CRT monitors they have replaced. The *contrast ratio* is the maximal luminance divided by the black level. In practice, when viewing clinical images in a room that is not completely dark, the minimal luminance achievable is determined not only by the black level, but also by the scattering of ambient light from the face of the monitor and by veiling glare. *Veiling glare* is stray light from the face of the monitor that occurs when an image is displayed. The amount of veiling glare at a specific location on the monitor's face is determined by the size and brightness of other areas of the displayed image and the distances from those areas. Veiling glare causes a reduction in image contrast. LCD monitors suffer less

---

[†]The word "photopic" refers to the normal daylight color vision of the human visual system. The photopic spectral sensitivity differs from the scotopic spectral sensitivity of dark-adapted night vision.

from veiling glare than do CRT monitors. In practice, monitors are not viewed in completely dark rooms. The diffuse reflection of ambient light from the face of the monitor reduces image contrast. The specular (mirror-like) reflection of light from bright objects imposes structured noise on the displayed image. The faces of LCD monitors reflect less ambient light than do those of CRT monitors.

Spatial linearity (freedom from spatial distortion) describes how accurately shapes and lines are presented on the monitor. Because the pixel matrix is physically built into LCD monitors, they provide excellent spatial linearity.

CRT monitors, whose images are formed by scanning electron beams, must refresh the image at a rate greater than a threshold to avoid the perception of flicker in the image. This threshold, called the flicker-fusion frequency, increases with the brightness of the image and the fraction of the visual field occupied by the image and varies from person to person; it ranges from about 60 to over 80 frames per second for very bright monitors. Active matrix LCD monitors, unlike CRT monitors, do not exhibit flicker when displaying stationary images and so the refresh rate is irrelevant in this situation. However, the refresh rate of an LCD monitor does matter when displaying dynamic images. The frame refresh rate needed to provide the appearance of continuous motion when viewing cine images is less than that needed to avoid the perception of flicker and may be as low as about 25 frames per second.[†] LCD monitors typically suffer more from lag in displaying dynamic images than do CRT monitors. The lag in LCD monitors is caused by the time required to change the electrical charges stored by the small capacitors in individual pixels. Monitors add both spatial and temporal noise to displayed images.

There are practical differences between LCD and CRT monitors. LCD monitors require much less space, are much lighter, consume less electrical power, and generate much less heat. A problem of LCD monitors is nonfunctional pixels or subpixels; these may be permanently off or permanently on. The fraction of nonfunctional pixels or subpixels should be small and they should not be grouped together. Another disadvantage of LCD monitors is limited viewing angle, which varies with the LCD technology. The luminance and apparent contrast are reduced if the monitor is not viewed from nearly directly in front. In distinction, CRT monitors permit very wide viewing angles. The lifetimes of LCD monitors, limited by the brightness of the fluorescent tubes in the backlights, exceed those of CRT monitors, limited by the electron guns and phosphor.

The spatial resolution of a display monitor is primarily described by its addressable pixel format (e.g., 1,280 by 1,024 pixels) with respect to the useful display area. An active matrix LCD monitor provides spatial resolution superior to a CRT monitor with the same addressable pixel format. Because the individual pixels are physical structures, LCD monitors provide uniform spatial resolution over their entire faces. Improvements in the performance of LCD monitors have resulted in their replacing CRT monitors.

The necessary dimensions of the active face of a display monitor and its pixel format (number of rows and columns of pixels or, equivalently, the pixel pitch, defined as the distance from the center of a pixel to the center of an adjacent pixel in the same row or column) depend upon the pixel matrix sizes of the images produced by the modalities whose images will be displayed, the distance from the viewer's eyes to the display surface, and the spatial resolution of the human visual system. Digital mammograms and radiographs contain many more pixels than other radiological images (Table 5-7) and are referred to as large matrix-size images.

It is desirable for a radiologist to view an entire image at or near maximal spatial resolution. To avoid a reduction in spatial resolution when an image is displayed, a monitor should have at least as many pixels in the horizontal and vertical directions as

---

[†]The standard for motion pictures in the United States is 24 frames per second.

TABLE 5-7   TYPICAL RADIOLOGIC IMAGE FORMATS

MODALITY	PIXEL FORMAT	BITS PER PIXEL
Scintillation camera planar	64^2 or 128^2	8 or 16
SPECT	64^2 or 128^2	8 or 16
PET	128^2 to 336^2	16
Digital fluoroscopy	512^2 or $1,024^2$	8 to 12
Digital radiography		
Fuji CR chest (200 µm)	$2,140 \times 1,760$	10 to 12
Trixell DR (143 µm)	$3,000 \times 3,000$	12 to 16
Mammography		
GE—24 × 31 cm (100 µm)	$2,394 \times 3,062$	12–16
Hologic—24 × 29 cm (70 µm)	$3,328 \times 4,096$	
X-ray CT	512^2	12
MRI	64^2 to $1,024^2$	12
Ultrasound	512^2	8

CT, computed tomography; MRI, magnetic resonance imaging; PET, positron emission tomography; SPECT, single photon emission computed tomography.

the image. On the other hand, it serves no purpose to provide spatial resolution that is beyond the ability of the viewer to discern. The distance from a person's eyes to the face of a display monitor of a workstation commonly ranges from about 50 to 60 cm. The viewer may lean closer to the monitor for short periods to see more detail, but viewing at a distance much closer than about 55 cm for long periods is uncomfortable.

To assess perceived contrast and spatial resolution, scientists studying human vision commonly use test images containing a sinusoidal luminance pattern centered in an image of constant luminance equal to the average luminance of the sinusoidal pattern (Fig. 5-10). Contrast may be defined as

$$C = (L_{max} - L_{min})/L_{avg},$$

where L_{max} is the maximal luminance in the pattern, L_{min} is the least luminance, and L_{avg} is the average luminance. The smallest luminance difference $(L_{max} - L_{min})$ that is detectable by half of a group of human observers is known as a *just noticeable difference* (JND). The threshold contrast is the JND divided by L_{avg}. Contrast sensitivity is defined as

■ FIGURE 5-10 Sinusoidal luminance test patterns are used by researchers to assess the perception of contrast as a function of spatial frequency and average luminance. **A.** Four different spatial frequencies with the background luminance equal to the average luminance of the pattern are shown. **B.** Four different contrast levels at a fixed frequency. Sinusoidal lines (in *blue*) above the patterns show the change in luminance as amplitude and frequency variations

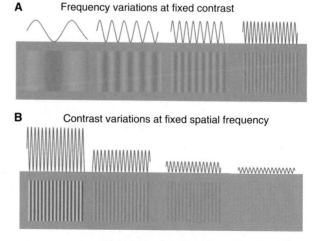

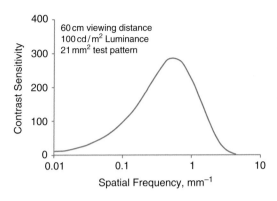

■ **FIGURE 5-11** Contrast sensitivity of the human visual system as a function of spatial frequency. Adapted from Flynn MG. Visual requirements for high-fidelity display. In: *Advances in digital radiography: categorical course in diagnostic radiology physics*. Oak Brook, IL: Radiological Society of North America, 2003:103–107.

the inverse of the threshold contrast. Figure 5-11 is a graph of contrast sensitivity as a function of spatial frequency (cycles per mm at a 60 cm viewing distance) from a typical experiment. Studies have shown that people with good vision perceive image contrast best at about five cycles per visual degree. The threshold contrast is reduced to about a tenth of the maximum at about 20 cycles per visual degree and reduced to less than one hundredth of the maximum at about 40 to 50 cycles per visual degree (Barten, 1999). At a 60-cm viewing distance, a visual degree is equivalent to a distance of 10.5 mm (10.5 mm = 60 cm $\times$ tan 1°) on the face of the monitor. Thus, at a 60-cm viewing distance, a person with good vision perceives contrast best at about half a cycle per mm, perceives contrast reduced to less than a tenth of this at about two cycles per mm, and perceives very little contrast beyond about four cycles per mm. Two cycles per mm is approximately equivalent to 4 pixels per mm, or a pixel pitch of 1 mm per 4 pixels = 0.25 mm and four cycles per mm is approximately equivalent to 8 pixels per mm, or a pixel pitch of 1 mm per 8 pixels = 0.125 mm.

Monitor Pixel Formats

Display monitors are available in many face sizes and pixel formats. Two common formats for commercial color monitors are 1,280 by 1,024 pixels and 1,600 by 1,200 pixels. Digital radiographs are typically stored in formats of about 2,000 by 2,500 pixels. A common active display size for monitors used to display radiographs, including mammograms, is 54 cm (21 inches) diagonal. The faces of the monitors typically have aspect ratios (width to height) of about 3 to 4 or 4 to 5. A common pixel format for these monitors is 2,560 pixels by 2,048 pixels; such monitors are commonly called "5 megapixel monitors." This pixel format permits the display of an entire large matrix image at near maximal resolution. Less-expensive 54-cm diagonal monitors have pixel formats of 2,048 by 1,536 pixels, commonly called "3 megapixel monitors," and 1,600 $\times$ 1,200 pixels, commonly called "2 megapixel monitors." A typical pixel pitch of a 5-megapixel monitor is 0.165 mm and that of a 3-megapixel monitor is 0.21 mm.

LCD monitors with 76 cm (30 inches) diagonal faces are available in ten-, 6-, and 4-megapixel formats. Such a monitor is intended to replace a pair of 54-cm diagonal monitors and permit the simultaneous side-by-side display of two radiographs or mammograms in full or near full spatial resolution.

A monitor orientated so that the horizontal field is greater than the vertical is called *landscape display*, whereas an orientation with the vertical field greater than the horizontal is called *portrait display*. Monitors used for the display of digital radiographs are usually used in the portrait orientation, although the newer 76 cm diagonal monitors that display two radiographs in full or near full resolution side-by-side are used in the landscape orientation.

When an entire image is displayed on a display monitor with a smaller number of horizontal or vertical pixels than the image itself, the image must be reduced to a smaller pixel format by averaging neighboring pixels in the stored image, causing a loss of spatial resolution. The zoom function permits a portion of the image to be displayed in full spatial resolution on such a monitor and the pan function on the workstation allows the viewing of different portions of the image.

Display of Image Contrast and Contrast Enhancement

A display system must be able to display a range of pixel values from the minimal pixel value to the maximal value in the image. For displaying the image, a range of light intensities is available, from the darkest to the brightest the display monitor is calibrated to produce. A great amount of choice exists in how the mapping from pixel value to light intensity is performed. A mapping can be selected that optimizes the contrast of important features in the image, thereby increasing their conspicuity. Alternatively, if this mapping is poorly chosen, the conspicuity of important features in the image can be reduced.

Lookup tables (LUTs) are commonly used by medical image processing and display computers to affect the display of image contrast. Such use of a LUT may be considered to be a method of image processing. However, it is intimately connected with displaying images and so is discussed here. A LUT is simply a table containing a value for each possible pixel value in an image. For example, if each pixel in an image could have one of 4,096 values, a LUT would have 4,096 elements. In practice, each pixel value in the transformed image is determined by selecting the value in the LUT corresponding to the pixel value in the unmodified image. For example, if the value of a pixel in the unmodified image is 1,342, the value of the corresponding pixel in the transformed image is the 1,342nd value in the LUT. Figure 5-12 illustrates the use of a LUT.

A LUT may be applied to transform image contrast at more than one point in the chain from image acquisition to image display. For example, a digital radiography system may use a LUT to modify the acquired pixel values, which are proportional to the detected x-ray signals, to cause the display of contrast to resemble that of a film (Fig. 5-13). Similarly, a medical grade image display system may employ a LUT to modify each pixel value before it is sent to the DAC and becomes an analog signal; this is commonly done to compensate for the different display functions of individual display monitors and is described below in this chapter. Figure 5-13 shows five LUTs in graphical form.

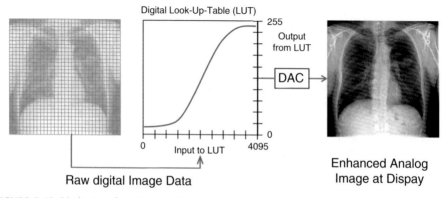

■ **FIGURE 5-12** Display interface showing function of a lookup table (LUT). An image is transferred to the memory of the display interface. The display interface selects pixel values in a raster pattern, and sends the pixel values, one at a time, to the LUT. The LUT produces a digital value indicating display intensity to the DAC. The DAC converts the display intensity from a digital value to an analog form (e.g., a voltage).

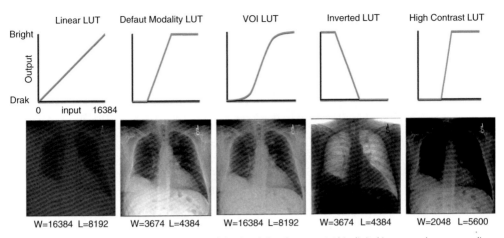

■ **FIGURE 5-13** Graphs of five digital lookup tables (LUT), for the same 14 bit digital image and corresponding "window" and "level" settings. From left to right, the first is a linear LUT that preserves the way the image was originally acquired. Typically, the *useful* image data occupies only a small range of values for this 14 bit image, and thus contrast is low. The second is the "default modality LUT" that is assigned by the modality, based upon an optimized grayscale range. Note that a large fraction of the range of the image is set to zero (*dark*) or largest output (maximal brightness), and that a small range of values is mapped from the dark to the bright values on the display. The third is the "Value of Interest" LUT (VOILUT), which encompasses the full range of input values and maps the output according to the capabilities of the display. Typically, this LUT is a sigmoidally-shaped curve, which softens the appearance of the image in the dark and bright regions. The fourth LUT inverts image contrast. Shown here is the inverted second image. The fifth image demonstrates windowing to enhance contrast in underpenetrated parts of the image by increasing the slope of the LUT. Note that this causes the loss of all contrast in the highly penetrated regions of the lung.

Windowing and leveling is a common method for contrast enhancement. It permits the viewer to use the entire range of display intensities to display just a portion of the total range of pixel values. For example, an image may have a minimal pixel value of 0 and a maximum of 200. If the user wishes to enhance contrast differences in the brighter portions of the image, a window from 100 to 200 might be selected. Then, pixels with values from 0 to 100 are displayed at the darkest intensity and so will not be visible on the monitor. Pixels with values of 200 will be displayed at the maximal brightness, and the pixels with values between 100 and 200 will be assigned intensities determined by the current LUT. Figure 5-13 (rightmost image) illustrates windowing.

Most display workstations have level and window controls. The level control determines the midpoint of the pixel values to be displayed and the window control determines the range of pixel values about the level to be displayed. Some nuclear medicine workstations require the user to select the lower level (pixel value below which all pixels are displayed at the darkest intensity) and the upper level (pixel value above which all pixel values are set to the brightest intensity):

$$\text{Lower level} = \text{Level} - \text{Window}/2$$

$$\text{Upper level} = \text{Level} + \text{Window}/2.$$

Windowing and leveling can be performed with a LUT or, equivalently, by calculation; if calculated, it is accomplished by subtraction of a number from each pixel, followed by multiplication by another number. If calculated, each pixel value equal to or below the lower level is set to zero and each equal to or above the upper level is set to the maximal pixel value possible. For each pixel whose value is between the lower and upper level, the windowed pixel value is calculated as

$$P_{i,j}' = (P_{ij} - \text{Lower level})\ (\text{maximal allowed pixel value}/\text{window}),$$

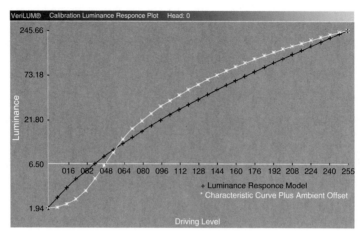

■ **FIGURE 5-14** A typical response function (digital driving level versus output luminance) of an LCD monitor is shown as the white "x" symbols. Note the nonlinear luminance response as a function of digital driving level. The black "+" symbols are the monitor luminance values that conform to the DICOM Grayscale Standard Display Function (GSDF), PS 3.14. For the noncalibrated monitor, the lower luminance areas of the image will be displayed suboptimally. (See Fig. 5-18 for a comparison of calibrated and uncalibrated monitors.) The Luminance Response Model in black is a portion of the DICOM GSDF curve shown in Figure 5-16.

where P_{ij} is a pixel value before windowing, $P_{i,j}'$ is the pixel value after windowing, "maximal pixel value" is the largest possible pixel value, and window = upper level – lower level.

Luminance Calibration of Display Systems

The *display function* of a display monitor describes the luminance produced as a function of the magnitude of the digital (sometimes called a "digital driving level") or analog signal sent to the monitor. The display function of a monitor can greatly affect the perceived contrast of the displayed image. The inherent display function of a monitor is nonlinear (increasing the input signal does not, in general, cause a proportional increase in the luminance), varies from monitor to monitor, and also changes with time. Figure 5-14 shows a display function of an LCD monitor (white curve). Furthermore, individual display monitors differ in maximal and minimal luminance.

A display monitor has controls labeled "brightness" and "contrast" that are used to adjust the shape of the display function. On most monitors used for medical image interpretation, they are not available to the user.

After acquisition of digital images by an imaging device, the pixel values may be adjusted automatically by the device's computer so that the displayed images have an appearance acceptable to radiologists (black curve in Fig. 5-14). For example, digital radiography systems, including digital mammography systems, modify the pixel values to give the images appearances similar to screen-film radiographs. Other processing may be performed, such as the automatic contrast equalization processing of some digital mammography systems (Chapter 8), to increase the conspicuity of structures of interest and to reduce the need for the interpreting physician to window and level the images. When these images are sent to a workstation for viewing, unless the display functions of the display devices were known to the designer of the imaging device, the images' contrast intended by the imaging device designer may not be achieved. Also, the images' appearance may also be modified by a technologist using a review workstation prior to transfer to the PACS. If the display system of the review workstation

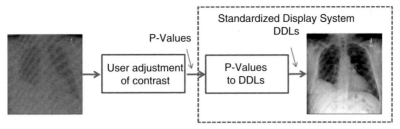

■ **FIGURE 5-15** This diagram shows the use of a lookup table (LUT), labeled "P-values to DDLs," with each display system, such as a display monitor, so that the net display function, provided by the LUT and display device, will conform to the DICOM Grayscale Standard Display Function (GSDF). The DICOM GSDF does not replace adjustment of contrast by the user. (Adapted from Digital Imaging and Communications in Medicine (DICOM) Part 14: Grayscale Standard Display Function, PS 3.14-2011, National Electrical Manufacturers Association, 2011.)

has a display function significantly different from that of the interpretation workstation, the interpreting physician may see contrast displayed quite differently than the technologist intended. Furthermore, if the monitors on display stations have different display functions, an image may have a different appearance on different display monitors, even when more than one monitor is attached to a single workstation.

To resolve this problem, the Digital Imaging and Communications in Medicine (DICOM) Grayscale Standard Display Function (GSDF)[§] was created to standardize the display of image contrast. The DICOM GSDF pertains to grayscale (monochrome) images, whether displayed on monitors or printed onto paper or onto film for viewing on a light box. It does not apply to color images, although it does pertain to grayscale images displayed by a color monitor. The goals of the DICOM GSDF are to

1. Provide applications with a predictable transformation of digital pixel values (called "presentation values," abbreviated as "P-values") to luminance
2. Insofar as possible, provide a similar display of contrast on display monitors and printed media
3. Insofar as possible, provide *perceptual linearization*, that is, equal differences in the pixel values received by the display system should be perceived as equal by the human visual system

The first two of these goals are met by the DICOM GSDF. In fact, on display monitors having identical minimal and maximal luminances, the DICOM GSDF will provide almost identical displays of contrast. The third goal, perceptual linearization, can likely not be perfectly achieved, given the complexity of the human visual system; nonetheless, the DICOM GSDF comes close to achieving it.

The display function of a monitor can be modified to any desired shape by the use of a LUT in the workstation or monitor, as described in earlier in this chapter. The LUT contains an output pixel value for each possible pixel value in an image. In the DICOM standards, the input pixel values provided to the LUT are called "presentation values," as shown in Figure 5-15, and the output values of the LUT that are provided to the display system are called "digital driving levels." Thus, by using a LUT for each monitor, the net display function (monitor and LUT) will conform to the DICOM GSDF.

Figure 5-16 shows the DICOM GSDF response model, which specifies luminance as a function of a parameter called "JND index"; "JND" is an acronym for "just-noticeable difference," discussed earlier in this section. DICOM PS 3-14, 2011, defines the JND index as "The input value to the GSDF, such that one step in JND

[§]The DICOM GSDF is part of the DICOM standards discussed later in this chapter.

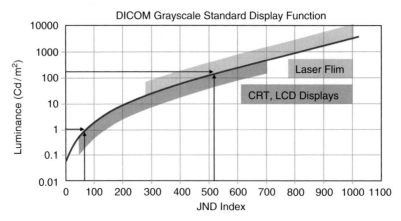

■ FIGURE 5-16 The DICOM Grayscale Standard Display Function. Only a segment of the curve from the minimum to the maximum luminance values of a display device, such as a CRT or LCD monitor or laser printed film, is used as the calibrated display function. For instance, the arrows point to the operating range of the LCD monitor whose response is shown in Figure 5-14. The maximum operating ranges for CRT or LCD displays and laser film in terms of luminance relative to the JND index are shown in red and blue highlights, respectively. A calibrated monitor or film response will fall along a subset of the ranges depicted above.

Index results in a Luminance difference that is a Just-Noticeable Difference." The shape of the GSDF is based on a model of the human visual system. A detailed explanation of this model is beyond the scope of this book; it is discussed in DICOM PS 3-14, 2011, and Flynn 2003.

Only a portion of the DICOM GSDF curve, that lies between the minimal and maximal calibrated luminances of a monitor, is used as the display function for that monitor. For example, as shown in Figure 5-16, if the minimal and maximal calibrated luminances of a display monitor are 2 and 250 cd/m², the portion of the DICOM GSDF contained in the segment encompassing 2 and 250 cd/m² is used as the display function. The presentation values p, from 0 to the maximal possible presentation value (typically $2^N - 1$, where N is the number of bits used for a presentation value), are linearly related to the values of JND index j for that segment:

$$j = j_{min} + p \, (j_{max} - j_{min})/p_{max,}$$

where j_{min} is the smallest JND index in the rectangle, j_{max} is the largest JND index in the rectangle, and p_{max} is the maximum possible presentation value. Thus, a presentation value of 0 is assigned the lowest luminance of the monitor, which is the lowest luminance in the part of the GSDF within the segment. The maximum possible presentation value p_{max} is assigned the maximal calibrated luminance of the monitor, which is the maximal luminance in the segment. Each intermediate presentation value p is assigned the luminance on the GSDF corresponding to the JND index j determined from the equation above.

The calibration of a display monitor to the DICOM GSDF is usually performed automatically by the workstation itself, using specialized software and a calibrated photometer that sends a digital luminance signal to the workstation. The photometer is aimed at a single point on the face of the monitor (Fig. 5-17). The software, starting with a digital driving level of zero, increases the digital driving levels provided to the display system in a stepwise fashion and the photometer sends to the software the measured luminance for each step, thereby measuring the display function of the

External

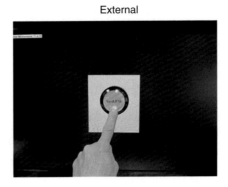

Internal

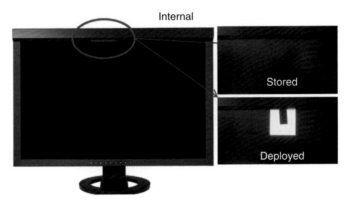

■ **FIGURE 5-17** A display monitor can be calibrated so its corrected display function conforms to the DICOM GSDF. This is accomplished by using a photometer that measures the luminance at the center of the monitor as a program varies the digital driving levels that control the luminance of pixels in a square area at the center of the monitor. The photometer sends the digitized luminance values to the computer. The program then calculates and stores values in a LUT to cause the monitor to conform to the GSDF. The upper picture shows a monitor with a photometer manually placed at the center of the monitor. The lower picture shows a medical-grade monitor with a built-in internal photometer that calibrates the display automatically

display system. The software then calculates the values to be placed in the LUT that will cause the LUT and display system, acting together, to conform to the DICOM GSDF. Some display monitors are equipped with photometers and can automatically assess monitor luminance and GSDF calibration (Fig. 5-17, bottom.).

The DICOM GSDF also can be applied to printed images, whether on transmissive media (film on a viewbox) or reflective media (e.g., an image printed on paper). Shown in Figure 5-18 is an image of a "Briggs" contrast test pattern for a display without luminance calibration (left) and luminance calibration conforming to the DICOM GSDF (right).

False Color Displays

As mentioned above, radiographic images do not inherently have the property of color. When color is used to display them, they are called *false color images*. Figure 5-19 shows how false color images are produced by nuclear medicine computer workstations. Common uses of false color displays include nuclear medicine, in which color is often used to enhance the perception of contrast, and ultrasound, in which color is used to superimpose flow information on images displaying anatomic information. False color displays

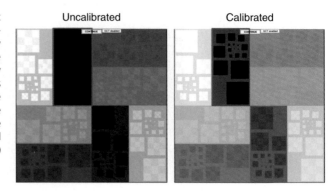

■ FIGURE 5-18 A Briggs contrast pattern. **Left**. The uncalibrated monitor display (its uncorrected display function is shown in Fig. 5-14 as the *white symbols*) shows the difficulty in resolving the contrast differences in the darker areas of the image (highlighted *red box*). **Right**. The calibrated monitor display (response to luminance variations is graphed in Fig. 5-14 as the *black symbols*) shows improved contrast response.

are also commonly used in image co-registration, in which an image obtained from one modality is superimposed on a spatially congruent image from another modality. For example, it is often useful to superimpose nuclear medicine images, which display physiology, but may lack anatomic landmarks, on CT or MRI images. In this case, the nuclear medicine image is usually superimposed in color on a grayscale MRI or CT image.

Performance of Diagnostic Monitors versus That of Consumer-Grade Monitors

Radiological images are displayed for interpretation using very expensive LCD monitors designed for medical image display instead of consumer-grade LCD monitors. Advantages of these diagnostic monitors commonly include

1. Much higher maximal luminance
2. More uniform luminance
3. Smaller pixels, providing higher spatial resolution
4. Wider viewing angles, due to different LCD technology

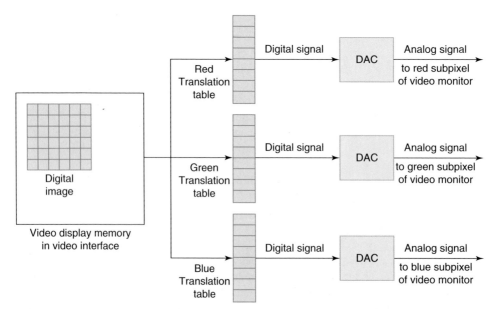

■ FIGURE 5-19 Creation of a false color display in nuclear medicine. Each individual pixel value in the image being displayed is used to look up a *red*, a *green*, and a *blue* intensity value. These are simultaneously displayed adjacent to one another within a single pixel of a color display monitor. The mix of these three colors creates the perception of a single color for that pixel.

5. More than 8 bits for digital driving levels (grayscale monitors) or more than 8 bits each for the digital driving levels for red, green, and blue (color monitors), to display subtle contrast differences

5. Automatic luminance stabilization circuits to compensate for changing backlight intensity

6. Hardware and software for implementing the DICOM GSDF

7. Ability to monitor display monitor luminance and GSDF calibration over a network

Cameras to Record Digital Images on Film

Despite the increasing capability to transfer and view medical images without the use of photographic film, there are still situations in which digital images must be recorded on film. For example, federal mammography regulations in effect require each facility performing full-field digital mammography to have such a capability. Today, images are commonly recorded on film by multiformat laser cameras, also known as laser imagers. The images are usually sent to the device by a computer network. These devices usually provide several formats (e.g., one image, four images, and six images per sheet). After exposure of the film, it is chemically developed and viewed on a light box. Although films with silver halide grains and wet chemical processing were once used, nearly all laser imagers today use silver-based film and a dry thermal development process to convert the latent images on the exposed film into visible images.

A laser camera typically contains a microprocessor; an image memory; an analog-to-digital converter; a laser with a modulator to vary the intensity of the beam; a rotating polygonal mirror to scan the laser beam across the film; and a film-transport mechanism to move the film in a linear fashion so the scanning covers the entire film. Each sweep of the laser beam across the film records a single row of pixel values. The lasers in most laser cameras emit red or infrared light, requiring the use of red- or infrared-sensitive film. Care must be taken not to handle this film under the normal red darkroom safelight.

5.6 Computer Networks

Definitions and Basic Principles

Computer networks permit the transfer of information between computers, allowing computers to share devices, such as printers, laser multiformat cameras, and information storage devices, and enabling services such as electronic transmission of messages (e-mail), transfer of computer files, and use of distant computers. Networks, based upon the distances they span, may be described as local area networks (LANs) or wide area networks (WANs). A *LAN* connects computers within a department, a building such as medical center, and perhaps neighboring buildings, whereas a *WAN* connects computers at large distances from each other. LANs and WANs evolved separately and a computer can be connected to a WAN without being part of a LAN. However, most WANs today consist of multiple LANs connected by medium or long distance communication links. The largest WAN is the Internet.

A *server* is a computer on a network that provides a service to other computers on the network. A computer with a large array of magnetic disks that provides data storage for other computers is called a file server. There are also print servers, application servers, database servers, e-mail servers, web servers, etc. A computer, typically a workstation, on a network that makes use of a server is called a *client*.

Two common terms used to describe client-server relationships are *thick client* and *thin client*. "Thick client" describes the situation in which the client computer provides most information processing and the function of the server is mainly to store information, whereas "thin client" describes the situation in which most information processing is provided by the server and the client mainly serves to display the information. An example would be the production of volume rendered images from a set of CT images. In the thin client relationship, the volume rendered images would be produced by the server and sent to a workstation for display, whereas in a thick client relationship, the images would be produced by software and/or a graphics processor installed on the workstation. The thin client relationship can allow the use of less capable and less expensive workstations and enable specialized software and hardware, such as a graphics processor, on a single server to be used by several or many workstations.

Networks have both hardware and software components. A physical connection must exist between computers so that they can exchange information. Common physical connections include coaxial cable, copper wiring, optical fiber cables, and radio, including microwave, communication systems. A coaxial cable is a cylindrical cable with a central conductor surrounded by an insulator that, in turn, is surrounded by a tubular grounded shield conductor. Coaxial cable and copper wiring carry electrical signals. Optical fiber cables use glass or plastic fibers to carry near-infrared radiation signals produced by lasers or light emitting diodes. Optical fiber cables have several advantages over cables or wiring carrying electrical signals, particularly when the cables must span long distances—optical fiber is not affected by electrical interference and thus usually has lower error rates; it can carry signals greater distances before attenuation, distortion, and noise require the use of repeaters to read and retransmit the signals; and it permits much greater information transmission rates. There are also layers of software between the application program with which the user interacts and the hardware of the communications link.

Network *protocols* are standards for communication over a network. A protocol provides a specific set of services. Both hardware and software must comply with established protocols to achieve successful transfer of information. Failure to conform to a common protocol would be analogous to a person speaking only English attempting to converse with a person speaking only Arabic. Several hardware and software protocols will be described later in this chapter.

In most networks, multiple computers share communication pathways. Most network protocols facilitate this sharing by dividing the information to be transmitted into *packets*. Packets may be called frames, datagrams, or cells. Some protocols permit packets of variable size, whereas others permit only packets of a fixed size. Each packet has a header containing information identifying its destination. In most protocols, a packet also identifies the sender and contains information used to determine if the packet's contents were garbled during transfer. The final destination computer reassembles the information from the packets and may request retransmission of lost packets or packets with errors.

Large networks usually employ switching devices to forward packets between network segments or even between entire networks. Each device on a network, whether a computer or switching device, is called a *node* and the communications pathways between them are called *links*. Each computer is connected to a network by a network adapter, also called a network interface, installed on the I/O bus of the computer or incorporated on the motherboard. Each interface between a node and a network is identified by a unique number called a *network address*. A computer usually has only a single interface, but a switching device connecting two or more networks may have an address on each network.

The maximal data transfer rate of a link or a connection is called the *bandwidth*, a term originally used to describe the data transfer capacities of analog communications channels. An actual network may not achieve its full nominal bandwidth because of overhead or inefficiencies in its implementation. The term *throughput* is commonly used to describe the maximal data transfer rate that is actually achieved. Bandwidth and throughput are usually described in units of megabits per second (10^6 bps = 1 Mbps) or gigabits per second (10^9 bps = 1 Gbps). These units should not be confused with megabytes per second (MBps) and gigabytes per second (GBps), commonly used to specify the data transfer rates of computer components such as magnetic and optical disks. (Recall that a byte consists of eight bits. Megabytes and gigabytes are defined in Table 5-3.) The *latency* is the time delay of a transmission between two nodes. In a packet-switched network, it is the time required for a small packet to be transferred. It is determined by factors such as the total lengths of the links between the two nodes, the speeds of the signals, and the delays caused by any intermediate repeaters and packet switching devices.

On some small LANs, all computers are directly connected, that is, all packets reach every computer. However, on a larger network, every packet reaching every computer would be likely to cause unacceptable network congestion. For this reason, most networks larger than a small LAN, and even many small LANs, employ *packet switching*. The packets are sent over the network. Devices such as switches and routers (to be discussed shortly) store the packets, read the destination addresses, and send them on toward their destinations, a method called "store and forward." In some very large packet-switched networks, individual packets from one computer to another may follow different paths through the network and may arrive out-of-order.

Networks are commonly designed in layers, each layer following a specific protocol. Figure 5-20 shows a model of a network consisting of five layers. Each layer in the stack provides a service to the layer above.

The top layer in the stack is the Application Layer (Layer 5 in Fig. 5-20). Application programs, commonly called *applications*, function at this layer. Applications are programs that perform useful tasks and are distinguished from systems software, such as an operating system. On a workstation, applications include the programs, such as an e-mail program, word processing program, web browser, or a program for displaying medical images, with which the user directly interacts. On a server, an application is a program providing a service to other computers on the network. The purpose of a computer network is to allow applications on different computers to exchange information.

Network communications begin at the Application Layer on a computer. The application passes the information to be transmitted to the next lower layer in the stack.

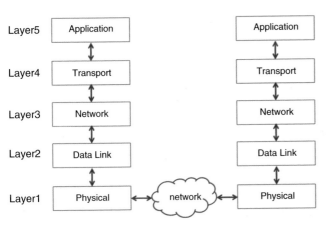

■ FIGURE 5-20 TCP/IP Network Protocol Stack. Another network model, the Open Systems Interconnection (OSI) model, is also commonly used to model networks. The OSI model has seven layers. The bottom four layers of the OSI model match the bottom four layers shown in this figure. The OSI model has two additional layers between the transport layer and the application layer.

The information is passed from layer to layer, with each layer adding information, such as addresses and error-detection information, until it reaches the Physical Layer (Layer 1 in Fig. 5-20). The Physical Layer sends the information to the destination computer, where it is passed up the layer stack to the application layer of the destination computer. As the information is passed up the layer stack on the destination computer, each layer removes the information appended by the corresponding layer on the sending computer until the information sent by the application on the sending computer is delivered to the intended application on the receiving computer.

The lower network layers (Layers 1 and 2 in Fig. 5-20) are responsible for transmission of packets from one node to another over a LAN or point-to-point link, and enable computers with dissimilar hardware and operating systems to be physically connected. The lowest layer, the Physical Layer, transmits physical signals over a communication channel (e.g., the copper wiring, optical fiber cable, or radio link connecting nodes). The protocol followed by this layer describes the signals (e.g., voltages, near-infrared signals, or radiowaves) sent between the nodes. Layer 2, the Data Link Layer, encapsulates the information received from the layer above into packets for transmission across the LAN or point-to-point link, and transfers them to Layer 1 for transmission. The protocol followed by Layer 2 describes the format of packets sent across a LAN or point-to-point link. It also describes functions such as media access control (determining when a node may transmit a packet on a LAN) and error checking of packets received over a LAN or point-to-point link. It is usually implemented in hardware.

Between the lower layers in the protocol stack and the Application Layer are intermediate layers that mediate between applications and the network interface. These layers are usually implemented in software and incorporated in a computer's operating system. Many intermediate level protocols are available, their complexity depending upon the scope and complexity of the networks they are designed to serve. Some functions of these intermediate layers will be discussed later in this chapter when the methods for linking multiple LANs are described.

Local Area Networks

LAN protocols are typically designed to permit the connection of computers over limited distances. On some small LANs, the computers are all directly connected and so only one computer can transmit at a time and usually only a single computer accepts the information. This places a practical limit on the number of computers and other devices that can be placed on a LAN without excessive network congestion. The congestion caused by too many devices on a LAN can be relieved by dividing the LAN into *segments* connected by packet switching devices, such as bridges, switches, and routers, that only transmit information intended for other segments.

Most types of LANs are configured in bus, ring, or star topologies (Fig. 5-21). In a *bus topology*, all of the nodes are connected to a single cable. One node sends a packet, including the network address of the destination node, and the destination node accepts the packet. All other nodes must wait. In a *ring topology*, each node is only directly connected to two adjacent nodes, but all of the nodes and their links form a ring. In a *star topology*, all nodes are connected to a central node, often called a hub.

Ethernet

The most commonly used LAN protocols are the various forms of Ethernet. Before transmission over Ethernet, information to be transmitted is divided into packets, each with a header specifying the addresses of the transmitting and destination

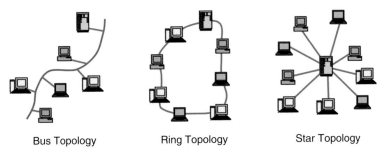

Bus Topology   Ring Topology   Star Topology

■ **FIGURE 5-21** Network topologies—bus, ring and star. Early forms of Ethernet used the bus topology; only one computer at a time could transmit packets. Other networks have used the ring topology. Modern forms of Ethernet use the star topology. The central node of the star is usually a packet switch that enables multiple pairs of nodes to simultaneously exchange packets. Multiple stars can be connected by connecting the central nodes.

nodes. Ethernet is contention based. A node ready to transmit a packet first "listens" to determine if another node is transmitting. If none is, it attempts to transmit. If two nodes inadvertently attempt to transmit at nearly the same moment, a collision occurs. In Ethernet, collisions are normal expected events. When a collision occurs, each node ceases transmission, waits a randomly determined but traffic-dependent time interval, and again attempts to transmit. This media access control protocol is called *carrier-sense multiple-access with collision detection* (CSMA/CD).

Ethernet has evolved greatly since its invention, resulting in several varieties of Ethernet (Table 5-8). In early forms of Ethernet, only a single node could transmit at a time on a LAN segment and usually only one node would receive and store the packets. All other nodes had to wait. Modern forms of Ethernet are configured in a star topology with a switch as the central node. The switch does not broadcast the

TABLE 5-8 COMMON LAN STANDARDS

TYPE	BANDWIDTH (MBPS)	PHYSICAL TOPOLOGY	MEDIUM	MAXIMAL RANGE
Switched Ethernet (10 Base-T)	10	star	UTP (common telephone wiring)	100 m from node to switch
Switched Fast Ethernet (100 Base-TX)	100	star	Category 5 UTP	100 m from node to switch
Gigabit Ethernet (1000 Base-CX and 1000 Base-T)	1,000	star	copper wiring	at least 25 m and perhaps 100 m
Gigabit Ethernet (1000 Base-SX and 1000 Base-LX)	1,000	star	optical fiber cable	550 m (multimode cable) and 3 km (single mode)
FDDI	100	ring	optical fiber cable	2 km (multimode) and 40 km (single mode) between each pair of nodes

Note: Early forms of Ethernet, which used the bus topology, are not listed. FDDI has largely been replaced by the various forms of Ethernet. In all but FDDI, the bandwidth is between each pair of nodes, with multiple nodes being able to simultaneously transmit. In FDDI, only a single node can transmit at a time.

packets to all nodes. Instead, it stores each packet in memory, reads the address on the packet, and then forwards the packet only to the destination node. Thus, the switch permits several pairs of nodes to simultaneously communicate at the full bandwidth (either 10 or 100 Mbps) of the network. 10Base-T Ethernet supports data transfer rates up to 10 Mbps. Fast Ethernet (100Base-TX) is like 10Base-T, except that it permits data transfer rates up to 100 Mbps over high-grade Category 5 UTP wiring. There are also optical fiber versions of Ethernet and Fast Ethernet. Gigabit Ethernet and Ten Gigabit Ethernet provide bandwidths of one and ten Gbps, respectively.

Other LAN Protocols

Many LAN protocols other than Ethernet have achieved wide implementation in the past. These include Token Ring, AppleTalk, and Fiber Distributed Data Interface (FDDI). These protocols have been largely replaced by the many forms of Ethernet.

Extended Local Area Networks

An extended LAN connects facilities, such as the various buildings of a medical center, over a larger area than can be served by a single LAN segment. An extended LAN is formed by connecting individual LAN segments. This is commonly performed by devices such as packet switches that only transmit packets when the addresses of the transmitting and destination nodes are on opposite sides of the device. Such a device operates at the Data Link Layer (Layer 2) of the network protocol stack. It stores each incoming packet in memory, reads its LAN destination address, and then forwards the packet toward its destination. Thus, in addition to extending a LAN, these devices segment it, thereby reducing congestion. Links, sometimes called "backbones," of high bandwidth media such as Gigabit or Ten Gigabit Ethernet, may be used to carry heavy information traffic between individual LAN segments.

Large Networks and Linking Separate Networks

It is often desirable to connect separate networks, which may use different hardware and software protocols. A network of networks is called an *internetwork* or *internet* (with a lower-case "i"). Today, most WANs are internets formed by linking multiple LANs (Fig. 5-22). There are several problems encountered when constructing an

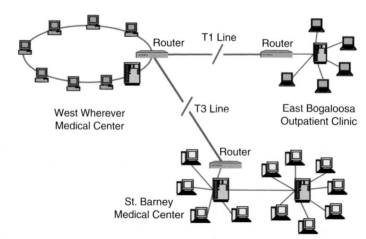

■ FIGURE 5-22 Wide area networks are commonly formed by linking together two or more local area networks using routers and links (e.g., T1 and T3 lines) leased from a telecommunications company.

internet. One is the routing of packets across the internet. LAN protocols are not designed for efficient routing of packets across very large networks. Furthermore, the addresses of nodes on a LAN, even though they may be unique, are not known to the nodes on other LANs. Additional problems are posed by the dissimilar protocols that may be used in individual LANs and point-to-point links.

WANs and separate networks are usually connected by devices called *routers* and long distance links provided by telecommunications companies, as shown in Figure 5-22. Routers are specialized computers or switches designed to route packets among networks. Routers perform packet switching—they store incoming packets, determine the intended destinations, and, by following directions in routing tables, forward the packets toward their destinations. Each packet may be sent through several routers before reaching its destination. Routers communicate among each other to determine optimal routes for packets.

Routers follow a protocol that assigns each interface in the connected networks a unique network address distinct from its LAN address. Routers operate at the Network Layer (Layer 3 in Fig. 5-20) of the network protocol stack. The dominant routable protocol today is the Internet Protocol (IP), described below. The function of a router is described in greater detail below.

The Internet Protocol Suite—TCP/IP

The Internet Protocol Suite, commonly called TCP/IP, is a packet-based suite of protocols used by many large networks and the Internet. TCP/IP permits information to be transmitted from one computer to another across a series of networks connected by routers. TCP/IP is specifically designed for internetworking, that is, linking separate networks that may use dissimilar lower-level protocols. TCP/IP operates at protocol layers above those of lower layer protocols such as Ethernet. The two main protocols of TCP/IP are the *Transmission Control Protocol (TCP)*, operating at the Transport Layer (Layer 4 in Fig. 5-20) and the *Internet Protocol (IP)*, operating at the Network Layer (Layer 3 in Fig. 5-20).

Communication begins when an application (at Layer 5 in Fig. 5-20) passes information to the Transport Layer, along with information designating the destination computer and the application on the destination computer, which is to receive the information. The Transport Layer, following TCP, divides the information into packets, attaches to each packet a header containing information such as a packet sequence number and error-detection information, and passes the packets to the Network Layer. The Network Layer, following IP, may further subdivide the packets. The Network Layer adds a header to each packet containing information such as the source address and the destination address. The Network Layer then passes these packets to the Data Link Layer (Layer 2 in Fig. 5-20) for transmission across the LAN or point-to-point link to which the computer is connected.

The Data Link Layer, following the protocol of the specific LAN or point-to-point link, encapsulates the IP packets into packets for transmission over the LAN or point-to-point link. Each packet is given another header containing information such as the LAN address of the destination computer. For example, if the lower level protocol is Ethernet, the Data Link Layer encapsulates each packet it receives from the Network Layer into an Ethernet packet. The Data Link Layer then passes the packets to the Physical Layer, where they are converted into electrical, infrared, or radio signals and transmitted.

Each computer and router is assigned an *IP address*. Under IP Version 4 (IPv4), an IP address consists of four 1-byte binary numbers, permitting over 4 billion distinct addresses. The first part of the address identifies the network and the latter part identifies the individual computer on the network. A new version of IP, IPv6, designed to ultimately replace IPv4, permits a much larger number of addresses. IP addresses do not have meaning to the lower network layers. IP defines methods by which a sending computer determines, for the destination IP address, the next lower layer address, such as a LAN address, to which the packets are to be sent by the lower network layers.

IP is referred to as a "connectionless protocol" or a "best effort protocol." This means that the packets are routed across the networks to the destination computer following IP, but some may be lost enroute. IP does not guarantee delivery or even require verification of delivery. On the other hand, TCP is a connection-oriented protocol providing reliable delivery. Following TCP, Network Layer 4 of the sending computer initiates a dialog with Layer 4 of the destination computer, negotiating matters such as packet size. Layer 4 on the destination computer requests the retransmission of any missing or corrupted packets, places the packets in the correct order, recovers the information from the packets, and passes it up to the proper application.

The advantages of designing networks in layers should now be apparent. LANs conforming to a variety of protocols can be linked into a single internet by installing a router in each LAN and connecting the routers with point-to-point links. The point-to-point links between the LANs can also conform to multiple protocols. All that is necessary is that all computers and routers implement the same WAN protocols at the middle network layers. A LAN can be replaced by one conforming to another protocol without replacing the software in the operating system that implements TCP/IP and without modifying application programs. A programmer developing an application need not be concerned with details of the lower network layers. TCP/IP can evolve without requiring changes to applications programs or LANs. All that is necessary is that each network layer conforms to a standard in communicating with the layer above and the layer below.

Routers

The packet switching performed by a router is different from that performed by Ethernet switches, which merely forward identical copies of received packets. On a LAN, the packets addressed to the router are those intended for transmission outside the LAN. The LAN destination address on a packet received by the router is that of the router itself.

A router performs the functions of the three lowest network levels shown in Figure 5-20. On the router, Layer 1 receives the signals forming a packet and passes the packet to Layer 2. Layer 2 removes the WAN packet from the lower level protocol packet in which it is encapsulated and passes it to Layer 3. Layer 3 reads the WAN address (in WANs conforming to the Internet Protocol Suite, an IP address) and, using a routing table, determines the optimal route for forwarding the packet. If the link for the next hop of the packet is part of a LAN, the router determines the LAN address of the next node to which the packet is to be sent. Layer 3 then sends the WAN packet and the LAN address of the next node to Layer 2, which encapsulates the WAN packet into a packet conforming to the lower level protocol for the next hop. Layer 2 passes this packet to Layer 1, which transmits the packet on toward its ultimate destination. Thus, the packets transmitted by a router may conform to a different lower level protocol than those received by the router.

The Internet

The *Internet* (with a capital letter "I") is an international network of networks using the TCP/IP protocol. A network using TCP/IP within a single company or organization is sometimes called an *intranet*.

The Internet is not owned by any single company or nation. The main part of the Internet consists of national and international backbone networks, consisting mainly of fiber optic links connected by routers, provided by major telecommunications companies. These backbone networks are interconnected by routers. Large organizations can contract for connections from their networks directly to the backbone networks. Individual people and small organizations connect to the Internet by contracting with companies called Internet service providers (ISPs), which operate regional networks that are connected to the Internet backbone networks.

IP addresses, customarily written as four numbers separated by periods (e.g., 152.79.110.12), are inconvenient. Instead, people use host names, such as www.ucdmc.ucdavis.edu, to designate a particular computer. The domain name system is an Internet service consisting of servers that translate host names into IP addresses.

Other Internet Protocols

The Internet Protocol Suite contains several protocols other than TCP and IP. These include application layer protocols such as File Transfer Protocol (FTP) for transferring files between computers; Simple Mail Transfer Protocol for e-mail; TELNET, which allows a person at a computer to use applications on a remote computer; and Hypertext Transfer Protocol (HTTP), discussed below.

A universal resource locator (URL) is a string of characters used to obtain a service from another computer on the Internet. Usually, the first part of a URL specifies the protocol (e.g., FTP, TELNET, or HTTP), the second part of the URL is the host name of the computer from which the resource is requested, and the third part specifies the location of the file on the destination computer. For example, in the URL http://www.ucdmc.ucdavis.edu/physics/text/, "http" is the protocol, "www.ucdmc.ucdavis.edu," is the host name, and "physics/text/" identifies the location of the information on the host computer.

The World Wide Web (WWW) is the largest and fastest growing use of the Internet. The WWW consists of servers connected to the Internet that store documents, called *web pages*, written in a language called Hypertext Markup Language (HTML). To read a web page, a person must have a computer, connected to the Internet, that contains an application program called a web browser such as Firefox or Microsoft Internet Explorer. Using the web browser, the user types or selects a URL designating the web server and the desired web page. The browser sends a message to the server requesting the web page and the server sends it, using a protocol called Hypertext Transfer Protocol (HTTP). When the browser receives the web page, it is displayed using the HTML instructions contained in the page. For example, the URL http://www.ucdmc.ucdavis.edu/physics/text/ will obtain, from a server at the U.C. Davis Medical Center, a web page describing this textbook.

Much of the utility of the WWW stems from the fact that a displayed web page may itself contain URLs. If the user desires further information, he or she can select a URL on the page. The URL may point to another web page on the same server or it may point to a web page on a server on the other side of the world. In either case, the web browser will send a message and receive and display the requested web page. WWW technology is of particular interest in PACS because it can be used to provide images and reports to clinicians.

Long Distance Telecommunications Links

Long distance telecommunication links are used to connect individual computers to a distant network and to connect distant LANs into a WAN. Most long distance telecommunication links are provided by telecommunications companies. In some cases, there is a fixed fee for the link, depending upon the maximal bandwidth and distance, regardless of the usage. In other cases, the user only pays for the portion of time that the link is used. Connections to the Internet are usually provided by companies called Internet service providers (ISPs). The interface to an ISP's network can be by nearly any of the telecommunications links described below.

The slowest but least expensive link is by the telephone *modem*. "Modem" is a contraction of "modulator/demodulator." A telephone modem converts digital information to a form for transmission over the standard voice-grade telephone system to another modem. Typical data transfer rates of modems are up to 56 kbps.

Digital subscriber lines (DSL) use modulation techniques similar to a modem to transfer digital information over local copper twisted-pair telephone lines to the nearest telephone company end office at speeds up to about 1.5 Mbps. At the telephone company's end office, the information is converted to another form suitable for the telephone company's or an ISP's network. DSL is usually used to connect computers or networks to the Internet. Some versions of DSL provide higher speeds downstream (to the customer) than upstream and are referred to as asymmetric DSL (ADSL). DSL is usually available only when the length of the copper telephone lines from the home or office to the nearest telephone company end office is less than about 5 km; the bandwidth decreases as the length of the line increases.

Cable modems connect computers to the Internet by analog cable television lines. Cable television lines usually support a higher bandwidth than do local telephone lines, often up to or beyond 2 Mbps. A disadvantage to using cable television lines is that the bandwidth is shared among the users of the line. If only a single computer is connected to the line, it can utilize the entire bandwidth; however, if several computers are connected, they share the bandwidth.

Some local telecommunication companies provide optical fiber cables directly to homes and small businesses. These usually provide higher bandwidth than DSL and cable modems. These lines will likely ultimately replace DSL and cable modems.

Point-to-point digital telecommunications links may be leased from telecommunications companies. A fixed rate is usually charged, regardless of the amount of usage. These links are available in various capacities (Table 5-9). The most common are T1, at 1.544 Mbps, and T3, at 44.7 Mbps. Although these links behave as dedicated lines between two points, they are really links across the telecommunications company's network. Optical carrier (OC) links are high-speed links that use optical fiber transmission lines.

The Internet itself may be used to link geographically separated LANs into a WAN. Encryption and authentication can be used to create a virtual private network (VPN) within the Internet. However, a disadvantage to using the Internet to link LANs into a WAN is the inability of today's Internet to guarantee quality of service. Disadvantages to the Internet today include lack of reliability, inability to guarantee bandwidth, and inability to give critical traffic priority over less important traffic. For critical applications, such as PACS and teleradiology, quality of service is the major reason why leased lines are commonly used instead of the Internet to link distant sites.

TABLE 5-9   LONG DISTANCE COMMUNICATIONS LINKS PROVIDED BY TELECOMMUNICATION COMPANIES

	DATA TRANSFER RATE	NOTE	POINT-TO-POINT?
Modem	28.8, 33.6, and 56 kbps	Digital signals over commercial telephone system	No. Can connect to any computer or ISP with modem.
DSL	Various, typically up to DS1.	Digital signals over local telephone wires	Typically provides connection to one ISP.
Cable modem	Various, typically 500 kbps to 10 Mbps	Signals over a cable television line	Typically provides connection to one ISP.
T1	DS1 (1.544 Mbps)	Leased line	Yes
T3	DS3 (44.7 Mbps)	Leased line	Yes
OC1	51.84 Mbps	Leased line	Yes
OC3	155 Mbps	Leased line	Yes
OC48	2,488 Mbps	Leased line	Yes

These can be used to connect an individual computer to a network or to link LANs into a WAN.

5.7 PACS and Teleradiology

Digital imaging technology and the falling costs and increasing capabilities of computer networks, workstations, storage devices and media, and display devices have spurred the implementation of picture archiving and communications systems (PACS) and teleradiology, with the goal of improving the utilization and efficiency of radiological imaging. For example, a PACS can replicate images at different display workstations simultaneously for the radiologist and referring physician, and be a repository for several years' images. The loss of images, once a major problem in teaching hospitals producing images on film, has been mostly eliminated. The transfer of images via teleradiology can bring subspecialty expertise to rural areas and smaller facilities and permit prompt interpretation of studies, particularly in trauma and other urgent cases, outside of normal working hours. Knowledge of the basic aspects of these systems is needed when obtaining or upgrading them; for their optimal use; and when purchasing imaging devices that will exchange information with them.

A PACS is a system for the storage, transfer, and display of radiological images. Teleradiology is the transmission of such images for viewing at a site or sites remote from where they are acquired. PACS and teleradiology are not mutually exclusive. Many PACS incorporate teleradiology. It is essential that PACS and teleradiology systems provide images suitable for the task of the viewer and, when the viewer is the interpreting physician, the images viewed must not be significantly degraded in either contrast or spatial resolution with regard to the acquired images.

Picture Archiving and Communications Systems

A PACS consists of a digital archive to store medical images, display workstations to permit physicians to view the images, and a computer network to transfer images and related information between the imaging devices and the archive and between the archive and the display workstations. There also must be a database program to track the locations of images and related information in the archive and software to permit interpreting, and perhaps referring, physicians to select and manipulate images. For efficiency of workflow and avoidance of errors, the PACS should exchange information with other information systems, such as the hospital information system (HIS), radiology information system (RIS), and electronic medical record (EMR) system. There may be additional components to the PACS, such as a film digitizer, a film printer, a CD or DVD "burner," and a web server to provide images to referring clinicians.

Today, PACS vary widely in size and in scope. On one hand, a PACS may be devoted to only a single modality at a medical facility. For example, a PACS may be limited to a nuclear medicine department, the ultrasound section, mammography, or a cardiac catheterization laboratory. Such a small single-modality PACS is sometimes called a *mini-PACS*. Mini-PACSs may exist in a large medical enterprise that has adopted an enterprise-wide PACS, if the enterprise PACS lacks functionality needed by specialists such as mammographers or nuclear medicine physicians. On the other hand, a PACS may incorporate all imaging modalities in a system of several medical centers and affiliated clinics (Fig. 5-23). Furthermore, a PACS may permit images to be viewed only by interpreting physicians or it may make them available to the ER, ICUs, and referring physicians as well. The goal, achieved at many medical centers today, is to store all images in a medical center or healthcare system on PACS, with images available to interpreting and referring clinicians through the EMR or thin-client workstations within the enterprise, with the PACS receiving requests for studies from the HIS and RIS, and with the PACS providing information to the HIS and RIS on the status of studies, and images available on the EMR. Another goal, far from being achieved, is to make medical images and related reports available nationwide, regardless of where they were acquired.

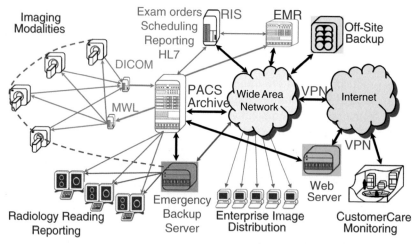

■ **FIGURE 5-23** Modern PACS uses a webserver connected to the Internet and a thin client paradigm to allow referring clinicians without access to the medical enterprise network to obtain images and reports over the Internet. Users within the medical enterprise have access through a LAN and WAN. The RIS provides the patient database for scheduling and reporting of image examinations through HL7 (Health Level 7) transactions and provides modality worklists (MWLs) with patient demographic information to the modalities, allowing technologists to select patient-specific scheduled studies to ensure accuracy. After a study is performed, the information is sent to the PACS in DICOM format, and reconciled with the exam-specific information (accession number). An emergency backup server ensures business continuity (red dotted line and highlights) in the event of unscheduled PACS downtime. Also depicted are an "off-site" backup archive for disaster recovery and real-time customer care monitoring to provide around the clock support. Not shown is the mirror archive, which provides on-site backup, with immediate availability, in cause of failure of the primary archive.

Teleradiology

Teleradiology can provide improved access to radiology for small medical facilities and improved access to specialty radiologists. For example, teleradiology can permit radiologists at a medical center to promptly interpret radiographs acquired at affiliated outpatient clinics. This requires devices producing digital radiographs or film digitizers at each clinic, leased lines to the medical center, and an interpretation workstation at the medical center. In another example, teleradiology can permit an on-call radiologist to interpret after-hours studies at home, avoiding journeys to the medical center and providing interpretations more promptly. This requires the radiologist to have an interpretation workstation at home, perhaps with a DSL or cable modem connection provided by a local telecommunications company, and the medical center to have images in a digital format and a matching communications connection. Image interpretation outside normal working hours may be provided by commercial "nighthawk" services consisting of radiologists with display workstations, sometimes located in countries such as Australia or India with time zones very different from those in the Americas, connected by high bandwidth links provided by telecommunications companies.

Acquisition of Digital Images

Most medical imaging devices today produce digital images. However, radiographic and mammographic images at some medical centers are still acquired using film-screen image receptors and older images may exist on film. Film images can be digitized by laser or charge-coupled device (CCD) digitizers.

Image Formats

The formats of digital radiological images are selected to preserve the clinical information acquired by the imaging devices. As mentioned earlier in this chapter, the numbers of rows and columns of pixels in an image are determined by the spatial resolution and the field-of-view of the imaging device, whereas the number of bits used for each pixel is determined by the contrast resolution of the imaging device. Thus, imaging modalities providing high spatial resolution (e.g., mammography) and with large fields of view (e.g., radiography) require large numbers of pixels per image, whereas modalities providing lower spatial resolution (e.g., CT) or small fields of view (e.g., ultrasound) can use fewer pixels. Modalities providing high contrast resolution (e.g., x-ray CT) require a large number of bits per pixel, whereas modalities with low contrast resolution (e.g., ultrasound) require fewer bits per pixel. Typical formats of digital images are listed in Table 5-7.

Film Digitizers

A film digitizer is a device that uses a light source and one or more light detectors to measure the light transmitted through individual areas of a film and form a digital image depicting the distribution of optical density in the film. The most common digitizer technology employs a collimated light source and a charge-coupled-device (CCD) linear array.

In a CCD digitizer (Fig. 5-24), the film is continuously moved across a lighted slit. A lens system focuses the transmitted light onto a CCD. A CCD, discussed in Chapter 7, is a solid-state integrated circuit with a rectangular array of light detectors. Each detector element of the CCD accumulates the signal from the transmitted light incident on it and stores the signal as an electrical charge until the CCD is read. When the CCD

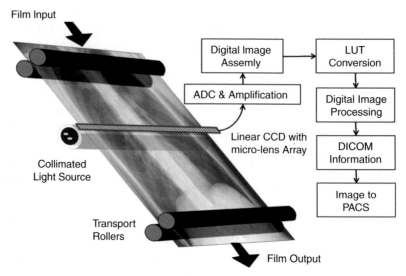

■ **FIGURE 5-24** CCD film digitizer. A linear array of light-emitting diodes is the typical illumination source and a CCD array at near contact to the film detects the transmitted light, which is then converted into a corresponding digital value, typically using 16 bits of quantization for modern CCD digitizers. In this configuration, the linear CCD photo-sensor, comprised of up to 4,000 pixels in a single row, produces electrons in proportion to the light transmitted through the film at a corresponding film location. The signal is proportional to the fraction of transmitted light.

is read, the analog signal from each element of the CCD is digitized by an analog-to-digital converter (ADC). The logarithm is taken of the intensity signal from each element of the CCD so that each pixel value in the digital image is proportional to the optical density (OD) of the corresponding portion of the film. (In Chapter 7, the optical density is defined as $OD = \log_{10}(I_o/I) = \log_{10}(I_o) - \log_{10}(I)$, where I is the intensity of the light transmitted through the film and I_o is the intensity if the film is removed.)

The role of film digitizers in PACS is likely to be transient, due to the decreasing use of screen-film image receptors. However, it is likely be several years before the film's role in recording and displaying images will be but a footnote in a future edition of this book.

Transfers of Images and Related Information

Computer networks, discussed in detail earlier in this chapter, permit exchanges of images and related information between the imaging devices and the PACS, between the PACS and display workstations, between the PACS and other information systems such as the RIS and HIS, and between various components of the PACS itself. A PACS may have its own local area network (LAN) or LAN segment, or it may share another LAN, such as a medical center LAN. The bandwidth requirements depend upon the imaging modalities and their workloads. For example, a LAN adequate for nuclear medicine or ultrasound may not be adequate for other imaging modalities. Network traffic typically varies in a cyclical fashion throughout the day. Network traffic also tends to be "bursty"; there may be short periods of very high traffic, separated by periods of low traffic. Network design must take into account both peak and average bandwidth requirements and the delays that are tolerable. Network segmentation, whereby groups of imaging, archival, and display devices that communicate frequently with each other are placed on separate segments, is commonly used to reduce network congestion. Network media providing different bandwidths may be used for various network segments. For example, a network segment serving nuclear medicine will likely have a lower bandwidth requirement than a network segment serving CT scanners.

Digital Imaging and Communications in Medicine

Connecting imaging devices to a PACS with a network, by itself, does not achieve transfer of images and related information. This would permit the transfer of files, but medical imaging equipment manufacturers and PACS vendors may use proprietary formats for digital images and related information. In the past, some facilities solved this problem by purchasing all equipment from a single vendor; others had custom software developed to translate one vendor's format into another's format. To help overcome problems such as these, the American College of Radiology and the National Electrical Manufacturers' Association jointly sponsor a set of standards called *Digital Imaging and Communications in Medicine* (DICOM) to facilitate the transfer of medical images and related information. Other professional societies work to develop medical specialty-specific DICOM standards. Many other national and international standards organizations recognize the DICOM standards.

DICOM includes standards for the transfer, using computer networks, of images and related information from individual patient studies between devices such as imaging devices and storage devices. DICOM specifies standard formats for the images and other information being transferred, services that one device can request from another, and messages between the devices. DICOM does not specify formats for the storage of information by a device itself, although a manufacturer may choose to use DICOM formats for this purpose. DICOM also includes standards for exchanging information regarding workflow; standards for the storage of images and related information on removable storage media, such as optical disks; and standards for the consistency and presentation of displayed images.

DICOM specifies standard formats for information objects, such as "patients," "images," and "studies." These are combined into composite information objects, such as the DICOM CT (computed tomography) image object, CR (computed radiography) image object, DX (digital x-ray) image object, MG (digital mammography x-ray) image object, US (ultrasound) image object, MR (magnetic resonance imaging) image object, and NM (nuclear medicine) image object. DICOM specifies standard services that may be performed regarding these information objects, such as storage, query and retrieve, storage commitment, print management, and media storage.

DICOM provides standards for workflow management, such as modality worklists (MWLs) listing patients to be imaged on specific imaging devices, and Performed Procedure Step, for communicating information about the status of a procedure. DICOM also provides standards, particularly Grayscale Standard Display Function (GSDF) and Presentation State, for the consistency and presentation of displayed and printed images. The DICOM GSDF was discussed earlier in this chapter.

DICOM Presentation State is a standard for capturing and storing a technologist's or a radiologist's adjustments of and annotations on key images. It records adjustments such as roaming and zooming, cropping, flipping, and windowing and leveling, and annotations such as arrows and clinical notes. These are stored with the image set on a PACS. When the images are viewed, the key images appear with the adjustments and annotations made by the technologist or radiologist.

DICOM is compatible with common computer network protocols. DICOM is an upper layer (Application Layer) standard and so is completely independent of lower layer network protocols, such as LAN protocols. DICOM adopts the Internet

Protocol Suite (TCP/IP). DICOM will function on any LAN or WAN, provided that the intermediate network layer protocol is TCP/IP.

Today, the products of nearly all vendors of medical imaging and PACS equipment permit exchanges of information that conform to parts of the DICOM standard. A *DICOM conformance statement* is a formal statement, provided by a vendor, describing a specific implementation of the DICOM standard. It specifies the services, information objects, and communications protocols supported by the implementation.

There are practical issues regarding DICOM that are worthy of emphasis. First, DICOM applies not just to a PACS, but also to each imaging device that exchanges information with the PACS. Hence, issues of DICOM conformance and functionality must be considered when purchasing individual imaging devices, as well as when purchasing or upgrading a PACS. Another issue is that DICOM is a set of standards, not a single standard. When purchasing an imaging device or a PACS, the contract should specify the specific DICOM standards with which conformance is desired. For example, support for DICOM Modality Worklists, Performed Procedure Step, and Storage Commitment should be provided in most cases, in addition to image store. Furthermore, there may be more than one DICOM standard that will permit information transfer, but all may not be equally useful. For example, digital radiographs may be transferred as the older DICOM CR image object or the newer DX image object. However, the old CR image object contains much less mandatory information regarding procedure, projection, laterality, etc. Also, the CR image object does not clearly define the meaning of pixel values. Even though use of the CR image object will permit image transfer, the lack of information about the image will hinder the use of automatic hanging protocols and optimal display of image contrast. For example, purchasers of PACS and CR and DR imaging systems should consider whether the systems support transfers using the CR image object or the newer DX image object and whether display workstations are able to use the additional information in the DX image object to provide automated hanging protocols (Clunie, 2003).

Communication with the Radiology Information System and Hospital Information System

It is advantageous to have communication among a PACS, the radiology information system (RIS), the hospital information system (HIS), and the electronic medical record (EMR, also known as the electronic patient record and electronic health record). A RIS is an information system that supports functions within a radiology department such as ordering and scheduling procedures, maintaining a patient database, transcription, reporting, and bill preparation. The RIS is not always a separate system—it may be part of the HIS or incorporated in the PACS. The RIS can provide worklists of scheduled studies to the operator's consoles of the imaging devices, thereby reducing the amount of manual data entry and the likelihood of improperly identified studies.

Communication among the RIS, HIS, EMR, and PACS is often implemented using a standard called HL7 (Health Level 7) for the electronic exchange of alphanumeric medical information, such as administrative information and clinical laboratory data. HL7 to DICOM translation, for instance, is a step in the RIS or HIS providing worklists to the imaging devices. HL7, like DICOM, applies to the Application Layer in the network protocol stack.

Modality worklists, supplied by the RIS, contain patient identifying information that helps to reduce a common problem in PACS—the inadvertent assignment of different patient identifiers to studies of a specific patient. This can arise from errors in manual data entry, for example, a technologist or clerk entering a single digit of a social security number incorrectly. Entering names differently (e.g., Samuel L. Jones, S. L. Jones, and Jones, Samuel) also may cause problems. These problems are largely obviated if the imaging technologists select patient identifiers from worklists, provided of course that the RIS and/or HIS furnishes unique patient identifiers. A "lost study" can still occur if the technologist mistakenly associates an imaging study with the wrong patient in a worklist.

Modality worklists also permit the prefetching of relevant previous studies for comparison by interpreting physicians. The network interfaces to the RIS and HIS can provide the interpreting physicians with interpretations of previous studies and the electronic patient record via the PACS workstation, saving the time that would be required to obtain this information on separate computer terminals directly connected to the RIS and/or HIS. These interfaces can also permit the PACS to send information to the RIS and/or HIS regarding the status of studies (e.g., study completed).

In a PACS, each patient study is commonly identified by a unique number called the accession number. The accession number is commonly assigned by the RIS.

Integrating the Healthcare Enterprise

As mentioned above, to provide optimal efficiency, the PACS and imaging devices must exchange information with other healthcare information systems. DICOM and HL7 provide standards for such exchanges of information, but they do not fully describe the optimal use of these standards within a healthcare system. *IHE* (Integrating the Healthcare Enterprise) is an initiative sponsored by the Radiological Society of North America and the Health Information Management Systems Society to improve the sharing of information by healthcare information systems. Under IHE, priorities for integration are identified and industry representatives achieve consensus on standards-based transactions to meet each identified clinical need. These decisions are recorded in documents called "integration profiles," the collection of which is called the "Technical Framework" and made freely available. Participating companies build into their systems the capability to support IHE transactions. Testing, performed during events called Connectathons, ensure a high degree of conformity with the Technical Framework. IHE does not provide standard formats for the exchange of information between pairs of devices. It instead describes the uses of existing standards such as DICOM, HL7, and the Internet Protocol Suite.

The most fundamental IHE integration profile for radiology is Radiology Scheduled Workflow. It defines the flow of information for the key steps in a typical patient imaging encounter (registration, ordering, scheduling, acquisition, distribution, and storage). If an imaging device or PACS conforms to the Scheduled Workflow Integration Profile, it will support DICOM store, modality worklist, performed procedure step, and storage commitment transactions. At the time of publication of this textbook, the IHE Technical Framework included about 20 integration profiles relevant to radiology that provide solutions to actual clinical problems. For example, significant hindrances to workflow can occur in mammography if the digital mammography system, the PACS or mammography mini-PACS, and interpretation workstation do not conform to the IHE Mammography Image Integration Profile in addition to the Radiology Scheduled Workflow Integration Profile. A major benefit of the IHE integration profiles is that a single integration profile can require conformance with several DICOM, HL7, and other standards and so a commitment by a vendor to support that integration profile will commit the vendor to conforming with the various standards included in that single integration profile.

Provision of Images and Reports to Attending Physicians and Other Healthcare Providers

WWW technology, described above, provides a cost-effective means for the distribution of images and other information over the HIS to noninterpreting physicians and other healthcare professionals. A web server, interfaced to the PACS, RIS, and HIS, maintains information about patient demographics, reports, and images. The server permits queries and retrievals of information from the PACS database. Physicians obtain images and reports from the web server using workstations with commercial web browsers. Information is sent from the PACS, typically in a study summary form containing just the images that are pertinent to a diagnosis. The full image set may be available as well. A major advantage to using WWW technology is that the workstations need not be equipped with specialized software for image display and manipulation; instead, these programs can be sent from the web server with the images or the server itself can provide this function. It is particularly desirable, for healthcare systems that have implemented electronic medical records, that relevant images can be accessed from the EMR.

Healthcare professionals at remote sites such as doctors' offices, small clinics, or at home can connect to the EMR using modems or leased lines. Alternatively, if the PACS web server is interfaced to the Internet, these clinicians can obtain images and reports over the Internet using DSL lines, cable modems, or fiber optic links provided by Internet service providers.

Storage of Images

The amount of storage required by a PACS archive depends upon the modality or modalities served by the PACS, on the workload, and the storage duration. The amounts of storage required for individual images and for typical studies from the various imaging modalities were discussed earlier in this chapter. For example, a medium size nuclear medicine department without PET/CT or SPECT/CT generates a few gigabytes (uncompressed) of image data in a year and so a single large-capacity magnetic disk and an optical disk drive for backup would suffice for a mini-PACS serving such a department. On the other hand, CT, MRI, and digitized radiographs from a medium size radiology department can generate several gigabytes of image data in a day and several terabytes (uncompressed) in a year, requiring a much larger and complex archival system. Ultrasound storage requirements strongly depend on the number of images in a study that are selected for archiving. For a medium-sized medical center, if 60 images per patient are selected for storage, then up to 0.5 TB per year may be generated. A cardiac catheterization laboratory may generate a few terabytes (uncompressed) in a year.

Storage Schemes

In a PACS, one of two storage schemes is commonly used. In a hierarchical storage scheme, recent images are stored on arrays of magnetic hard disk drives, and older images are stored on slower but more capacious archival storage media, such as optical disks and magnetic tape. In hierarchical storage schemes, the term *on-line storage* is used to describe storage, typically arrays of magnetic disks, used to provide nearly immediate access to studies. The term *near-line storage* refers to storage, such as automated libraries of optical disks or magnetic tape, from which studies may be retrieved within about a minute without human intervention. Optical disks have an advantage over magnetic tape cassettes for near-line storage because of shorter average access times, but magnetic tape is less expensive per unit storage capacity. *Off-line storage* refers to optical disks or magnetic tape cassettes stored on shelves or racks. Obtaining a study from off-line storage requires a person to locate the relevant disk, cartridge, or cassette and to manually load it into a drive. When hierarchical storage is used, if considerable delays in displaying older studies are to be avoided, the system must automatically copy ("prefetch") relevant older studies from near-line to online storage to be available for comparison when new studies are viewed.

An alternative to hierarchical storage is to store all images on arrays of magnetic hard disk drives. As these become full, more disk arrays are added to the system. This storage scheme has become feasible because of the increasing capacities of magnetic drives and the decreasing cost per unit storage capacity. This method is commonly referred to as "everything on line" storage.

Regardless of the storage scheme, the PACS must create and maintain a copy or copies of all information on separate storage devices for backup and disaster recovery. This is discussed later in this chapter in the section on security. The backup storage should be in a location such that a single plausible incident would not destroy both the primary and backup information.

Image Management

The PACS archive may be centralized, or it may be distributed, that is, stored at several locations on a network. In either case, there must be archive management software on a server. The archive management software includes a database program that contains information about the stored studies and their locations in the archive. The archive management software communicates over the network with imaging devices sending studies for storage and sends copies of the studies received from imaging devices to the storage devices, including to backup storage. The transfers between imaging devices and the PACS usually conform to the DICOM standard. The archive management software must also obtain studies from the storage devices and send either the studies or selected images from them to workstations requesting studies or images for display. In PACS with hierarchical storage, the archive management software transfers studies between the various levels of archival storage, based upon factors such as the recentness of the study and, when a new study is ordered, prefetches relevant older studies from near-line storage to online storage to reduce the time required for display.

In some PACS, studies or images from studies awaiting interpretation and relevant older studies are requested by viewing workstations from the PACS archive as needed ("on demand") during viewing sessions, but this can slow the workflow process of the interpreting physician. Alternatively, studies may be obtained ("prefetched") from the archive and stored on a display workstation or local file server, prior to the interpretation session, ready for the interpreting physician's use. The prefetch method requires the interpretation workstations or server to have more local storage capacity, whereas the on-demand method requires a faster archive and faster network connections between the archive and the interpretation workstations. An advantage to the on-demand method is that a physician may use any available workstation to view a particular study, whereas to view a particular study with the prefetch method, the physician must go to a workstation that has access to the locally stored study. When images are fetched on-demand, the first image should be available for viewing within about two seconds. Once images reside on the local workstation's disk or local server, they are nearly instantaneously available.

On-demand systems may send all the images in entire studies to the workstation, or they may just send individual images when requested by the viewing workstation.

The method of sending entire studies at once requires greater network bandwidth and much more magnetic disk storage capacity on the viewing workstation and causes greater delay before the first images are displayed, but once the images are stored on the viewing workstation's disk, they are nearly instantaneously available. On the other hand, providing only individual images upon request by the viewing workstation reduces the delay before the first image or images are displayed, but places more demand on the archive server to respond to frequent requests for individual images.

Image Compression

The massive amount of data in radiological studies (Table 5-10) poses considerable challenges regarding storage and transmission. Image compression reduces the number of bytes in an image or set of images, thereby decreasing the time required to transfer images and increasing the number of images that can be stored on a magnetic disk or unit of removable storage media. Compression can reduce costs by permitting the use of network links of lower bandwidth and by reducing the amount of required storage. Before display, the image must be decompressed (Fig. 5-25). Image compression and decompression can be performed by either a general-purpose computer or specialized hardware. Image compression and decompression are calculation-intensive tasks and can delay image display. The compression ratio is the number of bytes of the uncompressed image divided by the number of bytes of the compressed image.

There are two categories of compression: *reversible*, also called bit-preserving, lossless, or recoverable compression; and *irreversible*, also called lossy or nonrecoverable, compression. In reversible compression, the uncompressed image is identical to the original. Typically, reversible compression of medical images provides compression ratios from about two to three. Reversible compression takes advantage of redundancies in data. It is not possible to store random and equally likely bit patterns in less space without the loss of information. However, medical images incorporate considerable redundancies, permitting them to be converted into a more compact representation without loss of information. For example, although an image may have a dynamic range (difference between maximal and minimal pixel values) requiring 12 bits per pixel, pixel values usually change only slightly from pixel to adjacent pixel and so changes from one pixel to the next can be represented by just

TABLE 5-10   IMAGE STORAGE REQUIREMENTS FOR VARIOUS RADIOLOGICAL STUDIES, IN UNCOMPRESSED FORM

STUDY	TYPICAL STORAGE (MB)
Chest radiographs (PA and lateral, 2 × 2.5 k)	20
Standard CT series of the head (50 512^2 images)	26
Tl-201 myocardial perfusion SPECT study	1
Ultrasound (512^2, 60 images to PACS archive)	16
Cardiac cath lab study (coronary and LV images)	450–3,000
Digital screening mammograms (2 CC and 2 MLO)	60–132

Note: The number of images per study varies greatly depending on the type of study (e.g., CT cardiac angiography), number of acquisition phases, and whether thin slices for MPRs are necessary, which can increase the number of images by an order of magnitude. Storage is calculated as the product of the number of images and the size in bytes of an image.

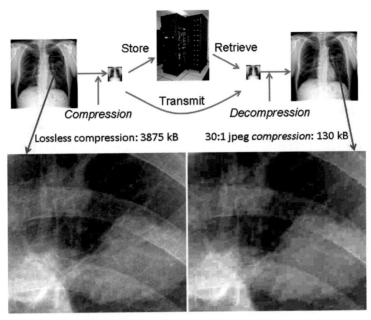

■ FIGURE 5-25 Image compression reduces the number of bytes in an image to reduce image storage space and image transmission times. At a display workstation, an image retrieved from the archive over the network require image decompression, which restores the images to full physical size (number of pixels) and number of bytes. Shown above is a chest image with lossless compression (**left**), and 30:1 jpeg lossy compression (**right**). Although the minified images (above) look similar, the magnified views (below) illustrate loss of image fidelity and nondiagnostic image quality with too much lossy compression.

a few bits. In this case, the image could be compressed without a loss of information by storing the differences between adjacent pixel values instead of the pixel values themselves. Dynamic image sequences, because of similarities from one image to the next, permit high compression ratios.

In irreversible compression, information is lost and so the uncompressed image will not exactly match the original image. However, irreversible compression permits much higher compression; ratios of 15-to-one or higher are possible with very little loss of image quality. Currently, there is controversy on how much compression can be tolerated. Research shows that the amount of compression is strongly dependent upon the type of examination, the compression algorithm used, and the way that the image is displayed (e.g., on film or display monitor). In some cases, images that are irreversibly compressed and subsequently decompressed are actually preferred by radiologists over the original images, due to the reduction of image noise. Legal considerations also affect decisions on the use of irreversible compression in medical imaging. The ACR *Technical Standard for Electronic Practice of Medical Imaging* (2008) states, "Data compression may be performed to facilitate transmission and storage. The type of medical image, the modality, and the objective of the study will determine the degree of acceptable compression. Several methods, including both reversible and irreversible techniques… may be used under the direction of a qualified physician or practitioner, with minimal if any reduction in clinical diagnostic image quality. If compression is used, algorithms recommended by the DICOM standard … should be used. The types and ratios of compression used for different imaging studies transmitted and stored by the system should be selected and periodically reviewed by the responsible physician to ensure appropriate clinical image quality."

However, at the time of printing, the US Food and Drug Administration (FDA), under the authority of the federal Mammography Quality Standards Act, restricts the use of lossy compression in mammography. In particular, the FDA does not permit mammograms compressed by lossy methods to be used for final interpretation, nor does it accept the storage of mammograms compressed by lossy methods to meet the requirements for retention of original mammograms. The FDA does permit interpretation of digital mammograms compressed by lossless methods and considers storage of such mammograms to meet the requirement for retention of original mammograms. The reader should refer to current guidance from the FDA on this topic.

Display of Images

Images from a PACS may be displayed on monitors or, less often, may be recorded by a laser imager on light-sensitive film, which is chemically developed, and then viewed on light boxes. The purpose of the display system is to present anatomic and/or physiologic information in the form of images to interpreting physicians and other clinicians.

Computer workstations equipped with display monitors are commonly used, instead of viewboxes and photographic film, to display radiological images for both interpretation and review. The various radiological modalities impose specific requirements on workstations. For example, a workstation that is suitable for the interpretation of nuclear medicine or ultrasound images may not be adequate for digital radiographs or mammograms.

As mentioned earlier in this chapter, the CRT monitors once used for radiological image display have been mostly replaced by high-quality LCD monitors. The physical principles and performance of these devices were described earlier in this chapter and only their use in medical imaging will be discussed here.

Display Workstations

Display Systems for Workstations

As mentioned above, the various imaging modalities impose specific requirements on workstations. An interpretation workstation for large matrix images (digital radiographs, including mammograms) is commonly equipped with two high-luminance 54-cm diagonal 3 or 5 megapixel grayscale monitors, in the portrait orientation, to permit the simultaneous comparison of two images in near full spatial resolution (Fig. 5-26). A "navigation" monitor is also present on a diagnostic workstation to provide access to the RIS database, patient information, reading worklist, digital voice dictation system, EMR, and the Internet. Such a workstation is also suitable for viewing CT and MRI images, unless surface and volume rendering are utilized, in which case color monitors are preferable. Such a workstation can also be used to view digital fluorographs and, if it has adequate cine capability, angiographic images. Three megapixel 54-cm diagonal color monitors are available with sufficient calibrated maximal luminances (400 to 500 cd/m^2) for viewing radiographs, and are now a typical choice for replacing older grayscale monitors. Another monitor format that is becoming popular is the 76-cm diagonal monitor, available with 4, 6, or 10 megapixels, designed to replace a pair of 54-cm

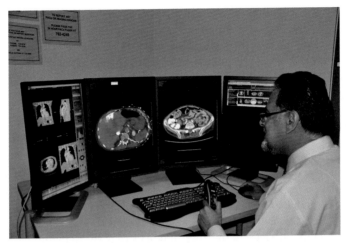

■ **FIGURE 5-26** Interpretation workstation containing two 1.5 by 2 k pixel (3 megapixel) portrait-format grayscale monitors for high resolution and high luminance image interpretation, flanked by two 1.9 by 1 k (2 megapixel MP) color "navigation" monitors (**left and right**) for PACS access, patient worklist, timeline, and thumbnail image displays; multipurpose display for 3D color rendering, digital voice dictation reporting, and EMR and RIS information access. The keyboard, mouse, and image navigation and voice dictation device assist Ramit Lamba, M.D., in his interpretation duties.

diagonal monitors. Such a monitor provides a seamless viewing area. However, when a pair of 54-cm monitors is used, each can be turned slightly inward to face the viewer, whereas, when a 76-cm monitor displays a pair of radiographs, the viewer must move his or her head from side to side to look directly at each radiograph.

Workstations for viewing CT and MRI images, fluorographs, and angiographic images can have smaller pixel format monitors. If surface or volume rendered images or co-registered PET/CT or SPECT/CT images are to be displayed, the workstation should be equipped with high-luminance color monitors. Workstations for interpretation of angiographic image sequences (e.g., cardiac angiograms and ventriculograms and digital subtraction angiograms) should be capable of displaying cine images (sequences of images acquired to depict temporal variations in anatomy or contrast material).

Workstations for the interpretation of nuclear medicine and ultrasound images should have color monitors and must be able to display cine images. A single color monitor with a pixel format on the order of 1,000 × 1,000 is sufficient for a nuclear medicine or ultrasound workstation.

Most noninterpreting physicians typically use standard commercial personal computers with consumer-grade color monitors, although some, such as orthopedic surgeons, may require specialized workstations with display systems similar to those of interpreting physicians.

An application program on the workstation permits the interpreting physician to select images, arrange them for display, and manipulate them. The way in which the program arranges the images for presentation and display is called a *hanging protocol*. The hanging protocols should be configurable to the preferences of individual physicians. Image manipulation capabilities of the program should include window and level, and zoom (magnify) and roam (pan). In particular, because the dynamic range of a display monitor is much less than that of film on a viewbox, windowing and leveling are needed to compensate. The program should also provide quantitative tools to permit accurate measurements of distance and the display of individual pixel values in modality-appropriate units (e.g., CT numbers). Image processing, such as smoothing and edge enhancement, may be provided. Modality-specific or physician specialty–specific tools may be needed. For example, ultrasound and nuclear medicine have specific display and tool requirements and orthopedic surgeons and cardiologists have specific requirements such as specific quantitative and angular measurements.

Ambient Viewing Conditions

Proper ambient viewing conditions, where interpretation workstations are used, are needed to permit the interpreting physicians' eyes to adapt to the low luminances of the monitors, to avoid a loss in contrast from diffuse reflections from the faces of the monitors, and to avoid specular reflections on the monitor's faces from bright objects. Viewing conditions are more important when monitors are used than when view-boxes are used, because of the lower luminances of the monitors. The faces of LCDs are flat and less reflective than those of CRTs and so LCDs are less affected by diffuse and specular reflections. The replacement of CRT monitors by LCD monitors has made ambient viewing conditions less critical. The photometric quantity *illuminance*, also discussed in Chapter 8, describes the rate of light energy, adjusted for the photopic spectral sensitivity of the human visual system, impinging on a surface, per unit area. In areas used for viewing clinical images from display monitors, the illuminance should be low (20–40 lux), but not so low as to interfere with other necessary tasks, such as reading printed documents, or to require a major adjustment in adaption when looking at a monitor after looking at another object, or vice versa. A reading room should have adjustable indirect lighting and should not have windows unless they can be blocked with opaque curtains or shutters. When more than one workstation is in a room, provisions should be made, either by monitor placement or by the use of partitions, to prevent monitors from casting reflections on each other. Particular care must be taken, if both conventional viewboxes and viewing workstations are used in the same room, to prevent the viewboxes from casting reflections on monitor screens and impairing the adaptation of physicians' eyes to the dimmer monitors.

Challenges of PACS

There are many challenges to implementing, using, maintaining, upgrading, and replacing PACS. An important goal is achieving efficient workflow. There are far too many issues regarding efficiency of workflow to be listed here; this paragraph merely lists several important objectives. Prior to image acquisition by an imaging device, little manual entry of information should be required by imaging technologists. This can be facilitated by utilizing "modality worklists" generated by the radiology information system and sent to the modality. Worklists of studies to be interpreted, arranged by factors such as modality and priority, should be provided to interpreting physicians. Images should be displayed promptly, ideally within two seconds, to referring and interpreting physicians. Little or no manipulation of images should be routinely necessary; automated hanging protocols should display the images in the order, orientation, magnification, and position on the monitor expected. Software tools should be available to technologists to help identify studies that are not assigned to the proper patient, are mislabeled, or require image manipulation. Image interpretation is made more efficient by a digital speech recognition system that promptly displays the dictated report for review and approval by the interpreting physician before he or she interprets the next study. These systems greatly decrease the turn-around-time of diagnostic reports, and are a major benefit to the referring physician and ultimately to the patient.

Major challenges include the following:

1. Initial and recurring equipment purchase or lease costs.
2. Expensive technical personnel to support the PACS.
3. Training new users in system operation.
4. Achieving communication among equipment from several vendors.
5. Achieving information transfer among digital information systems (PACS, RIS, HIS, EMR).
6. Maintaining security of images and related information and compliance with Health Insurance Portability and Accountability Act (HIPAA) Regulations (discussed in a later section).
7. Equipment failures can impede interpretation and distribution of images and reports.
8. Digital storage media longevity and obsolescence.
9. Maintaining access to images and data during PACS upgrades.
10. Maintaining access to archived images and related data if: converting to a new archival technology, the PACS vendor goes out of business, the PACS vendor ceases to support particular the PACS, or you replace the system with a PACS from another vendor.
11. Providing access to and display of legacy film images.
12. Conversion of film images into digital images. (Some facilities choose to not convert old film images to digital images.)
13. Completely eliminating the production of film images.
14. Locating misidentified studies.
15. Multiple PACS in a single healthcare enterprise.
16. Obtaining and importing images from outside your healthcare enterprise.
17. Providing images and reports to healthcare providers outside your healthcare enterprise.
18. Quality control program for display monitors.
19. Providing adequate software tools for specialists such as orthopedic surgeons and cardiologists.

This list is far from complete. Of course, the desirable strategy is to enhance the advantages and minimize the disadvantages. Benefits will expand as experience with these systems increases. Furthermore, the rapidly increasing capabilities and falling costs of the technology used in PACS will continue to increase their performance while reducing their cost.

Quality Control of PACS and Teleradiology Systems

PACS and teleradiology systems are part of the imaging chain and therefore require quality control monitoring. Although both analog and digital portions of the system can degrade images, the performance of digital portions (computer network, software, storage, etc.) regarding image quality does not usually change with time. The performance of analog portions (film digitizers, laser printers, and display monitors) changes with time and therefore requires monitoring. Quality control can be divided into acceptance testing, to determine if newly installed components meet desired performance specifications, and routine performance monitoring. Display monitors must be evaluated periodically to ensure all the monitors of a workstation have adequate maximal calibrated luminances and the same display characteristics.

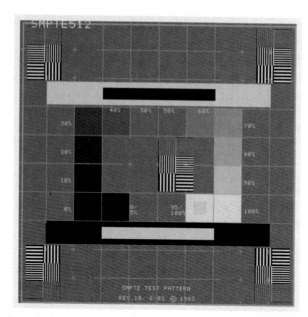

■ **FIGURE 5-27** Society of Motion Picture and Television Engineers (SMPTE) monitor test pattern. This pattern allows the inspection of spatial resolution in the center and at the corners of the image (high and low contrast line patterns in horizontal and vertical orientations), assessment of contrast differences over the entire range of luminance by the ten 10% intensity steps, contrast in the dark and bright areas of the image (5% patches in the 0% and 100% bright areas, when used with a linear LUT), brightness linearity across the range of grayscale values, geometric linearity grid pattern, and transitions from dark to bright and bright to dark.

In particular, the display functions of grayscale monitors and color monitors that display grayscale images should be evaluated to ensure that they conform to the DICOM GSDF. The maximal luminance of a display monitor degrades with the amount of time that the monitor is on and with the brightness of displayed images. Turning LCD monitors off when they will not be used for an extended period of time can significantly prolong their lives; however, monitors may take some time to stabilize from a cold start, so a common strategy is to place them into a "standby" mode. Monitors should be replaced when their maximal luminances become inadequate. Some medical grade LCD monitors can measure their own luminances and can send information on their maximal calibrated luminances and conformance to the DICOM GSDF across a network to a workstation, greatly simplifying the task of monitoring display monitor performance.

Test patterns, such as the Society of Motion Picture and Television Engineers (SMPTE) Test Pattern (Fig. 5-27) are useful for semi-quantitative assessments of display monitor performance. The American Association of Physicists in Medicine has available a set of test images for monitor quality control and evaluation.** Monitor faces should be cleaned frequently to remove fingerprints and other dirt to avoid image artifacts.

Another important quality assurance task is ensuring that acquired studies are properly associated with the correct patients in the PACS, RIS, and EMR. Problems can occur if an error is made in manually entering patient identifying information, if a technologist selects the wrong patient identifier from a modality worklist, an imaging

---

**http://aapm.org/pubs/reports/OR_03.pdf

study is performed on an unidentified patient, or if a patient's name is changed, such as after a marriage. These can result in imaging studies stored in a PACS that are not associated with the proper patients. Procedures should be established to identify such incorrectly associated studies and to associate them with the proper patients.

5.8 Image Processing

An important use of computers in medical imaging is to process digital images to display the information contained in the images in more useful forms. Digital image processing cannot add information to images. For example, if an imaging modality cannot resolve objects less that a particular size, image processing cannot cause such objects to be seen.

In some cases, the information of interest is visible in the unprocessed images and is merely made more conspicuous. In other cases, information of interest may not be visible at all in the unprocessed image data. X-ray CT is an example of the latter case; observation of the raw projection data fails to reveal many of the structures visible in the processed cross-sectional images. The following examples of image processing are described only superficially and will be discussed in detail in later chapters.

The addition or subtraction of digital images is used in several imaging modalities. Both of these operations require the images being added or subtracted to be of the same format (same number of pixels along each axis of the images) and produce a resultant image (sum image or difference image) in that format. In image subtraction, each pixel in one image is subtracted from the corresponding pixel in a second image to yield the corresponding pixel value in the difference image. Image addition is similar, but with pixel-by-pixel addition instead of subtraction. Image subtraction is used in digital subtraction angiography to remove the effects of stationary anatomic structures not of interest from the images of contrast-enhanced blood vessels and in nuclear gated cardiac blood pool imaging to yield difference images depicting ventricular stroke-volume and ventricular wall dyskinesis.

Spatial filtering is used in many types of medical imaging. Medical images commonly have a grainy appearance, called *quantum mottle*, caused by the statistical nature of the acquisition process. The visibility of quantum mottle can be reduced by a spatial filtering operation called *smoothing*. In most spatial smoothing algorithms, each pixel value in the smoothed image is obtained by a weighted averaging of the corresponding pixel in the unprocessed image with its neighbors. Although smoothing reduces quantum mottle, it also blurs the image. Images must not be smoothed to the extent that clinically significant detail is lost. Spatial filtering can also enhance the edges of structures in an image. Edge-enhancement increases the statistical noise in the image. Convolution filtering, the method used for most spatial filtering, is discussed in detail in Chapter 4.

A computer can calculate physiologic performance indices from image data. For example, the estimation of the left ventricular ejection fraction from nuclear gated cardiac blood pool image sequences is described in Chapter 18. In some cases, these data may be displayed graphically, such as the time-activity curves of a bolus of a radiopharmaceutical passing through the kidneys.

In x-ray and nuclear CT, sets of projection images are acquired from different angles about the long axes of patients. From these sets of projection images, computers calculate cross-sectional images depicting tissue linear attenuation coefficients (x-ray CT) or radionuclide concentration (SPECT and PET). The methods by which volumetric data sets are reconstructed from projection images are discussed in detail in Chapters 10 and 19.

In *image co-registration*, image data from one medical imaging modality is super-imposed on a spatially congruent image from another modality. Image co-registration is especially useful when one of the modalities, such as SPECT or PET, provides physiologic information lacking anatomic detail and the other modality, often MRI or x-ray CT, provides inferior physiologic information, but superb depiction of anatomy. When the images are obtained using two separate devices, co-registration poses formidable difficulties in matching the position, orientation, and magnification of one image to the other. To greatly simplify co-registration, PET and SPECT devices that incorporate x-ray CT systems have been developed and are discussed in Chapter 19.

Computer-Aided Detection

Computer-aided detection, also known as computer-aided diagnosis, uses a computer program to detect features likely to be of clinical significance in images. Its purpose is not to replace the interpreting physician, but to assist by calling attention to structures that might have been overlooked. For example, software is available to automatically locate structures suggestive of masses, clusters of microcalcifications, and architectural distortions in mammographic images (Chapter 8). Computer-aided detection can improve the sensitivity of the interpretation, but also may reduce the specificity. (Sensitivity and specificity are defined in Chapter 4.)

Display of Volumetric Image Data

High spatial resolution, thin slice tomographic imaging modalities (e.g., CT and MRI) provide image sets that can exceed a thousand images covering large volumes of patients. SPECT and PET, which have lower spatial resolution and therefore typically produce smaller image sets, are commonly co-registered on CT image sets. The display and interpretation of these massive image sets presents formidable challenges to display systems, interpreting physicians, and other clinicians.

Stack versus Tile Mode Display

Tomographic images were once recorded on film and displayed side by side on motorized light boxes. In early PACS systems, radiologists often replicated this side-by-side viewing by attempting to simultaneously display all images in a study. This side-by-side image display is referred-to as "tile-mode" display and early display workstations were commonly equipped with four or more video monitors for this purpose. Tile mode display became increasing impractical with thin slice image acquisitions and correspondingly larger numbers of transaxial images. Tile mode display has been largely replaced by stack mode display, in which only a single image is displayed at a time and, as the viewing clinician manipulates a pointing device or key on the keyboard, the computer successively replaces that image with the next adjacent image. Stack mode permits the viewer to follow blood vessels and organ boundaries while scrolling through the images.

Multiplanar Reformatting

Multiplanar reconstruction (MPR) is the reformatting of a volumetric dataset (e.g., a stack of axial images) into tomographic images by selecting pixel values from the dataset that correspond to the desired tomographic image planes. MPR is most commonly used to produce images that are parallel to one or more of the three orthogonal planes: axial, coronal, and sagittal. In many cases (especially CT), the data are acquired in the axial plane. A coronal image can be formed from such a dataset by selecting a specific row of pixel values from each axial image. Similarly, a sagittal image can be created by selecting a specific column of pixel values from each axial image. Oblique reconstructions (arbitrary planes that are not orthogonal to the axial plane), "slab" (thicker plane) presentations, and curved MPR images are also commonly produced. The latter are obtained along user-determined curved surfaces through the volumetric dataset that follow anatomic structures such as the spine, aorta, or a coronary artery. In MPR, particularly in creating oblique and curved images, some pixels of the MPR images may not exactly correspond to the locations of values in the volumetric dataset. In this case, the pixel values in the MPR images are created by interpolation of the values in the nearest pixels in the volumetric dataset. Figure 5-28 shows three MPR images.

Maximum Intensity Projection Images

Maximum intensity projection (MIP) is a method of forming projection images by casting "rays" through a volume dataset and selecting the maximal pixel value along each ray. The rays may be parallel or they may diverge from a point in space; in either case, each ray intersects the center of one pixel in the projection image. This method is extremely useful for depicting high signals in a volume (e.g., contrast CT or MRI studies) for vascular angiography or demonstrating calcified plaque in vasculature, for instance. A variation is thin or thick slab MIP, using MPR projections and a selectable number of image slices (a slab), displaying the maximum values obtained along rays projected through the slab. Figure 5-28 shows two thin-slab MIP images.

Volume Rendering

For some applications, there are advantages to providing a 2D image that contains depth cues to permit it to be viewed as a 3D object. Two approaches are shaded surface displays, also called surface rendering (not significantly used) and volume rendering. In both approaches, the first step is to segment the volume set into different structures (e.g., bones and soft tissue). Segmentation may be done entirely by the computer or with guidance by a person. Segmentation is simplest when there are large differences in the pixel values among the tissues or other objects to be segmented.

Shaded surface display (SSD) provides a simulated 3D view of surfaces of an object or objects in the volume dataset. First, the surfaces to be displayed must be identified. For instance, for bony structures on CT images, this can be by simple thresholding to exclude soft tissues. Alternatively, they may be identified by a gradient edge-detection technique. Surfaces are identified by marking individual voxels as belonging or not belonging to the surface, creating a binary dataset. Then the computer calculates the observed light intensity in the SSD image by calculating the reflections from simulated direct and diffuse light sources. The surface may be displayed in shades of gray or in color, such as flesh-tone for "fly-through" colonoscopy image sequences. Shaded surface display algorithms are computationally efficient; however, a major disadvantage of SSDs is that only a very small fraction of the information in the original image dataset is displayed. Furthermore, errors may occur in the identification of the surface to be displayed.

Volume rendering, in contrast to SSD and MIP, uses a more complete set of the voxels within the stacked axial images. In volume rendering, each voxel in the image volume of a stacked tomographic image set is assigned an opacity ranging from 0% to 100% and a color. A voxel assigned an opacity of 0% will be invisible in the final image and assigning a voxel an opacity of 100% will prevent the viewing of voxels behind it. A voxel with an opacity between 0% and 100% will be visible and will permit the viewing of voxels behind it. The voxels in the volume image set are segmented into those corresponding to various organs, tissues, and

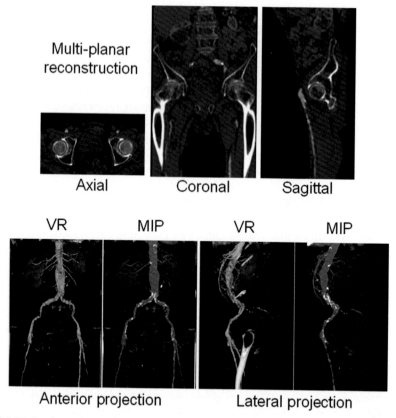

Multi-planar reconstruction

Axial   Coronal   Sagittal

VR   MIP   VR   MIP

Anterior projection   Lateral projection

■ **FIGURE 5-28** A volumetric view from a 3D tomographic dataset is depicted. **Top**. multiplanar reconstruction from axial images include coronal and sagittal views with 1.25 mm slice thickness; **Bottom**. volume rendered dataset from the full volume with bone removal, and corresponding thin-slab maximum intensity projection (MIP) images for the anterior and posterior projections.

objects (e.g., bone, soft tissue, contrast enhanced blood vessels, air, fat) based upon specific ranges of pixel values (e.g., CT numbers or MRI digital values), perhaps also using assumptions about anatomy and/or guidance by a person. Then, opacity values and colors are assigned to voxels containing specific tissues. The assignments of these artificial characteristics to the voxels containing specific tissues are selected from predefined templates for specific imaging protocols and organ systems (e.g., CT angiogram, pulmonary embolism, or fracture). Next, as in MIP image formation, a set of rays, parallel or diverging from a point, are cast through the volume dataset, with each ray passing through the center of a pixel in the volume rendered image. Each pixel value in the volume rendered image is calculated from the opacities and colors of the voxels along the ray corresponding to that pixel. Simulated lighting effects may be added. Volume rendering provides a robust view of the anatomy and depth relationships. On the other hand, it displays only a small fraction of the information in the initial image dataset, although much more that SSD or MIP. Furthermore, segmentation errors can occur, causing errors in the displayed anatomy. Additionally, the color assignments, while appearing realistic, are arbitrary and can be misleading because of erroneous tissue classification. Nevertheless, volume rendering is useful for surgical planning and provides images that are easy for referring physicians to understand. Figure 5-28 shows thin-slab MIP and volume rendered images.

5.9   Security, Including Availablility

An important issue regarding medical imaging, PACS, and teleradiology is information security. The main goals of information security are (1) privacy, (2) integrity, (3) authentication, (4) nonrepudiation, and (5) availability. Privacy, also called confidentiality, refers to denying persons, other than intended recipients, access to confidential information. Integrity means that information has not been altered, either accidentally or deliberately. Authentication permits the recipient of information to verify the identity of the sender and the sender to verify the identity of the intended recipient. Nonrepudiation prevents a person from later denying an action, such as approval of a payment or approval of a report. Availability means that information and services are available when needed.

Privacy is commonly achieved either by storing information in a secure location, such as locked room, or by encrypting the information into a code that only intended recipients can convert to its original form. Unintentional alteration of information can be detected by use of an error detecting code. A sending computer calculates the error detecting code from the information to be transmitted over a network and sends the code along with the transmitted information. The receiving computer calculates the error detecting code from the information it receives and compares the code it calculated to the code sent with information. If the two codes match, there is a high degree of assurance that the information was transmitted without error. Protection against intentional modification can be achieved by encrypting both the transmitted information and the error detecting code. Authentication is usually performed by the use of passwords, which are encrypted when transmitted across a network, or by using biometric methods, such as a scan of a person's fingerprint or retina. Measures to ensure availability are described later in this section.

The federal Health Insurance Portability and Accountability Act of 1996 (HIPAA) and associated federal regulations (45 CFR 164) impose security requirements for "electronic protected healthcare information." Goals of the HIPAA regulations are to

1. Ensure the confidentiality, integrity, and availability of all electronic protected healthcare information
2. Identify and protect against reasonably anticipated threats or hazards to the security or integrity of the information
3. Protect against reasonably anticipated impermissible uses or disclosures
4. Ensure compliance by the workforce

The security measures described below largely conform to HIPAA security regulations, but do not include all such requirements. Furthermore, the regulations are subject to change. Hence, a person responsible for a security program should refer to the current regulations.

A major danger in using a computer is that the operating system, applications programs, and important information are often stored on a single disk; an accident could cause all of them to be lost. The primary threats to information and software on digital storage devices or media are mechanical or electrical malfunction, such as a disk head crash; human error, such as the accidental deletion of a file or the accidental formatting of a disk (potentially causing the loss of all information on the disk); and malicious damage. To reduce the risk of information loss, important files should be copied ("backed up") onto magnetic disks, optical disks, or magnetic tape at regularly scheduled times, with the backup copies stored in a distant secure location.

Programs written with malicious intent are a threat to computers. The most prevalent of these are computer viruses. A virus is a string of instructions hidden in a program. If a program containing a virus is loaded into a computer and executed, the virus copies itself into other programs stored on mass storage devices. If a copy of an infected program is sent to another computer and executed, that computer becomes infected. Although a virus need not do harm, many deliberately cause damage, such as the deletion of all files on the disk on Friday the 13th. Viruses that are not intended to cause damage may interfere with the operation of the computer or cause damage because they are poorly written. A computer cannot be infected with a virus by the importation of data alone or by the user reading an e-mail message. However, a computer can become infected if an infected file is attached to an e-mail message and if that file is executed.

Malicious programs also include Trojan horses, programs that are presented as being of interest so people will load them onto computers, but have hidden purposes; worms, programs that automatically spread over computer networks; time bombs, programs or program segments that do something harmful, such as change or delete information, on a future date; key loggers, programs that record everything typed by a user, which can later be viewed for information of use, such as login names, passwords, and financial and personal information; and password grabbers, programs that ask people to log in and store the passwords and other login information for unauthorized use. A virus, worm, or Trojan horse may incorporate a time bomb or key logger. In 1988, a worm largely brought the Internet to a standstill. The primary way to reduce the chance of a virus infection or other problem from malicious software is to establish a policy forbidding the loading of storage media and software from untrustworthy sources. Commercial virus-protection software, which searches files on storage devices and files received over a network for known viruses and removes them, should be used. The final line of defense, however, is the saving of backup copies. Once a computer is infected, it may be necessary to reformat all disks and reload all software and information from the backup copies. A related threat is a denial of service attack, the bombardment of a computer or network with so many messages that it cannot function. Denial of service attacks are commonly launched from multiple computers that are being controlled by malicious software.

Sophisticated computer operating systems provide security features including password protection and the ability to grant individual users different levels of access to stored files. Measures should be taken to deny unauthorized users access to your system. Passwords should be used to deny access, directly and over a network or a modem. Each user should be granted only the privileges required to accomplish needed tasks. For example, technologists who acquire and process studies and interpreting physicians should not be granted the ability to delete or modify system software files or patient studies, whereas the system manager must be granted full privileges to all files on the system.

Security measures include administrative, physical, and technical safeguards. The following is a list of elements in a PACS and teleradiology security plan:

1. Perform a risk analysis.
2. Establish written policies and procedures for information security.
3. Train staff in the policies and procedures.
4. Backups—Maintain copies of important programs and information in case the data on a single device are lost. Backup copies should be stored in a secure location remote from the primary storage.
5. Install commercial anti-virus software on all computers to identify and remove common viruses and periodically update the software to recognize the signatures of recent viruses.

6. Forbid the loading of removable media (e.g., floppy and optical disks from the homes of staff) and programs from nontrustworthy sources and forbid activating attachments to unexpected e-mail messages.
7. Authenticate users, directly and over a network or a modem, by passwords. Use secure passwords.
8. Terminate promptly the access privileges of former employees.
9. "Log off" workstations, particularly those in nonsecure areas, when not in use.
10. Grant each user only sufficient privileges required to accomplish needed tasks and only access to information to which the user requires access.
11. Secure transfer—Encrypt information transferred over nonsecure networks.
12. Secure storage—Physically secure media (e.g., store it in a room to which access is controlled) or encrypt the information on it.
13. Erase information on or destroy removable media and storage devices before disposal or transfer for reuse. On most operating systems, deleting a file merely removes the listing of the file from the device directory. The information remains stored on the device or media.
14. Install "patches" to the operating system to fix security vulnerabilities.
15. Install "firewalls" (described below) at nodes where your LAN is connected to other networks.
16. Audit trails—Each access to protected healthcare information must be recorded.
17. Establish an emergency operations and disaster recovery plan.

The goal of availability is to ensure that acquired studies can be interpreted and stored images can be viewed at all times. Availability is achieved by the use of reliable components and media, fault-tolerant and risk-informed design and installation, provisions for prompt repair, and an emergency operation and disaster recovery plan. A design that continues to function despite equipment failure is said to be fault tolerant. The design of a PACS must take into account the fact that equipment will fail. Fault tolerance usually implies redundancy of critical components. Not all components are critical. For example, in a PACS with a central archive connected by a network to multiple workstations, the failure of a single workstation would have little adverse effect, but failure of the archive or network could prevent the interpretation of studies.

An essential element of fault tolerance is for the PACS to create and maintain copies of all information on separate and remote storage devices for backup and disaster recovery. Offsite storage for disaster recovery, perhaps leased from a commercial vendor, is an option. The value of a study declines with time after its acquisition and so, therefore, does the degree of protection required against its loss. A very high degree of protection is necessary until it has been interpreted.

The design of the PACS and the policies and procedures for its use should take into account the probability and possible consequences of risks, such as human error; deliberate attempts at sabotage, including computer viruses, worms, and denial of service attacks; fire; water leaks; and natural disasters such as floods, storms, and earthquakes. Examples are installing a redundant PACS archive far from the primary archive, preferably in another building, and, in an area vulnerable to flooding, not installing a PACS archive in a basement or ground floor of a building.

Provisions for repair of a PACS are important. A failure of a critical component is less serious if it is quickly repaired. Arrangements for emergency service should be made in advance of equipment failure.

Computer networks pose significant security challenges. Unauthorized persons can access a computer over the network and, on some LANs, any computer on the network can be programmed to read the traffic. If a network is connected to the Internet, it is vulnerable to attack by every "hacker" on the planet.

Not only must the confidentiality and integrity of information be protected during transmission across a network, but the computers on the network must be protected from unauthorized access via the network. A simple way to protect a network is to not connect it to other networks. However, this may greatly limit its usefulness. For example, at a medical center, it is useful to connect the network supporting a PACS to the main hospital network. The main hospital network typically provides a link to the Internet as well.

A *firewall* can enhance the security of a network or network segment. A firewall is a program, router, computer, or even a small network that is used to connect two networks to provide security. There are many services that can be provided by a firewall. One of the simplest is packet filtering, in which the firewall examines packets reaching it. It reads their source and destination addresses and the applications for which they are intended and, based upon rules established by the network administrator, forwards or discards them. For example, packet filtering can limit which computers a person outside the firewall can access and can forbid certain kinds of access, such as FTP and Telnet. Different rules may be applied to incoming and outgoing packets. Thus, the privileges of users outside the firewall can be restricted without limiting the ability of users on the protected network to access computers past the firewall. Firewalls also can maintain records of the traffic across the firewall, to help detect and diagnose attacks on the network. A firewall, by itself, does not provide complete protection and thus should merely be part of a comprehensive computer security program.

SUGGESTED READINGS

American Association of Physicists in Medicine Task Group 18, AAPM On-Line Report No. 03, *Assessment of display performance for medical imaging systems.* April 2005.

American College of Radiology, ACR Technical Standard for Electronic Practice of Medical Imaging. *ACR Practice Guidelines and Technical Standards,* 2007.

American College of Radiology. ACR—SIIM Practice Guideline for Electronic Medical Information Privacy and Security. *ACR Practice Guidelines and Technical Standards,* 2009.

Badano A. Principles of cathode ray tube and liquid crystal display devices. In: *Advances in digital radiography: categorical course in diagnostic radiology physics.* Oak Brook, IL: Radiological Society of North America, 2003:91–102.

Barten PGJ. *Contrast sensitivity of the human eye and its effects on image quality.* Bellingham, WA: SPIE Optical Engineering Press, 1999.

Branstetter BF IV. Basics of imaging informatics, part 1. *Radiology* 2007;243:656–667.

Clunie DA. DICOM implementations for digital radiography. In: *Advances in digital radiography: categorical course in diagnostic radiology physics.* Radiological Society of North America, 2003:163–172.

Code of Federal Regulations, 45 CFR Part 164, HIPAA Privacy and Security Regulations.

Cohen MD, Rumreich LL, Garriot KM, et al. Planning for PACS: a comprehensive guide to nontechnical considerations. *J Am Coll Radiol* 2005;2:327–337.

Cusma JT, Wondrow MA, Holmes DR. Image storage considerations in the cardiac catheterization laboratory. In: *Categorical course in diagnostic radiology physics: cardiac catheterization imaging.* Oak Brook, IL: Radiological Society of North America, 1998.

Digital Imaging and Communications in Medicine (DICOM) Part 1: Introduction and Overview, PS 3.1-2011, National Electrical Manufacturers Association, 2011.

Digital Imaging and Communications in Medicine (DICOM) Part 14: Grayscale Standard Display Function, PS 3.14-2011, National Electrical Manufacturers Association, 2011.

Flynn MG. Visual requirements for high-fidelity display. In: *Advances in digital radiography: categorical course in diagnostic radiology physics.* Radiological Society of North America, 2003:103–107.

Myers RL. *Display interfaces*: Fundamentals and Standards. John Wiley & Sons, Ltd, Chichester, UK, 2003.

Seibert JA, Filipow LJ, Andriole KP, eds. *Practical digital imaging and PACS.* Madison, WI: Medical Physics Publishing, 1999.

Tanenbaum AS, Wetherall DJ. *Computer networks.* 5th ed. Upper Saddle River, NJ: Prentice Hall PTR, 2010.

Wallis JW, Miller TR, *Three-dimensional display in nuclear medicine and radiology. J Nucl Med* 1991;32: 534–546.

SELECTED REFERENCES

Goo JM, Choi JY, et al. Effect of Monitor Luminance and Ambient Light on Observer Performance in Soft-Copy Reading of Digital Chest Radiographs. Radiology, September 2004, Volume 232 Number 3: 762-766

Krupinski EA. Technology and Perception in the 21st-Century Reading Room. *J Am Coll Radiol* 2006;3: 433-440.

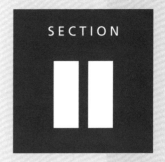

SECTION

II

Diagnostic Radiology

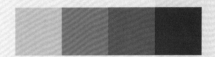

CHAPTER 6

X-ray Production, X-ray Tubes, and X-ray Generators

X-rays are produced when highly energetic electrons interact with matter, converting some of their kinetic energy into electromagnetic radiation. A device that produces x-rays in the diagnostic energy range typically contains an electron source, an evacuated path for electron acceleration, a target electrode, and an external power source to provide a high voltage (potential difference) to accelerate the electrons. Specifically, the *x-ray tube insert* contains the electron source and target within an evacuated glass or metal envelope; the *tube housing* provides protective radiation shielding and cools the x-ray tube insert; the *x-ray generator* supplies the voltage to accelerate the electrons; *x-ray beam filters* at the tube port shape the x-ray energy spectrum; and *collimators* define the size and shape of the x-ray field incident on the patient. The generator also permits control of the x-ray beam characteristics through the selection of voltage, current, and exposure time. These components work in concert to create a beam of x-ray photons of well-defined intensity, penetrability, and spatial distribution. In this chapter, the x-ray creation process, characteristics of the x-ray beam, and equipment components are discussed.

 ## 6.1 Production of X-rays

Bremsstrahlung Spectrum

X-rays are created from the conversion of kinetic energy of electrons into electromagnetic radiation when they are decelerated by interaction with a target material. A simplified diagram of an x-ray tube (Fig. 6-1) illustrates these components. For diagnostic radiology, a large electric potential difference (the SI unit of potential difference is the volt, V) of 20,000 to 150,000 V (20 to 150 kV) is applied between two electrodes (the cathode and the anode) in the vacuum. The *cathode* is the *source* of electrons, and the *anode,* with a positive potential with respect to the cathode, is the *target* of electrons. As electrons from the cathode travel to the anode, they are accelerated by the voltage between the electrodes and attain kinetic energies equal to the product of the electrical charge and potential difference (see Appendix A). A common unit of energy is the electron volt (eV), equal to the energy attained by an electron accelerated across a potential difference of 1 V. Thus, the kinetic energy of an electron accelerated by a potential difference of 50 kV is 50 keV. One eV is a very small amount of energy, as there are 6.24×10^{18} eV/J.

On impact with the target, the kinetic energy of the electrons is converted to other forms of energy. The vast majority of interactions are *collisional,* whereby energy exchanges with electrons in the target give rise to heat. A small fraction of the accelerated electrons comes within the proximity of an atomic nucleus and is influenced by its positive electric field. As discussed in Chapter 3, electrical (Coulombic) forces attract and decelerate an electron and change its direction, causing a loss of kinetic energy, which is emitted as an x-ray photon of equal energy (i.e., bremsstrahlung radiation).

171

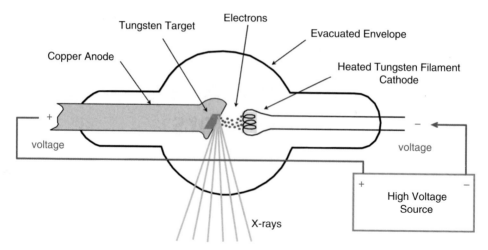

■ **FIGURE 6-1** Minimum requirements for x-ray production include a source and target of electrons, an evacuated envelope, and connection of the electrodes to a high-voltage source.

The amount of energy lost by the electron and thus the energy of the resulting x-ray are determined by the distance between the incident electron and the target nucleus, since the Coulombic force is proportional to the inverse of the square of the distance. At relatively large distances from the nucleus, the Coulombic attraction is weak; these encounters produce low x-ray energies (Fig. 6-2, electron no. 3). At closer interaction distances, the force acting on

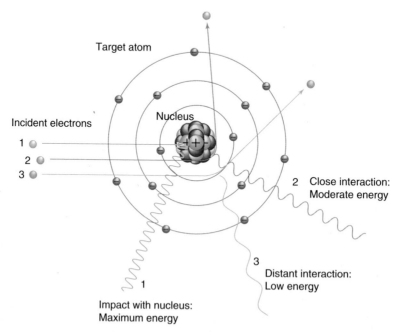

■ **FIGURE 6-2** Bremsstrahlung radiation arises from energetic electron interactions with an atomic nucleus of the target material. In a "close" approach, the positive nucleus attracts the negative electron, causing deceleration and redirection, resulting in a loss of kinetic energy that is converted to an x-ray. The x-ray energy depends on the interaction distance between the electron and the nucleus; it decreases as the distance increases.

the electron increases, causing a greater deceleration; these encounters produce higher x-ray energies (see Fig. 6-2, electron no. 2). A nearly direct impact of an electron with the target nucleus results in loss of nearly all of the electron's kinetic energy (see Fig. 6-2, electron no. 1). In this rare situation, the highest x-ray energies are produced.

The probability of electron interactions that result in production of x-ray energy E is dependent on the radial interaction distance, r, from the nucleus, which defines a circumference, $2\pi r$. With increasing distance from the nucleus, the circumference increases, and therefore the probability of interaction increases, but the x-ray energy decreases. Conversely, as the interaction distance, r, decreases, the x-ray energy increases because of greater electron deceleration, but the probability of interaction decreases. For the closest electron-atomic nuclei interactions, the highest x-ray energies are produced. However, the probability of such an interaction is very small, and the number of x-rays produced is correspondingly small. The number of x-rays produced decreases linearly with energy up to the maximal x-ray energy, which is equal to the energy of the incident electrons. A *bremsstrahlung spectrum* is the probability distribution of x-ray photons as a function of photon energy (keV). The *unfiltered* bremsstrahlung spectrum (Fig. 6-3A) shows an inverse linear relationship between the number and the energy of the x-rays produced, with the highest x-ray energy determined by the peak voltage (kV) applied across the x-ray tube. A typical *filtered* bremsstrahlung spectrum (Fig. 6-3B) has no x-rays below about 10 keV; the numbers increase to a maximum at about one third to one half the maximal x-ray energy and then decrease to zero as the x-ray energy increases to the maximal x-ray energy. Filtration in this context refers to the removal of x-rays by attenuation in materials that are inherent in the x-ray tube (e.g., the glass window of the tube insert), as well as by materials that are purposefully placed in the beam, such as thin aluminum and copper sheets, to remove lower energy x-rays and adjust the spectrum for optimal low-dose imaging (see Section 6.7).

Major factors that affect x-ray production efficiency include the atomic number of the target material and the kinetic energy of the incident electrons. The approximate ratio of radiative energy loss caused by bremsstrahlung production to

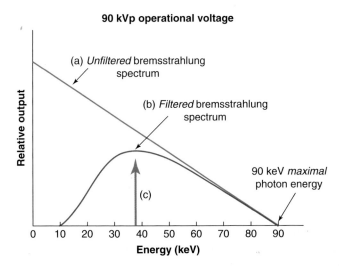

90 kVp operational voltage

(a) *Unfiltered* bremsstrahlung spectrum

(b) *Filtered* bremsstrahlung spectrum

90 keV *maximal* photon energy

(c)

Relative output

Energy (keV)

0 10 20 30 40 50 60 70 80 90

■ FIGURE 6-3 The bremsstrahlung energy distribution for a 90-kV acceleration potential difference. The unfiltered bremsstrahlung spectrum (a) shows a greater probability of low-energy x-ray photon production that is inversely linear with energy up to the maximum energy of 90 keV. The filtered spectrum (b) shows the preferential attenuation of the lowest-energy x-ray photons. The vertical arrow (c) indicates the average energy of the spectrum, which is typically 1/3 to 1/2 the maximal energy.

collisional (excitation and ionization) energy loss within the diagnostic x-ray energy range (potential difference of 20 to 150 kV) is expressed as follows:

$$\frac{\text{Radiative energy loss}}{\text{Collisional energy loss}} \cong \frac{E_K Z}{820,000} \qquad \text{[6-1]}$$

where E_K is the kinetic energy of the incident electrons in keV, and Z is the atomic number of the target electrode material. The most common target material is tungsten (W, Z = 74); in mammography, molybdenum (Mo, Z = 42) and rhodium (Rh, Z = 45) are also used. For 100-keV electrons impinging on tungsten, the approximate ratio of radiative to collisional losses is $(100 \times 74)/820,000 \cong 0.009 \cong 0.9\%$; therefore, more than 99% of the incident electron energy on the target electrode is converted to heat and nonuseful low-energy electromagnetic radiation. At much higher electron energies produced by radiation therapy systems (millions of electron volts), the efficiency of x-ray production is dramatically increased. However, Equation 6-1 is not applicable beyond diagnostic imaging x-ray energies.

Characteristic X-ray Spectrum

In addition to the continuous bremsstrahlung x-ray spectrum, discrete x-ray energy peaks called "characteristic radiation" can be present, depending on the elemental composition of the target electrode and the applied x-ray tube voltage. Electrons in an atom are distributed in shells, each of which has an electron binding energy. The innermost shell is designated the K shell and has the highest electron binding energy, followed by the L, M, and N shells, with progressively less binding energy. Table 6-1 lists the common anode target materials and the corresponding binding energies of their *K*, *L*, and *M* electron shells. The electron binding energies are "characteristic" of the elements. When the energy of an incident electron, determined by the voltage applied to the x-ray tube, exceeds the binding energy of an electron shell in a target atom, a collisional interaction can eject an electron from its shell, creating a vacancy. As discussed in Chapter 2, an outer shell electron with less binding energy immediately transitions to fill the vacancy, and a characteristic x-ray is emitted with an energy equal to the difference in the electron binding energies of the two shells (Fig. 6-4).

For tungsten, an *L*-shell (binding energy = 10.2 keV) electron transition to fill a *K*-shell (binding energy = 69.5 keV) vacancy produces a characteristic x-ray with a discrete energy of

$$E_{bK} - E_{bL} = 69.5 \text{ keV} - 10.2 \text{ keV} = 59.3 \text{ keV}$$

Electron transitions occur from adjacent and nonadjacent electron shells in the atom, giving rise to several discrete characteristic energy peaks superimposed on the

TABLE 6-1	ELECTRON BINDING ENERGIES (KeV) OF COMMON X-RAY TUBE TARGET MATERIALS		
ELECTRON SHELL	**TUNGSTEN**	**MOLYBDENUM**	**RHODIUM**
K	69.5	20.0	23.2
L	12.1/11.5/10.2	2.8/2.6/2.5	3.4/3.1/3.0
M	2.8–1.9	0.5–0.4	0.6–0.2

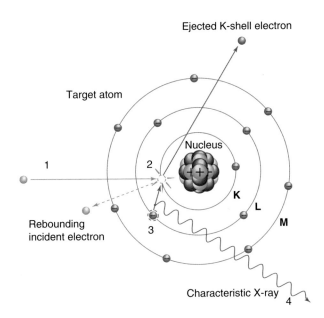

Ejected K-shell electron

Target atom

Nucleus

1

2

K

L

M

Rebounding
incident electron

3

Characteristic X-ray
4

■ **FIGURE 6-4** Generation of a characteristic x-ray in a target atom occurs in the following sequence: (1) The incident electron interacts with the *K*-shell electron via a repulsive electrical force. (2) The *K*-shell electron is removed (only if the energy of the incident electron is greater than the *K*-shell binding energy), leaving a vacancy in the *K*-shell. (3) An electron from the adjacent *L*-shell (or possibly a different shell) fills the vacancy. (4) A K_α characteristic x-ray photon is emitted with energy equal to the difference between the binding energies of the two shells. In this case, a 59.3-keV photon is emitted.

bremsstrahlung spectrum. Characteristic x-rays are designated by the shell in which the electron vacancy is filled, and a subscript of α or β indicates whether the electron transition is from an adjacent shell (α) or nonadjacent shell (β). For example, K_α refers to an electron transition from the *L* to the *K* shell, and K_β refers to an electron transition from the *M*, *N*, or *O* shell to the *K* shell. A K_β x-ray is more energetic than a K_α x-ray. Characteristic x-rays other than those generated by *K*-shell transitions are too low in energy for any useful contributions to the image formation process and are undesirable for diagnostic imaging. Table 6-2 lists electron shell binding energies and corresponding *K*-shell characteristic x-ray energies of W, Mo, and Rh anode targets.

Characteristic *K* x-rays are produced *only* when the electrons impinging on the target *exceed* the binding energy of a *K*-shell electron. x-Ray tube voltages must therefore be greater than 69.5 kV for W targets, 20 kV for Mo targets, and 23 kV for Rh targets to produce *K* characteristic x-rays. In terms of intensity, as the x-ray tube voltage increases, so does the ratio of characteristic to bremsstrahlung x-rays. For example, at 80 kV, approximately 5% of the total x-ray output intensity for a tungsten target is composed of characteristic radiation, which increases to about 10% at 100 kV. Figure 6-5 illustrates a bremsstrahlung plus characteristic radiation spectrum. In mammography, characteristic x-rays from Mo and Rh target x-ray tubes are particularly useful in optimizing image contrast and radiation dose (See Chapter 8 for further information).

TABLE 6-2   K-SHELL CHARACTERISTIC X-RAY ENERGIES (keV) OF COMMON X-RAY TUBE TARGET MATERIALS

SHELL TRANSITION	TUNGSTEN	MOLYBDENUM	RHODIUM
$K_{\alpha1}$	59.32	17.48	20.22
$K_{\alpha2}$	57.98	17.37	20.07
$K_{\beta1}$	67.24	19.61	22.72

Note: Only prominent transitions are listed. The subscripts 1 and 2 represent energy levels that exist within each shell.

■ **FIGURE 6-5** The filtered spectrum of bremsstrahlung and characteristic radiation from a tungsten target with a potential difference of 90 kV illustrates specific characteristic radiation energies from K_α and K_β transitions. Filtration (the preferential removal of low-energy photons as they traverse matter) is discussed in Section 6.5.

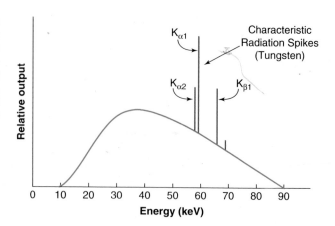

6.2 X-ray Tubes

The x-ray tube provides an environment for the production of bremsstrahlung and characteristic x-rays. Major tube components are the *cathode, anode, rotor/stator, glass or metal envelope, tube port, cable sockets,* and *tube housing,* illustrated in Figure 6-6. An actual x-ray tube showing the x-ray tube insert and part of the housing is shown in Figure 6-7. The x-ray generator (Section 6.3) supplies the power and permits selection of tube voltage, tube current, and exposure time. Depending upon the type of imaging examination and the characteristics of the anatomy being imaged, the *x-ray tube voltage* is set to values from 40 to 150 kV for diagnostic imaging, and 25 to 40 kV for mammography. The *x-ray tube current*, measured in milliamperes (mA), is proportional to the number of electrons per second flowing from the cathode to the anode, where 1 mA = 6.24×10^{15} electrons/s. For continuous fluoroscopy, the tube current is relatively low, from 1 to 5 mA, and for projection radiography, the tube current is set from 50 to 1,200 mA in conjunction with short exposure times (typically less than 100 ms). (In pulsed fluoroscopy, the tube current is commonly delivered in short pulses instead of being continuous; the average tube current is typically in the range of 10 to 50 mA, while the overall number of electrons delivered through the tube is about the same per image.) The kV, mA, and exposure time are the three major selectable parameters on the x-ray generator control panel that

■ **FIGURE 6-6** A diagram of the major components of a modern x-ray tube and housing assembly is shown.

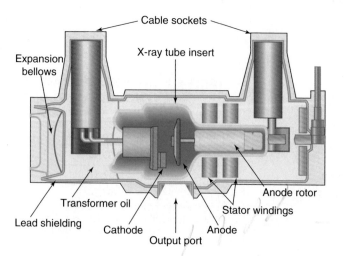

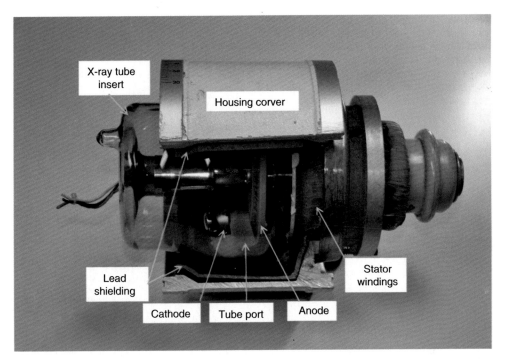

■ FIGURE 6-7 Picture of an x-ray tube insert and partially cut-away housing, shows the various components of the x-ray tube. For this housing, the lead shielding thickness is 2 mm.

determine the x-ray beam characteristics. Often, the product of the tube current and exposure time are considered as one entity, the mAs (milliampere-second; technically, mAs is a product of two units but, in common usage, it serves as a quantity). These parameters are discussed further in the following sections.

Cathode

The cathode is the negative electrode in the x-ray tube, comprised of a *filament* or filaments and a *focusing cup* (Fig. 6-8). A filament is made of tungsten wire wound in a helix, and is electrically connected to the filament circuit, which provides a voltage of approximately 10 V and variable current up to 7,000 mA (7 A). Most x-ray tubes for diagnostic imaging have two filaments of different lengths, each positioned in a slot machined into the focusing cup, with one end directly connected to the focusing cup, and the other end electrically insulated from the cup by a ceramic insert. Only one filament is energized for an imaging examination. On many x-ray systems, the small or the large filament can be manually selected, or automatically selected by the x-ray generator depending on the technique factors (kV and mAs).

When energized, the filament circuit heats the filament through electrical resistance, and the process of *thermionic emission* releases electrons from the filament surface at a rate determined by the filament current and corresponding filament temperature. Heat generated by resistance to electron flow in the filament raises the temperature to a point where electrons can leave the surface. However, electrons flow from the cathode to the anode *only when the tube voltage is applied between these electrodes*. The numbers of electrons that are available are adjusted by the filament current and filament temperature, as shown in Figure 6-9, where small changes in the filament current can produce relatively large changes in tube current. Output

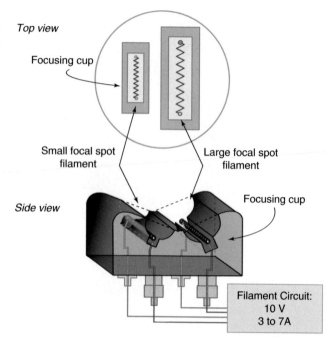

of the x-ray tube is *emission-limited*, meaning that the filament current determines the x-ray tube current; at any kV, the x-ray flux is proportional to the tube current. Higher tube voltages also produce slightly higher tube current for the same filament current. A filament current of 5 A at a tube voltage of 80 kV produces a tube current of about 800 mA, whereas the same filament current at 120 kV produces a tube current of about 1,100 mA.

In most x-ray tubes, the focusing cup is maintained at the same potential difference as the filament relative to the anode, and at the edge of the slot, an electric field exists that repels and shapes the cloud of emitted electrons from the filament surface. As a large voltage is applied between the cathode and anode in the correct polarity, electrons are accelerated into a tight distribution and travel to the anode, striking a small area called the focal spot (Fig. 6-10). The focal spot dimensions are determined by the length of the filament in one direction and the width of electron distribution in the perpendicular direction.

A *biased* x-ray tube has a focusing cup totally insulated from the filament wires so that its voltage is independent of the filament. Because high voltages are applied

■ **FIGURE 6-9** Relationship of tube current to filament current for various tube voltages shows a dependence of approximately $kV^{1.5}$. For tube voltages 40 kV and lower, a space charge cloud shields the electric field so that further increases in filament current do not increase the tube current. This is known as "space charge–limited" operation. Above 40 kV, the filament current limits the tube current; this is known as "emission-limited" operation.

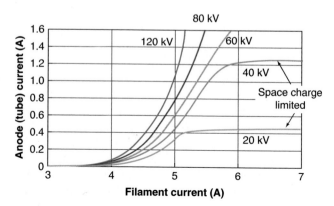

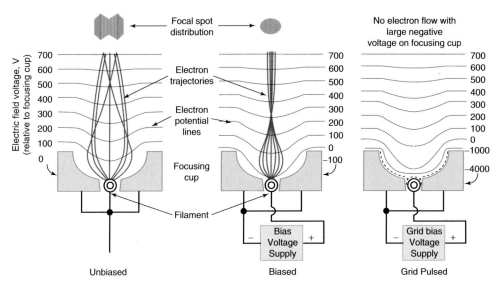

■ FIGURE 6-10 The focusing cup shapes the electron distribution when it is at the same voltage as the filament (**left**). Isolation of the focusing cup from the filament and application of a negative bias voltage (~ −100 V) reduces electron distribution further by increasing the repelling electric fields surrounding the filament and modifying the electron trajectories (**middle**). At the top are typical electron distributions incident on the target anode (the focal spot) for the unbiased and biased focusing cups. Application of −4,000 V on an isolated focusing cup completely stops electron flow, even with high voltage applied on the tube; this is known as a grid biased or grid pulsed tube (**right**).

to the cathode, electrical insulation of the focusing cup and the bias supply voltage is necessary, and can add significant expense to the x-ray system. A voltage of about 100 V negative is applied with respect to the filament voltage to further reduce the spread of electrons and produce a smaller focal spot width (Fig. 6-10 middle). Even greater negative applied voltage (about −4,000 V) to the focusing cup actually stops the flow of electrons, providing a means to rapidly switch the x-ray beam on and off (Fig. 6-10 right); a tube with this capability is referred to as a *grid-biased* x-ray tube. Grid-biased x-ray tube switching is used by more expensive fluoroscopy systems for pulsed fluoroscopy and angiography to rapidly and precisely turn on and turn off the x-ray beam. This eliminates the build-up delay and turnoff lag of x-ray tubes switched at the generator, which cause motion artifacts and produce lower average x-ray energies and unnecessary patient dose.

Ideally, a focal spot would be a point, eliminating geometric blurring. However, such a focal spot is not possible and, if it were, would permit only a tiny tube current. In practice, a finite focal spot area is used with an area large enough to permit a sufficiently large tube current and short exposure time. For magnification studies, a small focal spot is necessary to limit geometric blurring and achieve adequate spatial resolution (see Figure 6-16 and Chapter 7 on magnification).

Anode

The anode is a metal target electrode that is maintained at a large positive potential difference relative to the cathode. Electrons striking the anode deposit most of their energy as heat, with only a small fraction emitted as x-rays. Consequently, the production of x-rays, in quantities necessary for acceptable image quality, generates a large amount of heat in the anode. To avoid heat damage to the x-ray tube, the rate of x-ray production (proportional to the tube current) and, at large tube currents, the duration of x-ray production, must be limited. Tungsten (W, Z = 74) is the most widely used anode material because of its high melting point and high atomic number. A tungsten anode can handle substantial heat deposition without cracking or pitting of its surface. An alloy of 10% rhenium and 90% tungsten provides added resistance to surface damage. Tungsten provides greater bremsstrahlung production than elements with lower atomic numbers (Equation 6-1).

Molybdenum (Mo, Z = 42) and rhodium (Rh, Z = 45) are used as anode materials in mammographic x-ray tubes. These materials provide useful characteristic x-rays for breast imaging (see Table 6-2). Mammographic tubes are described further in Chapter 8.

Anode Configurations: Stationary and Rotating

A simple x-ray tube design has a stationary anode, consisting of a tungsten insert embedded in a copper block (Fig. 6-11). Copper serves a dual role: it mechanically supports the insert and efficiently conducts heat from the tungsten target. However, the small area of the focal spot on the stationary anode limits the tube current and x-ray output that can be sustained without damage from excessive temperature. Dental x-ray units and some low-output mobile x-ray machines and mobile fluoroscopy systems use fixed anode x-ray tubes.

Rotating anodes are used for most diagnostic x-ray applications, mainly because of greater heat loading and higher x-ray intensity output. This design spreads the heat over a much larger area than does the stationary anode design, permitting much larger tube currents and exposure durations. The anode is a beveled disk mounted on a *rotor* assembly supported by bearings in the x-ray tube insert (Fig. 6-12). The rotor consists of copper bars arranged around a cylindrical iron core. A donut-shaped *stator* device, comprised of electromagnets, surrounds the rotor and is mounted outside of the x-ray tube insert. Alternating current (AC), the periodic reversal of electron movement in a conductor, passes through the stator windings and produces a rotating magnetic field (see electromagnetic induction, Section 6.3). This induces an electrical current in the rotor's copper bars, which creates an opposing magnetic field that causes it to spin. Rotation speeds are 3,000 to 3,600 (low speed) or 9,000 to 10,000 (high speed) revolutions per minute (rpm). X-ray systems are designed such that the x-ray tube will not be energized if the anode is not at full speed; this is the cause for the short delay (1 to 2 s) when the x-ray tube exposure button is pushed.

Rotor bearings are heat sensitive and are often the cause of x-ray tube failure. Bearings require special heat insensitive, nonvolatile lubricants because of the vacuum inside the x-ray tube insert and also require thermal insulation from the anode, achieved by using a molybdenum (a metal with poor heat conductivity) stem attaching the anode to the rotor. Most rotating anodes are cooled by infrared radiation emission, transferring heat to the x-ray tube insert and to the surrounding oil bath

■ FIGURE 6-11 The anode of a fixed anode x-ray tube consists of a tungsten insert mounted in a copper block. Heat is removed from the tungsten target by conduction into the copper block.

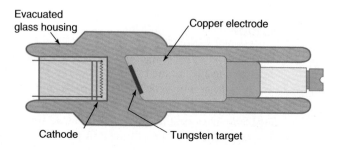

Evacuated glass housing

Copper electrode

Cathode

Tungsten target

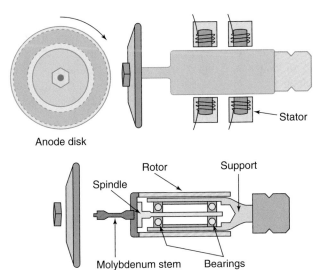

■ **FIGURE 6-12** The anode of a rotating anode x-ray tube is a tungsten disk mounted on a bearing-supported rotor assembly (front view, **top left**; side view, **top right**). The rotor consists of a copper and iron laminated core and forms part of an induction motor. The other component is the stator, which exists outside of the insert, **top right**. A molybdenum stem (molybdenum is a poor heat conductor) connects the rotor to the anode to reduce heat transfer to the rotor bearings (**bottom**).

and tube housing. In imaging situations demanding higher heat loads and more rapid cooling, such as interventional fluoroscopy and computed tomography (CT), sophisticated designs with externally mounted bearings and oil or water heat exchangers are employed (see special x-ray tube designs in this section).

The focal track area of the rotating anode is approximately equal to the product of the circumferential track length ($2\pi r$) and the track width (Δr), where r is the radial distance from the axis of the x-ray tube to the center of the track (Fig. 6-13). Thus, a rotating anode with a 5-cm focal track radius and a 1-mm track width provides a focal track with an annular area 314 times greater than that of a fixed anode with a focal spot area of 1 × 1 mm. The allowable instantaneous heat loading depends on

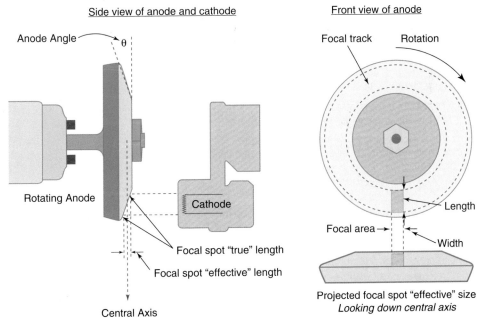

■ **FIGURE 6-13** The anode (target) angle, θ, is defined as the angle of the target surface in relation to the central ray. The focal spot length, as projected down the central axis, is foreshortened, according to the line focus principle (**lower right**).

the anode rotation speed and the focal spot area. Faster rotation distributes the heat load over a greater portion of the focal track area for short exposure times. A larger focal spot allows a greater x-ray beam intensity but causes a loss of spatial resolution that increases with distance of the imaged object from the image receptor. A large focal spot, which permits high x-ray output and short exposure times, should be used in situations where motion is expected to be a problem and geometric magnification is small (the object is close to the image receptor).

Anode Angle, Field Coverage, and Focal Spot Size

The anode angle is defined as the angle of the target surface with respect to the central ray (central axis) in the x-ray field (Fig. 6-13, left diagram). Anode angles in diagnostic x-ray tubes typically range from 7 to 20 degrees, with 12- to 15-degree angles being most common. Major factors affected by the anode angle include the effective focal spot size, tube output intensity, and x-ray field coverage provided at a given focal spot to detector distance.

The actual focal spot size is the area on the anode that is struck by electrons, and is primarily determined by the length of the cathode filament and the width of the focusing cup slot. However, the projected length of the focal spot area at the x-ray field central ray is much smaller, because of geometric foreshortening of the distribution from the anode surface. Thus, the effective and actual focal spot lengths are geometrically related as

$$\text{Effective focal length} = \text{Actual focal length} \times \sin \theta \qquad [6\text{-}2]$$

where θ is the anode angle. Foreshortening of the focal spot length at the central ray is called the *line focus principle*, as described by Equation 6-2. An ability to have a smaller effective focal spot size for a large actual focal spot increases the power loadings for smaller effective focal spot sizes.

EXAMPLE 1: The actual anode focal area for a 20-degree anode angle is 4 mm (length) by 1.2 mm (width). What is the projected focal spot size at the central axis position?

Answer: Effective length = actual length $\times$ sin θ = 4 mm $\times$ sin 20 degrees = 4 mm $\times$ 0.34 = 1.36 mm; therefore, the projected focal spot size is 1.36 mm (length) by 1.2 mm (width).

EXAMPLE 2: If the anode angle in Example 1 is reduced to 10 degrees and the actual focal spot size remains the same, what is the projected focal spot size at the central axis position?

Answer: Effective length = 4 mm $\times$ sin 10 degrees = 4 mm $\times$ 0.174 = 0.69 mm; thus, the smaller anode angle results in a projected size of 0.69 mm (length) by 1.2 mm (width) for the same actual target area.

As the anode angle decreases (approaches 0 degrees), the *effective* focal spot becomes smaller for the same *actual* focal area, providing better spatial resolution of the object when there is geometric image magnification. Also, for larger actual focal areas, greater x-ray output intensity with shorter exposure times is possible. However, a small anode angle limits the usable x-ray size at a given source to image receptor distance, because of cutoff of the beam on the anode side of the beam. *Field coverage* is also less for short focus-to-detector distances (Fig. 6-14). Therefore, the optimal anode angle depends on the clinical imaging application. A small anode angle (~7 to 9 degrees) is desirable for small field-of-view devices, such as some small fluoroscopy detectors, where field coverage is limited by the image receptor diameter

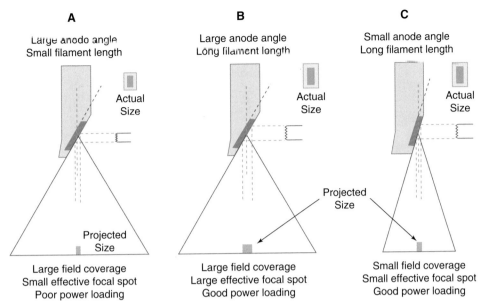

A
Large anode angle
Small filament length

Actual Size

Projected Size

Large field coverage
Small effective focal spot
Poor power loading

B
Large anode angle
Long filament length

Actual Size

Large field coverage
Large effective focal spot
Good power loading

C
Small anode angle
Long filament length

Actual Size

Projected Size

Small field coverage
Small effective focal spot
Good power loading

■ **FIGURE 6-14** Field coverage and effective focal spot length vary with the anode angle. **A.** A large anode angle provides good field coverage at a given distance; however, to achieve a small effective focal spot, a small actual focal area limits power loading. **B.** A large anode angle provides good field coverage, and achievement of high power loading requires a large focal area; however, geometric blurring and image degradation occur. **C.** A small anode angle limits field coverage at a given distance; however, a small effective focal spot is achieved with a large focal area for high power loading.

(e.g., 23 cm). Larger anode angles (~12 to 15 degrees) are necessary for general radiographic imaging to achieve sufficiently large field area coverage at typical focal spot-to-detector distances such as 100 cm.

The effective focal spot length varies with the position in the image plane, in the anode-cathode (A–C) direction. Toward the anode side of the field, the projected length of the focal spot shortens, whereas it lengthens towards the cathode side of the field (Fig. 6-15). The width of the focal spot does not change appreciably with position in the image plane. Nominal focal spot size (width and length) is specified at the central ray of the beam, from the focal spot to the image receptor, perpendicular to the anode-cathode axis and bisecting the plane of the image receptor. x-Ray mammography is an exception, where "half-field" geometry is employed, as explained in Chapter 8.

Measurement and verification of focal spot size can be performed in several ways. Common tools for measuring focal spot size are the pinhole camera, slit camera, star pattern, and resolution bar pattern (Fig. 6-16). The *pinhole camera* uses a very small circular aperture (10 to 30 μm diameter) in a thin, highly attenuating metal (e.g., lead, tungsten, or gold) disk to project a magnified image of the focal spot onto an image receptor. With the pinhole camera positioned on the central axis between the x-ray source and detector, an image of the focal spot is recorded. Figure 6-16E shows magnified (2×) pinhole pictures of the large (top row) and small (bottom row) focal spots with a typical "bi-gaussian" intensity distribution. Correcting for the known image magnification allows measurement of the focal spot dimensions. The *slit camera* consists of a highly attenuating metal (usually tungsten) plate with a thin slit, typically 10 μm wide. In use, the slit camera is positioned above the image receptor, with the center of the slit on the central axis, and with the slit either parallel or perpendicular to the A-C axis. Measuring the width of the x-ray distribution in the image and correcting for magnification yields one dimension of

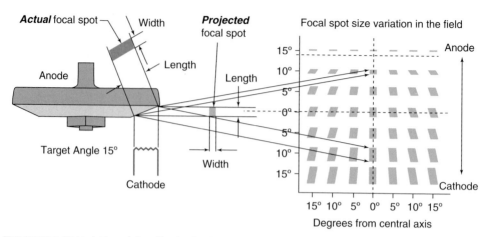

■ **FIGURE 6-15** Variation of the effective focal spot size in the image field occurs along the anode-cathode direction. Focal spot distributions are plotted as a function of projection angle in degrees from the central axis, the parallel (vertical axis), and the perpendicular (horizontal axis).

the focal spot. A second radiograph, taken with the slit perpendicular to the first, yields the other dimension of the focal spot, as shown in Figure 6-16F. The *star pattern* test tool (Fig. 6-16G) contains a radial pattern of lead spokes of diminishing width and spacing on a thin plastic disk. Imaging the star pattern at a known magnification and measuring the distance between the outermost blur patterns (location of the outermost unresolved spokes as shown by the arrows) on the image allows the calculation of the effective focal spot dimensions in the directions perpendicular and parallel to the A-C axis. A large focal spot will have a greater blur diameter than a small focal spot, as shown in the figure. A resolution bar pattern is a simple tool for evaluation of focal spot size (Fig. 6-16H). Bar pattern images demonstrate the effective resolution parallel and perpendicular to the A-C axis for a given magnification geometry, determined from the number of the bar pattern that can be resolved.

The National Electrical Manufacturers Association (NEMA) has published tolerances for measured focal spot sizes. For focal spot nominal (indicated) sizes less than 0.8 mm, the measured focal spot size can be larger by 50% (e.g., for a 0.6-mm focal spot, the measured size can be up to 0.9 mm), but not smaller than the nominal size. For focal spots between 0.8 and 1.5 mm nominal size, the measured focal spot size can be 0% smaller to 40% larger; and for focal spots greater than 1.5 mm, 0% smaller to 30% larger.

Focal spot "blooming" is an increase in the size of the focal spot resulting from high tube current (mA), and is caused by electron repulsion in the electron beam between the cathode and anode. It is most pronounced at low kVs. Focal spot "thinning" is a slight decrease in the measured size with increasing kV (electron repulsion and spreading in the x-ray tube is reduced). NEMA standards require measurement at 75 kV using 50% of the maximal rated mA for each focal spot.

Heel Effect

The *heel effect* refers to a reduction in the x-ray beam intensity toward the anode side of the x-ray field (Figure 6-17), caused by the greater attenuation of x-rays directed toward the anode side of the field by the anode itself. The heel effect is less prominent with a longer source-to-image distance (SID). Since the x-ray beam intensity is greater on the cathode side of the field, the orientation of the x-ray tube cathode over thicker parts of the patient can result in a better balance of x-ray photons transmitted

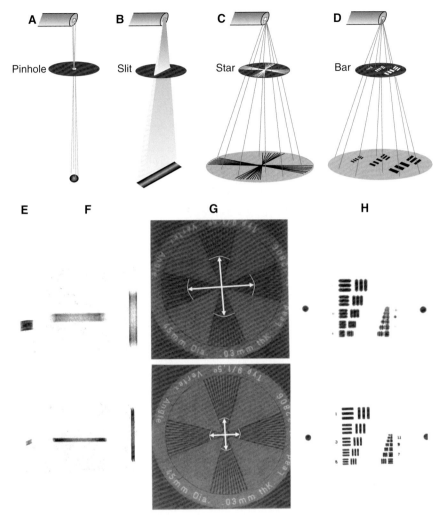

■ **FIGURE 6-16** Various tools allow measurement of the focal spot size, either directly or indirectly. **A** and **E**: Pinhole camera and images. **B** and **F**: Slit camera and images. **C** and **G**: Star pattern and images. **D** and **H**: Resolution bar pattern and images. For **E–H**, the top row of images represents the measurements of the large focal spot (1.2 mm × 1.2 mm), and the bottom row the small focal spot (0.6 mm × 0.6 mm). The star and bar patterns provide an "equivalent" focal spot dimension based upon the resolvability of the equivalent spatial frequencies.

through the patient and onto the image receptor. For example, the preferred orientation of the x-ray tube for a chest x-ray of a standing patient would be with the A-C axis vertical, and the cathode end of the x-ray tube down.

Off-Focal Radiation

Off-focal radiation results from electrons that scatter from the anode, and are re-accelerated back to the anode, outside of the focal spot area. These electrons cause low-intensity x-ray emission over the entire face of the anode, as shown in Figure 6-18, increasing patient exposure, causing geometric blurring, reducing image contrast, and increasing random noise. A small lead collimator aperture placed near the x-ray tube output port can reduce off-focal radiation by intercepting x-rays that are produced away from the focal spot. An x-ray tube that has a metal enclosure and the anode at electrical ground potential will have less off-focal radiation, because many of the scattered electrons are attracted to the metal envelope instead of the anode.

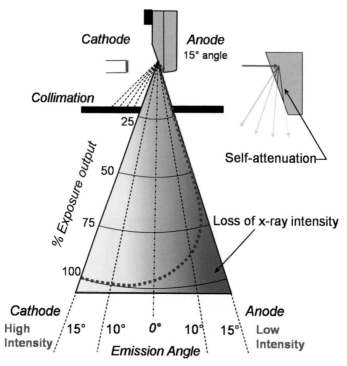

FIGURE 6-17 The heel effect is a loss of intensity on the anode side of the x-ray field of view. It is caused by attenuation of the x-ray beam by the anode. Upper right is an expanded view that shows electrons interacting at depth within the anode and the resultant "self attenuation" of produced x-rays that have a trajectory towards the anode side of the field.

X-ray Tube Insert

The *x-ray tube insert* contains the cathode, anode, rotor assembly, and support structures sealed in a glass or metal enclosure under a high vacuum. The high vacuum prevents electrons from colliding with gas molecules and is necessary in most electron beam devices. As x-ray tubes age, trapped gas molecules percolate from

FIGURE 6-18 Off-focal radiation is produced from back-scattered electrons that are re-accelerated to the anode outside the focal spot. This causes a low-intensity, widespread radiation distribution pattern. Hotspots outside the focal spot indicate areas where the electrons are more likely to interact.

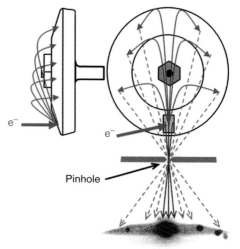

tube structures and degrade the vacuum. A "*getter*" circuit is used to trap gas in the insert and to maintain the vacuum.

X-rays are emitted in all directions from the focal spot; however, the x-rays that emerge through the *tube port* constitute the useful beam. Except for mammography and special-purpose x-ray tubes, the port is typically made of the same material as the tube enclosure. Mammography tubes use beryllium (Z = 4) in the port to minimize absorption of the low-energy x-rays used in mammography.

X-ray Tube Housing

The x-ray tube housing supports, insulates, and protects the x-ray tube insert from the environment. Between the x-ray tube insert and housing is oil that provides heat conduction and electrical insulation. In many radiographic x-ray tubes, an expanding bellows inside the housing accommodates oil expansion due to heat absorption during operation. If the oil heats excessively, a microswitch disables the operation of the x-ray tube until sufficient cooling has occurred. X-ray tubes used in interventional fluoroscopy and CT commonly have heat exchangers to allow prolonged operation at high output.

Lead shielding inside the housing attenuates nearly all x-rays that are not directed to the tube port (see Fig. 6-7 for the typical lead sheet thickness and location within the housing). A small fraction of these x-rays, known as leakage radiation, penetrates the housing. Federal regulations (21 CFR 1020.30) require manufacturers to provide sufficient shielding to limit the leakage radiation exposure rate to 0.88 mGy air kerma per hour (equivalent to 100 mR/h) at 1 m from the focal spot when the x-ray tube is operated at the leakage technique factors for the x-ray tube. Leakage techniques are the maximal operable kV (kV_{max}, typically 125 to 150 kV) at the highest possible continuous current (typically 3 to 5 mA at kV_{max} for most diagnostic tubes). Each x-ray tube housing assembly has a maximal rated tube potential that must not be exceeded during clinical operation of the x-ray tube source assembly. The x-ray equipment is designed to prevent the selection of x-ray tube kV greater than the maximal rating.

Collimators

Collimators adjust the size and shape of the x-ray field emerging from the tube port. The collimator assembly typically is attached to the tube housing at the tube port with a swivel joint. Two pairs of adjustable parallel-opposed lead shutters define a rectangular x-ray field (Fig. 6-19). In the collimator housing, a beam of light reflected by a mirror of low x-ray attenuation mimics the x-ray beam. Thus, the collimation of the x-ray field is identified by the collimator's shadows. Federal regulations (21 CFR 1020.31) require that the light field and x-ray field be aligned so that the sum of the misalignments, along either the length or the width of the field, is within 2% of the SID. For example, at a typical SID of 100 cm (40 inches), the sum of the misalignments between the light field and the x-ray field at the left and right edges must not exceed 2 cm, and the sum of the misalignments at the other two edges also must not exceed 2 cm.

Positive beam limitation (PBL) collimators automatically limit the field size to the useful area of the detector. Mechanical sensors in the film cassette holder detect the cassette size and location and automatically adjust the collimator blades so that the x-ray field matches the cassette dimensions. Adjustment to a smaller field area is possible; however, a larger field area requires disabling the PBL circuit.

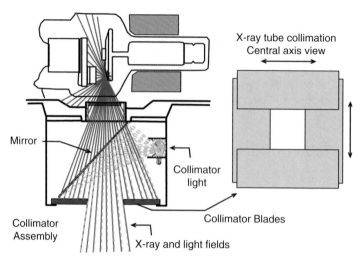

■ FIGURE 6-19 The x-ray tube collimator assembly is attached to the housing at the tube port, typically on a collar that allows it to be rotated. A light source, positioned at a virtual focal spot location, illuminates the field from a 45-degree angle mirror. Lead collimator blades define both the x-ray and light fields.

Special X-ray Tube Designs

A grid-biased tube has a focusing cup that is electrically isolated from the cathode filament and maintained at a more negative voltage. When the bias voltage is sufficiently large, the resulting electric field stops the tube current. Turning off the grid bias allows the tube current to flow and x-rays to be produced. Grid biasing requires approximately –4,000 V applied to the focusing cup with respect to the filament to switch the x-ray tube current off (see Fig. 6-10). The grid-biased tube is used in applications such as pulsed fluoroscopy and cine-angiography, where rapid x-ray pulsing is necessary. Biased x-ray tubes are significantly more expensive than conventional, nonbiased tubes.

Mammography tubes are designed to provide the low-energy x-rays necessary to produce optimal mammographic images. As explained in Chapter 8, the main differences between a dedicated mammography tube and a conventional x-ray tube are the target materials (molybdenum, rhodium, and tungsten), the output port (beryllium versus glass or metal insert material), the smaller effective focal spot sizes (typically 0.3 and 0.1 mm nominal focal spot sizes), and the use of grounded anodes.

X-ray tubes for interventional fluoroscopy and CT require high instantaneous x-ray output and high heat loading and rapid cooling. Furthermore, in CT, with the fast x-ray tube rotation (as low as 0.3 s for a complete rotation about the patient) and the tremendous mechanical forces it places on the CT tube, planar surface cathode emitter designs different than the common helical filaments and enhanced bearing support for the rotating anode are often used. One manufacturer's CT tube incorporates a novel design with the cathode and the anode as part of a metal vacuum enclosure that is attached to externally mounted bearings and drive motor to rotate the assembly as shown in Figure 6-20. Dynamic steering of the electron beam within the tube is achieved by external electromagnetic deflection coils to direct the electrons to distinct focal spots on the anode, which can produce slightly different projections and improve data sampling during the CT acquisition (refer to Chapter 10 on CT). Direct anode cooling by oil circulating within the housing provides extremely high cooling rates, and eliminates the need for high anode heat storage capacity. The cessation of imaging during clinical examinations to allow anode cooling is seldom necessary when using these advanced x-ray tubes.

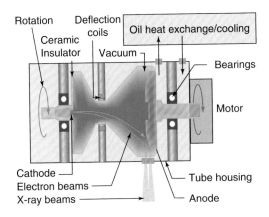

■ **FIGURE 6-20** Diagram of an advanced CT x-ray tube, showing the anode and the planar cathode within a rotating vacuum enclosure. The bearings are mounted outside of the vacuum enclosure. Deflection coils magnetically direct the electron beam to specific areas on the target. Circulating oil rapidly removes excess heat from the anode. The electron beam can be rapidly deflected between two focal spots; this is known as a "flying focal spot."

Recommendations to Maximize X-ray Tube Life

X-ray tubes eventually must be replaced, but a long lifetime can be achieved with appropriate care and use. Several simple rules are discussed here. (1) Minimize filament boost "prep" time (the first detent of two on the x-ray exposure switch) especially when high mA is used. If applied for too long, filament life will be shortened, unstable operation will occur, and evaporated tungsten will be deposited on the glass envelope. (2) Use lower tube current with longer exposure times to arrive at the desired mAs if possible. (3) Avoid extended or repeated operation of the x-ray tube with high technique (kV and mAs) factors because, even though the x-ray generator has logic to prohibit single exposure settings that could damage the x-ray tube, multiple exposures could etch the focal track, resulting in less radiation output; transmit excessive heat to the bearings; and cause outgassing of the anode structure that will cause the tube to become unstable. (4) Always follow the manufacturer's recommended warm-up procedure. Do not make high mA exposures on a cold anode, because uneven expansion caused by thermal stress can cause cracks. (5) Limit rotor start and stop operations, which can generate significant heating and hot spots within the stator windings; when possible, a 30 to 40 s delay between exposures should be used.

Filtration

As mentioned earlier, filtration is the removal of x-rays as the beam passes through a layer of material. Filtration includes both the inherent filtration of the x-ray tube and added filtration. Inherent filtration includes the thickness (1 to 2 mm) of the glass or metal insert at the x-ray tube port. Glass (primarily silicon dioxide, SiO_2) and aluminum have similar attenuation properties ($Z_{Si} = 14$ and $Z_{Al} = 13$) and effectively attenuate all x-rays in the spectrum below about 15 keV. Dedicated mammography tubes, on the other hand, require beryllium ($Z = 4$) to permit the transmission of low-energy x-rays. Inherent filtration includes attenuation by housing oil and the field light mirror in the collimator assembly.

Added filtration refers to sheets of metal intentionally placed in the beam to change its effective energy. In general diagnostic radiology, added filters attenuate the low-energy x-rays in the spectrum that have almost no chance of penetrating the patient and reaching the x-ray detector. Because the low-energy x-rays are absorbed by the filters instead of the patient, radiation dose is reduced by beam filtration. Aluminum (Al) is the most commonly used added filter material. Other common filter materials include copper and plastic (e.g., acrylic). An example of the patient dose savings obtained with extra tube filtration is described in Section 6.5, point no. 4, beam filtration. In mammography, thin filters of Mo, Rh, and silver (Ag) are used to transmit bremsstrahlung x-rays in the intermediate energy range (15 to 25 keV), including characteristic radiation from Mo and Rh, and also to highly attenuate lowest and highest x-ray energies in the spectrum (see Chapter 8). Some have advocated using rare earth elements (K-absorption edges of 39 to 65 keV) such as erbium in filters in radiography to reduce patient dose and improve image contrast when contrast materials are used.

Compensation (equalization) filters are used to change the spatial pattern of the x-ray intensity incident on the patient, so as to deliver a more uniform x-ray exposure to the detector. For example, a trough filter used for chest radiography has a centrally located vertical band of reduced thickness and consequently produces greater x-ray fluence in the middle of the field. This filter compensates for the high attenuation of the mediastinum and reduces the exposure latitude incident on the image receptor. Wedge filters are useful for lateral projections in cervical-thoracic spine imaging, where the incident fluence is increased to match the increased tissue thickness encountered (e.g., to provide a low incident flux to the thin neck area and a high incident flux to the thick shoulders). "Bow-tie" filters are used in CT to reduce dose to the periphery of the patient, where x-ray paths are shorter and fewer x-rays are required. Compensation filters are placed close to the x-ray tube port or just external to the collimator assembly.

 ## 6.3 X-ray Generators

The principal function of an x-ray generator is to provide current at a high voltage to an x-ray tube. Electrical power available to a hospital or clinic provides up to about 480 V, much lower than the 20,000 to 150,000 V needed for x-ray production. Transformers are principal components of x-ray generators; they convert low voltage into high voltage through a process called *electromagnetic induction.*

Electromagnetic Induction and Voltage Transformation

Electromagnetic induction is a phenomenon in which a changing magnetic field induces an electrical potential difference (voltage) in a nearby conductor and also in which a voltage is induced in a conductor moving through a stationary magnetic field. For example, the changing magnetic field from a moving bar magnet induces a voltage and a current in a nearby conducting wire (Fig. 6-21A). As the magnet moves in the opposite direction away from the wire, the induced current flows in the opposite direction. The magnitude of the induced voltage is proportional to the rate of change of the magnetic field strength.

Electrical current, such as the electrons flowing through a wire, produces a magnetic field whose magnitude (strength) is proportional to the magnitude of the current (see Fig. 6-21B). For a coiled wire geometry, superimposition of the magnetic fields from adjacent turns of the wire increases the amplitude of the overall magnetic field (the magnetic fields penetrate the wire's insulation), and therefore the magnetic field strength is proportional to the number of wire turns. A constant current flowing through a wire or a coil produces a constant magnetic field, and a varying current produces a varying magnetic field. With an AC and voltage, such as the standard 60 cycles/s (Hz) AC in North America and 50 Hz AC in most other areas of the world, the induced magnetic field alternates with the current.

A Changing magnetic field induces electron flow:

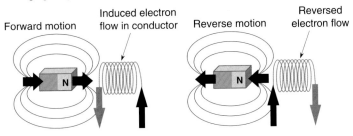

B Current (electron flow) in a conductor creates a magnetic field; its *amplitude and direction* determines magnetic field strength and polarity

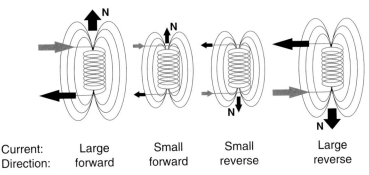

Current:	Large	Small	Small	Large
Direction:	forward	forward	reverse	reverse

■ **FIGURE 6-21** Principles of electromagnetic induction are illustrated. **A.** Induction of an electrical current in a wire conductor coil by a moving (changing) magnetic field. The direction of the current is dependent on the direction of the magnetic field motion. **B.** Creation of a magnetic field by the current in a conducting coil. The polarity and magnetic field strength are determined by the amplitude and direction of the current.

A wire or a wire coil with a changing current will induce a voltage in a nearby wire or wire coil, and therefore, an AC applied to a wire or a wire coil will induce an alternating voltage in another wire or wire coil by electromagnetic induction. However, when a constant current, like that produced by a chemical battery, flows through a wire or a wire coil, although it creates a constant magnetic field, electromagnetic induction does not occur, and so it does not induce a voltage or current in a nearby conductor.

Transformers

Transformers use the principle of electromagnetic induction to change the voltage of an electrical power source. The generic transformer has two distinct, electrically insulated wires wrapped about a common iron core (Fig. 6-22). Input AC power produces an oscillating magnetic field on the "primary winding" of the transformer, where each turn of the wire amplifies the magnetic field that is unaffected by the electrical insulation and permeates the iron core. Contained within the core, the changing magnetic field induces a voltage on the "secondary winding," the magnitude of which is amplified by the number of turns of wire. The voltage induced in the second winding is proportional to the voltage on the primary winding and the ratio of the number of turns in the two windings, as stated by the *Law of Transformers*,

$$\frac{V_P}{V_S} = \frac{N_P}{N_S}$$ [6-3]

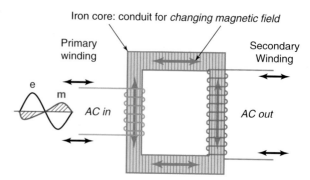

■ **FIGURE 6-22** The basic transformer consists of an iron core, a primary winding circuit, and a secondary winding circuit. An AC flowing through the primary winding produces a changing magnetic field, which permeates the core and induces an alternating voltage on the secondary winding. This mutual electromagnetic induction is mediated by the containment of the magnetic field in the iron core and permeability through wire insulation.

where N_p is the number of turns in the primary coil, N_s is the number of turns in the secondary coil, V_p is the amplitude of the input voltage on the primary side of the transformer, and V_s is the amplitude of the output voltage on the secondary side.

A transformer can increase, decrease, or isolate input voltage, depending on the ratio of the numbers of turns in the two coils. For $N_s > N_p$, a "step-up" transformer increases the secondary voltage; for $N_s < N_p$, a "step-down" transformer decreases the secondary voltage; and for $N_s = N_p$, an "isolation" transformer produces a secondary voltage equal to the primary voltage. Configurations of these transformers are shown in Figure 6-23. An input AC waveform is supplied to a transformer in order to produce a changing magnetic field and induce a voltage in the secondary winding. A step-up transformer circuit provides the high voltage necessary (20 to 150 kV) for a diagnostic x-ray generator.

For electrons to be accelerated to the anode in an x-ray tube, the voltage at the anode must be positive with respect to the cathode, but alternating waveforms change between negative and positive voltage polarity each half cycle. For continuous production of x-rays, the anode must be continuously at a positive voltage with respect to the cathode. However, this occurs only half of the time if an alternating voltage waveform is provided directly to the x-ray tube. A basic electrical component known as a *rectifier* will allow current to flow in one direction only. For instance, the x-ray tube itself can act as a rectifier, since current usually will flow only when the anode

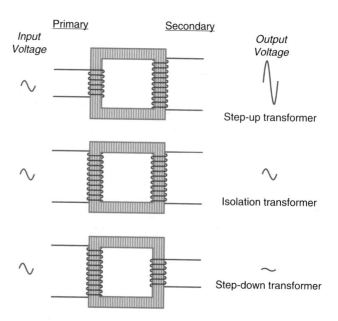

■ **FIGURE 6-23** Transformers increase (step up), decrease (step down), or leave unchanged (isolate) the input voltage depending on the ratio of primary to secondary turns, according to the Law of Transformers. In all cases, the input and the output circuits are electrically isolated.

has positive and the cathode has negative polarity; however, if the anode becomes very hot from use and the accelerating voltage is applied with reverse polarity (tube cathode positive and anode negative), electrons can be released from the hot anode and accelerated into the cathode, possibly damaging it. A diode is a device with two terminals. When a voltage is applied between the terminals with a specific polarity, there is very little resistance and a large current flows; when the same voltage is applied with the opposite polarity, little or no current flows. Diodes come in all sizes, from large, x-ray tube–sized devices down to microscopic, solid-state components on an integrated circuit board. Clever use of diodes arranged in a *bridge rectifier circuit* can route the flow of electrons through an AC circuit to create a direct current (DC), a unidirectional movement of electrons in which the voltage polarity never reverses. Rectification is an important function of the x-ray generator.

Power is the rate of energy production or expenditure per unit time. The SI unit of power is the watt (W), defined as 1 joule (J) of energy per second. For electrical devices, power is equal to the product of voltage and current.

$$P = I\,V \tag{6-4}$$

Because a volt is defined as 1 joule per coulomb and an ampere is 1 coulomb per second,

$$1\ \text{watt} = 1\ \text{volt} \times 1\ \text{ampere}$$

For an ideal transformer, because the power output is equal to the power input, the product of voltage and current in the primary circuit is equal to that in the secondary circuit

$$V_P I_P = V_S I_S \tag{6-5}$$

where I_P is the input current on the primary side and I_S is the output current on the secondary side. Therefore, a decrease in current must accompany an increase in voltage, and vice versa. Equations 6-3 and 6-5 describe ideal transformer performance. Power losses in an actual transformer due to inefficient coupling cause both the voltage and current on the secondary side of the transformer to be less than those predicted by these equations.

EXAMPLE: The ratio of primary to secondary turns is 1:1,000 in a transformer. If an input AC waveform has a peak voltage of 50 V, what is the peak voltage induced in the secondary side?

$$\frac{V_P}{V_S} = \frac{N_P}{N_S}; \frac{50}{V_S} = \frac{1}{1000}; V_S = 50 \times 1,000 = 50,000\ \text{V} = 50\text{kV}$$

What is the secondary current for a primary current of 10 A?

$$V_P\,I_P = V_S\,I_S; 50\ \text{V} \times 10\ \text{A} = 50,000\ \text{V} \times I_S; I_S = 0.001 \times 10\ \text{A} = 10\,\text{mA}$$

The high-voltage section of an x-ray generator contains a step-up transformer, typically with a primary-to-secondary turns ratio of 1:500 to 1:1,000. Within this range, a tube voltage of 100 kV requires an input line voltage of 200 to 100 V, respectively. The center of the secondary winding is usually connected to ground potential ("center tapped to ground"). Ground potential is the electrical potential of the earth. Center tapping to ground does not affect the maximum potential difference applied between the anode and cathode of the x-ray tube, but it limits the maximum voltage at any point in the circuit relative to ground to one half of the peak voltage applied to the tube. Therefore, the maximum voltage at any point in the circuit for a center-tapped transformer of 150 kV is −75 kV or +75 kV, relative to ground. This reduces electrical insulation requirements and improves electrical safety. In some x-ray tube designs (e.g., mammography and CT), the anode is maintained at the same potential as the body of the insert, which is maintained at ground potential. Even though this places the cathode at peak negative voltage with respect to ground, the low kV (less than 50 kV) used in mammography does not present a big electrical insulation problem, while in modern CT systems (up to 140 kV) the x-ray generator is placed adjacent to the x-ray tube in the enclosed gantry.

X-ray Generator Modules

Modules of the x-ray generator (Fig. 6-24) include the high-voltage power circuit, the stator circuit, the filament circuit, the focal spot selector, and automatic exposure control (AEC) circuit. Generators typically have circuitry and microprocessors that monitor the selection of potentially damaging overload conditions in order to protect the x-ray tube. Combinations of kV, mA, and exposure time delivering excessive power to the anode are identified, and such exposures are prohibited. Heat load monitors calculate the thermal loading on the x-ray tube anode, based on kV, mA, and exposure time, and taking cooling into account. Some x-ray systems are equipped with sensors that measure the temperature of the anode. These systems protect the x-ray tube and housing from excessive heat buildup by prohibiting exposures that would damage them. This is particularly important for CT scanners and high-powered interventional fluoroscopy systems.

Operator Console

For radiographic applications, a technologist at the operator's console can select the tube voltage (kV), the tube current (mA), the exposure time (s), or the product of mA and time (mAs), the AEC mode, the AEC sensors to be used, and the focal spot.

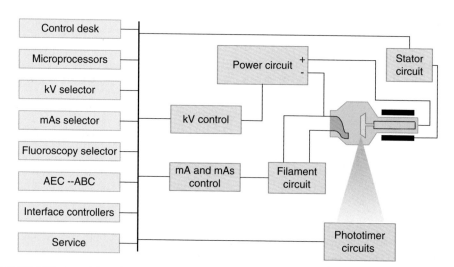

■ FIGURE 6-24 A modular schematic view shows the basic x-ray generator components. Most systems are now microprocessor controlled and include service support diagnostics.

If AEC is used, exposure time is not set. The focal spot size (i.e., large or small) is usually determined by the mA setting; low mA selections allow the small focal spot to be used, and higher mA settings require the use of the large focal spot due to anode heating concerns. On some x-ray generators, preprogrammed techniques can be selected for various examinations (e.g., chest; kidneys, ureter and bladder; cervical spine; and extremities). For fluoroscopic procedures, although kV and mA can be manually selected, the generator's automatic exposure rate control circuit, sometimes called the automatic brightness control (ABC), is commonly activated. It automatically sets the kV and mA from feedback signals from a sensor that indicates the radiation intensity at the image receptor. All console circuits have relatively low voltages and currents to minimize electrical hazards.

High-Frequency X-ray Generator

Several x-ray generator circuit designs are in use, including single-phase, three-phase, constant potential, and high-frequency inverter generators. The high-frequency generator is now the contemporary state-of-the-art choice for diagnostic x-ray systems. Its name describes its function, whereby a high-frequency alternating waveform (up to 50,000 Hz) is used for efficient conversion of low to high voltage by a step-up transformer. Subsequent rectification and voltage smoothing produce a nearly constant output voltage. These conversion steps are illustrated in Figure 6-25. The operational frequency of the generator is variable, depending on the exposure settings (kV, mA, and time), the charge/discharge characteristics of the high-voltage capacitors on the x-ray tube, and the frequency-to-voltage characteristics of the transformer.

Figure 6-26 shows the components and circuit diagram of a general-purpose high-frequency inverter generator. Low-frequency, low-voltage input power (50 to 60 cycles/s AC) is converted to a low voltage, direct current. Next, an inverter circuit creates a high-frequency AC waveform, which supplies the high-voltage transformer to create a high-voltage, high-frequency waveform. Rectification and smoothing produces high-voltage DC power that charges the high-voltage capacitors placed across the anode and cathode in the x-ray tube circuit. Accumulated charge in the capacitors will produce a voltage to the x-ray tube according to the relationship V = Q/C, where V is the voltage (volts), Q is the charge (coulombs), and C is the capacitance (farads). During the x-ray exposure, feedback circuits monitor the tube voltage

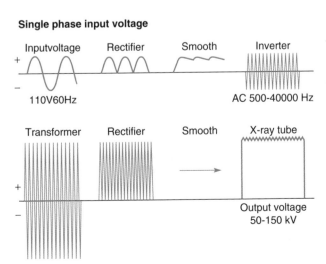

Single phase input voltage

Inputvoltage   Rectifier   Smooth   Inverter
110V60Hz   AC 500-40000 Hz

Transformer   Rectifier   Smooth   X-ray tube
                                       Output voltage
                                       50-150 kV

■ FIGURE 6-25 In a high-frequency inverter generator, a single- or three-phase AC input voltage is rectified and smoothed to create a DC waveform. An inverter circuit produces a high-frequency AC waveform as input to the high-voltage transformer. Rectification and capacitance smoothing provide the resultant high-voltage output waveform, with properties similar to those of a three-phase system.

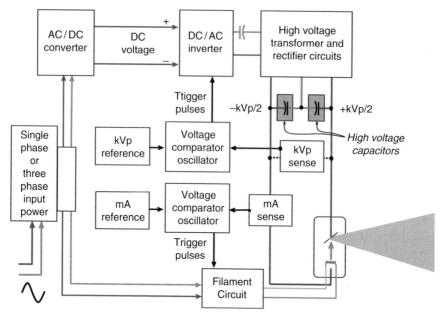

■ FIGURE 6-26 Modular components and circuits of the high-frequency generator. The selected high voltage across the x-Ray tube is created by charging high voltage capacitors to the desired potential difference. During the exposure when the x-ray circuit is energized, tube current is kept constant by the "mA sense" circuit that maintains the proper filament current by sending trigger pulses to the filament circuit , and tube voltage is kept constant by the "kV sense" circuit that sends trigger pulse signals to the DC/AC inverter to maintain the charge of high voltage capacitors.

and tube current and continuously supply charge to the capacitors as needed to maintain a nearly constant voltage.

For kV adjustment, a voltage comparator measures the difference between the reference voltage (a calibrated value proportional to the requested kV) and the actual kV measured across the tube by a voltage divider (the kV sense circuit). Trigger pulses generated by the comparator circuit produce a frequency that is proportional to the voltage difference between the reference signal and the measured signal. A large discrepancy in the compared signals results in a high trigger-pulse frequency, whereas no difference produces few or no trigger pulses. For each trigger pulse, the DC/AC inverter circuit produces a corresponding output pulse, which is subsequently converted to a high-voltage output pulse by the transformer. The high-voltage capacitors store the charge and increase the potential difference across the x-ray tube. When the requested x-ray tube voltage is reached, the output pulse rate of the comparator circuit settles down to a constant value, and recharging of the high-voltage capacitors is constant. When the actual tube voltage drops below a predetermined limit, the pulse rate increases. The feedback pulse rate (generator frequency) strongly depends on the tube current (mA), since the high-voltage capacitors discharge more rapidly with higher mA, thus actuating the kV comparator circuit. Because of the closed-loop voltage regulation, input line voltage compensation is not necessary, unlike older generator designs.

The mA is regulated in an analogous manner to the kV, with a resistor circuit sensing the actual mA (the voltage across a resistor is proportional to the current) and comparing it with a reference voltage. If the mA is too low, the mA comparator circuit increases the trigger frequency, which boosts the power to the filament to raise its temperature and increase the thermionic emission of electrons. The feedback circuit eliminates the need for space charge compensation circuits and automatically corrects for filament aging effects.

There are several advantages to the high-frequency inverter generator. Single-phase or three-phase input voltage can be used. Closed-loop feedback and regulation circuits ensure reproducible and accurate kV and mA values. Transformers operating at high frequencies are efficient, compact, and less costly to manufacture than those in other generator designs such as single-phase, three-phase, or constant-potential generators. Modular and compact design makes equipment installation and repairs relatively easy.

The high-frequency inverter generator is the preferred system for all but a few applications (e.g., those requiring extremely high power, extremely fast kV switching, or submillisecond exposure times provided by a *constant-potential* generator, which is very costly and requires more space).

Voltage Ripple

Ideally, the voltage applied to an x-ray tube would be constant. However, variations occur in the high voltage produced by an x-ray generator and applied to the x-ray tube. In an electronic waveform, voltage ripple is defined as the difference between the peak voltage and the minimum voltage, divided by the peak voltage and multiplied by 100%:

$$\% \text{ voltage ripple} = \frac{V_{max} - V_{min}}{V_{max}} \times 100 \qquad [6\text{-}6]$$

The voltage ripple for various types of x-ray generators is shown in Figure 6-27. In theory, a single-phase generator, whether one-pulse or two-pulse output, has 100% voltage ripple. Actual voltage ripple for a single-phase generator is less than 100% because of cable capacitance effects (longer cables produce a greater capacitance, whereby the capacitance "borrows" voltage from the cable and returns it a short time later, smoothing the peaks and valleys of the voltage waveform). Three-phase 6-pulse and 12-pulse generators (not discussed in this chapter) have voltage ripples of 3% to 25%. High-frequency generators have a ripple that is kV and mA dependent, typically

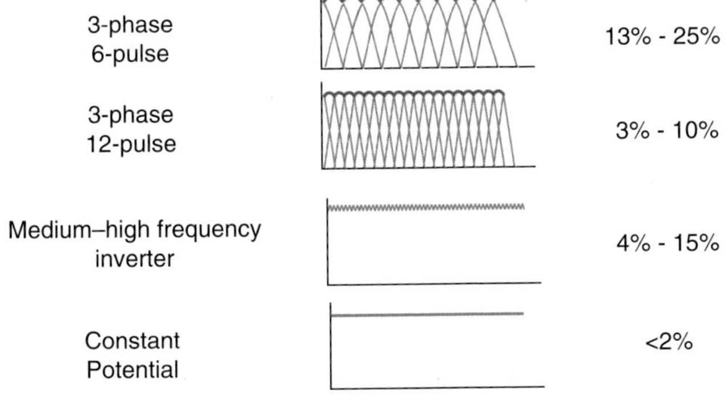

Generator type	Typical voltage waveform	kV ripple
Single-phase 1-pulse (self rectified)		100%
Single-phase 2-pulse (full wave rectified)		100%
3-phase 6-pulse		13% - 25%
3-phase 12-pulse		3% - 10%
Medium–high frequency inverter		4% - 15%
Constant Potential		<2%

■ **FIGURE 6-27** Typical voltage ripple for various x-ray generators used in diagnostic radiology varies from 100% voltage ripple for a single-phase generator to almost no ripple for a constant-potential generator.

similar to a three-phase generator, ranging from 4% to 15%. Higher kV and mA settings result in less voltage ripple for these generators. Constant-potential generators have an extremely low ripple, less than 2%, but are expensive and bulky.

Timers

Digital timers have largely replaced electronic timers based on resistor-capacitor circuits and charge-discharge timers in older systems. Digital timer circuits have extremely high reproducibility and microsecond accuracy, but the precision and accuracy of the x-ray exposure time depends chiefly on the type of switching (high voltage, low voltage, or x-ray tube switching) employed in the x-ray system. A countdown timer, also known as a backup timer, is used as a safety mechanism to terminate the exposure in the event of an exposure switch or timer failure.

Switches

The high-frequency inverter generator typically uses electronic switching on the primary side of the high-voltage transformer to initiate and stop the exposure. A relatively rapid response resulting from the high-frequency waveform characteristics of the generator circuit allows exposure times as short as 2 ms.

Alternatively, a grid-controlled x-ray tube can be used with any type of generator to switch the exposure on and off by applying a bias voltage (about ~4,000 V) to the focusing cup. This is the fastest switching method, with minimal turn-on–turnoff "lag"; however, there are extra expenses and high-voltage insulation issues to be considered.

Phototimer—Automatic Exposure Control

The phototimer, also known as the automatic exposure control (AEC) system, is often used instead of manual exposure time settings in radiography. Phototimers measure the actual amount of radiation incident on the image receptor (i.e., screen-film or digital radiography detector) and terminate x-ray production when the proper radiation exposure is obtained. Compensation for patient thickness and other variations in attenuation are achieved at the point of imaging. A phototimer system consists of one or more radiation detectors, an amplifier, a film density or digital SNR variable selector, a signal integrator circuit, a comparator circuit, a termination switch, and a backup timer safety shutoff switch (Fig. 6-28). X-rays transmitted through the patient and antiscatter grid, if present, generate ion pairs in one to three selectable ionization chambers positioned prior to the detector. An amplifier boosts the signal, which is fed to a voltage comparator and integration circuit. When the accumulated signal equals a preselected reference value, an output pulse terminates the exposure. A user-selectable "film density" or "SNR" selector on the generator control panel increases or decreases the reference voltage about 10% to 15% per step to modify the total accumulated x-ray exposure. For general diagnostic radiography, the phototimer sensors are placed in front of the image receptor to measure the transmitted x-ray flux through the patient (see Fig. 6-28). Positioning in front of the image receptor is possible because of the high transparency of the ionization chambers at the high kV values (greater than 50 kV) used for diagnostic radiography exams. In the event of a phototimer detector or circuit failure, the backup timer safety switch terminates the x-ray exposure after a preset "on" time.

To facilitate radiography of various anatomic projections, wall-mounted chest and table cassette stands and DR image receptors typically have three photocells arranged as shown in Figure 6-28 (front view). The technologist can select which photocells are used for each radiographic application. For instance, in posteroanterior chest

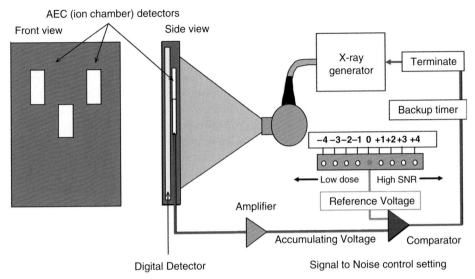

■ **FIGURE 6-28** AEC detectors measure the radiation incident on the detector and terminate the exposure according to a preset optical density or signal-to-noise ratio achieved in the analog or digital image. A front view (**left**) and side view (**middle**) of a chest cassette stand and the locations of ionization chamber detectors are shown. The desired signal to the image receptor and thus the signal-to-noise ratio may be selected at the operator's console with respect to a normalized reference voltage.

imaging, the two outside chambers are usually activated, and the x-ray beam transmitted through the lungs determines the exposure time. This prevents signal saturation in the lung areas, which can occur when the transmitted x-ray flux is otherwise measured under the highly attenuating mediastinum with the center chamber.

6.4 Power Ratings and Heat Loading and Cooling

The *power rating* of an x-ray tube or generator is the maximal power that an x-ray tube focal spot can accept or the generator can deliver. General diagnostic x-ray tubes and x-ray generators use 100 kV and the maximum ampere rating available for a 0.1 s exposure as the benchmark, as

$$\text{Power (kW)} = 100 \text{ kV} \times I \text{ (A}_{\text{max}} \text{ for a 0.1 s exposure)} \qquad [6\text{-}7]$$

For instance, a generator that can deliver 800 mA (0.8 A maximum) of tube current at 100 kV for 0.1 second exposure has a power rating of 80 kW according to Equation 6-7. For applications such as computed tomography and interventional fluoroscopy, higher- power x-ray generators are specified, typically of 80 to 100 kW or higher. However, this power capability must be matched to the power deposition capability of the focal spot; otherwise, the power cannot be realized without exceeding the x-ray tube heat limitations. Focal spot dimensions of approximately 1.2 mm × 1.2 mm, large diameter anodes, and fast rotation speeds are necessary to achieve 80 to 100 kW of power deposition. Most medium focal spot dimensions (0.6 mm × 0.6 mm) have moderate power ratings (30 to 50 kW), and smaller focal spots (0.3 mm × 0.3 mm) have low power ratings (5 to 15 kW), but power ratings are dependent on several engineering, operational, and x-ray tube design factors. For instance, in modern CT x-ray tubes, a shallow anode angle (7°), bearings mounted outside of the vacuum of the insert, and heat exchangers allow for extended high power operation (e.g., continuous operation at 800 mA at 120 kV for minutes). X-ray generators have circuits or programs to prohibit combinations of kV, mA, and exposure time that will exceed the single-exposure power deposition tolerance of the focal spot.

X-ray generator power ratings vary considerably. The highest generator power ratings (80 to 120 kW) are found in interventional radiology and cardiovascular fluoroscopic imaging suites, while modern multirow detector CT scanners have 85- to 100-kW generators. General radiographic or radiographic/fluoroscopic systems use generators providing 30 to 80 kW. Lower powered generators (5 to 30 kW) are found in mobile radiography and fluoroscopy systems, dental x-ray systems, and other systems that have fixed anode x-ray tubes. When purchasing an x-ray generator and x-ray tube system, the clinical application must be considered, as well as the matching of the power ratings of the x-ray tube large focal spot and the x-ray generator. Otherwise, there will be a mismatch in terms of capability, and most likely needless expense.

Heat Loading

The Heat Unit

The heat unit (HU) is a traditional unit that provides a simple way of expressing the energy deposition on and dissipation from the anode of an x-ray tube. The number of HU can be calculated from the parameters defining the radiographic technique

$$\text{Energy (HU)} = \text{peak voltage (kV)} \times \text{tube current (mA)} \times \text{exposure time (s)} \quad [6\text{-}8]$$

Although Equation 6-8 is correct for single-phase generator waveforms, it underestimates the energy deposition of three-phase, high-frequency, and constant-potential generators because of their lower voltage ripple and higher average voltage. A multiplicative factor of 1.35 to 1.40 compensates for this difference, the latter value being applied to constant-potential waveforms. For example, an exposure of 80 kV, 250 mA, and 100 ms results in the following HU deposition on the anode:

$$\text{Single-phase generator: } 80 \times 250 \times 0.100 = 2,000 \text{ HU}$$
$$\text{Three-phase or high-frequency inverter generator: } 80 \times 250$$
$$\times 0.100 \times 1.35 = 2,700 \text{ HU}$$

For continuous x-ray production (fluoroscopy), the HU/s is defined as follows:

$$\text{HU} / \text{s} = \text{kV} \times \text{mA} \quad\quad\quad [6\text{-}9]$$

Heat accumulates by energy deposition and simultaneously disperses by anode cooling. The anode cools faster at higher temperatures, so that for most fluoroscopic and long CT procedures, steady-state equilibrium exists and Equation 6-9 will overestimate the heat energy delivered to the anode. This is taken into consideration by the anode thermal characteristics chart for heat input and heat output (cooling) curves.

The Joule

The joule (J) is the SI unit of energy. One joule is deposited by a power of one watt acting for 1 s (1 J = 1 W × 1 s). The energy, in joules, deposited in the anode is calculated as follows:

$$\text{Energy (J)} = \text{Voltage (V)} \times \text{Tube current (A)} \times \text{Exposure time(s)} \quad [6\text{-}10]$$

The root-mean-square voltage, V_{RMS}, is the constant voltage that would deliver the same power as a varying voltage waveform (e.g., for a single phase generator), which would be substituted for V, and, from Equation 6-8 and 6-10, the relationship between the deposited energy in joules and HU can be approximated as

$$\text{Energy (HU)} \cong 1.4 \times \text{Heat input (J)} \qquad \text{[6-11]}$$

Anode Heating and Cooling Chart

Multiple x-ray exposures, continuous x-ray tube operation with CT, and prolonged fluoroscopy in interventional procedures deliver significant heat energy to the anode. An *anode heating and cooling chart* (Fig. 6-29) shows the anode heat loading for various input powers (kW or HU/s) as the x-ray tube is operating, taking into account the cooling that simultaneously occurs. For low-input power techniques, the heat loading increases to a plateau, where the cooling rate equals the heating rate. At higher power inputs, heating exceeds cooling, and after a certain time, a limit is reached where x-ray production must be stopped and anode cooling must be allowed prior to using the x-ray tube again. With larger anode heat capacities, the anode cooling curve is steeper because higher temperatures result in more rapid cooling (the "black-body" effect, where the radiative cooling rate is proportional to T^4, for absolute temperature T). The maximal anode heat capacity is indicated by the peak value of the cooling curve on the y-axis (0 time) of the chart. Each anode heating and cooling chart is specific to a particular x-ray tube and housing assembly. Some high-powered x-ray tubes for CT exceed 8 MHU anode heat loading with extremely high anode and x-ray tube housing cooling rates, achieved through advanced anode, rotor bearing, and housing designs. An example

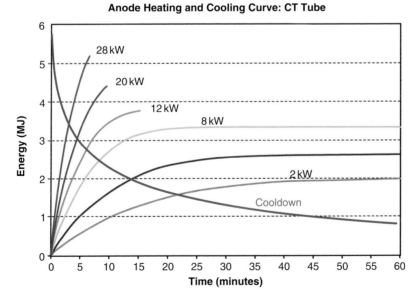

Anode Heating and Cooling Curve: CT Tube

■ FIGURE 6-29 Anode heating and cooling curve chart for a CT scanner plots *energy* in megajoules (MJ) on the vertical axis and *time* in minutes on the horizontal axis. A series of power input curves from low (2 kW) to high (28 kW) are determined by the kV and mA settings with continuous x-ray tube operation as a function of time. The cooling curve shows the rate of cooling and indicates faster cooling with higher anode heat load (temperature). In this example the maximum capacity is 5.7 MJ. For low power inputs, heating and cooling rates eventually equilibrate and reach a steady state, as shown for the 2, 4, and 8 kW curves.

of a heating and cooling chart for a modern x-ray CT tube, with a maximum anode heat capacity of 5.7 megajoules (MJ) (equivalent to 8.0 MHU), is shown in Figure 6-29. If the x-ray technique is high or a large number of sequential or continuous exposures have been taken (e.g., during operation of a CT scanner), it can be necessary to wait before reenergizing the x-ray tube to avoid damage to the anode. Use of the specific anode cooling curve can determine how long to wait, based upon the total amount of accumulated heat, the simultaneous cooling that occurs, and the amount of power that will be deposited during the next acquisition. Modern x-ray systems have sensors and protection circuits to prevent overheating.

6.5   Factors Affecting X-ray Emission

The output of an x-ray tube is often described by the terms quality, quantity, and exposure. *Quality* describes the penetrability of an x-ray beam, with higher energy x-ray photons having a larger half-value layer (HVL) and higher "quality." (The HVL is discussed in Chapter 3.) *Quantity* refers to the number of photons comprising the beam. *Exposure,* defined in Chapter 3, is nearly proportional to the energy fluence of the x-ray beam. X-ray production efficiency, exposure, quality, and quantity are determined by six major factors: x-ray tube target material, tube voltage, tube current, exposure time, beam filtration, and generator waveform.

1. **Anode target material** affects the *efficiency* of bremsstrahlung radiation production, with output exposure roughly proportional to atomic number. Incident electrons are more likely to have radiative interactions in higher-Z materials (see Equation 6-1). The energies of characteristic x-rays produced in the target depend on the target material. Therefore, the target material affects the quantity of bremsstrahlung photons and the quality of the characteristic radiation.

2. **Tube voltage** (kV) determines the maximum energy in the bremsstrahlung spectrum and affects the quality of the output spectrum. In addition, the efficiency of x-ray production is directly related to tube voltage. Exposure is approximately proportional to the square of the kV in the diagnostic energy range.

$$\text{Exposure} \propto kV^2 \qquad\qquad [6\text{-}12]$$

For example, according to Equation 6-12, the relative exposure of a beam generated with 80 kV compared with that of 60 kV for the same tube current and exposure time is calculated as follows:

$$\left(\frac{80}{60}\right)^2 \cong 1.78$$

Therefore, the output exposure increases by approximately 78% (Fig. 6-30). *An increase in kV increases the efficiency of x-ray production and the quantity and quality of the x-ray beam.*

Changes in the kV must be compensated by corresponding changes in mAs to maintain the same exposure. At 80 kV, 1.78 units of exposure occur for every 1 unit of exposure at 60 kV. To achieve the original 1 unit of exposure, the mAs must be adjusted to 1/1.78 = 0.56 times the original mAs, which is a *reduction* of 44%. An additional consideration of technique adjustment concerns the x-ray attenuation characteristics of the patient. To achieve equal transmitted exposure through a typical patient (e.g., 20-cm tissue), the compensatory mAs varies with approximately the fifth power of the kV ratio

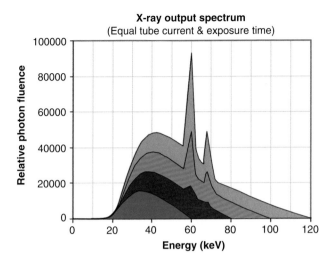

X-ray output spectrum
(Equal tube current & exposure time)

Relative photon fluence (y-axis): 0, 20000, 40000, 60000, 80000, 100000

Energy (keV) (x-axis): 0, 20, 40, 60, 80, 100, 120

■ **FIGURE 6-30** x-Ray tube output intensity varies as the square of tube voltage (kV). In this example, the same tube current and exposure times (mAs) are compared for 60 to 120 kV. The relative area under each spectrum roughly follows a squared dependence (characteristic radiation is ignored).

$$\left(\frac{kVp_1}{kVp_2}\right)^5 \times \; mAs_1 = mAs_2 \qquad\qquad [6\text{-}13]$$

According to Equation 6-13, if a 60-kV exposure requires 40 mAs for a proper exposure through a typical adult patient, at 80 kV the adjusted mAs is approximately

$$\left(\frac{60}{80}\right)^5 \times 40 \; mAs \cong 9.5 \; mAs$$

or about one fourth of the original mAs. The value of the exponent (between four and five) depends on the thickness and attenuation characteristics of the patient.

3. **Tube current** (mA) is proportional to the number of electrons flowing from the cathode to the anode per unit time. The exposure of the beam for a given kV and filtration is proportional to the tube current. Also the exposure time is the duration of x-ray production. The quantity of x-rays is directly proportional to the product of tube current and exposure time (mAs), as shown in Figure 6-31.

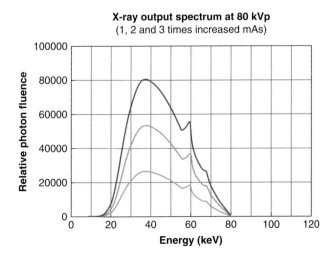

X-ray output spectrum at 80 kVp
(1, 2 and 3 times increased mAs)

Relative photon fluence (y-axis): 0, 20000, 40000, 60000, 80000, 100000

Energy (keV) (x-axis): 0, 20, 40, 60, 80, 100, 120

■ **FIGURE 6-31** X-ray tube output intensity is proportional to the mAs (tube current and exposure time). Shown is the result of increasing the mAs by a factor of two and three, with a proportional change in the number of x-rays produced.

■ FIGURE 6-32 X-ray tube output intensity decreases and spectral quality (effective energy) increases with increasing thickness of added tube filters. Shown are spectra with added filtration at the same kV and mAs.

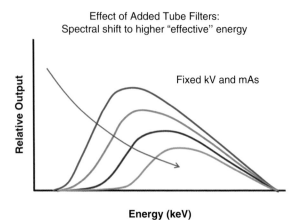

Effect of Added Tube Filters:
Spectral shift to higher "effective" energy

Fixed kV and mAs

Relative Output

Energy (keV)

4. **Beam filtration** modifies the quantity and quality of the x-ray beam by preferentially removing the low-energy photons in the spectrum. This reduces the number of photons (quantity) and increases the average energy, also increasing the quality (Fig. 6-32). For highly filtered beams, the mAs required to achieve a particular x-ray intensity will be much higher than for lightly filtered beams; therefore, it is necessary to know the HVL of the beam and the normalized x-ray tube intensity per mAs (in addition to the geometry) to calculate the incident exposure and radiation dose to the patient. One cannot simply use kV and mAs for determining the "proper technique" or to estimate the dose to the patient without this information. In the United States, x-ray system manufacturers must

TABLE 6-3   MINIMUM HVL REQUIREMENTS FOR X-RAY SYSTEMS IN THE UNITED STATES (21 CFR 1020.30)

DESIGNED OPERATING RANGE	MEASURED X-RAY TUBE VOLTAGE (kV)	MINIMUM HVL (mm OF ALUMINUM)
<51 kV	30	0.3
	40	0.4
	50	0.5
51–70 kV	51	1.3
	60	1.5
	70	1.8
>70 kV	71	2.5
	80	2.9
	90	3.2
	100	3.6
	110	3.9
	120	4.3
	130	4.7
	140	5.0
	150	5.4

Note: This table refers to systems manufactured after June 2006. It does not include values for dental or mammography systems.

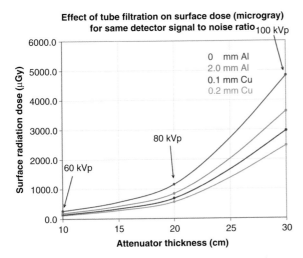

Effect of tube filtration on surface dose (microgray) for same detector signal to noise ratio

■ **FIGURE 6-33** Added x-ray tube filters can significantly reduce patient dose. Compared are measured entrance doses (air kerma with backscatter) to 10, 20, and 30 cm sheets of PMMA when using photo-timed exposures at 60, 80, and 100 kV, respectively. The top curve represents the nominal beam condition, then 2.0 mm Al, 0.1 mm Cu + 1 mm Al, and 0.2 mm Cu + 1 mm Al for the lowest curve. For constant signal-to-noise ratio, the mAs is increased to compensate for added filter attenuation, as listed in Table 6-4.

comply with minimum HVL requirements specified in the Code of Federal Regulations, 21CFR 1020.30 (Table 6-3), which have been adopted by many state regulatory agencies. A pertinent clinical example of the radiation dose savings achievable with added filtration compared to the minimum filtration is shown in Figure 6-33, comparing the surface entrance radiation dose to the *same signal* generated in the detector for 0 mm Al (minimum filtration), 2 mm Al, 0.1 mm Cu, and 0.2 mm Cu. With more filtration, the dose savings become greater. For instance, as listed in Table 6-4, the comparison of 30 cm polymethylmethacrylate (PMMA) at 100 kV indicates a dose savings of 49% when a 0.2 mm Cu filter is added to the beam. To achieve this requires an increase in mAs of 37%, from 14.5 to 19.8 mAs at 100 kV. Even though the acquisition technique is much higher, the entrance dose is much lower, without any loss of image quality, particularly for digital imaging devices where image contrast and brightness enhancements are easily applied. Using added filtration in a modern x-ray collimator assembly is as

TABLE 6-4 TUBE FILTRATION, MEASURED CHANGES IN REQUIRED mAs, AND MEASURED SURFACE DOSE (μGy) FOR EQUIVALENT SIGNAL IN THE OUTPUT DIGITAL IMAGE

	10 cm PMMA (60 kV)				20 cm PMMA (80 kV)				30 cm PMMA (100 kV)			
	TUBE CURRENT		DOSE (μGy)		TUBE CURRENT		DOSE (μGy)		TUBE CURRENT		DOSE (μGy)	
FILTRATION	mAs	% Δ	DOSE	% Δ	mAs	% Δ	DOSE	% Δ	mAs	% Δ	DOSE	% Δ
0 mm Al	3.8	0	264	0	6.8	0	1,153	0	14.5	0	4,827	0
2 mm Al	5.0	32	188	−29	8.2	21	839	−27	16.5	14	3,613	−25
0.1 mm Cu + 1 mm Al	6.2	63	150	−43	9.3	37	680	−41	17.6	21	2,960	−39
0.2 mm Cu + 1 mm Al	8.8	132	123	−53	11.2	65	557	−52	19.8	37	2,459	−49

Note: % Δ indicates the percentage change from the *no added filtration* measurement. For mAs, there is an increase in the mAs required to compensate for increased attenuation of the beam by the added filters. For surface dose, there is a decrease in the percentage surface dose change with more added filters for equivalent absorbed signal in the detector because of less attenuation of the beam in the object.

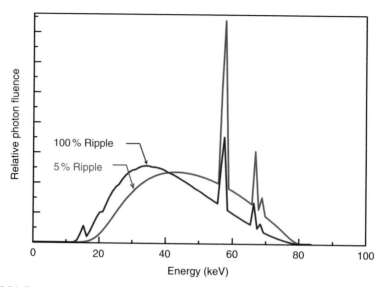

■ FIGURE 6-34 Output intensity (bremsstrahlung) spectra for the same tube voltage (kV) and the same tube current and exposure time (mAs) demonstrate the higher effective energy and greater output of a three-phase or high-frequency generator voltage waveform (~5% voltage ripple), compared with a single-phase generator waveform (100% voltage ripple).

simple as pushing the filter selection button, or automatically selecting the filter with anatomical programming.

5. **Generator waveform** affects the quality of the emitted x-ray spectrum. For the same kV, a single-phase generator provides a lower average potential difference than does a three-phase or high-frequency generator. Both the quality and quantity of the x-ray spectrum are affected (Fig. 6-34).

The x-ray *quantity* is approximately proportional to $Z_{target} \times kV^2 \times mAs$. The x-ray *quality* depends on the kV, the generator waveform, and the tube filtration. Exposure depends on both the quantity and quality of the x-ray beam. Compensation for changes in kV with radiographic techniques requires adjustments of mAs on the order of the fourth to fifth power of the kV ratio, because kV determines quantity, quality, and transmission through the object, whereas mAs determines quantity only. Added filters to the x-ray tube can significantly lower patient dose by selectively attenuating the low energy x-rays in the bremsstrahlung spectrum, but require a compensatory increase in the mAs.

In summary, x-rays are the basic radiologic tool for a majority of medical diagnostic imaging procedures. Knowledge of x-ray production, x-ray generators, and x-ray beam control is important for further understanding of the image formation process and the need to obtain the highest image quality at the lowest possible radiation exposure.

SUGGESTED READING

Krestel E, ed. *Imaging systems for medical diagnostics*. Berlin/Munich, Germany: Siemens Aktiengesellschaft, 1990.

McCollough CH. The AAPM/RSNA physics tutorial for residents: x-ray production. *Radiographics* 1997;17:967–984.

Seibert JA. The AAPM/RSNA physics tutorial for residents: x-ray generators. *Radiographics* 1997;17: 1533–1557.

CHAPTER 7

Radiography

7.1 Geometry of Projection Radiography

Radiography is the production of a two-dimensional image from a three-dimensional object, the patient (Fig. 7-1). The procedure projects the x-ray shadows of the patient's anatomy onto the detector and is often called *projection radiography*. The source of radiation in the x-ray tube is a small spot, and x-rays that are produced in the x-ray tube diverge as they travel away from this spot. Because of beam divergence, the collimated x-ray beam becomes larger in area and less intense with increasing distance from the source. Consequently, x-ray radiography results in some magnification of the object being radiographed. Radiography is performed with the x-ray source on one side of the patient, and the detector is positioned on the other side of the patient. During the exposure, incident x-rays are differentially attenuated by anatomical structures in the patient. A small fraction of the x-ray beam passes through the patient unattenuated and is recorded on the radiographic detector, forming the latent radiographic image.

The geometry of projection transmission imaging is described in Figure 7-2. Magnification can be defined simply as

$$M = \frac{L_{image}}{L_{object}} \qquad [7\text{-}1]$$

where L_{image} is the length of the object as seen on the image and L_{object} is the length of the actual object. Due to similar triangles, the object magnification can be computed using the source to object distance (a) and the object to detector distance (b)

$$M = \frac{a+b}{a} \qquad [7\text{-}2]$$

The magnification will always be greater than 1.0 but approaches 1.0 when a relatively flat object (such as a hand in radiography) is positioned in contact with the detector, where $b \approx 0$. The magnification factor changes slightly for each plane perpendicular to the x-ray beam axis in the patient, and thus different anatomical structures are magnified differently. This characteristic means that, especially for thicker body parts, an AP (anterior-posterior) image of a patient will have a subtly different appearance to an experienced viewer than a PA (posterior-anterior) image of the same patient. Knowledge of the magnification in radiography is sometimes required clinically, for example, in angioplasty procedures where the diameter of the vessel must be measured to select the correct size of a stent or angiographic balloon catheter. In these situations, an object of known dimension (e.g., a catheter with notches at known spacing) is placed near the anatomy of interest, from which the magnification can be determined and a correction factor calculated.

Radiographic detectors, both screen-film and digital, should be exposed to an x-ray intensity within a relatively small range. X-ray technique factors such as the applied tube voltage (kV), tube current (mA), and exposure time will be discussed

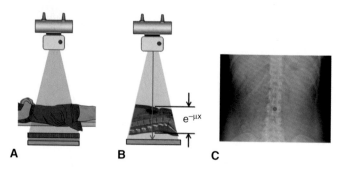

A   **B**   **C**

■ **FIGURE 7-1** The basic geometry of radiographic imaging is illustrated. The patient is positioned between the x-ray tube and the detector system (**A**), and the radiograph is acquired. The photocell (seen between the grid and detector) determines the correct exposure levels to the detector (phototiming). In transmission imaging (**B**), the x-rays pass through each point in the patient, and the absorption of all the structures along each ray path combine to produce the primary beam intensity at that location on the detector. The density at each point in the image (**C**) reflects the degree of x-ray beam attenuation across the image. For example, the gray scale under the red dot on (**C**) corresponds to the total beam attenuation along the line shown in (**B**).

later, but an important parameter that should be kept consistent is the distance between the x-ray source and the detector. For most radiographic examinations, the source to imager distance (SID) is fixed at 100 cm, and there are usually detents in the radiographic equipment that help the technologists to set this distance. An exception to the 100-cm (40 inches) SID is for upright chest radiography, where the SID is typically set to 183 cm (72 inches). The larger SID used for chest radiography reduces the differential magnification in the lung parenchyma.

The focal spot in the x-ray tube is very small but is not truly a point source, resulting in magnification-dependent resolution loss. The blurring from a finite x-ray source is dependent upon the geometry of the exam, as shown in Figure 7-3. The length of the edge gradient (L_g) is related to the length of the focal spot (L_f) by

$$L_g = L_f \frac{b}{a},$$

[7-3]

■ **FIGURE 7-2** The geometry of beam divergence is shown. The object is positioned a distance *a* from the x-ray source, and the detector is positioned a distance (*a* + *b*) from the source. From the principle of similar triangles,

$$m = \frac{L_{image}}{L_{object}} = \frac{a+b}{a}$$

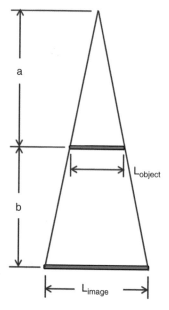

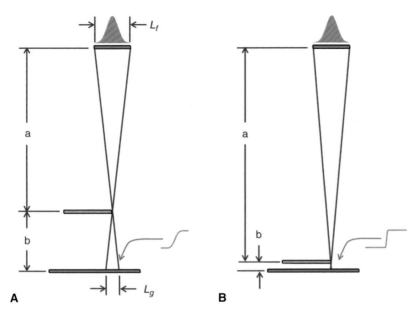

■ **FIGURE 7-3** The magnification of a sharp edge in the patient will result in some blurring of that structure because of the use of a focal spot that is not truly a point source. For a focal spot with width L_f, the intensity distribution across this distributed (nonpoint) source will result in the edge being projected onto the image plane. The edge will no longer be perfectly sharp, but rather its shadow will reflect the source distribution. Most sources are approximately gaussian in shape, and thus the blurred profile of the edge will also appear gaussian. The length of the blur in the image is related to the width of the focal spot by $L_g = \dfrac{b}{a} L_f$.

where $\dfrac{b}{a}$ represents the magnification of the focal spot. The "edge gradient" is measured using a highly magnified metal foil with a sharp edge. In most circumstances, higher object magnification increases the width of the edge gradient and reduces the spatial resolution of the image. Consequently, in most cases, the patient should be positioned as close as possible to the detector to reduce magnification. For thin objects that are placed in contact with the detector, the magnification is approximately 1.0, and there will be negligible blurring caused by the finite dimensions of the focal spot. In some settings (e.g., mammography), a very small focal spot is used intentionally with magnification. In this case, the small focal spot produces much less magnification-dependent blur, and the projected image is larger as it strikes the detector. This intentional application of magnification radiography is used to overcome resolution limitations of the detector, and increases spatial resolution.

7.2 Screen-Film Radiography

Screen-film radiography defined the field of radiology for most of the 20th century. As other digital modalities such as CT and MRI became routinely used, picture archiving and communication systems (PACS) evolved. Radiography and then mammography were the last modalities to become assimilated into the digital arena, due to the large display monitors and storage requirements for large-format, high-resolution digital radiographic images. Nevertheless, screen-film radiography still is used in low-volume clinics and other niche areas.

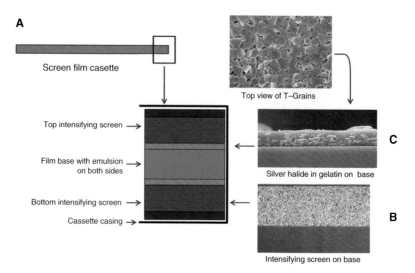

■ **FIGURE 7-4** **A.** A diagram showing the various layers in a double-sided screen-film cassette is shown, with the dual emulsion film laying inside the screen with two intensifying screens. **B.** A micrograph of the intensifying screen phosphor, attached to a plastic base, is shown. The scintillating layer consists of small (~25 μm) crystals of phosphor (i.e., Gd_2O_2S:Eu), packed with a binder into a screen. This is an unstructured or amorphous intensifying screen. **C.** A micrograph of the emulsion layer is shown. The individual grains of silver halide are seen within the gelatin layer.

Screens

In screen-film radiography, a sheet of film with a light-sensitive emulsion on both sides is sandwiched between two intensifying screens (Fig. 7-4). A light-tight cassette encapsulates the screens and film. The intensifying screens are composed of a scintillator, such as Gd_2O_2S crystals, held together by a binder material (Fig. 7-4 shows a micrograph of a screen). The scintillator in the intensifying screen converts incident x-ray photons to visible light, which then exposes the silver halide emulsion on the film. Close physical contact between the screen and film is very important, as gaps promote excessive lateral light propagation, which blur the image. The screens in a cassette are mounted on compressible foam backing, which presses the screens against the film to maintain good screen-film contact. The intensifying screen is composed of high Z compounds that have high absorption efficiency for x-rays. $CaWO_4$ initially was used; more common today are the rare-earth scintillators Gd_2O_2S, LaOBr, and $YTaO_4$. Thicker intensifying screens absorb more x-ray photons than thinner screens, but the scintillation light that is emitted in a thicker screen diffuses greater distances to reach and expose the film emulsion (Fig. 7-5). This results in more light spread, which reduces the spatial resolution of the screen. For very high-resolution screen-film systems (some extremity cassettes and nearly all mammography systems), only one screen is used in conjunction with a single emulsion film. Intensifying screens are discussed in more detail later in this chapter.

Film

Film is composed of a thin plastic base coated on one or both sides with a layer of light-sensitive emulsion consisting of silver halide (about 95% AgBr and 15% AgI) crystals held in water-soluble gelatin (Fig. 7-4 shows a micrograph). The shapes of the silver halide crystals incorporated in radiographic film are engineered in a tabular

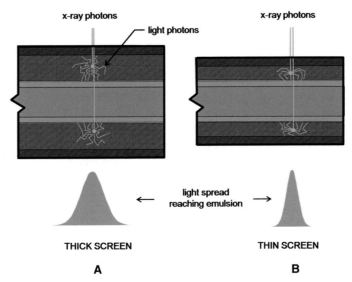

■ FIGURE 7-5 The indirect detection process is illustrated, with a thick screen (**A**) and a thinner screen (**B**). X-ray photons are incident on both screen-film systems, interact in both the upper and lower screens, and the light photons that are created by scintillation then diffuse by scattering through the screen matrix, until some eventually reach the film emulsion. The thicker screen creates a geometry where the light photons can travel farther laterally, and this increases the width of the light distribution reaching the emulsion, compared to the thinner screen. Thus, thicker screens absorb more photons (are more sensitive) but have reduced spatial resolution compared to thinner screens. Not shown in this diagram is the fact that exponentially more x-ray photons are deposited in the upper screens as compared to the lower screens, due to the exponential manner in which x-rays are absorbed.

"T" grain shape (see Fig. 7-4) to increase surface area for improving light capture efficiency and reducing silver content to save cost. Silver halide grains have a small amount of AgS that introduces defects in the ionic crystal structures, where the negative charge (from Br– and I–) builds up on the surfaces and a net positive charge (Ag^+) is more central in the crystals. A *sensitivity speck*, induced by the lattice defects caused by AgS, is a protrusion of the positive charge that reaches the surface of the crystal. When a silver halide grain is exposed to visible light, a small number of Ag^+ ions are reduced (gain electrons) and are converted into metallic Ag ($Ag^+ + e^- \rightarrow Ag$). If ≥ 5 Ag^+ ions are reduced, which depends on the incident light intensity, a stable *latent image center* is formed. An exposed film that has not been chemically developed contains a latent image consisting of a pattern of invisible silver halide grains with latent image centers. There is also a slight intensity *rate* effect, giving rise to slight differences in film density depending on the exposure rate (called *reciprocity law failure*).

Film Processing

The gelatin layer is permeable to aqueous solutions, which is necessary for the aqueous developing chemicals to come into contact with the silver crystals. When the film is developed in an aqueous chemical bath containing a reducing agent, called the developer, the metallic Ag atoms at the latent image centers act as a catalyst, causing the remaining silver ions in that grain to be reduced. A grain of reduced metallic silver atoms appears as a black speck on the film.

After the film has passed through the developer, it passes through a bath of an aqueous oxidizing solution called *fixer* that dissolves the remaining (inactivated) silver halide from the emulsion layer areas that were not exposed (or were underexposed) to light. The film is then rinsed with water to remove residual developer and fixer, and is dried.

In this way, the visible light striking the film emulsion acts locally to cause film darkening. The film appears darker to the human eye as a result of an increasing density of microscopic black silver grains in the emulsion layer. Thus, when the film is placed on a light box, a gray scale image is produced that is darker where the x-ray beam incident on the screen-film detector was more intense (where x-ray attenuation in the patient was lower), and the film is lighter where the x-ray beam was less intense (where the attenuation in the patient was higher). Film radiographs are negative images—higher exposure to the detector produces darker images.

The details of film processing are outside the scope of this chapter. However, it is worth noting that the catalytic reaction that is promoted by the sensitivity speck in the presence of a strong reducing agent results in an approximately 10^9 gain in optical density on the film with very little added noise—this is a chemical amplification process that few electronic detector systems can match.

The Characteristic Curve

Although the intensifying screen responds linearly to incident x-ray exposure (e.g., twice the x-ray fluence results in twice the visible light output), the response of the film emulsion to light results in a nonlinear characteristic curve for screen-film systems. An "H and D" curve (for Hurter and Driffield) shown in Figure 7-6, is a plot of the log of the relative exposure on the x-axis and the optical density (OD) of the processed film on the y-axis. This figure illustrates that the optical density (OD) of film changes nonlinearly with the x-ray exposure level. The OD is defined as the negative of the base-10 logarithm of the transmittance (T) of the film

$$OD = -\log_{10}(T),$$

[7-4]

In Eq. 7-4, T is defined as the fraction of visible light passing through the film from a light source:

$$T = \frac{I}{I_o},$$

[7-5]

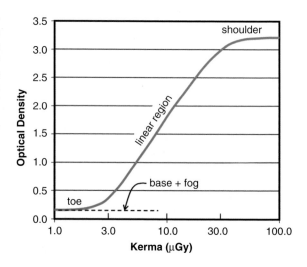

■ **FIGURE 7-6** A characteristic curve for screen-film is shown. This is also called the "H and D" curve after Hurter and Driffield's early work. The H and D curve is typically shown as the OD as a function of log-relative exposure. The curve shows low contrast in the toe and shoulder regions, and a higher contrast (higher slope) in the linear region. If an unexposed film is developed, its OD will be the base + fog level.

In Eq. 7-5, I is the intensity of light that passes through the film and I_o is the intensity of the light source at the same point with the film removed. From the above equations, a film of OD=1 transmits 10%, OD=2 transmits 1% and OD=3 transmits 0.1% of the intensity of a light source from a fluorescent light box. Since the human eye responds approximately logarithmically to light intensity, a film OD of 1.0 appears to be two times brighter than an OD of 2.0, and three times brighter than an OD of 3.0. The inverse of the relationship given in Eq. 7-4 is given by:

$$10^{-OD} = T. \tag{7-6}$$

Radiography has many clinical applications, and both the screen characteristics and film characteristics can be changed to optimize the detector for different clinical demands. Screen-film sensitivity can be adjusted as shown in Figure 7-7A. Systems can be more sensitive (and have higher "speed"), which means that less x-ray radiation is required to produce a given OD. "Slower" screen-film systems require more radiation to produce a given level of film darkening, which results in more radiation dose, but because more x-ray photons are used to make the image, the statistical integrity of the image is better (lower quantum noise). A change in screen-film speed is seen as a lateral shift of the H and D curve (Fig. 7-7A). Screen-film systems can also be adjusted to deliver different image contrast, as seen in Figure 7-7B. Contrast is adjusted by altering the grain size and other parameters in the film emulsion. While high contrast is desirable, the compromise is that dynamic range (called *latitude* in radiography) is reduced.

High contrast films are not suitable for all applications. For example, a large difference in x-ray fluence to the detector occurs in chest radiography, because of the highly attenuating mediastinum and the highly transmissive lung fields—a low-contrast, wide-latitude film is required for this setting, otherwise the heart silhouette would be too white and the lung fields would be too dark on the processed film. Moreover, very high contrast films require more precise exposure levels to maintain

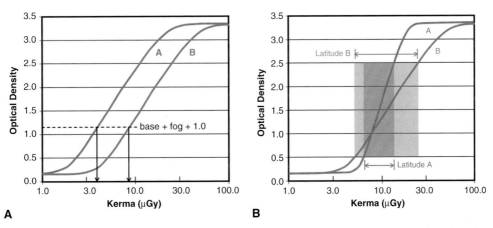

A   **B**

■ **FIGURE 7-7 A.** Two characteristic curves are shown, one for a more sensitive system (curve A), and one for a system with lower sensitivity (curve B). The *speed* of a screen-film system relates to how much exposure is required to deliver a specific OD, typically OD = 1 + base + fog. Curve A requires less radiation to reach this OD, and hence it is *faster*. **B.** With these two characteristic curves, the speed is approximately the same; however, the slopes of these curves are different. Curve A has a steeper slope, and therefore has higher contrast, but the exposure latitude is narrow—the exposure levels striking the screen-film system are optimally kept to within this range. Curve B has less slope, and will produce less *radiographic contrast,* but it has a wider exposure latitude. For examinations where a lot of subject contrast is expected (such as the chest radiograph), wider latitude screen-film systems are required.

proper optical density on the film, and failure to achieve such precision may require more studies to be repeated. For mammography, on the other hand, the compressed breast is almost uniformly thick and thus the x-ray fluence striking the detector (under the breast anatomy) is relatively uniform, and thus a very high contrast (but narrow latitude) film can be used (system A in Fig. 7-7B).

The concepts of changing the characteristics of screen film systems are discussed above, however in actual practice screen film characteristics are fixed by the manufacturer. The user typically discusses the needs of their imaging facility with the film vendor, and purchases the screen film system or systems appropriate for their needs.

 ## 7.3 Computed Radiography

Computed radiography (CR) refers to photostimulable phosphor detector (PSP) systems, which are historically housed in a cassette similar to a screen-film cassette. Traditional scintillators, such as Gd_2O_2S and cesium iodide (CsI), emit light promptly (nearly instantaneously) when irradiated by an x-ray beam. When x-rays are absorbed by photostimulable phosphors, some light is also promptly emitted, but a fraction of the absorbed x-ray energy is trapped in the PSP screen and can be read out later using laser light. For this reason, PSP screens are also called *storage phosphors*. CR was introduced in the 1970s, saw increasing use in the late 1980s, and was in wide use at the turn of the century as many departments installed PACS.

Most CR imaging plates are composed of a mixture of BaFBr and other halide-based phosphors, often referred to as barium fluorohalide. A CR plate is a flexible screen that is enclosed in a light-tight cassette. The CR cassette is exposed to x-rays during the radiographic examination and is subsequently placed in a CR reader. Once placed in the CR reader, the following steps take place:

1. The cassette is moved into the reader unit, and the imaging plate is mechanically removed from the cassette.
2. The imaging plate is translated vertically in the (y) direction by rollers across a moving stage and is scanned horizontally in the (x) direction by a laser beam of approximately 700 nm wavelength.
3. Red laser light stimulates the emission of trapped energy in a tiny area (x,y location) of the imaging plate, and blue-green visible light is emitted from the storage phosphor as energetic electrons drop down to their ground state.
4. The light emitted through photostimulated luminescence is collected by a fiber optic light guide and strikes a photomultiplier tube (PMT), where it produces an electronic signal.
5. The electronic signal is digitized and stored as a pixel value. For every spatial location (*x, y*) on the imaging plate, a corresponding gray scale value is determined that is proportional to the locally absorbed x-ray energy.
6. The plate is exposed to bright white light to erase any residual trapped energy.
7. The imaging plate is returned to the cassette and is ready for reuse.

The digital image that is generated by the CR reader is stored temporarily on a local hard disk. Once acquired, the digital radiographic image undergoes image processing by the CR reader. The image is then typically sent to a PACS for interpretation by a radiologist and long-term archiving.

The imaging plate itself is a completely analog device, but it is read out by analog and digital electronic techniques, as shown in Figure 7-8.

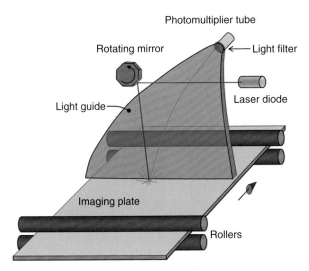

■ FIGURE 7-8 The readout mechanics of a CR system are shown. The imaging plate is translated through the mechanism by a series of rollers, and a laser beam scans horizontally across the plate. The rotating multifaceted mirror causes the laser beam to scan the imaging plate in a raster fashion. The light released by laser stimulation is collected by the light guide and produces a signal in the PMT. The red light from the laser is filtered out before reaching the PMT.

The light that is released from the imaging plate is a different color than the stimulating laser light (Fig. 7-9). Indeed, the blue light that is emitted from the screen has shorter wavelength and higher energy per photon than the stimulating red light. This is energetically feasible only because the energy associated with the emitted blue light was actually stored in the screen from the absorption of very energetic x-ray photons, and the red light serves only to release this energy from the storage phosphor. To eliminate detection by the PMT of the scattered excitation laser light, an optical filter that is positioned in front of the PMT transmits the blue light and attenuates the red laser light.

Figure 7-10 illustrates how photostimulable phosphors work. A small mass of screen material is shown being exposed to x-rays. Typical imaging plates are composed of about 85% BaFBr and 15% BaFI, activated with a small quantity of europium. The CR screen is amorphous (lacks structure); the barium fluorohalide crystals are small and are held together by an inert, optically transparent binder. The nomenclature BaFBr:Eu indicates that the BaFBr phosphor is activated by europium. This activation procedure, also called *doping*, creates defects in the BaFBr crystals that allow electrons to be trapped more efficiently. The defects in the crystalline lattice caused by the europium dopant give rise to so-called F-centers.

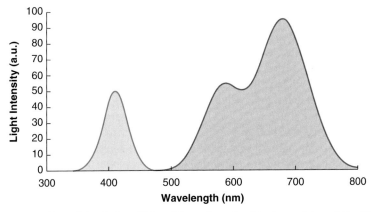

■ FIGURE 7-9 The red laser light (600 to 700 nm) is used to stimulate the emission of the blue light (400 to 450 nm); the intensity of the blue light is proportional to the x-ray exposure to the region of the detector illuminated by the laser light.

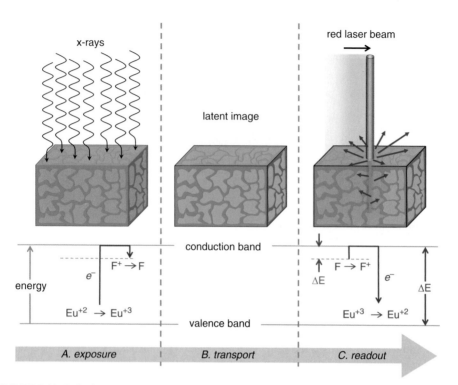

■ **FIGURE 7-10 A.** During exposure, x-rays are absorbed in the storage phosphor and some of the electrons reach the conduction band, where they may interact with an F-center, causing the reduction of europium (Eu) ions. **B.** The electrons are trapped in this high-energy, metastable state, and can remain there for minutes to months. **C.** During readout, the phosphor is scanned by a red laser, which provides the trapped electrons enough energy to be excited into the conduction band. Here, some fraction of electrons will drop down to the valence band, emitting blue light during the transition. When the F-center releases a trapped electron, the trivalent europium (Eu^{+3}) is converted back to its divalent state. (Eu^{+2}).

When x-ray energy is absorbed by the BaFBr phosphor, the absorbed energy excites electrons associated with the europium atoms, causing divalent europium atoms (Eu^{+2}) to be oxidized and changed to the trivalent state (Eu^{+3}). The excited electrons become mobile, and a fraction of them interact with F-centers. The F-centers trap these electrons in a higher-energy, metastable state, where they can remain for minutes to weeks, with only slight fading over time. The latent image that is encoded on the imaging plate after x-ray exposure, but before readout, exists as billions of electrons trapped in F-centers. The number of trapped excited electrons per unit area of the imaging plate is proportional to the intensity of x-rays incident at each location of the detector during the x-ray exposure.

When the red laser light scans the exposed imaging plate, some energy is absorbed at the F-center and transferred to the electrons. A proportional fraction of electrons gain enough energy to reach the conduction band, become mobile, and then drop to the ground energy state, and thus Eu^{+3} is converted back to Eu^{+2}. Emission of the blue emitted light is captured by a light guide and is then channeled to the PMT (Fig. 7-10).

The first readout of the imaging plate does not release all of the trapped electrons that form the latent image; indeed, a plate can be readout a second time and a third time with only slight degradation. To erase the latent image so that the imaging plate can be reused for another exposure without ghosting, the plate is exposed to a very bright light source, which flushes almost all of the metastable electrons to their ground state, emptying most of the F-centers.

Charge-Coupled Device and Complementary Metal-Oxide Semiconductor detectors

Charge-coupled device (CCD) detectors form images from visible light (Fig. 7-11A). CCD detectors are used in commercial-grade television cameras and in scientific applications such as astronomy. The CCD chip itself is an integrated circuit made of crystalline silicon, as is the central processing unit of a computer. A CCD chip has an array of discrete detector electronics etched into its surface. Linear arrays are configured with single or multiple rows in a wide selection, such as 1 × 2048 detector elements (dexels), or 96 × 4096 dexels in a rectangular format for line scan detection (e.g, movement of a slot-scan detector with a narrow fan-beam collimation). Area arrays have a 2.5 × 2.5-cm dimension with 1,024 × 1,024 or 2,048 × 2,048 detector elements on their surface. Larger chips and larger matrices spanning 6 × 6 cm are available, but are very expensive, and ultimately the size is limited by the dimensions of crystalline silicon wafers. Another limitation is the requirement for a small dexel (e.g., 20 μm dimension and smaller) to achieve charge transfer efficiency of 99.99% to keep additive electronic noise low. The silicon surface of a CCD chip is photosensitive—as visible light falls on each dexel, electrons are liberated and build up in the dexel. More electrons are produced in dexels that receive more intense light. The electrons are confined to each dexel because there are electronic barriers (voltage) on each side of the dexel during exposure.

Once the CCD chip has been exposed, the electrical charge that resides in each dexel is read out. The readout process is akin to a bucket brigade (Fig. 7-11B). Along one column of the CCD chip, the electronic charge is shifted dexel by dexel

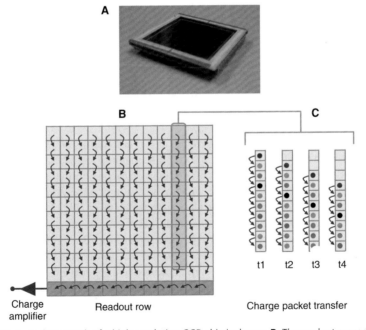

■ FIGURE 7-11 **A.** A photograph of a high-resolution CCD chip is shown. **B.** The readout procedure in a CCD chip is illustrated. After exposure, electrodes in the chip shift the charge packets for each detector element by switching voltages, allowing the charge packets to move down by one detector element at a time. Charge from the bottom element of each column spills onto the readout row, which is rapidly read out horizontally. This process repeats itself until all rows in each column are read out. **C.** This illustration shows the shift of a given pattern of exposure down one column in a CCD chip in four (t1–t4) successive clock cycles.

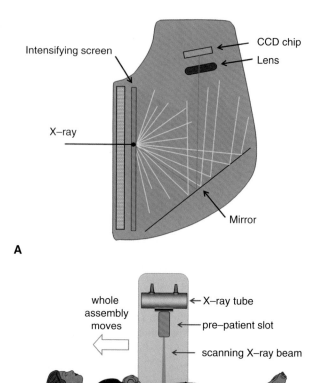

■ **FIGURE 7-12 A.** A CCD-based DR system is shown. The x-ray is converted to visible light in the intensifying screen, which propagates through the light-tight enclosure. A small fraction of the light photons will strike the mirror and be redirected to the lens to ultimately be detected in the CCD chip. **B.** A CCD-based Time Delay and Integration (TDI) system is shown. As the x-ray tube / slit-slot / detector assembly moves at velocity V (to the left in this figure), the CCD chip is read-out at a velocity $-V$ (to the right). By synchronizing the velocity of the read out with the scanning motion, the signal region under an object in the patient travels across the entire field of view of the detector, and its contrast signal is built up across all of the dexels in the TDI CCD chip.

by appropriate control of voltage levels at the boundaries of each dexel. The charge packet from each dexel in the entire column is shifted simultaneously, in parallel. For a two-dimensional CCD detector, the charges on each column are shifted onto the bottom row of electronics, that entire row is read out horizontally, then the charge packets from all columns are shifted down one detector element (Fig. 7-11C), and so on.

CCD detectors are small, whereas the field of view in most medical imaging applications is large. Unfortunately, it is impossible to focus the light emitted from a large scintillation screen (~43 × 43 cm) onto the surface of the CCD chip (~4 × 4 cm) without losing a large fraction of light photons due to optical lens coupling inefficiency. The amount of light transferred to the CCD is determined by the directionality of light emitted by the scintillator, the lens characteristics (f number, the ratio of the focal length of a lens to its effective diameter), and the demagnification factor, m, required to focus the image from the screen onto the CCD array. For a typical scintillator material (so-called lambertian emitter), the amount of light recorded is inversely proportional to the square of the f number times the square of the demagnification factor. Even with an excellent lens (e.g., f number = 1) and a demagnification of 10, less than 1% of the light produced by x-ray interactions will reach the CCD array. (Fig. 7-12A).

Many x-ray imaging systems are multi-stage, where the signal is converted from stage to stage. For example, in a CCD system, x-rays are converted to visible light in the scintillator, and then the light is converted to electrons in the CCD chip. X-ray photons, visible photons, and electrons are all forms of *quanta*. The *quantum sink* refers to the stage where the number of quanta is the lowest and therefore where the statistical integrity of the signal is the worst. Ideally, in a radiographic image, the quantum sink should be at the stage where the x-ray photons are absorbed in the converter (scintillator or solid state detector). This is referred to as an *x-ray quantum limited detector*. However, if there is a subsequent stage where the number of quanta are less than the number of absorbed x-rays, the image statistics and consequently the image noise will be dominated by this stage, and a secondary quantum sink will occur. Although an image can be produced, an x-ray detector system with a secondary quantum sink will have image quality that is not commensurate with the x-ray dose used to make the image. Large field of view CCD-based radiographic detectors have a secondary quantum sink due to the very low coupling efficiency of the lens system. Despite this, higher doses can be used to create acceptable quality images. These systems are relatively cost-effective and are sold commercially as entry-level digital radiographic systems. Higher end area CCD radiography systems typically make use of CsI input screens with improved x-ray detection efficiency and light capture efficiency, while less costly systems use Gd_2O_2S screens. For a typical 43 × 43 cm FOV, 3,000 × 3,000-pixel CCD camera (4 × 4 cm area with ~13 μm dexels) and ~10:1 demagnification, the pixel dimensions in the resulting images are approximately 140 to 150 μm.

Linear CCD arrays optically coupled to an x-ray scintillator by fiberoptic channel plates (a light guide made of individual light conducting fibers), often with a de-magnification taper of 2:1 to 3:1, are used in *slot-scan* x-ray systems. These systems operate using a narrow x-ray fan beam with pre-and post-patient collimators, acquiring an image by scanning the beam over the anatomy for several seconds. An advantage of this geometry is the excellent scatter rejection achieved, allowing the elimination of the anti-scatter grid and the associated dose penalty (see section 7–12 in this chapter). Coupling of the scintillator to the linear CCD array requires less demagnification than with a two dimensional CCD system, reducing the secondary quantum sink problem. A readout process known as Time-Delay and Integration (TDI) can deliver high dose efficiency and good signal to noise ratio. TDI readout is a method that electronically integrates signal information from the stationary patient anatomy by compensating for the velocity V of the x-ray/detector assembly by reading out the CCD in the opposite direction at a velocity $-V$. (Fig 7-12B). The transmitted x-ray beam passes through the same object path during the dwell time of the scan over the area. Disadvantages of slot-scan systems include the longer exposure time required for the scan, increasing the potential for motion artifacts, and substantially increased x-ray tube loading. Imaging systems using slot-scan acquisition have shown excellent clinical usefulness in x-ray examinations of the chest and in full-body trauma imaging.

Complementary Metal-Oxide Semiconductor (CMOS) light sensitive arrays are an alternative to the CCD arrays discussed above. Based upon a crystalline silicon matrix, these arrays are essentially random access memory "chips" with built-in photo-sensitive detectors, storage capacitors, and active readout electronics, operating at low voltage (3 to 5 volts). Inherent in the CMOS design is the ability to randomly address any detector element on the chip in a read or read and erase mode, enabling unique opportunities for built-in automatic exposure control (AEC) capabilities that are not easily performed with a CCD photo detector. A major issue with CMOS has been electronic noise from both acquisition (storage) and readout / reset noise sources. Correlated sampling methods can reduce the electronic reset noise common to multiple measurements. Construction of a large area detector is a hurdle, due to the maximum dexel size currently achievable (on the order of 50 μm). CMOS detector applications for radiography are currently limited to small FOV (10 × 15 cm) applications such as specimen tissue imaging of surgery samples.

7.5 Flat Panel Thin-Film-Transistor Array Detectors

Flat panel Thin-Film-Transistor (TFT) array detectors (Fig. 7-13) make use of technology similar to that used in flat panel displays, and much of this has to do with the wiring requirements of a huge number of individual display elements. Instead of producing individual electrical connections to each one of the elements in a flat panel display, a series of horizontal and vertical electrical lines is used which, when combined with appropriate readout logic, can address each individual display element. This signal modulates light transmittance from a backlit liquid crystal display element in the flat panel display. With this approach, only 2000 connections between the display and the electronics are required for a 1000 × 1000 display, instead of 1,000,000 individual connections. For a flat panel display, the wiring is used to send signals from the computer graphics card to each display element, whereas in an x-ray detector the wiring is used to measure the signal generated in each detector element.

Flat-panel TFT arrays are made of amorphous silicon, where lithographic etching techniques are used to deposit electronic components and connections necessary for x-ray detector operation. The large area TFT array is divided into individual detector elements (dexels), arranged in a row and column matrix. Electronic components

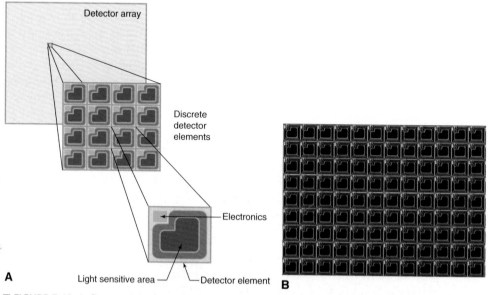

■ **FIGURE 7-13 A.** flat panel detector systems are pixelated descrete detector systems. The detector array is comprised of a large number of individual detector elements (dexels). Each dexel has a light sensitive region and a light-insensitive area where the electronic components are located. **B.** A photomicrograph of an actual TFT system is shown. The electronics component can be seen in the upper left corner of each dexel (Image courtesy John Sabol and Bill Hennessy, GE Healthcare).

within each dexel include a TFT, a charge collection electrode, and a storage capacitor. The TFT is an electronic switch that is comprised of three connections: gate, source, and drain. Gate and drain lines connect the source and drain of the TFT's along the row and columns, respectively.

The gate is the transistor's "on" – "off" switch, and is attached to the gate conductor line along each row of the array. The source is attached to the storage capacitor, and the drain is attached to the drain conductor line running along each column of the array. The charge collection electrode captures the charge produced by incident x-ray energy deposited over the area of the dexel (either by indirect or direct conversion, as discussed below), and the storage capacitor stores it. During x-ray exposure, the TFT switch is closed, allowing charge in each dexel to be accumulated and stored. After the exposure is completed, sequential activation of the TFT array occurs one row at a time, by sequentially turning on the gate line to every dexel in the row (Fig 7-14). This allows the accumulated charge in each dexel capacitor to flow through the transistor to the drain line, and subsequently to the connected charge amplifier. The charge amplifiers are positioned outside of the panel active area. They amplify the charge, convert it to a proportional voltage, and digitize the voltage level, resulting in a gray scale value for each dexel in the row. This sequence is repeated row by row, to fully read out the array. The speed of the detector readout is governed by the intrinsic electronic characteristics of the x-ray converter material and the TFT array electronics.

Indirect Detection TFT Arrays

Indirect x-ray conversion TFT arrays use a scintillator to convert x-rays to light with optical coupling of the scintillator to the active matrix. The scintillator is layered on the front surface of the flat panel array. Thus the light emanating from the *back* of the scintillator layer strikes the flat panel and, because x-ray interactions are more likely to occur toward the front of the scintillator layer, the light that is released in the scintillation layer has to propagate relatively large distances, which can result in appreciable "blurring" and a loss of spatial resolution (Fig. 7-15A). To improve

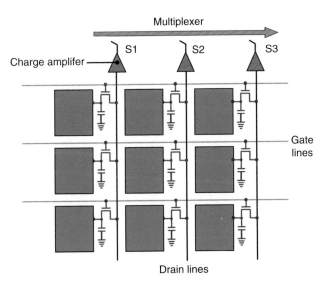

■ **FIGURE 7-14** This diagram shows circuitry for a TFT flat panel detector system. The readout process is described in the text.

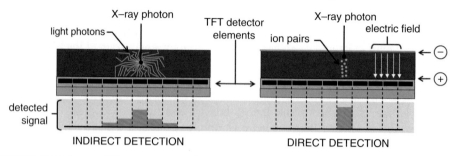

FIGURE 7-15 Indirect and direct detector TFT–based x-ray detectors are shown. **A**. Photons in the indirect system propagate laterally, compromising resolution. The detected signal shown for the indirect detector shows this lateral spread in the signal from one x-ray photons interaction. **B**. For the direct detector system, the ion pairs liberated by x-ray interaction follow the electric field lines (electron holes travel upwards, electrons travel downwards) and have negligible lateral spread. Here, the detected electronic signal from one x-ray photons interaction is collected almost entirely in one detector element, and therefore better spatial resolution is achieved.

this situation, most flat panel detector systems for general radiography use a CsI scintillator instead of Gd_2O_2S. CsI is grown in columnar crystals, and the columns act as light pipes to reduce the lateral spread of light. The reduction of the lateral propagation of light helps to preserve spatial resolution.

Because the electronics requires a certain amount of area on the dexel, the entire surface area is not photosensitive. This reduces the geometrical efficiency of light collection of each dexel to less than 100%. The *fill factor* refers to the percent of the area of each dexel that is photosensitive. The fill factor is typically about 80% for dexel dimensions of 200 μm × 200 μm, and much less (40% to 50%) for smaller dexel dimensions. Fill factor issues place limitations on how small dexels in a TFT array can be made, and currently the smallest indirect detector dexel size is about 100 μm. Technological advances are now overcoming fill-factor penalties by stacking the electrical components of each dexel in lithographic layers under the photosensitive layer.

Direct Detection TFT Arrays

Direct x-ray conversion TFT arrays use a semiconductor material that produces electron-hole pairs in proportion to the incident x-ray intensity. Absorbed x-ray energy is directly converted into charge in the detector - there is no intermediate step involving the production of visible light photons. Amorphous selenium (*a*-Se) is the semiconductor most widely used, and is layered between two surface-area electrodes connected to the bias voltage and a dielectric layer. The dielectric layer prevents overcharging dexels, which could damage the TFT array. Ion pairs are collected under applied voltage across the solid state converter (10–50 V/mum of thickness). This electric field in the converter almost completely eliminates lateral spreading of the charges during transit through the semiconductor, resulting in high spatial resolution (Fig. 7-15B). Even though Se has a relatively low atomic number and consequently low absorption efficiency, the Se layer can be made thick (0.5 to 1.0 mm) to improve detection efficiency and still maintain excellent spatial resolution. Fill factor penalties are not as significant with direct conversion TFT systems compared to indirect conversion TFT arrays. This is because the electrical potential field lines are designed to bend and thereby direct charge carriers to the collection electrode, avoiding the insensitive regions of the dexel. In addition to selenium, other materials such as mercuric iodide (HgI_2), lead iodide (PbI_2), and cadmium telluride (CdTe) are being studied for use in direct detection flat panel systems.

7.6 Technique Factors in Radiography

The principal x-ray technique factors used for radiography include the tube voltage (the kV), the tube current (mA), the exposure time, and the x-ray source-to-image distance, SID. The SID is standardized to 100 cm typically (Fig. 7-16), and 183 cm for upright chest radiography. In general, lower kV settings will increase the dose to the patient compared to higher kV settings for the same imaging procedure and same body part, but the trade-off is that subject contrast is reduced with higher kV. The kV is usually adjusted according to the examination type—lower kVs are used for bone imaging and when iodine or barium contrast agents are used; however, the kV is also adjusted to accommodate the thickness of the body part. For example, in bone imaging applications, 55 kV can be used for wrist imaging since the forearm is relatively thin, whereas 75 to 90 kV might be used for L-spine radiography, depending on the size of the patient's abdomen. The use of the 55-kV beam in abdominal imaging would result in a prohibitively high radiation dose. Lower kVs emphasize contrast due to the photoelectric effect in the patient, which is important for higher atomic number (Z) materials such as bone ($Z_{calcium} = 20$) and contrast agents containing iodine (Z = 53) or barium (Z = 56). Conversely, for chest radiography, the soft tissues of the cardiac silhouette and pulmonary anatomy are of interest, and the ribs obscure them. In this case, high kV is used (typically 120 kV) in order to decrease the conspicuity of the ribs by reducing photoelectric interactions.

With the SID and kV adjusted as described above, the overall x-ray fluence is then adjusted by using the mA and the time (measured in seconds). The product of the mA and time (s) is called the *mAs*, and at the same kV and distance, the x-ray fluence is linearly proportional to the mAs—double the mAs, and the x-ray fluence doubles. Modern x-ray generators and tubes designed for radiography can operate at relatively high mA (such as 500 to 800 mA), and higher mA settings allow the exposure time to be shorter, which "freezes" patient motion.

Manual x-ray technique selection was used up until the 1970s in radiography, whereby the technologist selected the kV and mAs based on experience and in-house "technique charts". Some institutions required technologists to use large calipers to measure the thickness of the body part to be imaged, to improve the consistency of the radiographic film optical density. Today, radiography usually makes use of *automatic exposure control* (AEC), which informally is called *phototiming*. The mA is set to a high value such as 500 mA, and the exposure time (and hence the overall mAs) is determined by the AEC system. In general radiography, an air-ionization photocell is located behind the patient and grid, but in front of the x-ray detector (Fig. 7-16).

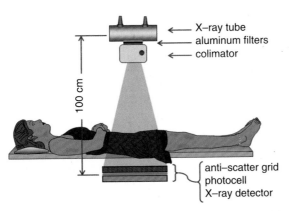

■ FIGURE 7-16 The standard configuration for radiography is illustrated. Most table-based radiographic systems use a SID of 100 cm. The x-ray collimator has a light bulb and mirror assembly in it, and (when activated) this casts a light beam onto the patient that allows the technologist to position the x-ray beam relative to the patient's anatomy. The light beam is congruent with the x-ray beam. The x-rays that pass through the patient must pass through the antiscatter grid and the photocell (part of the AEC system) to then strike the x-ray detector.

During exposure, the AEC integrates the exposure signal from the photocell in real time until a preset exposure level is reached, and then the AEC immediately terminates the exposure. The preset exposure levels are calibrated by the service personnel, and the sensitivity of the radiographic detector is taken into account in the calibration procedure. For screen-film radiography, the AEC is set to deliver proper film darkening. For a digital radiographic system, the AEC is adjusted so that the exposure levels are both in the range of the detector system and produce images with good statistical integrity based on a predetermined signal-to-noise ratio. This means that a trade-off between radiation dose to the patient and noise in the digital image should be reached. For some digital imaging systems, the signal from the detector itself can be used as the AEC sensor.

7.7   Scintillators and Intensifying Screens

An indirect x-ray detector system uses a scintillator to convert the x-ray fluence incident on the detector into a visible light signal, which is then used to expose the emulsion in screen-film radiography or a photoconductor in digital radiographic systems. Over the long history of screen-film radiography, a number of scintillators were developed. Most intensifying screens are comprised of fine-grain crystalline scintillating powders (also called phosphors), formed into a uniformly thick intensifying screen that is held together by a binder. During production, the phosphor power is mixed with the binder material at high temperature, and then this molten mixture is layered onto a metallic sheet, where rollers spread the material into a uniform thickness. The material hardens as it cools, and the intensifying screen is cut to the desired dimensions. The binder is usually a white powder, and intensifying screens appear white to the naked eye. Intensifying screens are considered *turbid* media—they are not strictly transparent to optical light (in such case they would be clear in appearance), but instead the visible light that is produced in the screen from x-ray interactions undergoes many scattering events as it propagates through the intensifying screen. The light photons have a certain probability of being absorbed as well. Most intensifying screens are amorphous (lack structure), and are comprised of billions of tiny crystals of the scintillator randomly embedded in the inert binder layer. Because the index of refraction of the binder is different than the scintillator crystals, the facets of these tiny crystals are sites where light scattering (and absorption) occurs. Each light photon that is produced by x-ray interaction inside a scintillator crystal propagates in any direction in the screen, refracting off thousands of small surfaces until it either exits the screen matrix or is absorbed. Consequently, a burst of perhaps 2,000 light photons produced at the point of x-ray interaction propagates inside the screen matrix undergoing many scattering and absorption events, and eventually about 200 photons reach the surface of the screen where they can interact with the photodetector.

In thicker screens, the packet of photons diffuses a greater thickness before emerging from the phosphor layer, and this results in more spreading of light reaching the light detector (see Fig. 7-5). The extent of lateral light spread is also governed by the design of the phosphor screen itself—the relative coefficients of optical scattering and optical absorption affect the amount of blurring, and the overall sensitivity of the screen. Increasing the optical absorption reduces light spread, improving spatial resolution for the same screen thickness, but less light reaches the surface.

Some crystalline scintillators such as CsI form in long columnar crystals, which are tiny natural light pipes, and this structured crystal tends to reduce lateral light spread and preserve spatial resolution for a given screen thickness. CsI is a salt, chemically similar to NaCl, and is hygroscopic (absorbs moisture from the air). It therefore must be sealed to keep out moisture; it may be kept in a vacuum or encapsulated in a plastic layer. CsI is too fragile and expensive for screen-film radiography applications.

7.8   Absorption Efficiency and Conversion Efficiency

Because of the dynamics of indirect x-ray detection described above, there are two factors that are important in x-ray detectors. The first is the absorption efficiency in the phosphor layer, which is determined by the phosphor composition (its effective Z and density), and the screen thickness. The absorption efficiency is also dependent on the x-ray beam energy. The term *quantum detection efficiency* is used to describe how well x-ray detectors capture the incident x-ray photon beam, but because this metric does not consider x-ray fluorescence (where a considerable fraction of the detected photon energy is re-emitted by the detector), the *energy absorption efficiency* is perhaps a better metric, given that most x-ray detectors are *energy integrators*, not *photon counters*. Thicker, denser phosphor layers absorb more of the incident x-ray beam (Fig. 7-17), and increased absorption efficiency is always desirable. However, increasing the screen thickness has to be balanced with the concomitant increase in blurring and loss of spatial resolution that results in thicker screens.

A second factor relates to how efficiently the optical signal is conveyed from the scintillator to the silicon photodetector, and how it is then amplified and converted to signal in the image (i.e., gray scale value or digital number). *Conversion Efficiency* (CE) includes x-ray to light photon energy transfer in scintillators, the light to charge

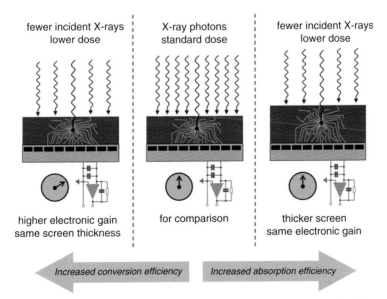

■ **FIGURE 7-17** The center panel is used for comparison, and here a higher exposure level is used as represented by the larger number of x-ray photons incident on the detector system. By increasing the absorption efficiency (**right panel**) using a thicker screen by a factor G (G>1), the x-ray beam can be reduced to 1/G and the same number of x-ray photons will be absorbed in the detector, yielding the same image noise as before. By increasing the conversion efficiency (**left panel**) by a factor G, the x-ray beam intensity is turned down to 1/G to compensate but because the absorption efficiency has not changed in this case, the number of absorbed photons is decreased, and this increases the image noise.

conversion efficiency for photodiodes, the light to OD in film, geometry and lens efficiency in optically coupled detectors, and the electronic gain in a digital detector (see Fig. 7-17). To reduce the radiation dose (i.e., use fewer photons to make the image), but to keep the same gray scale (or OD) in the image, if the conversion efficiency is increased by a factor G (where $G > 1$) for a system with the same absorption efficiency, the x-ray fluence must be reduced by a factor of G to deliver the same gray scale value. This would result in $1/G$ of the photons being absorbed in the detector, and hence a $\sqrt{G}$ increase in relative quantum noise would result.

If, on the other hand, the absorption efficiency is increased by the factor G, the x-ray fluence is decreased by the AEC by this same factor. The increase in absorption is balanced by the reduction in x-ray fluence (saving dose), in order to get the same gray scale. In this case, the same number of x-rays are absorbed by the detector (i.e., $G \times 1/G = 1$), and the quantum noise therefore is not changed. So, for a discussion where *the same signal levels in the image are being compared*, increasing the speed of the detector (and lowering the radiation dose) by increasing the conversion efficiency *increases* image noise, whereas increasing absorption efficiency can reduce dose but has no detrimental effect on quantum noise in the image.

7.9 Other Considerations

The choice of a digital detector system requires a careful assessment of the needs of the facility. CR is often the first digital radiographic system installed in a hospital, because it can directly replace screen-film cassettes in existing radiography units and in portable, bedside examinations, where the cost of retakes in both technologist time and money is high. A benefit of CR over TFT-based digital radiographic technology is that the relatively expensive CR reader is stationary, but because the CR imaging plates themselves are relatively inexpensive, several dozen plates may be used in different radiographic rooms simultaneously. The number of rooms that one CR reader can serve depends on the types of rooms, workload, and proximity. Typically, one multi-cassette CR reader can handle the workload of three radiographic rooms. The cost of an individual flat panel detector is high, and it can only be in one place at one time. The obvious use for flat panel detectors or other solid-state digital radiographic systems is for radiographic suites that have high patient throughput, such as a dedicated chest room. Because no cassette handling is required and the images are rapidly available for technologist approval, the throughput in a single room using flat panel detectors can be much higher than for CR systems, where manual cassette handling is required. Recent introduction of portable TFT flat panel cassettes using wireless technology is an alternative to the portable CR detectors that have historically been used in portable radiography, however, the consequences of the technologist dropping the fragile flat panel cassette can be expensive.

7.10 Radiographic Detectors, Patient Dose, and Exposure Index

In traditional screen-film radiography, film OD serves as an exposure indicator, and direct feedback is obtained by simple visual inspection of the processed film image (Fig. 7-18, left). CR and DR detectors have wide exposure latitude and with image post-processing, these systems produce consistent image gray scale even with

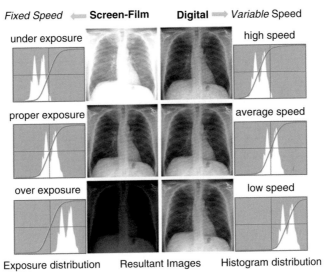

Fixed Speed ⇐ **Screen-Film   Digital** ⇒ *Variable* Speed

under exposure   high speed

proper exposure   average speed

over exposure   low speed

Exposure distribution   Resultant Images   Histogram distribution

■ **FIGURE 7-18** Response of a screen-film detector with fixed radiographic speed and a digital detector with variable radiographic speed to underexposure, correct exposure, and overexposure are shown. For screen-film, to the left of each radiograph is a distribution representing the x-ray exposure absorbed by the screen and converted to OD on the film. Note that the characteristic curve translating exposure to OD is fixed on the exposure axis. For digital detectors, to the right of each radiograph is a distribution representing the frequency of digital values (a histogram) linear with exposure absorbed by the detector and converted to a digital value. Note that the look-up table curve translating the digital values to brightness and contrast on a display monitor is variable and adjusts to the histogram to achieve optimal rendering of the image contrast.

underexposed and overexposed images (Fig. 7-18, right). With the capability of automatically adjusting the gray scale on digital radiographic images, the checks and balances provided to the technologist from the immediate feedback of film density are lost. Underexposed DR images use fewer absorbed x-rays, and can be recognized by increased image noise, but overexposed images can easily go unnoticed, resulting in unnecessary overexposure to the patient. Furthermore, underexposed images are likely to be criticized by radiologists for excessive image noise, whereas overexposed images will likely be of high quality; this may lead to a phenomenon known as "dose creep," whereby technologists tend to use unnecessarily high exposures. Dose creep is most likely to occur in examinations such as portable radiography in which automatic exposure control is not feasible and manual technique factors must be chosen.

In most digital radiographic systems, image-processing algorithms are used to align measured histogram values (after exposure) with a predetermined look-up table, to make image gray scale appear similar to screen-film images. The measured histogram distribution on each radiograph is used to determine the incident radiation exposure to the detector, and to provide an "exposure index" value. Anatomically relevant areas of the radiograph are segmented (parts of the image corresponding to no patient attenuation—high values, and collimated regions—low values, are excluded), a histogram is generated from the relevant image area, and it is compared to an examination-specific (e.g. chest, forearm, head, etc.) histogram shape. The gray scale values of the raw image are then digitally transformed using a look-up-table (LUT) to provide desirable image contrast in the "for presentation" image.

TABLE 7-1 MANUFACTURER, CORRESPONDING SYMBOL FOR EI, AND CALCULATED EI FOR THREE INCIDENT EXPOSURES TO THE DETECTOR

MANUFACTURER	SYMBOL	50 μGy	100 μGy	200 μGy
Canon (Brightness = 16, contrast = 10)	REX	50	100	200
Fuji, Konica	S	400	200	100
Kodak (CR, STD)	EI	1,700	2,000	2,300
IDC (ST = 200)	F#	−1	0	1
Philips	EI	200	100	50
Siemens	EI	500	1,000	2,000

The median value of the histogram is used in many systems to determine a proprietary exposure index (EI) value, which is dependent on each manufacturer's algorithm and detector calibration method. This exposure index indicates the amount of radiation reaching the detector and is not an indicator of dose to the patient. Unfortunately, widely different methods to calculate the EI value have evolved, as shown in Table 7-1.

An international standard for an exposure index for digital radiographic systems has been published by the International Electrotechnical Commission (IEC), IEC 62424-1. This standard describes "Exposure Indices" and "Deviation Indices," along with a method for placing these values in the DICOM header of each radiographic image. The manufacturer's responsibility is to calibrate the imaging detector according to a detector-specific procedure, to provide methods to segment pertinent anatomical information in the relevant image region, and to generate an EI from histogram data that is proportional to detector exposure.

This dose index standard for radiography requires staff to establish *target exposure index* (EI_T) values for each digital radiographic system and for each type of exam; for instance, the EI_T for a skull radiographic will, in general, differ from that of a chest radiograph. Feedback to the user on whether an "appropriate" exposure has been achieved is given by the *deviation index* (DI), calculated as

$$DI = 10 \log_{10} (EI / EI_T) \qquad [7\text{-}6]$$

The DI provides feedback to the operator with a value that is equal to 0 (zero) when the intended exposure to the detector is achieved (i.e., EI = EI_T), a positive number when an overexposure has occurred, and a negative number when an underexposure has occurred. A DI of +1 indicates an overexposure of about 26%; a value of −1 indicates an underexposure of 20% less than desired. The acceptable range of DI values is approximately from +1 to −1. When the DI is in the desired range, the radiographic system is considered to be working well and is able to deliver the EI_T values set up by the institution. Tracking DI values with respect to equipment and technologist can be useful in maintaining high image quality for radiography at an institution.

7.11 Dual-Energy Radiography

As mentioned in Chapter 4, anatomical noise can contribute to a loss of conspicuity in radiological imaging. Dual-energy radiographic techniques have been developed, which can in some instances reduce anatomical noise and thereby produce an image that has better information content. Dual-energy chest radiography is a good example of this and will be used to illustrate the concept.

Figure 7-19A shows the attenuation characteristics of iodine, bone, and soft tissue as a function of x-ray photon energy. The curves have different shapes, and thus the energy dependencies of bone, iodine, and soft tissue attenuation are different. The reason for these differences is that higher atomic number materials (i.e., bone, with effective $Z \approx 13$, or iodine, with $Z = 53$) have higher photoelectric absorption levels than lower atomic materials such as soft tissue (effective $Z \approx 7.6$). The photoelectric interaction component of the linear attenuation coefficient has an energy dependency of E^{-3}, as opposed to very little energy dependency for the Compton scattering component in the x-ray energy range used for diagnostic imaging. Because of the different energy dependencies in tissue types, the acquisition of two radiographic images at two different effective energy levels (i.e., different kVs), enables either the bone component or the soft tissue component in the image to be removed by image post-processing. The general algorithm for computing dual-energy subtracted images on each pixel (x,y) is

$$DE(x, y) = \alpha + \beta \left[Ln\{(I_{HI}(x, y)\} - R \ Ln\{I_{LO}(x, y)\} \right] \qquad \text{[7-7]}$$

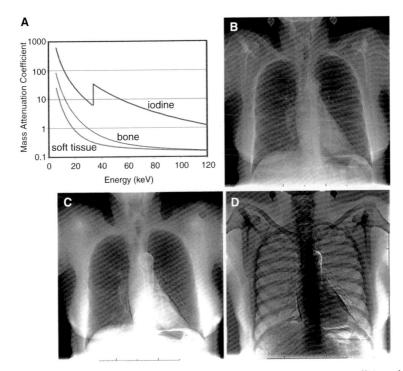

■ **FIGURE 7-19** Dual-energy chest radiography is illustrated. **A.** The linear attenuation coefficients for soft tissue, bone, and iodine are shown. **B.** The single-energy (120 kV) radiograph is shown. **C.** The bone-subtracted, soft tissue–only image is illustrated. This image shows the lung parenchyma and mediastinum, which are the principal organs of interest on most chest radiographs. **D.** The soft tissue–subtracted, bone-only image is illustrated. Note that the earrings, which are made of metal and are more similar to bone than soft tissue in terms of composition, show up on the bone-only image.

where $DE(x,y)$ is the gray scale value in the dual-energy image, $I_{HI}(x,y)$ is the corresponding gray value in the acquired high-energy image, and $I_{LO}(x,y)$ is the corresponding gray scale value in the acquired low-energy image. The value of R is selected to isolate bone, iodine, or soft tissue in the subtraction, and α and β scale the output image for brightness and contrast for optimal display. Equation 7-7 represents *logarithmic weighted subtraction*.

Figure 7-19B shows a standard single-energy chest radiograph for comparison, and Figure 7-19C and 7-19D illustrate the soft tissue and bone-only images, respectively. Notice on the tissue-only image (Fig. 7-19C), the ribs are eliminated and the soft tissue parenchyma of the lungs and mediastinum are less obscured by the ribs. On the bone-only image, bones are of course better depicted. Interestingly, one can also see the metallic earrings on this patient, whereas they are not visible on the soft tissue–only image. The metal earrings have attenuation properties more like bone than soft tissue.

 ## 7.12 Scattered Radiation in Projection Radiographic Imaging

The basic principle of projection x-ray imaging is that x-rays travel in straight lines. However, when x-ray scattering events occur in the patient, the resulting scattered x-rays are not aligned with the trajectory of the original primary x-ray, and thus the straight-line assumption is violated (Fig. 7-20). Scattered radiation that does not strike the detector has no effect on the image; however, scattered radiation emanating from the patient is of concern for surrounding personnel due to the associated radiation dose. If scattered radiation is detected by the image receptor, it does have an effect on the image and can be a significant cause of image degradation. Scattered radiation generates image gray scale where it does not belong, and this can significantly reduce contrast in screen-film radiography. Because contrast can be increased in digital images by window/leveling or other adjustment schemes, on

■ **FIGURE 7-20** This illustration demonstrates that when x-rays are scattered in the patient and reach the detector, they stimulate gray scale production, but since they are displaced on the image, they carry little or no information about the patient's anatomy.

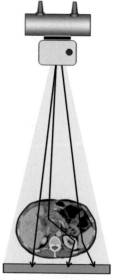

primary x-ray   scattered x-rays

digital radiographic images, scatter acts chiefly as a source of noise, degrading the signal-to-noise ratio.

The amount of scatter detected in an image is characterized by the scatter-to-primary ratio (SPR) or the scatter fraction. The SPR is defined as the amount of energy deposited in a specific location in the detector by scattered photons, divided by the amount of energy deposited by primary (non-scattered) photons in that same location. Thus,

$$SPR = \frac{S}{P} \qquad [7\text{-}8]$$

For an SPR of 1, half of the energy deposited on the detector (at that location) is from scatter—that is, 50% of the information in the image is largely useless. The scatter fraction (F) is also used to characterize the amount of scatter, defined as

$$F = \frac{S}{P + S} \qquad [7\text{-}9]$$

The relationship between the SPR and scatter fraction is given by

$$F = \frac{SPR}{SPR + 1} \qquad [7\text{-}10]$$

The vast majority of x-ray detectors integrate the x-ray energy and do not count photons (which is typical in nuclear medicine). Thus, the terms S and P in this discussion refer to the energies absorbed in the detector from the scattered and primary photons, respectively.

If uncorrected, the amount of scatter on an image can be high (Fig. 7-21). The SPR increases typically as the volume of tissue that is irradiated by the x-ray beam increases. Figure 7-21 illustrates the SPR as a function of the side of a square field of view, for different patient thicknesses. The SPR increases as the field size increases and as the thickness of the patient increases. For a typical 30 × 30 abdominal radiograph in a 25-cm-thick patient, the SPR is about 4.5—so 82% (the scatter fraction) of the information in the image is essentially useless, if scatter correction methods are not used.

The Anti-scatter Grid

The anti-scatter grid, or sometimes just called a scatter grid, is the most widely used technology for reducing scatter in radiography, fluoroscopy, and mammography. The

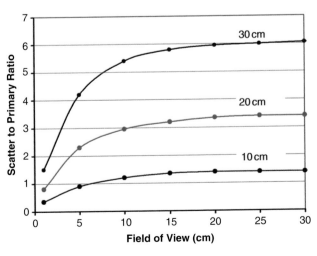

■ FIGURE 7-21 The SPR is shown as a function of the side dimension of a square field of view, for three different patient thicknesses. For example, the 20-cm point on the x-axis refers to a 20 × 20-cm field. The SPR increases with increasing field size and with increasing patient thickness. Thus, scatter is much more of a problem in the abdomen as compared to extremity radiography. Scatter can be reduced by aggressive use of collimation, which reduces the field of view of the x-ray beam.

■ FIGURE 7-22 The antiscatter grid is located between the patient, who is the principal source of scatter, and the detector. Grids are geometric devices, and the interspace regions in the grid are aligned with the x-ray focal spot, which is the location where all primary x-ray photons originate from. Scattered photons are more obliquely oriented, and as a result have a higher probability of striking the attenuating septa in the grid. Hence, the grid allows most of the primary radiation to reach the detector, but prevents most of the scattered radiation from reaching it.

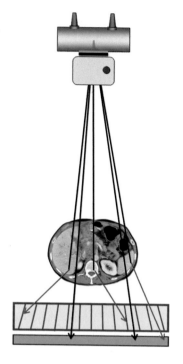

grid is placed between the detector and the patient (Fig. 7-22). Ideally, it would allow all primary radiation incident upon it to pass, while absorbing all of the scattered radiation. The scatter grid has a simple geometric design, in which open interspace regions and alternating x-ray absorbing septa are aligned with the x-ray tube focal spot. This alignment allows x-ray photons emanating from the focal spot (primary radiation) to have a high probability of transmission through the grid (thereby reaching the detector), while more obliquely angled photons (scattered x-rays emanating in the patient) have a higher probability of striking the highly absorbing grid septa (Fig. 7-23). The alignment of the grid with the focal spot is crucial to its efficient

■ FIGURE 7-23 The basic dimensions of a 10:1 antiscatter grid are shown. The grid is manufactured from alternating layers of interspace material and septa material. This illustration shows parallel grid septa; however, in an actual grid, the septa and interspace are focused (and thus would be slightly angled).

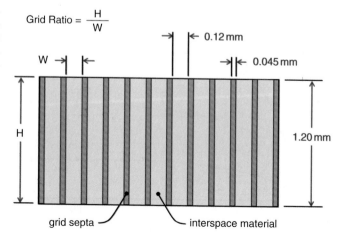

Grid Ratio = $\dfrac{H}{W}$

0.12 mm

0.045 mm

1.20 mm

grid septa — — interspace material

operation, and errors in this alignment can cause reduced grid performance or artifacts in the image.

There are several parameters that characterize the anti-scatter grid. In the clinical imaging environment (practical radiographic imaging), the following grid parameters are important:

Grid Ratio

The grid ratio (see Fig. 7-23) is the ratio of the height of the *interspace material* to its width—the septa dimensions do not affect the grid ratio metric. Grid ratios in general diagnostic radiology are generally 6, 8, 10, 12, or 14, with the central three values used most commonly. Grid ratios are lower (~5) in mammography. The grid septa in a grid are typically manufactured from lead ($z = 82$, $\rho = 11.3$ g/cm^3). The grid ratio is the most fundamental descriptor of the grid's construction.

Interspace Material

Ideally, air would be the interspace material; however, the lead septa are very malleable and require support for structural integrity. Therefore, a solid material is placed in the interspace in the typical linear grid used in general radiography to keep the septa aligned. Low-cost grids in diagnostic radiology can have aluminum ($z = 13$, $\rho = 2.7$ g/cm^3) as the interspace material, but aluminum can absorb an appreciable number of the primary photons (especially at lower x-ray energies), and so, carbon fiber interspaced grids are more common in state-of-the-art imaging systems. Carbon fiber ($z = 6$, $\rho = 1.8$ g/cm^3) has high primary transmission due to the low atomic number of carbon fiber and its lower density, and thus is a desirable interspace material.

Grid Frequency

The grid frequency is the number of grid septa per centimeter. Looking at the grid depicted in Figure 7-23, the septa are 0.045 mm wide and the interspace is 0.120 mm wide, resulting in a line pattern with 0.165 mm spacing. The corresponding frequency is 1/0.165mm = 6 lines/mm or 60 lines/cm. Grids with 70 or 80 lines/cm are also available, at greater cost. For imaging systems with discrete detector elements, a stationary high-frequency grid can be used instead of grid motion (no Bucky mechanism). For example, a 2,048 × 1,680 chest radiographic system has approximately 200 μm detector elements, and thus a grid with 45-μm-wide grid septa (see Fig. 7-23) should be largely invisible because the grid bars are substantially smaller than the spatial resolution of the detector.

Grid Type

The grid pictured in Figure 7-23 is a linear grid, which is fabricated as a series of alternating septa and interspace layers. Grids with crossed septa are also available but seldom are used in general radiography applications. Crossed grids are widely used in mammography (Chapter 8).

Focal Length

The interspace regions in the antiscatter grid should be aligned with the x-ray source, and this requires that the grid be focused (see Fig. 7-22). The focal length of a grid is typically 100 cm for most radiographic suites and is 183 cm for most upright chest imaging units. If the x-ray tube is accidentally located at a different distance from the grid, then *grid cutoff* will occur. The focal distance of the grid is more forgiving for lower grid ratio grids, and therefore high grid ratio grids will have more grid cutoff if the source to detector distance is not exactly at the focal length. For systems where the source-to-detector distance can vary appreciably during the clinical examination (fluoroscopy), the use of lower grid ratio grids allows greater flexibility and will suffer less from off-focal grid cutoff, but will be slightly less effective in reducing the amount of detected scattered radiation.

Moving Grids

Grids are located between the patient and the detector, and for high-resolution detector systems such as screen-film receptors, the grid bars will be seen on the image if the grid is stationary. Stationary grids were common in upright screen-film chest radiography systems, and the success of this approach suggests that the radiologist is quite adroit at "looking through" the very regularly spaced grid lines on the image. A **Bucky** grid is a grid that moves with a reciprocating motion during the x-ray exposure, causing the grid bars to be blurred by this motion and not visible in the image. The motion is perpendicular to the long axis of the linear septa in the grid.

Bucky Factor

The Bucky factor, not to be confused with the moving Bucky grid, describes the relative increase in x-ray intensity or equivalently, mAs, needed when a grid is used, compared to when a grid is not used. The Bucky factor essentially describes the radiation dose penalty of using the grid—and typical values of the Bucky factor for abdominal radiography range from 3 to 8. The Bucky factor is relevant in screen-film radiography, but less so with digital imaging systems. In screen-film radiography, the use of the grid slightly reduces the amount of detected primary radiation and substantially reduces the amount of scattered radiation detected, and both of these effects reduce the OD of the resulting film. Thus, the x-ray technique has to be increased by the Bucky factor to replace this lost radiation, in order to deliver films of the same OD. Digital systems, however, have much wider dynamic ranges than screen-film systems in general, and therefore the x-ray technique does not *have to* be increased to replace the lost x-ray exposure to the detector, which was mostly scattered radiation anyway. In practice, since digital imaging systems have replaced our century-long experience with screen-film image receptors, the exposures used in digital systems largely follow the trends of what was used in the screen-film era. Nevertheless, these considerations suggest that DR systems may be used to provide lower dose examinations than in the screen-film era.

It should be noted that for thin anatomical structures, there is very little scattered radiation, and the use of a grid is not necessary. For example, for hand or forearm radiography, scatter levels are low and the technologist will usually place the limb to be imaged directly on the detector, with no grid (if it is removable).

There are other parameters that characterize the performance of the anti-scatter grid, which are used primarily in the scientific evaluation of grid performance. These parameters are less important to x-ray technologists and radiologists, but are of interest to those engaged in designing grids or optimizing their performance. These metrics are discussed below.

Primary Transmission Factor

T_p is the fraction of primary photons that are transmitted through the grid, and ideally it would be 1.0. In Figure 7-23, the grid bars cover 27% of the field (0.045/[0.045 + 0.120]) and primary x-rays striking the top of the septa (parallel to their long axis) will be mostly attenuated. For that grid, then, the primary transmission would at most be 73%, and this does not consider the attenuation of the interspace material. Values of T_p typically run from 0.50 to 0.75 with modern grids, and this value is kV-dependent due to the penetration of the interspace material.

Scatter Transmission Factor

T_s is the fraction of scattered radiation that penetrates the grid. Ideally, it would be 0. The value of T_s can range substantially depending on the amount of scatter in the field, the x-ray energy, and the grid design. Typical values of T_s run approximately from 0.05 to 0.20 in general diagnostic radiography.

Selectivity

Selectivity (Σ) is simply defined as

$$\Sigma = \frac{T_P}{T_S} \qquad [7\text{-}11]$$

Contrast Degradation Factor

The contrast degradation factor (CDF) refers to the reduction in contrast due to scattered radiation. It can be shown that contrast is reduced by

$$CDF = \frac{1}{1 + SPR} \qquad [7\text{-}12]$$

However, because digital images can be adjusted to enhance contrast, CDF is of less importance in digital radiography than in film-screen radiography.

Other Methods for Scatter Reduction

While the anti-scatter grid is by far the most ubiquitous tool used for scatter reduction, air gaps and scan-slot techniques have been studied for years (Fig. 7-24). The principle of the air gap is that by moving the patient away from the detector, less of the scatter that is emitted from the patient will strike the detector. The concept is

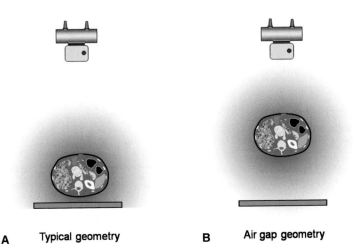

A   Typical geometry   B   Air gap geometry

■ **FIGURE 7-24** The air gap technique has been used to reduce scattered radiation, and this figure shows the air gap geometry. The scattered radiation that might strike the detector in the typical geometry (**A**) has a better probability of not striking the detector as the distance between the patient and the detector is increased. (**B**) While often discussed, the air gap technique suffers from field coverage and magnification issues, and is used only rarely in diagnostic radiography.

similar to the inverse square law (radiation intensity decreases as the square of the distance from the source), except that for an extended source of radiation (scatter from the patient does not originate from a point, but instead a large volume), the scattered x-ray intensity with air gap distances is not proportional to $1/r^2$, but rather approaches $1/r$. Increasing the air gap distance also increases the magnification of the patient's anatomy (see Fig. 7-2). Thus, practical factors limit the utility of the air gap method for scatter reduction—as magnification of the patient anatomy increases, the coverage of a given detector dimension is reduced, and there is a loss in spatial resolution due to the increased blurring of the finite focal spot with magnification (see Fig. 7-3).

The scan-slot system for scatter reduction (Fig. 7-25) is one of the most effective ways of reducing the detection of scattered x-rays, and the images that result from scan-slot systems are often noticeably better in appearance due to their excellent contrast and signal-to-noise ratio. Scan-slot radiography can be regarded as the gold standard in scatter reduction methods. The method works because a very small field is being imaged at any point in time (see Fig. 7-21), most scatter is prevented from reaching the image receptor, and the image is produced by scanning the small slot across the entire field of view. In addition to excellent scatter rejection, slot-scan radiography also does not require a grid and therefore has the potential to be more dose efficient. The dose efficiency of scan-slot systems is related to the geometric precision achieved between the alignment of the prepatient slit and the postpatient slot. If the postpatient slot is collimated too tightly relative to the prepatient slit, primary radiation that has passed through the patient will be attenuated, and this will reduce dose efficiency. If the postpatient slot is too wide relative to the prepatient slit, then more scatter will be detected.

Despite the excellent scatter reduction from these systems, there are limitations. The scanning approach requires significantly longer acquisition times, and the potential for patient motion during the acquisition increases. The narrow aperture for scanning requires a high x-ray tube current and the longer scan time requires significant heat loading of the x-ray tube anode. Alignment of mechanical systems is always a source of concern, and complex mechanical systems invariably require more attention from service personnel.

■ FIGURE 7-25 The scanning slit (or "slot-scan") method for scatter reduction is illustrated. The prepatient slit is aligned with the postpatient slot, and these two apertures scan across the field of view together. The challenge is to keep the slot aligned with the slit, and this can be done electronically or mechanically. This geometry was deployed for an early digital mammography system, but is also commercially available for radiography applications. Excellent scatter reduction can be achieved using this method.

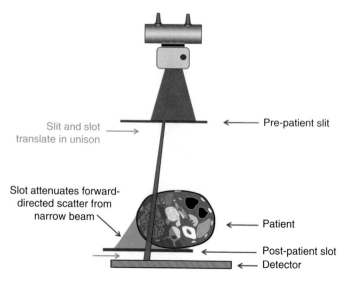

Slit and slot translate in unison →

Slot attenuates forward-directed scatter from narrow beam

← Pre-patient slit

← Patient

← Post-patient slot
← Detector

SUGGESTED READING

Alvarez RE, Seibert JA, Thompson SK. Comparison of dual energy detector system performance, *Med Phys* 2004;31:556–565.

Amis ES, Butler PF, Applegate KE, et al, American College of Radiology White paper on radiation dose in medicine. *JACR* 2007;4:272–284.

Chan H-P, Doi K. Investigation of the performance of antiscatter grids: Monte Carlo simulation studies, *Phys Med Biol* 1982;27:785–803.

Chan H-P, Higashida Y, Doi K. Performance of antiscatter grids in diagnostic radiology: Experimental measurements and Monte Carlo simulations studies, *Med Phys* 1985;12:449–454.

International Electrotechnical Commission, Report IEC 62424-1 (2008).

Shepard SJ, Wang J, Flynn M, et al. An exposure indicator for digital radiography: AAPM Task Group 116 (Executive Summary), *Med Phys* 2009;36:2989–2914.

CHAPTER **8**

Mammography

Mammography is a radiographic examination that is designed for detecting breast pathology, particularly breast cancer. Breast cancer screening with mammography assists in detecting cancers at an earlier, more treatable stage, and is an important clinical procedure because approximately one in eight women will develop breast cancer over their lifetimes. Technologic advances over the last several decades have greatly improved the diagnostic sensitivity of mammography. Early x-ray mammography was performed with direct exposure film (intensifying screens were not used), required high radiation doses, and produced images of low contrast and poor diagnostic quality. Mammography using the xeroradiographic process was very popular in the 1970s and early 1980s, spurred by high spatial resolution and edge-enhanced images; however, its relatively poor sensitivity for breast masses and higher radiation dose compared to screen-film mammography led to its demise in the late 1980s. Continuing refinements in screen-film technology and digital mammography, which entered the clinical arena in the early 2000s, further improved mammography (Fig. 8-1).

The American College of Radiology (ACR) mammography accreditation program changed the practice of mammography in the mid-1980s, with recommendations for minimum standards of practice and quality control (QC) that spurred improvements in technology and ensured quality of service. The federal Mammography Quality Standards Act (MQSA) was enacted in 1992. The law, and associated federal regulations (Title 21 of the Code of Federal Regulations, Part 900) issued by the US Food and Drug Administration (FDA), made many of the standards of the accreditation program mandatory. For digital mammography systems, many of the regulatory requirements entail following the manufacturer's recommended QC procedures.

Breast cancer screening programs depend on x-ray mammography because it is a low-cost, low–radiation dose procedure that has the sensitivity to detect early- stage breast cancer. Mammographic features characteristic of breast cancer are masses, particularly ones with irregular or "spiculated" margins; clusters of microcalcifications; and architectural distortions of breast structures. In screening mammography as practiced in the United States, two x-ray images of each breast, in the mediolateral oblique and craniocaudal views, are acquired. Whereas *screening mammography* attempts to identify breast cancer in the asymptomatic population, *diagnostic mammography* procedures are performed to assess palpable lesions or evaluate suspicious findings identified by screening mammography. The diagnostic mammographic examination may include additional x-ray projections, magnification views, spot compression views, ultrasound, magnetic resonance imaging (MRI), or mammoscintigraphy.

Ultrasound (Chapter 14) is often used to differentiate cysts (typically benign) from solid masses (often cancerous) and is also used when possible for biopsy needle guidance. MRI (Chapters 12 and 13) has excellent tissue contrast sensitivity and with contrast enhancement can differentiate benign from malignant tumors; it is used for diagnosis, staging, biopsy guidance, and, in some cases, screening. The clinical utility of mammoscintigraphy utilizing Tc-99m sestamibi is in the evaluation

Screen-film (2006)   Digital (2009)   Digital tomosynthesis (2010)

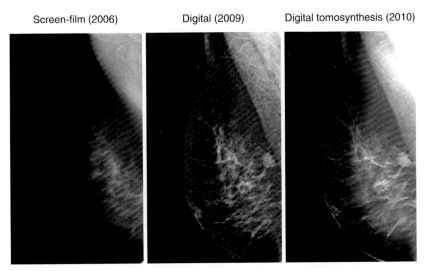

■ **FIGURE 8-1** Improvements in mammography. Images of a medial-lateral oblique view of the breast are shown. On the left is a state-of-the-art screen-film image (2006); in the middle is a corresponding digital mammogram (2008) demonstrating excellent exposure latitude and the skin line not seen in the film image; and on the right is one of approximately 50 digital tomosynthesis images (2010), which reduce superposition of anatomy in the projection image at about the same dose as a screen-film mammogram. Today, digital imaging equipment is used in the majority of mammography clinics.

of suspected breast cancer in patients for whom mammography is nondiagnostic, equivocal, or difficult to interpret (e.g., the presence of scar tissue, mammographically dense breast tissue, implants, or severe dysplastic disease). It is also used to assist in identifying multicentric and multifocal carcinomas in patients with tissue diagnosis of breast cancer.

The morphological differences between normal and cancerous tissues in the breast and the presence of microcalcifications require the use of x-ray equipment designed specifically to optimize breast cancer detection. As shown in Figure 8-2A, the attenuation differences between normal and cancerous tissue are extremely small. Subject contrast, shown in Figure 8-2B, is highest at low x-ray energies (10 to 15 keV) and reduced at higher energies (e.g., greater than 30 keV). Low x-ray

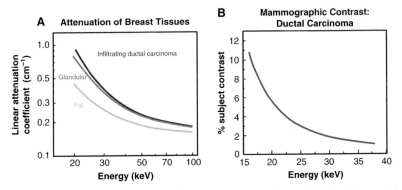

■ **FIGURE 8-2** **A.** Attenuation of breast tissues as a function of energy, showing fat, glandular, and ductal carcinoma linear attenuation coefficients. Comparison of the three tissues shows a very small difference between the glandular and the cancerous tissues. **B.** Calculated percentage contrast of the ductal carcinoma relative to the glandular tissue declines rapidly with energy; contrast is optimized by the use of a low-energy, nearly monoenergetic x-ray spectrum (Adapted from Yaffe MJ. Digital mammography. In: Haus AG, Yaffe MJ, eds. *Syllabus: a categorical course in physics: technical aspects of breast imaging.* Oak Brook, IL: RSNA, 1994:275–286.)

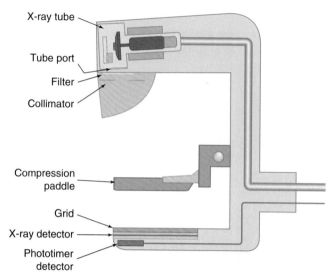

X-ray tube

Tube port

Filter

Collimator

Compression paddle

Grid

X-ray detector

Phototimer detector

■ **FIGURE 8-3** A dedicated mammography system has many unique attributes. Major components of a typical system, excluding the generator and user console, are shown.

energies provide the best differential attenuation between the tissues; however, the high absorption results in higher radiation doses and long exposure times. Detection of small calcifications in the breast is also important because microcalcifications are in some cases early markers of breast cancer. Thus, mammography requires x-ray detectors with high spatial resolution that function best at higher doses. Enhancing contrast sensitivity, reducing dose, and providing the spatial resolution necessary to depict microcalcifications impose extreme requirements on mammographic equipment and detectors. Therefore, dedicated x-ray equipment, specialized x-ray tubes, breast compression devices, antiscatter grids, x-ray detectors (screen-film or digital), and phototimer detector systems are essential for mammography (Fig. 8-3). Strict QC procedures and cooperation among the technologist, radiologist, and medical physicist are necessary to ensure that high-quality mammograms are achieved at the lowest possible radiation doses. With these issues in mind, the technical and physical considerations of mammographic x-ray imaging are discussed below. Many of the basic concepts regarding image quality, x-ray production, and radiography are presented in Chapters 4, 6, and 7, respectively. The applications of these concepts to mammography, together with many new topics specific to mammography, are presented below.

8.1 X-ray Tube and Beam Filtration

A dedicated mammography x-ray tube has more similarities than differences when compared to a conventional x-ray tube. Therefore, this section highlights the differences between mammography and general radiography x-ray tubes.

Cathode and Filament Circuit

The mammography x-ray tube is configured with dual filaments in the focusing cup to produce 0.3- and 0.1-mm focal spot sizes, with the latter used for magnification studies to reduce geometric blurring, as discussed later in this chapter. An important distinction between mammography and conventional x-ray tube operation is the low operating voltage, below 40 kV, which requires feedback circuits in the x-ray generator to adjust the filament current as a function of kV to deliver the desired tube current because of the nonlinear relationship between filament current and tube current as described in Chapter 6. In addition, the filament current is restricted to limit the tube current, typically to 100 mA for the large (0.3 mm) focal spot and 25 mA for the small (0.1 mm) focal spot so as to not overheat the Mo or Rh targets due to the small interaction areas. Higher filament currents and thus tube currents, up to and beyond 200 mA for the large focal spot and 50 mA for the small focal spot, are possible with tungsten anodes chiefly due to a higher melting point compared to Mo and Rh anodes.

Anode

Molybdenum is the most common anode target material used in mammography x-ray tubes, but Rh and increasingly tungsten (W) are also used as targets. Characteristic x-ray production is the major reason for choosing Mo (K-shell x-ray energies of 17.5 and 19.6 keV) and Rh (20.2 and 22.7 keV) targets, as the numbers of x-rays in the optimal energy range for breast imaging are significantly increased by characteristic x-ray emission. With digital detectors, W is becoming the target of choice. Increased x-ray production efficiency, due to its higher atomic number, and improved heat loading, due to its higher melting point, are major factors in favor of W. Digital detectors have extended exposure latitude, and because post-acquisition image processing can enhance contrast, characteristic radiation from Mo or Rh is not as important in digital mammography as it is with screen-film detectors.

Mammography x-ray tubes have rotating anodes, with anode angles ranging from 16 to 0 degrees, depending on the manufacturer. The tubes are typically positioned at a source-to-image receptor distance (SID) of about 65 cm. In order to achieve adequate field coverage on the anterior side of the field, the x-ray tube must be physically tilted so that the *effective anode angle* (the actual anode angle plus the physical tube tilt) is at least 22 degrees for coverage of the 24 × 30-cm field area. A tube with a 0-degree anode angle requires a tube tilt of about 24 degrees to achieve an effective anode angle of 24 degrees (Fig. 8-4A). A 16-degree anode angle requires a tube tilt of 6 degrees for an effective angle of 22 degrees (Fig. 8-4B).

The intensity of the x-rays emitted from the focal spot varies within the beam, with the greatest intensity on the cathode side of the projected field and the lowest intensity on the anode side, a consequence of the *heel effect* (Chapter 6). Positioning the cathode over the chest wall of the patient and the anode over the anterior portion (nipple) achieves better uniformity of the *transmitted* x-rays through the breast (Fig. 8-5). Orientation of the tube in this way also decreases the equipment bulk near the patient's head. The anode is kept at ground potential (0 voltage), and the cathode is set to the highest negative voltage to reduce *off-focal radiation* (Chapter 6).

Focal Spot Considerations

Focal spot nominal sizes of 0.3 to 0.4 mm for contact mammography (breast compressed against the grid and image receptor) and 0.10 to 0.15 mm for magnification imaging (breast compressed against a magnification stand, which supports the breast at a distance from the image receptor to provide geometric image magnification)

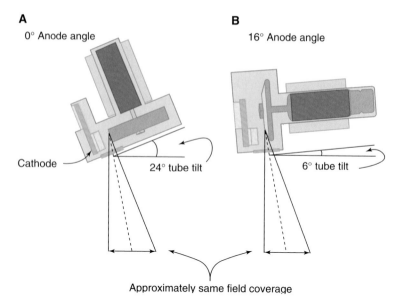

A

0° Anode angle

Cathode

24° tube tilt

B

16° Anode angle

6° tube tilt

Approximately same field coverage

■ **FIGURE 8-4** Design of a dedicated mammography system includes unique geometry and x-ray tube design. A "half-field" geometry is implemented with the x-ray beam central axis perpendicular to the plane of the image receptor at the center edge of the field at the chest wall, and centered horizontally. To provide full-area x-ray beam coverage over the large FOV (24 × 30 cm) at the 60- to 70-cm SID, a tube tilt of about 20 to 24 degrees is necessary. **A.** An anode angle of 0 degrees requires a tube tilt of 24 degrees. **B.** An anode angle of 16 degrees requires a tube tilt of about 6 degrees.

■ **FIGURE 8-5** Orientation of the cathode-anode direction of the x-ray tube is from the chest wall side of the breast (over the cathode) to the anterior side of the breast (over the anode). Variation of x-ray beam intensity is caused by the heel effect, a result of anode self-filtration of x-rays directed toward the anode side of the field, with a significant reduction in x-ray intensity. The thickest part of the breast (at the chest wall) is positioned below the cathode, which helps equalize x-ray intensities reaching the image receptor that are transmitted through the breast in the cathode-anode direction.

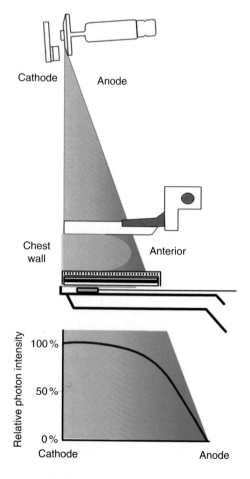

Cathode   Anode

Chest wall   Anterior

Relative photon intensity

100%

50%

0%

Cathode   Anode

reduce geometric blurring so that microcalcifications can be resolved. A consequence of using small focal spots is reduced maximal tube current (e.g., for a Mo target, 100 mA for the large focal spot and 25 mA for the small focal spot) and correspondingly longer exposure times.

In order to avoid exposure of the patients' torsos and to maximize the amount of breast tissue near the chest wall that is imaged, all dedicated mammography systems utilize a "half-field" x-ray beam geometry, which is achieved by fixed collimation at the x-ray tube head. As a result, the central axis of the x-ray beam is directed at the chest wall edge of the receptor and perpendicular to the plane of the image receptor. Furthermore, by convention, the nominal focal spot size is measured at the *reference axis*, which bisects the x-ray field along the chest wall—anterior direction of the x-ray field (Fig. 8-6A).

The sum of the target angle and tube tilt is equal to θ, and ϕ represents the reference angle. At the reference axis, the focal spot length, a_{ref}, is foreshortened compared to the focal spot length at the chest wall, $a_{chest\ wall}$, given by the relationship

$$a_{ref} = a_{chest\ wall} \left(1 - \frac{\tan(\theta - \phi)}{\tan \theta} \right)$$ [8-1]

Nominal focal spot size and tolerance limits for the width and length are listed in Table 8-1. As a consequence of the effective focal spot size variation in the field (the line focus principle), sharper image detail is rendered on the anode (anterior) side of the field toward the nipple, which is more evident with magnification examinations, as described in Section 8.3.

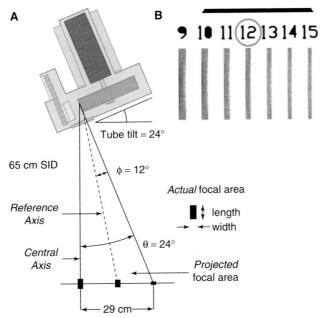

A.

Tube tilt = 24°

65 cm SID

$\phi = 12°$

Actual focal area

Reference Axis

$\updownarrow$ length

$\rightarrow \leftarrow$ width

Central Axis

$\theta = 24°$

Projected focal area

29 cm

B. 9 10 11 (12) 13 14 15

■ **FIGURE 8-6 A.** The projected focal spot size varies along the cathode-anode axis, and the nominal focal spot size is specified at a *reference axis* at an angle ϕ from a line perpendicular to the cathode-anode axis (*dashed line*, ϕ = 12 degrees). The actual focal area is the electron distribution area on the anode (width × length), and the projected length is foreshortened according to the line focus principle. **B.** A resolution bar pattern with object magnification measures overall system resolution including that of the focal spot. Bars of 12 line pairs per mm are resolved for this particular system (magnification = 1.5×, 0.1-mm focal spot).

TABLE 8-1   NOMINAL FOCAL SPOT SIZE AND MEASURED TOLERANCE LIMITS OF MAMMOGRAPHY X-RAY TUBES SPECIFIED BY NEMA AND MQSA REGULATIONS

NOMINAL FOCAL SPOT SIZE (mm)	WIDTH (mm)	LENGTH (mm)
0.10	0.15	0.15
0.15	0.23	0.23
0.20	0.30	0.30
0.30	0.45	0.65
0.40	0.60	0.85
0.60	0.90	1.30

National Electrical Manufacturers Association publication XR-5, and MQSA regulations 21 CFR 900.

Focal spot resolvability with or without magnification is measured by imaging a high-resolution bar pattern with up to 20 line pairs/mm. For conventional breast imaging, the bar pattern is placed 4.5 cm above the breast support surface near the chest wall; for magnification imaging, it is placed 4.5 cm above the magnification platform. Orientation of the bar pattern parallel and perpendicular to the cathode-anode direction yields measurements of overall *effective* resolution that reflect the effects of the focal spot dimensions, the acquisition geometry, and the detector sampling characteristics. A resolution bar pattern is shown in Figure 8-6B for a magnification study using the 0.1-mm focal spot. The resolving capability of the imaging system is limited by the component that causes the most blurring. In magnification mammography, this is generally the focal spot, whereas in contact mammography, it may be the detector element size, and at other times patient motion.

Tube Port, Tube Filtration, and Beam Quality

The tube port and added tube filters play an important role in shaping the mammography x-ray energy spectrum. The tube port window is made of beryllium. The low atomic number (Z=4) of beryllium and the small thickness of the window (0.5 to 1 mm) allow the transmission of all but the lowest energy (less than 5 keV) bremsstrahlung x-rays. In addition, Mo and Rh targets produce beneficial K-characteristic x-ray peaks at 17.5 and 19.6 keV (Mo) and 20.2 and 22.7 keV (Rh) (see Chapter 6, Table 6-2), whereas tungsten targets produce a large fraction of unwanted L-characteristic x-rays at 8 to 10 keV. Figure 8-7 shows a bremsstrahlung, characteristic, and composite x-ray spectrum from an x-ray tube with a Mo target and Be window operated at 30 kV.

Added x-ray tube filtration improves the energy distribution of the mammography output spectrum by selectively removing the lowest and highest energy x-rays from the x-ray beam, while largely transmitting desired x-ray energies. This is accomplished by using elements with *K-absorption edge* (Chapter 3) energies between 20 and 27 keV. Elements that have these K-shell binding energies include Mo, Rh, and Ag, and each can be shaped into thin, uniform sheets to be used as added x-ray tube filters. At the lowest x-ray energies, the attenuation of added filtration is very high. The attenuation decreases as the x-ray energy increases up to the K-edge of the filter element. For x-ray energies just above this level, photoelectric absorption interactions dramatically increase attenuation as a step or "edge" function (Fig 8-8A). At higher x-ray energies, the attenuation decreases. The result is the selective transmission of x-rays in a narrow band of energies from about 15 keV up to the K-absorption edge of the filter.

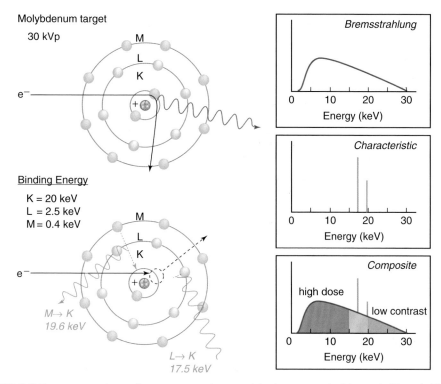

Molybdenum target
30 kVp

Binding Energy
K = 20 keV
L = 2.5 keV
M = 0.4 keV

$M \rightarrow K$
19.6 keV

$L \rightarrow K$
17.5 keV

■ FIGURE 8-7 The x-ray spectrum of a mammography x-ray tube is composed of bremsstrahlung (with a continuous photon energy spectrum) and characteristic (discrete energies) radiation (see Chapter 6 for more details). A Mo anode tube operated at 30 kV creates the continuous spectrum as well as characteristic radiation with photon energies of 17.5 and 19.6 keV. On the lower right, the "unfiltered" composite spectrum transmitted through 1 mm of Be (tube port material) has a large fraction of low-energy x-rays that will deposit high dose without contributing to the image, and a substantial fraction of high-energy x-rays that will reduce subject contrast of the breast tissues. The ideal spectral energy range is from about 15 to 25 keV, depending on breast tissue composition and thickness.

In Figure 8-8B, the unfiltered Mo target spectrum and a superimposed attenuation curve for a Mo filter are shown. Importantly, the characteristic x-ray energies produced by the Mo target occur at the lowest attenuation of the filter in this energy range.

With a Mo target, a 0.030-mm-thick Mo filter or a 0.025-mm Rh filter is typically used, and for a Rh target, a 0.025-mm Rh filter is used. A variety of filters are used with W targets, including Rh (0.05 mm), Ag (0.05 mm), and Al (0.7 mm).

The spectral output of a Mo target and 0.030-mm-thick Mo filter is shown in Figure 8-9A, illustrating the selective transmission of Mo characteristic radiation and significant attenuation of the lowest and highest x-rays in the transmitted spectrum. Tuning the spectrum to achieve optimal effective x-ray energy for breast imaging is accomplished by selecting the anode material, added filtration material, and kV. Screen-film detectors most often use a Mo target and 0.03-mm Mo filtration with a kV of 24 to 25 kV for thin, fatty breasts and up to 30 kV for thick, glandular breasts. For thicker and denser breasts, a Mo target and Rh filter are selected with higher voltage, from 28 to 32 kV, to achieve a higher effective energy and more penetrating beam (Fig. 8-9B, right graph). Some systems have Rh targets, which produce Rh characteristic x-ray energies of 20.2 and 22.7 keV, achieving an even higher effective energy x-ray beam for a set kV (Fig. 8-10A). A Mo filter should *never* be used with a Rh target, because Rh characteristic x-rays are attenuated significantly as their energies are above the Mo K-absorption edge (Fig. 8-10B).

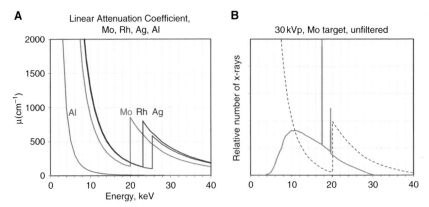

■ **FIGURE 8-8 A**. The linear attenuation coefficients of Al, Mo, Rh, and Ag are plotted as a function of energy. A low-attenuation "window" exists below the K-absorption edge energy for the higher Z elements. **B**. An unfiltered Mo target spectrum generated at 30 kV shows a large fraction of low- and high-energy photons. Superimposed at the same energy scale is a *dashed line* illustrating a Mo filter attenuation as a function of energy.

W targets are now used for many digital mammography systems because of their higher bremsstrahlung production efficiency and higher tube loadings than Mo and Rh targets. K-edge filters can optimize the output energy spectrum for breast imaging. However, an unfiltered W spectrum contains a huge fraction of unwanted L x-rays in the 8- to 12-keV range (Fig. 8-11A). Therefore, minimum filter thicknesses of 0.05 mm for Rh and Ag are needed to attenuate the L-x-rays to negligible levels, as shown in Figure 8-11B. In some applications, an Al filter is used, but because of its low Z and lack of a useful K-absorption edge, a thickness of 0.7 mm is necessary to attenuate the L x-rays. In digital tomosynthesis, in which contrast is largely provided by the tomographic image reconstruction process (Section 8.5), breast dose can be reduced by the use of Al filtration, which yields a larger fraction of high-energy x-rays.

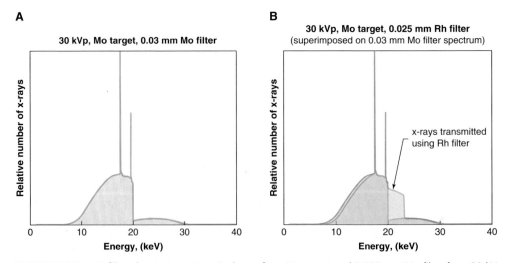

■ **FIGURE 8-9 A**. A filtered output spectrum is shown for a Mo target and 0.030-mm Mo filter for a 30-kV tube voltage, with prominent characteristic peaks at 17.5 and 19.6 keV. This is a common spectrum for less dense and thinner breast tissues, particularly with lower operating tube voltages (25 to 28 kV). **B**. A filtered output spectrum is shown for a Mo target and 0.025-mm Rh filter, superimposed on the Mo/Mo spectrum in (A), indicating the transmission of higher energy bremsstrahlung x-rays up to the K absorption edge of Rh at 23.2 keV. The spectrum, including the Mo characteristic x-rays, is more energetic and penetrating, and is preferable for imaging thicker and denser breast tissues.

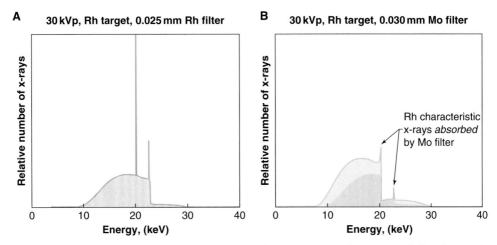

■ **FIGURE 8-10 A.** A filtered output spectrum is shown for a Rh target and 0.025-mm Rh filter for a 30-kV tube voltage, with prominent Rh characteristic x-rays at 20.2 and 22.7 keV. This spectrum provides a higher effective energy than a Mo target—Rh filter x-ray beam at the same kV, due to the higher energy characteristic x-rays. **B.** A combination of a Rh target and Mo filter *is inappropriate*, as the Rh characteristic x-rays are strongly attenuated as shown.

Half-Value Layer

The half-value layer (HVL) of a mammography x-ray beam ranges from 0.3 to 0.7-mm Al for the kV range and combinations of target material, filter material, and filter thickness used in mammography (Fig. 8-12). The HVL depends on the target material (Mo, Rh, W), kV, filter material, and filter thickness. Measurement of the HVL is usually performed with the compression paddle in the beam, using 99.9% pure Al sheets of 0.1-mm thickness. A Mo target, 0.03-mm Mo filter, 28 kV, and a 1.5 mm Lexan compression paddle produce a HVL of about 0.35-mm Al, whereas a W target, 0.05-mm Rh filter, and 30 kV produce a HVL of about 0.55-mm Al. HVLs vary

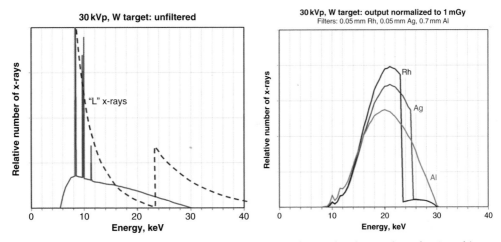

■ **FIGURE 8-11 A.** An unfiltered W target spectrum generated at 30 kV shows a large fraction of lower energy L-Characteristic x-rays at 8 to 11.5 keV. Superimposed at the same energy scale is a *dashed line* illustrating the high- and low-attenuation characteristics of a Rh filter. **B.** Filtered W-target x-ray spectra by Rh (0.05 mm), Ag (0.05 mm), and Al (0.7 mm) are normalized to the same exposure output.

■ FIGURE 8-12 The HVL (including the compression paddle attenuation) versus kV is plotted for Mo targets with Mo and Rh filters, and for W targets with Rh, Ag, and Al filters. HVL measurements are representative of an average of a number of evaluations on various mammography systems at the UC Davis Health System and are generally within +/− 0.05 mm of the values shown.

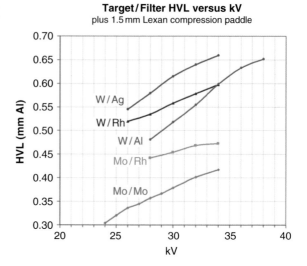

from machine to machine because of slight variation in actual filter thicknesses and kV. The HVL of breast tissue is highly dependent on tissue composition (glandular, fibrous, or fatty) and the HVL of the incident x-ray beam. Usually, the HVL for breast tissues is from 1 to 3 cm.

Minimum HVL limits, listed in Table 8-2, are prescribed by MQSA regulations to ensure that a beam of adequate effective energy is achieved. Maximum HVL limits are recommended by the ACR accreditation guidelines, as listed in Table 8-3. An x-ray beam that is "harder" than optimal indicates too much filtration or a pitted anode or aged tube and can result in reduced output and poor image quality. Estimates of the radiation dose to the breast require accurate assessment of the HVL (see Section 8.6).

Tube Output and Tube Output Rate

Tube output is a measure of the intensity of the x-ray beam, typically normalized to mAs or to 100 mAs, at a specified distance from the source (focal spot). Common units of tube output are mGy (air kerma)/100 mAs and mR (exposure)/mAs. The kV, target, filter material and thickness, distance from the source, and focal spot size must be specified. Figure 8-13 shows the output at a 50-cm distance from Mo and W

TABLE 8-2   REQUIREMENTS FOR MINIMUM HVL IN THE MQSA REGULATIONS (21 CFR PART 1020.30); ACR: WITH COMPRESSION PADDLE

TUBE VOLTAGE (kV)	MQSA: kV/100	ACR: kV/100 + 0.03
24	0.24	0.27
26	0.26	0.29
28	0.28	0.31
30	0.30	0.33
32	0.32	0.35

ACR, American College of Radiology; CFR, Code of Federal Regulations; MQSA, Mammography Quality Standards Act.

TABLE 8-3 ACR SPECIFICATIONS FOR MAXIMUM HVL: MAXIMUM HVL (mm Al) = kV/100 + C FOR TARGET-FILTER COMBINATIONS

TUBE VOLTAGE (kV)	Mo/Mo C = 0.12	Mo/Rh C = 0.19	Rh/Rh C = 0.22	W/Rh C = 0.30
24	0.36	0.43	0.46	0.54
26	0.38	0.45	0.48	0.56
28	0.40	0.47	0.50	0.58
30	0.42	0.49	0.52	0.60
32	0.44	0.51	0.54	0.62

ACR Accreditation Program requirements as specified in the Medical Physics testing section, http://www.acr.org

target x-ray tubes with a variety of tube filter materials and thicknesses. Even though W targets are more efficient at producing x-rays, the thicker filters needed to attenuate the L-characteristic x-rays result in lower tube output per mAs compared to the Mo target. However, W spectra have higher HVLs and greater beam penetrability, allow higher tube current, and result in comparable exposure times to a Mo target and filter for a similar breast thickness.

X-ray tube output values are useful for calculating the free-in-air incident air kerma (or exposure) to the breast for a mammography system's target and filter combination, kV, mAs, and source-to-breast surface distance. The source-to-breast surface distance is determined from the known SID, breast platform to detector distance, and compressed breast thickness. For instance, assume that a mammography system with a Mo target and Rh filter uses 30 kV and 160 mAs for a SID of 65 cm, compressed breast thickness of 6 cm, and a breast platform to detector distance of 2 cm. The entrant breast surface to the source is closer by 8 cm, and is therefore 57 cm from the source. From Figure 8-13, the tube output is 16 mGy/100 mAs for 30 kV at a distance of 50 cm. Calculation of incident air kerma considers tube output at a specific kV, the mAs used, and inverse square law correction from 50 to 57 cm:

$$16 \text{ mGy/100 mAs} \times 160 \text{ mAs} \times [50.0/57.0]^2 = 19.7 \text{ mGy}$$

Calculation of the average glandular dose to the breast is determined from the measured incident air kerma value and other parameters as discussed in Section 8.6.

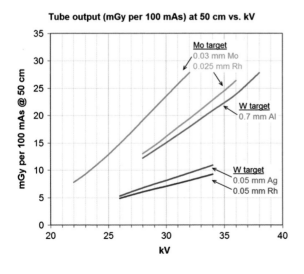

Tube output (mGy per 100 mAs) at 50 cm vs. kV

■ **FIGURE 8-13** Tube output (mGy/100 mAs at 50-cm distance from the source with compression paddle in the beam) for two clinical mammography units is measured at 2-kV intervals, and the data are smoothed. A Mo target with 0.030-mm Mo and 0.025-mm Rh filter, and a W target with 0.05-mm Rh, 0.05-mm Ag, and 0.7-mm Al filters are plotted.

Tube output rate is the air kerma rate at a specified distance from the x-ray focal spot and is a function of the tube current achievable for an extended exposure time (typically ~300 mAs for an exposure time greater than 3 s). To ensure the ability to deliver a sufficient x-ray beam fluence rate to keep exposure times reasonable, MQSA regulations require that systems be capable of producing an air kerma rate of at least 7.0 mGy/s, when operating at 28 kV in the standard (Mo/Mo) mammography mode, at any SID for which the system is designed to operate for screen-film detectors. Digital systems have requirements specified by the manufacturers' QC manuals.

X-ray Tube Alignment and Beam Collimation

Alignment of the x-ray tube and collimator are crucial to ensure that the x-ray beam central axis is perpendicular to the plane of the image receptor and intercepts the center of the chest wall edge of the image receptor. This will protect the patient from unnecessary radiation exposure to the lungs and torso and include as much breast tissue as possible in the image. Tube alignment with respect to the image receptor must be verified during acceptance testing of the system and after x-ray tube replacements.

Collimation of the x-ray beam is achieved by the use of fixed-size metal apertures or adjustable shutters. For most screen-film examinations, the field size is automatically set to match the film cassette dimensions (e.g., 18 × 24 cm or 24 × 30 cm). For a large area digital detector (24 × 30 cm), when operating with the smaller field area (18 × 24 cm), one of three active acquisition areas is used: center, left shift, and right shift, which requires the collimator assembly to restrict the x-ray field to the corresponding active detector area. Field shifts are used for optimizing the oblique projections for subjects with smaller breasts to accommodate positioning of the arm and shoulder at the top edge of the receptor. Collimation to the full active detector area is the standard of practice (see Section 8.4: "Film-Viewing Conditions"). There is no disadvantage to full-field collimation compared to collimation to the breast only, as the tissues are fully in the beam in either case. However, for magnification and spot compression studies, manually adjusted shutters allow the x-ray field to be more closely matched to the volume being imaged.

The projected x-ray field must extend to the chest wall edge of the image receptor without cutoff, but not beyond the receptor by more than 2% of the SID. If the image shows evidence of collimation of the x-ray field on the chest wall side or if the chest wall edge of the compression paddle is visible in the image, service must be requested. A collimator light and mirror assembly visibly display the x-ray beam area. Between the tube port and the collimator is a low-attenuation mirror that directs light from the collimator lamp through the collimator opening to emulate the x-ray field area. Similar to conventional x-ray tube collimator assemblies, the light field must be congruent with the actual x-ray field to within 2% overall, which is achieved by adjustment of the light and mirror positions. MQSA regulations require repairs to be made within 30 days if the light/x-ray field congruence, x-ray field-image receptor alignment, or compression paddle alignment is out of tolerance as described above.

8.2   X-ray Generator and Phototimer System

X-ray Generator

A dedicated mammography x-ray generator is similar to a conventional x-ray generator in design and function. Differences include the lower voltages supplied to the x-ray tube, space charge compensation, and automatic exposure control (AEC) circuitry. In most cases, AEC is employed for mammography screening and diagnostic examinations, although there are instances when the technologist will use manual controls to set the tube current - exposure duration product (mAs). Like most contemporary x-ray imaging systems, high-frequency generators are used for mammography due to low voltage ripple, fast response, easy calibration, long-term stability, and compact size. There are circuits that prohibit x-ray exposures if the setup is incomplete (e.g., insufficient compression, cassette not in the tunnel, or digital detector not ready to capture an image).

Automatic Exposure Control

The AEC employs a radiation sensor or sensors, a charge amplifier, and a voltage comparator to control the exposure (Fig. 8-14). For cassette-based image receptors (screen-film *and* computed radiography [CR]), the phototimer sensor is located *underneath* the cassette, and consists of a single ionization chamber or an array of three or more semiconductor diodes. X-rays transmitted through the breast, antiscatter grid (if present), and the image receptor generate a signal in the detector. The signal is accumulated (integrated) and, when the accumulated signal reaches a preset value, the exposure is terminated. The preset value corresponds to a specified signal-to-noise ratio (SNR) in a digital mammography unit or an acceptable optical density (OD) if a film-screen system is used. For an active matrix flat-panel imager, the detector array itself can be used to measure the x-rays transmitted through the breast and the antiscatter grid.

Phototimer algorithms use several inputs to determine the radiographic technique, including compressed breast thickness, phototimer adjustment settings on the generator console, the kV, the tube anode selection (if available), and the tube filter to achieve the desired film OD or digital SNR in the acquired image. The operator typically has two or three options for AEC: (a) a fully automatic AEC mode that sets the optimal kV and filtration (and target material on some systems) from a short test exposure of approximately 100 ms to determine the penetrability of the breast; (b) automatic kV with a short test exposure, with user-selected target and filter values; and (c) automatic time of exposure using manually set target, filter, and

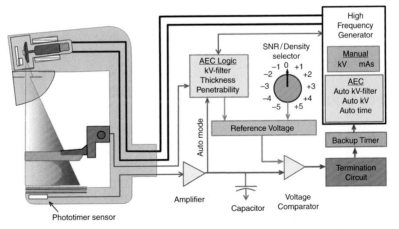

■ **FIGURE 8-14** The AEC (phototimer) circuits use algorithms with input from the breast thickness (from the compression paddle), breast density (via a test exposure), density setting (operator density selector), and exposure duration (reciprocity law failure issues) to determine overall exposure time. In fully automatic modes, the kV, beam filter, and target are also determined, usually from a short (100 ms) exposure to determine attenuation characteristics of the breast.

kV values. For most patient imaging, the fully automatic mode is used, but, for QC procedures, the automatic exposure time adjustment mode with other parameters manually selected by the user is often employed.

At the generator control panel, an exposure adjustment selector modifies the AEC response to permit adjustments for unusual imaging circumstances such as imaging breasts with implants, magnification, or for radiologist preference in film OD or digital image SNR. Usually, eleven steps (-5 to 0 [neutral] to $+5$) are available to increase or decrease exposure by adjusting the AEC comparator switch. Each step provides a difference of 10% to 15% positive (greater exposure) or negative (lesser exposure) per step from the baseline (0) setting.

An x-ray exposure that is not stopped by the AEC circuit and exceeds a preset time (e.g., greater than 5 s) is terminated by a *backup timer*. This can occur if there is a malfunction of the AEC system or if the kV is set too low with insufficient x-ray transmission. In the latter situation, the operator must select a *higher* kV to achieve greater beam penetrability and shorter exposure time to correct the problem.

Inaccurate phototimer response, resulting in an under- or overexposed film or digital image, can be caused by breast tissue composition (adipose versus glandular) heterogeneity, compressed thickness beyond the calibration range (too thin or too thick), a defective cassette, a faulty phototimer detector, or an inappropriate kV setting. Screen-film response to very long exposure times, chiefly in magnification studies caused by the low mA capacity of the small focal spot, results in *reciprocity law failure* (Chapter 7), whereby the resultant OD is less than would be predicted by the amount of radiation delivered to the screen-film cassette; consequently, insufficient film OD results, and extension of the exposure time is added to compensate. For extremely thin or fatty breasts, the phototimer circuit and x-ray generator can be too slow in terminating the exposure, causing film overexposure. In situations where the exposure is terminated too quickly, grid-line artifacts will commonly appear in the image due to lack of complete grid motion during the short exposure.

The position of the phototimer detector (e.g., under dense or fatty breast tissue) can have a significant effect on film density but has much less of an impact on digital images because of postprocessing capabilities, even though the SNR will vary. Previous mammograms can aid the technologist in selecting the proper position for the phototimer detector to achieve optimal film density or optimal SNR for glandular areas of the breast. Most systems allow phototimer positioning in the chest wall to anterior direction, while some newer systems also allow side-to-side positioning to provide flexibility for unusual circumstances.

Technique Chart

Technique charts are useful guides to help determine the appropriate kV and target-filter combinations for specific imaging tasks, based on breast thickness and breast composition (fatty versus glandular tissue fractions). Most mammographic techniques use phototiming, and the proper choice of kV is essential for a reasonable exposure time, defined as a range from approximately 0.5 to 2.0 s to achieve an OD of 1.5 to 2.0 for film, or the desired SNR for digital images. Too short an exposure can cause visible grid lines to appear on the image, whereas too long an exposure can result in breast motion, either of which degrades the quality of the image. Table 8-4 lists kV recommendations for screen-film detectors to meet the desired exposure time range for breast thickness and breast composition using a Mo target and 0.030-mm Mo filter, determined from computer simulations and experimental

TABLE 8-4   RECOMMENDED kV, AS A FUNCTION OF BREAST COMPOSITION AND THICKNESS

BREAST COMPOSITION	BREAST THICKNESS (cm)						
	2	3	4	5	6	7	8
Fatty	24	24	24	24	25	27	30
50/50	24	24	24	25	28	30	32
Glandular	24	24	26	28	31	33	35

The goal is an exposure time between 0.5 and 2.0 s. This chart is for a Mo target and 0.030-mm Mo filter using a 100-mA tube current and screen-film detector. These kVs may not be appropriate for other target/filter combinations or for digital detectors. The kV values were determined by computer simulations and clinical measurements.

measurements. Techniques for digital detector systems are more flexible, and because of postprocessing and contrast enhancement capabilities, will often use a wider range of kV settings. A technique chart example for an amorphous selenium (Se) flat panel detector system using a Mo target, a W target, or a W target (without a grid for a digital tomosynthesis acquisition) and corresponding tube filtration is listed in Table 8-5.

 8.3   Compression, Scattered Radiation, and Magnification

Compression

Breast compression is an important part of the mammography examination, whether using screen-film or digital detectors. Firm compression reduces overlapping anatomy, decreases tissue thickness, and reduces inadvertent motion of the breast (Fig. 8-15A). It results in fewer scattered x-rays, less geometric blurring of anatomic structures, and lower radiation dose to the breast tissues. Achieving a uniform breast thickness lessens exposure dynamic range and allows the use of higher contrast film, or allows more flexibility in image processing enhancement of the digital image.

Compression is achieved with a compression paddle, a Lexan plate attached to a mechanical assembly (Fig. 8-15B). The full area compression paddle matches the size of the image receptor (18 × 24 cm or 24 × 30 cm) and is flat and parallel to the breast support table. An alternative to the flat compression paddle is the "flex" paddle

TABLE 8-5   TECHNIQUE CHART FOR A DIGITAL MAMMOGRAPHY SYSTEM WITH SELENIUM DETECTOR FOR 50% GLANDULAR 50% ADIPOSE COMPOSITION

THICKNESS (cm)	DIGITAL, Mo TARGET, CELLULAR GRID			DIGITAL, W TARGET, CELLULAR GRID			DIGITAL TOMOSYNTHESIS, W TARGET, NO GRID		
	FILTER	kV	mAs	FILTER	kV	mAs	FILTER	kV	mAs
<3	Mo 30 μm	24	35	Rh 50 μm	25	40	Al 700 μm	26	35
3–5	Mo 30 μm	27	75	Rh 50 μm	28	80	Al 700 μm	29	50
5–7	Mo 30 μm	31	100	Rh 50 μm	31	150	Al 700 μm	33	65
>7	Rh 25 μm	33	150	Ag 50 μm	32	200	Al 700 μm	38	85

■ **FIGURE 8-15 A.** Compression is essential for mammographic studies to reduce breast thickness (less scatter, reduced radiation dose, and shorter exposure time) and to spread out superimposed anatomy. **B.** Suspicious areas often require "spot" compression to eliminate superimposed anatomy by further spreading the breast tissues over a localized area. **C.** Example of image with suspicious finding (**left**). Corresponding spot compression image shows no visible mass or architectural distortion (**right**).

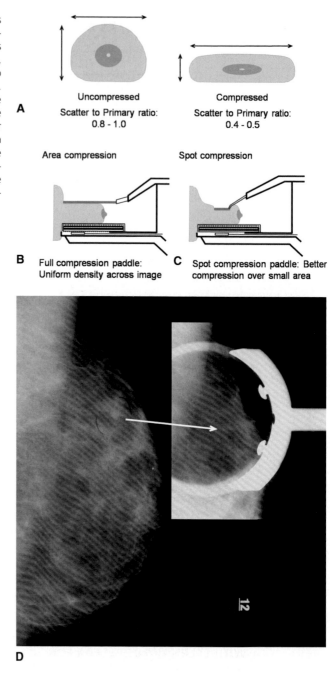

A

Uncompressed
Scatter to Primary ratio:
0.8 - 1.0

Compressed
Scatter to Primary ratio:
0.4 - 0.5

Area compression

Spot compression

B
Full compression paddle:
Uniform density across image

C
Spot compression paddle: Better
compression over small area

D

that is spring loaded on the anterior side to tilt and accommodate variations in breast thickness from the chest wall to the nipple, providing more uniform compression of the breast. A compression paddle has a right-angle edge at the chest wall to produce a flat, uniform breast thickness when an adequate force of 111 to 200 newtons (25 to 44 lb) is applied. A smaller "spot" compression paddle (~5-cm diameter) reduces the breast thickness further over a specific region and redistributes the tissue for improved contrast and reduced anatomic overlap (Fig. 8-15C,D).

Typically, a hands-free (e.g., foot-pedal operated), motor-driven compression paddle is used, which is operable from both sides of the patient. In addition, a mechanical adjustment knob near the paddle holder allows fine manual adjustments of compression. While firm compression is not comfortable for the patient, it is often necessary for a clinically acceptable image.

Scattered Radiation and Antiscatter Grids

X-rays transmitted through the breast contain primary and scattered radiation. Primary radiation carries information regarding the attenuation characteristics of the breast and delivers the maximum possible subject contrast to the detector. Scattered radiation is an additive, gradually varying radiation distribution that degrades subject contrast and adds random noise. If the maximum subject contrast without scatter is C_0 and the maximum contrast with scatter is C_s, then the contrast degradation factor (CDF) is approximated as

$$CDF = \frac{C_s}{C_0} = \frac{1}{1 + SPR}$$ [8-2]

where SPR is the scatter-to-primary ratio (Chapter 7). X-ray scatter increases with increasing breast thickness and breast area, with typical SPR values shown in Figure 8-16. A breast of 6-cm compressed thickness will have an SPR of approximately 0.6 and a calculated scatter degradation factor of $(1/(1+0.6)) = 0.625 = 62.5\%$. Without some form of scatter rejection, therefore, only a fraction of the inherent subject contrast can be detected.

In digital mammography, unlike screen-film mammography, the main adverse effect of scattered x-rays is not a reduction of contrast. Contrast can be improved by any desired amount by post-acquisition processing, such as windowing. The main adverse effect of scatter in digital mammography is that scattered photons add random noise, degrading the signal to noise ratio.

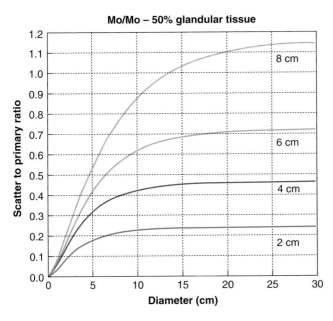

■ **FIGURE 8-16** X-ray scatter reduces the radiographic contrast of the breast image. Scatter is chiefly dependent on breast thickness and field area, and largely independent of kV in the mammography energy range (25 to 35 kV). The scatter-to-primary ratio is plotted as a function of the diameter of a semicircular field area aligned to the chest wall edge, for several breast thicknesses of 50% glandular tissue.

Scattered radiation reaching the image receptor can be greatly reduced by the use of an *antiscatter grid* or *air gap*. (Antiscatter grids are described in Chapter 7.) For contact mammography, an antiscatter grid is located between the breast and the detector. Mammography grids transmit about 60% to 70% of primary x-rays and absorb 75% to 85% of the scattered radiation. Linear focused grids with grid ratios (height of the lead septa divided by the interspace distance) of 4:1 to 5:1 are common (e.g., 1.5 mm height, 0.30-mm distance between septa, 0.016-mm septa thickness), with carbon fiber interspace materials (Fig. 8-17A). Grid frequencies (number of lead septa per cm) of 30/cm to 45/cm are typical. To avoid grid-line artifacts, the grid must oscillate over a distance of approximately 20 lines during the exposure. Excessively short exposures are the cause of most grid-line artifacts because of insufficient grid motion.

A cellular grid, made of thin copper septa, provides scatter rejection in two dimensions (Fig. 8-17B). Specifications of this design include a septal height of 2.4 mm, 0.64-mm distance between septa (3.8 ratio), a septal thickness of 0.03 mm, and 15 cells/cm. During image acquisition, a specific grid motion is necessary for complete blurring, so specific exposure time increments are necessary and are determined by AEC logic evaluation of the first 100 ms of the exposure. Because of two dimensional scatter rejection and air interspaces, the cellular grid provides a better contrast improvement factor than the linear grid.

Grids impose a dose penalty to compensate for loss of primary radiation that would otherwise contribute to SNR in the digital image or for x-ray scatter and primary radiation losses that would otherwise contribute to film optical density in film-screen mammography. As discussed in Chapter 7, the *Bucky factor* is the ratio of exposure with the grid compared to the exposure without the grid to achieve the same film optical density. For mammography grids, the Bucky factor is 2 to 3, so the breast dose is doubled or tripled, but the benefit is improvement of image contrast by up to 40%. For digital acquisitions, there is no similar "Bucky factor" definition, but the loss of signal in the digital image from primary radiation being attenuated by the grid strips will increase the exposure needed to achieve a similar SNR. Typically,

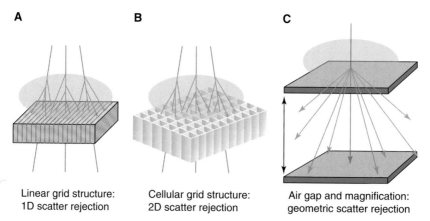

Linear grid structure: 1D scatter rejection

Cellular grid structure: 2D scatter rejection

Air gap and magnification: geometric scatter rejection

■ **FIGURE 8-17** Antiscatter devices commonly employed in mammography include (**A**) the linear grid of approximately 5:1 grid ratio and carbon fiber interspace material, (**B**) a cellular crosshatch grid structure made of copper sheet of approximately 3.8 grid ratio with air interspaces and scatter rejection in two dimensions, and (**C**) the air gap intrinsic to the magnification procedure. Note: while the illustration depicts 100% scatter rejection by the grid, approximately 15% of scattered x-rays are transmitted.

the extra radiation needed for a digital detector is less than the Bucky factor for screen-film, perhaps by one half or more. Grid performance is far from ideal, but digital acquisition and image processing can somewhat mitigate the dose penalty incurred by the use of the antiscatter grid and analog screen-film detectors.

An air gap reduces scatter by increasing the distance of the breast from the detector, so that a large fraction of scattered radiation misses the detector (Fig. 8-17C). The consequences of using an air gap, however, are that the field of view (FOV) is reduced, the magnification of the breast is increased, and the dose to the breast is increased. However, use of a sufficiently large air gap can render the antiscatter grid unnecessary, thus reducing dose to the breast by approximately the same factor.

Magnification Techniques

Geometric magnification (Chapter 7) is used to improve system resolution, typically for better visualization of microcalcifications. In magnification studies, geometric magnification is achieved by placing a breast support platform (a magnification stand) at a fixed distance above the detector, selecting the small (0.1 mm) focal spot, removing the antiscatter grid, and using a compression paddle (Fig. 8-18). Most dedicated mammographic units offer magnifications of 1.5×, 1.8×, or 2.0×. Advantages of magnification include (a) increased effective resolution of the image receptor by the magnification factor; (b) reduction of image noise relative to the objects being rendered; and (c) reduction of scattered radiation. Geometric magnification of the x-ray distribution pattern relative to the inherent unsharpness of the image receptor improves effective resolution, as long as the loss of resolution by geometric blurring is mitigated with the small 0.1-mm nominal focal spot. Since there are more x-rays per object area in a magnified image, the effective quantum noise is reduced, compared to the standard contact image. The distance between the breast support surface of the magnification stand and the image receptor reduces scattered radiation reaching the image receptor, thereby improving image contrast and reducing random noise and making an antiscatter grid unnecessary.

Magnification has several limitations, the most significant being geometric blurring caused by the finite focal spot area. Even with a small 0.1-mm focal spot, spatial resolution will be less on the cathode side of the x-ray field (toward the chest

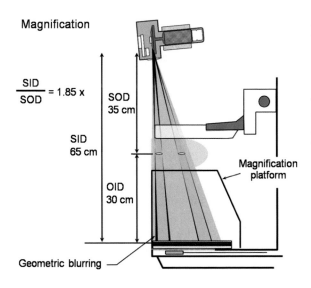

Magnification

$$\frac{SID}{SOD} = 1.85 \text{ x}$$

SOD 35 cm

SID 65 cm

OID 30 cm

Magnification platform

Geometric blurring

■ FIGURE 8-18 Geometric magnification. A support platform positions the breast closer to the source focal spot, resulting in 1.5× to 2.0× image magnification. A small focal spot (0.1-mm nominal size) reduces geometric blurring. Variation of effective focal spot size along the cathode-anode axis (large to small effective size) is accentuated with magnification and increased penumbra width. Best resolution and detail in the image exist on the anode side of the field. SID: source to image distance; SOD: source to object (midplane) distance; OID: object to image distance.

wall), where the effective focal spot length is largest. In addition, the small focal spot has a tube current limit of about 25 mA for a Mo target, so a 100-mAs technique requires 4 s exposure time. Even slight breast motion will result in image blurring, which is exacerbated by the magnification. For screen-film detectors and long exposure times, reciprocity law failure requires additional radiation exposure to achieve the desired film OD. Regarding breast dose, the elimination of the grid reduces dose by a factor of 2 to 3, but the shorter distance between the x-ray focal spot and the breast increases dose by about the same factor due to the inverse square law. Therefore, in general, the average glandular dose delivered to the breast with magnification is similar to that from contact mammography. However, the smaller irradiated FOV justifies collimating the x-ray beam to only the volume of interest, which reduces radiation scatter and breast dose.

8.4 Screen-Film Cassettes and Film Processing

Screen-film detectors in mammography have been a proven technology over the last 30 years; in fact, the 2001–2005 study comparing screen-film and digital mammography detectors showed that screen-film detectors are comparable to digital detectors in terms of diagnostic accuracy as a means of screening for breast cancer. Digital mammography has been shown to be more accurate for women under the age of 50 years, women with radiographically dense breasts, and premenopausal or peri-menopausal women compared to screen-film mammography (Pisano et al. 2005). While digital mammography has reduced the use of screen-film mammography, for some low-volume mammography clinics and those clinics not yet able to transition to digital technology, screen-film detectors remain a reasonable and cost-effective technology.

Design of Mammographic Screen-Film Systems

A mammographic screen-film detector is comprised of a cassette, intensifying screen or screens, and a light-sensitive film. Most cassettes are made of low-attenuation carbon fiber and have a single high-definition phosphor screen used in conjunction with a single emulsion film. Terbium-activated gadolinium oxysulfide (Gd_2O_2S:Tb) is the most commonly used screen phosphor. This scintillator emits green light, requiring a green-sensitive film emulsion. Intensifying screen-film speeds and spatial resolution are determined by screen phosphor particle size, number of phosphor particles per volume, light-absorbing dyes in the phosphor matrix, and phosphor layer thickness. Mammography screen-film systems have their own speed ratings and are classified as regular (100 or par speed) and medium (150 to 190 speed), whereby the 100-speed screen-film system requires 120 to 150 µGy incident air kerma to achieve the desired film OD. For comparison, a conventional "400-speed" screen-film cassette for general diagnostic imaging requires about 5-µGy air kerma.

The intensifying screen is positioned in the *back* of the cassette so that x-rays travel through the cassette cover and the film before interacting with the phosphor. Exponential attenuation in the phosphor results in a greater fraction of x-ray interactions near the phosphor surface closest to the film emulsion. At shallow depths in the phosphor, absorbed x-rays produce light distributions that have minimal light spread prior to interacting with the film, thus preserving spatial resolution. X-ray absorption occurring at greater depth in the screen produces a broader light distribution and reduces spatial resolution (Fig. 8-19), but the number of interactions

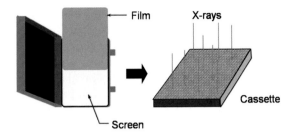

Single Emulsion Film and Single Phosphor Screen

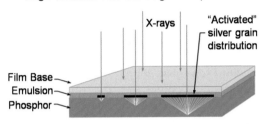

■ **FIGURE 8-19** Nearly all screen-film systems used in mammography employ a single phosphor screen with a single emulsion film and are "front-loaded" (x-rays pass through the film to the screen). Light spread varies with the depth of x-ray absorption, as depicted in the lower diagram. Most x-rays interact in the layers of the screen closest to the film, preserving spatial resolution because of reduced spread of the light distribution.

decreases exponentially with depth. For a "100-speed" mammography screen-film cassette, the limiting spatial resolution is 15 to 20 lp/mm.

Selection of a screen-film combination requires consideration of measures such as spatial resolution and radiographic speed, as well as factors such as screen longevity, cassette design, film base color, film contrast characteristics, radiologist's preference, and cost. In today's market, there is no single best choice; hence, most screen-film receptors, when used as recommended with particular attention to film processing, provide excellent image quality for mammography imaging.

Film Recording and Film Processing

Mammography films are sensitized by x-ray–induced light from the phosphor screen. Light produces latent image centers on microscopic light-sensitive silver halide grains in the emulsion layered on a film substrate. (See Chapter 7 for more information.) Intensity variations in the light produce corresponding variations in the number of sensitized grains per area. Chemical processing in a bath of developer solution renders the invisible latent image into a visible image by reducing the sensitized grains to elemental silver. Unsensitized grains in the film emulsion are not reduced and are dissolved and washed away by the fixer solution. Subsequent rinsing and drying complete the film processing. Film is thus a two-dimensional recording of the incident light patterns encoded by silver grains on the substrate that produce an image with varying light intensities when the film is placed on a lightbox. Film opacity is the degree of the obstruction of light transmission (the inverse of transmittance), and optical density (OD), equal to the base ten logarithm of the opacity, is used as the metric of film response, as the eye responds linearly to variations in OD (e.g., an OD = 2 appears to be twice as "dark" as an OD = 1, although 10 times more light is attenuated with an OD = 2 compared to OD = 1). The useful OD levels on a mammography film range from about 0.2 up to about 3.

Film processing is a critical step in the mammographic imaging chain for screen-film detectors and is performed by automatic film processors. Film characteristics such as film speed (an indication of the amount of incident radiation required to achieve a specified OD on the film) and film contrast (the rate of change of OD for a known difference in incident radiation) are consistently achieved by following the manufacturer's recommendations for developer formulation, development time, developer temperature, developer replenishment rate, and processor maintenance. If the developer temperature is too low, the film speed and film contrast will be reduced, requiring a compensatory increase in radiation dose. If the developer temperature is too high or immersion time too long, an increase in film speed occurs, permitting a lower dose; however, the film contrast is likely to be reduced because film fog and quantum mottle are increased. Stability of the developer may also be compromised at higher-than-recommended temperatures. The manufacturer's guidelines for optimal processor settings and chemistry specifications should be followed. Also, because mammographic films must be retained for years, fixer retention on the film must be measured when evaluating the processor. If film washing is incomplete and fixer is retained, the films will oxidize and image quality will deteriorate over time.

Film Response, Sensitometry, and Quality Control

A film characteristic curve, also referred to as an *H* and *D curve*, represents the relationship between the incident x-ray exposure (proportional to light intensity on the film) and the resulting OD in the processed film. As shown in Figure 8-20A, a film characteristic curve is a graph of the OD as a function of the logarithm of the relative exposure and has three major sections: (a) the *toe* has a low OD that changes very little with incident exposure up to a threshold; (b) the *linear section* represents increasing OD with increasing incident exposure, with subject contrast mapped as optical densities that render the radiographic contrast; and (c) the *shoulder* represents saturation of the film, where increases in incident exposure do not significantly increase the OD. A film's characteristic curve is determined by both the design of the film and the film processing. Another way of displaying the film's response is the gradient curve, shown in Figure 8-20B. The gradient curve is a graph of the change of OD per unit change in the incident exposure, as a function of the logarithm of the relative exposure. The gradient is the rate of change of the characteristic curve, that is, the film contrast. The Film contrast changes with incident exposure and has a value near the maximum only over a narrow range of incident exposures.

Because of the high sensitivity of mammography film quality to slight changes in processor performance, routine monitoring of film contrast, speed, and base plus fog OD is important. A film-processor QC program is required by the MQSA

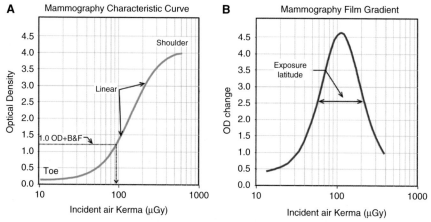

■ **FIGURE 8-20** **A.** The film characteristic curve is a graph of the OD as a function of the logarithm of incident air kerma, μGy (or exposure, mR). **B.** The gradient curve (the rate of change of the characteristic curve) indicates the contrast as a function of the logarithm of air kerma (exposure). The maximal value of the gradient curve is achieved for an exposure of about 120 μGy (14 mR), which is OD of about 2.0 for this exposure. Thus, the maximal contrast (change in OD for a change in exposure) is achieved at an OD of about 2.0.

regulations, and daily sensitometric tests must be performed before the first clinical images to verify acceptable performance. This requires the use of a sensitometer and a densitometer. A sensitometer is a device that emulates a range of incident radiation exposures by using a constant light source and calibrated optical attenuation steps to expose a mammographic film to known relative light intensities. Developing the film produces a range of numbered OD steps known as a *film sensitometric strip*. A densitometer is a device that measures the light transmission through a small area of the film and calculates the OD. Additionally, a thermometer is used to measure the temperature of the developer solution in the processor and monitoring chart are tools used to complete the processor evaluation. A chart is used to record and monitor the quality control measurements.

A box of film is reserved for QC testing; using films from a single box eliminates variations among different lots of film from the manufacturer. Daily, in the darkroom prior to the first case of the day, a film is exposed using a calibrated sensitometer and is then developed (Fig. 8-21A). On the processed film, optical densities on the sensometric strip are measured with a film densitometer (Fig. 8-21B). Data, which are plotted on a processor QC chart, are the base plus fog OD (measured at an area on the film that was not subjected to light exposure), a mid-density speed index step, and a density difference (an index of contrast) between two steps. The mid-density OD step and the two steps for calculating the density difference are selected from 5 day average ODs when the QC program is established. The mid-density step is the one whose OD is closest to, but does not exceed 1.2; the density difference steps are those whose ODs are closest to but not exceeding 0.45 and closest to 2.20. Action limits, determined from the initial 5-day averages, define the range of acceptable processor performance; they are *base* + *fog density* not exceeding +0.03, *middensity* ± 0.15 OD, and *density difference* ± 0.15 OD. If the test results fall outside of these limits, corrective action must be taken prior to patient imaging.

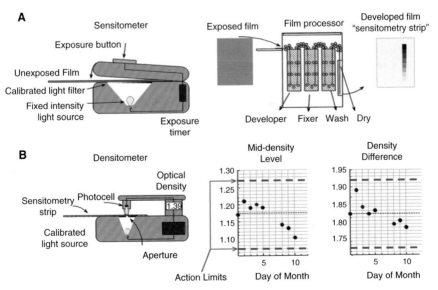

■ **FIGURE 8-21 A**. Film-processor testing requires a calibrated sensitometer to "flash" an unexposed film to a specified range of light intensities using an optical step wedge. The film is then developed. **B**. The corresponding optical densities on the processed film are measured with a densitometer, and Base + Fog (the lowest OD value), the mid-density level step (a measurement indicating relative speed), and the density difference value, calculated by the subtraction of a low OD step from a high OD step (indicating the relative contrast response), are plotted to verify processor performance before patients are imaged.

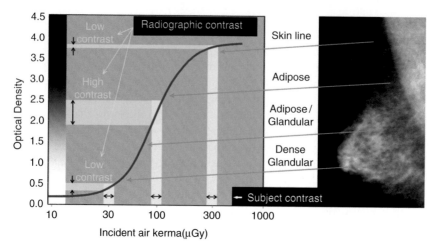

■ **FIGURE 8-22** Equal x-ray subject contrast (range of transmitted relative exposures) generated in the breast are manifested with variable contrast in the film image, resulting from the nonlinear characteristic curve. Areas in the breast that have high transmitted exposure, such as the skin line, and low transmitted exposure, such as glandular tissue, will have reduced radiographic contrast. Only over a small range of exposures is the radiographic contrast high.

Variability of Screen-Film Contrast Response

Radiographic contrast (i.e., OD differences on the developed film) results from variations in subject contrast (x-ray transmission differences due to anatomy) translated into these OD differences according to the film's characteristic curve. Therefore, the radiographic contrast varies depending upon the incident exposure to each area on the film-screen cassette. The best recording of subject contrast occurs on areas of the film where the exposure corresponds to the steepest part of the film characteristic curve. Significant reduction of contrast occurs on parts of the film where the exposures correspond to the toe and shoulder segments of the curve. Unfortunately, not all important anatomical information is rendered with optimal contrast, particularly in dense glandular breast tissues and at the skin line, as illustrated in Figure 8-22.

Film Viewing Conditions

Viewing conditions are very important so that the information on the film is visualized well by the radiologist. Subtle lesions on the mammographic film may be missed if viewing conditions are suboptimal. Since mammography films are exposed to high optical densities to achieve high contrast, view boxes in the mammography reading area must provide high *luminance* (a measure of brightness as described in Chapter 5). Mammography view boxes should have minimum luminances of at least 3,000 cd/m^2, and luminances exceeding 6,000 cd/m^2 are common. (Note: the luminance of 1 cd/m^2 is approximately the luminous intensity of the sky at the western horizon on a clear day, 15 min after sunset.) In comparison, the luminance of a view box in diagnostic radiology is typically about 1,500 cd/m^2.

A high-intensity "bright" light should be available in the reading room to penetrate high OD regions of the film, such as the skin line and the nipple area. Furthermore, the use of a magnifying glass improves the visibility of fine detail in the image, such as microcalcifications.

Film masking (blocking clear portions of the film and areas of the view box that are not covered by film to prevent extremely bright light from degrading the

Collimated to Breast   Collimated to Film

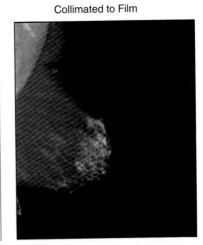

 FIGURE 8-23 Optimal viewing of film mammograms requires that the entire area of the film be exposed to radiation to darken the background surrounding the breast image; otherwise, light cannot easily be masked when viewing the films on a viewbox. For digital acquisitions, the background area location in each image is determined, and "pixel padding" is performed so that the background is dark, even when digitally inverting contrast.

radiologist's visual adaptation to the range of luminances displayed by the images) is essential for preserving perceived radiographic contrast. The film must be fully darkened in background areas around the breast (Fig. 8-23) by collimating the x-ray beam to the full area of the detector (see Section 8.1: "Collimation"). Most dedicated mammography view boxes have adjustable shutters for masking to the film size.

The ambient light intensity (as measured by the *illuminance*) in a mammography reading room must be reduced to eliminate reflections from the film and to improve perceived radiographic contrast. Illuminance is the luminous flux incident upon a surface per unit area, measured in lux or lumens/m². For example, the full moon in a clear night sky produces about 1 lux, whereas normal room lighting generates 100 to 1,000 lux. Subdued room lighting providing an illuminance of about 20-40 lux is acceptable for the viewing and interpretation of mammograms.

8.5 Digital Mammography

Digital acquisition devices became available in mammography in the early 1990s in the form of small field-of-view digital biopsy systems. In early 2000, a full-field digital mammography system was first approved by the FDA; it had a thin-film-transistor (TFT) indirect detection flat panel array with an 18 × 23-cm active area. Since that time, several digital mammography systems have been approved by the FDA in the United States and, in 2010, 70% of all clinical mammography machines in the United States were digital systems.

Full-Field Digital Mammography

There are compelling advantages to digital mammography, the most important of which is the ability to overcome the exposure latitude limitations of screen-film detectors and produce better image quality at lower doses. Other reasons include

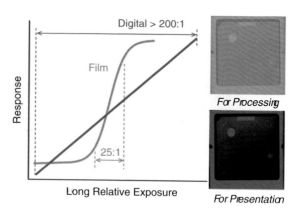

■ FIGURE 8-24 A comparison of the response of a screen-film and digital radiography detector to variations in relative exposure shows the large differences in exposure latitude and image response. The *For Processing* image (DICOM term for a raw image that has been corrected for flaws and detector non-uniformities) is linearly related to incident exposure; the *For Presentation* image is postprocessed by contrast and spatial resolution enhancements for viewing.

increased technologist productivity through rapid acquisition and evaluation of digital images; reduced patient waiting time, particularly for diagnostic studies; and improved image quality and conspicuity of lesions.

Screen-film detectors for mammography are excellent image capture devices, and the film serves as both the display device and the storage media, but the major drawbacks are the limited exposure dynamic range and narrow latitude, which are necessary to achieve high radiographic contrast (Fig. 8-24). A highly glandular breast can produce exposure latitude that exceeds 200:1, causing underexposed film areas corresponding to the glandular tissue, and overexposed film areas corresponding to the skin line and thinner parts of the breast. Digital flat panel and digital cassette (CR) detectors have exposure dynamic ranges greater than 1,000:1, which result in images showing little contrast when the entire ranges of pixel values are displayed. The full exposure data is contained in the the raw, *For Processing* image shown in Figure 8-24. With mammography-specific image postprocessing, high image contrast can be rendered over all exposure levels (e.g., from the high detector exposure at the skin line to the low detector exposure behind dense glandular areas of the breast), as shown in the processed *For Presentation* image. Postprocessing image enhancement is a key element in producing an optimized digital mammogram.

Flat panel detector arrays, which became clinically available in the mid to late 1990s for general radiography (see Chapter 7), are the major detector technologies used in digital mammography. An active matrix, thin film transistor (TFT) array collects the local signal (electric charge) generated during the x-ray exposure, absorption, and conversion process; stores the charge in a capacitor attached to each detector element; and actively reads the array immediately afterward to produce the image (Fig. 8-25). Key components in each detector element include a transistor (which serves as an "on-off" switch), a charge collection electrode, and a storage capacitor. During image acquisition, the transistor, controlled by the gate line, is in the "off" position, and the charge collected by the electrode from incident x-rays is stored in the capacitor. Immediately after the exposure, readout occurs by activating each gate line, one row at a time, which turns on the transistors along each row, allowing charge transfer via the drain lines along each column to a series of charge amplifiers and digitizers. The digital image is then stored in computer memory. In some "fast" flat panel designs, readout of the whole array is performed in hundreds of milliseconds, allowing near real-time acquisition of data for applications such as digital tomosynthesis.

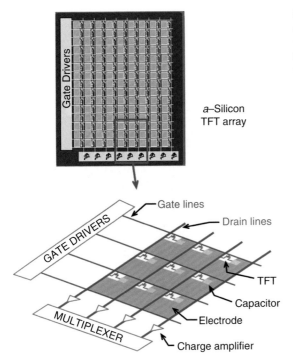

a–Silicon
TFT array

■ **FIGURE 8-25** The flat panel array is a two-dimensional matrix of individual detector elements lithographed on an amorphous silicon substrate. Each detector element is comprised of an electronic switch (the TFT), a charge collection electrode, and a storage capacitor. The gate and drain lines provide the mechanism to extract the locally stored charge by activating gate lines row by row, and collecting charge down each column. Charge amplifier and digitizers convert the signals to corresponding digital values for transfer to the digital image matrix.

Common to all flat panel TFT arrays is the amorphous silicon circuit layer (Fig. 8-26A). At present, approved digital mammography systems are based on four technologies. The first is an indirect x-ray conversion TFT flat panel array receptor with 100-μm sampling pitch and 18 × 23-cm or 24 × 31-cm FOV (Fig. 8-26B). A structured cesium iodide (CsI) phosphor converts x-rays into light; the light is emitted onto a photodiode in each detector element, from which the charge is generated and stored in the local capacitor. *Indirect conversion* describes absorption of x-rays in the CsI, the production of secondary light photons directed to a photodiode, and the generation of the charge, which is stored on the storage capacitor in that detector element.

A second technology is based on a direct x-ray conversion TFT detector with 70-μm sampling pitch and 24 × 29-cm FOV (Fig. 8-26C). A semiconductor x-ray converter, Se, is uniformly deposited between two electrodes, with a large voltage placed across the Se layer. Incident x-rays absorbed by the Se directly produce electron-hole pairs; the applied voltage causes the electrons to travel to one electrode and the holes to the opposite electrode. The local storage capacitor captures the charge from the collection electrode. *Direct conversion* refers to the direct generation of charge by x-rays within the photoconductor and capture by the electrode without intermediate signals.

A third technology approved for digital mammography is a cassette-based, dual-side readout CR photostimulable storage phosphor (PSP) imaging plate detector and reader system. Cassettes of 18 × 24 cm and 24 × 30 cm are used in place of screen-film cassettes (Fig. 8-27), whereby x-rays absorbed in the phosphor raise electrons to higher energy levels in the PSP material, where a fraction of them are caught in semi-stable electron traps. An exposed imaging plate is subsequently processed by a reader system that scans the plate with a laser beam with an effective spot size of 50 microns. The laser beam provides energy to free the stored excited electrons from the traps; these electrons fall to a lower energy state with the emission of light, a process called "stimulated luminescence." Some of the light reaches a photomultiplier tube (PMT), which produces and amplifies an electrical current

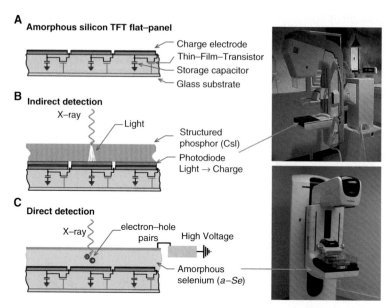

■ **FIGURE 8-26 A**. TFT flat panel arrays have a common underlying amorphous silicon structure, but there are two types of TFT detectors, determined by the conversion of the x-rays into electrical signals. **B**. "Indirect x-ray conversion" TFT arrays have an additional photodiode layer placed on the charge collection electrode of each detector element. The photodiodes are optically coupled to a layer of a phosphor, such as CsI, that produces light when irradiated by x-rays. The light produced by x-ray absorption in the phosphor in turn creates mobile electric charge in the photodiode. The charge is collected by the electrode and stored in the capacitor. **C**. A "Direct x-ray conversion" TFT array has a semiconductor layer of approximately 0.5 mm thickness between the surface electrode extending over the detector area and each detector element electrode, under a potential difference of approximately 10 V/μm. As hole-electron pairs are created in the semiconductor layer by x-rays, the electrons and holes migrate to the positive and negative electrodes, with minimal lateral spread. A proportional charge is stored on the capacitor. The outward appearances of the indirect and direct detectors are similar, shown by the pictures on the right.

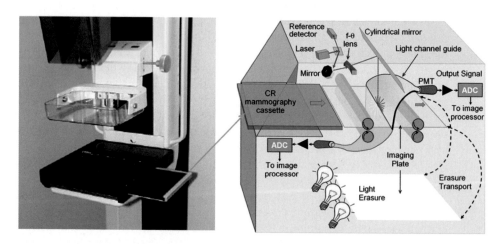

Cassette-based digital detector and "dual-side" readout of imaging plate

■ **FIGURE 8-27** The CR digital mammography detector uses a cassette that contains a PSP imaging plate, compatible with screen-film cassette sizes. Workflow is similar to screen film, but the AEC settings require independent calibration. When exposed to x-rays, the storage phosphor contains a "latent image" of trapped, excited electrons. Subsequent imaging plate processing uses dual-side readout (Fig. 8-27, **right**) by a scanning 0.050-mm laser beam, plate translation, and approximately 60-s readout time. Stimulated luminescence produces a light signal at each point on the imaging plate that is detected and digitized to create the digital image. Erasure of the imaging plate after the readout eliminates residual signals prior to next use.

proportional to the light intensity. The signal from the PMT is digitized to provide pixel values of the digital image. Typical turnaround time of an imaging plate is on the order of 60 to 90 s, similar to the batch mode processing of screen-film images.

The fourth technology approved for digital mammography uses a narrow 22 cm long charge-coupled-device (CCD)-detector array, optically coupled to a CsI phosphor x-ray converter, to capture x-ray signals in a highly collimated x-ray beam configuration (a "slot"). The moving collimator slot sweeps a narrow x-ray beam across the breast. The detector moves across the image plane to stay aligned with the scanning-slot x-ray beam. The scan acquires data in the medial to lateral directions in about 5 s, with 50-μm sampling over a 22 × 29-cm FOV. A major advantage of the scanning-slot fan-beam system is that very little scattered radiation from the breast reaches the detector. This technology is not being manufactured at the present time.

All current full-field digital mammography detectors have similar attributes with respect to exposure latitude. In terms of spatial resolution, the direct conversion TFT detector achieves the best intrinsic spatial resolution due to active charge collection and minimal signal spread in the semiconductor material, the signal being acquired onto each 70 μm × 70 μm detector element (dexel). The indirect conversion TFT detector uses a CsI(Tl)-structured phosphor to reduce lateral spread of the light photons onto a 100 μm × 100 μm dexel, and the CR system uses a 50-μm scanning laser beam and plate translation speed to maintain an effective 50 μm × 50 μm dexel. In terms of detective quantum efficiency (DQE—defined in Chapter 4), the indirect TFT array has better performance at low to intermediate spatial frequencies, and the direct TFT array has better performance at higher spatial frequencies. For cassette-based CR mammography detectors, the image quality and SNR at a given incident radiation exposure to the detector is lower than that of the TFT array detectors. In general, mammography technique factors and the corresponding average glandular doses are lowest for the indirect TFT detectors and highest for the cassette-based CR detectors. In most situations (with appropriate calibration of the AEC), use of digital detector systems will result in lower doses than screen-film detectors, particularly for thick, dense breast tissues.

Due to high-spatial resolution requirements, digital mammography images are quite large. A digital mammography system with a 0.07-mm pixel, 2 bytes per pixel, and a 24 × 29-cm active detector area, produces a 27-MB image. One screening study (4 images) will therefore contain 108 MB of data and, if 3 years of prior images are reviewed, 432 MB of data will be required per patient reading session. The network overhead and storage required for the picture archiving and communications system are very large and even larger with the increased number of images in a diagnostic exam. In addition, if *For Processing* images are stored, another factor of two increase is incurred. Typical digital image sizes for mammography systems are listed in Table 8-6.

TABLE 8-6   DIGITAL IMAGE SIZE FOR MAMMOGRAPHY SCREENING EXAMS

DETECTOR TYPE	FOV (cm)	PIXEL SIZE (mm)	IMAGE SIZE (MB)	EXAM SIZE (MB)	+3 Y PRIORS (MB)
Indirect TFT	19 × 23	0.10	9	35	140
Indirect TFT	24 × 31	0.10	15	60	240
Direct TFT	18 × 24	0.07	18	70	280
Direct TFT	24 × 29	0.07	27	108	432
CR	18 × 24	0.05	32	128	512
CR	24 × 30	0.05	50	200	800

Currently, the recommendation regarding mammography image compression to reduce file size is to not use lossy compression algorithms—that is, an exact (lossless) image must be reproduced during the decompression step. For most digital mammograms, there is a significant background area that is "pixel-padded" with a constant value number in the *For Presentation* image. On average, a compression factor of 3 to 5 can be achieved using lossless compression, depending on the fraction of the image matrix area comprising the breast. FDA regulations require that facilities maintain mammography films, digital images, and reports in a permanent medical record of the patient for a period of not less than 5 years and not less than 10 years if no additional mammograms of the patient are performed at the facility. A longer retention period may be mandated by state or local law. Many considerations are described in the ACR practice guideline, "Determinants of Image Quality in Digital Mammography" available on the ACR website, http://www.acr.org.

Processing and Viewing Digital Mammograms

Even the best digital detectors have malfunctioning detector elements, column and line defects, and variation in gain across the detector area. Without corrections, these artifacts would result in unacceptable image quality and interfere with the diagnostic interpretation. Manufacturers use "preprocessing" algorithms to correct these defects. First, the locations of inoperative detector elements and line defects are determined, and these data are interpolated from nearest-neighbor pixels. Next, a uniform beam of x-rays exposes the detector and generates an image, showing the variable gain from the detector submodule electronics. Multiple images are averaged together to create a *flat-field* correction image, which is normalized and inverted as an inverse-gain map. When applied to an uncorrected image on a pixel-by-pixel basis, the gain variations are canceled, and the corrected "raw" image is defect-free (see Chapter 4). In practice, flat-field gain maps for various acquisition conditions are measured, stored on the system, and applied to each clinical image that is acquired under similar conditions.

The output *For Processing* image has wide latitude, digital signals that are proportional to the detector exposure or the logarithm of exposure, and very low contrast (Fig. 8-28A). While not useful for diagnosis by the radiologist, this is the preferred image for *Computer-Assisted Detection* (CADe) programs, which use computer algorithms to identify image features that may indicate the presence of breast cancer. Contrast enhancement of the *For Processing* image is shown in Figure 8-28B, which looks similar to a screen-film image. Nonlinear postprocessing algorithms applied to the *For Processing* image data identify the skin line of the mammogram, modify the local-area pixel values, and equalize the response in the high-signal, low-attenuation skin area to the other areas of the breast. Contrast and spatial resolution enhancements are then applied to create the *For Presentation* image for viewing and diagnosis. Unlike film radiographic contrast, which is variable in the areas corresponding to the thinnest and thickest parts of the breast image (see Fig. 8-22), image contrast is equalized across the entire the digital image (Fig. 8-28C). Each manufacturer has proprietary methods of image processing; the radiologist must to adopt a particular "look" for viewing current and prior digital mammograms for consistency. The *For Processing* images should be saved in addition to the *For Presentation* images as part of a patient's examination if CAD algorithms will be used in possible subsequent applications, or if other image processing algorithms are to be applied, since *For Presentation* images cannot be "unprocessed." The disadvantage to saving the *For Processing* images is the extra storage required.

It is strongly recommended that diagnostic interpretation of digital mammograms be performed on display monitors approved by the FDA for mammography having a minimum of 5 million pixels (5 MP) and a calibrated, sustained maximal luminance

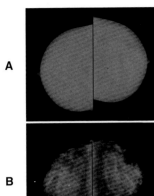

Detector corrections,
gain map corrections,
no enhancement,
"For Processing"

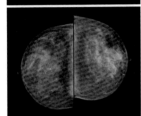

Simple linear contrast &
brightness corrections,
no advanced processing

Skin equalization
processing and non-
linear enhancement
"For Presentation"

■ **FIGURE 8-28 A**. The *For Processing* images of the right and left cranial-caudal breast projection images have detector and gain map corrections applied with unity radiographic contrast. **B**. Linear contrast and brightness adjustments are applied. Appearance is similar to a screen-film image. **C**. Nonlinear processing identifies the breast skin line and densest parts of the image, to equalize the response of the processed image, with contrast and spatial resolution enhancement.

of at least 450 cd/m^2 (per ACR guidelines for digital mammography), but preferably at 600 cd/m^2. Monitors of lower luminance make reading conditions more susceptible to poor ambient lighting and illuminance conditions. A typical workstation has two large-format portrait-oriented LCD monitors (each 54 cm diagonal, 34 cm width, 42 cm height) with 2,560 × 2,048 pixels at a pixel pitch of approximately 0.165 mm and a contrast ratio (ratio of brightest to darkest luminance) greater than 350:1. The optimal viewing distance for the resolution provided by the 0.165-mm pixel is about 50 cm (slightly less than arm's length). A lower resolution, smaller format "navigation" monitor is used for patient lists and operating system access. All monitors should be calibrated to conform to the DICOM Grayscale Standard Display Function, as described in Chapter 5, to ensure image contrast is consistently and optimally displayed.

To optimize the workflow of the radiologist, mammography workstations should provide automated *mammography-specific hanging protocols* that present the images in a useful and sequential way for review and diagnosis according to view, laterality, magnification, and prior examination comparisons. Demographic overlays (patient name, technique factors, and details of the exam) should be mapped in areas outside of the breast anatomy. It is important to display images in *true size* at one point in the diagnostic review (as close as possible to a magnification of 1, *independent of the detector pixel dimension* so that measurements can be made directly on the monitor if necessary) and to effectively handle images of different size from different manu-facturers to appear the same size on the workstation when direct comparisons are made. Also, viewing of *all* mammograms at one image pixel to one monitor pixel ensures that the monitor does not limit the intrinsic resolution of the image. This requires a "zoom and pan" procedure for each image. Sometimes, radiologists will use a magnifying glass on a displayed digital mammogram to overcome limitations of the human visual system acuity; this is reasonable as long as the image (or portion of) is displayed at full resolution. However, a digital magnification by pixel replication and interpolation to enlarge the image directly on the monitor is preferable. Issues confronting digital mammography workflow and hanging protocols are addressed in the Integrating the Healthcare Enterprise Mammography Image Integration Profile*. Even after solving many of the display concerns, image appearance may be considerably different between the manufacturers' proprietary processing algorithms, which can make comparisons challenging.

An alternative to "soft-copy" reading of digital mammograms is the use of an FDA-approved laser printer to record all digital studies on film, an unlikely scenario. However, there is FDA requirement to have the capability of printing film images from digital mammograms at each facility to be able to provide hard-copy images to patients upon request. QC procedures must be performed on the printer periodically, as described in the printer manufacturer's QC manual for digital mammography printers.

Computer-Aided Detection and Computer-Assisted Diagnosis Systems

A computer-aided detection (CADe) system is a computer-based set of algorithms that incorporates pattern recognition and uses sophisticated matching and similarity rules to flag possible findings on a digital mammographic image, which may be a digitized film mammogram. The computer software searches for abnormal areas of density, mass, calcifications, and/or structural patterns (e.g., spiculated masses, architectural distortion) that may indicate the presence of cancer. The CADe system then marks these areas on the images, alerting the radiologist for further analysis. For digitally acquired mammograms, the CADe algorithms require the use of linear, *For Processing* images for analysis, as the algorithms are trained on these images and evaluation of processed images would result in lower performance in terms of sensitivity and specificity.

Computer-assisted diagnosis (CADx) devices include software that provides information beyond identifying suspicious findings; this additional information includes an assessment of identified features in terms of the likelihood of the presence or absence of disease, or disease type. For instance, a CADx system for mammography will not only identify clusters of microcalcifications and masses on digital mammograms but also provide a probability score of the disease or malignancy to the radiologist for each potential lesion. Currently, CADe and CADx systems are widely used by radiologists who interpret mammography studies in addition to other duties. The fraction of False-positive marks (marks placed on image features that do not correspond to malignancy) can be high and is one of the downsides of using these systems. Many expert mammography radiologists avoid using CAD for this reason.

Stereotactic Breast Biopsy

Stereotactic breast biopsy systems provide the capability to localize breast lesions in three dimensions and physically sample them with a targeted biopsy instrument. Generally, these systems are used for targeting microcalcifications associated with lesions, whereas localization and biopsy of masses and areas of architectural distortion are performed either with ultrasound guidance or MRI. Figure 8-29A shows a prone-geometry stereotactic imaging system. The image receptors of these systems are CCD cameras coupled to x-ray phosphor screens of 5 cm × 5-cm FOV by either lens optics or fiber optics. A 1,000 × 1,000 detector element matrix, with an

---

*http://www.ihe.net/Resources/handbook.cfm)

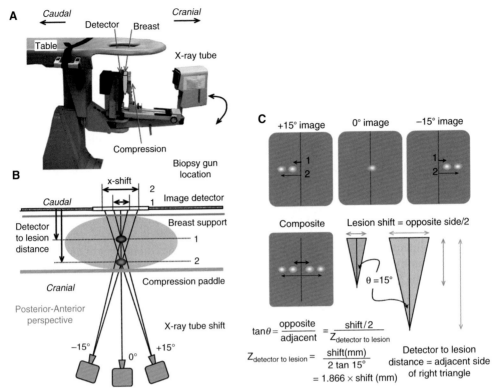

FIGURE 8-29 A. A stereotactic biopsy system with a prone positioning system is shown. The patient's pendulant breast is positioned on the detector platform and compressed by an open-access paddle. The x-ray tube pivots about a fulcrum point to acquire digital images at +15-, and −15-degree projections within the 5 × 5-cm detector FOV. **B.** Breast lesions positioned more cranially (toward the tube) will have a greater shift in the image pair than lesions closer to the detector. **C.** Trigonometric relationships allow the determination of lesion depth from the measured shift distance in the images. A frame of reference calibration between the images on the computer and the biopsy gun placed on rails between the x-ray tube and breast allows a trajectory calculation and needle orientation under computer control.

effective detector element size of 50 μm (0.05 mm), which is equivalent to 10 lp/mm, is deemed sufficient to visualize microcalcifications. Image acquisition is performed by integrating light from x-ray exposure of the phosphor screen on the CCD photodetector, reading the detector element array one line at a time after the exposure, amplifying the electronic signal, and digitizing the output.

The breast is aligned and compressed by an open-area paddle. After verification with a scout image, two images of the breast are acquired, at +15 and −15 degrees from the normal, causing the lesion projections to shift on the detector, as shown in Figure 8-29B. The shift distance is measured (Fig. 8-29C) from trigonometry relationships, the opposite sides of two right triangles, and the common adjacent side, each with a 15-degree angle (30 degrees total). The adjacent side represents the lesion distance from the detector, and since Opposite/Adjacent = tan(θ = 15 degrees), the lesion distance from the detector (mm) is calculated as 1.866 × shift (mm). Trajectory information is determined by the position of the marked points in the images correlated with the frame of reference of the biopsy device, which is positioned and activated to capture the tissue samples.

Digital add-on biopsy units with larger FOVs (e.g., 8 × 8 cm) using CCDs or other photosensitive detectors that fit into the cassette assemblies of the standard mammography units are alternatives to the prone biopsy table, as well as full-field digital mammography units that can provide similar capabilities.

Breast Digital Tomosynthesis

Digital radiographic imaging offers postacquisition processing capabilities that are not possible with conventional analog imaging systems. One of the major problems with conventional projection imaging is that overlying and underlying anatomy are superimposed on the pathology, often obscuring the visualization and detection of the cancer or other abnormality. A method for reducing this superimposition is to acquire multiple low-dose images at several angular positions as the x-ray tube moves in an arc about the breast. Each image projects the content in the breast volume with different shifts depending on the distance of the object from the detector. With high-speed digital readout, several projection images can be acquired in under 10 s, and each image set is processed with a limited-angle reconstruction algorithm to synthesize a tomogram (in-focus plane) at a given depth in the breast. Many tomograms representing incremental depths within the volume are produced, and in-focus planes throughout the breast can assist in enhanced detection of pathology (e.g., tumor) or elimination of superimposed anatomy that mimics pathology. Even though many more images must be reviewed by the radiologist, digital tomosynthesis technology can lead to a superior diagnosis that might save a patient an unneeded biopsy or provide guidance for early treatment of a cancer.

Digital tomosynthesis for breast imaging is made possible with fast readout TFT arrays by acquiring many sequential images (11 to 51) over a limited angle ($\pm$ 7.5 to $\pm$ 50 degrees) in a short time span (4 to 20 s). For one vendor's implementation, 15 projection images of the compressed breast are acquired over a range of 15 degrees (1 image per degree) in 4s (270 ms per image), using a W target with 0.7-mm Al filtered x-ray beam, 32 to 38 kV, with no antiscatter grid, and 2 $\times$ 2 pixel binning of the digital detector array (140-μm sampling). The image acquisition process is illustrated in Figure 8-30A. Average glandular dose (discussed below) for 15 image acquisitions is approximately 2 mGy for the accreditation phantom. Larger breast thicknesses will require larger doses for tomosynthesis acquisition, but the dose is similar to that of a single view mammogram of the same compressed thickness. The 15 images are used in the reconstruction process to create 1-mm focal plane images (tomograms), where the location of the reconstructed plane depends on the reconstruction algorithm, and the number of reconstructed images depends on the compressed breast thickness. Reconstruction can be performed in several ways: (a) "shift and add" method shown in Figure 8-30B is the simplest; (b) filtered backprojection; (c) simultaneous algebraic reconstruction techniques; and (d) maximum likelihood algorithms. More sophisticated methods require longer reconstruction times but provide enhancement by further reducing out-of-plane signals.

A series of approximately 60 tomograms was reconstructed from a volunteer patient who was imaged in the cranial-caudal and medial-lateral oblique projections; four images from that dataset, at the entrance and exit points of the x-ray beam and at two depths, are shown in Figure 8.30C. Rapid "stack mode" viewing helps the perception of otherwise undetected lesions with good conspicuity. Investigations of breast tomosynthesis have demonstrated that its advantages are greater for masses and architectural distortion, than for calcifications. The current role of tomosynthesis is to supplement full-field digital mammography exams; however, future limited-angle acquisition techniques and processing algorithms are expected to provide both the tomosynthesis images at in-focal planes throughout the breast and a high-quality reconstructed conventional projection mammogram from the same image dataset.

A *Image Acquisition*:
Multiple angular views
11 – 25 images, < 5 s

B *Image Reconstruction*:
Shift images to select plane
Add images to create tomograms

Left ⟶ ⎸⟵   ⟶⎸ ⟵ Right

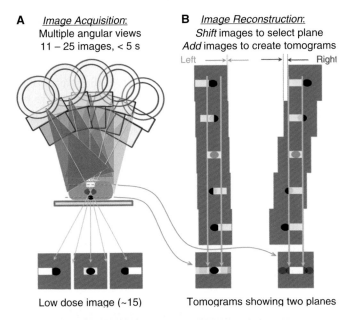

Low dose image (~15)

Tomograms showing two planes

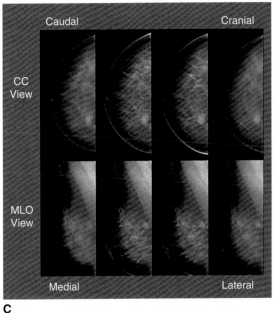

Caudal   Cranial

CC
View

MLO
View

Medial   Lateral

C

■ **FIGURE 8-30 A**. Digital tomosynthesis images are acquired using low-dose techniques over a limited projection angle, from ±7.5 degrees up to ± 30 degrees, with 15 to 40 images comprising the dataset. Illustrated are a "square" and "circle" at two depths within the breast **B**. Reconstruction of tomogram images at 1-mm incremental planes in the breast is performed by shifting the acquired images a known amount, summing the images by projection and normalizing the output. In-focus images are shown for two depths, illustrating the ability to blur the underlying and overlying signals for the white rectangle and black circle. **C**. Tomosynthesis images from a volunteer patient are shown for the cranial-caudal and medial-lateral oblique projections at 4 depths. The overall breast dose is similar to that from a single projection mammogram.

8.6 ## Radiation Dosimetry

X-ray mammography is the technique of choice for detecting nonpalpable breast cancers. However, the risk of carcinogenesis from the radiation dose to the breast is of concern, particularly in screening, because of the very large number of women receiving the exams. Thus, the optimization of breast dose is important and dose monitoring is required yearly as specified by the MQSA regulations.

The glandular tissue is the site of carcinogenesis, and thus the preferred dose index is the *average glandular dose*. Because the glandular tissues receive varying doses depending on their depths from the skin entrance site of the x-ray beam, estimating the dose is not trivial. The *midbreast dose,* the dose delivered to the plane of tissue in the middle of the breast, was the radiation dosimetry benchmark until the late 1970s. The midbreast dose is typically lower than the average glandular dose and does not account for variation in breast tissue composition.

Average Glandular Dose

The average glandular dose, D_g, is calculated from the equation

$$D_g = D_{gN} \times X_{ESAK}$$

where X_{ESAK} is the entrance skin air kerma (ESAK) in mGy, and D_{gN} is an air kerma to average glandular dose conversion factor with units of mGy dose/mGy incident air kerma. An air ionization chamber is used to measure the air kerma for a given kV, mAs, and beam quality. Previously, this calculation involved a roentgen to rad conversion, where the units of the D_{gN} were mrad/R.

The conversion factor D_{gN} is determined by computer simulation methods and depends on radiation quality (kV and HVL), x-ray tube target material, filter material, breast thickness, and tissue composition. Table 8-7 lists D_{gN} values for a 50% adipose, 50% glandular breast that is 4.5-cm thick. The coefficients are shown as a function of HVL and kV for a Mo/Mo target-filter combination. For a 26-kV technique with a HVL of 0.35-mm Al, the average glandular dose is approximately 19% of the measured ESAK (Table 8-7). For higher average x-ray energies (e.g., Mo/Rh, Rh/Rh, W/Rh, W/Ag), conversion tables specific to the generated x-ray spectrum must be used, as the D_{gN} values increase due to the higher effective energy of the beam. D_{gN} values decrease with an increase in breast thickness for constant beam quality and breast composition. This is because the glandular tissues furthest from the beam entrance receive much less dose in the thicker breast due to attenuation (e.g., D_{gN} = 0.220 mGy dose/mGy air kerma for 3-cm thickness versus 0.110 mGy dose/mGy air Kerma for 6-cm thickness). However, the lower D_{gN} coefficients for the thicker breast do not mean that larger breasts receive less dose. The lower D_{gN} values are more than offset by a large increase in the entrance kerma necessary to achieve the desired OD on the film or SNR in a digital image. Measured average glandular doses for 50% glandular/50% adipose tissue of 2 to 8-cm tissue thicknesses using AEC are shown in Figure 8-31 for screen-film and direct-detection digital systems.

Factors Affecting Breast Dose

Many variables affect breast dose. The speed of the screen-film receptor, the film OD, and the digital detector SNR level are major factors. Breast thickness and tissue composition strongly affect x-ray absorption. Higher kV (higher HVL)

TABLE 8-7 D_{gN} CONVERSION FACTOR (mGy AVERAGE GLANDULAR DOSE PER mGy INCIDENT AIR KERMA) AS A FUNCTION OF HVL AND kV FOR Mo TARGET AND FILTER, 4.5-cm BREAST THICKNESS OF 50% GLANDULAR AND 50% ADIPOSE BREAST TISSUE COMPOSITION

HVL (mm)	kV							
	25	26	27	28	29	30	31	32
0.25	0.140							
0.26	0.144	0.147						
0.27	0.149	0.151	0.153					
0.28	0.153	0.156	0.158	0.159				
0.29	0.159	0.161	0.163	0.164	0.165			
0.30	0.164	0.166	0.167	0.168	0.169	0.171		
0.31	0.168	0.171	0.172	0.173	0.174	0.175	0.176	
0.32	0.173	0.175	0.176	0.177	0.179	0.181	0.182	0.183
0.33	0.177	0.180	0.181	0.182	0.183	0.185	0.187	0.188
0.34	0.183	0.184	0.185	0.187	0.188	0.190	0.191	0.192
0.35	0.188	0.190	0.191	0.192	0.194	0.195	0.196	0.197
0.36	0.192	0.195	0.196	0.197	0.198	0.199	0.200	0.202
0.37		0.199	0.200	0.202	0.203	0.204	0.204	0.205
0.38		0.205	0.206	0.207	0.208	0.208	0.210	
0.39			0.211	0.212	0.213	0.213	0.214	
0.40				0.216	0.218	0.219	0.220	

Adapted from ACR QC Manual, 1999; converted from mrad per R using 0.01 mGy/mrad and 0.1145 mGy air Kerma/R

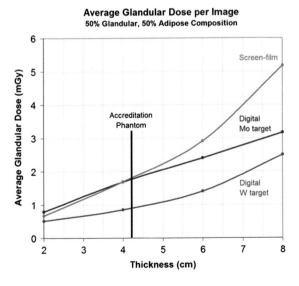

Average Glandular Dose per Image
50% Glandular, 50% Adipose Composition

Screen-film

Accreditation Phantom

Digital Mo target

Digital W target

Average Glandular Dose (mGy)

Thickness (cm)

■ **FIGURE 8-31** Approximate average glandular doses (25 to 35 kV using AEC acquisition) are shown for a screen-film detector with Mo target and Mo/Rh filtration (green), a digital system using a-Se direct conversion detector with Mo target and Mo/Rh filtration (purple), and a digital system using a-Se direct conversion detector with W target and Rh/Ag filtration (blue). The accreditation phantom (4.5 cm thickness) is indicated with the vertical black bar for comparison of average glandular dose noted in MQSA reports.

TABLE 8-8 AVERAGE GLANDULAR DOSE IN mGy WITH TWO TISSUE COMPOSITIONS OF THE BREAST USING kV VALUES IN TABLE 8-4[a] FOR SCREEN-FILM AND TABLE 8-5[b] FOR DIGITAL ACQUISITIONS

DETECTOR: BREAST COMPOSITION	BREAST THICKNESS (cm)			
	2	4	6	8
Screen-Film: 100% Adipose	0.50	1.25	3.00	4.30
Screen-Film: 50/50	0.65	1.80	3.80	5.20
Digital Selenium, W target: 100% Adipose	0.50	0.75	1.55	2.45
Digital Selenium, W target: 50/50	0.60	1.00	2.40	4.20

[a]Mo/Mo target/filter, 5:1 grid, and film OD = 1.80 (Fuji AD-M film and AD-fine screens).
[b]W/Rh (2, 4, 6 cm); W/Ag (8 cm) for selenium detector.

increases beam penetrability (lower ESE and therefore lower average glandular dose) but also decreases subject contrast. Antiscatter grids improve subject and radiographic contrast, but increase radiation dose by the Bucky or digital technique compensation factor (~2×). Table 8-8 lists measured average glandular doses for a contemporary clinical screen-film mammography system with a film OD of 1.8, a Mo/Mo target/filter, and a kV recommended in Table 8-4, compared to a digital mammography system utilizing a W/Rh or W/Ag target/filter combination with kV recommended in Table 8-5. Digital acquisition with higher effective energy beams is shown to substantially reduce average glandular dose over that of screen-film systems.

The MQSA regulations limit the average glandular dose for a compressed breast thickness of 4.2 cm and a breast composition of 50% glandular and 50% adipose tissue (the MQSA-approved mammography phantom) to 3 mGy per film or digital image (6 mGy for two films or images). If the average glandular dose exceeds 3 mGy for this size breast, mammography may not be performed. The average glandular dose using screen-film receptors is typically about 2 mGy per view or 4 mGy for two views. For full-field digital mammography systems, the dose is lower, typically from 1.2 to 1.8 mGy per view.

Mammography image quality strongly depends on beam energy, quantum mottle, and detected x-ray scatter. Faster screen-film detectors can use a lower dose, but often at the expense of spatial resolution. Digital detectors with higher quantum detection efficiency can deliver significantly reduced dose; the tradeoff for reduced dose can be a loss of SNR and contrast-to-noise ratio (CNR) and potentially less diagnostic information. Higher energy beams (e.g., Rh target Rh filter or W target Rh filter or Ag filter) can reduce the dose to thick or dense glandular breasts with little or no loss of image quality.

8.7 Regulatory Requirements

Regulations mandated by the MQSA of 1992 specify operational and technical requirements necessary to perform mammography in the United States. These regulations are contained in Title 21 of the Code of Federal Regulations, Part 900.

Accreditation and Certification

Accreditation and certification are two separate processes. For a facility to perform mammography legally under the MQSA, it must be accredited and certified. To begin the process, the facility must first apply for accreditation from an accreditation body (the ACR or one of several states if located in one of those states). The accreditation body verifies that the mammography facility meets standards set forth by the MQSA to ensure safe, reliable, high-quality, and accurate mammography. These include the initial qualifications and continuing experience and education of interpreting physicians, technologists, and physicists involved in the mammography program. Existence of an active QC program and image quality standards are verified and validated. *Certification* is the approval of a facility by the US FDA to provide mammography services and is granted when accreditation is achieved.

Specific Technical Requirements and Quality Control

For screen-film mammography systems, requirements are largely unchanged from the 1999 FDA regulations. Tables 8-9 and 8-10 summarize the annual QC tests performed by the technologist and physicist, respectively, as required by MQSA regulations.

Under FDA rules, facilities using x-ray systems other than screen-film mammography must maintain a QA and QC program that is substantially equivalent to the program recommended by the manufacturer. This has created a number of unique tests that the technologist and physicist must understand and perform according to the manufacturer's manuals and procedural methods. In addition, QC procedures for the diagnostic review workstation monitor and the laser printer for producing hard-copy film are also under the auspices of the manufacturer.

Federal regulations specify that whenever QC test results fall outside of the action limits *for image receptor modalities other than screen-film*, the source of the problem shall be identified and corrective action taken before any further examinations are performed. However, an alternative QC standard lists three different categories in which specific action requirements are detailed.

Category A QC tests and action levels are specific to the digital acquisition system and, when outside of the prescribed limits, the source of the problem must be identified and corrective action taken before any examinations can be performed. These tests include system resolution, breast dose, image quality evaluation, SNR/CNR, flat-field calibration, and compression.

Category B QC tests and action levels are specific to the performance of a diagnostic device used for mammographic interpretation, including the review workstation and laser film printer. When tests produce results that fall outside of the action limits specified by the manufacturer, the source of the problem shall be identified and corrective action taken before that specific device can be used for interpretation. Image acquisition can continue, as long as there are alternate approved diagnostic devices available for interpretation.

Category C QC tests and action levels evaluate performance of components other than the digital image receptor or diagnostic devices for interpretation. When test results are outside the action limits specified by the manufacturer, the source of the problem shall be identified and corrective action shall be taken within 30 days of the test date. Clinical imaging and mammographic image interpretation can continue during this period. Applicable QC tests include collimation assessment, artifact evaluation,

TABLE 8-9 PERIODIC TESTS PERFORMED BY THE QC TECHNOLOGIST FOR SCREEN-FILM DETECTOR SYSTEMS

TEST AND FREQUENCY	REQUIREMENTS FOR ACCEPTABLE OPERATION	DOCUMENTATION GUIDANCE	TIMING OF CORRECTIVE ACTION
Daily: Processor Base + fog density Middensity Density difference	Established operating level $\leq +0.03$ OD ± 0.15 OD ± 0.15 OD	QC records 12 mo QC films 30 d	Before any clinical film processing is performed
Weekly: Phantom Center OD Reproducibility Density difference between disk and background Phantom scoring	Established operating level OD ≥ 1.20 ± 0.20 OD ± 0.05 OD Four fibers, three speck groups, three masses	QC records 12 mo Phantom images 12 wk	Before any further exams are performed
Quarterly: Fixer retention; quarterly Repeat analysis; quarterly	Residual fixer no $>5\mu g/cm^2$ <2% change up or down from previous	QC records since last inspection	30 d
Semiannually: Darkroom fog Screen-film contact Compression device	OD difference ≤ 0.05 40 mesh copper screen with no obvious artifacts Compression force ≥ 111 newtons (25 lb)	QC records since last inspection QC records since last inspection, three previous contact tests QC records since last inspection or past three tests	Before any clinical film processing Before any further exams performed using cassettes Before exams performed using compression device

kV accuracy, HVL assessment, AEC performance and reproducibility, radiation output rate, and compression thickness indicator.

An effort to standardize QC in digital mammography is underway, under the auspices of the ACR, based upon review of QC test results and findings from the multi-institutional Digital Mammography Imaging Screening Trial completed in 2005.

The Mammography Accreditation Phantom

The mammography accreditation phantom simulates the radiographic attenuation of an average-size compressed breast and contains structures that model very basic image characteristics of breast parenchyma and cancer. Its role is to help determine the adequacy of the overall imaging system (including film processing and digital processing) in terms of detection of subtle radiographic findings, and to assess the reproducibly of image characteristics (e.g., contrast and OD or SNR and CNR) over time. It is composed of a poly-methyl-methacrylate (PMMA) block, a wax insert, and a PMMA disk (4-mm thick, 10-mm diameter) attached to the top of the phantom, and is intended to mimic the attenuation characteristics of a "standard breast" of 4.2-cm compressed breast thickness of 50% adipose and 50% glandular tissue composition. The wax insert contains six

TABLE 8-10 SUMMARY TABLE OF ANNUAL QC TESTS BY THE MEDICAL PHYSICIST FOR SCREEN-FILM DETECTOR SYSTEMS

TEST	REGULATORY ACTION LEVELS	TIMING OF CORRECTIVE ACTION
AEC	OD exceeds the mean by >0.30 (over 2–6 cm range) or the phantom image density at the center is <1.20	30 d
kV	>5% of indicated or selected kV; C.O.V. > 0.02	30 d
Focal spot	See Table 8.1	30 d
HVL	See Tables 8.2 and 8.3	30 d
Air kerma and AEC reproducibility	Reproducibility C.O.V.[a] > 0.05	30 d
Dose	>3.0 mGy per exposure	Immediate, before any further exams
X-ray field/light field congruence	>2% SID at chest wall	30 d
Compression device alignment	Paddle visible on image	30 d
Screen speed uniformity	O.D. variation >0.30 from the maximum to minimum	30 d
System artifacts	Determined by physicist	30 d
Radiation output	<6.1 mGy/s (700 mR/s)	30 d
Automatic decompression control	Failure of override or manual release	30 d
Any applicable annual new modality tests	To be determined	Immediate, before any further exams

Note: documentation requires the inclusion of two most recent reports
[a]C.O.V., coefficient of variation, equal to the standard deviation of a series of measurements divided by the mean.
AEC, automatic exposure control; SID, source-to-image distance.

cylindrical nylon fibers of decreasing diameter, five simulated calcification groups with simulated calcifications (Al_2O_3 specks) of decreasing size, and five low contrast disks of decreasing diameter and thickness that simulate masses (Fig. 8-32A). Identification of the smallest objects of each type that are visible in the phantom image indicates system performance. To pass the MQSA image quality standards for screen-film mammography, at least four fibers, three calcification groups, and three masses must be clearly visible (with no obvious artifacts) at an average glandular dose of less than 3 mGy. Further details on other parameters can be found in the MQSA regulations.

For digital mammography, each manufacturer has set the criteria for meeting an acceptable performance level in terms of qualitative visibility of the objects in the accreditation phantom, as well as specific tests using the quantitative evaluation of regions of interest (ROI) to calculate SNR and CNR. The "direct flat panel" detector manufacturer, for instance, requires the visibility of five fibers, four speck groups, and four masses, whereas the "indirect flat panel" and the cassette-based CR detector manufacturers require the visibility of four fibers, three speck groups, and three masses. Quantitative evaluation for one manufacturer includes the evaluation of the signal under the added acrylic disk and in the background area using ROIs of a specified size

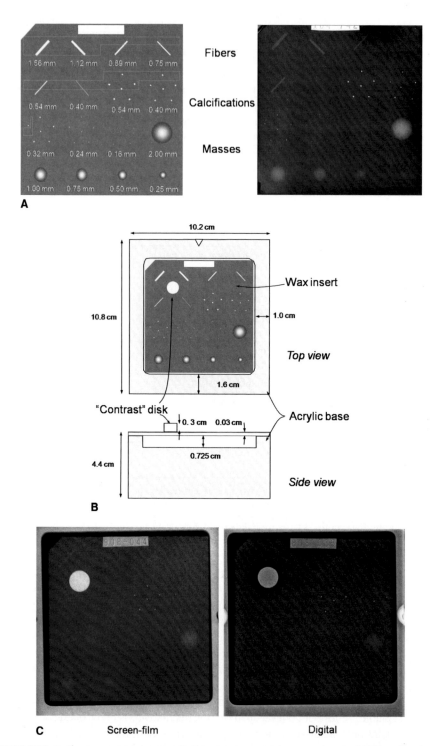

■ **FIGURE 8-32 A.** The mammography accreditation phantom contains a wax insert which has six nylon fibers, five aluminum oxide speck groups (six specks in each group), and five disks simulating masses. Mean diameters of the objects are indicated. The corresponding radiograph of the wax insert shows their "undegraded" radiographic appearance. **B.** The wax insert is placed into a cutout in a clear acrylic phantom with dimensions listed in the diagram. The phantom is intended to mimic the attenuation characteristics of a "standard breast" of 4.2-cm compressed breast thickness of 50% adipose and 50% glandular tissue composition. Note the "contrast disk" on top of the phantom, which generates a signal for evaluation of contrast. **C.** Mammographic image of the composite phantom with scatter and noise illustrates the loss of image quality.

and locations, while another uses the largest mass in the ACR phantom and an adjacent background area. The SNR is calculated as the average signal in the background ROI divided by its standard deviation. The CNR is determined as the difference of the average signals from the object and background, divided by the standard deviation in the background ROI. Each manufacturer requires the mammography site technologist to measure the SNR and CNR weekly using the accreditation phantom, and to verify that the calculated values are within the manufacturer's established limits. When found out of tolerance, the system may not be used clinically until the causes of the failures are determined and the corrections are implemented and verified with subsequent tests.

Quality Assurance

Mammography is a very demanding imaging procedure, in terms of equipment performance, and in regards to technical competence of the radiologist, technologist, and medical physicist. Achieving the full potential of the mammography examination requires careful optimization of the technique and equipment. Even a small change in equipment performance, film processing, digital image SNR or CNR, image artifacts, patient setup, or image-viewing conditions can decrease the sensitivity and specificity of mammography.

Ultimate responsibility for mammography quality assurance rests with the radiologist in charge of the mammography practice, who must ensure that all interpreting radiologists, mammography technologists, and the medical physicist meet the initial qualifications and maintain the continuing education and experience required by the MQSA regulations. Records must be maintained of employee qualifications, quality assurance, and the physicist's tests. Clinical performance and QC issues should be periodically reviewed with the entire mammography staff.

The technologist performs the examinations, that is, patient positioning, compression, image acquisition, and film processing and/or evaluation of digital image quality. The technologist also performs the daily, weekly, monthly, and semiannual QC tests. The medical physicist is responsible for equipment performance measurements before first clinical use, annually thereafter, and following major repairs, and for oversight of the QC program performed by the technologist.

SUGGESTED READING

ACR Mammography Quality Control Manual, 1999. American College of Radiology, Reston, VA.

ACR Practice Guideline for the Performance of Screening and Diagnostic Mammography. 2008. American College of Radiology, Reston, VA. Document is available at: http://www.acr.org/SecondaryMainMenuCategories/quality_safety/guidelines/breast/Screening_Diagnostic.aspx

Food and Drug Administration Mammography Program (MQSA). The MQSA regulations and other documentation are available on the Web at http://www.fda.gov/cdrh/mammography

Integrating the Healthcare Enterprise (IHE) Radiology Technical Framework. Mammography image (MAMMO) profile. Document is available at: http://www.ihe.net/Technical_Framework/upload/IHE_Rad1344TF_Suppl_MAMMO_T1_2006-04-13.pdf

Pisano E, Gatsonis C, Hendrick E, et.al. Performance of digital versus film mammography for breast-cancer screening. *N Engl J Med* 2005;353:1773–1783.

Practice Guideline for Determinants of Image Quality in Digital Mammography. 2007. American College of Radiology, Reston, VA. Document is available at: http://www.acr.org/SecondaryMainMenuCategories/quality_safety/guidelines/breast/image_quality_digital_mammo.aspx

CHAPTER **9**

Fluoroscopy

Fluoroscopy systems produce projection x-ray images and allow real-time x-ray viewing of the patient with high temporal resolution. They are commonly used to position the imaging system for the recording of images (e.g., angiography) and to provide imaging guidance for interventional procedures (e.g., angioplasty). Before the late 1950s, fluoroscopy was performed in a darkened room with the radiologist viewing the faint scintillations from a thick fluorescent screen. Modern fluoroscopic systems use image intensifiers (IIs) coupled to digital video systems or flat panel digital detectors as image receptors. Fluoroscopy has undergone much technological advancement in recent years. The II has increased in size from the early 15-cm (6-inch)-diameter field of view (FOV) systems to 40-cm (16-inch) systems available today. Analog television (TV) cameras have been replaced with high-resolution, low-noise, digital charge-coupled device (CCD) or complementary metal-oxide semiconductor (CMOS) cameras. Flat panel detector technology has led to larger rectangular FOV systems (e.g. 48 cm) with high spatial resolution and improved image fidelity, and will gradually replace II detectors. Improvements in fluoroscopic systems with increased x-ray beam filtration, higher x-ray detection efficiency phosphors, lower acquisition frame rates, and electronic image guidance and enhancement have led to lower dose operation. Now, dose-monitoring technology is a component of all interventional fluoroscopy systems manufactured since June 10, 2006.

9.1 Functionality

"Real-time" imaging is usually considered to be 30 frames per second (FPS), equivalent to older analog television frame rates in the United States, and sufficient to provide the appearance of continuous motion. Modern general-purpose fluoroscopy systems use a pulsed x-ray beam in conjunction with digital image acquisition, which commonly allows variable frame rates ranging from 3 to 30 FPS. Lower frame rates reduce radiation dose when high temporal resolution is not needed. Digital fluoroscopy systems allow the recording of a real-time sequence of digital images (digital video) that can be played back as a movie loop with subsequent archiving in the patient's electronic file in the picture archiving and communications system (PACS). Unrecorded fluoroscopy sequences are used for advancing a catheter (*positioning*) during angiographic procedures and, once the catheter is in place, an image sequence is recorded using high frame rate pulsed fluorography as x-ray contrast material is injected through the catheter into the vessels (e.g., angiography) or the body cavity of interest. In gastrointestinal fluoroscopy, much of the diagnosis is formulated during the unrecorded fluoroscopy sequence; however, fluorographic images are acquired for documenting the study and illustrating important diagnostic findings. Imaging the heart at rates of 15 to 60 FPS, formerly obtained with cine cameras on the optical distributor of the II, using 35 mm continuous roll photographic film is now achieved by using digital cameras or directly with flat-panel detectors.

9.2 Fluoroscopic Imaging Chain Components

A standard fluoroscopic imaging chain is shown in Figure 9-1. The added filtration in fluoroscopy systems has increased in recent years, as pulsed systems with high mA capabilities have replaced older continuous fluoroscopy systems. Copper filtration combined with lower kV values allows angiography systems to provide lower dose operation while still delivering high image contrast for angiographic applications. Collimators on fluoroscopy systems utilize circular diaphragms for II-based systems and rectangular collimation for flat panel fluoroscopy systems. The collimators on fluoroscopy systems are motorized, which allows the collimated x-ray beam to change size in response to adjustment of the source-to-image distance (SID) or when the FOV is electronically changed (see magnification mode in Section 9.3).

In addition to added filtration and beam collimation, some fluoroscopy systems also have operator adjustable attenuating wedges to provide additional attenuation at specified locations in the x-ray field, such as the pulmonary space between the heart and chest wall, where excessive x-ray penetration of the pulmonary structures can lead to bright regions in the image. The use of wedges can reduce the glare from these areas, equalize the x-ray beam incident on the image receptor, and lower radiation dose to the patient.

The principal feature of the imaging chain that distinguishes fluoroscopy from radiography is the ability to produce real-time x-ray images with high frame rates and a low-dose per image. In general, five configurations of fluoroscopy systems are available: gastrointestinal/genitourinary (GI/GU) systems (with the x-ray tube under the patient table); remote fluoroscopy (over-table x-ray tube); interventional vascular (vascular surgery, radiology); cardiology and interventional electrophysiology, and mobile C-arm configurations (surgery, pain medicine). All configurations have the same basic components.

The basic product of a fluoroscopic imaging system is a projection x-ray image; however, a 10-minute "on time" fluoroscopic procedure, if conducted at 30 FPS, produces a total of 18,000 individual images! Due to the extremely large number of images required to depict motion and to achieve positioning, fluoroscopic systems must produce each usable image with about one thousandth of the x-ray dose of radiography, for radiation dose reasons. Consequently, a very sensitive low-noise

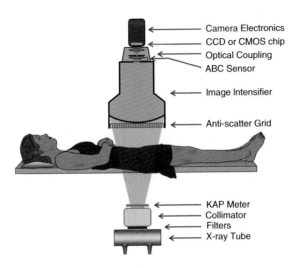

■ **FIGURE 9-1** The fluoroscopic imaging chain is illustrated, with the patient in the supine position. This figure shows an II as the detector, but flat panel detector systems are common as well. The detector in fluoroscopy is more sensitive than radiography to enable low-dose, real-time, longer duration studies. The x-ray system includes a collimator with motorized blades to adjust to the FOV, and a Kerma Air Product (KAP) meter to monitor radiation output for each patient is often available on interventional and cardiac catheterization fluoroscopic systems.

Camera Electronics
CCD or CMOS chip
Optical Coupling
ABC Sensor

Image Intensifier

Anti-scatter Grid

KAP Meter
Collimator
Filters
X-ray Tube

detector is needed. IIs and fluoroscopic flat panel detectors operate in a mode that is several thousand times more sensitive than a standard radiographic detector and, in principle, can produce images using several thousand times less radiation. In practice, standard fluoroscopy uses about 9 to 17 nGy (~1 to 2 μR) incident upon the detector per image, whereas a computed radiography (CR) system requires an exposure of about 5 to 9 μGy (~0.6 to 1 mR) to the detector.

9.3 Fluoroscopic Detector Systems

The Image Intensifier, Based Fluoroscopy Systems

A diagram of a modern II is shown in Figure 9-2. There are four principal components of an II: (a) a vacuum housing to keep air out and allow unimpeded electron flow, (b) an input layer that converts the absorbed incident x-rays into light, which in turn releases electrons, (c) an electron optics system that accelerates and focuses the electrons emitted by the input layer onto the output layer, and (d) an output phosphor that converts the accelerated electrons into a visible light image. When appropriate, an antiscatter grid is mounted adjacent to the input layer on the housing.

Input Screen

The input screen of the II consists of four different layers, as shown in Figure 9-3. The first layer is the vacuum window, a thin (typically 1 mm) aluminum window that is part of the vacuum containment vessel. The vacuum window keeps the air out of the II, and its curvature is designed to withstand the force of the air pressing against it. The vacuum window of a large FOV (35-cm) II supports over a ton of force from atmospheric air pressure. A vacuum is necessary in all devices in which electrons are accelerated across open space. The second layer is the support layer, which supports the input phosphor and photocathode layers. The support, commonly 0.5 mm of aluminum, is the first component in the electronic lens system, and its curvature is designed for accurate electron focusing.

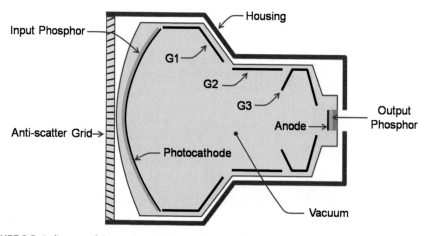

■ **FIGURE 9-2** A diagram of the modern II is shown. X-rays strike the input phosphor, producing light that stimulates the photocathode to emit electrons, which are ejected into the electronic lens system. The electronic lens system is comprised of the cathode, anode, and three additional focusing electrodes (G1, G2, and G3). Energetic electrons strike the output phosphor, generating light that is then imaged by a digital camera system.

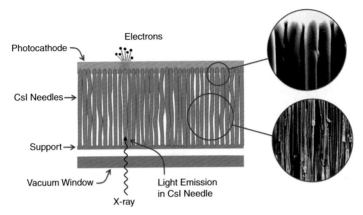

Electrons

Photocathode

CsI Needles→

Support→

Vacuum Window

X-ray

Light Emission in CsI Needle

■ **FIGURE 9-3** A detailed view of the input window of an II is shown. Incident x-rays pass through the antiscatter grid (not shown), and must also pass through the vacuum support window (~1 mm Al) and the support for the input phosphor (~0.5 mm Al). X-rays are absorbed by the CsI input phosphor, producing green light that is channeled within the long CsI needles to the antimony trisulfide photocathode, which then ejects electrons into the vacuum space of the II. Scanning electron micrographs illustrate the crystalline needle–like structure of CsI.

After passing through the Al input window and substrate, x-rays strike the input phosphor, whose function is to absorb the x-rays and convert their energy into visible light. The input phosphor must be thick enough to absorb a large fraction of the incident x-rays, but thin enough to not significantly degrade the spatial resolution of the image by the lateral dispersion of light through the phosphor. Virtually all modern IIs use cesium iodide (CsI) for the input phosphor. With proper deposition techniques, CsI can be made to form in long, columnar crystals (Fig. 9-3). The long, thin columns of CsI function as light pipes, channeling the visible light emitted within them toward the photocathode with less lateral spreading than an amorphous phosphor. As a result, the CsI input phosphor can be quite thick and still produce high resolution. The CsI crystals are approximately 400 μm tall and 5 μm in diameter and are formed by vacuum deposition of CsI onto the substrate. The CsI crystals have a trace amount of sodium, causing it to emit blue light. For a 60-keV x-ray photon absorbed in the phosphor, approximately 3,000 light photons (at about 420 nm wavelength) are emitted. The *K*-edges of cesium (36 keV) and iodine (33 keV) are well positioned with respect to the fluoroscopic x-ray spectrum, which contribute to high x-ray absorption efficiency.

The fourth layer of the input screen is the photocathode, which is a thin layer of antimony and alkali metals (such as Sb_2S_3) that emits electrons when struck by visible light. With 10% to 20% conversion efficiency, approximately 400 electrons are released from the photocathode for each 60-keV x-ray photon absorbed in the phosphor.

Electron Optics

X-rays are converted into light which then ejects electrons from the input screen into the evacuated volume of the II. The electrons are accelerated by a large electric field created by a high voltage- between the anode and the cathode. Focusing the electrons is accomplished by the several electrodes in the electron optics chain. The kinetic energy of each electron is dramatically increased by acceleration due to the voltage difference between the cathode and anode, resulting in *electronic gain*. The spatial pattern of electrons released at the photocathode (Fig. 9-3) is maintained at the output phosphor, albeit minified. The curved surface of the input screen, necessary for proper electron

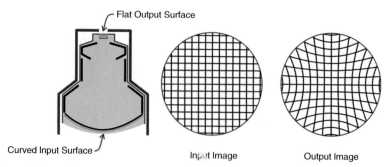

■ **FIGURE 9-4** The input phosphor/photocathode surface is curved to accommodate the physics of electronic focusing, and the output phosphor is planar. Because the image is produced on a curved surface and projected onto a plane surface, a characteristic *pincushion distortion* results in the output image.

focusing, causes unavoidable *pincushion distortion* of the image (Fig. 9-4). The G1, G2, and G3 electrodes (Fig. 9-2), along with the input phosphor substrate (the cathode) and the anode just proximal to the output phosphor, comprise the five-component ("pentode") electronic lens system of the II. The electrons are released from the photocathode with very little kinetic energy, but under the influence of the 25,000 to 35,000 V electric field, they are accelerated and arrive at the anode with high velocity and considerable kinetic energy. The intermediate electrodes (G1, G2, and G3) shape the electric field, focusing the electrons properly onto the output layer, where the energetic electrons strike the output phosphor and cause visible light to be emitted.

The Output Phosphor

The output phosphor (Fig. 9-5) is made of zinc cadmium sulfide doped with silver (ZnCdS: Ag), which has a green (~530 nm) emission spectrum. The ZnCdS phosphor particles are very small (1 to 2 μm), and the output phosphor is quite thin (4 to 8 μm), to preserve high spatial resolution. The anode is a very thin (0.2 μm) coating of aluminum on the vacuum side of the output phosphor, which is electrically conductive to carry away the electrons once they deposit their kinetic energy in the phosphor. Each electron causes the emission of approximately 1,000 light photons from the output phosphor.

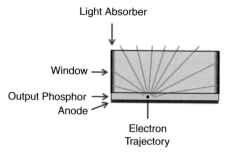

■ **FIGURE 9-5** The output window of the II is shown. The electron strikes the very thin (0.2 μm or 200 nm) anode and phosphor, and the impact of this high-velocity charged particle causes a burst of green light in the phosphor, which is very thin (1 to 2 μm). The light exits the back side of the phosphor into the thick glass window. Light photons that hit the side of the window are scavenged by the black light absorber, but a high fraction of photons that reach the distal surface of the window will be focused using an optical lens and captured by a digital camera. Light propagates by diffusion (multiple scatter interactions) in a turbid phosphor medium, but in the clear glass window, light travels in straight lines until surfaces are reached, and then standard optics principles (the physics of lenses) are used for focusing.

The image is much smaller at the output phosphor than it is at the input phosphor, because the 15- to 35-cm-diameter input image is focused onto a 2.5-cm (1 inch)-diameter circle. To preserve a resolution of 5 line pairs/mm at the input plane, the output phosphor must deliver resolution in excess of 70 line pairs/mm. This is why a very fine grain phosphor is required at the output phosphor. The reduction in image diameter also leads to light intensity amplification, since, for example, the electrons produced on the 410 cm^2 area of the 23-cm-diameter input phosphor are concentrated onto the 5-cm^2 output phosphor. By analogy, a magnifying glass collects light over its lens surface area and can focus it onto a small spot, and in the process, the light intensity is amplified enough to start a fire using only sunlight. The so-called *minification gain* of an II is simply the ratio of the area of the input phosphor to that of the output phosphor. The ratio of areas is equal to the square of the ratio of diameters, so a 23-cm-diameter II (with a 2.5-cm-diameter output phosphor) has a minification gain of $(22.8/2.55)^2 = 81$, and in 17-cm mode it is 49.

The last stage in the II that the image signal passes through is the output window (Fig. 9-5). The output window is part of the vacuum enclosure and must be transparent to the emission of light from the output phosphor. The output phosphor is coated directly onto the output window. Some fraction of the light emitted by the output phosphor is reflected inside the glass window. Such stray light reflecting inside the output window contributes to *veiling glare,* which can reduce image contrast. This glare is reduced by using a thick (about 14 mm) clear glass window, in which internally reflected light eventually strikes the side of the window, which is coated with a black pigment to absorb the scattered light.

Optical Coupling to the Video Camera

A light-sensitive camera such as an analog vidicon or a solid-state CCD or CMOS system is optically coupled to the output screen of the II and is used to relay the output image to a video monitor for viewing by the operator. The lenses used in fluoroscopy systems focus light emitted at the output phosphor onto the focal plane of the video camera. The lens assembly includes an adjustable aperture, basically a small hole positioned between individual lenses. Adjusting the size of the hole changes how much light gets through the lens system. The *f-number* is inversely related to the *diameter* of the hole (f = focal length/aperture diameter), but it is the *area* of the hole that determines how much light gets through. Standard f-numbers increment by multiples of $\sqrt{2}$: 1.0, 1.4, 2.0, 2.8, 4.0, 5.6, 8, 11, and 16. Changing the diameter of the hole by a factor of $\sqrt{2}$ changes its area by a factor of 2, and thus, increasing the f-number by one *f-stop* reduces the amount of light passing through the aperture by a factor of 2. At f/16, the aperture is tiny, little light gets through, and the overall gain (signal amplification of the light by minification gain and electron acceleration) of the II and combined optics is reduced. At f/5.6, more light gets through, and the overall gain of the II-optics subsystem is eight times higher than at f/16.

Adjustment of the lens aperture on II-based fluoroscopy systems markedly changes the gain of the system, which has an important effect on its performance. By lowering the gain of the II and associated optics by increasing the f-number, a higher x-ray exposure rate will result, producing lower noise images and higher patient dose. Increasing the gain reduces the x-ray exposure rate and lowers the dose, but reduces image quality. This will be discussed more fully below (see Section 9.4).

IIs absorb x-ray photons and emit light photons, just as an intensifying screen does, but the amplification of the II produces orders-of-magnitude more light. It is this electronic gain that creates a very sensitive detector, which produces a viewable output image using much less radiation compared to a radiographic detector.

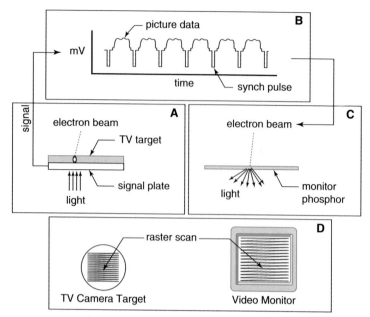

■ FIGURE 9-6 A diagram illustrating the closed circuit analog TV system used in older fluoroscopy systems is illustrated. At the TV camera (**A**), an electron beam is swept in raster fashion on the TV target (e.g. $SbSO_3$). The TV target is a photoconductor, whose electrical resistance is modulated by varying levels of light intensity. In areas of more light, more of the electrons in the electron beam pass across the TV target and reach the signal plate, producing a higher video signal in those lighter regions. The video signal (**B**) is a voltage versus time waveform which is communicated electronically by the cable connecting the video camera to the video monitor. Synchronization pulses are used to synchronize the raster scan pattern between the TV camera target and the video monitor. Horizontal sync pulses (shown) cause the electron beam in the monitor to laterally retrace and prepare for the next scan line. A vertical sync pulse (not shown) has different electrical characteristics and causes the electron beam in the video monitor to reset at the top of the screen. Inside the video monitor (**C**), the electron beam is scanned in raster fashion, and the beam current is modulated by the video signal. Higher beam current at a given location results in more light produced at that location by the monitor phosphor (**D**). The raster scan on the monitor is done in synchrony with the scan of the TV target.

Video Cameras

The operation of a legacy fully-analog electron-beam (vidicon) video camera is shown schematically in Figure 9.6. In the video camera, patterns of light (the image data) are incident upon the TV target (Fig. 9.6A). The target is swept by a scanning electron beam in a raster scan pattern. The TV target is made of a photoconductor, which has high electrical resistance in the dark, but becomes less resistive as the light intensity striking it increases. As the electron beam (electrical current) scans each location on the target, the amount of current that crosses the TV target and reaches the signal plate depends on the resistance of the target at each location, which in turn is related to the local light intensity. Thus the electrical signal is modulated by the local variations in light intensity, and that is physically how the video system converts the optical image incident upon it into to an electronic signal. Note that this is a process of sampling in time described as temporal sampling frequency with units of cycles/s, with the unit hertz (Hz).

The video signal, which is represented as voltage versus time (Figure 9.6B), is transferred by wire to the video monitor. Synchronization pulses are electronically added to the signal to synchronize the raster scanning in the video camera and video monitor. At the monitor, the raster scan pattern on the target is replicated by an electron beam scanning the monitor phosphor,. The video signal voltage modulates the beam current in the monitor, which in turn modulates the luminance at that location on the monitor (Figure 9.6C). The raster scan on the monitor is done in synchrony with the scan of the TV target. (Figure 9.6D).

Vidicon video systems typically operate at 30 FPS in an *interlaced* scanning mode to reduce *flicker*, the perception of the image flashing on and off. The human eye-brain system can detect temporal fluctuations slower than about 47 images/s, and therefore at 30 FPS, flicker would be perceptible. With interlaced systems, each frame is composed of two *fields* (called *odd* and *even* fields, corresponding to every other row in the raster, with the odd field starting at row 1, and the even field starting at row 2), and each field is refreshed at a rate of 60 FPS (although with only half the information), which is fast enough to avoid the perception of flicker. One drawback of interlaced scanning is the inability to uniformly read out a short pulsed exposure (less than 33 ms), since the scanning electron beam occupies distributed profile on the TV target, which causes some of the photoconductive charge patterns to be removed from the alternate field when the other field is scanned. Because light is not continuously incident on the target, the first field that is read will have a much larger video signal (and therefore greater brightness on a monitor) than the second field, and when interlaced, a bright/dark flicker pattern will be present. (This was a common presentation problem with pulsed cardiac angiography studies in legacy systems).

Charge coupled device (CCD) and complementary metal oxide semiconductor (CMOS) photosensitive cameras are solid-state electronic arrays that convert a projection image into a digital image and then into a video signal. Such a device uses photodiode semiconductor materials in an array to convert incident light intensity incident into corresponding electronic charge (electrons), and locally store the charge for electronic readout. Both CCD and CMOS cameras have very small pixel dimensions, on the order of 10–20 micron (0.01 to 0.02 mm), incorporated into a 2.5 × 2.5 cm area that replaces an analog TV camera. The typical matrix comprises 1,000 × 1,000 or 2,000 × 2,000 detector elements, but there is a wide variety and selection of sizes that a manufacturer might choose to include in a system. Unlike analog photoconductive targets, which have a non-linear response to light, CCD and CMOS cameras have a linear characteristic response over a very wide brightness range. Both CCD and CMOS systems can integrate light produced from intermittent pulsed exposures, or continuously read out fluoroscopic images in real time (30 FPS). The CCD reads out the stored charge in a "bucket brigade" fashion, as discussed in Chapter 7, causing locally stored electrons to be transferred from one row to the next row, along defined columns, to eventually be deposited onto a charge amplifier at the end of each column. The signals from the column amplifiers are synchronized and convert each row of accumulated charge into a corresponding digital value in the digital frame buffer. The CMOS device has independent detector elements, each comprised of a storage capacitor and transistor switch. The signal from a CMOS device is accessed, as is the signal from a TFT flat panel detector, as discussed in chapter 7. In either output (CCD or CMOS) a digital projection image is produced, and then converted to a video signal that is used to drive one or more monitors in the fluoroscopy suite. Solid-state cameras are preferred because of their stability, reproducibility, and linearity.

Characteristics Unique to Image Intensifier Systems

Brightness Gain

The brightness gain is the product of the electronic and minification gains of the II. The electronic gain of an II is roughly about 50, and the minification gain is variable depending on the electronic magnification (see magnification mode in Section 9.5). For a 30-cm (12-inch) diameter II, the minification gain is 144, but in 23-cm (9-inch) mode it is 81, and in 17-cm (7-inch) mode it is 49. The overall brightness gain, therefore, ranges from about 2,500 to 7,000. As the effective diameter (FOV) of the input phosphor decreases (increasing magnification), the brightness gain *decreases*.

Pincushion Distortion

Pincushion distortion was mentioned previously and is the result of projecting the image with a curved input phosphor to the flat output phosphor (Fig. 9-4). Pincushion distortion worps the image by stretching the physical dimensions in the periphery of the image. Therefore, for improved accuracy with distance measurements, it is best to position the desired anatomy in the central area of the FOV.

S Distortion

S distortion is a spatial warping of the image in an S shape through the image. This type of distortion is usually subtle, if present, and is the result of stray magnetic fields and the earth's magnetic field affecting the electron trajectory from the cathode to the anode inside the II. On fluoroscopic systems capable of rotation, the S distortion will generally shift in the image during rotation due to the change in the II's orientation with respect to the earth's magnetic field.

Flat Panel Detector Based Digital Fluoroscopy Systems

Flat panel detectors are comprised of thin film transistor (TFT) arrays of individual detector elements (dexels) that are packaged in a square or rectangular area. A more complete discussion of TFT arrays can be found in Chapter 7. Both indirect and direct x-ray conversion modes are used with TFT panels for fluoroscopy applications. In both types of systems, each detector element has a capacitor, which accumulates and stores the signal as an electrical charge, and a transistor which serves as a switch. For indirect detection TFT systems, in which the absorbed x-rays are initially converted to light in the adjacent layered phosphor, each dexel has a transistor and a capacitor, in addition to a photodiode, which converts the x-ray induced light from the phosphor into a corresponding charge. For direct detection fluoroscopy detectors, the semiconductor (selenium) produces x-ray induced charge directly, which is collected under a voltage to ensure that the signal is captured within the same dexel as the x-ray absorption event. In either detector type, while a frame is being acquired, the electrical charge proportional to the x-ray flux incident on that dexel is accumulated and stored by the capacitor. Later, when the image receptor is "read", a signal is sent to all the transistors in a row of dexels and the signals from the capacitors in the dexels of that row are simultaneously read as the charge from the capacitor is sent down a corresponding "drain" line along each column of the array to a charge amplifier. Reading the array discharges the capacitors and readies them for acquiring the next frame. This is performed row by row until the full frame is read. Even in continuous fluoroscopic acquisitions, the charge continues to be stored in each capacitor in a steady-state situation so that x-ray information is always collected as the flat-panel image receptor provides real-time fluoroscopic presentation of image data.

For fluoroscopic applications, the flat panel image receptor replaces the II, lenses, and camera system, and directly records the real-time fluoroscopic image sequence. The size of a detector element (dexel) in fluoroscopy is usually larger than in radiography, and some flat panel systems have the ability to adjust the dexel size by binning four dexels into one larger dexel. For example, four 100-μm detector elements are grouped together ("binned") electronically to form an effective 200 μm × 200 μm dexel. Such dual-use systems have dexels small enough for high-resolution radiography (e.g., 100 to 150 μm), but the dexels can be binned to provide a detector useful for fluoroscopy (e.g., 200 to 300 μm).

In some fluoroscopic flat-panel detectors, larger dexels (providing less spatial resolution) are necessary for fluoroscopy because data transfer rate ("bandwidth") limitations restrict the amount of image data that can be displayed at 30 FPS. The 2 × 2 binning reduces the amount of data by a factor of four, making real-time display feasible. In addition, the low doses per frame used in fluoroscopy results in significant quantum noise, and ultimately the poor statistical integrity (low SNR) limits the ability to see small objects. Therefore, larger dexel and poorer spatial resolution are sometimes necessary for fluoroscopic operation. In other flat panel detectors for fluoroscopy, the detector is read out always with full resolution, and to the extent that the number of pixels in the digital image exceeds those on the display monitor, real-time video processors interpolate and average the information as displayed to the fluoroscopist. The effect of this averaging on the video monitor results in an image presentation that appears similar to the binning method, but in image playback mode the full image resolution can be viewed with image zoom, unlike the systems that implement directly on the detector binning. Flat panel receptors replace the II, optics, video camera, digital spot film device, and cine camera in a much lighter and smaller package. A cover comprised of carbon fiber (~1 mm) instead of ~1.5 mm Al in an II input screen reduces x-ray attenuation and improves the quantum detection efficiency compared to the II (Fig. 9-7).

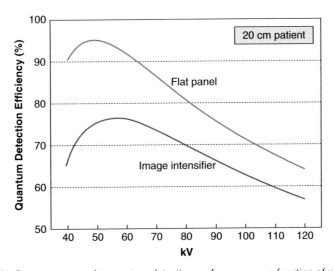

■ **FIGURE 9-7** This figure compares the quantum detection performance as a function of x-ray beam energy (kV of a polyenergetic spectrum hardened by a 20-cm-thick patient). In an II system, an x-ray has to penetrate about 1.5 mm of aluminum before reaching the actual phosphor. A considerable fraction of incident photons will be attenuated, reducing QDE, especially at lower kV values. The flat panel detector system also uses a CsI phosphor, but only a carbon fiber cover is in the x-ray beam path, which acts as physical protection and as a light shield to the detector.

9.4 Automatic Exposure Rate Control

The exposure rates in modern fluoroscopic systems are controlled automatically. The purpose of the *automatic exposure rate control* (AERC) circuit (formerly referred to as Automatic Brightness Control – ABC) is to keep the signal-to-noise ratio (SNR) of the image constant when possible. It does this by regulating the x-ray exposure rate incident on the input phosphor of the II or flat panel detector. When the system is panned from a region of low attenuation to one of greater attenuation (e.g., thin to a thick region of soft tissue) of the patient, fewer x-rays strike the detector. An AERC sensor (Fig. 9-1) measures the x-ray intensity and the AERC sends a signal to the x-ray generator to increase the x-ray exposure rate. The AERC circuitry strives to keep the detected photon fluence used for each fluoroscopic frame at a constant level, keeping the SNR of the image approximately constant regardless of the thickness of the patient. It also increases the exposure rate when magnification modes are used, so that the detected photon fluence per pixel is approximately constant as the effective pixel area on the displayed image becomes larger. The AERC circuitry in the x-ray generator is capable of changing the mA and the kV in continuous fluoroscopy mode. For pulsed fluoroscopy systems, the AERC circuitry may regulate the pulse width (the time duration) or pulse height (the mA) of the x-ray pulses as well as kV (to increase or decrease penetrability of the beam).

For large patients, the x-ray exposure rate may reach a regulatory limit, discussed later in this chapter, yet the image will still not be appropriately bright. Some II-based fluoroscopic systems employ AERC circuitry, which can modulate the lens aperture to increase the conversion efficiency (i.e., gain) of the system when the exposure rate reaches regulatory limits. With current technology flat-panel detectors for fluoroscopy, the charge amplifier gain is fixed (although variable gain, avalanche detector technologies are in the development stage). When x-ray exposure rates reach a maximum (e.g., 87 mGy/min (10 R/min) maximum tabletop exposure rate) the visible noise in the image will be very apparent. Special activation controls (175 mGy/min [20 R/min] tabletop exposure) can be utilized in such circumstances to reduce excessive noise when absolutely necessary.

For AERC, the x-ray generator changes the mA and the kV in a predetermined manner; however, this varies with different models of generators and is often selectable on a given fluoroscopic system. How the mA and kV change as a function of patient thickness has an important influence on the compromise between patient dose and image quality. When the fluoroscopist pans to a thicker region of the patient, the AERC circuit requests more x-rays from the generator. When the generator responds by increasing the kV, the subject contrast decreases, but the dose to the patient is kept low because more x-rays penetrate the patient at higher kV. In situations where contrast is crucial (e.g., angiography), the generator can increase the mA instead of the kV; this preserves subject contrast at the expense of higher patient dose. In practice, the mA and kV are increased together, but the curve that describes this can be designed to aggressively preserve subject contrast, or alternately, to favor a lower dose examination (Fig. 9-8). Many fluoroscopy systems have "low dose," "conventional", or "high contrast" selections on the console, which select the different mA-kV curves shown in (Fig. 9-8).

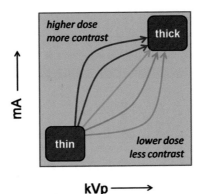

■ **FIGURE 9-8** AERC circuitry adjusts the x-ray output in response to the thickness of the patient. X-ray output can be increased for thick regions by increasing the mA, kV, or both. Increasing kV increases the dose rate but contrast is reduced, whereas increasing mA raises the dose rate but preserves contrast. Different AERC curves can be used on some systems (five are shown, typically fewer are available), which allow the user to select the low-dose or high-contrast AERC logic, depending on the clinical application.

 9.5 ## Fluoroscopy Modes of Operation

Modern x-ray generators and imaging systems are controlled by computers, resulting in a great deal of flexibility regarding operational modes compared to the availability in the 1990s and earlier. A brief description of various fluoroscopy modes, analog and digital, is given below.

Continuous Fluoroscopy

Continuous fluoroscopy produces a continuous x-ray beam typically using 0.5 to 6 mA (depending on patient thickness and system gain). A camera displays the image at 30 FPS, so that each fluoroscopic frame is displayed for 33 ms (1/30 s). Any motion that occurs within the 33-ms acquisition blurs the fluoroscopic image. This mode is the most basic approach to fluoroscopy acquisition, is typically used on all analog systems, and was the standard operating mode for image-intensified fluoroscopy up until the 1980s. The TV camera-based systems typically operated with either 525 line or 1,000 (1023, 1024) line video output in an interlaced scanning format. Modern fluoro systems may permit operation in this mode and some very simple mobile "mini-C-arm" systems for extremity use only work in this mode.

Variable Frame Rate Pulsed Fluoroscopy

In pulsed fluoroscopy, the x-ray generator produces a series of short x-ray pulses (Fig. 9-9). The pulsed fluoroscopy system can generate 30 pulses/s, but each pulse can be very short in time. With pulsed fluoroscopy, the exposure time ranges from about 3 to 10 ms instead of 33 ms, which reduces blurring from patient motion (e.g., pulsatile vessels and cardiac motion) in the image. Therefore, in fluoroscopic procedures where object motion is high (e.g., positioning catheters in highly pulsatile vessels), pulsed fluoroscopy offers better image quality at the same average dose rates.

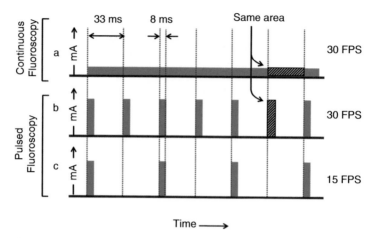

■ **FIGURE 9-9** This figure illustrates three different pulse sequences for fluoroscopy. The top (a) is continuous fluoroscopy, which was the standard operating mode for fluoroscopy for decades. The 33-ms frame integration time led to motion blurring in highly pulsatile regions of the patient. The middle sequence (b) shows a pulsed fluoroscopy sequence at 30 FPS. Here, the pulse width is 8 ms instead of 33, while the mA is increased by the factor 33/8, to deliver images of similar image quality (same dose) but with less motion blurring. The bottom sequence (c) shows a 15-FPS sequence, which reduces not only the temporal sampling but also the radiation dose by a factor of 2. To reduce dose, the fluoroscopist should use the lowest frame rate that is practical for the clinical task at hand. The hatched areas shown in sequences a and b illustrate that the area of each pulse is the product of the time (s) and mA and hence is the mAs per fluoroscopic frame.

During much of a fluoroscopic procedure, temporal resolution with high frame rate is not required. For example, in a carotid angiography procedure, initially guiding the catheter from the femoral artery access to the aortic arch might allow the use of 7.5 FPS—reducing the radiation dose for that portion of the study to 25% (7.5/30). Pulsed fluoroscopy at selectable frame rates (typically 30, 15, 7.5 and 3.75 FPS) allows the fluoroscopist to reduce temporal resolution when it is not needed, sparing dose. At low frame rates, the fluoroscopic image would demonstrate intolerable flicker if not displayed with continuous refresh during the time intervals between the pulses. However, all modern fluoroscopy systems use a digital refresh memory, where each image is captured digitally and is displayed continuously at the refresh rate of the fluoroscopy display monitor. (e.g., 60 to 72 Hz or faster) until it is refreshed with the next x-ray pulse and newer digital image. In this way, a slightly jerky temporal progression of images may be seen by the human observer at low frame rates, but the image does not suffer from overt on-and-off flicker that would occur if the displayed image flickered off and on synchronously with the x-ray pulse.

Field of View and Magnification Modes

IIs are available in different sizes, commonly 23-, 30-, 35-, and 40-cm diameter FOV. Large IIs are appropriate for GI/GU work, where it is useful to image the entire abdomen. For cardiac imaging, the 23-cm (9-inch) II is adequate for imaging the heart, and its smaller size allows closer positioning in a typically biplane configuration and craniocaudad tilt without moving the center of the image receptor far from the patient.

In addition to the largest FOV, which is determined by the physical size of the II, most IIs have several *magnification modes,* which yield higher spatial resolution for a smaller field of view. Magnification is produced by changing the voltages applied to the electrodes in the II, resulting in electron focusing from a smaller central area of the

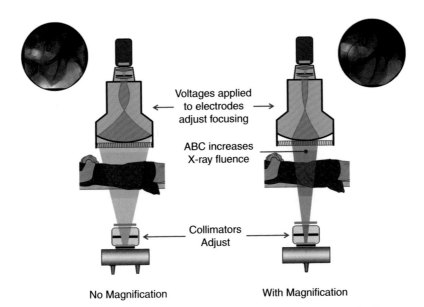

Voltages applied
to electrodes
adjust focusing

ABC increases
X-ray fluence

Collimators
Adjust

No Magnification   With Magnification

■ **FIGURE 9-10** No-magnification (**left**) and magnification (**right**) modes are illustrated. When the magnification mode is selected, the electrode voltages in the II are changed such that the electrons are focused to a smaller FOV. The motorized collimator blades also constrict the x-ray field to the smaller region. The AERC senses a loss of light immediately after switching to the magnification mode, and increases the exposure rate.

II's input screen to the entire output phosphor. As the magnification factor increases, a smaller area on the input of the II is seen (Fig. 9-10). When the magnification mode is engaged, the x-ray beam collimator automatically adjusts to match the x-ray beam dimensions to the smaller FOV.

As discussed previously, the brightness gain (and hence the overall gain) of the II decreases as the magnification increases. The AERC circuitry compensates for the lower signal by boosting the x-ray exposure rate. The increase in the exposure rate is commonly equal to the ratio of FOV areas, although the user can deviate from this algorithm to lower the radiation dose to the patient at the expense of greater quantum noise in the image. Consider a 30-cm II, which may have 23- and 18-cm magnification modes. Switching from the 30-cm mode to the 23-cm mode will increase the x-ray exposure rate by a factor of $(30/23)^2 = 1.7$, and going from the 30-cm FOV to the 17-cm FOV will increase the exposure rate by a factor of $(30/17)^2 = 3.1$. Image-intensified fluoroscopy systems use a sensor at the output of the II to drive the AERC, so the overall gain of the II and optics systems drives the AERC feedback operation.

Flat panel fluoroscopy systems can provide similar exposure rate adjustment as a function of field size as IIs; however, the exposure rate is controlled by system logic and is explicitly calibrated into the fluoroscopy system. In designing fluoroscopy systems using flat panel detector systems, it is logical that the same approximate dose rate-versus-FOV performance as with II systems should be used, since that is what users are familiar with.

In comparing image quality between imaging intensifiers and flat panel detector systems, although the rectangular format, compact design, and intrinsic digital attributes of flat panel systems enhance functionality, the electronic gain circuitry in the II produces images with very little added electronic noise. Flat panel systems, however, have amplifier systems that work at the very limit of what compact digital electronics can deliver, and consequently, there is appreciably more electronic noise in most flat panel fluoroscopy systems. Thus, flat panel fluoroscopy detectors are calibrated to use slightly higher exposures per frame compared to IIs of similar area. Electronic noise is far less of an issue in flat panel detectors when they are used in higher dose fluorographic and radiographic acquisition modes.

To minimise patient dose, the fluoroscopist should use the least magnification and smallest collimation area that facilitates the diagnostic task at hand.

Frame Averaging

Fluoroscopy systems provide excellent temporal resolution, a feature that is the basis of their clinical utility. However, fluoroscopy images are also relatively noisy, and under certain circumstances it is appropriate and beneficial to (reduce) temporal resolution for lower quantum noise. This can be accomplished by averaging a series of images, as shown in Figure 9-11. Appreciable frame averaging can cause noticeable image *lag* with reduced temporal resolution. The compromise depends on the specific fluoroscopic application and the preferences of the user. Aggressive use of frame averaging can provide lower dose imaging in many circumstances. Mobile fluoroscopy systems use x-ray tubes with limited output, and consequently temporal frame averaging is a common feature.

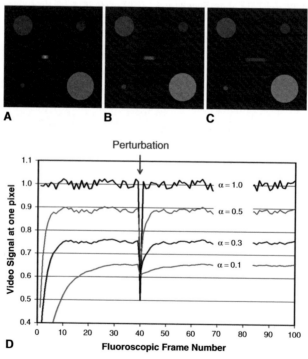

■ **FIGURE 9-11 A.** This image shows the trade-off between temporal blurring and noise. Frame A integrates five frames, and there is minimal blurring of the moving central object, but the image is overall noisier. Frame **B** shows 10-frame blurring, with a considerably broader central object but lower noise in the static areas of the image. Frame **C** (20-frame averaging) shows dramatic blurring of the central, moving object but enjoys a very high SNR in the static regions of the image. **D.** This figure shows the influence of different recursive filters for temporal averaging. A parameter (α) setting of 1.0 results in no temporal filtering, and a noisy trace at this one (arbitrary) pixel is seen. As the value of α is lowered, the amount of temporal lag is increased and the trace becomes smoother. However, the rounded leading edges (at $t = 1$ and $t = 40$) show the increased lag that occurs in the signal.

Different temporal averaging algorithms can be used, but a common approach to frame averaging is called *recursive filtering*. In this approach, the image just acquired, I_n, is added together with the last displayed image (I_{n-1}) using

$$I_{displayed} = \alpha I_n + (1 - \alpha)I_{(n-1)}$$ [9-1]

The parameter α ranges from 0 to 1; as α is reduced, the contribution of the current image (I_n) is reduced, the contribution of the previous displayed image is enhanced, and the amount of lag is increased. As α is increased, the amount of lag is reduced, and at $\alpha = 1$, no lag occurs. The current displayed image $I_{displayed}$ becomes the I_{n-1} image for the next frame, and the weighted image data from an entire sequence of images (not just two images) is included (Fig. 9-11). For example, for $\alpha = 0.3$, if the x-rays are abruptly turned off, the signal in the displayed image would be less than 1% after 17 blank (no input) frames at 30 FPS, or about 0.56 s.

Last-Frame-Hold, Last-Sequence-Display

When the fluoroscopist steps off the pedal and deactivates fluoroscopy, rather than seeing a blank monitor, *last-frame-hold* continuously displays the last acquired image or set of images on the fluoroscopy monitor. Last-frame-hold is a standard feature on modern fluoroscopy systems, and is achieved by continuously digitizing images in real time and temporarily storing them in a digital video frame memory. When the fluoro pedal is released, are displayed the last bright image or images on the monitor. Rather than orienting oneself with patient anatomy while the fluoroscopy pedal is depressed and x-rays are on, last-frame-hold allows the fluoroscopist to examine the image on the monitor for as long as necessary, using no additional radiation. A playback of the last sequence of images, programmable over several seconds, is available on many advanced fluoro systems with larger video buffer memories, and can be useful for complicated procedures. Last-frame-hold is a necessary feature for dose reduction, especially at training institutions.

Road Mapping

Road mapping is a software- and video-enhanced variant of the last-frame-hold feature and is useful for angiography procedures. Two different approaches to road mapping can be found on fluoroscopic systems. Some systems employ side-by-side video monitors, and allow the fluoroscopist to capture an image (usually with a small volume of injected contrast media), which is then shown on the monitor next to the live fluoroscopy monitor. In this way, the path of the vessel can be seen on one monitor, while the angiographer advances the catheter viewing in real-time on the other monitor. Another approach to road mapping is to capture a contrast injection image or subtracted image, and use this as an overlay onto the live fluoroscopy monitor. In this way, the angiographer has the vascular "road map" superimposed on the fluoroscopy image and can orient the guidewire or catheter tip to negotiate the patient's vascular anatomy. Road mapping is useful for advancing catheters through tortuous vessels.

C-Arm CT

Some modern C-arm fluoroscopic systems for angiography have computed tomography (CT) acquisition modes (Fig. 9-12). The C-arm is capable of motorized rotation of about 220 degrees around the patient, which allows two-dimensional projection

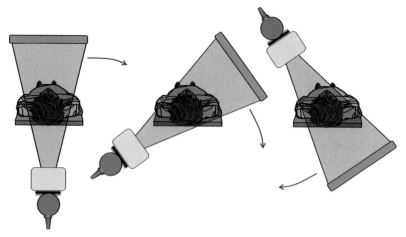

■ **FIGURE 9-12** C-arm CT on an angiographic system makes use of a motorized rotating C-arm, and acquires image data over about a 220-degree arc around the patient.

images to be acquired at many different angles around the patient. This data is then reconstructed using cone beam reconstruction algorithm. Images from such a cone-beam CT acquisition have poorer image quality compared to a conventional CT scanner, but can be of value in applications such as angiography. Details on CT and cone beam reconstruction are discussed in Chapter 10. The fidelity of the images is not as good as with whole body CT scanners, because the rotational axis on the C-arm system is not as rigid, and the cone beam geometry results in the detection of much higher scatter levels compared to whole body CT systems. Nevertheless, C-arm CT provides tomographic capability during interventional procedures, and this provides interventionalists an important additional tool in validating the success of the procedure. Dose levels during these procedures are high, and so physicians should use this acquisition mode sparingly.

9.6 Image Quality in Fluoroscopy

Spatial Resolution

For routine quality control testing in fluoroscopy, a visual assessment of a resolution test object imaged with minimal geometric magnification is commonly used to assess spatial resolution (Fig. 9-13). The intrinsic limiting resolution of modern fluoroscopy detectors is quite high, ranging from 3 to 5 cycles/mm; however, the limiting resolution of the entire system is most often governed by the video device and the effective sampling matrix size across the FOV, the latter determining the pixel dimension in the displayed image. A 23 cm FOV II/TV system with a 1024 × 1024 matrix will have a pixel dimension of 230 mm / 1024 = 0.22 mm, which translates to about 2.2 cycles/mm (Table 9-1). Higher magnification modes provide better resolution; for example, an 11-cm mode may have a limiting resolution up to 3.5 cycles/mm.

Flat panel detectors for fluoroscopy are designed to deliver similar or better spatial resolution as image-intensifier systems. Arrays with detector elements having similar dimensions as II/TV systems with or without pixel binning are being used. In many systems, the full sampling resolution of the flat panel is maintained,

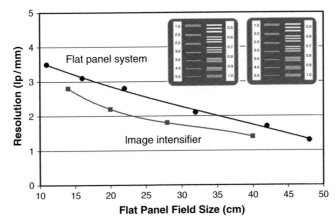

FIGURE 9-13 The spatial resolution in fluoroscopy for an II based fluoro system and a flat panel system is shown. As the field size decreases, magnification increases, and the spatial resolution increases commensurately. The resolution template is shown before (**left**) and after (**right**) image blurring.

independent of the displayed FOV. Spatial resolution in this instance is limited by the monitor's display matrix size and the software which interpretates and scales the full FOV image onto the monitor. With image zoom and panning, however, the full inherent spatial resolution of the acquired image can be obtained, regardless of the mode of operation. For systems with detector element binning, the intrinsic resolution is reduced by the binning factor (e.g., 2×2 binning reduces resolution by a factor of 2.

The theoretical intrinsic resolution of fluoroscopy cannot exceed the Nyquist frequency, $F_N = 1/2\Delta$, where Δ is the size of a detector element. Thus, for a system with a 30-cm FOV and $1{,}024 \times 1{,}024$ imaging matrix, $\Delta = 300$ mm$/ 1{,}024 = 0.29$ mm; $F_N = 1/(0.29 \times 2) = 1.7$ line pairs/mm.

The Nyquist frequency describes the maximum possible resolution in a digitally sampled imaging system; Overall spatial resolution is also determined by the calibration of electronic and optical focusing of the II/TV system, pincushion distortion of the II at the periphery of the image, and the size of the focal spot.

Geometric magnification, when used in conjunction with a small focal spot, is sometimes useful in overcoming the spatial resolution limitations of a fluoroscopy system, and is achieved by moving the detector away from the patient. Downsides to geometric magnification are the large increase in dose nesessary to address the increase in source to detector distance and the reduced anatomical coverage for a given detector field at view.

TABLE 9-1 TYPICAL LIMITING SPATIAL RESOLUTION IN FLUOROSCOPY

FOV: cm (inches)	525 LINE VIDEO LINE PAIRS/mm	1023 LINE VIDEO LINE PAIRS/mm	FLAT PANEL 0.157 mm LINE PAIRS/mm
14 (5.5)	2.7	1.4	3.2
20 (7.9)	2.0	1.0	2.8
27 (10.6)	1.6	0.7	2.5
40 (15.7)	1.3	0.5	1.8

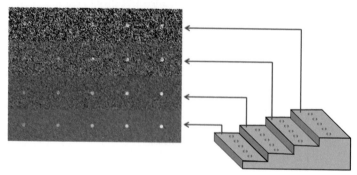

■ **FIGURE 9-14** Contrast resolution in fluoroscopy is essentially a measure of image noise. Many different types of phantoms (and testing procedures) are used, but shown here is a step wedge with holes of different depths drilled into each of the steps. The thicker step attenuates more x-rays, resulting in a noisier image. The noise differences between steps in this example were amplified for the purposes of this demonstration.

Contrast Resolution

The contrast resolution of fluoroscopy compared to radiography is low, chiefly due to the low SNR. Contrast resolution is usually measured subjectively by viewing contrast-detail phantoms under fluoroscopic imaging conditions (Fig. 9-14). When higher exposure rates are used contrast resolution increases, but dose to the patient also increases. The use of exposure rates consistent with the image quality needs of the fluoroscopic examination is an appropriate guiding principle. Fluoroscopic systems with different dose settings (selectable at the console) allow the user flexibility from patient to patient to adjust the compromise between contrast resolution and patient dose.

Scattered radiation from the patient also has a significant impact on contrast resolution, and therefore the use of an antiscatter grid in front of the fluoroscopy detector is employed in most situations other than pediatric and extremity imaging. The antiscatter grid selectively removes contrast-degrading scatter and preferentially allows primary radiation to pass, improving contrast sensitivity. However, the use of a grid causes a 2 to 4 times increase in radiation dose to the patient because of compensation by AERC due to the attenuation of x-rays by the grid (both scatter and primary). Grids with grid ratios of 6:1 to 12:1 and short (100 cm or less) focal distances are used in fluoroscopic examinations. In some systems, the grid can be moved in and out of the beam by the fluoroscopist. It is important that this feature be employed, particularly in the case of smaller-size pediatric patients.

Temporal Resolution

The excellent temporal resolution and its ability to provide real-time images are the advantages of fluoroscopy in comparison to radiography. As mentioned previously, temporal blurring is typically called image *lag*. Lag implies that a fraction of the image data from one frame carries over into the next frame, and this can be intentionally affected using algorithms such as recursive filtering (Equation 9-1). By blurring together several temporal frames of image data, a higher SNR is realized, because the x-ray photons from the several images are combined into one image. In addition to the lag of the fluoroscopic system, the photoreceptors in the human eye produce a lag of about 0.2 s. At 30 FPS, this means that approximately six frames are averaged together by the lag of the human eye-brain system. An image with six times the x-ray photons increases the SNR by $\sqrt{6} \approx 2.5$ times, and thus the contrast resolution improves at the expense of temporal resolution. Whereas some lag is usually beneficial for unrecorded fluoroscopic viewing, for recording dynamic events such as in digital subtraction angiography, lag is undesirable and recursive filtering modes are disabled. The significantly higher exposure per frame (and higher SNR) in DSA negate the need for intentional lag.

9.7 Fluoroscopy Suites

The clinical application strongly influences the type of fluoroscopic equipment that is needed. Although smaller facilities may use one fluoroscopic system for a wide variety of procedures, larger hospitals have several fluoroscopic suites dedicated to specific applications, such as GI/GU, cystography, peripheral vascular and cardiac angiography, cardiac electrophysiology, and neurovascular imaging procedures.

Genitourinary

In GI fluoroscopic applications, the radiographic/fluoroscopic room (commonly referred to as an "*R and F room*") has a large table that can be rotated from horizontal to vertical to put the patient in a head-down (Trendelenburg) or head-up position (Fig.9-15A). The detector is typically mounted over the table, with the x-ray tube under the table. The table has a large metal base that hides the fluoroscopic x-ray tube and provides radiation shielding. For radiography, an overhead x-ray tube is mounted on a ceiling crane in the room. The table may have a Bucky tray for use with screen-film, CR and portable DR cassette detectors. Typically the cassette holder has a moving antiscatter grid and has the capability of being aligned with the overhead x-ray tube. Alternately, a DR detector system can be built directly into the table.

Remote Fluoroscopy Rooms

A remote fluoroscopy room is designed for remote operation by the physician in charge of the examination (e.g., a radiologist or urologist). The fluoroscopic system is motorized and is controlled by the operator sitting in a shielded control booth. In addition to the normal operation of the detector (pan, zoom, up, down, magnification), a remote room typically has a motorized compression paddle that is used to remotely palpate the patient, to manipulate contrast agent in the upper or lower GI tract. Remote rooms use a reverse geometry, with the x-ray tube above the table and the detector system below the table. These systems reduce the radiation exposure to the physician operating it and reduce fatigue by allowing the procedure to be performed sitting down and without a lead apron on. However, because of the remote operation, these rooms require more operator experience. Remote rooms with over-table x-ray tubes should not be used with the operator in the room, as a GI/GU would be used. The x-ray scatter from the patient is most intense on the entrant side of the patient and, with the over-table x-ray tube geometry, that means

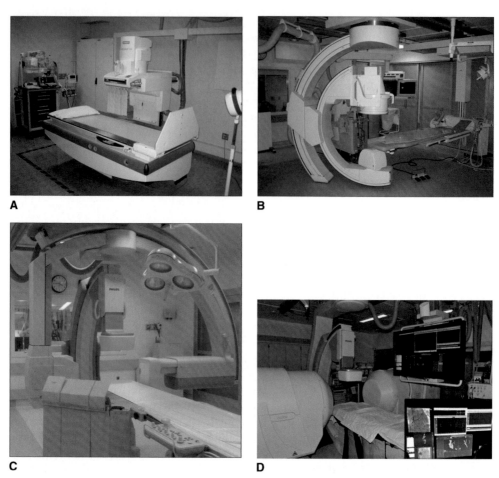

FIGURE 9-15 A. An II-based fluoroscopy system for GI/GU applications is shown. This system has a foot board to allow the patient to be tilted upright in a standing position, in order to move barium contrast agent in the GI track. **B**. An II-based angiography system with a floating table is shown. This is a body angiography system with a relatively large (40 cm) II. **C**. A flat panel–based, biplane, cardiac catheterization laboratory is shown. The smaller format of the flat panel detectors permits tighter positioning. Notice the lead drape system mounted on the table for radiation protection. **D**. Electrophysiology lab with permanent magnet and steerable catheter system that allows the operator to map cardiac functions remotely, outside the room.

that the highest scattered radiation levels will strike a person standing next to the table in his or her upper body and face.

Peripheral Angiography Suites

In the angiographic setting, the table does not rotate but rather "floats"—it allows the patient to be moved from side to side and from head to toe (Fig. 9-15B). The fluoroscopy imaging chain (the x-ray tube and detector) can also be panned around the stationary patient. The fluoroscopic system is typically mounted on a C-arm apparatus, which can be rotated and skewed, and these motions provide considerable flexibility in providing standard posteroanterior, lateral, and oblique projections. Because of the routine use of iodinated contrast media, power injectors (for injecting intravenous or intra-arterial iodinated contrast material) are often table- or ceiling-mounted in angiographic suites. For peripheral angiography and body work, the detector dimensions run from 30 to 44 cm. For neuroangiography rooms, 23- to 30-cm detector dimensions are commonly used.

Cardiology Catheterization Suite

The cardiac catheterization suite is very similar to an angiography suite, but typically smaller (~23 cm) flat panel detectors are used (Fig. 9-15C). The smaller detectors permit more tilt in the cranial caudal direction, as is typical in cardiac imaging. High frame rate (15 to 60 FPS) pulsed x-ray cineradiography operation is mandatory to capture injected contrast medium as it moves through the vessels in the rapidly beating heart. Because multiple cine acquisitions are acquired, many cardiac catheterization systems are *biplane* (see below) to reduce the amount of contrast material that must be administered.

Cardiology Electrophysiology Laboratory

Interventional cardiac electrophysiology (EP) studies chiefly use fluoroscopy to guide pacing and recording electrodes that are introduced into the heart to stimulate and measure the electrical properties of various cardiac control functions. These studies can sometimes take hours, and therefore it is important that the interventional system be tuned for very low fluoroscopy dose rates by using heavy beam filtration, very low pulsed fluoroscopy frame rates (3.75 or 7.5 FPS), and high sensitivity fluoroscopy detectors. Advanced EP laboratories use remote fluoroscopy capabilities coupled with high-field strength magnets that can steer intracardiac catheters to target locations in the heart with excellent accuracy. (Fig 9.15D)

Biplane Angiographic Systems

Biplane angiographic systems are systems with one patient table but with two complete imaging chains; there are two generators, two fluoroscopic detectors, and two x-ray tubes (Fig. 9-15C). Two complete x-ray tube-detector systems are used to simultaneously record two approximately orthogonal views following a single injection of contrast material. The additional complexity and cost of a biplane system is to reduce the amount of iodinated contrast agent that is injected, to avoid or reduce contrast reactions, and to allow more vessels to be evaluated. Two imaging chains allow two orthogonal (or oblique) views of the area of interest to be acquired simultaneously with one contrast injection. During biplane angiography, the x-ray pulse sequence of each plane is staggered so that scattered radiation from one imaging plane is not imaged by the other plane. Biplane suites usually allow one of the imaging chains to be swung out of the way when single plane operation is desired.

Mobile Fluoroscopy—C Arms

Mobile fluoroscopy systems are C-arm devices, and are used frequently in operating rooms and intensive care units. These systems plug into a standard wall plug for power, and therefore are relatively low power. Most C-arm systems use 15- to 23-cm detector systems. The typical system has two movable units, one is the C-arm and base itself, and the other unit (which can be connected by cables to the C-arm unit) contains the fluoroscopic controls and display monitors.

Radiation Dose

Patient Dose Rate

The US Food and Drug Administration (FDA) regulates the manufacture of medical equipment and fluoroscopic equipment in the u.s. The maximum permissible entrance exposure rate to the patient for normal fluoroscopy is 87.3 mGy/m or (10 R/m). For specially activated fluoroscopy, the maximum exposure rate allowable is 175 mGy/m (20 R/min). These dose rates limits are assessed at specified positions – for systems in which the x-ray tube is below the patient table, the measurement position is one cm above the table; for C-arm fluoroscopes, this position is 30 cm from the image receptor toward the x-ray source along the central axis of the beam. Most states impose similar regulations on the users of fluoroscopes in their states. However, neither the FDA nor the states provide dose limits for image recording. Typical entrance exposure rates for fluoroscopic imaging are about 8.7 to 17 mGy/m (1 to 2 R/min) for thin body parts and 26 to 44 mGy/m (3 to 5 R/min) for the average patient. The dose rate may be much larger for oblique and lateral projections and for obese patients. The entrance exposure rate to the skin of a patient can also substantially exceed these values if the skin of the patient is much closer to the x-ray source than the dose reference point.

Dose rates are evaluated in fluoroscopy by using a tissue-equivalent phantom made of a material such as polymethyl methacrylate (PMMA, also known as Lucite or Perspex) placed in the field, with an ionization chamber positioned in front of it to measure the entrance skin dose (Fig. 9-16). Dose rates are measured with the

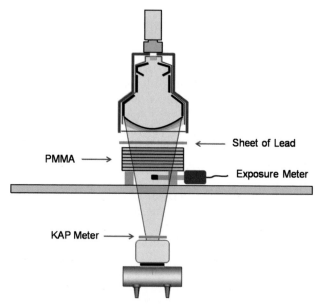

■ **FIGURE 9-16** This figure shows the procedure for measuring the entrance dose rates on a fluoroscopy system. The exposure meter is positioned under the PMMA using blocks, and different thicknesses of PMMA are used to assess the dose rate over a range of magnification factors and operating modes (different fluoro schemes, cine, DSA, etc.) of the system. To determine the maximum tabletop exposure rate, a sheet of lead is positioned in the back of the PMMA—this drives the system to maximum output and allows the measurement of maximum exposure rates.

fluoroscopic system operating in all typical modes (e.g., magnification modes, low dose/high contrast, cine, DSA, etc), with the antiscatter grid in. Dose rates also are measured using different thicknesses of PMMA to determine the entrance dose as a function of "patient" thickness, for example, using 10, 20, and 30 cm of PMMA. To determine the maximum exposure rate, a sheet of lead is placed between the PMMA and the detector system to attenuate the x-ray beam and drive the AERC system to its maximum output. The geometry shown in Figure 9-16 includes the measurement of backscatter, because the ionization chamber is very close to the PMMA attenuator.

The overall sensitivity of the fluoroscopic system in a particular operating mode can be characterized directly, and this approach is used when service personnel calibrate the fluoroscopic systems during installation and service. The grid is removed, and all objects are removed from the FOV, including the table. A sheet of approximately 0.5 - 1.2 mm of copper is taped to the x-ray tube port to provide some beam hardening so that the x-ray beam spectrum striking the detector is roughly similar that used during patient imaging. An ionization chamber is placed over the detector, and the exposure rate is measured at the surface of the detector. Typical entrance kerma rates for fluoroscopic detectors range from 8.7 nGy (1 μR) to 44 nGy (5 μR) per frame. Figure 9-17 shows the dose rate at the detector, as a function of field size, for several fluoroscopic systems. For the II, these data are simply a computed curve with $1/x^2$ performance normalized to 17 nGy/frame for a 23-cm-diameter II. The other curves shown correspond to exposure rates measured on flat panel fluoroscopic systems. These data fit curves with exposure rate dependencies of $1/x^{1.9}$, $1/x^{1.7}$, and $1/x^{1.5}$, respectively, where x is the side dimension of the rectangular FOV.

Dose to Personnel

Occupational exposures of physicians, nurses, technologists, and other personnel who routinely work in fluoroscopic suites can be high. As a rule of thumb, standing 1 m from the patient, the fluoroscopist receives from scattered radiation (on the

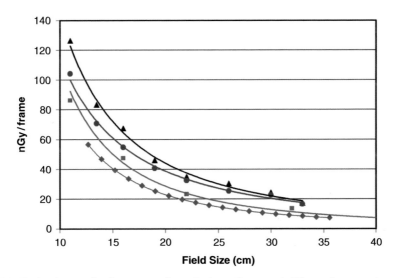

■ **FIGURE 9-17** The dose to the detector per frame is shown for several different fluoroscopic systems. The curve with diamond symbols shows an II-based fluoroscopy system, while the other curves correspond to different flat panel imaging systems. It is seen that the flat panel system response, which is calibrated into the system, closely matches that of the II.

outside of his or her apron) approximately 1/1,000 of the exposure incident upon the patient. To reduce radiation exposure in fluoroscopy, everyone in the fluoroscopy suite should wear radiation attenuating aprons, always. Movable lead shields should be available for additional protection to staff members observing or participating in the procedure. The dose to personnel is reduced when the dose to the patient is reduced, so measures such as reducing the total fluoroscopy time, using variable rate pulsed fluoroscopy at low pulse rates, and aggressive beam collimation are beneficial to everyone. Stepping back from the radiation field helps reduce dose to the fluoroscopist and other staff, particularly during image recording when dose rates are typically higher. In addition to the protective apron, lead eyeglasses, a thyroid shield, and the use of ceiling-mounted and table-mounted radiation shields can substantially reduce the radiation doses to personnel in the fluoroscopy suite.

Stray radiation, comprised of both leakage and scatter radiation, has a distinctly non-uniform distribution, chiefly due to backscattered radiation from the entrant beam surface. A factor of 10 or more scatter difference exists between the entry and exit locations on the patient, as shown in Figure 9-18.

Dose Monitoring

Patient Dose Monitoring

Active monitoring of doses to patients by fluoroscopy systems is routinely performed during exams that can lead to large skin dose levels, such as interventional neuroangiography and cardiology procedures. The purposes of patient dose monitoring are to assess risks to individual patients and for quality assurance. With large radiation doses delivered in a short time for these types of procedures, deterministic effects, including skin injury, hair loss, and cataract formation, can occur (See Chapter 20 on Radiation Biology). One would like to know the peak skin dose or have a map of skin doses, as in some cases the x-ray tube and detector move over a considerable area of the body (e.g., cardiac catheterization, while in other procedures, the x-ray tube movement is limited (e.g., interventional neuroangiography).

Dose monitoring may make use of ion chambers placed over the x-ray tube and collimator assembly, as illustrated in Figure 9-1. These systems have various acronyms such as kerma-area-product (KAP), roentgen-area-product, and dose-area-product meters. These systems are large ion chambers that are located after the collimator, and so the meter does not indicate exposure or kerma rate, because the entire chamber is not exposed as the collimator changes dimensions during fluoroscopy. Consequently, KAP meters typically report output in the units of mGy-cm^2. If field area in cm^2 is known for a particular exposure (e.g., at the skin surface, then the incident accumulated air kerma in mGy at that point can be calculated by simply dividing the KAP measurement by the area. For the same exposure rate, the KAP will give a larger value with a larger collimator setting. Since the collimated beam dimensions, patient position, and x-ray technique factors are constantly changing during most fluoroscopy and examinations, the KAP reading is useful metric of accumulated dose, especially to the skin. This in turn can be useful in managing the followup of patients who may reach dose levels that can cause deterministic effects.

Active dose monitoring is important in interventional procedure rooms (typically cardiac and neuroangiography suites) to alert physicians when skin dose levels are getting so high as to potentially cause erythema. It is typically the responsibility of the x-ray technologist or other personnel to monitor these dose levels during the

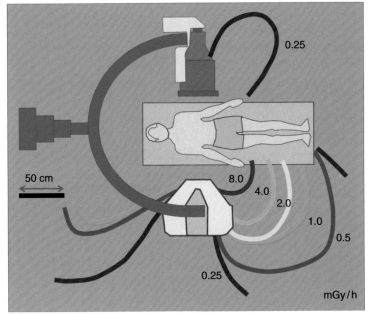

A   90 degree LAO projection, 100 cm

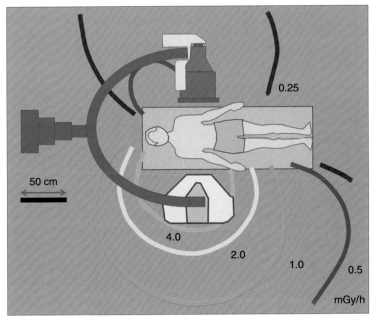

B   60 degree LAO projection, 100 cm

■ **FIGURE 9-18** Stray (scatter plus leakage) radiation distributions surrounding the patient are not uniformly distributed, as shown for three common projections used in cardiac catheterization procedures. **A.** 90 degree LAO projection; **B.** 60 degree LAO projection.

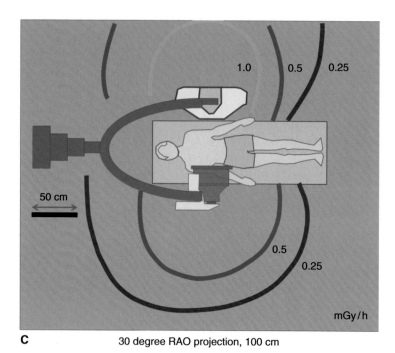

C   30 degree RAO projection, 100 cm

■ **FIGURE 9-18** (*Continued*) **C.** 30 degree RAO projection. "Isokerma" maps at the plane of the tabletop are for one manufacturer's equipment and for a given patient size. These do not represent the stray radiation levels for a general situation. The intent is to depict the factor of 10 and more difference between stray radiation between the entry port and exit port of the beam on the patient for different projections, where backscatter predominates the distribution. Figures are adapted from NCRP report 168, "Radiation Dose Management for Fluoroscopically–Guided Interventional Procedures," The National Council on Radiation Protection and Measurements, Bethesda, MD, 2011. LAO: Left Anterior Oblique; RAO: Right Anterior Oblique.

procedure. A *procedural pause* is required by some institutions when the integrated skin dose reaches predefined levels, in order to evaluate the benefits and risk of continuing with the procedure.

Fluoroscopy systems manufactured on or after June 10, 2006 are required to display the cumulative air kerma (commonly in the units of mGy) at a reference point. For a C-arm fluoroscope, this reference point is on the beam axis, 15 cm from the isocenter, toward the x-ray tube. The cumulative air kerma provides an actual dose value that will have more meaning to most users. To avoid the additional cost of active dose monitors, it is also possible (with proper calibration) to compute the cumulative air kerma from the mA, time, kV, and SID used during the fluoroscopic procedure—no physical dose monitoring is necessary.

The cumulative air kerma may significantly over or underestimate the actual peak skin dose for three reasons: (1) The cumulative air kerma does not account for backscattered radiation. Due to back scatter, the actual skin dose will exceed the air kerma at that location by a factor of about 1.25 to 1.5, depending upon the kV, beam filtration, and x-ray field size. (2) The x-ray beam may be incident upon a single area on the skin, or may be incident on multiple areas. If these areas do not overlap, the dose is spread over the multiple areas. (3) The skin may closer or farther from the x-ray tube than the reference point at which the cumulative air kerma is specified. If the skin is much closer to the x-ray tube, the skin dose may greatly exceed the cumulative air kerma.

Dosimeters are available that may be placed on a patient's skin. Some are read after the procedure and some give readings of cumulative dose during the procedure.

Monitoring of Doses to Personnel

Personnel who are routinely involved in interventional fluoroscopic procedures usually wear personal dosimeters to measure their exposures. A number of technologies such as thermoluminescent dosimeters, film, and other dose integrating materials can be used; these are discussed in Chapter 21. Doses are reported monthly or quarterly, to ensure that these individuals do not exceed dose limits defined by the institution or state and to assess the effectiveness of dose-reduction measures. It is customary to wear a single dosimeter at the collar level, in front of the protective apron. A second dosimeter may be worn on the body under the apron. Methods are available to estimate the effective doses from the readings from the dosimeters (NCRP Report No. 122). A finger dosimeter may be worn to monitor the dose to the hand likely to receive the largest exposure. Furthermore, a self-reading dosimeter may be worn on the collar outside the apron to monitor the dose from individual procedures.

Dose Reduction

Actively employing dose reduction techniques has immediate benefit to the patient on the fluoroscopic table but also benefits the physicians and other personnel who spend considerable time in the fluoroscopic suite. Techniques to minimize the dose include heavy x-ray beam filtration (e.g., 0.2-mm copper), aggressive use of low frame rate pulsed fluoroscopy, and use of low-dose (higher kV, lower mA) AERC options.

The x-ray tube should be kept as far from the patient's skin as possible. Aggressive beam collimation should be used. Although collimation does not reduce the skin dose, it does limit the area irradiated, reduces the effective dose to the patient, improves image quality by reducing the amount of scattered radiation, and reduces dose to staff in the room. Removing the antiscatter grid is a selection on some fluoroscopy systems, and should be chosen when imaging patients of smaller size, particularly young pediatric patients and extremities. Using the lowest magnification mode that is clinically acceptable reduces the higher dose that accompanies these modes. Patient positioning is important: when possible, ensure that the patient's arms are out of the beam when using lateral projections; when the patient is supine, keep the x-ray tube under the table to spare dose to the lenses of the eye and breast tissue in women; and if possible, use dose spreading by varying the location of the x-ray entrance field on the patient. The most effective way to reduce patient dose during fluoroscopy is to use less fluoroscopy time. The fluoroscopist should learn to use fluoroscopic imaging sparingly, only to view motion in the image, and should release the fluoroscopy pedal frequently. The last-frame-hold feature helps to reduce fluoroscopy time. Radiation dose during fluoroscopy procedures is not only from fluoroscopy *per se*, but also from radiographic acquisitions: DSA sequences in the angiography suite, digital spot images in the GI/GU fluoroscopy suite, and cineradiography runs in the cardiac catheterization laboratory. Reducing the number of radiographic images, consistent with the diagnostic requirement of the examination, is an excellent way of reducing patient dose. During cine and DSA radiographic acquisitions, when possible, all personnel should stand behind portable lead shields or other radiation barriers in the room, as these provide more protection than just a lead apron. A summary of how changes in these operational factors affect image quality and radiation dose to the patient and staff is given in Table 9-2.

TABLE 9-2   SUMMARY OF OPERATIONAL FACTORS THAT AFFECT IMAGE QUALITY AND RADIATION DOSE TO THE PATIENT AND STAFF

	EFFECT ON IMAGE QUALITY & RADIATION DOSE		
OPERATIONAL CHANGE	IMAGE QUALITY	RADIATION DOSE TO THE PATIENT	RADIATION DOSE TO THE STAFF
Increase in patient size	Worse (increased scatter fraction)	Higher	Higher
Increase in tube current (mA) with constant kV (i.e., AERC off)	Better (lower image noise)	Higher	Higher
[1]Increase in tube potential (kV) with AERC active	Soft tissue: Better (lower noise) Bone & contrast material: Worse: (decreased subject contrast)	Lower	Lower
Increase in tube filtration with AERC active	Little change	Lower	Lower
Increase in source to skin distance	Slightly better	Lower	Little change
[2]Increase in Skin to image receptor Distance	Slightly better (less scatter)	Higher	Higher
Increase in Magnification Factor	Better (improved spatial resolution)	Higher	Higher
Increase in Collimator opening	Worse (increased scatter fraction)	Little change (however higher integral and effective dose)	Higher
Increase Beam on time	No effect	Higher	Higher
Increase in pulsed fluroscopy frame rate	Better (improved temporal resolution)	Higher	Higher
Grid is used	Better (decreased scatter fraction)	Higher	Higher
Image recording modes (cine, DSA, radiographic)	Better (lower noise, higher resolution)	Higher	Higher

[1]When kV is increased with AERC activated, the system decreases the mA to maintain a constant signal level at the image receptor.
[2]Fixed source to skin distance.

Dose Recording and Patient Follow-up

Records of doses to the patient from each procedure should be kept for quality assurance purposes. Records of doses may also be entered into the patient's medical record; these doses should always be recorded when they are sufficiently large to potentially cause tissue reaction. In high dose procedures, the stored information should include the estimated skin doses and their locations on the patient's skin.

If the estimated skin doses are large enough to cause skin injury, arrangements should be made for clinical follow-up of the patient. Such large skin doses are most likely to be imparted by prolonged fluoroscopically-guided interventional procedures such as angioplasties, cardiac radiofrequency ablations, transjugular intrahepatic portosystemic shunt (TIPS) procedures, and vascular embolizations, particularly in procedures on large patients. If erythema does not appear approximately 10 to 15 days after the procedure or if moist desquamation does not appear within 8 weeks, further follow-up is likely unnecessary (see chapter 20).

DICOM and IHE standards (discussed in Chapter 5) will ultimately permit the automatic transfer of patient dose information from fluoroscopes to the PACS or other information system. Ideally, software will become available providing maps of doses on each patient's skin. Today, it is common practice to establish a cumulative air kerma threshold (e.g., 3 or 5 gray) and arrange for follow-up of each patient whose procedure exceeds that threshold. For older fluoroscopes that do not display cumulative air kerma, similar thresholds should be established for fluoroscopy time.

SUGGESTED READING

American Association of Physicist in Medicine Radiation Protection Task Group no. 6. *Managing the use of fluoroscopy in medical institutions.* AAPM Report No. 58. Madison, WI: Medical Physics, 1998.

Code of Federal Regulations 21 Food and Drugs. 21 CFR §1020.32, Office of the Federal Register National Archives and Records Administration. April 1, 1994.

Medical Exposure of Patients in *Ionizing Radiation Exposure of the Population of the United States* NCRP publication no. 160. Bethesda, MD: National Council on Radiation Protection and Measurement, March 2009.

Proceedings of the ACR/FDA Workshop on Fluoroscopy, Strategies for Improvement in Performance, Radiation Safety and Control. American College of Radiology, Reston, VA, October 16–17, 1992.

Radiation Dose Management for Fluoroscopically-Guided Interventional Procedures, NCRP Report No. 168. Bethesda, MD: National Council on Radiation Protection and Measurement, July 2010.

Schueler BA. The AAPM/RSNA physics tutorial for residents: general overview of fluoroscopic imaging. *RadioGraphics* 2000;20:1115–1126.

Van Lysel MS. The AAPM/RSNA physics tutorial for residents: fluoroscopy: optical coupling and the video system. *RadioGraphics* 2000;20:1769–1786.

Wagner LK, Archer BR. *Minimizing risks from fluoroscopic x-rays: bioeffects, instrumentation and examination,* 4th ed. Woodlands, TX: RM Partnership, 2004.

Wang J, Blackburn TJ. The AAPM/RSNA physics tutorial for residents: x-ray image intensifiers for fluoroscopy. *RadioGraphics* 2000;20:1471–1477.

CHAPTER 10

Computed Tomography

10.1 Clinical Use

From the first 80×80 matrix, 3-bit computed tomography (CT) images of the early 1970s, CT scanner capabilities and image quality have grown steadily over the past 40 years. Scanner rotation times have plummeted from the early 4.5-min scans to sub–half-second scanner rotation of today, a greater than 500-fold increase in the mechanical speed of gantry rotation. Increased gantry rotation speed combined with an increasing number of detector arrays on the CT gantry has led to the acquisition times *per CT image* going from 135 *seconds per image* in 1972 to greater than 200 *images per second* today. The reduced scan time, increased x-ray tube power, and advanced reconstruction algorithms have led to significant advances in CT image quality, as shown in Figure 10-1. Once called computed axial tomography ("CAT") scanners, modern CT systems can provide isotropic spatial resolution resulting in excellent three-dimensional (3D) image data sets, including axial, coronal, and sagittal images (Fig. 10-2).

Due to the advances in image quality and reduction in acquisition time, CT has experienced enormous growth in clinical use over the past three decades. Most reports put the number of CT scans performed annually in the United States between 70 and 80 million. The speed of CT image acquisition increased with the introduction of helical (or spiral) scanning in the late 1980s, and another large increase in scanner speed occurred when multislice CT scanners became available in the late 1990s. Each of these advances led to pronounced increases in the utilization rates as seen in Figure 10-3. Utilization rates (the slope of the curve shown in Figure 10-3) increased as CT scanner acquisition speed increased, because reducing scan time increases the number of clinical applications for CT imaging. Reduced scan time also means that one CT scanner can image more patients per day.

10.2 CT System Designs

Gantry Geometries

Figure 10-4 shows a pediatric patient undergoing a head CT scan. For most CT scans, a full 360-degree rotation of the CT gantry is used to collect data. The gantry is the moving part of the scanner apparatus; however, there is a large housing that surrounds the moving gantry to prevent mechanical injury to patients due to the rapidly rotating hardware. In earlier scanners, electrical cables were connected from the stationary frame to the moving frame, and the outer rim of the gantry served as a cable take-up spool. These cables connected the stationary x-ray generator to the rotating x-ray tube, and the signal data from the detector arrays were transferred

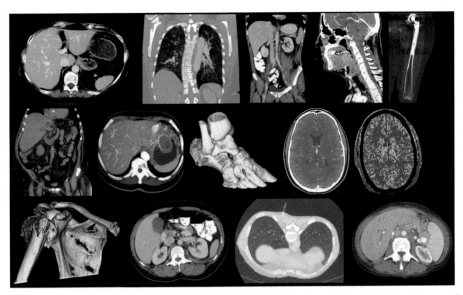

■ **FIGURE 10-1** A collection of CT images is shown, demonstrating the wide use of CT and the excellent anatomical detail that CT provides.

off of the rotating gantry via cables as well. All modern CT scanners use a slip ring connection (Fig. 10-5) between the stationary and the rotating frames, allowing the gantry to rotate freely, untethered to the stationary frame.

The patient table is an intrinsic component of the CT scanner as well. The CT computer controls table motion using precision motors with telemetry feedback, for patient positioning and CT scanning. The patient table (or couch) can be removed from the bore of the CT gantry and lowered to allow the patient to comfortably get on the table, usually in the supine position as shown in Figure 10-6A. Under the technologist's control, the system then moves the table upward and inserts the table

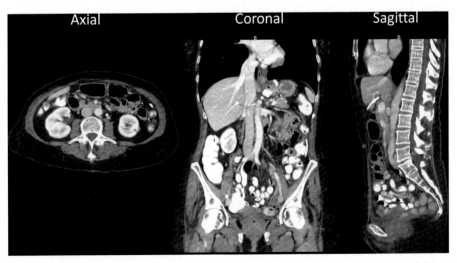

■ **FIGURE 10-2** Multiple detector array CT has led to a drastic reduction in slice thickness, and this means that the spatial resolution of CT is nearly isotropic. Thus, in addition to the natively reconstructed axial images, high-resolution coronal and sagittal images are routinely produced and used.

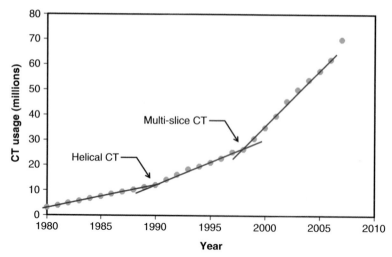

■ **FIGURE 10-3** The excellent image quality and rapid acquisition time of CT has led to a dramatic increase in utilization rates in recent years. Major technological advances in CT including the introduction of helical (spiral) and multidetector array CT led to reductions in scan time, opening up CT for more clinical applications. Hence, the use of CT in the United States has grown steadily over the past three decades. (Courtesy SE McKenney.)

with the patient into the bore of the scanner (Fig. 10-6B). A series of laser lights provide reference to allow the patient to be centered in the bore and to adjust the patient longitudinally. The cranial caudal axis of the patient is parallel to the z-axis of the CT scanner (Fig. 10-7). The scanner field of view (FOV) is a circle in the x-y

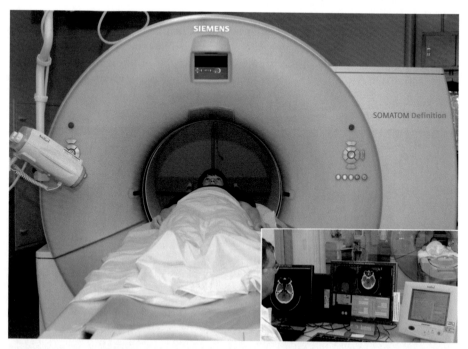

■ **FIGURE 10-4** This figure illustrates a pediatric patient in position to receive a head CT scan. Control pads are located on either side of the gantry to allow the CT operator to position the patient. The operator console (**inset**) is positioned behind a large lead glass window, providing an excellent view of the scanner and the patient. A power injector is seen to the patient's right side, hanging from the ceiling. Photo credit: Emi Manning UC Davis Health System

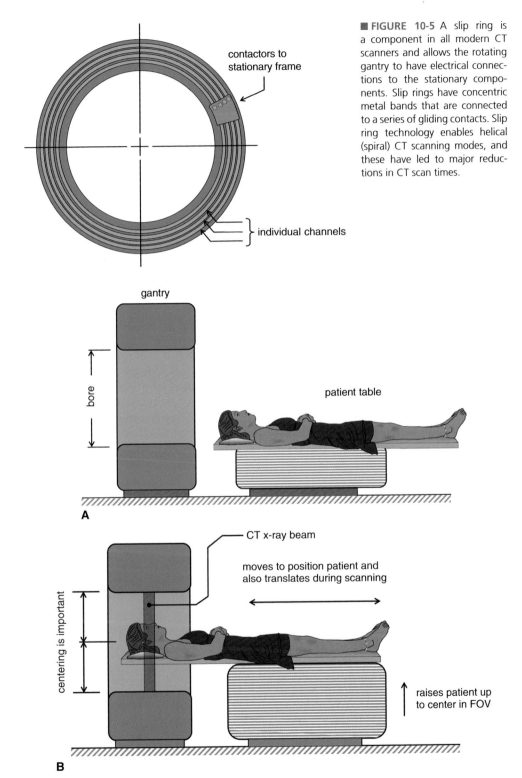

■ **FIGURE 10-5** A slip ring is a component in all modern CT scanners and allows the rotating gantry to have electrical connections to the stationary components. Slip rings have concentric metal bands that are connected to a series of gliding contacts. Slip ring technology enables helical (spiral) CT scanning modes, and these have led to major reductions in CT scan times.

individual channels

gantry

bore

patient table

A

CT x-ray beam

moves to position patient and also translates during scanning

centering is important

raises patient up to center in FOV

B

■ **FIGURE 10-6** **A.** The gantry is comprised of the imaging hardware, and the patient table can move up and down and translate. The gantry is lowered to allow the patient to get on or off. **B.** The patient table is raised and translated, allowing the patient to be inserted into the bore of the scanner. Laser lights are used for patient positioning, in all three orthogonal planes. During the actual scan, the CT imaging hardware rotates inside the gantry cover, and the table and patient translate through the bore of the gantry.

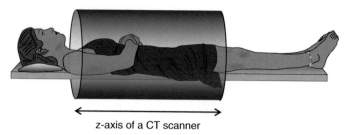

z-axis of a CT scanner

■ **FIGURE 10-7** The CT image is a circle inside of the square 512 × 512 image matrix. The circular field of view over the length of the patient forms a volume field of view that is cylindrical in shape. Most CT scanners have a maximum circular field of view of 50 to 70 cm in diameter, but there are few restrictions in terms of the scan length (in z).

plane but can extend considerably along the z-axis, essentially forming a cylindrical FOV, which envelopes the patient.

In the first years of CT, the x-ray tube and detectors used a linear scanning trajectory, as illustrated in Figure 10-8. The data that were collected in this scanning pattern correspond to attenuation measurements that are parallel to each other, and this geometry is called a *parallel beam* projection. Parallel beam projection is a more general geometrical concept, and it has utility in some nuclear and x-ray tomography geometries till today. For example, some modern scanners reorganize their acquired data in order to use parallel ray algorithms for image reconstruction. A *projection* refers to the data collected at a specific angle of interrogation of the object, and this term is synonymous with the terms *profile* or *view*. Rays are individual attenuation measurements that correspond to a line through the object defined at one end by the x-ray source and at the other end by a detector. A projection is a collection of rays.

Fan beam projection is shown in Figure 10-9. For a single detector array CT scanner, the geometry shown in Figure 10-9 is a true fan beam geometry. The individual rays in this geometry each correspond to a line integral that spans between the x-ray source and the x-ray detector; however, there are a lot more detectors in the fan beam geometry compared to the parallel beam geometry. The "true fan beam" geometry caveat refers to the 2D geometry shown in the figure, where there is only minimal divergence of the x-ray beam trajectory in and out of the plane of the figure. Figure 10-10 shows a more accurate depiction of a modern multislice CT scanner, where the fan angle defines the "fan beam geometry," but there is nonnegligible x-ray

■ **FIGURE 10-8** In earlier CT scanners, the x-ray tube and detector(s) translated to cover the patient, and this geometry lead to the formation of parallel beam geometry. Although scanners no longer use this acquisition geometry, the concept of the parallel beam geometry remains useful in the science of reconstruction. A *projection* is a collection of *rays*.

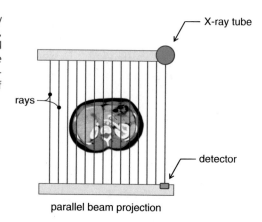

X-ray tube

rays

detector

parallel beam projection

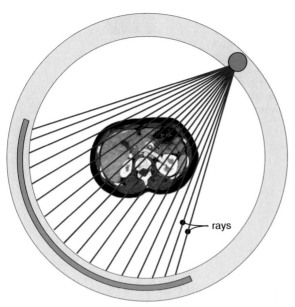

■ FIGURE 10-9 A fan beam projection refers to a fan of data that converges on a vertex, and using rotate-rotate geometry as shown in this figure, the apex of the fan is the x-ray tube. The individual rays correspond to each detector measurement. The collection of rays in this geometry is a fan beam projection.

fan beam projection

beam divergence in the orthogonal direction, which gives rise to the concept of narrow *cone beam* geometry. For typical 64 to 128 detector array CT scanners, the fan angle is approximately 60 degrees, while the full cone angle is about 2.4 degrees.

Most clinical CT scanners have detector arrays that are arranged in an arc relative to the x-ray tube, as shown in Figure 10-10. This arc is efficient from several standpoints—firstly, by mounting the detector modules on a support structure that is aligned along a radius of curvature emanating from the x-ray source, there is very little difference in fluence to the detectors due to the inverse square law. Very importantly, the primary x-rays strike the detector elements in a nearly normal manner, and so there are effectively no lateral positioning errors due to x-ray beam parallax.

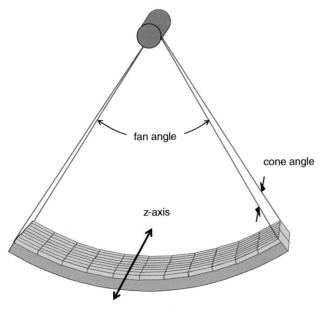

■ FIGURE 10-10 As modern scanners use more detector arrays, their width in the z-axis dimension gives rise to a narrow cone beam geometry, as illustrated here. Cone beam reconstruction algorithms are used on all modern MDCT scanners.

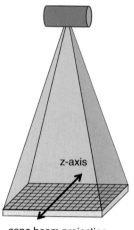

■ **FIGURE 10-11** Some commercial cone beam CT scanners use flat panel detectors, and these systems may be considered as *true* cone beam scanners, with cone half angles approaching 10 degrees. These systems are used for image guidance on radiation therapy treatment machines, for cone beam dental CT, and for other niche CT applications such as breast, extremity, and SPECT/CT systems.

z-axis

cone beam projection

Some niche CT scanners make use of flat panel detectors for the detector array, and this is shown in Figure 10-11. This geometry represents a full cone beam geometry, where the cone angle is almost as great as the fan angle. The use of the planar flat panel detector system leads to a 2D bank of detectors, which has no curvature, and so correction methods are needed for the different distances from source to detector, giving rise to inverse square law and heel effect–based differences in fluence to each detector element in the 2D array. There is also some parallax that occurs in this geometry. The cone angle that exists in some true cone beam scanners can be appreciable; for example, using a standard 30 × 40 cm flat panel detector at a source-to-detector distance of 90 cm, the fan angle spans about 25 degrees and the cone angle spans about 19 degrees. Flat panel detectors are used for cone beam systems in dental and maxillofacial CT systems, breast CT systems, and in radiation therapy imaging applications where the cone beam CT system is mounted orthogonally to the high-energy linear accelerator treatment beam.

Basic Concepts and Definitions

Figure 10-12 illustrates some basic geometry pertinent to CT scanners. The isocenter is the center of rotation of the CT gantry, and in most cases (but not all), the isocenter is also the center of the reconstructed CT image—that is, pixel (256, 256) on the 512 × 512 reconstructed CT image. The maximum FOV is defined by the physical extent of the curved detector arrays (the fan angle). The source-to-isocenter distance is illustrated as A in Figure 10-12, and the source-to-detector distance is labeled B. The magnification factor from the isocenter to the detectors is then given by M = B/A. If the (minimum) CT slice thickness is quoted on a scanner as, for example, 0.50 mm, the actual detector width is larger by the magnification factor M. Thus, if B ≈ 95 cm and A ≈ 50 cm, M = 1.9 and the physical width of the detector arrays is M × 0.50 mm = 0.95 mm. Hence by convention, most dimensions in CT are related to the plane of the isocenter.

Figure 10-12B illustrates the rotation of the gantry around the circular FOV. Almost all modern CT scanners have a design where the x-ray tube and detector are attached rigidly to the rotating gantry, and this leads to a so-called third-generation or "rotate-rotate" geometry. Thus, as the gantry rotates, the x-ray tube and detector arrays stay in a rigid alignment with each other. This fixed geometry allows the use

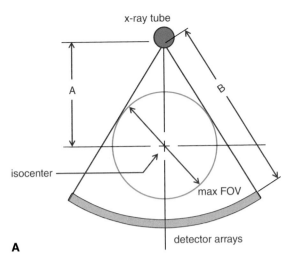

x-ray tube

A

B

isocenter

max FOV

detector arrays

A

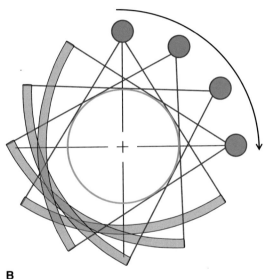

B

■ FIGURE 10-12 **A.** The general geom-etry of a CT scanner is illustrated, with the source-to-detector distance of B and the source-to-isocenter distance A. The magni-fication factor at the scanner's isocenter is M = B/A. Detector dimensions in CT are gen-erally referred to their size as projected to the isocenter. The maximum field of view (FOV) is shown, although scanners routinely recon-struct smaller FOVs for heads and smaller patients. **B.** The majority of modern MDCT systems use a rotate-rotate (third generation) geometry, where the x-ray tube and detec-tor arrays are mounted rigidly onto the same rotating platform and rotate in unison.

of an antiscatter grid in the detector array, as shown in Figure 10-13. The grid septa are aligned with the dead space between individual detectors, in an effort to preserve the geometrical detection efficiency of the system. As the width of the x-ray beam has increased with multidetector array CT (to 40, 80 mm, and larger), there is greater need for more aggressive scatter suppression. At least one manufacturer uses a 2D grid on its large multidetector array CT system.

X-ray Tubes, Filters, and Collimation

X-ray tubes for CT scanners have much more power than tubes used for radiography or fluoroscopy, and consequently, they are quite expensive. It is not unusual to replace an x-ray tube every 9 to 12 months on CT systems. CT x-ray tubes have a power rat-ing of about 5 to 7 megaJoule (MJ), whereas a standard radiographic room may use a 0.3- to 0.5-MJ x-ray tube. There were many advancements in x-ray tube power during the decade of the 1990s. With the advent of multidetector array CT in the late 1990s, x-ray tube power issues abated somewhat because multislice CT scanners

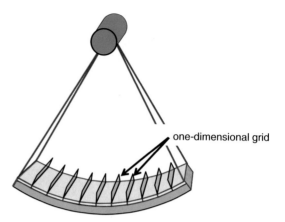

■ FIGURE 10-13 Most CT systems use some form of antiscatter technology such as the grid pictured here. The grid septa are aligned with the detector dead spaces to reduce impact on detection efficiency. A one-dimensional grid is shown here, although some manufacturers use a two-dimensional grid. This figure shows the concept, actual grid spacing on CT systems, is much tighter.

one-dimensional grid

make much more efficient use of the x-ray tube output by opening up the collimation. In changing from a 10-mm collimated beam width to a 40-mm beam width, a four-fold increase (400%) in effective x-ray beam output results (Fig. 10-14).

CT gantry rotation speeds are approaching 5 rotations per second (0.20 s rotation time), and these high angular velocities create enormous g-forces on the components that rotate. The x-ray tube is mounted onto the gantry such that the plane of the anode disk is parallel to the plane of gantry rotation (Fig. 10-14A), which is necessary to reduce gyroscopic effects that would add significant torque to the rotating anode if mounted otherwise. Furthermore, this configuration means that the anode-cathode axis and thus the heel effect run parallel to the z-axis of the scanner. This eliminates heel effect–induced spectral changes along the fan angle, which is important. The angular x-ray output from an x-ray tube can be very wide in the dimension parallel to the anode disk but is quite limited in the anode-cathode dimension (Fig. 10-15), and so this x-ray tube orientation is necessary given the approximately 60-degree fan beam of current scanners.

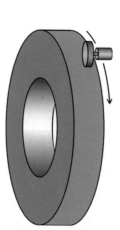

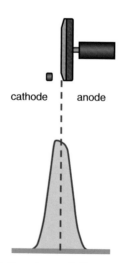

cathode   anode

A. tube position relative to gantry   **B.** X-ray beam profile along z

■ FIGURE 10-14 **A.** The x-ray tube rotates on the gantry as shown in this figure. This tube orientation is required to reduce gyroscopic effects. The anode-cathode axis runs parallel to the z-axis. **B.** The x-ray beam profile in the z-dimension of the scanner includes the heel effect, since this is the direction of the anode-cathode axis.

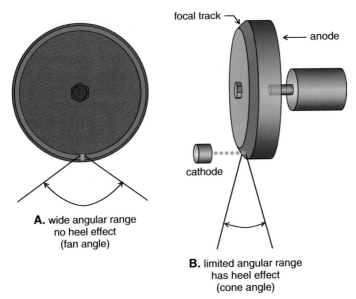

focal track

anode

cathode

A. wide angular range
no heel effect
(fan angle)

B. limited angular range
has heel effect
(cone angle)

■ **FIGURE 10-15** This figure demonstrates the angular coverage of an x-ray tube. In the plane of the fan angle (**A**), the x-ray beam coverage is quite wide, whereas in the direction parallel to the z-axis (**B**), the coverage is limited due to the anode angle and resulting heel effect.

Most modern CT scanners use a continuous output x-ray source; the x-ray beam is not pulsed during the scan (some exceptions are described later). The detector array sampling time in effect becomes the acquisition interval for each CT projection that is acquired, and the sampling dwell times typically run between 0.2 and 0.5 ms, meaning that between 1,000 and 3,000 projections are acquired per 360-degree rotation for a ½-s gantry rotation period. For a typical CT system with about a 50-cm source-to-isocenter distance, the circle that defines the x-ray tube trajectory is about 3,140 mm ($2\pi r$) in circumference. Therefore, using a 2-kHz detector sampling rate, for example, the x-ray focal spot moves about $3,140/2,000 \approx 1.5$ mm along the circumference of the circle per sample. While the x-ray detectors are moving in unison with the x-ray source, the patient is stationary, and thus the 1.5-mm circumferential displacement of the x-ray source over the time it takes to acquire one projection can lead to motion blurring and a loss of spatial resolution. To compensate for this, some scanners use a magnetic steering system for the electrons as they leave the cathode and strike the anode. With clockwise rotation of the x-ray tube in the gantry (Fig. 10-16A), the electron beam striking the anode is steered counterclockwise in synchrony with the detector acquisition interval (Fig. 10-16B), and this effectively stops the motion of the x-ray source and helps to preserve spatial resolution. Notice that given the 1- to 2-mm overall dimensions of an x-ray focal spot in a CT scanner x-ray tube, steering the spot a distance of approximately 1.5 mm is realistic in consideration of the physical dimensions of the anode and cathode structures.

One CT manufacturer also uses a focal spot steering approach to provide oversampling in the z-dimension of the scan. This x-ray tube design combines high power with the ability to stagger the position of the x-ray focal spot inside the x-ray tube, as illustrated in Figure 10-17A. The electron beam is steered using magnetic fields provided by steering coils, and due to the steep anode angle, modulating the electron beam landing location on the focal track causes an apparent shift in the source position along the z-axis of the scanner. Another manufacturer uses a different magnetic electron beam steering approach (Figure 10-17B) to achieve a similar effect.

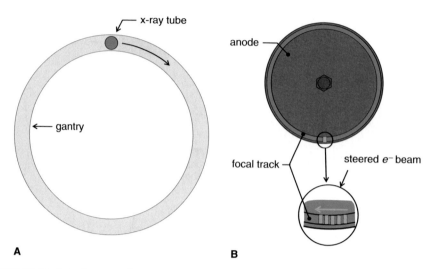

■ **FIGURE 10-16 A.** As the x-ray tube and detector rotate around the table and patient, they can travel on the order of 1 to 2 mm per acquisition cycle, leading to potential motion artifacts. Some manufacturers compensate for this motion by steering the electron beam (**B**) between the cathode and the anode to rotate the focal spot in the opposite direction, partially correcting for gantry motion.

For helical (spiral) scans, this approach leads to an oversampling in the z-dimension, which leads to Nyquist—appropriate sampling in z (see Chapter 4).

X-ray CT scanners typically run at 120 kV for generic scanning; however, more recently, the tube voltage has been used more aggressively to optimize the trade-off between image quality and radiation dose to the patient. The high kV combined with the added filtration in the x-ray tube leads to a relatively "hard" x-ray spectrum. The tube voltage options in CT depend on the vendor; however, 80- 100- 120- and 140-kV spectra are typical (but not exclusive) in the industry (Fig. 10-18). The high x-ray energy used in CT is important for understanding what physical properties of

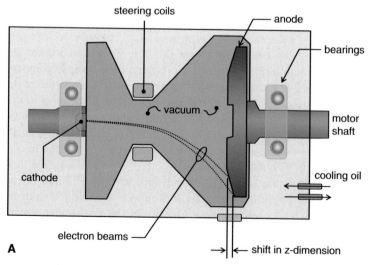

■ **FIGURE 10-17 A.** As the table advances through the gantry, the x-ray beam is rapidly shifted along z using the x-ray design shown in this figure. The magnetic steering coils in the tube assembly shift the electron beam trajectory, resulting in a different location for the focal spot. This design allows oversampling in the z-dimension, improving the spatial resolution in z. Using N actual detectors arrays (in z), with two focal spot positions (about a half detector width apart), a total of 2N detector *channels* are formed.

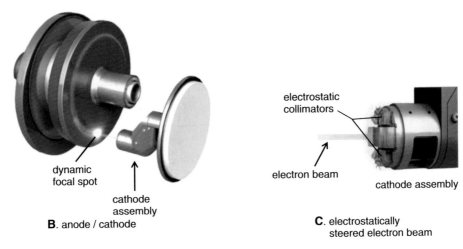

dynamic
focal spot

cathode
assembly

B. anode / cathode

electrostatic
collimators

electron beam

cathode assembly

C. electrostatically
steered electron beam

■ **FIGURE 10-17** (*Continued*) **B.** The alignment of the anode and cathode is shown. **C.** Another vendor approach to focal spot steering uses a more conventional x-ray tube geometry, where electrostatic collimators are used to steer the electron beam to alter its trajectory from cathode to anode. (courtesy J. Hsieh).

tissue are being displayed on CT images. The effective energy of the 80-kV spectrum is about 40 keV, while that of the 140-kV spectrum is approximately 60 keV. The range of effective x-ray energies in typical CT spectra is shown in Figure 10-19, overlaid on the mass attenuation coefficients for soft tissue. In this region, it is seen that Rayleigh scattering has the lowest interaction probability and the Compton scatter interaction has the highest interaction probability. For the 120- to 140-kV spectra, the Compton scattering interaction is 10-fold more likely than the photo-electric effect *in soft tissue*. For soft tissue, the CT image depicts physical properties for which Compton scattering is most dependent on electron density. As discussed in Chapter 3, the Compton scatter linear attenuation coefficient is proportional to

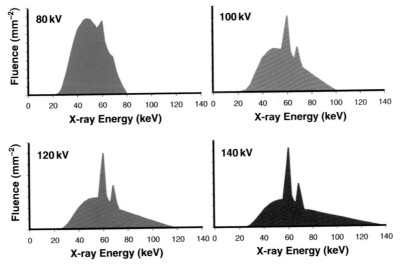

■ **FIGURE 10-18** This figure illustrates typical x-ray spectra that are used by several of the CT manufacturers. Tube voltages of 90, 130, and other slight variations are used by some vendors. The x-ray spectra in CT scanners are hardened using significant thicknesses (5 to 10 mm Al) of added filtration, in addition to the beam shaping filters.

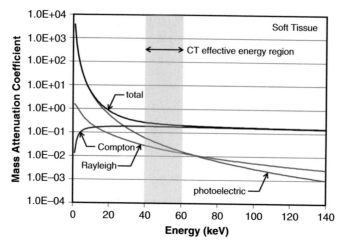

■ FIGURE 10-19 The mass attenuation coefficient for soft tissue is shown as a function of x-ray beam energy, and the various interaction cross sections are shown. For the energy region of CT (~40 to 60 keV effective energy), it is seen that the Compton scatter interaction cross section is much higher than the Rayleigh or photoelectric cross sections. Hence, for soft tissue, the CT image is essentially a map of the parameter that primarily impacts the Compton scatter cross section—electron density.

$$\mu_{Compton} \propto \rho \, N \, \frac{Z}{A} \qquad [10\text{-}1]$$

where $\mu_{Compton}$ is the linear attenuation coefficient for the Compton scattering interaction, ρ is the mass density of the tissue in a voxel, N is Avogadro's number (6.023×10^{23}), Z is the atomic number, and A is the atomic mass. The primary constituents of soft tissue are carbon, hydrogen, oxygen, and nitrogen. It is interesting to note that in all of these elements except hydrogen, the ratio (Z/A) is ½ for commonly occurring isotopes. For hydrogen, the Z/A ratio is 1. While this would imply that hydrogenous tissues such as adipose tissue would have a higher $\mu_{Compton}$, in reality, the range of fluctuation in hydrogen content in tissues is small and the lower density of adipose ($\rho \approx 0.94$ g/cm^3) relative to soft tissue ($\rho \approx 1$) tends to dominate Equation 10-1 when it comes to the difference between soft tissue and adipose tissues. Consequently, adipose tissue appears darker (has a lower $\mu_{Compton}$) than soft tissues such as liver or other organ parenchyma.

Figure 10-19 illustrates the attenuation characteristics of soft tissue, but the relative attenuation coefficients for soft tissue, bone, and iodine are shown in Figure 10-20. Also shown is the range of effective energies for most CT spectra. Because of the higher proportion of photoelectric interactions (relative to Compton) in bone and iodine due to their higher Z, the overall mass attenuation coefficients are higher. The mass attenuation coefficient is defined at unit density, and the higher density of bone ($\rho \approx 2$ to 3) relative to soft tissue further increases the linear attenuation coefficient μ (the linear attenuation coefficient μ is the product of the mass attenuation coefficient [μ/ρ] and density, ρ). Hence, it is clear from Figure 10-20 that bone and pure iodine have larger μ values than soft tissue, water, or adipose.

The gray scale in CT images is a quantitatively meaningful value, unlike any other clinical imaging modality used today. The gray scale values in CT are called Hounsfield units (HUs), in honor of Sir Godfrey Hounsfield who was one of the principal innovators of CT technology in its early days. The HU is defined as

$$HU(x, y, z) = 1000 \frac{\left(\mu(x, y, z) - \mu_w \right)}{\mu_w} \qquad [10\text{-}2]$$

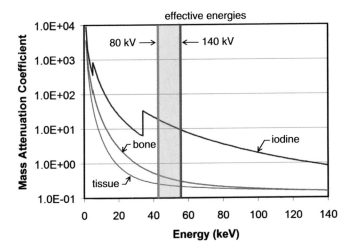

■ FIGURE 10-20 This figure shows the mass attenuation coefficient for bone, tissue, and iodine as a function of x-ray energy. The attenuation coefficient is much greater for bone and greater still for 100% iodine. Typically, tissues have much lower concentrations of iodine. This figure illustrates the basis for contrast in CT between bone-, tissue-, and contrast-enhanced CT.

where $\mu(x,y,z)$ is the average linear attenuation coefficient for a volume element ("voxel") of tissue in the patient at location (x,y,z) (Fig. 10-21). $HU(x,y,z)$ represents the gray scale CT images in the same (x,y,z) spatial coordinates, and μ_w is the linear attenuation coefficient of water for the x-ray spectrum used. Note that when $\mu(x,y,z)$ corresponds to a voxel of water, then the numerator in Equation 10-2 is zero, and $HU = 0$. Because $\mu(x,y,z)$ is essentially zero for air, the ratio on the right in Equation 10-2 becomes -1, and therefore $HU = -1,000$ for air. The HU range is defined only at these two points—water and air. In practice, adipose tissues typically range from $HU = -80$ to -30, and most organ parenchyma runs from approximately $HU = +30$ to $+220$. Tissue with iodinated contrast and bone can run much higher, to a maximum of $HU = 3,095$ for most 12-bit CT scanners. Because urine in the urinary bladder is predominately water, it should be close to $HU = 0$. At all x-ray tube voltages, $HU_{water} \equiv 0$ and $HU_{air} \equiv -1,000$; however, due to energy-dependent attenuation, the HU values of adipose and soft tissues will shift slightly with different tube voltages. This shift should be most apparent for bone and iodine contrast.

The CT reconstruction process converts the raw acquired data from the CT scanner to a series of CT images, usually reconstructed as a series of contiguous axial images. While each of the individual CT images is 2D, in the patient's body that image corresponds to a 3D cross section of tissue as shown in Figure 10-21A. Hence, when referring to the location in the body, the term *volume element* (voxel) is used. Axial and

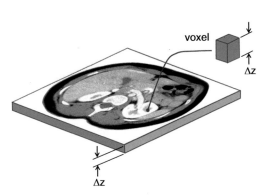

■ FIGURE 10-21 **A.** The dimensions of the in-plane (Δx, Δy) and the slice thickness in the z-axis (Δz) are combined to form the volume element or *voxel*. In modern MDCT scanners, the dimensions of the voxel are approximately equal on thin-slice reconstructions, where $\Delta x = \Delta y \approx \Delta z$.

A. in the patient

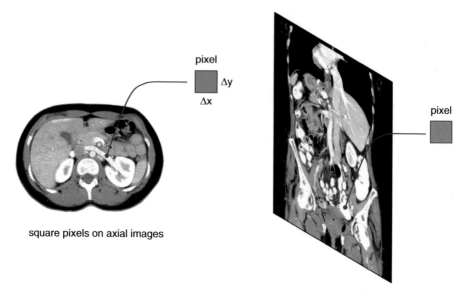

square pixels on axial images

rectangular pixels on coronal images

B. in the images

■ **FIGURE 10-21** (*Continued*) **B.** Despite the three-dimensional nature of most CT scan data, the individual images are fundamentally two dimensional. Like all digital images, each picture element is called a *pixel*. The pixel on an axial image (x,y) is square; however, the coronal image (x, z) and sagittal image (y, z) usually have rectangular pixel which can be resampled along z such that $\Delta x = \Delta y = \Delta z$.

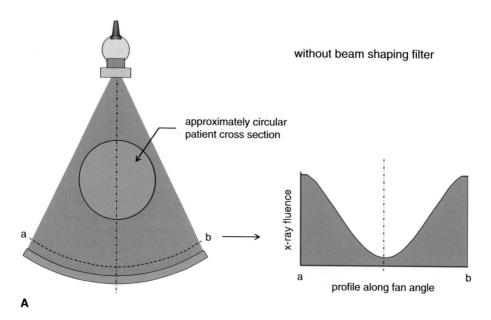

A

■ **FIGURE 10-22 A.** Most body areas scanned by a CT scanner are circular in cross section, and this gives rise to an uncorrected x-ray fluence at the detector that is high at the edges and low in the center, as seen in the profile. A beam shaping filter, also called a bow tie filter, is used on all whole body CT scanners and is located in the x-ray tube assembly. The shape of the filter is designed to attenuate more toward the periphery of the field, which tends to make the signal levels at the detector more homogeneous.

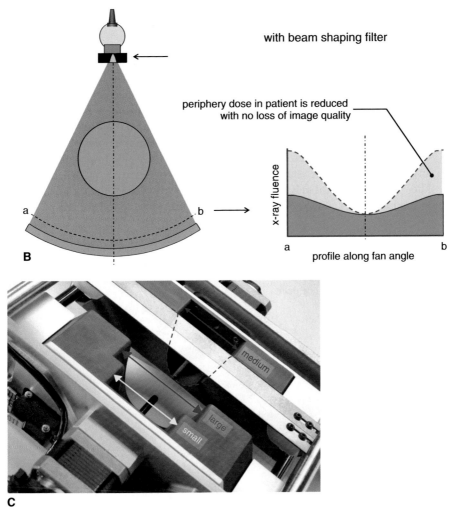

with beam shaping filter

periphery dose in patient is reduced
with no loss of image quality

x-ray fluence

a   b

B

profile along fan angle

medium

large

small

C

■ **FIGURE 10-22** (*Continued*) **B.** This creates the opportunity to reduce dose to the patient with no loss of image quality. **C.** A photograph of a beam shaping filter assembly from a commercial CT scanner is shown. This assembly has three different bow tie filters, as labeled. (Courtesy J. Hsieh.)

coronal CT images are illustrated in Figure 10-21B with one *picture element* (pixel) indicated. The 2D pixels in each image correspond to 3D voxels in the patient.

The vast majority of CT scans are either of the head or of the torso, and the torso is typically broken up into the chest, abdomen, and pelvis. These exams represent over three fourths of all CT procedures in a typical institution. All of these body parts are either round or approximately round in shape. Figure 10-22A shows a typical scan geometry where a circular body part is being scanned. The shape of the attenuated (primary) x-ray beam, which reaches the detectors after attenuation in the patient, is shown in this figure as well, and this shape is due to the attenuation of the patient when no corrective measures are taken. Figure 10-22B shows how the x-ray beam striking the detector array is made more uniform when a beam shaping filter is used. The beam shaping filter, often called a bow tie filter due to its shape, reduces the intensity of the incident x-ray beam in the periphery of the x-ray field where the attenuation path through the patient is generally thinner. This tends to equalize or flatten the x-ray fluence that reaches the detector array. An assembly from a commercial whole body CT scanner employing three different bow tie filters is illustrated in Figure 10-22C.

The bow tie filter has consequences both on patient dose and on image quality. Figure 10-23A shows a central ray (C) and a peripheral ray (P) with no bow tie filter in place. The dose at the entrance points for these two rays is only slightly different due to the slight differences in distance from the x-ray source (i.e., the inverse square law). The dose at the exit points in the central and peripheral rays can be markedly different, however, due to the much longer attenuation path in the central ray compared to that of the peripheral ray. Thus, the dose at the exit point of the peripheral ray is much greater. When these factors are applied and the dose distribution from an entire rotation of the x-ray tube around the patient is considered, when no bow tie filter is used, increased radiation dose at the periphery of the patient results, as shown in Figure 10-23B. An ideal bow tie filter equalizes dose to the patient perfectly, as

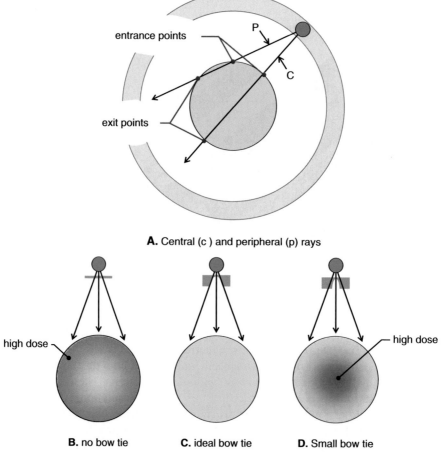

A. Central (c) and peripheral (p) rays

B. no bow tie   **C.** ideal bow tie   **D.** Small bow tie

■ FIGURE 10-23 **A.** The peripheral ray (marked P) passes through a shorter path of tissue to reach the exit point than the central ray (C) on a circular object, and thus the dose at the exit point for ray P is greater than for ray C. When the source is rotated 360 degrees around the object, this consideration leads to higher dose levels at the periphery (**B**) for larger cylindrical objects when no beam shaping filter is used. **C.** With an ideal bow tie filter, the attenuation thicknesses of the object are exactly compensated for, producing a nearly homogeneous dose distribution in the patient. **D.** If a bow tie filter designed for a small cylinder is used for a larger cylinder (such as using a head bow tie for a body scan), the dose will be too concentrated toward the center of the fan angle, and higher doses will result centrally.

shown in Figure 10-23C. If the bow tie filter has too much peripheral beam attenuation, then it will concentrate the radiation toward the center of the patient and lead to higher central doses as in Figure 10-23D.

Since CT images are reconstructed from many projection data acquired around the patient, the image noise at a given pixel in the CT image is the consequence of the noise from all of the projection data which intersect that pixel. The noise variance (σ^2) at a point in the CT image results from the propagation of noise variance from the individual projections (p1, p2, ..., pN). A simplified mathematical description of the noise propagation is given by

$$\sigma^2_{CTimage} = \sigma^2_{p1} + \sigma^2_{p2} + \sigma^2_{p3} + ... \sigma^2_{pN} \qquad [10\text{-}3]$$

For the peripheral beams (such as P in Fig. 10-23A), in the absence of a bow tie filter, the x-ray fluence striking the detectors is high, and thus the noise variance is low. However, because the noise in the CT image results from all the views, some of the projections through any point in the CT image will be from central rays (ray C in Fig. 10-23A), and these rays have lower x-ray fluence and higher statistical variance. Thus, the noise in the reconstructed CT image will be dominated by these higher noise central rays. Consequently, the higher dose that is delivered to the periphery of the patient is essentially wasted and does not contribute to better image quality (i.e., lower noise). Hence, the bow tie filter is a very useful tool because it reduces patient dose with no loss of image quality. The bow tie filter is used in all commercial whole body CT scanners and in all CT acquisition scenarios.

The standard adult head is about 17 cm in diameter, whereas the standard adult torso ranges from 24 up to 45 cm or greater, with an average diameter ranging between 26 and 30 cm. Because of these large differences, all commercial CT scanners make use of a minimum of two bow tie filters—a head and a body bow tie. The head bow tie filter is also used in pediatric body imaging on most scanners.

Detector Arrays

All modern multidetector array CT scanners use indirect (scintillating) solid-state detectors. Intensifying screens used for radiography are composed of rare earth crystals (such as Gd_2O_2S) packed into a binder, which holds the screen together. To improve the detection efficiency of the scintillator material for CT imaging, the scintillation crystals (Gd_2S_2O and other materials as well) are *sintered* to increase physical density and light output. The process of sintering involves heating up the phosphor crystals to just below their melting point for relatively long periods of time (h), and there are many other details to the process. In the end, densification occurs, and the initial scintillating powder is converted into a high-density ceramic. The ceramic phosphor is then scored with a saw or laser to create a number of individual detector elements in a detector module, for example, 64 × 64 detector elements. An opaque filler is pressed into the space between detector elements to reduce optical cross talk between detectors. The entire fabrication includes a photodiode in contact with the ceramic detector (Fig. 10-24).

The detector module sits on top of a larger stack of electronic modules, which provide power to the detector array and receive the electronic signals from each photodiode (Fig. 10-25). The electronics module has gain channels for each detector in the module and also contains the analog-to-digital converter, which converts the amplified electronic signal to a digital number. The detector array modules are mounted onto an aluminum frame on the mechanical gantry assembly.

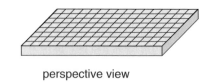

perspective view

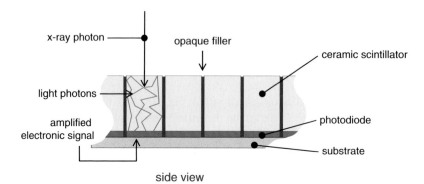

x-ray photon

opaque filler

ceramic scintillator

light photons

amplified
electronic signal

photodiode

substrate

side view

■ **FIGURE 10-24** The detectors in modern CT are fabricated as detector modules (perspective view). A side view of the modern CT detector shows individual detector elements coupled to photodiodes that are layered on substrate electronics. Spaces between detector elements are scored out creating a small void, which is filled with an optical filler material to reduce detector cross talk. CT detectors are much more expensive than those used in radiography and make use of sintered phosphors resulting in high-density ceramic detector arrays. The increased density improves x-ray detection efficiency.

The aluminum frame forms an approximate radius of curvature from the position of the x-ray source. Each detector module can be removed and exchanged on the gantry for rapid repair, when necessary.

Figure 10-26 illustrates cross sections through the x-ray beam and detector array for three different models of CT scanners—a single array CT (for comparison),

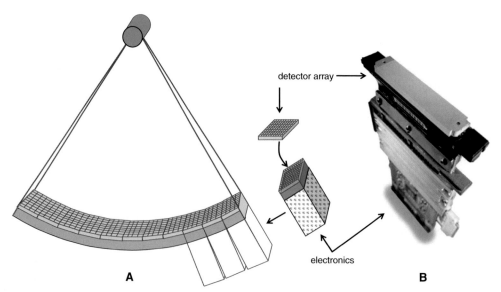

detector array

electronics

A

B

■ **FIGURE 10-25 A.** The detector arrays are mounted on electronics module, which includes power supplies for the amplifiers, amplification circuits for the detector module, and analog-to-digital converter systems. **B.** A photograph of a detector module with electronics from a commercial CT scanner is shown. (Photograph courtesy J. Hsieh.)

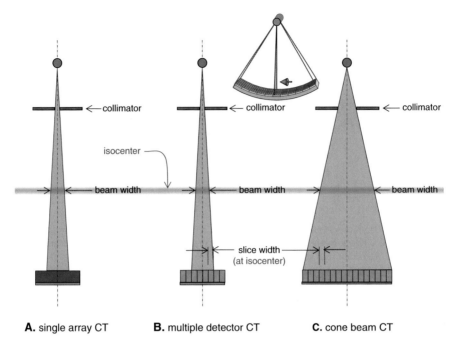

A. single array CT   **B.** multiple detector CT   **C.** cone beam CT

■ **FIGURE 10-26 A.** A cross section (see inset figure showing orientation) of a single array CT scanner is shown. Adjustment of slice thickness in single detector CT involved the relatively simple manipulation of the x-ray beam width using the collimator. **B.** Multiple detector array CT (MDCT) systems result in a divorce between slice thickness and x-ray beam width. The detector array width (T) determines the minimum CT slice width, while the overall x-ray beam thickness (>nT) is determined by the collimator. **C.** Cone beam CT systems are essentially MDCT systems that have a very large number of detector arrays. While typical state-of-the-art MDCT systems may use 64 to 128 detector channels, some manufacturers have expanded this to 256 to 320 element detector arrays (T = 0.5 mm), which give rise to a collimated beam width of 160 mm.

a small multiple detector array CT (MDCT), and a larger MDCT system. In a single detector array scanner, the detectors were 13 to 16 mm wide, and the x-ray beam collimation was used to determine the slice thickness. Collimator settings ranged from 1 mm (thin slice) to 10 mm (thick slice) or larger. The single detector array system integrated the x-ray signal over the entire width of each detector, and so changing slice thickness was solely a function of the collimation. Thin slices could be acquired, but a greater number of CT acquisitions were required to interrogate a given length of the patient's anatomy. For example, to scan 20 cm in the abdomen with contiguous images, a total of 100 CT images need to be acquired for 2-mm slice thicknesses (t = 2 mm). For a typical 1-s scan time, this would require 100 s of actual scan time (longer in practice due to breathing gaps). That was generally too long to be practical, and thus 7- or 10-mm slices would typically be acquired, requiring 28 scans (28 s) or 20 scans (20 s), respectively.

With MDCT, the slice thickness and x-ray beam width are decoupled. The slice thickness is determined by the detector configuration, and the x-ray beam width is determined by the collimator. In the standard vernacular of CT, the detector thickness is T (measured at isocenter) and the number of detectors is n. For one manufacturer's 64 slice (n) scanner, $T = 0.625$ mm and so the collimated x-ray beam width is $nT = 40$ mm. For contiguous images, the 20-cm section of abdomen discussed in the paragraph above could be acquired in just 5 scans (5 × 40 mm = 200 mm), and a total of 256 CT images, each 0.625 mm thick, would be acquired. So compared to the single slice CT system, the scan time in this example went from 100 to 5 s,

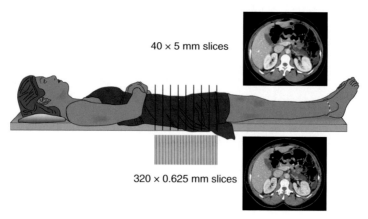

40 × 5 mm slices

320 × 0.625 mm slices

■ **FIGURE 10-27** Slice thickness plays an important role in regard to the relationship between radiation dose and CT image noise. Although very thin CT images can be produced by all modern MDCT scanners, the user needs to balance this advantage of spatial resolution in the z-dimension with the clinical necessity for low-dose CT imaging. One CT acquisition can produce thin-section relatively noisy images (0.625) that have high z-axis resolution, and thick-section lower noise images can also be produced for primary interpretation.

and the slice thickness went from 2 to 0.625 mm. These capabilities underscore the advances that MDCT offers—faster scans and thinner slices.

Dose and Image Noise Consequences of CT Section Thickness

Take an example where a top of the line MDCT (64 slice or larger) scans 200 mm of anatomy with $nT = 40$ mm. Five gantry rotations (pitch = 1, as discussed later) are required[*], and with a 0.5-s scan, this takes 2.5 s. A total of 320 very thin (0.625 mm) CT scans can be reconstructed, delivering excellent spatial resolution along the z-axis of the patient. Compare this to combining the acquired projection data from 8 contiguous detectors (8 × 0.625 mm = 5 mm), and reconstructing 5-mm thick CT images, which would lead to 40 images covering the same 200-mm section of anatomy (Fig. 10-27). For a fixed technique (e.g., 120 kV, 300 mA, and pitch = 1.0 for a helical scan), the radiation dose to the patient will be the same. Indeed, the two image data sets described above were reconstructed from the same physical CT acquisition, so of course the dose was the same. However, the thinner $T = 0.625$ mm images are eight times thinner than the $T = 5$ mm images, and consequently each thin CT image makes use of eight times fewer detected x-ray photons. The $T = 0.625$ mm images provide more spatial resolution in the z-axis. However, the use of an eightfold reduction in photons means that they are a factor of $\sqrt{8} = 2.8$ times noisier. This can be seen in Figure 10-27. One can acquire thin $T = 0.625$ mm images with the same noise levels as the 5-mm images, by increasing the dose by a factor of 8. For example, at 120 kV as before, increase the mA to 600 (2×), increase the scan time from 0.5 to 1.0 s (2×), and go to a pitch of 0.5 (2×). However, given heightened concerns about the radiation dose levels in CT, using thicker CT slices for interpretation is a good way to reduce noise while keeping dose levels low.

The message of the above observations is this: Even though MDCT scanners allow a vast number of thin images to be reconstructed, there is a trade-off in terms of image noise, patient dose, and z-axis resolution, and that trade-off needs to balance patient dose with image quality (resolution and noise).

---

[*]Actually six rotations are required in helical mode on some systems, as discussed later.

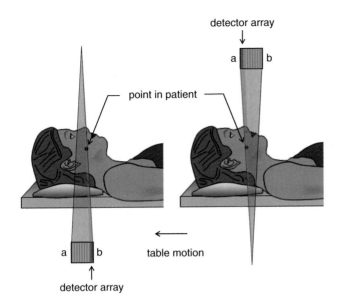

detector array

a b

point in patient

a b   table motion

detector array

■ FIGURE 10-28 In MDCT scanners operating in helical (spiral) acquisition mode with the pitch near 1.0, essentially all of the detector arrays contribute to the raw data acquisition for each CT image. Because of this, the beam profile for all detector arrays needs to be approximately the same, otherwise, artifacts will result. This means that the x-ray beam penumbra needs to be located outside of the active detector array, resulting in some dose inefficiencies with MDCT.

Overbeaming and Geometrical Efficiency

For helical (spiral) scanning on a MDCT system, a given voxel in the patient is reconstructed from the data acquired by most or all of the detector arrays as the patient's body translates through the gantry. Figure 10-28 shows how the rightmost detector array (b) acquires the x-ray projection of a given point in the patient, but as the table advances through the gantry and as the gantry rotates, a different detector array (a) acquires the x-ray projection through this point in the patient. If the z-axis beam width or shape differed significantly from detector array to detector array in the system, then the projection data used to reconstruct each CT image would differ around 360 degrees and artifacts would occur. The artifact would be most pronounced when there is an abrupt change in attenuation in the z-dimension such as at the end of a bone. The x-ray beam has relatively constant intensity throughout its center, but the consequences of the finite focal spot and the highly magnified collimator give rise to a penumbra at the edges of the beam (Fig. 10-29). Because the beam shape is so different in the penumbra region compared to the center of the beam, the penumbra region is to be avoided, and hence the penumbra is positioned outside of the active detector arrays—those x-rays essentially strike lead shielding on the sides of the detector assembly or inactive detectors. This is called *overbeaming*. Note that for a single detector array scanner, this is not necessary. The consequence of overbeaming is that for MDCT scanners, the geometrical efficiency is less than the 100% geometrical efficiency of a single detector array scanner. In the early days of MDCT scanners when 4 or 8 detector arrays were used, the geometrical efficiency was quite low (~70%), and consequently there was a considerable radiation dose penalty (~30%) that resulted. As more detector arrays were used and as the beam width in the z-dimension consequently increased, the penumbra region of the beam became a smaller fraction of the overall x-ray beam flux, and the geometrical efficiency increased as a result. With state-of-the-art MDCT scanners ($\geq$64 detector channels), the geometrical efficiency is greater than 95%.

Selection of CT Slice Width

As mentioned previously (Fig. 10-26), for single detector array CT, the slice width was selected by adjusting the collimator width. With MDCT, the collimator adjusts

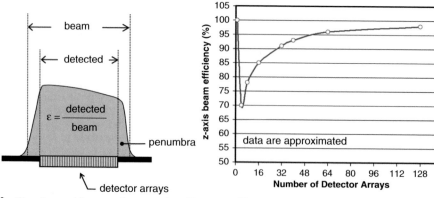

A. The shape of the x-ray beam and position of x-ray detector arrays are illustrated

B. The relative geometric dose efficiency as a function of detector arrays is shown

■ **FIGURE 10-29** **A.** The z-axis dose profile of a typical MDCT scanner is illustrated and the influence of heel effect is seen. The beam profile slopes off dramatically in the penumbra, and therefore the penumbra edge is placed outside the active detector arrays. The x-ray beam that does not strike active detectors represents a reduction of geometrical dose efficiency. **B.** The dose efficiency is shown as a function of the number of the detector arrays. In the early days of MDCT systems with only a few detector arrays (n ≈ 4 to 16), the wasted dose in the penumbra was a considerable fraction (up to 30%) of the total x-ray beam. As detector arrays become wider, the fraction of the beam represented by the penumbra is reduced, giving rise to very acceptable geometrical efficiencies for MDCT systems with more numerous arrays.

the overall beam width (nT) and the slice thickness is governed by the width of the detector arrays (T). For a state-of-the-art scanner (typically ≥64 detector channels), each detector array has its own data channel and all of the detector array signals are recorded during a CT scan. Let's use the example of a 64-slice scanner with 0.5-mm-wide detector arrays (at isocenter). All of the data are recorded, and so the system can be instructed to reconstruct 64 × 0.50 mm slices, or 32 × 1.0 mm, 16 × 2.0 mm, 8 × 4.0 mm, 4 × 8.0 mm, etc. Any combination of signals from adjacent detector arrays is possible, although the actual selections on commercial scanners are limited to standard, usable combinations. So assuming that the acquired raw data exist on the CT scanner console, one can go back days later and re-reconstruct the CT slice thickness to any selectable value on the scanner. However, the raw CT data only reside on the scanner's computer for a period of time until it is overwritten with new data—how long that is depends on how large the data drive is and how many CT scans are performed with the system in a day—in busy settings, the raw data are available for a day or less. With these scanners, it is typical to reconstruct 5.0-mm axial slices for radiologist interpretation, and 0.50- to 0.625-mm axial slices to be used for reformatting to coronal or sagittal data sets.

In older MDCT scanners with 4 to 32 detector arrays, the number of data acquisition channels in many cases was less than the number of detector arrays. For example, one vendor's 16-detector scanner had only 4 data channels. In this setting, the desired slice thickness had to be selected *prior* to the CT scan. For the 1.25-mm detector width, the user could acquire 4 × 1.25 mm for a total collimated beam width of 5.0 mm. The signals from adjacent detector arrays can be combined, and so by "binning" together signals from two adjacent detector arrays, the scanner could acquire 4 × 2.5 mm data (10.0-mm collimation). By binning 3 and 4 adjacent detector signals, 4 × 3.75 (15-mm collimation) or 4 × 5.0 mm (20-mm collimation) could also be acquired, respectively (Fig. 10-30).

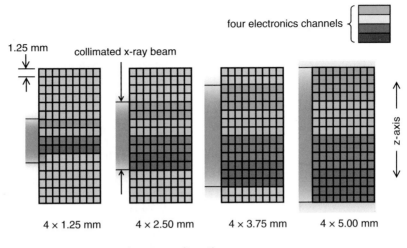

■ **FIGURE 10-30** For the early MDCT systems, the number of electronics channels was less than the number of detector arrays, and so a decision of CT slice thickness had to be made *prior* to acquisition. For a standard 16-slice CT scanner as illustrated here, with 4 channels of electronics, the detectors could be used individually (4 × 1.25 mm data sets) or could be binned to produce thicker slices and better CT coverage (e.g., 4 × 5.0 mm data sets).

10.3 Modes of CT Acquisition

Scanned Projection Radiograph

Once the patient is on the table and the table is moved into the gantry bore, the technologist performs a preliminary scan called the CT radiograph. This image is also called the scout view, topogram, scanogram, or localizer; however, some of these terms are copyrighted to specific vendors. The CT radiograph is acquired with the CT x-ray tube and detector arrays stationary, the patient is translated through the gantry, and a digital radiographic image is generated from this line-scan data. CT systems can scan anterior-posterior (AP), posterior-anterior (PA), or lateral. It is routine to use one CT radiograph for patient alignment; however, some institutions use the lateral localizer as well to assure patient centering. The PA CT radiograph is preferred over the AP to reduce breast dose in women and girls.

Using the CT radiograph, the CT technologist uses the software on the CT console to set up the CT scan geometry (Fig. 10-31). The process for doing this is specific to each vendor's CT scanner; however, a common theme is to place guidelines to define each end of the CT scan. It is at this point in the scanning procedure that all the CT scan parameters are set, usually using preset protocols. For a basic CT scan, these parameters include kV, mA, gantry rotation time(s), type of scan (helical or axial), direction of scan, pitch, detector configuration, reconstruction kernels(s), mA modulation parameters, if used, and so on. Complexity increases for more advanced scanning protocols.

Basic Axial/Sequential Acquisition

The axial (also called sequential) CT scan is the basic step-and-shoot mode of a CT scanner (Fig. 10-32). The gantry rotates at typical rotation speeds of 0.5 s or so, but

■ FIGURE 10-31 The CT radiograph, known by a number of other names, is typically acquired first and is used by the technologist to set up the extent of the CT exam. Bounding lines for an abdominal pelvis CT scan are shown.

CT radiograph

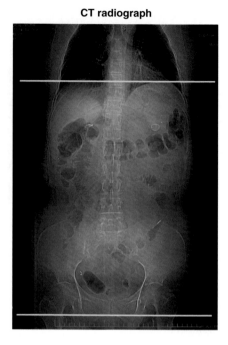

the x-ray tube is not turned on all the time. The table is stationary during the axial data acquisition sequences. The system acquires 360 degrees of projection data with the x-ray tube activated, the tube is deactivated, the table is moved with the x-ray beam off, another scan is acquired, and so on. This process is repeated until the entire

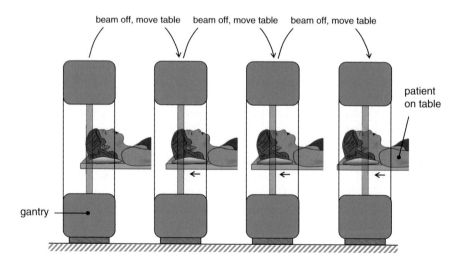

beam off, move table   beam off, move table   beam off, move table

patient on table

gantry

Axial or Sequential CT Acquisition

■ FIGURE 10-32 Axial (also called sequential) CT scanning is the basic step-and-shoot mode of the CT scanner—the x-ray beam is not "on" while the patient is being translated between acquisition cycles. For MDCT systems, the table advance between each scan is designed to allow the production of contiguous CT images in the z-axis direction. Thus, for a scanner with 64 (*n*) detector arrays with width *T* = 0.625 mm, the table is moved a distance of about *nT* between axial acquisitions—about 40 mm in this example.

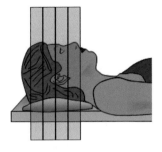

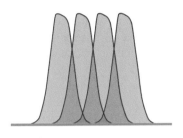

■ FIGURE 10-33 For axial (or sequential) CT imaging with contiguous spacing, (**A**) while the table increment results in contiguous images, because the x-ray beam is slightly wider than the beam width (*nT*), there is overlap of the x-ray beam (**B**) between locations that increases the radiation dose to the patient in these regions.

A. contiguous axial imaging   **B.** dose overlap between scans

anatomical area is covered. Because the table and patient are stationary during an axial scan, the x-ray tube trajectory defines a perfect circle around the patient. Due to the table's start/stop sequence, axial CT requires more acquisition time than helical scanning (described below). With the advent of MDCT, it is common to acquire *contiguous* CT images during an axial acquisition. This implies that between each axial acquisition, the table moves a distance D, which is essentially equal to the width of the detector array at isocenter (nT). This results in a series of images in the CT volume data set, which are contiguous and evenly spaced along the z-direction. In practice, the x-ray beam width is slightly wider than the distance nT, and so the series of axial scans results in some x-ray beam overlap between the axial acquisitions (Fig. 10-33).

Helical (Spiral) Acquisition

With helical (also called spiral) scanning, the table moves at a constant speed while the gantry rotates around the patient. This geometry results in the x-ray source forming a helix around the patient, as shown in Figure 10-34. The advantage of helical

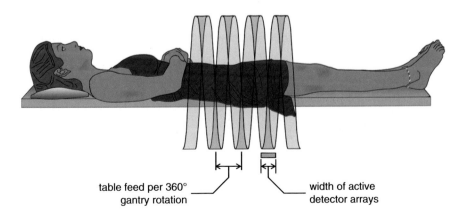

table feed per 360°
gantry rotation

width of active
detector arrays

Helical or Spiral CT Acquisition

■ FIGURE 10-34 With helical (or spiral) CT scanning, the x-ray tube has a helical trajectory around the patient's body, as illustrated. There is an important relationship between the width of the active detector arrays used during the scan and the table feed per rotation of the gantry—this relationship is defined at the *pitch*.

scanning is speed—by eliminating the start/stop motion of the table as in axial CT, there are no inertial constraints to the procedure. Similar to the threads on a screw, the *pitch* describes the relative advancement of the CT table per rotation of the gantry. The pitch of the helical scan is defined as

$$pitch = \frac{F_{table}}{nT} \qquad [10\text{-}4]$$

where F_{table} is the table feed distance per 360-degree rotation of the gantry and nT is the nominal collimated beam width. For example, for a 40-mm (nT) detector width in z and a 0.5-s rotation time for the gantry, a pitch of 1.0 would be obtained if the table moved 80 mm/s. For most CT scanning, the pitch can range between 0.75 and 1.5; however, some vendors give more flexibility in pitch selection than others. A pitch of 1.0 corresponds in principle to contiguous axial CT. A pitch lower than 1.0 (Fig. 10-35B) results in overscanning the patient and hence higher radiation dose to the patient than a pitch of 1.0, all other factors being equal. A pitch greater than 1.0 represents underscanning (Fig. 10-35C), and results in lower radiation dose to the patient. The relationship between relative dose and pitch is given by

$$dose \propto \frac{1}{pitch} \qquad [10\text{-}5]$$

Pitch settings near 1.5 allow for faster scanning and are used for thoracic or pediatric CT scanning where speed is important. Low pitch values are used in cardiac imaging, or when a very large patient is to be scanned and the other technique factors (kV and mAs) are already maximized.

Because the table is moving along the z-axis during helical acquisition, there is a slight motion artifact that reduces the spatial resolution very slightly. However, this concern is generally balanced by the speed of the helical CT scan and the corresponding reduction in patient motion blurring that results. This is especially important in the torso, where the beating heart and churning intestines cannot be voluntarily stopped in even the most compliant of patients.

The acquired data at the very beginning and end of a helical scan do not have sufficient angular coverage to reconstruct artifact-free CT images. Consequently, along the z-direction, helical scans start ½ nT before an axial scan would start, and stop ½ nT after an axial scan would end. For example, for a scan where nT = 20 mm and there is a desired scan length of 200 mm, an axial scan would scan only the desired

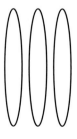 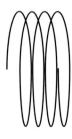 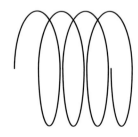

A. axial / sequential   **B.** low pitch helical / spiral   **C.** high pitch helical / spiral

■ **FIGURE 10-35 A.** A series of axial or sequential CT scans results in a number of circular x-ray tube trajectories around the patient, requiring the x-ray tube to be turned off between each axial scan. For helical (or spiral) scanning, the helix can be "tight" corresponding to a low-pitch study (**B**), or it can be "loose" corresponding to a high-pitch CT study (**C**). Pitch values in conventional (noncardiac) CT scanning run typically between 0.75 and 1.5.

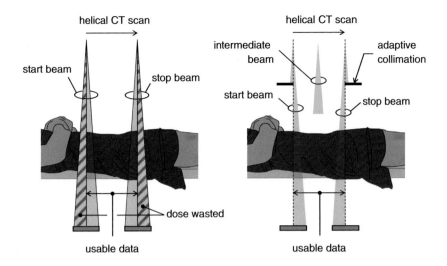

A. no adaptive beam collimation   **B.** adaptive beam collimation

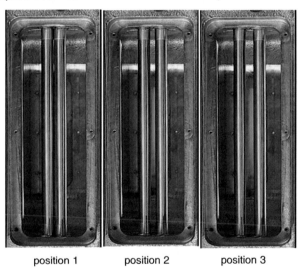

position 1   position 2   position 3
C. adaptive beam collimators

■ **FIGURE 10-36** For helical (or spiral) CT scanning without adaptive beam collimation (**A**), half of the x-ray beam width at both ends of the scan is not used because those data do not have sufficient angular sampling to produce high-quality CT images, and this results in dose inefficiency. The inefficiency is worse for wider x-ray beams and for shorter scan lengths. **B.** With adaptive beam collimation, collimators are used to eliminate patient exposure at the edges of the scan, improving the dose efficiency of the helical CT acquisition. **C.** Adaptive beam collimators are illustrated in these photographs. The vertical rods are cam shaped, and independent rotation provides the effect illustrated in (**B**). (Courtesy J. Hsieh.)

200 mm, but a helical scan would require 220 mm of acquisition to reconstruct that same 200 mm of image data. Thus, in this example, 10% of the radiation dose to the patient is essentially wasted. Newer helical systems, however, have adaptive beam collimation (various trade names exist) as shown in Figure 10-36. With this shielding, the wasted dose at the outer edges of a helical scan is collimated out. The amount of dose that is saved as a percentage of the overall dose increases for scans of smaller scan length, and for CT scanners with larger collimated beam widths (nT). Some manufacturers achieve adaptive beam collimation using an additional

set of motorized collimators in the x-ray tube head assembly, while others use a cam-shaped collimator, which can rotate to achieve the same effect (Fig. 10-36C).

The speed of a CT scan using a modern CT system is quite remarkable, and this is one of the key reasons why CT is so widely used for clinical diagnosis. An example will illustrate this. An abdomen-pelvis CT scan requires a scan length of 48 cm on a tall patient. Using a modern MDCT scanner with a collimated nominal beam width of 40 mm, a pitch of 1.0, and a gantry rotation time of 0.5 s, the scan can be completed in 6 s, well within a breath-hold for most patients.

Cone Beam Acquisition

All top of the line (≥64 detector channels) CT systems are technically cone beam CT systems, as the reconstruction algorithm used for converting the raw data into CT images takes into account the cone angle. However, most conventional CT systems still make use of only slight cone angles on the order of 2 degrees (cone half-angle). Some vendors, however, have developed what could be called true cone beam CT scanners— where the half cone angle approaches 10 degrees. For example, one vendor has a 320-detector array system with 0.5-mm detectors, so the entire z-axis coverage is 16 cm (Fig. 10-37). There are of course benefits and tradeoffs with such a wide cone beam design. The challenges of wide cone beam imaging include increased x-ray scatter and increased cone beam artifacts. The benefit of this design, however, is that whole organ imaging can be achieved without table motion—so for CT angiography (CTA) or perfusion studies, the anatomical coverage is sufficient for most organs (head, kidneys, heart, etc.), and so whole organ perfusion imaging with high temporal resolution is possible.

Cardiac CT

The challenges of imaging the heart have to do with temporal resolution. With a typical heart rate of 60 beats per minute, one cardiac cycle is about 1 s. To freeze cardiac motion, an image acquisition time window of 100 ms or less is required. With that as

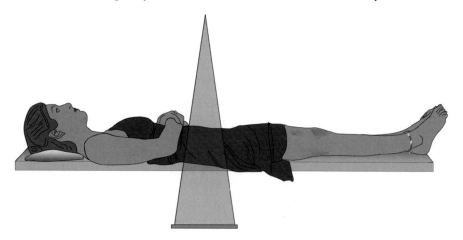

Full Cone Beam CT Acquisition

■ FIGURE 10-37 For some CT scanners such as the 320-detector system, which has a 160-mm-wide x-ray beam at the isocenter of the scanner, cone beam acquisition strategies are used for whole organ imaging. This is essentially an axial CT scan that is capable of acquiring the entire data set along z, without table translation, owing to the very large detector array and cone angle. Other full cone beam systems used in radiation oncology and dental CT use flat panel detectors that extend up to 300 mm in width.

a goal, scientists in the 1980s developed an electron beam CT (EBCT) scanner, which could image the heart with a scan time of about 50 ms. This scanner had a series of semicircular tungsten rings below the patient. An electron beam accelerated at approximately 120 kV was magnetically steered, such that it rotated around the tungsten rings very rapidly, forming a dynamically moving x-ray source for the EBCT scanner. An annular array of detectors was mounted above the patient. For true CT reconstruction, data only need to be acquired 180 degrees plus the fan angle. For the heart, the fan angle is small, and so the requirements are essentially 180 to 190 degrees for a properly centered patient. This unconventional EBCT scanner set the standards for high-speed CT imaging in an era when contemporary CT technology required 3- to 5-s CT scans per image. However, modern third-generation CT systems have developed to the point where cardiac imaging can be performed on more conventional CT hardware.

To image the entire heart using most current rotate-rotate (third-generation) CT scanners, cardiac gating techniques are required. With cardiac gating methods, the image data for CT reconstruction are acquired over several cardiac cycles. Gating methods are made more challenging if the cardiac cycle changes from cycle to cycle, and thus patients with regular heat beats are the ideal candidates for cardiac CT. To steady the heart rate of patients with irregular heart beat, beta-blockers can be administered prior to imaging, and this has been found to produce high-quality cardiac CT images in many settings.

Figure 10-38A shows the general imaging geometry for cardiac imaging. When third-generation cardiac scanners were introduced, it was common to use retrospective gating techniques (Fig. 10-38B). With this approach, the heart was imaged continuously with the rapidly rotating CT scanner, and the electrocardiogram (ECG) data were recorded in synchrony with the CT data acquisition. Because the heart is longer in the z-dimension than what many MDCT scanners can image (nT), the procedure for imaging the heart requires data acquisition at several table positions, so that the entire length of the heart is imaged. As long as the cardiac cycle is not in complete synchrony with the scanner's gantry rotation speed, after several cardiac cycles, enough data would be acquired over different phases of the cardiac cycle to reconstruct the heart. With retrospective reconstruction, projection data are acquired

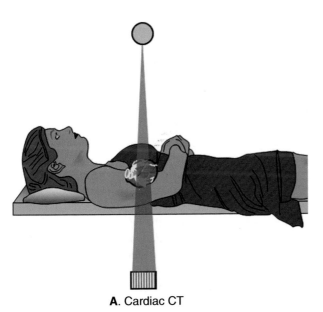

■ FIGURE 10-38 **A.** Cardiac CT systems use multiple rotations of data acquisition over time to acquire the data necessary for reconstructing high-quality images of the heart.

A. Cardiac CT

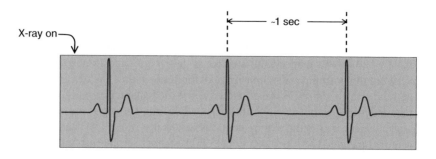

B. retrospective cardiac gating

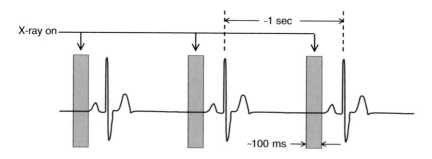

C. prospective cardiac gating

■ **FIGURE 10-38** (*Continued*) **B.** Early cardiac CT acquisition modes used retrospective gating, where the CT scanner acquires data while it also records the electrocardiogram (ECG) information. This allowed the acquired projection data to be selected at various time points in the cardiac cycle ("gated"), and these projection data are then combined and used to reconstruct cardiac CT images—with retrospective gating, CT images could be produced throughout the cardiac cycle, resulting in the generation of a 3D movie of the beating heart. However, this acquisition mode results in high dose to the patient and there is only occasional need for cardiac imaging throughout the entire cardiac cycle. **C.** In prospective cardiac gating modes, the ECG is used to trigger the x-ray tube such that projection data are only acquired during the most quiescent part of the cardiac cycle, end-diastole. This mode reduces dose to the patient considerably and produces one cardiac CT image that is useful for assessing coronary artery stenosis and other anatomical anomalies in the heart.

over the entire cardiac cycle. Therefore, CT images can be synthesized using the ECG gating information over the entire cardiac cycle, and a rendered "beating heart" image can be produced. In clinical practice, however, most of the interest in cardiac CT imaging is in identifying blockages in the coronary arteries, as these represent the greatest risk to the patient. For the evaluation of coronary stenoses, a temporal depiction of the heart is not necessary and only the end-diastole images are necessary. While the dynamic information achieved from retrospective cardiac imaging is visually dramatic, it represents a high-dose procedure.

Most cardiac CT systems have advanced, so that prospective gating techniques can be used (Fig 10-38C). With prospective gating, the ECG triggers the x-ray tube such that projection data are acquired only during the end-diastolic period of the cardiac cycle—this is the point in the cardiac cycle where the heart is the most stationary. The benefit of prospective cardiac CT is that the radiation dose to the patient is significantly less than with retrospective gating. The downside of prospective gating is that a full temporal record of the beating heart is not acquired, only one snapshot during end-diastole, but as mentioned previously, this image is usually sufficient for evaluation of coronary artery disease. Another downside of prospective gating is that if the patient's heart beat is irregular during the scan, the acquisition may lead to an incomplete CT data set, which may not be recoverable. An alternative to a full prospective mode (Fig. 10-38C) is to use higher mA during the end-diastole periods as shown in Figure 10-38C, but to use a lower mA during the rest of the cardiac cycle, so that images (albeit of higher noise) could be reconstructed even when an irregular cardiac cycle is encountered during the scan.

One CT vendor has taken a more aggressive approach toward building a cardiac CT scanner, by building a CT system that has two entire imaging chains on it (Fig. 10-39). There is a large FOV imaging chain comprising an x-ray tube (Tube A) and a full fan beam gantry, and a second imaging chain with another x-ray tube (Tube B) and a smaller detector array is mounted almost orthogonal to the first system. The B-imaging chain has a smaller FOV because of space limitations on the gantry. Furthermore, the FOV required for imaging the relatively small heart does not have to be as large as a standard FOV for imaging the body. The reason why this system is well suited for cardiac imaging is described in the next paragraph.

True CT reconstruction requires only 180 degrees plus the fan angle, and as mentioned previously, due to the small dimensions of the heart, the fan angle is small as well. The full 360-degree gantry rotation of the dual source CT (DSCT) system is 0.33 s, and so a 180-degree rotation requires $\frac{1}{2} \times 0.33$ s = 166 ms. With two redundant x-ray systems configured approximately 90 degrees with respect to each other, a quarter of a rotation of the gantry results in a full 180-degree acquisition data set when the projection data from both imaging chains are combined. The 90-degree rotation of the gantry requires just $\frac{1}{4} \times 330$ ms = 83 ms. Hence, with the speed of gantry rotation combined with the two redundant x-ray imaging systems, the DSCT scanner can acquire data fast enough during end-diastole to freeze the motion of the heart and provide an excellent diagnostic tool for the diagnosis of coronary artery stenosis.

It is noted that cardiac CT requires only an intravenous injection of contrast agent, while the competing technology coronary angiography requires intra-arterial contrast injection, a far more invasive procedure. So for *diagnostic* cardiac procedures, CT techniques offer the patient and their physician a less invasive diagnostic procedure. However, for cardiac *interventional* procedures involving balloon angioplasty with or without the placement of coronary stents, coronary angiography is still required.

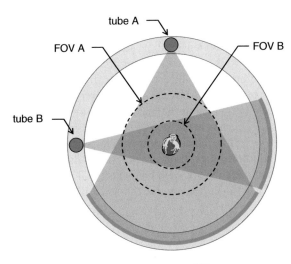

dual source CT

■ FIGURE 10-39 The dual source CT system was developed specifically for cardiac imaging. This system has two full x-ray imaging systems—two x-ray tubes and two sets of detector arrays; however, due to space issues, the B imaging chain has a smaller detector array resulting in a smaller field of view, but still well tailored to the imaging requirements for the heart. Due to the approximately 90-degree juxtaposition of the two imaging chains, a 90-degree rotation of the gantry results in the acquisition of projection data over 180 degrees, which is sufficient for true CT reconstruction at the center of the field of view. With a 330-ms period for 360-degree gantry rotation, the 90-degree rotation requires 330/4 = 83 ms. Thus, it is a short enough time period to acquire a full projection data for CT reconstruction within a fraction of the typical cardiac cycle.

Dual Energy CT

In his original notes on CT, Hounsfield predicted the use of CT for dual energy decomposition methods to separate density from the elemental composition of materials. The initial experimental work on dual energy x-ray imaging was performed on a CT scanner in the mid-1970s, as this was the only platform at that time that could conveniently produce digital images. Dual energy CT is similar conceptually to dual energy projection imaging discussed in Chapter 7.

The concept of using CT for dual energy imaging has been known in the research arena for decades, but it is likely that the dual source CT scanner described above for cardiac imaging launched the most recent clinical interest in dual energy CT. The DSCT scanner was designed primarily for cardiac imaging; however, the availability of two complete x-ray systems on the same gantry clearly lends itself to the acquisition of a low and high kV data set during the same CT acquisition. On single source CT systems, other manufacturers have developed the ability to rapidly switch the kV to achieve dual energy acquisition in a single acquisition. However, it is more difficult to switch the tube current (mA) with high temporal frequency since the tube current is determined by the x-ray tube filament temperature, which cannot be modulated at kilohertz rates due to the thermal inertia of the filament. This is an issue because optimization studies of dual energy CT imaging demonstrate that the low kV (80 kV) needs higher output levels than the high kV (140 kV) setting. However, at the same mA, the x-ray tube is far more efficient at x-ray production at high energies. Averaged across four major CT manufacturers, the output (air kerma) at the isocenter of the scanner at the same mAs is about 3.3 times higher at the highest kV setting (135 to 140 kV) compared to the lowest kV setting (80 to 90 kV). To overcome this, single tube CT scanners increase the temporal pulse width at the lower kV setting to increase the relative signal levels at the lower tube potential.

There are trade-offs for dual energy CT between the dual source and single source approaches. The dual source system has a smaller Tube B FOV, which limits the FOV of the dual energy reconstruction. Also, because both x-ray systems are operational simultaneously on a DSCT system, scatter from one imaging chain impacts the other and this requires correction techniques, which ultimately result in more noise in the data. On the other hand, DSCT systems have two distinct x-ray imaging chains and so additional added filtration can be added to the higher kV source, which increases energy separation and improves the energy subtraction.

There are two approaches to reconstructing dual energy CT images—the raw dual energy image data sets for each projection angle can be subjected to logarithmic weighted subtraction techniques, similar to those used in projection radiography, and then the dual energy subtracted projection data can be used to reconstruct dual energy CT images. Alternatively, the low kV and high kV data sets can be reconstructed separately and subtraction techniques or other digital image manipulation can be applied directly to the reconstructed CT images. In clinical practice, the latter technique is most widely used. Note that the HU values in CT are already linear with respect to the linear attenuation coefficient, and so no additional logarithms are necessary. Ultimately, the dual energy image is a linear combination of the low- and high-energy CT images. Figure 10-40 illustrates the mapping of HU values between the 80- and 140-kV images.

CT Angiography

CT has higher contrast resolution than traditional angiography, and consequently requires only venous access as opposed to more invasive arterial access for

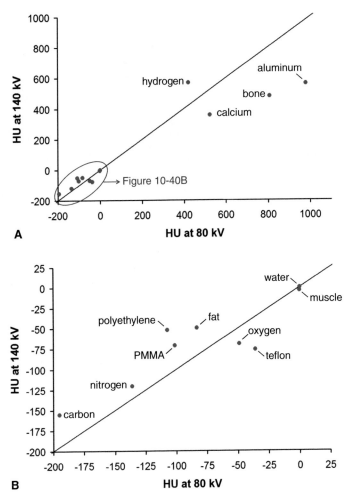

■ **FIGURE 10-40** This figure shows the Hounsfield units for a number of elements, biological compounds, and tissues *at unit density*. The 80 kV HU values are plotted on the horizontal axis, while the 140 kV HU values are plotted on the vertical axis. **A.** A plot covering large HU values is shown. It is noted that higher Z materials are below the line of identity. The Zs of hydrogen, aluminum, and calcium are 1, 13, and 20, respectively. The HU of calcium assumes 10% density. **B.** This plot zooms in on HU values in a range closer to water. Water has an effective Z of 7.42, and materials with a lower effective Z than water are above the line of identity, while materials with a higher effective Z are below the line of identify. The Zs of carbon, nitrogen, and oxygen are 6, 7, and 8, respectively. Z_{eff} of Teflon (CF_2) is 8.4, polyethylene is 5.4, PMMA is 6.5, and muscle is approximately 7.6.

fluoroscopy-based angiography. CTA is really just contrast-enhanced CT where the images have been processed to highlight the vascular anatomy using image processing techniques (Fig. 10-41). In general, maximum intensity projection procedures produce excellent CTA images. Some image rendering techniques use pseudocolor to add realism to the images.

CT Perfusion

CT perfusion imaging is used to evaluate vascular perfusion and other physiological parameters related to blood flow to a specific organ. While most often used to evaluate stroke or vasospasm in the brain, CT perfusion is also used for abdominal organ imaging, especially in the oncologic setting. CT perfusion is a high radiation dose

■ **FIGURE 10-41** CT angiography (CTA) is used with increasing frequency instead of fluoroscopy-based angiography. For diagnostic procedures, the venous access for contrast agent injection is far less invasive than penetrating the (high-pressure) arterial system for iodine injection. CTA images of the arteries in the leg and the head are shown, with false color rendering.

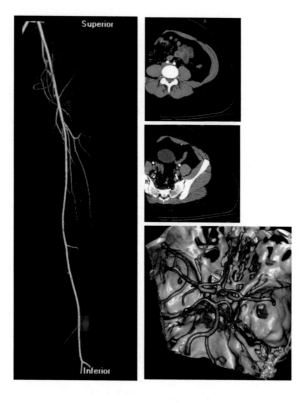

study—the CT scanner acquires images of an organ repeatedly in real time to quantify the flow of iodine-based contrast agent through that organ. Typical head CT perfusion protocols call for the acquisition of about 40 CT images, each using a 1-s acquisition, resulting in about 40 s of scanning in the same area of tissue (Fig. 10-42A). CT perfusion takes advantage of the wide collimated beam width (20 to 160 mm) of top of the line scanners ($\geq$64 data channels) to image a volume of tissue in the same region of the body repeatedly. The CT scan starts prior to the intravenous injection of contrast, and hence the scanner produces a number of CT images prior to the arrival of the contrast bolus to the organ of interest. This is necessary because the mathematical models (Patlak, etc.) that are used to compute the parametric maps require an input function (HU versus time), typically the artery supplying blood to the organ of interest. From this data set of temporal CT scans, and with physician demarcation of the location of the input function, parametric maps are computed with high resolution. In addition to the raw gray scale CT images, most commercial perfusion software packages compute a number of different parametric 3D volume data sets of pseudocolored images, showing for example blood volume, tissue perfusion, and time to peak enhancement (Fig. 10-42B). Perfusion CT is an example of where the well-appreciated anatomical capabilities of CT are combined with the high temporal resolution capabilities of the modality to produce physiologically meaningful, quantitative, functional images.

Shuttle Mode CT

Shuttle mode allows a CT scanner to repeatedly image a volume of tissue that is wider than the detector array (nT). The table rocks back and forth a prescribed distance, during the temporal acquisition procedure (Fig. 10-43). This mode allows CT perfusion analysis to be performed over a larger section of tissue. The temporal resolution

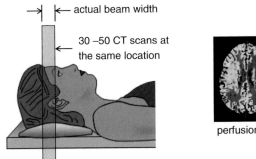

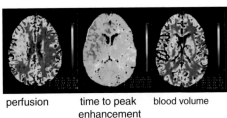

perfusion   time to peak   blood volume
                   enhancement

A. perfusion imaging   **B.** computed parametric images

■ **FIGURE 10-42** CT perfusion is an extension of CT angiography, where a relatively long time sequence of repeated CT images is acquired for physiologic assessment of various organs (**A**). Typically on the order of 40 full CT data sets are acquired for brain perfusion studies, requiring about 40 seconds. From these data and some user input, (**B**) physiological metrics such as vascular perfusion, time to peak enhancement, and blood volume can be computed using software designed for this purpose.

is lower in shuttle mode, but adequate physiological information can in general be derived. Due to the change in direction of the table, shuttle mode results in image data being acquired during table acceleration and deceleration, which implies that the reconstruction algorithm needs to accommodate for the changing pitch.

Dose Modulation

Some body regions in the patient are rounder than other regions. An elliptical cross section of a patient is shown in Figure 10-44A. With fixed x-ray tube current and hence

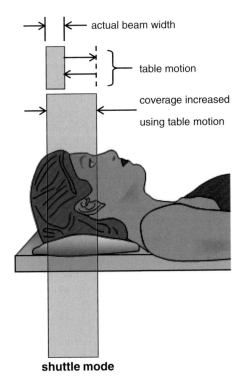

shuttle mode

■ **FIGURE 10-43** Shuttle mode imaging is a hybrid between CT perfusion and helical CT imaging—the table shuttles back and forth over a relatively small (e.g., 100 to 200 mm) predefined region in the patient, allowing temporal imaging and hence CT perfusion assessment to be made over a wider length of anatomy than the width (*nT*) of an MDCT field of view.

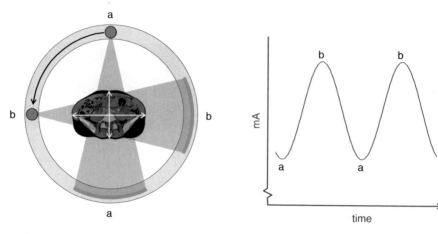

A. Tube rotation around oval patient   **B.** mA modulation

■ **FIGURE 10-44** Tube current modulation is illustrated. **A.** As the x-ray tube and detector array rotate around the patient, the x-ray path length is determined either by attenuation measurements or from the CT radiograph, or both. The tube current (mA) is modulated to optimize the use of radiation in the patient. The mA is increased when the beam is projected through thicker regions, and it is decreased as the x-ray beam traverses thinner projections through the patient. **B.** For an elliptical shaped body part such as in the pelvis, the mA modulation scheme is approximately sinusoidal as the gantry rotates around the patient.

constant x-ray flux, the detectors will receive more primary x-rays when the gantry is in position *a* compared to gantry position *b*, due to the increased attenuation path in position *b*. However, as we have already seen in the context of the bow tie filter, the noise variance in the projection data propagates into the reconstructed CT image in a manner that is more optimal when the projection data variance levels are nearly matched (Equation 10-3). Hence, the higher signal levels (higher dose and lower signal variance) in position *a* are essentially wasted when combined with those in position *b* during CT image reconstruction. When the mA is modulated, the mA is reduced in position *a* compared to position *b* as shown in Figure 10-44B. When mA modulation is performed, lower radiation dose levels can be used to achieve the same image quality.

The mA modulation scheme shown in Figure 10-44 occurs as the x-ray gantry rotates once around the patient. However, as the patient translates through the gantry over greater distances in z, the shape and size of the patient's body can change appreciably. Therefore, modulation also can be applied along the z-axis of the patient. The average mAs values are shown as a function of position along a patient's torso in Figure 10-45. The angular modulation as a function of gantry angle is quasi-sinusoidal in elliptical body parts and constant in round body regions, and these fluctuations occur over relatively shorter distances as highlighted in Figure 10-45. The impact of mA modulation is illustrated on CT images in Figure 10-46, where the average mAs per CT image are indicated.

The role of mA modulation in CT is analogous to that of automatic exposure control in radiography and automatic exposure rate control in fluoroscopy. mA modulation is implemented differently for different CT vendors. One scanner manufacturer uses the attenuation data measured by the detectors near the central ray in the scanner to adjust the target mA for 180 degrees later in the scan. Manufacturers also use the attenuation data measured during the acquisition of the CT radiograph to plan the mA modulation scheme for each patient. Figures 10-44 and 10-45 demonstrate the relative mA values used, but mA modulation technology is also used to set the absolute mA levels (and hence the patient's radiation dose) for the scan.

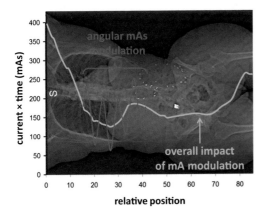

■ **FIGURE 10-45** Tube current modulation occurs as the gantry rotates around the patient to address the different x-ray path lengths between the AP and the lateral projections, but it also is active along the z-dimension of the patient. As the scanner images the patient's thorax, abdomen, and pelvis, the tube current is modulated to optimize the image quality through the entire extent (along z) of the patient scan. The overall mAs per slice along the z-axis of the patient is shown in this figure, and the oscillatory nature of the angular mAs modulation is also shown. (Courtesy SE McKenney.)

Different scanner manufacturers employ very different concepts for the selection of the overall dose levels in CT, and this can and does lead to confusion in the clinical environment. The details are beyond the scope of this book; however, a general description is in order here. One approach is to set the actual noise level in the reconstructed CT image, and this value is used to guide the overall dose levels (by adjusting the mA levels used). With this approach, when *lower* noise levels are selected, the mA values and resulting radiation doses are *higher*. Maximum and minimum mA values can be set as a precaution. A different approach to mA modulation is to set a

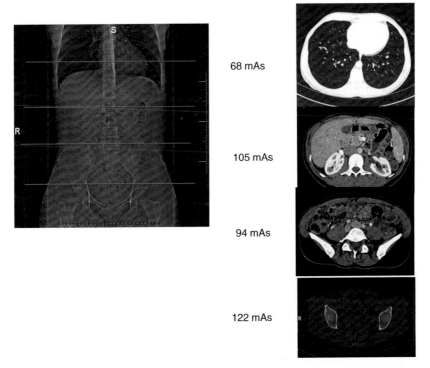

■ **FIGURE 10-46** The overall effect of tube current modulation is to use different radiation levels for regions in the body with different overall attenuation, and most tube current modulation schemes result in a more homogeneous distribution of CT noise in the patient images along the z-axis. Here, the mAs values used for the various body regions are indicated.

nominal mA level that the system uses as guidance for the overall dose settings, but in this situation, *higher* nominal mA values result in higher mA settings and *higher* radiation dose to the patient. When used correctly, mA modulation techniques produce excellent CT images at near-optimal radiation dose levels. Therefore, it is an important feature of modern CT scanners that should be used, especially in body imaging. However, when the responsibility of adjusting something as important as the radiation dose in CT is turned over to the CT computer, it is important that the operators (technologists, radiologists, medical physicists) are well educated in the use of the mA modulation technology on each CT scanner they use.

CT Protocols

A typical CT scanner may have 100 to 300 different preset protocols loaded on it. The CT operator usually starts a patient scan procedure by selecting the CT protocol appropriate to the scan for that patient. The CT protocol encompasses a wide variety of parameters, which can be set, including CT acquisition parameters such as kV, mA, rotation time, slice thickness, and pitch, but also the reconstruction kernel(s) used, the timing, volume, and injection rate of the contrast injection scheme (if used), the default window/level settings for the reconstructed CT images, and what computer to send the images to when they are ready. The protocol is the starting point in the scanning procedure, and once the patient is on the table and the CT scan is about to commence, it is the role of the experienced CT technologist to modify the protocol in some cases. For example, for very large patients, the mAs (or maximum mAs for dose modulation schemes) need to be increased to produce a diagnostic quality CT examination.

10.4 CT Reconstruction

Preprocessing

There are a number of preprocessing procedures that are applied to the actual acquired projection data prior to CT image reconstruction. The details of these steps are proprietary to each vendor; however, some general observations can be made. During routine calibration of the CT scanner, the influence of the bow tie filter is characterized by performing air scans. The air scans also characterize differences in individual detector response, which may be due to differences in photodiode or amplifier gain. The measured projection data for a given CT scan to be reconstructed are normalized by the calibration scans, and this procedure corrects for previously identified inhomogeneities in the field. In some scanners, a small fraction of the detector elements may be "dead," and these are routinely identified using software for this purpose. A dead pixel correction algorithm is applied, which replaces dead pixel data with interpolated data from surrounding pixels. Scatter correction algorithms generally need to be applied before the logarithm of the data is applied. Adaptive noise filtration methods can be applied; for example, the scanner can invoke algorithms, which identify regions in the projection data that correspond to low signal areas, and these areas have high noise and after backprojection will correspond to locations of high noise on the CT images. To reduce the impact of noise, some algorithms identify these low signal areas and then apply smoothing or other data processing steps to reduce the noise in these areas.

After preprocessing, the projection data undergo logarithmic transformation and normalization, in order to correct for the exponential attenuation characteristics of x-ray interaction. Each projection measurement through the patient corresponds to a discrete measurement of I_j at detector element j, where

$$I_j = g_j I_o \, e^{-(\mu_1 t + \mu_2 t + \mu_3 t + \dots \mu_n t)} \qquad [10\text{-}6]$$

The signal in a reference detector I_r located outside the FOV of the patient is also measured during the CT scan:

$$I_r = g_r I_o \qquad [10\text{-}7]$$

It is known during the calibration air scans that the ratio of the gains between a detector j and the reference detector r is given by $\beta = g_r/g_j$. This ratio can not only compensate for differences in actual gain between detectors, but also correct for differences in bow tie filter thickness, distance from the x-ray source (i.e., inverse square law), etc.

$$P_j = \ln\left\{\frac{I_r}{\beta I_j}\right\} = t\left(\mu_1 + \mu_2 + \mu_3 + \dots \mu_n\right) \qquad [10\text{-}8]$$

From Equation 10-8, we see that the projection measurements, P_j, after preprocessing and logarithmic conversion, correspond to linear sums of the linear attenuation coefficients through the patient and along the path of the ray, and this is illustrated in Figure 10-47 as well.

Simple Backprojection

To start the discussion as to how the CT image is computed from the projection data sets, let's examine a simplified but realistic example of the problem (Fig. 10-48). As discussed above, the logarithm converts the exponential nature of x-ray absorption into a linear problem, and we will therefore deal with this example as a linear problem. The 3 × 3 grid of numbers in the central boxes in Figure 10-48 are the data of interest—these numbers represent the object, and the image of the object. Four projections through this "patient" are shown, *a–d*. It can be seen that the projected value through each line passing through the patient is the linear sum of the voxel values that each ray intersects. Creating the projections from the central data is called forward projection, and that is what the CT scanner hardware does physically. Mathematical forward projection is used in iterative reconstruction techniques and many other reconstruction processes as well. The problem that is posed by Figure 10-48

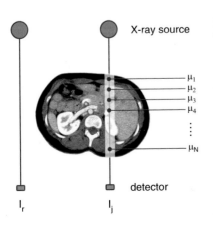

X-ray source

detector

I_r I_j

μ_1
μ_2
μ_3
μ_4
⋮
μ_N

■ **FIGURE 10-47** The reference detector is positioned to detect the output of the CT scanner with no patient anatomy in the measurement, resulting in I_r. A large number of ray measurements I_j are made for detector elements $j = 1$, N. The ray measurements sample a number of individual linear attenuation (μ) values along the beam path, as illustrated. While x-ray attenuation is an exponential process, logarithmic processing as described in the text converts the measured data to linear projections of μ.

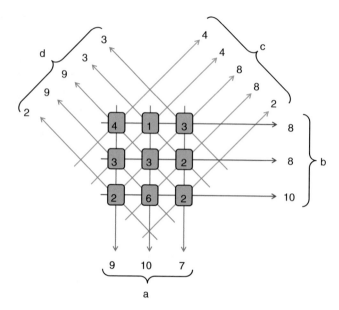

■ **FIGURE 10-48** The 3 × 3 grid in the center of this figure represents the actual attenuation values (scaled to integer values for demonstration), and the projection data (***a, b, c,*** and ***d***) show how the attenuation values are summed in this very simplified example. The ***a–d*** projections are the acquired data in a CT scan, and the reconstruction challenge is to determine the values in the nine elements in the 3 × 3 grid. For this simple example, the process is similar to Sudoku. The reader is challenged to use the projection values (only) to find a solution for the values in the gold rectangles.

is, if you erase the nine values in the 3 × 3 box, can you figure out what they are from the projection data? This looks very much like a Sudoku problem at this point, and given the simplicity of the 3 × 3 problem, it can be solved by trial and error. However, in a CT scanner, the matrix is typically 512 × 512, and the task of reconstructing the values in the image from the projection values is more formidable.

We saw that to produce the projection values, knowing the contents of the image, the straightforward process of forward projection is used. The reverse problem, computing the image matrix from the projection values, can be solved (almost) by backprojection. With backprojection, the measured projection values are simply smeared back into the image matrix to compute the backprojected image. Figure 10-49 shows an example of forward projection of a simple circular object at the center of the field, and therefore the projections at each angle are identical in shape. The projection of a circle is a parabola, and that is seen in Fig 10-49A. If that same (uncorrected) projection shape was used to backproject the CT image from all projection angles (Fig. 10-49B), the resulting image would have a characteristic blurring as shown in the isometric plot in Figure 10-49C. The take-home message is this: Using *simple* backprojection as described above, the reconstructed image has a characteristic 1/r blurring that results from the geometry of backprojection. To correct for this, a mathematical filtering operation is required, and that leads to the discussion of *filtered backprojection* in the next section.

Filtered Backprojection

In the case of simple backprojection, the process of summing projections from a large number of angles around 360 degrees results in the 1/r blur function as seen graphically in Figure 10-49C. The mathematical function 1/r is illustrated in Figure 10-50A.

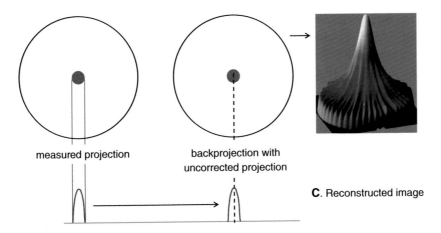

A. Measured projection   **B.** Backprojection reconstruction

■ **FIGURE 10-49** For actual CT data sets, the challenge is to reconstruct a total of 206,000 cells ($\pi \times 256^2$). In this figure, a simple circle at the center of the image is "imaged," producing the *measured projection* in **A**. If these same measured projection data are used in backprojection (**B**), the image will experience a characteristic 1/r blurring as illustrated in **C**.

It is possible to correct for the impact of the 1/r function using image processing procedures. The mathematical operation of *convolution* describes such a procedure, and convolution is discussed in more detail in Chapter 4, and in Appendix F. When "undoing" an effect caused by convolution, *deconvolution* is used. Deconvolution is mathematically identical to convolution, except that the deconvolution kernel is (by definition) designed to *undo* a specific effect. The convolution process is defined mathematically as

$$p'(x) = \int_{x'=-\infty}^{\infty} p(x)\ h(x - x')\ dx' = p(x) \otimes h(x) \qquad [10\text{-}9]$$

where $p(x)$ is each measured projection, $h(x)$ is the deconvolution kernel, and $p'(x)$ is the corrected projection value, which is used in filtered backprojection. The right-hand side of Equation 10-9 shows the short hand notion for convolution, where $\otimes$ is the mathematical symbol for convolution.

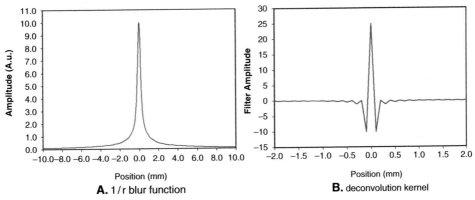

A. 1/r blur function   **B.** deconvolution kernel

■ **FIGURE 10-50 A.** The 1/r blurring function is illustrated. The blurring caused by the geometry of backprojection can be corrected by deconvolving the measured projection data prior to backprojection, resulting in the process of *filtered backprojection*. **B.** The discrete implementation of the deconvolution kernel is illustrated.

The deconvolution kernel that is designed to undo the 1/r blurring shown in Figure 10-50A is shown in Figure 10-50B. The oscillatory nature of the deconvolution kernel in Figure 10-50B is a result of the discrete nature of the operation, as applied in a computer. As mentioned in Chapter 4, when a convolution kernel has negative values such as that shown in Figure 10-50B, in general it "sharpens" an image. The kernel in Figure 10-50B is a 1D function, and it is used to deconvolve the measured 1D projection values prior to backprojection, as illustrated in Figure 10-51. Here it is seen that when all of the measured projections of the object are deconvolved with the appropriate kernel, subsequent backprojection results in a faithful representation of the object. An actual example of this is shown for a test object in Figure 10-52. The convolution operation described here is a form of mathematical filtering, and this is why the procedure is called filtered backprojection. Convolution backprojection as described in Equation 10-9 can be considered as a specific implementation of filtered backprojection.

Fourier-Based Reconstruction

Convolution as described in Equation 10-9 can be performed quicker using properties of the Fourier transform. Specifically, Equation 10-9 can be recast as

$$p'(x) = FT^{-1}\left\{FT[p(x) \times FT[h(x)]\right\} \qquad [10\text{-}10]$$

where $FT[]$ refers to the forward Fourier transform operation and $FT^1[]$ is the inverse Fourier transform. Equation 10-10 is mathematically equivalent to Equation 10-9; however, the Fourier transform approach can be performed faster in a computer. Therefore, the Fourier approach is used in commercial scanners more often than the convolution approach. Notice that the Fourier transform of the convolution kernel $h(x)$ is performed in Equation 10-10; however, because $h(x)$ does not change for a given CT reconstruction filter, its Fourier transform is precomputed. Because of this, it is very common in CT to discuss $FT\{h(x)\}$—more so than discussing $h(x)$ itself.

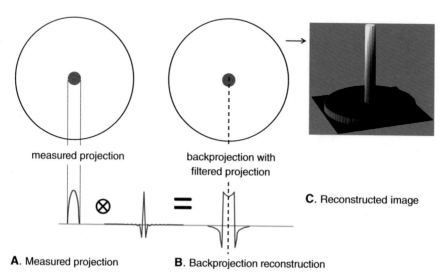

measured projection   backprojection with
                                   filtered projection

C. Reconstructed image

A. Measured projection   **B.** Backprojection reconstruction

■ **FIGURE 10-51** This figure shows the same object and projection data (**A**) as with Figure 10-49A; however, here the measured projection data are deconvolved with the kernel illustrated in Figure 10-50B. The resulting filtered projection data (**B**) are used for backprojection, and this results in an image that reflects the properties of the original object (**C**).

sinogram   reconstructed image

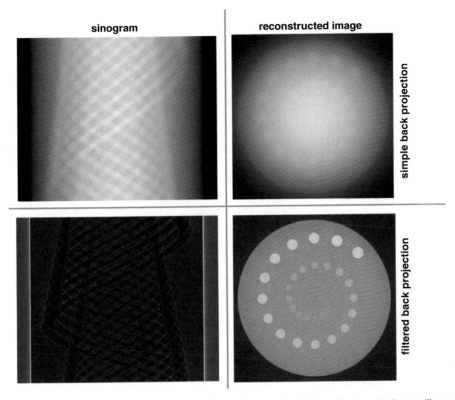

■ **FIGURE 10-52** The properties of simple backprojection (top row) and filtered backprojection are illustrated, (bottom row). The sinogram—the plot of the raw data showing rays horizontally and angles vertically—is shown on the left; the sinogram on the bottom has been filtered (horizontally) and the high-pass character-istics of the filtering process are evident. Backprojection of the filtered sinogram data results in an image that closely matches the characteristics of the object that was scanned, while the upper reconstructed image shows significant blurring.

Figure 10-53 shows the Fourier transform of the deconvolution kernel illustrated in Figure 10-50B, and this is the "ramp" filter labeled in Figure 10-53. The incredibly simple shape of the frequency domain filter FT{h(x)} is also perhaps why it is so widely discussed in the CT reconstruction setting.

Why is the ramp filter *the* filter that we start with in filtered backprojection? Figure 10-50A shows the 1/r blurring effect that results from simple backprojection, and it turns out that this is a 1/f effect in the frequency domain. So, if you have an image that has a 1/f dependency that you want to correct for, the correction process would involve multiplying the image by a function that has an f dependency, which is described mathematically as

$$H(f) = \alpha \times f \qquad [10\text{-}11]$$

where α is simply a scaling factor. The correction process results in $f \times 1/f$, which eliminates any frequency dependency. It should be recognized that Equation 10-11 defines the ramp filter seen in Figure 10-53, with some very minor caveats that are beyond the scope of this text.

As mentioned above, the ramp function $H(f)$ shown in Figure 10-53 is the *starting point* in designing the shape of the filter in filtered backprojection. It would work well in the case of an image where there was very little statistical noise in the projection image data sets (the measured data during CT reconstruction). However, because we

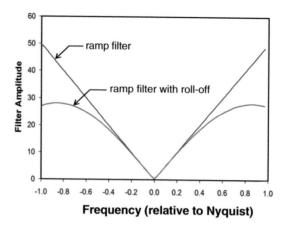

Frequency (relative to Nyquist)

■ **FIGURE 10-53** The kernel shown in Figure 10-50B is the convolution kernel that can be used in the spatial domain to correct the measured projection values prior to backprojection. In practice, the convolution process is implemented using Fourier-based mathematics, as described in the text. The Fourier transform of the deconvolution kernel in Figure 10-50B is shown in this figure as the ramp filter. While the ramp filter restores the blurring that occurs during backprojection, it amplifies high frequencies and can exacerbate quantum noise in the image. Hence, most clinical CT systems use a number of different reconstruction filters that include some "roll-off," which reduces the noise amplification effect of the ramp filter at the higher spatial frequencies. One filter is illustrated here, but there are a large number of reconstruction filters that are available on commercial CT scanners.

seek to reduce the radiation dose to patients in all x-ray imaging procedures including CT, the dose levels are set intentionally low, and as a result, the measured data sets are in fact noisy. Notice the shape of the ramp filter in Figure 10-53; it has high values at high spatial frequencies, and therefore significantly amplifies the high spatial frequencies in the projection data—and this is the frequency region where quantum noise tends to dominate. Consequently, if one were to use only the ramp filter in filtered backprojection, the reconstructed CT image would in most cases be unacceptably noisy. Therefore, it is customary to apply a function that "rolls off" the amplitude of the reconstruction filter at high spatial frequencies, as shown in Figure 10-53. The roll-off reduces the high frequency component of the reconstructed image, and tends to abate the noise as a result. The specific roll-off function varies for the specific application in CT. In the mathematical reconstruction literature, the names of specific roll-off filters include Shepp-Logan, Hamming, Cosine, etc. Some commercial CT manufacturers give these mathematical filters application-specific names such as soft tissue, bone, or standard filters. Other companies use numerical designations for their filters, such as H47 or H50 for head filters and B40 or B70 for body filters.

Cone Beam Reconstruction

Cone beam reconstruction algorithms are similar to standard fan beam reconstruction algorithms, but they keep track of the beam divergence in the z-direction (the cone angle direction, as illustrated in Figures 10-10 and 10-11). Backprojection occurs as described above; however, the algorithm computes the backprojection angles in both the fan and the cone angles. The basic cone beam reconstruction process, often referred to as the Feldkampt algorithm or FDK, reconstructs the entire volume data set (a series of CT images of a given thickness) simultaneously. Cone beam reconstruction violates mathematical requirements for sampling Fourier space, and for extreme cone beam geometries used in flat panel detectors (as in Fig. 10-11) or other very wide cone beam CT systems, this can lead to cone beam artifacts (discussed later).

Iterative Reconstruction in CT

Filtered backprojection was the primary method for reconstructing CT images for many decades; however, advancements in algorithm design coupled with fast computer hardware have led to the use of clinically useful iterative reconstruction algorithms for CT images. Iterative reconstruction is numerically intensive and has been used clinically for smaller data sets as with nuclear medicine applications such as single photon emission computed tomography (SPECT) for many years. However, by comparison, CT scanners acquire far more raw data than do SPECT systems, and the matrix size is much larger (512×512) versus (64×64) for most SPECT systems. It is observed that a 512^2 matrix has a factor of 64 more pixels than a 64^2 matrix.

The fundamental problem in CT image reconstruction is shown in Figure 10-54, where projection data sets are shown with a CT image. The projection data are what is *known*, and the CT image is the *unknown* and therefore needs to be reconstructed. The projection data sets are used to reconstruct the CT image as illustrated in Figure 10-54, but if the CT image (or an approximation of it) is known, then the projection data can be computed using forward projection. Note that in Figure 10-54 only three projection data sets are illustrated, but in clinical CT, a large number of projection data are acquired (1,000 to 4,000 projections).

Iterative reconstruction techniques go through a series of iterations in the process of CT reconstruction, as illustrated in Figure 10-55. The first image may start as a guess, a constant image, or as a filtered backprojection image. The iteration process then goes through a series of updates (iterations), which drive the CT image toward a final, accurate depiction of the object that was scanned. Most iterative algorithms use similar fundamental logic—the current estimate of the image is used to generate forward projections, which are then compared to the actual measured projections (during acquisition) as shown in Figure 10-55. The difference between the forward projection and the measured projection is the error matrix, which is computed for all projections measured around 360 degrees. Each specific iterative algorithm (there are many) uses the error matrix to update the next iteration of the image, with the intent of reducing the error matrix in the subsequent iteration. There is a balance between reconstructing

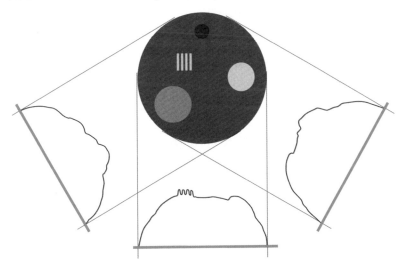

■ FIGURE 10-54 This figure shows an object and three projections through the object, illustrating a small subset of the measured projection data acquired during CT scanning. These projection data are in principle physically measured using the detector hardware on the scanner, but if a guesstimate of the image data is known, the projections can also be computed (as forward projections) using relatively simple mathematics (sines and cosines) in a computer.

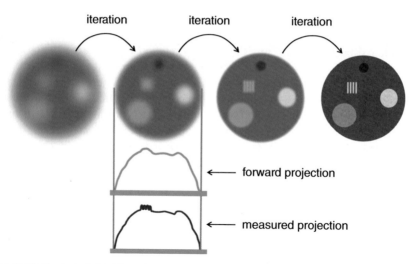

■ **FIGURE 10-55** The logic behind iterative CT image reconstruction is illustrated in this figure. The reconstruction process begins with an initial estimate of what the object may "look like." This guess is used to compute forward projection data sets, which are then compared with the measured projection data sets. The difference between the mathematical projections and the physical measurements creates an error matrix for each projection. Each type of iterative algorithm for reconstruction uses the error matrix and then updates the next iteration of the image. The process continues for a number of iterations until the error matrix is minimized, and the CT image at that point should be a good estimate of the actual object that was scanned.

the anatomical information and the noise in the image. The many different iterative algorithms use the error matrix to update the next iteration in a different manner. After a certain number of iterations, the estimated image becomes an excellent depiction of the object that was scanned. It is recognized that iterative algorithms can model many of the physical parameters that filtered backprojection cannot, such as the x-ray spectrum, the blurring of the focal spot, etc., and therefore, in principle, iterative algorithms can make better use of the acquired data—they can produce images with higher signal-to-noise ratio (SNR) at the same dose, or they can produce images of similar SNR at lower doses. Figure 10-56 illustrates comparisons between images reconstructed using filtered backprojection images and iterative methods, and the iteratively reconstructed images show a distinct advantage. Iterative methods for reconstruction do not explicitly use the filtering methods as described above, and consequently the noise texture in the images can be quite different than with filtered backprojection images.

All major CT manufacturers have implemented iterative reconstruction techniques on their CT scanners; however, at present, this capability is an optional feature. Because of the demonstrated benefit of potential dose reduction using iterative reconstruction techniques, CT reconstruction methods will gradually shift toward iterative methods in order to derive better image quality—lower noise CT images—using lower radiation doses.

10.5 Image Quality in CT

Spatial Resolution

Spatial resolution in CT results from the fundamental resolution properties of the image acquisition, as well as the resolution characteristics of the reconstruction filter that is used. Factors that determine the ultimate resolution include the focal spot

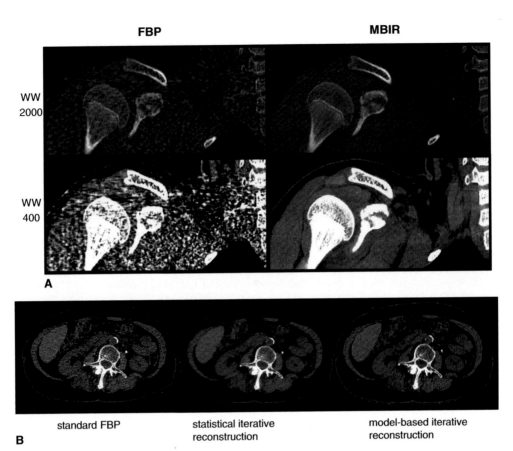

FBP   **MBIR**

WW 2000

WW 400

A

standard FBP   statistical iterative   model-based iterative
B   reconstruction   reconstruction

■ **FIGURE 10-56** Iterative reconstruction in CT is made possible by algorithms that are computationally efficient and require very few iterations. The iterative technique for reconstruction can in most cases extract more
signal-to-noise ratio from the acquired data set, resulting in higher SNR reconstructed images compared to
filtered backprojection techniques. Here, two images are illustrated showing the comparison from a clinical CT
system, where the interactive reconstruction methods resulted in superior noise properties compared to filtered
backprojection of the same acquired projection data. **A.** Filtered backprojection (FBP) is compared with model-
based iterative reconstruction (MBIR) in this figure. **B.** This figure shows the same image produced by standard
FBP, statistical iterative reconstruction, and model-based iterative reconstruction. (Courtesy J. Hsieh.)

size and distribution, the detector dimensions, the magnification factor, whether or
not gantry motion is compensated for, patient motion, etc. Because CT images are
the result of an elaborate mathematical reconstruction process, their resolution is
also very dependent on the characteristics of the reconstruction algorithm and any
mathematical filters used.

Spatial Resolution in the Reconstruction (x,y) Plane

The in-plane CT image is a direct product of the CT reconstruction, and by far most
clinical CT images are acquired and then natively reconstructed in the axial plane.
Some variations in patient positioning (e.g., bent neck with head tilted forward) lead to
occasional exceptions to this. Spatial resolution has historically been measured in the
clinical environment in CT using bar patterns, as illustrated in Fig 10-57. These images
were acquired using the American College of Radiology (ACR) accreditation phantom,
which has eight different bar pattern modules around the periphery of the 20-cm
diameter phantom. The bar phantom has modules corresponding to spatial frequencies of 0.4, 0.5, 0.6, 0.7, 0.8, 0.9, 1.0, and 1.2 line pairs per mm (lp/mm). Note that in

ACR phantom –spatial resolution section

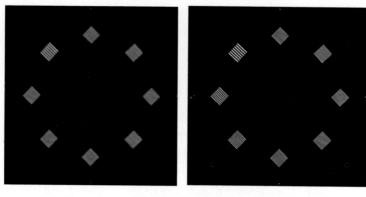

A. soft tissue kernel **B**. bone kernel

■ **FIGURE 10-57** In the field measurements of spatial resolution in CT still rely on visual assessment of bar phantoms—in this figure, the resolution module from the American College of Radiology (ACR) CT accreditation phantom is shown, imaged with (**A**) a soft tissue reconstruction filter and (**B**) with a bone filter. The same CT acquisition can produce different images depending on which reconstruction filters are used.

most commercial CT literature, the resolution is quoted in *line pairs per cm* instead of the *line pairs per mm* as is typical in the rest of x-ray imaging. Here, we use lp/mm for consistency, recognizing that lp/cm = 10 × lp/mm—thus, 12 lp/cm = 1.2 lp/mm.

The images shown in Figure 10-57 were generated from the same CT acquisition, and the differences in spatial resolution are the result of the reconstruction filter used. For the soft tissue image (Figure 10-57A), three of the bar patterns can be easily resolved corresponding to a limiting spatial resolution of 0.6 lp/mm. The CT image reconstructed with the bone kernel (Fig. 10-57B) allows six of the modules to be resolved, for a limiting spatial resolution of 0.9 lp/mm.

The modulation transfer function (MTF) is a more scientific measure of the spatial resolution characteristics of an imaging system, as discussed in Chapter 4. The MTF can be measured using a wire or plane of metal foil scanned on a CT scanner, and the *MTF(f)* is computed from the measured line spread function, *LSF(x)*. Five *MTF(f)* curves are shown in Figure 10-58, corresponding to a specific manufacturer's reconstruction filters, as listed in the figure. It is quite apparent from this figure that the reconstruction kernel has a significant influence on the *MTF(f)* and hence on the resolving power of the images. It is noted that the limiting resolution of each kernel is approximately at the 10% MTF level, and the limiting spatial resolutions seen in Figure 10-57 are corroborated by the MTF curves seen in Figure 10-58.

Spatial Resolution along the Z-axis

Historically, the spatial resolution along the z-axis of the CT data set (the slice thickness direction) has been measured using the *slice sensitivity profile* (SSP—Fig. 10-59A). The SSP is defined as the shape of the system response to a point input in the z-dimension. In standard image science vernacular, the SSP is the LSF along the z-dimension in the CT scanner. In the ACR phantom, there are a series of high contrast wires spaced 0.5 mm apart in the z-dimension (Fig. 10-59A). Counting the number of visible "lines" and multiplying by 0.5 mm results in a field measurement of the slice thickness. Images were reconstructed at nominal slice thicknesses of 4.8 mm (Fig. 10-59B) and 2.4 mm (Fig. 10-59C), and the ACR test suggests that these slice thicknesses measure about 5 and 3 mm, respectively.

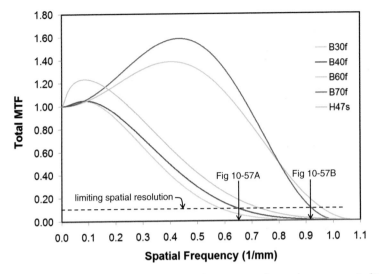

■ **FIGURE 10-58** Scientific evaluation of the resolution of CT images relies on the assessment of the modulation transfer function (MTF), as shown in this figure. This figure shows the dramatic impact on the MTF that various reconstruction filters have. (Courtesy K. Krzymyk.)

The typical reconstructed slice thickness in the mid-1990s was approximately 7 mm, and the SSP was routinely used in that era to characterize the "slice thickness." Today it is routine to reconstruct images with 0.5- to 0.625-mm slice thicknesses, rivaling or even finer than the voxel dimensions in the (x,y) plane. Therefore, it is useful to use the MTF metric to characterize the spatial resolution in the z-dimension as illustrated in Figure 10-60. For image data sets that are reconstructed into thicker sections (e.g., T = 2.5 mm), the $MTF(f)$ degrades as expected. It is noted that the z-dimension in an axially acquired CT data set can routinely have higher spatial resolution as compared to the (x,y) axial in-plane geometry. The reconstruction filter

ACR phantom –slice thickness section

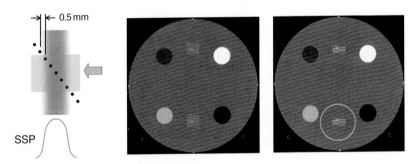

A. measurement concept   **B.** 4.8-mm slice thickness   **C.** 2.4-mm slice thickness

■ **FIGURE 10-59** The spatial resolution in the z-dimension of the CT image has been traditionally measured by the slice sensitivity profile, SSP. The ACR phantom has a series of small wires positioned at 0.5-mm intervals along the z-axis of the phantom (**A**). After scanning the phantom, the number of visible wires is counted and multiplied by 0.5 mm, to estimate slice thickness. **B.** A 4.8-mm nominal CT scan of the ACR phantom is showed, and 10 wires are visible suggesting that the slice thickness is approximately 5.0 mm. **C.** A 2.4-mm nominal image through the ACR phantom is illustrated, with 6 wires visible suggesting a 3.0-mm measured slice thickness.

■ **FIGURE 10-60** The method of estimating CT slice thickness using the ACR phantom is a discrete implementation of the traditional measurement of the slice sensitivity profile. The SSP is simply the line spread function (LSF) in the z-axis of the CT scan. So, measuring the SSP and then computing the Fourier transform of that results in the MTF for the z-axis of the CT scanner, as shown in this figure. The MTF shows higher spatial resolution along z for thinner slice images, and the z-axis resolution degrades (the MTF amplitude is reduced) as the reconstructed slice thickness increases.

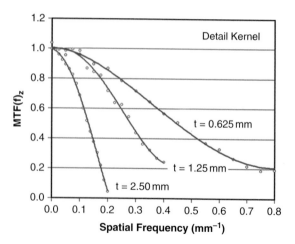

affects the resolution in the (x,y) plane, but it does not in the z-dimension. For this reason, coronal and sagittal CT images have the potential for better spatial resolution than axial CT images.

The spatial resolution in the z-axis dimension refers to the ability to see detail in the CT images; however, it should be recognized that the dose distribution in the z-dimension is an independent parameter. As mentioned previously, the width of the x-ray beam in all modern multidetector array CT scanners is wider than the actual detector array, in order to exclude the penumbra region from contributing to the images and causing artifacts. The dose profile in the z-dimension can be measured using various film products or a computed radiography (CR) plate, as illustrated in Figure 10-61. Isometric plots

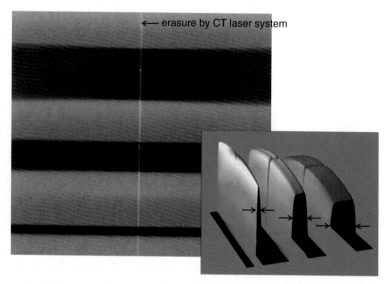

■ **FIGURE 10-61** The slice sensitivity profile, its discrete implementation in the ACR phantom, and the z-axis MTF all are measures of the z-axis *image* resolution. However, the overall dose profile along the z-axis can only be measured using an external device such as film or a computed radiography (CR) plate, the latter of which was used to generate the image data shown here. Various nominal collimated slice thicknesses (as set on the CT console) were used to scan a CT plate taken out of the cassette; the CR plate was moved along z to sequentially measure the dose profiles for different nominal slice thicknesses. The image data from the CR plate are plotted as isometric plots on the inset image. These plots show the dose profile along z for several different collimation thicknesses.

shown in the figure demonstrate the estimated width of the dose profiles—for the largest width shown, the dose profile was about 14% wider than the active detector array.

Noise Assessment in CT

Contrast Detectability Phantom: Visual Assessment

The traditional method for quantifying contrast resolution in CT is to visually assess a contrast detail phantom, as shown in Figure 10-62. These images were produced from the ACR phantom. The image on the left was produced using four times the radiation as the image on the right, and the number of visible low-contrast circles is far greater. The test objects on this phantom are designed to have 6 HU greater density (0.6%), than the background but they vary in diameter. The smaller circular test objects have lower SNR and therefore are theoretically and experimentally more difficult to see. This visual assessment of the low contrast resolution of a CT scanner is a relatively insensitive measure of the noise characteristics of a CT scanner; however, it is currently the industry standard.

Image Noise in CT: The Standard Deviation σ

The CT image of a region of the phantom that is homogeneous in composition can be used to quantify the noise directly, using software available on virtually any CT scanner or PACS system. The standard deviation σ, the direct measurement of "noise," is computed using the root mean square method:

$$\sigma = \sqrt{\frac{\sum_{i=1}^{N}\left(HU_i - \overline{HU}\right)^2}{N-1}} \qquad [10\text{-}12]$$

ACR phantom – low contrast detectability section

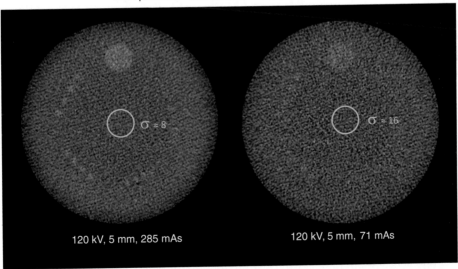

120 kV, 5 mm, 285 mAs   120 kV, 5 mm, 71 mAs

■ **FIGURE 10-62** CT images of the low-contrast module of the ACR phantom are illustrated, for radiation dose levels varying by about a factor of 4 (285 mAs/71 mAs ≈ 4.0). The circles visible in the phantom correspond to 0.6% differences in contrast (6 HU), and different rows of the circles have different diameters, which result in different signal-to-noise ratios (SNRs) of the circles. It is clear that more of the circular test objects are visible in the higher dose image on the left. The standard deviation, σ, is measured using software on most CT scanners or PACS systems. The standard deviation is seen to vary by a factor of two, for these images that used a fourfold difference in radiation dose, illustrating the Poisson relationship that image noise is relative to the square root of the dose.

As expected in Figure 10-62, the noise in the right image is about twice that of the left image since the radiation levels were reduced by a factor of 4. This underscores the relationship in quantum limited imaging where the noise (σ) is proportional to the square root of the dose—for example, double the dose and the noise goes down by 40%, quadruple the dose and the noise goes down by a factor of 2.

Noise Texture in CT: The Noise Power Spectrum

The $MTF(f)$ described above characterizes how efficiently *signal* propagates through an imaging system, while the noise power spectrum (NPS) describes how the *noise* propagates through an imaging system. The $NPS(f)$ is a spatial frequency–dependent function as is the $MTF(f)$. While the standard deviation σ measures the overall noise level in a region of the image, the $NPS(f)$ describes both the overall noise level and the noise *texture*—a term referring to the frequency dependence of the noise in an image. The NPS describes how the noise at one point in the image is correlated to the noise in the surrounding points of the image. Noise correlation occurs for a variety of reasons, but the point spread function of the imaging system tends to be a primary culprit in causing noise correlation—and because the PSF has "tails" that extend from one voxel location in the image to many other voxel locations in the image data set. Noise in the central region of the PSF is likely to therefore propagate to surrounding areas where the PSF extends. Another way to visualize this is to realize that the resolution cell in CT is not defined by a single voxel, but extends like a cloud to a number of voxels in the x-, y-, and z-dimensions. CT numbers (HUs) within this cloud have a tendency to influence each other.

Noise correlation in the (x,y) plane in CT is largely due to the filtered back-projection reconstruction kernel typically used in CT. Clearly, backprojection smears the projection data across the image, and therefore the noise in the backprojected data impacts a large swath of pixels in the reconstructed image. In the days of the single detector array CT scanners, however, there was little noise correlation in the z-dimension, because adjacent images (in z) were acquired using a completely different CT scan, separated in time and space. The multiple detector arrays of modern CT scanners combined with helical (and cone beam) CT reconstruction techniques give rise to physical mechanisms for noise correlation in the z-dimension (in addition to x and y). Electronic cross talk as well as PSF effects across the detector *arrays* in the z-dimension clearly can induce noise correlation in z. Because of the noise correlation, which exists in all three dimensions in CT, it is necessary to talk about the 3D NPS, which can be denoted as $NPS(f_x, f_y, f_z)$. To measure the 3D NPS, a volume of data that extends some distance in x, y, and z needs to be assessed. The NPS is measured by evaluating areas of an image that are generated from homogeneous sections of a phantom. In practice, the 3D NPS is determined by computing the 3D Fourier transform of data acquired from a 3D *volume of interest* (VOI) in the CT image data set. The mathematical details of NPS computation are beyond the scope of this chapter; however, they are discussed in Chapter 4 and Appendix G.

In most cases, the NPS in the (x,y) plane can be approximated to be rotational symmetric, and therefore it is possible to collapse the 2D $NPS(f_x, f_y)$ data into 1D using

$$f_{xy} = \sqrt{f_x^2 + f_y^2} \qquad [10\text{-}13]$$

This allows the depiction of the $NPS(f_{xy}, f_z)$, as illustrated in Figure 10-63. The family of NPS curves shown in Figure 10-63A illustrate the NPS as a function of frequency on the x-axis, where this axis corresponds to the f_{xy} frequency as described in Equation 10-13. There are a number of different NPS curves as a function of the

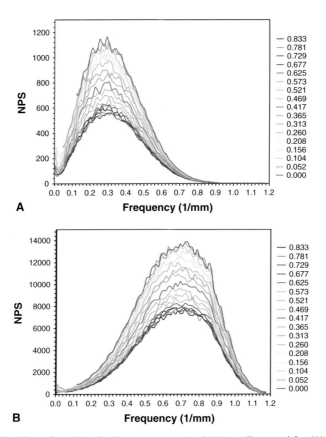

■ **FIGURE 10-63** The three-dimensional noise power spectra (NPS) are illustrated for (**A**) a standard body kernel. These data were computed computing the 3D Fourier transform from volumes of interest (VOIs) in a homogeneous region of a polyethylene phantom. The family of curves illustrates the z-axis dependency of the NPS, with the f_z values listed in the legend on the right. The figure on the right (**B**) illustrates similar data for the higher bandpass (bone) reconstruction kernel. (Courtesy SE McKenney.)

z-dimension, and the labels on the right side of the figure describe (using colors) the spatial frequency in the z-dimension. Figure 10-63A shows the 3D NPS for a CT data set reconstructed with a relatively smooth reconstruction filter (one with a lot of roll-off, for instance for soft tissue imaging), and Fig. 10-63B shows the 3D NPS for a higher bandpass reconstruction kernel (for instance, for bone imaging).

While the 3D NPS provides a rich description of the noise characteristics in a CT scanner, the use of the NPS as a practical tool in clinical CT image quality assessment is only now emerging. The NPS is a measure of noise power, and therefore the integral over all frequencies of the $NPS(f_x, f_y, f_z)$ will yield the noise variance of the CT image − σ^2.

MTF and NPS measurements on CT images assume that the images were produced using a linear system. When filtered backprojection is used to reconstruct the images, this results in a loose approximation for a linear system. However, when iterative reconstruction methods are used, it is likely that the CT image data strays significantly from the definition of a linear system. It is observed that the resolution of a CT image when reconstructed using iterative methods differs depending on the local noise levels, and therefore the PSF is not the same from region to region, and the system is not stationary (Chapter 4). Therefore, the MTF and NPS may not be valid analytical methods in this context. Other than the subjective visual observation methods described above, there are no obvious candidates for replacement of the MTF and NPS metrics when iterative reconstruction is used.

Primary Factors That Affect Spatial Resolution in CT

X-ray Tube Focal Spot Distribution

The focal spot plays a role in reducing the spatial resolution in CT, as the object is highly magnified relative to projection radiography. Also, CT systems run at very high mA typically, and this can increase the size of the x-ray focus (focal spot "blooming").

Gantry Motion

The x-ray source and detector array are moving relative to the stationary patient, both in the angular dimension and along the z-dimension for helical acquisition. Methods to compensate for gantry motion such as focal spot rastering (in both directions) can reduce this source of spatial resolution reduction.

Detector Size and Sampling

The detector width and sampling influence the resolution (width) and the Nyquist limitations (sampling) to resolution. Smaller detector dimensions and oversampling methods can improve spatial resolution.

Reconstruction Filter

Much of the reduction in spatial resolution is done intentionally, by the selection of a reconstruction filter with significant roll-off at high spatial frequencies, in an effort to reduce the appearance of image noise. CT images can be reconstructed multiple times with no dose penalty to the patient, producing both high spatial resolution and low noise image data sets.

Primary Factors That Affect Contrast Resolution (Noise) in CT

Technique Factors

The kV, mA, time, and pitch are fundamental determinants of the dose levels used for CT scanning, and they fundamentally impact the noise levels in the CT images. mA and time (and hence mAs) have a linear relationship with dose, while kV does not have a linear relationship with noise.

Slice Thickness

Thicker images combine signals from more detected x-ray quanta and therefore are less noisy than thinner images acquired at the same technique levels. A slice thickness of 5 mm has 40% less noise $\left(\sqrt{5.0 \div 2.5}\right)$ than a 2.5-mm slice thickness.

Reconstruction Filter (Filtered Backprojection)

The choice of reconstruction filter results in a fundamental and important trade-off between spatial resolution and image noise.

Reconstruction Method

The use of iterative CT reconstruction methods can significantly reduce image noise in comparison to filtered backprojection reconstruction. This means that lower dose images using iterative reconstruction techniques will be equivalent to higher dose studies using only filtered backprojection.

CT Image Artifacts

Beam Hardening

Standard filtered backprojection reconstruction algorithms do not fully address the polyenergetic nature of the x-ray spectrum used in CT, but rather treat the thickness-dependent attenuation using the notion of the effective linear attenuation coefficient. In rays that pass through a great deal of dense tissue, such as the petrous bone illustrated in the CT image inset in Figure 10-64, the high degree of attenuation causes the x-ray spectrum to become hardened. A "hard" x-ray spectrum refers to one with higher average x-ray energies, and a "soft" spectrum has lower average x-ray energies. Because the presence of dense (and higher z) structures such as bones in the x-ray path cause the lower energies in the x-ray spectrum to be preferentially attenuated compared to the higher x-ray energy photons, the beam undergoes a upward shift in average x-ray energy as it passes through greater thicknesses of bone. The curve in Figure 10-64 illustrates this, and the two x-ray spectra shown illustrate the relative removal of the lower x-ray energy photons at greater bone thicknesses.

In CT, to reduce artifacts caused by beam hardening, the x-ray beam is prehardened with significant thicknesses of added filtration (up to 10 mm of added aluminum, for example). However, beam hardening artifacts can occur, especially when dense objects such as bones or metal implants exist. Figure 10-65 illustrates beam hardening in a woman with bilateral hip implants. The x-ray beam corresponding to the paths that intersect both metallic hip implants are exceptionally hardened, and the angular artifact seen in the CT image (Fig. 10-65) results from this scan geometry. CT scanners do typically use simple methods for correcting for beam hardening; however, due to the simplicity of the most basic approach, artifacts can and do still occur. It is possible to use a two-pass reconstruction method that can yield almost complete correction for beam hardening; however, such algorithms are not usually applied in most clinical settings.

Streak Artifacts

Streak artifacts (Fig. 10-66) occur when the attenuation levels of a region in the patient are excessive, which can exceed the dynamic range of the detector systems or the effective linear range of the detectors. Metallic fillings in the teeth are a common source for streak artifacts, as are most implanted devices (e.g., cardiac pace-

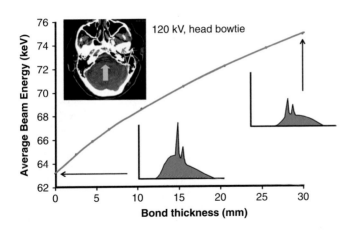

■ **FIGURE 10-64** The concept of beam hardening is illustrated. As the CT beam traverses greater thicknesses of highly attenuating material such as bone, the average x-ray energy changes as the graph demonstrates. The x-ray spectrum undergoes attenuation, and lower energy x-rays are preferentially attenuated, resulting in a characteristic right shift in the spectrum, as shown on the inset spectral diagrams. Beam hardening results in artifacts that appear as webbing between dense regions in the image (*inset image with arrow*).

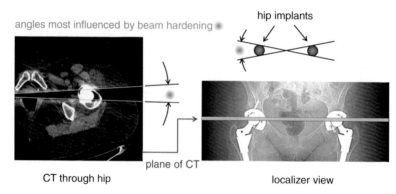

angles most influenced by beam hardening

hip implants

plane of CT

CT through hip

localizer view

■ **FIGURE 10-65** An extreme example of beam hardening is illustrated, from a women with two metallic hip implants as seen in the localizer view. The CT reconstruction through one hip shows the characteristic wedge artifact, which corresponds to the angles defined by the two metallic hips, as illustrated in the diagram.

makers, neurostimulators) that have significant metal components. Bullets and other high-density foreign bodies also can cause considerable streaking.

Streak artifacts are exacerbated by any motion of the high-density object; Although the head lends itself to excellent immobilization externally, during the CT scan, the patient will sometimes swallow or move their jaw, amplifying the streak artifacts that tend to emanate from metallic fillings.

View Aliasing

View aliasing refers to the use of too few projection images acquired to reconstruct high-frequency objects in the image. Figure 10-67A illustrates this effect on CT images of the head of a mouse. Most commercial CT scanners collect enough views such that view aliasing rarely occurs; however, for some very high frequency (sharp) objects (such as resolution test objects, Fig. 10-67B), view aliasing can occur.

Partial Volume

Partial volume artifacts occur (Fig. 10-68) when the CT voxels are large enough to encompass several types of tissue, such as bone and tissue or tissues from different organs. While partial volume artifacts can still occur, the dramatic reduction in the volume of a voxel in the past decade has substantially reduced the role that partial volume artifacts play in the diagnosis in modern CT examinations. Partial volume

■ **FIGURE 10-66** Streak artifacts from high-density, high atomic number dental fillings are seen in this image. Streak artifacts are amplified in effect if there is slight motion of the high-density object. Patients' who move their jaw or swallow during a head CT can generate significant artifacts due to this.

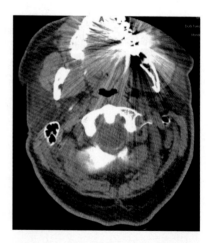

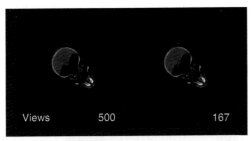

Views   500   167

A. Image of mouse with different numbers of views

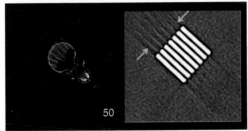

50

B. ACR resolution section

■ **FIGURE 10-67** View aliasing is the term given to CT reconstructions that do not have proper view sampling to render the sharper objects in the image. **A.** Images of a mouse head are shown, which were reconstructed using different numbers of views (as labeled). Most clinical CT scanners used a fixed, large number of views (950 to 3,000) for CT image reconstruction. View aliasing on commercial CT scanners is sometimes visible (**B**) when imaging high-contrast periodic structures, such as the resolution module on the ACR phantom.

artifacts arise essentially from reconstructing low resolution images, typically thick slice images. In many institutions, multiple reconstructions are used to produce two axial data sets, one thick slice and one thin slice. The thin slice images can be evaluated if partial volume effects are observed by the radiologist in reading the thicker slice images. Another method for reducing the impact of partial volume artifacts is to reconstruct multiple CT projections, such as the axial and coronal projections. What appears as a partial volume artifact in one projection can usually be ruled out by visualizing the same region in the other projection.

Cone Beam Artifacts

Cone beam acquisition strategies can lead to undersampling in the cone angle dimension, and this can cause a well-known cone beam artifact (Fig. 10-69). The Defrise phantom, which is a stack of attenuating disks separated by low density material (Fig. 10-69A), can be used to evaluate cone beam artifacts. In a well-sampled

5-mm section thickness   1.25-mm section thickness

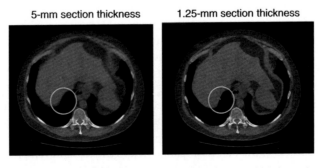

■ **FIGURE 10-68** Partial volume artifacts occur when the reconstructed voxel dimension is large relative to structures in the patient. With the advent of MDCT systems, images can be reconstructed with very small slice thicknesses, and in most cases, this eliminates partial volume artifacts. **A.** A 5-mm thick CT image through the lungs are shown, and a very small lesion is seen (circle) that has lower HU values consistent with lung cancer. **B.** When the same lesion is seen with thin section (1.25 mm) reconstruction, the contrast of the lesion is not diluted due to partial volume averaging, and the high HU values are evident, consistent with a benign diagnosis. (Courtesy R. Lamba.)

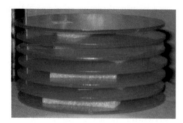

A. Defrise phantom

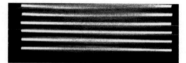

B. Some cone beam artifacts

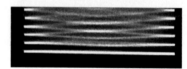

C. pronounced cone beam artifacts

■ **FIGURE 10-69** Cone beam artifacts are accentuated by using a phantom that has alternating stacks of high-attenuation and low-attenuation material, as pictured in **A**. This concept was originally described by Michael Defrise. In a system with good sampling along z (**B**), only minimal cone beam artifacts are seen. However, for a true cone beam CT scanner (**C**), the connections between the dense areas in the image demonstrate the cone beam artifact, which arises due to undersampling the object in Fourier space.

environment, cone beam artifacts can be kept to a minimum (Fig. 10-69B); however, the use of large cone angles can lead to considerable artifacts (Fig. 10-69C). Cone beam artifacts are a result of fundamental deficits in the acquired data, and the most obvious solution for these artifacts is to acquire a more complete data set.

10.7 CT Generations

Knowledge of the development of CT is useful because it demonstrates how engineering challenges were gradually overcome as new technology became available. In addition, it is common to refer to various acquisition geometries by their "generation" in CT, and so this section also provides the reader with the necessary vernacular used in the CT field.

Translate-Rotate: First- and Second-Generation CT

The first CT scanner used clinically was the EMI Mark 1, offered in 1972. By today's standards, the scanner would be virtually unusable with an 80 × 80 array of 2.4-mm pixels, and a 3-bit (8 shades of gray) image. But 40 years ago, CT provided physicians the nascent ability to see 3D anatomy within the body that did not require open surgery.

This first scanner was a head scanner only. An x-ray tube was mounted in a fixed relationship with the two detector array (the first multislice CT scanner!), and 80 parallel rays were acquired as the assembly translated across the FOV. The system rotated 1 degree, and then the x-ray tube/detector assembly translated in the other direction (Fig. 10-70). This scanning pattern continued until 180 degrees of data were acquired. This rotate-translate geometry using the pencil beam is referred to as the first-generation CT. The scan required over 4 minutes and image reconstruction ran overnight.

The success of the first EMI scanner led to the rapid development of the second-generation CT—which used the same rotate-translate motion as before; however, more detectors were added and so the initial pencil beam geometry became a narrow fan beam. A detector array using 30 detectors meant that more data could be acquired in a given scan (Fig.10-71) , and so this led to a shorter scan time and a larger, 160 × 160 matrix, reconstructed image.

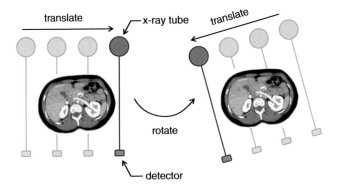

Translate-Rotate
First & Second Generation CT

■ **FIGURE 10-70** First- and second-generation CT systems used a translate-rotate motion for scanning the patient. The x-ray tube and detector assembly translate in one direction acquiring a series of rays that were parallel to each other, the system rotated 1 degree, and then the x-ray tube/detector translated back in the other direction. This scanning procedure continued until a total of 180 degrees of projection data was acquired.

Rotate-Rotate: Third-Generation CT

It was recognized by engineers at the time that the translate-rotate geometry of the first- and second-generation CT could never lead to rapid scanning, due to the large inertial forces involved in stopping the translation in one direction, and then reversing direction. For faster scanning, the translational motion had to go. Hence, with third-generation CT, the x-ray tube and detector array are mounted in a fixed position with respect to each other on a rotating gantry; however, the detector array is now long enough to allow angular sampling over the entire FOV. The rotate-rotate geometry of the third-generation CT (Fig. 10-72A) is still the most widely used geometry on modern scanners. With a detector array which sweeps out a fan angle of α, and a CT system with a source to isocenter distance of S, the diameter of the FOV is given by

$$FOV = 2S \, \sin(\alpha / 2)$$ [10-14]

For a practical body CT scanner, the FOV should be about 50 cm in diameter, and with a source to isocenter distance of 50 cm, the fan angle α needs to be about 60 degrees. Most modern CT scanners have geometries that roughly ($\pm 20\%$) adhere to these values.

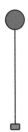

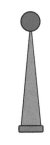

■ **FIGURE 10-71** The first-generation CT system had just two detectors, offset in z—so this first CT scanner was really a multiple detector system. The second-generation CT used more detectors arranged in the x-y plane, which produced better sampling for the CT reconstruction.

Pencil Beam
First Generation CT

Narrow Fan Beam
Second Generation CT

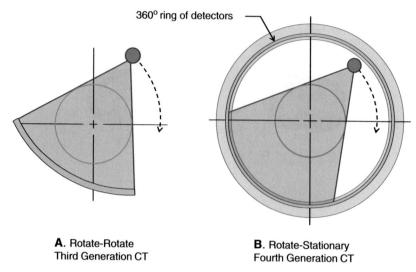

A. Rotate-Rotate
Third Generation CT

B. Rotate-Stationary
Fourth Generation CT

■ **FIGURE 10-72 A.** Third-generation CT is characterized by a gantry with rigidly mounted x-ray system and detector arrays, in which both systems rotate together around the patient—resulting in the rotate-rotate motion **B.** Fourth-generation CT systems used an entire 360-degree ring of detectors mounting in the stationary frame, with a rotating x-ray tube resulting in rotate-stationary acquisition.

Cable Spools and Inertial Limitations

Earlier third-generation CT scanners required cable spools to accommodate the cables, which connected the rotating components to the stationary components—the largest cable was the thick high-tension cable that ran between the stationary x-ray generator and the x-ray tube, which was on the rotating gantry, but power to motors (fans, collimator motors, etc.) and other rotating components (detectors, computers, etc.) also had to be provided, and the signals from the detectors had to be conveyed off of the moving gantry. These cable connections between the rotating and stationary frame required that the gantry accelerate fast, perform the scan, and then decelerate rapidly before cable lengths were exceeded. Much of the engineering involved cable handling systems. The cable-connected third-generation CT scanner had no inertial limitations during the acquisition of a single CT image (unlike first- and second-generation geometry); however, large acceleration and deceleration cycles existed between the acquisition of each CT image, and thus CT scan times (which involve the acquisition of many CT images) were several minutes. The minimum scan time on scanners with cable connections was about 3 s.

The introduction of the slip ring scanner (Fig. 10-5 shows a slip ring) has eliminated the cable connections between the stationary and rotating frames. However, because the x-ray tube is powered at electrical potentials of up to 140,000 V, the slip ring scanner requires that the x-ray transformer be located on the rotating frame to avoid the arcing problems that a 140-kV slip ring connection would cause. To convey sufficient power across the slip ring, very high current is required. The slip ring allows the CT gantry to rotate freely and therefore eliminates the need to deal with gantry inertia between scans. Allowing the table to move continuously as in helical (spiral) scanning eliminated patient inertia issues, and the elimination of inertial barriers during the entire examination led to the 0.3- to 0.5-s gantry rotation periods of modern CT scanners.

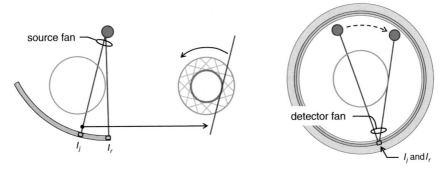

A. Third Generation CT   **B**. Ring artifact formation   **C**. Fourth Generation CT

■ **FIGURE 10-73** The rigid alignment of the x-ray source and detector array in third-generation CT (**A**) gives rise to the potential for ring artifact generation when the CT detectors are not properly calibrated with respect to each other (**B**). In fourth-generation CT, the alignment of the x-ray tube changes with respect to the detector array and the CT data are computed from the so-called detector fan (**C**). Because in fourth-generation CT each detector serves as its own reference detection, changes in detector sensitivity are factored out in the computation of the projection data sets—eliminating ring artifacts.

Rotate-Stationary: Fourth-Generation CT

The third-generation CT geometry leads to the potential for ring artifact production, due to the fixed angular relationship between the detectors and the x-ray source on the gantry. Fourth-generation CT scanners were designed primarily to address this issue. A fourth-generation CT scanner has a rotating x-ray tube but the entire detector array is stationary (Fig. 10-72B); hence, these systems have a rotate-stationary geometry. The major observation with fourth-generation scanners is that an entire 360-degree array of detectors is needed, instead of the 60-degree detector array of a third-generation scanner. Thus, a factor of six more detector elements is required, adding significant cost.

The rationale for the fourth-generation geometry is seen in Figure 10-73. Third-generation scanners (Fig. 10-73A) use a *source fan* geometry where the signal from two different detectors is used to make the two x-ray intensity measurements (I_r and I_j) necessary to compute a projection value, as described in Equation 10-8. If one detector drifts in terms of its calibration with respect to the other detector, the error in the projection measurement P_j will be propagated throughout the backprojection process, leading to a ring artifact (Fig. 10-73B). With the fourth-generation CT, a *detector fan* geometry is used (Fig. 10-73C). The same detector is used to make both measurements necessary to compute the projection value, and therefore any drift in the detector will be intrinsically factored out since the I_r and I_j measurements are made by the exact same detector element. This fundamentally eliminates the production of ring artifacts in the reconstructed CT image.

Fourth-generation CT geometry was devised in the 1970s as a method to combat ring artifacts with third-generation CT. Since that time, however, there have been enormous improvements in detector stability and in algorithms that monitor and correct for electronic gain fluctuations in the detector hardware. In addition to these preprocessing steps to reduce ring artifacts, algorithms have been developed that can correct for ring artifacts in the reconstructed CT images. These correction procedures have all but eliminated the ring artifact problem in modern third-generation CT systems.

SUGGESTED READING

Boone JM. Determination of the pre-sampled MTF in computed tomography. *Med Phys* 2001;28: 356–360.

Defrise M, Townsend D, Geissbuhler A. Implementation of three-dimensional image reconstruction for multi-ring positron tomographs. *Phys Med Biol.* 1990;35(10):1361–1372.

Feldkamp LA, Davis LC, Kress JW. Practical Cone-beam algorithm. *JOSA A.* 1984;1:612–619.

Joseph PM, Spital RD. A method for correcting bone induced artifacts in computed tomography scanners. *J Comput Assist Tomogr* 1978;2(1):100–108.

Kalender WA. *Computed Tomography: Fundamentals, System Technology, Image Quality, Applications,* 3rd Edition, Publics Publishing, Erlangen, Germany 2011.

Kalender WA, Seissler W, Klotz E, Vock P. Spiral volumetric CT with single-breath-hold technique, continuous transport, and continuous scanner rotation. *Radiology.* 1990 Jul;176(1):181–183.

Seidensticker PR, Hofmann LK. *Dual source CT imaging.* Heidelberg, Germany: Springer, 2008.

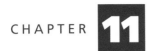
X-ray Dosimetry in Projection Imaging and Computed Tomography

11.1 Attenuation of X-rays in Tissue

When x-rays are used to image a patient, the *primary* x-ray beam is incident upon the entrant tissues of the patient and is attenuated at depth. For a depth x of tissue, the attenuation of the primary x-ray beam is determined by

$$D(x) = D_o \ e^{-\mu_{eff} x} \qquad [11\text{-}1a]$$

where D_o is the dose at the skin surface, $D(x)$ is the dose at greater distances from the skin, and μ_{eff} is the effective linear attenuation coefficient. The effective linear attenuation coefficient is that value that most closely matches the attenuation profile of a polyenergetic x-ray spectrum. Whereas Equations 11-1a and 11-1b is suitable for most cases, a more complete mathematical description of primary x-ray beam attenuation for a narrow beam geometry when an x-ray spectrum $\phi(E)$ is used is given by

$$D(x) = \int_{E=E\min}^{E\max} dE \ \phi(E) \ e^{-\mu(E)x}, \qquad [11\text{-}1b]$$

Figure 11-1 illustrates the intensity of the x-ray beam as a function of tissue thickness of the patient. X-ray beams are attenuated exponentially (i.e., Equations 11-1a and 11-1b), and this is plotted on a log-linear graph (Fig. 11-1). At 80 kV (2.5 mm added Al), only 1 out of 118 photons survives to a depth of 20 cm, and only 1 out of 353 photons survives to 25 cm. At 120 kV, only one out of 190 x-ray photons in the beam penetrates a 25-cm thickness of tissue and exits the patient toward the detector. These numbers illustrate that primary x-ray photons that exit the patient are relatively rare, and therefore structures that attenuate postpatient primary photons (patient table, detector covers, anti-scatter grid, etc.) should be designed to be minimally attenuating.

As a primary x-ray beam strikes an object and undergoes attenuation, many of the interaction events occur as Rayleigh or Compton scattering. Equations 11-1a and 11-1b describe the attenuation of *primary* x-rays but do not and cannot accurately describe what happens to the *scattered* x-ray photons that occur from primary photon scattering interactions. It has been observed that scattered photons can undergo subsequent scattering events. To accurately account for scattered photon dose deposition, Monte Carlo techniques, described later, are necessary.

Although attenuation leads to the deposition of radiation dose in the patient, attenuation is necessary for creating a projection image. In the absence of attenuation, no dose would be deposited but there would be no useful image either. In diagnostic radiology, x-rays interact by a combination of complete absorption events (photoelectric absorption) and scattering events (Compton and Rayleigh scattering).

375

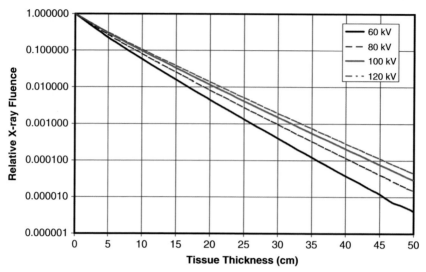

■ **FIGURE 11-1** The attenuation profiles for x-ray spectra at four different tube voltages are shown. The vertical axis is logarithmic, which compresses the actual magnitude of the attenuation.

Only the photoelectric effect and Compton scatter lead to dose deposited in tissue. Scattered radiation has an important role in redistributing the primary beam dose deposition patterns, and consequently, tissues outside the collimated (primary) x-ray beam receive some radiation dose due to scattered radiation. To the extent that x-ray scattering results in a fraction of x-ray photons *leaving* the patient's body, scatter represents a physical mechanism by which radiation dose to the patient is slightly reduced. However, in imaging procedures such as fluoroscopy where staff are near the patient, the scattered x-rays leaving the patient then become a source of radiation dose for the personnel in the fluoroscopic suite. All of the photon attenuation mechanisms mentioned above, as well as many of the dose terms discussed below, were introduced in Chapter 3.

Dosimetry in x-ray imaging is fundamentally related to x-ray attenuation, and the effective penetration of the x-ray spectrum has an important role to play in regard to attenuation (Fig. 11-1). The position of the x-ray field on the patient, the size of the x-ray field, the thickness and composition of the patient along the direction of the x-ray beam, and whether or not the x-ray beam changes position during the acquisition (as with tomography) are the patient and geometrical factors that influence overall dose and the pattern of dose deposition in the patient.

Absorbed dose, or simply "dose," is defined as

$$Absorbed\ Dose = \frac{Energy\ Imparted}{Mass} \qquad [11\text{-}2]$$

When *Energy Imparted* has the units of *joule*, and *Mass* is in *kilograms*, the dose unit is the gray (joule/kg). Thus, a millijoule deposited in a gram of tissue leads to a gray of dose. One gray is equal to 100 rads, and most (but not all) x-ray imaging procedures result in absorbed doses from tenths of mGy to a few tens of mGy.

Over the years, there have been a number of dosimetry metrics that have been used to estimate the radiation dose to patients for x-ray imaging. As a result, there are several different *surrogate* dose metrics that the practitioner should be aware of, in addition to absorbed dose. This chapter outlines some of the most commonly used figure of merits, as well as currently accepted dosimetry methods.

11.2 Dose-Related Metrics in Radiography and Fluoroscopy

For a projection image such as an abdominal radiograph, the magnitude of the dose changes dramatically with depth in the patient. This huge heterogeneity in dose makes an accurate dose assessment difficult. Figure 11-2 underscores this. Even across the distance of a fist-sized organ such as the kidney, the dose can change by as much as a factor of 3. In order to estimate organ doses, the exponential nature of the dose distribution must be taken into consideration.

While it is relatively difficult to compute various tissue doses in projection radiography, it is relatively easy to estimate the kerma at the skin surface—the entrance skin kerma (ESK). In order to estimate the entrance skin dose (ESD), the air kerma at the skin layer must be estimated.

X-ray Tube Output: mGy per 100 mAs

Most periodic quality control procedures performed on radiographic systems involve the measurement of the air kerma as a function of mAs at a specified distance from the x-ray source, over a range of kVs. Typically, the air kerma (mGy per 100 mAs at 100 cm) is measured (in the past, exposure in the units of mR per mAs was measured). An example of such information is shown in Figure 11-3. The output values (also listed in Table 11-1) are valid for the specific x-ray system in which the data were measured, and other x-ray systems will have slight-to-substantial variations from these values depending primarily on the amount of inherent filtration there is in the x-ray beam.

X-ray Imaging Geometry: Source-to-Skin Distance (SSD)

Referring to Figure 11-4, the distance from the x-ray tube's focal spot to the entrance skin layer—the source-to-skin distance (SSD)—needs to be estimated. Since most

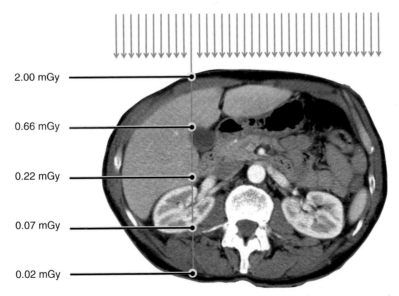

■ FIGURE 11-2 This figure shows the typical attenuation values as the x-ray beam penetrates the tissues in the body, represented here by an axial CT image. The x-ray dose at the surface of the patient is 2.0 mGy, and this value is attenuated to just 0.02 mGy at the exit surface, demonstrating that the x-ray intensity is reduced by a factor of 100 in this example.

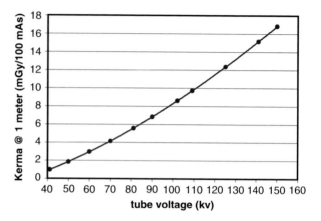

■ **FIGURE 11-3** The output kerma for a typical x-ray tube is illustrated. X-ray tube output efficiency increases slightly with tube voltage, as the upward curve of this graph illustrates.

radiography is performed at a source-to-detector distance of 100 cm (chest radiography at 183 cm), the SSD can be estimated by knowing the approximate thickness of the patient. For example, for a 25-cm-thick patient, with a 2-cm separation between the patient and the detector, the SSD is computed as SSD = 100 − [25 + 2] = 73 cm.

TABLE 11-1 HALF-VALUE LAYER AND OUTPUT LEVELS AS A FUNCTION OF kV FOR A TYPICAL GENERAL DIAGNOSTIC X-RAY SYSTEM

kV	HVL (mm Al)	OUTPUT (mGy per 100 mAs)
40	1.15	1.1
45	1.36	1.7
50	1.57	2.3
55	1.79	2.9
60	2.00	3.5
65	2.22	4.3
70	2.43	5.0
75	2.65	5.8
80	2.86	6.7
85	3.08	7.5
90	3.29	8.5
95	3.50	9.5
100	3.71	10.5
105	3.92	11.6
110	4.12	12.7
115	4.32	13.9
120	4.51	15.1
125	4.71	16.4
130	4.89	17.8
135	5.08	19.2
140	5.25	20.6

Output was measured free in air at a distance of 100 cm from the x-ray source, along the central beam. Multiply output column by 1.45 to get mR/mAS.

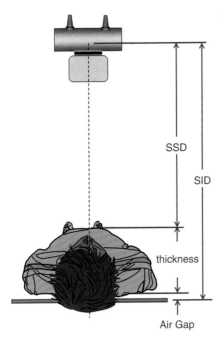

■ **FIGURE 11-4** The standard imaging geometry in radiography is illustrated, here for an anterior-posterior (AP) projection image. The source to detector distance (SID) is typically 100 cm for radiography, except it is 183 cm for upright chest radiography. The source to skin distance (SSD) can be estimated by knowing the SID, the thickness of the patient, and the dead space between the cover of the detector and the actual detector surface ("air gap" in this figure).

Estimation of Entrance Skin Kerma

Let us say that a radiograph was acquired using 80 kV and 82 mAs, and the SSD in Figure 11-4 was estimated to be 73 cm. Table 11-1 shows that at 80 kV, the output of this x-ray system is 6.7 mGy per 100 mAs at a distance of 100 cm from the source. The x-ray tube output at a given kV is linearly proportional to the mAs. For example, double the mAs and the air kerma will double. For the 82 mAs used in the example, the output kerma K is

$$K_{82mAs} = \frac{82}{100} K_{100mAs} \qquad \text{[11-3a]}$$

where K_{100mAs} is determined from Table 11-1 for 80 kV (6.7 mGy per 100 mAs), and thus, the kerma for this technique at 100 cm is 5.5 mGy. Correction for the inverse square law is necessary to compute the entrance kerma at the 73-cm SSD:

$$ESK = \left[\frac{100\,cm}{73\,cm} \right]^2 K_{82\,mAs} \qquad \text{[11-3b]}$$

As determined from Equation 11-3a, K_{82mAs} at 100 cm was 5.5 mGy. The inverse square correction in this example equates to a factor of 1.88, resulting in an ESK of 10.3 mGy (1.18 R).

Calculations as described above make use of so-called *free-in-air* measurements of kerma, and thus, x-ray scattering in tissue does not contaminate the estimate. Free-in-air measurements are also known as "without backscatter." If one were to actually measure the kerma by placing an ionization chamber in front of a tissue-equivalent phantom, the probe would measure both the incident primary beam and a considerable amount of scattered radiation from the phantom; because this scatter is directed back toward the x-ray source, it is called backscatter. When backscatter is included, depending on the beam energy and geometry, the measurement would be about 15% to 30% higher than a free-in-air measurement at the same position and with the same x-ray technique factors. It is common to refer to ESK measurements as "with backscatter" or "without backscatter," to clarify the measurement methodology. In general, most tabulated dose data (but not all) are computed for *free-in-air* measurements, as will be discussed below.

The ESK (formerly the quantity *entrance skin exposure* was used, involving different units) is a *surrogate measure* of the dose used in projection radiography. The ESK is *not* an accurate estimate of tissue dose but has evolved as an informal metric for comparing doses among radiographic procedures. For example, in the example of abdominal radiography given above, the ESK was computed as 10.3 mGy. A chest radiographic procedure may have an ESK of about 0.09 mGy or 90 µGy, but this is one of the lowest dose radiographic procedures performed. The abdominal radiograph requires more kerma because the abdomen (mostly solid tissue) at typically 80 kV attenuates considerably more than the lung parenchyma in the chest radiograph at 120 kV.

Estimation of Skin Dose in Radiography

The ESK represents the radiation intensity as the x-ray beam impinges on the surface of the skin. The skin dose, at the very surface of the skin where no attenuation has occurred, is computed as

$$ESD = \frac{\left(\dfrac{\mu_{en}}{\rho}\right)_{tissue}}{\left(\dfrac{\mu_{en}}{\rho}\right)_{air}} \; ESK \qquad [11\text{-}4]$$

Equation 11-4 is strictly correct only for a narrow entrance beam of primary photons. As the x-ray beam striking the surface of the skin gets larger, the role of scatter increases and for large beams a "backscatter factor" should be included. The ratio of the mass energy attenuation coefficients in Equation 11-4 has a numerical value of about 1.06 for general diagnostic x-ray energies.

Skin Dose in Fluoroscopy

The computation of skin dose in fluoroscopy uses Equation 11-4, but slightly different methods are used to estimate ESK. In fluoroscopy, the *kerma rate* is a function of the mA and kV, and the mA fluctuates during the procedure depending on the positioning of the fluoroscopic system relative to the patient's body and on the mode settings of the fluoroscopy system. The automatic brightness control system on all modern fluoroscopy systems modulates the mA based on the radiation intensity striking the fluoroscopic detector. A common way to estimate this is to use the setup shown in Chapter 9 (Fig. 9-15). Various thicknesses of an attenuator such as polymethyl methacrylate (PMMA) are positioned in the beam as the kerma rate is measured at the detector surface. The kerma rate is measured as a function of the thickness of the PMMA over a range of possible patient thicknesses, and these measurements can be used to estimate the entrance kerma rate to the patient, as shown in Figure 11-5. If the chamber is positioned close to the scatter material, then the measurements will be "with backscatter." Alternatively, the radiation meter can be positioned well away from the attenuator (i.e., closer to the x-ray tube), which would reduce the contribution of scatter to the measurement such that it is "without backscatter." In this later

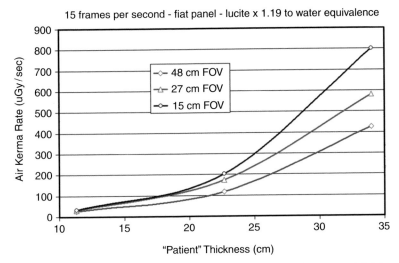

■ **FIGURE 11-5** In fluoroscopy, the measured x-ray flux at the detector drives the automatic brightness control circuitry, and the air kerma rate is controlled by the mA and kV of the system. In-field measurements of patient dose make use of plastic phantoms of varying thickness. The field of view also affects the gain of the detector system, and so measurements are made as a function of field of view. The data shown in this plot are for a flat panel detector–based fluoroscopic system.

case, the inverse square law is then used to calculate the measured kerma rates at the entrant surface of the "patient."

Modern fluoroscopy systems have the ability to automatically record the total fluoroscopy time used (in minutes) for a procedure, and the total fluoroscopy time is converted to seconds and multiplied by the kerma rate to determine the total ESK. From this, Equation 11-4 can then be applied to compute ESD. This calculation assumes that the entrance beam is located at the same position on the patient, such that the same patch of skin was exposed during the entire fluoroscopic procedure. When the fluoroscopy system is positioned at a number of different positions such that different areas of skin receive the entrance beam (as when both PA and lateral projections are used), the total time for each position must be estimated for the calculation of ESD in each location.

Many fluoroscopic systems employ Kerma-Area-Product (KAP) meters. These devices are mounted between the x-ray source and the patient (Fig. 9-15), and monitor the total KAP during a fluoroscopic procedure. If radiographic images are acquired, the doses from these are also included in the KAP value. The value of KAP is the product of the total air kerma exiting the x-ray tube housing and the area of the beam, and hence the units are mGy-cm². A calibration procedure can be performed to convert the KAP value into an estimate of ESK. Newer KAP meters also are required to provide a center "point kerma" reading. This value can be used directly to estimate the ESK, with the caveats mentioned above in regard to variable positioning of the beam on the patient. Because of the relative consistency of output of modern fluoroscopic systems combined with the comprehensive digital design of the systems (i.e., where SSD is known), for a well-engineered system, the ESK can be *inferred* (estimated), forgoing the need for a physical KAP meter.

The estimate of skin dose is useful primarily when fluoroscopic, cinefluorographic, and fluorographic procedures are performed and combine to produce high skin doses with potential deterministic effects. Deterministic effects in fluoroscopy are rare and usually occur in only the most lengthy procedures involving complicated cardiac or vascular interventional procedures. Estimates of skin dose will help to gauge whether dermatological effects such as epilation or erythema may occur, and to determine if the patient should be monitored for such effects. While the skin dose is the highest dose in the patient for projection radiographic procedures such as fluoroscopy and radiography, it is not an accurate measurement of the entire patient dose—that is discussed in the next sections.

11.3 Monte Carlo Dose Computation

Most modern x-ray dosimetry is based upon *Monte Carlo* calculations, with reference to the stochastic nature of gambling in the principality of Monaco. Monte Carlo. Monte Carlo procedures use computer simulation to study the dose deposition during an x-ray exposure. Computer programs can be used to produce random numbers, similar conceptually to flipping a coin, except that the output of the *random number generator* is usually a continuous variable between 0 and 1. Using these values, any probability distribution can be produced. Using the known physics of x-ray interaction in tissues, the known probabilities of scattering events (both Rayleigh and Compton scattering) as a function of angle and x-ray energy, a geometrical model of the simulated patient, and the random number generator, Monte Carlo calculations compute the three-dimensional dose distribution for a given exposure geometry (Fig. 11-6). The power of modern computers allows Monte Carlo simulations to be performed using many simulated photons, which reduces statistical uncertainty in the computation. Typically, 10^6 to 10^8 photons are simulated and their individual trajectories and interactions are tracked by the Monte Carlo program, photon by photon and interaction by interaction. Even though millions of photons (i.e., 10^6) can be

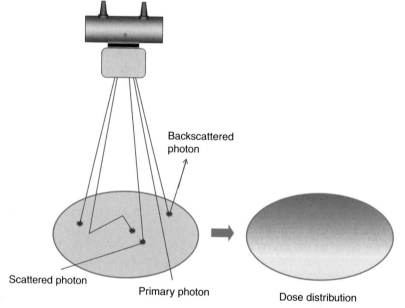

Backscattered photon

Scattered photon

Primary photon

Dose distribution

■ **FIGURE 11-6** Monte Carlo dosimetry is based on tracking the trajectory and energy deposition of x-ray photons through a mathematical phantom with a defined geometry and composition. Millions to billions of photons are typically simulated to produce a computed dose distribution in the phantom; using realistic mathematical models of patient anatomy, organ doses can be estimated with excellent accuracy.

TABLE 11-2 ORGAN CONVERSION FACTORS FOR SELECTED RADIOGRAPHIC PROCEDURES

	μ Gy PER mGy ENTRANCE KERMA				
	HVL FOR ENTRANT X-RAY BEAM (mm Al)				
	1.0	2.0	3.0	4.0	5.0
Lungs	2.4	9.6	17.2	24.0	28.6
Active bone marrow	7.4	30.9	59.5	85.9	109.9
Thyroid	0.0	0.1	0.2	0.3	0.3
Trunk tissue	68.7	137.4	187.8	224.4	253.0
Ovaries	59.5	183.2	296.6	385.9	453.4
Uterus	83.6	249.6	395.0	506.1	586.2

Adapted from Table 41 (AP Abdominal Radiography) 100 cm SID, 35 × 43 cm field of view, in *Handbook of Selected Tissue Doses for Projections Common in Diagnostic Radiology*, HEW publication (FDA) 89-8031 (1989).

simulated in Monte Carlo programs, the number of simulated photons is still much lower than that which occurs in a physical radiographic acquisition. For example, for a typical x-ray beam used in chest radiography (a very low dose examination), a total of about 1.6×10^{11} photons are incident upon the patient. For Monte Carlo calculations, the organ doses are normalized per incident kerma so that the results can be calibrated to the photon intensities used in actual imaging procedures.

Typically, Monte Carlo calculations are performed over a range of x-ray energies (e.g., 10 to 140 keV by 1 keV), and then the results are normalized for a given x-ray spectrum. X-ray spectra can be generated by computer models, or tabulated measured spectra can be used. Energy deposited in tissue from x-ray interactions is tallied when a photoelectric interaction occurs (in such cases, essentially all of the x-ray energy is deposited locally in tissue), or when a Compton scattering event takes place (the energy deposited at the site of a Compton interaction is the difference in energy between the incident x-ray photon and the scattered photon). Rayleigh scattering results in a slight redirection of the x-ray photon, but no energy is absorbed and so no dose is conveyed. After millions or even billions of x-ray interactions are simulated, the deposited energy is combined with the known mass of each small tissue volume and the absorbed dose can then be computed.

For radiography, Monte Carlo simulations have been performed for a comprehensive set of standard imaging projections, such as the chest radiograph (AP and lateral), skull (AP and lateral), and so on. Typically, the doses to the individual organs in the mathematical model are computed individually. A number of publications are available that contain tables that describe the organ dose for each radiographic projection. The data tables are provided over a range of x-ray spectra or beam qualities for each projection. An example for abdominal radiography is given in Table 11-2.

11.4 Equivalent Dose

In industries such as nuclear power or isotope projection facilities, particles such as neutrons, alpha particles, and energetic ions can be sources of radiation dose. Various types of particulate radiations at different energies do not produce the same biological damage per unit absorbed dose as x-ray or gamma-ray photons. The relative biological effectiveness of these heavy charged particle radiations to that of x-ray or gamma photons (and the energetic electrons they produce) is represented by the radiation weighting factor w_R. When the absorbed dose D to a tissue is known, the equivalent dose H can be computed using

$$H = D w_R \qquad [11\text{-}5]$$

When the units of D are milligray (mGy), and the unit of H are millisievert (Sv), the units of w_R are mSv mGy^{-1}. Biological effects are discussed in more detail in Chapter 20.

The radiation weighting factor w_R for x-rays and γ-rays is 1.0, and although the *equivalent dose* can in principle be computed with x-rays or γ-rays using this factor of 1.0 (resulting in the units of mSv), this practice is discouraged in x-ray dosimetry as it can lead to confusion with *effective dose* (E), which is discussed below.

11.5 Organ Doses from X-ray Procedures

Because the radiosensitivity of each organ is different, the computation of organ doses for x-ray dosimetry is considered the most accurate way in which to assess the overall radiation dose. A comprehensive understanding of organ doses also allows the radiation risks to be estimated for the *generic* patient. Dose assessments to the generic patient do not take into consideration patient age, gender, or body size. A complete assessment of organ doses also allows one to compute cancer detriment or E, as discussed later. A list of organs and tissues that affect the radiation risk profile is provided in Table 11-3.

TABLE 11-3 TISSUE WEIGHTING FACTORS (W_t) FOR VARIOUS TISSUES AND ORGANS (ICRP 103)

TISSUE	W_t
Gonads	0.08
Bone marrow	0.12
Colon	0.12
Lung	0.12
Stomach	0.12
Bladder	0.04
Breast	0.12
Liver	0.04
Esophagus	0.04
Thyroid	0.04
Skin	0.01
Bone surface	0.01
Brain	0.01
Salivary glands	0.01
Remainder	0.12
Total	1.00

W_t values are in the units of mSv/mGy.

This list of organs clearly is biased toward the visceral organs in the abdomen, and consequently, for the same absorbed dose levels, abdominal x-ray imaging is associated with higher risks than for similar radiation dose levels to the head or lower extremities.

Organ doses can be estimated in radiography or fluoroscopy using a series of Monte Carlo–derived tables for each radiographic projection, and similar concepts hold for computed tomography as well. These will be discussed below.

11.6 Effective Dose

A comprehensive estimation of organ dose is the first step in a complete description of stochastic risk to a generic "patient". Once organ doses to each of the organs listed in Table 11-3 are computed (in many imaging procedures, some organs will have zero dose), then it is straightforward to compute the E. The equivalent dose concept discussed above described weighting factors w_R, for different types of radiation, but E uses *tissue* weighting factors (w_T). Notice that in Table 11-3, the sum of the tissue weighting factors is 1.000, and the E concept can be thought of as a method of computing radiation detriment for partial body exposures, typical of medical imaging procedures—for example, if a patient received X amount of radiation dose to a tissue T, the whole-body dose that has the same risk would be calculated as $w_T \times$ X. Conversely, if a person were to receive a homogeneous whole body x-ray radiation exposure where all organs received the same absorbed dose D, then the E would be $E = 1.00$ Sv/Gy $\times D$. The SI unit of E is the sievert (Sv). In medical imaging, the units of effective dose typically encountered are mSv or μSv, and the units of absorbed dose D are mGy or μGy, thus w_T has units of mSv mGy^{-1}.

The tissue weighting factors listed in Table 11-3 were defined by a scientific committee (International Commission on Radiation Protection—ICRP 103), in their evaluation of epidemiological data from radiation exposure in humans, primarily the A-bomb survivors in Japan during World War II.

Cautionary Notes in the Use of Effective Dose

The utility and interpretation of E can be complicated, and there are some necessary caveats that need to be understood in regard to E. First, despite common practice (especially in CT), the use of E was never intended to be used for assigning risk to a specific patient—that is, a specific patient who has undergone a particular radiological procedure. The organ-specific radiation risks that are embedded in the w_T coefficients were calculated for a generic person, not a specific individual. Any specific patient may have a completely different risk profile than a generic individual—for instance, the patient may be 5 years old, or he or she may be 85 years old. The patient may be female, where risks are generally greater than for male patients. The patient may weigh 40 or 140 kg—each with profoundly different radiation doses and corresponding risk profiles than the average radiation worker. The patient may also have had a disease such as cancer, where risks of cancer induction are likely heightened by potential genetic predisposition chemotherapy, radiation therapy.

Where E is useful in radiological imaging is for comparing various radiological imaging procedures. For example, the radiation risk between a chest radiograph and a thoracic CT can be assessed, and the relative risk can be computed. Pediatric head radiography can be compared to a modified low-dose head CT procedure for evaluation of chronic sinus inflammation—there are many examples. Such a calculation may be useful in optimizing clinical imaging for a generic patient.

11.7 Absorbed Dose in Radiography and Fluoroscopy

The most straightforward way to compute the absorbed dose to a patient from a radiographic procedure is to determine the ESK and x-ray beam quality, and then locate the appropriate table for the radiographic projection (e.g., Table 11-2). These tables were produced using Monte Carlo simulations. A series of simple calculations then allows the computation of individual organ doses. Some tables provide direct conversion from entrance surface dose to E for radiographic projections, and an example of that for chest radiography is given in Table 11-4.

Since the introduction of the E concept in 1977, the organs selected for use in computing E and the w_T value assigned to them have changed twice (1991 and 2007) as the ICRP has refined their models and updated their recommendations. Consequently, the usefulness of some of the E estimation tables may be limited by the E formalism that was in effect at the time the table was created.

Other forms of direct dose estimation are possible. If one is interested in the point dose from *primary* radiation at a certain depth d in the patient from a radiographic projection, such as with fetal dose calculations, it is necessary to keep in mind that the x-ray beam experiences both tissue attenuation and a reduction in intensity from the inverse square law at depth. For an x-ray beam with an effective tissue linear attenuation coefficient of μ_{eff}, a known SSD, a known ESD (per Equation 11-4), and a depth d beyond the skin surface (along the direction of the x-ray beam), the point dose can be estimated as

TABLE 11-4

X-RAY POTENTIAL (kV)	FILTRATION (mm OF Al)	ANTEROPOSTERIOR (mSv/mGy)	POSTEROANTERIOR (mSv/mGy)	LATERAL (mSv/mGy)
90	2	0.176	0.116	0.074
90	3	0.196	0.131	0.084
90	4	0.210	0.143	0.091
100	2	0.190	0.128	0.081
100	3	0.208	0.143	0.091
100	4	0.222	0.155	0.098
110	2	0.201	0.139	0.088
110	3	0.219	0.154	0.097
110	4	0.232	0.165	0.104
120	2	0.211	0.149	0.094
120	3	0.228	0.163	0.103
120	4	0.240	0.174	0.110

Note: This table is an example for chest radiography, where the ED (msv) per entrance surface dose (mGy) is given for three different radiographic projections. The kV and filtration levels allow adjustment for different x-ray technique factors used for the procedure. Effective dose per entrance surface dose (mSv per mGy) for chest radiology 183 cm SID.
Source: From Estimation of effective dose in diagnostic radiology from entrance surface dose and dose-area product measurements. National Radiation Protection Board of Great Britain, 1994, Table 7.

$$D_d = \left(\frac{SSD}{SSD + d}\right)^2 e^{-\mu_{eff} d} \; ESD \qquad\qquad [11\text{-}6]$$

When the dose from scattered radiation is not considered, as in the above example, the estimates should be considered accurate to within an order of magnitude. The most common method to accommodate for scattered radiation is to use Monte Carlo simulation techniques or tables derived from them.

11.8 CT Dosimetry and Organ Doses

CT dosimetry is in a time of flux. As CT scanners have become more complicated and more capable, there are numerous operational modes that place challenges on the accuracy of dosimetry. Herein, a basic overview of CT dosimetry is provided.

Organ Doses in CT

Organ dosimetry in computed tomography is commonly performed using table lookup as with radiography; however, the normalization process is not the same. In radiography and fluoroscopy, the ESK is computed and used with the tables to compute organ dose. In CT, the concept of ESK is ambiguous due to the rotation of the x-ray source around the patient. The solution in this case is to compute the air kerma at the isocenter of the scanner—that is, at the center of rotation of the gantry with nothing in the beam. Most tables for CT organ doses are normalized to the air kerma at the isocenter. As with radiography, these tables are typically generated using Monte Carlo methods. There are a number of commercially available dose computation packages that are used by medical physicists to expedite organ dose computation in CT It is very important to remember that organ dose computation in CT using tables generally assumes that the entire organ has been irradiated. For CT angiography and perfusion studies and other CT acquisition protocols, this may not be the case. Dose in CT angiography and perfusion is discussed below.

Due to the rotational irradiation geometry used in CT, the radiation dose distribution in the patient is far more homogeneous than in radiography or fluoroscopy. The use of a beam-shaping filter further reduces heterogeneity in the dose distribution. Thus, in CT, the dose gradients are very slight, and the distribution depends on the diameter and shape of the patient and on the beam quality (kV).

In helical (spiral) acquisition, most modern CT scanners have dose modulation modes that adjust the x-ray tube output (by varying the mA) as the gantry rotates around the patient and as the table translates the patient through the rotating x-ray beam. Dose modulation modes generally increase the mA (and hence dose rate) as the x-ray beam is aligned along thicker x-ray paths through the patient, and the mA is reduced for thinner x-ray path lengths through the patient. The changing mA in dose modulation mode slightly reduces the accuracy of table lookup CT dosimetry.

Computed Tomography Dose Index, CTDI

The computed tomography dose index (CTDI) was originally designed as an *index*, not as a direct dosimetry method for patient dose assessment. Over the years, there have been enhancements and modifications to the original CTDI concept that have attempted to make it a more accurate patient dosimetry method, with mixed results.

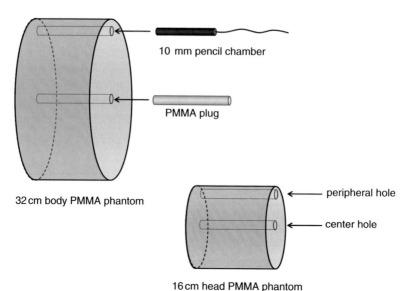

10 mm pencil chamber

PMMA plug

32 cm body PMMA phantom

peripheral hole

center hole

16 cm head PMMA phantom

■ FIGURE 11-7 The computed tomography dose index (CTDI) is measured using either a 16-cm or 32-cm-diameter polymethyl methacrylate (PMMA) phantom. The dosimeter is placed serially in the center hole and the peripheral hole, and the measurements are combined to produce the weighted CTDI, as described in the text.

Despite limitations that will be discussed later, CTDI-based dosimetry is the current worldwide standard for estimation of patient dose in CT.

The basic $CTDI_{100}$ measurement involves the use of a 100-mm-long cylindrical ("pencil") chamber, approximately 9 mm in diameter, inserted into either the center or a peripheral hole of a PMMA phantom. There are two standard PMMA dosimetry phantoms; the body phantom (Fig. 11-7) is 32 cm in diameter and 15 cm long, and the head phantom is 16 cm in diameter and 15 cm long (Fig. 11-7). The head phantom also serves as a pediatric torso phantom. With the pencil chamber located at the center (in the z-dimension) of the phantom and also at the center of the CT gantry, a single axial (also called *sequential*) CT scan is made (using no table translation).

An ionization chamber can only produce an accurate dose estimate if its entire sensitive volume is irradiated by the x-ray beam. Therefore, for the partially irradiated 100-mm CT pencil chamber, the nominal beam width (i.e., the total collimated x-ray beam width as indicated on the CT console) is used to correct the chamber reading for the partial volume exposure. The 100-mm chamber length is useful for x-ray beams from thin slices (e.g., 5 mm) to thicker beam collimations such as 40 mm. The correction for partial volume is essential and is calculated using

$$K_{corrected} = \frac{100\,mm}{B} K_{measured} \qquad [11\text{-}7]$$

where B is the total collimated beam width, in mm, for a single axial scan. The value of B is the product of the width of an individual CT detector projected to the scanner's isocenter (T) and the number of active detectors, n, and so typically $B = nT$. For example on a 64 channel CT scanner (n = 64) with each detector channel measuring 0.625 mm (T = 0.625 mm), $B = 64 \times 0.625$ mm = 40.0 mm.

The $CTDI_{100}$ is defined as

$$CTDI_{100} = \frac{1}{nT} \int_{L=-50\ mm}^{+50\ mm} D(z)\ dz \qquad [11\text{-}8]$$

The $CTDI_{100}$ in the above equation describes the measurement of the dose distribution, $D(z)$, along the z-axis, from a single circular (axial or sequential) rotation of the scanner with a nominal x-ray beam width of nT, where the primary and scattered radiation are measured over a 100-mm length, and where the center of the x-ray beam is at $z = 0$. The nominal beam width refers to the beam width as reported by the scanner, not the actual measured beam width, which is generally slightly wider. As mentioned previously, $CTDI_{100}$ measurements are made for both the center ($CTDI_{100,center}$) and periphery ($CTDI_{100,periphery}$). Combining the center and peripheral measurements using a 1/3 and 2/3 weighting scheme provides a good estimate of the average dose to the phantom (at the central CT slice along z), giving rise to the weighted CTDI, $CTDI_w$:

$$CTDI_w = \tfrac{1}{3}\ CTDI_{100,center} + \tfrac{2}{3}\ CTDI_{100,periphery} \qquad [11\text{-}9]$$

In helical (also called spiral) CT scanning, the CT dose is inversely related to the helical pitch used, that is,

$$dose \propto \frac{1}{pitch} \qquad [11\text{-}10]$$

where the pitch is defined as the table translation distance (mm) during a full rotation (360 degrees) of the gantry, divided by the nominal beam width nT (in mm). Because of this relationship, the $CTDI_w$ is converted to the volume CTDI ($CTDI_{vol}$) using

$$CTDI_{vol} = \frac{CTDI_w}{pitch} \qquad [11\text{-}11]$$

Most scanners have the ability to display the $CTDI_{vol}$ on the CT scanner console *prior* to the actual scan. The value can be displayed because the CT manufacturer has measured $CTDI_{vol}$ in the factory over the range of kV values for that model of scanner, and then that stored value, scaled appropriately by the mAs and pitch, is displayed on the console.

The product of the $CTDI_{vol}$ and the length of the CT scan along the z-axis of the patient, L, is the dose length product (DLP):

$$DLP = CTDI_{vol} \times L \qquad [11\text{-}12]$$

It has been shown that the DLP is approximately proportional to effective dose (E). The slope of the E versus DLP relationship is called the k value, and there are different k values for various CT examinations, as given in Table 11-5.

Limitations of CTDI$_{vol}$

The most important limitation of $CTDI_{vol}$ is that it is a dose *index*, and was not initially meant to be a measurement of dose *per se*. CTDI concepts were meant to enable medical physicists to compare the output between different CT scanners and were not

TABLE 11-5   CONVERSION FACTORS ("k FACTORS") FOR ESTIMATION OF EFFECTIVE DOSE (IN mSv) FROM DOSE-LENGTH PRODUCT (IN mGy-cm), FOR VARIOUS CT EXAMINATION TYPES (FROM AAPM REPORT 96)

CT EXAM TYPE	k FACTOR (mSv/mGy-cm)
Head	0.0021
Chest	0.014
Abdomen	0.015
Abdomen-pelvis	0.015
Pelvis	0.015

originally intended to provide patient-specific dosimetry information. The body $CTDI_{vol}$ as reported by the CT scanner, or as measured on a CT scanner, is a dose index that results from air kerma measurements at two locations to a very large (32-cm diameter) cylinder of PMMA plastic with a density of 1.19 g/cm³. In terms of human dimensions, the 32-cm-diameter PMMA body phantom corresponds to a person with a 119 cm (47") waistline—a large individual, indeed. For smaller patients, the actual doses are larger than the $CTDI_{vol}$ for the same technique factors—thus, the $CTDI_{vol}$ tends to underestimate dose to most patients. In light of this limitation, researchers have recently shown that patient size conversion factors can be used with the $CTDI_{vol}$ reported on a given CT scanner to produce size specific dose estimates (SSDEs). These conversion factors for the $CTDI_{vol}$ measured on a 32-cm-diameter phantom are illustrated graphically in Figure 11.8. The conversion factors described in AAPM Report 204 may be used to more accurately estimate size-corrected doses from the $CTDI_{vol}$, and these conversion factors are (to a first approximation) independent of scanner manufacturer and tube voltage. However, some CT scanner models use the $CTDI_{vol}$ value measured using the 16-cm-diameter PMMA phantom, and caution is needed to ensure that the correction factors specific to the appropriate reference phantom are used.

Another fundamental limitation of the $CTDI_{vol}$ is that it is computed, as defined in Equations 11-8 to 11-11, as the dose (in air) at the center of a 100-mm-long CT scan. However, because scattered radiation is a considerable component of radiation dose to

■ **FIGURE 11-8** This figure shows data taken from AAPM Report 204. This curve shows the conversion factors as a function of the effective diameter of the patient, relative to the 32-cm-diameter $CTDI_{vol}$ phantom. The data from this curve can be used to adjust the displayed $CTDI_{vol}$ when the effective diameter of the patient is known. More detailed information is provided in AAPM Report 204.

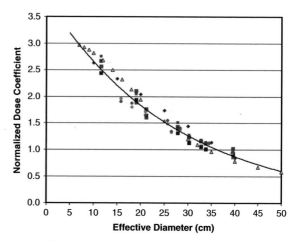

the patient in CT, the scattered dose distribution is important. The dose from scattered radiation in CT tends to be most intense along the z-axis close to the primary beam, and decreases as the distance along z from the primary CT beam increases. The notion of the dose spread function, similar to the line spread function, has been described, and dose spread functions are illustrated in Figure 11-9. The important observation in this figure is the fact that the scatter tails are low-amplitude, long-range functions that extend significant distances in the ±z-dimensions. Because of this, the dose tends to build up (both inside and outside the primary CT scan volume) as the scan length of the CT scan increases. The dose at the center (along z) of the scanned region in the patient builds up the most, and so the dose at the edge of the scanned field is smaller than the dose in the center. These trends are shown in Figure 11-10, where the dose profiles in the z-dimension are illustrated for a number of different CT scan lengths. The amplitude of the primary beam was the same for all dose profiles shown in Figure 11-10, and the dramatic increase in dose at the center of the field of view illustrates the consequence of summing those low-amplitude, long-ranged scatter tails.

As the scan length approaches the range of the scattered radiation tails, the dose at the center of the scan no longer increases and the dose at the center then becomes asymptotic—it no longer increases as the scan length increases. This is shown in Figure 11-11, which is a graph of the dose at the center of the scanned field of view as a function of scan length (or beam width in cone beam CT systems). This figure shows

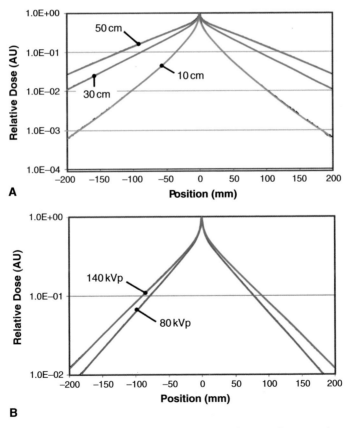

■ **FIGURE 11-9** The long-range, low-amplitude tails from scattered radiation in the CT are shown in this figure. **A.** the scatter tails are shown as a function of distance from the center (narrow) CT slice, for three different cylinder diameters. **B.** This curve shows that higher tube voltages generate scatter tails with greater range. At 200 mm from the narrow beam primary source, the scatter intensity is about 1/100 compared to the center of the beam.

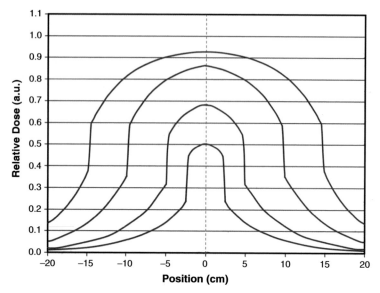

■ **FIGURE 11-10** The relative dose as a function of the position along the z-axis of a CT scan is shown, for different scan lengths. Dose profiles for scan lengths of 5, 10, 20, and 30 cm are shown, and the dose at the center of the field (see *vertical dashed line*) increases dramatically as the scan length increases.

that lower doses are delivered when the scan length is shorter than the equilibrium scan length. Indeed, Figure 11-11 suggests that the known scan length of a specific CT procedure can be used to correct for the radiation dose value at the center of the beam.

The measurement procedure that is used to acquire the data shown in Figure 11-11 is modified from the standard $CTDI_{100}$ methods, and is described by the report of AAPM Task Group 111 (TG-111). Instead of using a 100-mm pencil chamber and measuring the dose to a partially irradiated chamber, a smaller chamber is used and the helical (spiral) mode of the scanner is used to scan a given scan length, L, of the scanner. A series of such measurements on scans of different scan lengths is performed using the geometry illustrated in Figure 11-12. Using an integrating ion chamber located at the center of each scan, each point on the curve can be measured using a helical CT scan through a very long phantom. If a real-time radiation meter is used, the measurement can be made with one helical scan—the real-time chamber is positioned at the center of the field of view, and a helical scan is performed that interrogates the

■ **FIGURE 11-11** This figure shows the "rise to dose equilibrium" curve. This curve is essentially a plot of the data points along the vertical dashed line shown in Figure 11-10, as a function of scan length. The dose at the center of the field increases and reaches an asymptotic value once the scan length (or beam width for cone beam CT systems) approaches the width of the scatter tails.

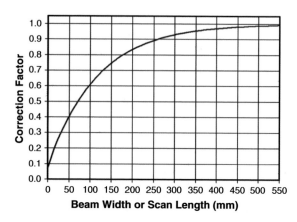

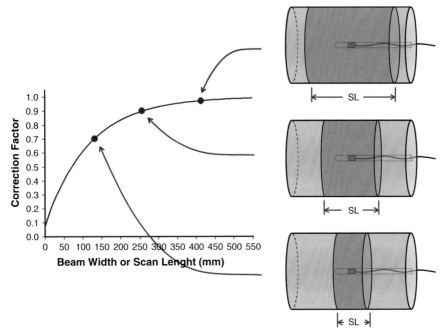

■ **FIGURE 11-12** The rise to equilibrium curve can be measured using an integrating dosimeter, and CT scans of different scan length are made to measure points along the curve. This figure illustrates AAPM Report 111 methodology.

entire length of the phantom (Fig. 11-13A). The probe measures a profile as shown in Figure 11-13B, as a function of time. The velocity of the table is used to convert the time axis of the probe read out to position along the phantom. The dose profile (Fig. 11-13B) shows a physical measurement of the scatter tails for a given set of imaging parameters, and this curve can be integrated for various scan lengths to derive the "rise

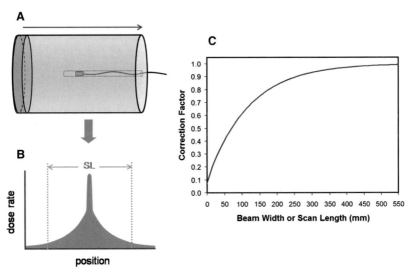

■ **FIGURE 11-13** If a dosimeter capable of real-time read-out is used, only one acquisition is needed as the phantom and x-ray chamber traverse (**A**) through the x-ray beam. The measured trace (**B**) shows the dose rate as a function of position (idealized), and (**C**) shows the rise to equilibrium curve that can be determined from the data in (**B**). This approach is the ICRU addendum to AAPM Report 111.

to dose equilibrium" curve (Fig. 11-13C). The benefit of the ICRU approach shown is Fig 11-13 is that only one scan through the phantom is required to determine the entire equilibrium dose curve. The "rise to dose equilibrium" curve shown in Figure 11-11 essentially provides a series of correction factors that can be used for specific scan lengths. Note that the correction factors would be dependent on scan parameters and the data shown in Figure 11-11 should not be used for patient dosimetry.

Dose in CT perfusion

CT perfusion studies are used for evaluating vascular function in organs, primarily the brain. Using a CT scanner with a reasonably wide coverage along the z-axis (such as 30 to 40 mm), the scanner repeatedly interrogates the organ during the injection of contrast agent—scanning typically at 1 scan per second for 40 to 50 seconds. The real-time imaging capability of the scanner is used with mathematical modeling equations applied in software to derive a number of functional parameters in regard to the imaged volume, including vascular permeability, time to peak enhancement, blood flow rate, and blood volume. The application of CT perfusion studies is primarily for the assessment of stroke or vasospasm, and this procedure generally uses no table movement and so the same tissue receives the radiation dose corresponding to about 40 or more CT scans, all in one procedure. Some scanners have a *shuttle* mode (see CT chapter for details), which allows the table to move back and forth repeatedly, and this allows the assessment of tissue perfusion over a larger region of tissue. The dosimetry methods pertinent to CT perfusion studies are different from that of routine head CT, primarily because the entire brain is not scanned. When the entire organ is not scanned (as with the brain in this procedure but this applies in general), the tissue weighting coefficients, w_t, are not accurate, and thus standard effective dose calculations can be misleading. Concerns in CT perfusion studies are primarily with the dose to the skin and the dose to the lenses of the eyes, and thus other dosimetry methods will in general be required. The details of such methods are beyond the scope of this text (see Bauhs 2008, Zhang 2011).

11.9 Computation of Radiation Risk to the Generic Patient

The estimation of radiation risk from a medical imaging procedure is typically computed by first computing the organ doses from the procedure. Organ dose assessment is usually performed using a generic-sized patient, and the dose deposition is computed using Monte Carlo procedures based on the medical imaging procedure being performed. Typically a mathematical phantom such as the MIRD* phantom is used, and this phantom simulates each organ as a mathematical shape in a standard-size "body" (Fig. 11-14). So-called *voxelized* phantoms have also been used, and these are full CT scans of humans, where each organ has been outlined so that organ dose can be estimated after the Monte Carlo procedure. In these Monte Carlo exercises, the dose for each organ is computed, for various entrance x-ray beam geometries. Organ doses are computed in the units of absorbed dose (mGy), usually normalized to ESK in radiography or to air kerma at isocenter in computed tomography. Such tables allow the estimation of organ doses for given radiological imaging procedures that use different technique factors. For example, in Table 11-2 for abdominal radiography, the organ dose coefficients for different beam qualities (half-value layers) are provided.

Neglecting the special risk issues from deterministic effects from very high dose procedures such as fluoroscopically-guided interventional procedures, the risk from

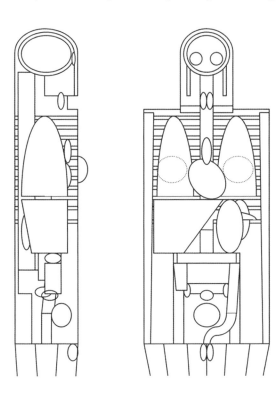

■ **FIGURE 11-14** The MIRD phantom is shown. This phantom uses mathematically defined organs and lends itself to Monte Carlo dosimetry simulations.

the vast majority of medical imaging examinations is the stochastic risk associated with cancer induction. In the generic patient, which is assumed in the notion of E, there is a risk coefficient that is used to weight each tissue type (Table 11-3), as discussed previously. The product of the organ dose (in mGy) and the organ (or tissue)-specific weighting factor is the E (in mSv) for that organ. The E for a given medical imaging procedure is then the sum of all of the organ-specific E. The E from a number of imaging procedures (such as may occur during a trauma workup) can be summed across all procedures as well.

Instead of performing an organ-by-organ assessment of dose, as discussed in the paragraph above, tables are provided in many reference publications that have already performed this computation and these charts provide estimates of E for various radiological procedures (e.g., chest radiography, pelvic CT, and mammography). For example, Table 11-4 provides coefficients for chest radiography, and this table includes coefficients for various chest radiographic views (AP, PA, lateral) and for different x-ray beam energies (half-value layers). Each value is normalized as the E (mSv) per unit ESK (mGy). This allows the user to compute the E for the specific technique factors used on the equipment that was used to image the patient. Table 11-5 illustrates the conversion factors for calculating E in CT—here, the table lists the E (mSv) as a function of the dose-length product (DLP, in mGy-cm) of the CT scan. This difference in the normalization reflects the differences in the geometry between CT and projection radiography.

Let us use the example of a thoracic CT scan, and compute the generic patient dose using the E coefficient listed in Table 11-5. The hypothetical thoracic CT scan was performed at 120 kV, 75 mAs, with a pitch of one and the scan length was 40 cm. The reported $CTDI_{vol}$ on the scanner was 5.5 mGy, and the DLP was 219 mGy-cm. Table 11-5 shows that for a chest CT, the *k factor* is 0.017 mSv per mGy-cm. Thus, the ED for this study is computed as 219 (mGy-cm) × 0.017 (mSv/mGy-cm) = 3.7 mSv.

Note that the conversion factor (0.017 mSv mGy^{-1} cm^{-1}) did not take into account the patient's age, gender, or body size. Hence, this estimation is considered to be for the generic member of the population.

The generally accepted risk (from BEIR VII) of a radiation-induced cancer fatality is 0.057 per 1000 mSv for a general population. So, the 3.7 mSv E from the CT scan estimated in the above paragraph results in a risk of induced cancer death of 0.0002109 = (0.057 × [3.7/1000]), or one fatal cancer induced for every 4742 patients having this procedure.

11.10 Computation of Patient-Specific Radiation Risk Estimates

Many scientists in the radiological community question the value of dose calculations for a specific patient, because every individual is different and has a unique propensity for cancer induction, which likely varies from organ to organ and from age to age. Calculations of cancer induction risk based on large cohorts are unlikely to capture a specific individual's risks with accuracy. Nevertheless, as awareness of the harms from ionizing radiation received during medical imaging procedures has increased due to press coverage, patients or their physicians sometimes require an estimate of "dose" from an imaging procedure. Beyond the radiation dose, the real issue relates to what the risk may be from that imaging procedure.

As mentioned in the above section, the notion of E cannot specifically address individual dosimetry. Using the example of CT, where this issue comes up most often, the first step in risk estimation for an individual is to refine his or her physical dose estimation by correcting the dose for the actual patient diameter (Fig. 11-8 and AAPM Report 204) and also by adjusting the estimate for the actual scan length (Fig. 11-11 and related discussion).

Once the organ dose estimates are adjusted to the patient size and scan length, then the Table 12D-2 in BEIR VII can be used to make relative risk calculations. The age-dependent and gender-dependent incidence of radiation-induced cancer deaths are illustrated in Figure 11-15. Here, the same case as mentioned in the section above (5.5 mGy dose due to thoracic CT scan) will be used to demonstrate age and gender dependencies in risk estimates. Computing the doses to each organ, and then summing the cancer fatality rate for each organ, the relative risk of this CT scan was estimated for male patients and was 0.00025 for a 10-year-old, 0.00012 for a 40-year-old, and 0.000063 for a 70-year-old person. Not surprisingly, the risk for a 10-year-old child is four times that of a 70-year-old, since younger patients are likely to live longer than older patients and manifest a radiogenic cancer. For female patients, the risks were calculated as 0.000423, 0.00019, and 0.0001 for the 10-, 40-, and 70-year-old patients, respectively. These differences in relative risk are reflected in Figure 11-15. The sensitivity of women to radiogenic stochastic effects is greater than that of men, and the increases in relative risk are estimated to be 1.62, 1.50, and 1.60 greater than male patients at ages 10, 40, and 70.

Absolute risks are small numbers with many zeros ofter the decimal point. Consequently, it is typical to invert these numbers—for example, a risk of 0.0010 equates to a risk of 1.0 per 1000. Table 11-6 provides these data for the example given above. Notice that when age and gender are considered, the values for this example range from risks of 1 in 400 to 1 in 2685. The concept of effective dose was not used for these computations, which used the tables from BEIR VII (Table 11-7).

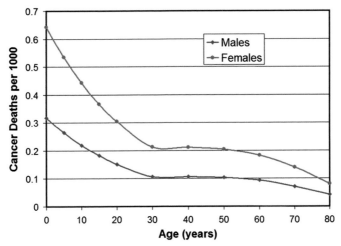

■ **FIGURE 11-15** The cancer death rate (per 1000 individuals exposied to 10 mGy) is shown as a function of age at irradiation, for men and women. Women and younger patients demonstrate higher cancer mortality from the risks of radiation exposure. (Data taken from BEIR VII Table 12D-2.)

For the case of the generic patient discussed in the previous section, the value was 1 fatality in 4742 CT exams, which was well within the range computed using BEIR VII techniques.

 ## Diagnostic Reference Levels

Now that virtually all radiological imaging procedures are digital, it is possible to automatically record estimates of the radiation levels used during each examination in radiography, fluoroscopy, mammography and computed tomography procedures. There are ongoing activities by the American College of Radiology, National Council on Radiation Protection, and other organizations to develop an infrastructure which would tally these dose metrics at each institution, for the purposes of comparing the dose levels between institutions. Dose statistics (such as mean dose for a chest radiograph, or mean effective dose for abdominal CT) would be compiled at each institution and compared against national norms. This exercise permits radiology managers to better understand how well their x-ray

TABLE 11-6

	10 y	40 y	70 y
Male risk	0.000254	0.000122	0.0000626
Male (1/risk)	1 in 3940	1 in 8208	1 in 15973
Female Risk	0.000423	0.000186	0.000101
Female (1/risk)	1 in 2364	1 in 5373	1 in 9850

Note: The relative risks, expressed in absolute fractions and as inverted fractions are listed. These data were calculated for a thoracic CT scan, 35 cm in length, as discussed in the text.

TABLE 11-7   ATTRIBUTABLE RISKS FOR CANCER FATALITY

LIFETIME ATTRIBUTABLE RISK OF CANCER MORTALITY[a]

CANCER SITE	AGE AT EXPOSURE (YEARS)										
	0	5	10	15	20	30	40	50	60	70	80
Male patients											
Stomach	41	34	30	25	21	16	15	13	11	8	4
Colon	163	139	117	99	84	61	60	57	49	36	21
Liver	44	37	31	27	23	16	16	14	12	8	4
Lung	318	264	219	182	151	107	107	104	93	71	42
Prostate	17	15	12	10	9	7	6	7	7	7	5
Bladder	45	38	32	27	23	17	17	17	17	15	10
Other	400	255	200	162	134	94	88	77	58	36	17
All solid	1028	781	641	533	444	317	310	289	246	181	102
Leukemia	71	71	71	70	67	64	67	71	73	69	51
All cancers	1099	852	712	603	511	381	377	360	319	250	153
Female patients											
Stomach	57	48	41	34	29	21	20	19	16	13	8
Colon	102	86	73	62	53	38	37	35	31	25	15
Liver	24	20	17	14	12	9	8	8	7	5	3
Lung	643	534	442	367	305	213	212	204	183	140	81
Breast	274	214	167	130	101	61	35	19	9	5	2
Uterus	11	10	8	7	6	4	4	3	3	2	1
Ovary	55	47	39	34	28	20	20	18	15	10	5
Bladder	59	51	43	36	31	23	23	22	22	19	13
Other	491	287	220	179	147	103	97	86	69	47	24
All solid	1717	1295	1051	862	711	491	455	415	354	265	152
Leukemia	53	52	53	52	51	51	52	54	55	52	38
All cancers	1770	1347	1104	914	762	542	507	469	409	317	190

Note: Number of deaths per 100,000 persons exposed to a single dose of 0.1 Gy.
[a]These estimates are obtained as combined estimates based on relative and absolute risk transport and have been adjusted by a DDREF of 1.5, except for leukemia, which is based on linear-quadratic model.
Source: Adapted From BEIR VII Table 12D-2.

techniques compare with other institutions, with the notion that institutions producing high dose levels would reduce their dose levels to national norms.

Although recommendations vary, it is thought that institutions who find themselves in the top quartile of doses for a given radiological procedure should implement dose reduction policies to bring their facility into line with mainstream practice.

As discussed in Chapter 5 (Informatics), the DICOM header contains a great deal of information and in recent years radiation dose information has been included in the DICOM standards. This allows the automated extraction of dose data by computer systems which are designed for this. Using this approach, at a busy institution a large amount of dose data can be acquired in a short period of time, depending on procedure volume. Although setting up the infrastructure for dose monitoring requires initial resources as well as ongoing maintenance and analysis, the use of reference dose levels has been embraced both nationally and internationally, and has already demonstrated its utility in dose reduction.

 ## Increasing Radiation Burden from Medical Imaging

NCRP 160 recently reported that the average effective dose per person due to medical imaging in the United States rose from 0.53 mSv in 1987 to 3.0 mSv in 2006. The bulk of the increased dose from medical procedures was from the increased used of computed tomography, which was thought to contribute about 50% of the ionizing radiation used for diagnostic imaging. Nuclear medicine procedures accounted for about 25% of medical radiation. The current average U.S. background radiation level is 3.1 mSv per year, so medical imaging now contributes about the same as background. Obviously these numbers represent averages, and many people have no radiological procedures in a year, while others may have a number of imaging procedures. Table 11-8 describes the breakdown of the effective doses from various medical imaging procedures.

TABLE 11-8   TYPICAL EFFECTIVE DOSES FOR VARIOUS RADIOGRAPHIC PROCEDURES

PROCEDURE	AVERAGE EFFECTIVE DOSE (mSv)
Radiographic Procedures	
Skull	0.1
Cervical Spine	0.2
Thoracic Spine	1.0
Lumbar Spine	1.5
PA and Lateral Chest	0.1
Mammography	0.4
Abdomen	0.7
Pelvis	0.6
Hip	0.7
Shoulder	0.01
Knee	0.005
Upper GI series[a]	6
Barium Enemaa[a]	8
CT Procedures	
Head	2
Chest	7
Abdomen	8
Pelvis	6
Three phase Liver	15
Spine	6
CT Colonography	10

[a]Includes dose from fluoroscopy.
From Mettler et al. *Radiology* 2008;248:254–263.

Summary: Dose Estimation in Patients

Dose estimation in radiography and fluoroscopy can be performed using a number of metrics, and comparisons or "rule of thumb" dose estimates may use ESD as a surrogate indicator of approximate dose levels. In fluoroscopy, the need for dose estimation is often in regard to skin dose, and skin dose estimates can be made relatively accurately when the exposure conditions and geometry are known. A computation of radiation dose to an individual organ in the patient from radiography and fluoroscopy requires the use of published tables to convert entrance kerma levels to organ doses, along with the known exposure conditions and techniques.

There are a number of accurate methods for computing the dose in CT, for the purposes of technique optimization and for monitoring patient dose levels. In most cases, the estimation of radiation absorbed dose (in mGy) to a model patient with dimensions approximate to an actual patient is sufficiently accurate. Dose estimates for a specific patient can be made by including corrections for patient diameter (Fig. 11-8) and corrections for the actual scan length used (Fig. 11.11). The figures shown in this chapter are meant to illustrate concepts, and these data should not be used for dose calculations on patients. Instead, the readers should refer to root documents and other literature for more specific details on dose estimation in CT.

SUGGESTED READING

Bauhs JA, Vrieze TJ, Primak AN, et al. CT dosimetry: comparison of measurement techniques and devices. *Radiographics* 2008;28(1):245–253. Review.

Boone JM. The trouble with CTDI100. *Med Phys* 2007;34(4):1364–1371.

Boone JM, Buonocore MH, Cooper VN III. Monte Carlo validation in diagnostic radiological imaging. *Med Phys* 2000;27:1294–1304.

Boone JM, Cooper VN, Nemzek WR, et al. Monte Carlo assessment of computed tomography dose to tissue adjacent to the scanned volume. *Med Phys* 2000;27:2393–2407.

DeMarco JJ, Cagnon CH, Cody DD, et al. A Monte Carlo based method to estimate radiation dose from multidetector CT (MDCT): cylindrical and anthropomorphic phantoms. *Phys Med Biol* 2005;50(17):3989–4004.

DeMarco JJ, Cagnon CH, Cody DD, et al. Estimating radiation doses from multidetector CT using Monte Carlo simulations: effects of different size voxelized patient models on magnitudes of organ and effective dose. *Phys Med Biol* 2007;52(9):2583–2597.

Dixon RL. A new look at CT dose measurement: beyond CTDI. *Med Phys* 2003;30(6):1272–1280.

Huda W, Scalzetti EM, Roskopf M. Effective doses to patients undergoing thoracic computed tomography examinations. *Med Phys* 2000;27(5):838–844.

Jarry G, DeMarco JJ, Beifuss U, et al. A Monte Carlo-based method to estimate radiation dose from spiral CT: from phantom testing to patient-specific models. *Phys Med Biol* 2003;48(16):2645–2663.

Khursheed A, Hillier MC, Shrimpton PC, et al. Influence of patient age on normalized effective doses calculated for CT examinations. *BJR* 2002;75:819–830.

Linton OW, Mettler FA. National conference on dose reduction in CT, with an emphasis on pediatric patients. *Am J Roentgenol* 2003;181:321–329.

McCollough CH. CT dose: how to measure, how to reduce. *Health Phys* 2008;95(5):508–517.

McCollough CH, Bruesewitz MR, Kofler JM Jr. CT dose reduction and dose management tools: overview of available options. *Radiographics* 2006;26(2):503–512. Review.

McCollough CH, Primak AN, Braun N, et al. Strategies for reducing radiation dose in CT. *Radiol Clin North Am* 2009;47(1):27–40. Review.

McCollough CH, Primak AN, Saba O, et al. Dose performance of a 64-channel dual-source CT scanner. *Radiology* 2007;243(3):775–784. [Epub 2007 Apr 19.]

McNitt-Gray MF. AAPM/RSNA physics tutorial for residents: topics in CT. Radiation dose in CT. *Radiographics* 2002;22(6):1541–1553. Review.

Menke J. Comparison of different body size parameters for individual dose adaptation in body CT of adults. *Radiology* 2005;236:565–571.

Mettler FA Jr, Wiest PW, Locken JA, et al. CT scanning: patterns of use and dose. *J Radiol Prot* 2000;20(4):353–359.

Shope T, Gagne R, Johnson G. A method for describing the doses delivered by transmission x-ray computed tomography. *Med Phys* 1981;8:488–495.

Turner AC, Zankl M, DeMarco JJ, et al. The feasibility of a scanner-independent technique to estimate organ dose from MDCT scans: using CTDIvol to account for differences between scanners. *Med Phys* 2010;37(4):1816–1825.

Zhang D, Cagnon CH, Villablanca JP, Cody DD, et. al. Peak Skin and Eye Lens Dose from Brain Perfusion CT Examinations based on monte carlo simulations, in press. *AJR*, 2011

Zhou H, Boone JM. Monte Carlo evaluation of CTDI(infinity) in infinitely long cylinders of water, polyethylene, and PMMA with diameters from 10 mm to 500 mm. *Med Phys* 2008;35:2424–2431.

Patient dosimetry for x-rays used in medical imaging. *J ICRU* Report 74 (2005).

Ionizing radiation exposure to the population of the United States, NCRP Report 160, 2008.

CHAPTER 12

Magnetic Resonance Basics: Magnetic Fields, Nuclear Magnetic Characteristics, Tissue Contrast, Image Acquisition

Nuclear magnetic resonance (NMR) is the spectroscopic study of the magnetic properties of the *nucleus* of the atom. The protons and neutrons of the nucleus have a *magnetic* field associated with their nuclear spin and charge distribution. *Resonance* is an energy coupling that causes the individual nuclei, when placed in a strong external magnetic field, to selectively absorb, and later release, energy unique to those nuclei and their surrounding environment. The detection and analysis of the NMR signal has been extensively studied since the 1940s as an analytic tool in chemistry and biochemistry research. NMR is not an imaging technique but rather a method to provide spectroscopic data concerning a sample placed in a small volume, high field strength magnetic device. In the early 1970s, it was realized that magnetic field gradients could be used to localize the NMR signal and to generate images that display magnetic properties of the proton, reflecting clinically relevant information, coupled with technological advances and development of "body-size" magnets. As clinical imaging applications increased in the mid-1980s, the "nuclear" connotation was dropped, and magnetic resonance imaging (MRI), with a plethora of associated acronyms, became commonly accepted in the medical community.

MR applications continue to expand clinical relevance with higher field strength magnets, improved anatomic, physiologic, and spectroscopic studies. The high contrast sensitivity to soft tissue differences and the inherent safety to the patient resulting from the use of nonionizing radiation have been key reasons why MRI has supplanted many CT and projection radiography methods. With continuous improvements in image quality, acquisition methods, and equipment design, MRI is often the modality of choice to examine anatomic and physiologic properties of the patient. There are drawbacks, however, including high equipment and siting costs, scan acquisition complexity, relatively long imaging times, significant image artifacts, patient claustrophobia, and MR safety concerns.

This chapter reviews the basic properties of magnetism, concepts of resonance, tissue magnetization and relaxation events, generation of image contrast, and basic methods of acquiring image data. Advanced pulse sequences, illustration of image characteristics/artifacts, MR spectroscopy, MR safety, and biologic effects, are discussed in Chapter 13.

12.1 Magnetism, Magnetic Fields, and Magnets

Magnetism

Magnetism is a fundamental property of matter; it is generated by moving charges, usually electrons. Magnetic properties of materials result from the organization and motion of the electrons in either a random or a nonrandom alignment of magnetic "domains," which are the smallest entities of magnetism. Atoms and molecules have electron orbitals that can be paired (an even number of electrons cancels the magnetic field) or unpaired (the magnetic field is present). Most materials do not exhibit overt magnetic properties, but one notable exception is the permanent magnet, in which the individual magnetic domains are aligned in one direction.

Unlike the monopole electric charges from which they are derived, magnetic fields exist as dipoles, where the north pole is the origin of the magnetic field lines and the south pole is the return (Fig. 12-1A). One pole cannot exist without the other. As with electric charges, "like" magnetic poles repel and "opposite" poles attract. *Magnetic field strength, B* (also called the magnetic flux density), can be conceptualized as the number of magnetic lines of force per unit area, which decreases roughly as the inverse square of the distance from the source. The SI unit for B is the Tesla (T). As a benchmark, the earth's magnetic field is about $1/20,000 = 0.00005$ T $= 0.05$ mT. An alternate (historical) unit is the gauss (G), where 1 T $= 10,000$ G.

Magnetic Fields

Magnetic fields can be induced by a moving charge in a wire (e.g., see the section on transformers in Chapter 6). The direction of the magnetic field depends on the sign and the direction of the charge in the wire, as described by the "right hand rule": The fingers point in the direction of the magnetic field when the thumb points in the direction of a moving positive charge (i.e., opposite to the direction of electron movement). Wrapping the current-carrying wire many times in a coil causes a superimposition of the magnetic fields, augmenting the overall strength of

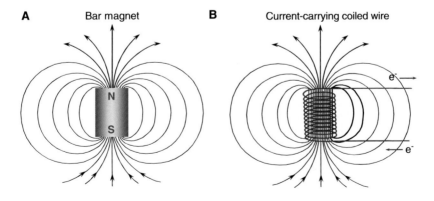

Dipole magnetic field

■ **FIGURE 12-1 A.** The magnetic field has two poles with magnetic field lines emerging from the north pole (*N*), and returning to the south pole (*S*), as illustrated by a simple bar magnet. **B.** A coiled wire carrying an electric current produces a magnetic field with characteristics similar to a bar magnet. Magnetic field strength and field density are dependent on the amplitude of the current and the number of coil turns.

the magnetic field inside the coil, with a rapid falloff of field strength outside the coil (see Fig. 12-1B). Amplitude of the current in the coil determines the overall magnitude of the magnetic field strength. The magnetic field lines extending beyond the concentrated field are known as fringe fields.

Magnets

The magnet is the heart of the MR system. For any particular magnet type, performance criteria include field strength, temporal stability, and field homogeneity. These parameters are affected by the magnet design. Air core magnets are made of wire-wrapped cylinders of approximately 1-m diameter and greater, over a cylindrical length of 2 to 3 m, where the magnetic field is produced by an electric current in the wires. When the wires are energized, the magnetic field produced is parallel to the long axis of the cylinder. In most clinically designed systems, the magnetic field is horizontal and runs along the cranial–caudal axis of the patient lying supine (Fig. 12-2A). Solid core magnets are constructed from permanent magnets, a wire-wrapped iron core "electromagnet," or a hybrid combination. In these solid core designs, the magnetic field runs between the poles of the magnet, most often in a vertical direction (Fig. 12-2B). Magnetic fringe fields extend well beyond the volume of the cylinder in air core designs. Fringe fields are a potential hazard, and are discussed further in Chapter 13.

To achieve a high magnetic field strength (greater than 1 T) requires the electromagnet core wires to be superconductive. Superconductivity is a characteristic of certain metals (e.g., niobium–titanium alloys) that when maintained at extremely low temperatures (liquid helium; less than 4°K) exhibit no resistance to electric current.

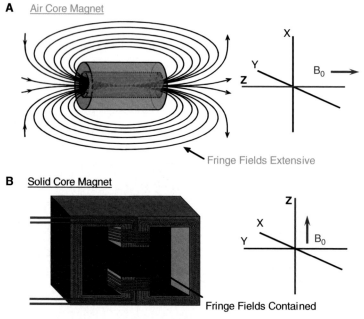

■ FIGURE 12-2 A. Air core magnets typically have a horizontal main field produced in the bore of the electrical windings, with the z-axis (B_0) along the bore axis. Fringe fields for the air core systems are extensive and are increased for larger bore diameters and higher field strengths. **B.** The solid core magnet has a vertical field, produced between the metal poles of a permanent or wire-wrapped electromagnet. Fringe fields are confined with this design. In both types, the main field is parallel to the z-axis of the Cartesian coordinate system.

Superconductivity allows the closed-circuit electromagnet to be energized and ramped up to the desired current and magnetic field strength by an external electric source. Replenishment of the liquid helium must occur continuously, because if the temperature rises above a critical value, the loss of superconductivity will occur and resistance heating of the wires will boil the helium, resulting in a "quench." Superconductive magnets with field strengths of 1.5 to 3 T are common for clinical systems, and 4 to 7 T clinical large bore magnets are currently used for research applications, with possible future clinical use.

A cross section of the internal superconducting magnet components shows integral parts of the magnet system including the wire coils and cryogenic liquid containment vessel (Fig. 12-3). In addition to the main magnet system, other components are also necessary. *Shim coils* interact with the main magnetic field to improve homogeneity (minimal variation of the magnetic flux density) over the volume used for patient imaging. *Radiofrequency (RF) coils* exist within the main bore of the magnet to transmit energy to the patient as well as to receive returning signals. *Gradient coils* are contained within the main bore to produce a linear variation of magnetic field strength across the useful magnet volume.

A magnetic field gradient is obtained by superimposing the magnetic fields of two or more coils carrying a direct current of specific amplitude and direction with a precisely defined geometry (Fig. 12-4). The bipolar gradient field varies over a predefined field of view (FOV), and when superimposed upon B_0, a small, continuous variation in the field strength occurs from the center to the periphery with distance from the center point (the "null"). Interacting with the much, much stronger main magnetic field, the subtle linear variations are on the order of 0.005 T/m (5 mT/m) and are essential for localizing signals generated during the operation of the MR system.

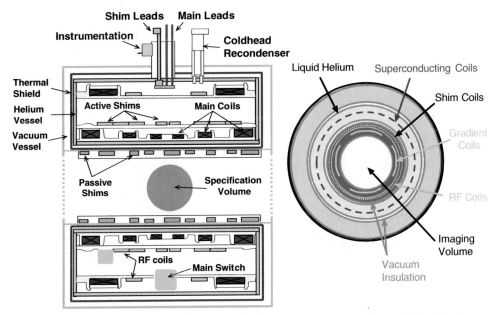

■ **FIGURE 12-3** Internal components of a superconducting air-core magnet are shown. On the left is a cross section through the long axis of the magnet illustrating relative locations of the components, and on the right is a simplified cross section across the diameter.

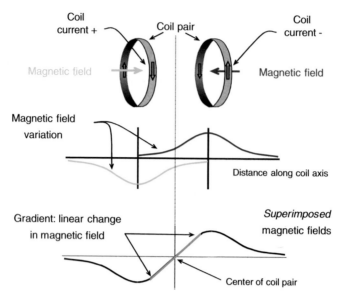

■ **FIGURE 12-4** Gradients are produced inside the main magnet with coil pairs. Individual conducting wire coils are separately energized with currents of opposite direction to produce magnetic fields of opposite polarity. Magnetic field strength decreases with distance from the center of each coil. When combined, the magnetic field variations form a linear change between the coils, producing a linear magnetic field gradient, as shown in the lower graph.

The MR System

The MR system is comprised of several components including those described above, orchestrated by many processors and control subsystems, as shown in Figure 12-5. Detail of the individual components, methods of acquiring the MR signals and reconstruction of images are described in the following sections. But first, characteristics of the magnetic properties of tissues, the resonance phenomenon, and geometric considerations are explained.

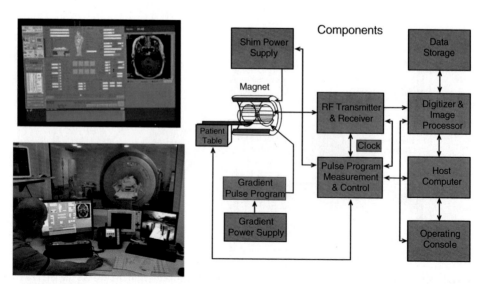

■ **FIGURE 12-5** The MR system is shown **(lower left)**, the operators display **(upper left)**, and the various subsystems that generate, detect, and capture the MR signals used for imaging and spectroscopy.

Magnetic Properties of Materials

Magnetic *susceptibility* describes the extent to which a material becomes magnetized when placed in a magnetic field. Induced internal magnetization opposes the external magnetic field and lowers the local magnetic field surrounding the material. On the other hand, the internal magnetization can form in the same direction as the applied magnetic field, and increase the local magnetic field. Three categories of susceptibility are defined: *diamagnetic, paramagnetic*, and *ferromagnetic*, based upon the arrangement of electrons in the atomic or molecular structure. Diamagnetic elements and materials have slightly negative susceptibility and oppose the applied magnetic field, because of paired electrons in the surrounding electron orbitals. Examples of diamagnetic materials are calcium, water, and most organic materials (chiefly owing to the diamagnetic characteristics of carbon and hydrogen). Paramagnetic materials, with unpaired electrons, have slightly positive susceptibility and enhance the local magnetic field, but they have no measurable self-magnetism. Examples of paramagnetic materials are molecular oxygen (O_2), deoxyhemoglobin, some blood degradation products such as methemoglobin, and *gadolinium*-based contrast agents. Locally, these diamagnetic and paramagnetic agents will deplete or augment the local magnetic field (Fig. 12-6), affecting MR images in known, unknown, and sometimes unexpected ways. Ferromagnetic materials are "superparamagnetic"—that is, they augment the external magnetic field substantially. These materials, containing iron, cobalt, and nickel, exhibit "self-magnetism" in many cases, and can significantly distort the acquired signals.

Magnetic Characteristics of the Nucleus

The nucleus, comprising protons and neutrons with characteristics listed in Table 12-1, exhibits magnetic characteristics on a much smaller scale than for atoms/molecules and their associated electron distributions. Magnetic properties are influenced by spin and charge distributions intrinsic to the proton and neutron. A magnetic dipole is created for the proton, with a positive charge equal to the electron charge but of opposite sign, due to nuclear "spin." Overall, the neutron is electrically uncharged, but subnuclear charge inhomogeneities and an associated nuclear spin result in a magnetic field of opposite direction and approximately the same strength as the proton. Magnetic characteristics of the nucleus are described by the *nuclear magnetic moment*, represented as

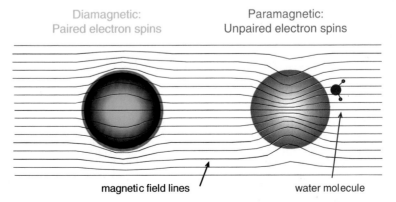

Diamagnetic:
Paired electron spins

Paramagnetic:
Unpaired electron spins

magnetic field lines   water molecule

■ FIGURE 12-6 The local magnetic field can be changed in the presence of diamagnetic (depletion) and paramagnetic (augmentation) materials, with an impact on the signals generated from nearby signal sources such as the hydrogen atoms in water molecules.

TABLE 12-1 PROPERTIES OF THE NEUTRON AND PROTON

CHARACTERISTIC	NEUTRON	PROTON
Mass(kg)	1.674×10^{-27}	1.672×10^{-27}
Charge (coulomb)	0	1.602×10^{-19}
Spin quantum number	½	½
Magnetic moment (J/T)	-9.66×10^{-27}	1.41×10^{-26}
Magnetic moment (nuclear magneton)	−1.91	2.79

a vector indicating magnitude and direction. For a given nucleus, the nuclear magnetic moment is determined through the pairing of the constituent protons and neutrons. If the sum of the number of protons (P) and number of neutrons (N) in the nucleus is even, the nuclear magnetic moment is essentially zero. However, if N is even and P is odd, or N is odd and P is even, the resultant noninteger nuclear spin generates a nuclear magnetic moment. A single nucleus does not generate a large enough nuclear magnetic moment to be observable, but the conglomeration of large numbers of nuclei ($\sim 10^{15}$) arranged in a nonrandom orientation generates an observable nuclear magnetic moment of the sample, from which the MRI signals are derived.

Nuclear Magnetic Characteristics of the Elements

Biologically relevant elements that are candidates for producing MR signals are listed in Table 12-2. Key features include the strength of the nuclear magnetic moment, the physiologic concentration, and the isotopic abundance. Hydrogen, having the largest magnetic moment and greatest abundance, chiefly in water and fat, is by far the best element for general clinical utility. Other elements are orders of magnitude less sensitive. Of these, ^{23}Na and ^{31}P have been used for imaging in limited situations, despite their relatively low sensitivity. Therefore, the nucleus of the hydrogen atom, the proton, is the principal focus for generating MR signals.

TABLE 12-2 MAGNETIC RESONANCE PROPERTIES OF MEDICALLY USEFUL NUCLEI

NUCLEUS	SPIN QUANTUM NUMBER	% ISOTOPIC ABUNDANCE	MAGNETIC MOMENT[b]	% RELATIVE ELEMENTAL ABUNDANCE[a]	RELATIVE SENSITIVITY
^{1}H	½	99.98	2.79	10	1
^{3}He	½	0.00014	−2.13	0	−
^{13}C	−½	0.011	0.70	18	−
^{17}O	⁵⁄₂	0.04	−1.89	65	9×10^{-6}
^{19}F	½	100	2.63	<0.01	3×10^{-8}
^{23}Na	³⁄₂	100	2.22	0.1	1×10^{-4}
^{31}P	½	100	1.13	1.2	6×10^{-5}

[a]moment in nuclear magneton units = 5.05×10^{-27} J T^{-1}.
[b]Note: by mass in the human body (all isotopes).

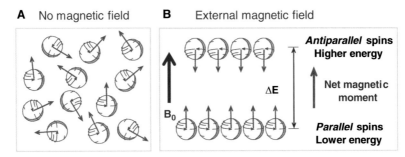

A No magnetic field   **B** External magnetic field

Antiparallel **spins Higher energy**

ΔE

Net magnetic moment

B_0

Parallel **spins Lower energy**

■ **FIGURE 12-7** Simplified distributions of "free" protons without and with an external magnetic field are shown. **A.** Without an external magnetic field, a group of protons assumes a random orientation of magnetic moments, producing an overall magnetic moment of zero. **B.** Under the influence of an applied external magnetic field, B_0, the protons assume a nonrandom alignment in two possible orientations: parallel and antiparallel to the applied magnetic field. A slightly greater number of protons exist in the parallel direction, resulting in a measurable *net magnetic moment* in the direction of B_0.

Magnetic Characteristics of the Proton

The spinning proton or *"spin"* (spin and proton are used synonymously herein) is classically considered to be a tiny bar magnet with north and south poles, even though the magnetic moment of a single proton is undetectable. Large numbers of unbound hydrogen atoms in water and fat, those unconstrained by molecular bonds in complex macromolecules within tissues, have a random orientation of their protons (nuclear magnetic moments) due to thermal energy. As a result, there is no observable magnetization of the sample (Fig. 12-7A). However, when placed in a strong static magnetic field, B_0, magnetic forces cause the protons to align with the applied field in parallel and antiparallel directions at two discrete energy levels (Fig. 12-7B). Thermal energy within the sample causes the protons to be distributed in this way, and at equilibrium, a slight majority exists in the low-energy, parallel direction. A stronger magnetic field increases the energy separation of the low- and high-energy levels and the number of excess protons in the low-energy state. At 1.0 T, the number of excess protons in the low-energy state is approximately 3 protons per million (3×10^{-6}) at physiologic temperatures. Although this number seems insignificant, for a typical voxel volume in MRI, there are about 10^{21} protons, so there are $3 \times 10^{-6} \times 10^{21}$, or approximately 3×10^{15} more protons in the low-energy state! This number of excess protons produces an observable "sample" nuclear magnetic moment, initially aligned with the direction of the applied magnetic field.

In addition to energy separation of the parallel and antiparallel spin states, the protons also experience a torque in a perpendicular direction from the applied magnetic field that causes *precession*, much the same way that a spinning top wobbles due to the force of gravity (Fig. 12-8). The precession occurs at an angular frequency (number of rotations/sec about an axis of rotation) that is proportional to the magnetic field strength B_0. The *Larmor equation* describes the dependence between the magnetic field, B_0, and the angular precessional frequency, ω_0:

$$\omega_0 = \gamma \, B_0$$

where γ is the gyromagnetic ratio unique to each element. This is expressed in terms of linear frequency as

■ **FIGURE 12-8** A single proton *precesses* about its axis with an angular frequency, ω, proportional to the externally applied magnetic field strength, according to the *Larmor* equation. A well-known example of precession is the motion a spinning top makes as it interacts with the force of gravity as it slows.

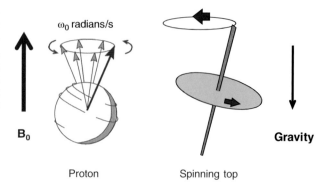

Precessional frequency

$$f_0 = \frac{\gamma}{2\pi} B_0$$

where $\omega = 2\pi f$ and $\gamma/2\pi$ is the *gyromagnetic ratio*, with values expressed in millions of cycles per second (MHz) per Tesla, or MHz/T.

Each element with a nonzero nuclear magnetic moment has a unique gyromagnetic ratio, as listed in Table 12-3.

Energy Absorption and Emission

The protons precessing in the parallel and antiparallel directions result in a quantized distribution (two discrete energies) with the net magnetic moment of the sample at equilibrium equal to the vector sum of the individual magnetic moments in the direction of B_0 as shown in Figure 12-9. The magnetic field vector components of the sample in the perpendicular direction are randomly distributed and sum to zero. Briefly irradiating the sample with an electromagnetic RF energy pulse tuned to the Larmor (resonance) frequency promotes protons from the low-energy, parallel direction to the higher energy, antiparallel direction, and the magnetization along the direction of the applied magnetic field shrinks. Subsequently, the more energetic sample returns to equilibrium conditions when the protons revert to the parallel direction and release RF energy at the

TABLE 12-3   GYROMAGNETIC RATIO FOR USEFUL ELEMENTS IN MAGNETIC RESONANCE

NUCLEUS	$\gamma/2\pi$ (MHz/T)
^{1}H	42.58
^{13}C	10.7
^{17}O	5.8
^{19}F	40.0
^{23}Na	11.3
^{31}P	17.2

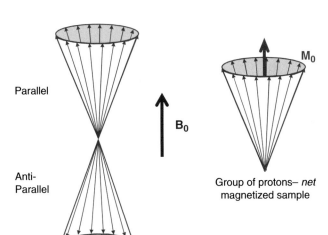

■ **FIGURE 12-9** A group of protons in the parallel and antiparallel energy states generates an equilibrium magnetization, M_0, in the direction of the applied magnetic field B_0. The protons are distributed randomly over the surface of the cone, and produce no magnetization in the perpendicular direction.

Parallel

Anti-Parallel

B_0

M_0

Group of protons– *net* magnetized sample

same frequency. This energy emission is detected by highly sensitive antennas to capture the basic MR signal.

Typical magnetic field strengths for MR systems range from 0.3 to 4.0 T. For protons, the precessional frequency is 42.58 MHz/T, and increases or decreases with an increase or decrease in magnetic field strength, as calculated in the example below. Accuracy of the precessional frequency is necessary to ensure that the RF energy will be absorbed by the magnetized protons. Precision of the precessional frequency must be on the order of cycles/s (Hz) out of millions of cycles/s (MHz) in order to identify the location and spatial position of the emerging signals, as is described in Section 12.6.

EXAMPLE: What is the frequency of precession of ¹H and ³¹P at 0.5 T? 1.5 T? 3.0 T? The Larmor frequency is calculated as $f_0 = (\gamma/2\pi)B_0$.

	FIELD STRENGTH		
ELEMENT	0.5 T	1.5 T	3.0 T
¹H	42.58 × 0.5 = 21.29 MHz	42.58 × 1.5 = 63.87 MHz	42.58 × 3.0 = 127.74 MHz
³¹P	17.2 × 0.5 = 8.6 MHz	17.2 × 1.5 = 25.8 MHz	17.2 × 3 = 51.6 MHz

The differences in the gyromagnetic ratios and corresponding precessional frequencies allow the selective excitation of one element from another in the same magnetic field strength.

Geometric Orientation, Frame of Reference, and Magnetization Vectors

By convention, the applied magnetic field B_0 is directed parallel to the z-axis of the three-dimensional Cartesian coordinate axis system and perpendicular to the x and y axes. For convenience, two frames of reference are used: the *laboratory frame* and the *rotating frame*. The laboratory frame (Fig. 12-10A) is a stationary reference frame from the observer's point of view. The sample magnetic moment vector precesses about the

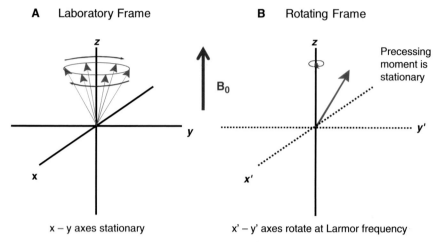

A Laboratory Frame   **B** Rotating Frame

B_0

Precessing moment is stationary

x – y axes stationary   x' – y' axes rotate at Larmor frequency

■ **FIGURE 12-10 A.** The *laboratory frame of reference* uses stationary three-dimensional Cartesian coordinates: x, y, z. The magnetic moment precesses around the z-axis at the Larmor frequency as the illustration attempts to convey. **B.** The *rotating frame of reference* uses rotating Cartesian coordinate axes that *rotate about the z-axis* at the Larmor precessional frequency, and the other axes are denoted: x' and y'. When precessing at the Larmor frequency, the sample magnetic moment is stationary.

z-axis in a circular geometry about the x-y plane. The rotating frame (Fig. 12-10B) is a *spinning* axis system, whereby the x'-y' axes rotate at an angular frequency equal to the Larmor frequency. In this frame, the sample magnetic moment vector appears to be stationary when rotating at the resonance frequency. A slightly higher precessional frequency is observed as a slow clockwise rotation, while a slightly lower precessional frequency is observed as a slow counterclockwise rotation. The magnetic interactions between precessional frequencies of the tissue magnetic moments with the externally applied RF (depicted as a rotating magnetic field) can be described more clearly using the rotating frame of reference, while the observed returning signal and its frequency content is explained using the laboratory (stationary) frame of reference.

The net magnetization vector of the sample, M, is described by three components. *Longitudinal magnetization,* M_z, along the z direction, is the component of the magnetic moment parallel to the applied magnetic field, B_0. At equilibrium, the longitudinal magnetization is maximal and is denoted as M_0, the *equilibrium magnetization*. The component of the magnetic moment perpendicular to B_0, M_{xy}, in the x-y plane, is *transverse magnetization*. At equilibrium, M_{xy} is zero. When the protons in the magnetized sample absorb energy, M_z is "tipped" into the transverse plane, and M_{xy} generates the all-important MR signal. Figure 12-11 illustrates this geometry.

12.2 The Magnetic Resonance Signal

Application of RF energy synchronized to the precessional frequency of the protons causes absorption of energy and displacement of the sample magnetic moment from equilibrium conditions. The return to equilibrium results in the emission of energy proportional to the number of excited protons in the volume. This occurs at a rate that depends on the structural and magnetic characteristics of the sample. Excitation, detection, and acquisition of the signals constitute the basic information necessary for MRI and and MR spectroscopy (MRS).

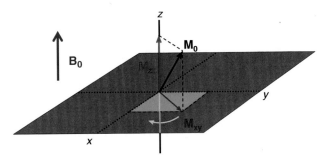

M_z: Longitudinal Magnetization: in z-axis direction

M_{xy}: Transverse Magnetization: in x-y plane

M_0: Equilibrium Magnetization: maximum magnetization

■ **FIGURE 12-11** *Longitudinal magnetization,* M_z*,* is the vector component of the magnetic moment in the z direction. *Transverse magnetization,* M_{xy}*,* is the vector component of the magnetic moment in the x-y plane. *Equilibrium magnetization,* M_0*,* is the maximal longitudinal magnetization of the sample, and is shown displaced from the z-axis in this illustration.

Resonance and Excitation

Displacement of the equilibrium magnetization occurs when the magnetic component of the RF excitation pulse, known as the B_1 field, is precisely matched to the precessional frequency of the protons. The *resonance* frequency corresponds to the energy separation between the protons in the parallel and antiparallel directions.

The **quantum mechanics model** considers the RF energy as photons (quanta) instead of waves. Protons oriented parallel and antiparallel to the external magnetic field, separated by an energy gap, ΔE, will transition from the low- to the high-energy level only when the RF pulse is equal to the precessional frequency. The number of protons that undergo an energy transition is dependent on the amplitude and duration of the RF pulse. M_z changes from the maximal positive value at equilibrium, through zero, to the maximal negative value (Fig. 12-12). Continued

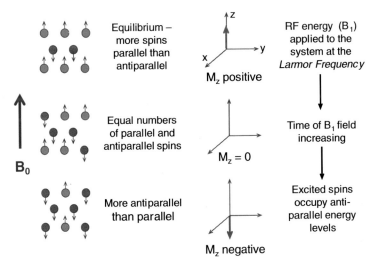

■ **FIGURE 12-12** A simple quantum mechanics process depicts the discrete energy absorption and the time change of the longitudinal magnetization vector as RF energy equal to the energy difference of the parallel and antiparallel spins is applied to the sample (at the Larmor frequency). Discrete quanta absorption changes the proton energy from parallel to antiparallel. With continued application of the RF energy at the Larmor frequency, M_z is displaced from equilibrium, through zero, to the opposite direction (high energy state).

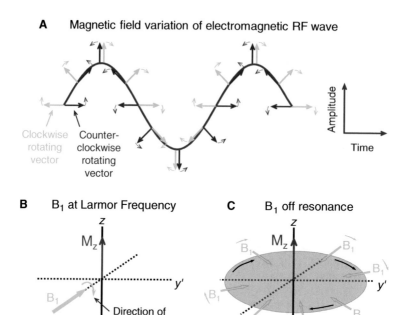

■ **FIGURE 12-13 A.** A classical physics description of the magnetic field component of the RF pulse (the electric field is not shown). Clockwise (*solid*) and counterclockwise (*dotted*) rotating magnetic vectors produce the magnetic field variation by constructive and destructive interaction. At the Larmor frequency, one of the magnetic field vectors rotates synchronously in the rotating frame and is therefore stationary (the other vector rotates in the opposite direction and does not synchronize with the rotating frame). **B.** In the *rotating frame*, the RF pulse (B_1 field) is applied at the Larmor frequency and is stationary in the x'-y' plane. The B_1 field interacts at 90 degrees to the sample magnetic moment and produces a torque that displaces the magnetic vector away from equilibrium. **C.** The B_1 field is not tuned to the Larmor frequency and is not stationary in the rotating frame. No interaction with the sample magnetic moment occurs.

irradiation can induce a return to equilibrium conditions, when an incoming RF quantum of energy causes the reversion of a proton in the antiparallel direction to the parallel direction with the energy-conserving spontaneous emission of two excess quanta. While this model shows how energy absorption and emission occurs, there is no clear description of how M_{xy} evolves, which is better understood using classical physics concepts.

In the **classical physics model**, the linear B_1 field is described with two magnetic field vectors of equal magnitude, rotating in opposite directions, representing the sinusoidal variation of the magnetic component of the electromagnetic RF wave as shown in Figure 12-13. One of the two rotating vectors is synchronized to the precessing protons in the magnetized sample, and in the rotating frame is stationary. If the RF energy is not applied at the precessional (Larmor) frequency, the B_1 field will not interact with M_z. Another description is that of a circularly polarized B_1 transmit field from the body coil that rotates at the precessional frequency of the magnetization.

Flip Angles

Flip angles represent the degree of M_z rotation by the B_1 field as it is applied along the x'-axis (or the y'-axis) perpendicular to M_z. A torque is applied on M_z, rotating it from the longitudinal direction into the transverse plane. The rate of rotation occurs

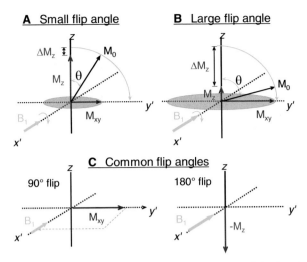

■ **FIGURE 12-14** Flip angles are the result of the angular displacement of the longitudinal magnetization vector from the equilibrium position. The rotation angle of the magnetic moment vector is dependent on the duration and amplitude of the B_1 field at the Larmor frequency. Flip angles describe the rotation of M_z away from the z-axis. **A.** Small flip angles (less than 45 degrees) and **B.** Large flip angles (75 to 90 degrees) produce small and large transverse magnetization, respectively.

at an angular frequency equal to $\omega_1 = \gamma B_1$, as per the Larmor equation. Thus, for an RF pulse (B_1 field) applied over a time t, the magnetization vector displacement angle, θ, is determined as $\theta = \omega_1 t = \gamma B_1 t$, and the product of the pulse time and B_1 amplitude determines the displacement of M_z. This is illustrated in Figure 12-14.

Common flip angles are 90 degrees ($\pi/2$) and 180 degrees (π), although a variety of smaller and larger angles are chosen to enhance tissue contrast in various ways. A 90-degree angle provides the largest possible M_{xy} and detectable MR signal, and requires a known B_1 strength and time (on the order of a few to hundreds of μs). The displacement angle of the sample magnetic moment is linearly related to the product of B_1 field strength and time: For a fixed B_1 field strength, a 90-degree displacement takes half the time of a 180-degree displacement. With flip angles smaller than 90 degrees, less time is needed to displace M_z, and a larger transverse magnetization per unit excitation time is achieved. For instance, a 45-degree flip takes half the time of a 90 degrees yet creates 70% of the signal, as the magnitude of M_{xy} is equal to the sine of 45 degrees, or 0.707. With fast MRI techniques, small displacement angles of 10 degrees and less are often used.

12.3 Magnetization Properties of Tissues

Free Induction Decay: T2 Relaxation

After a 90-degree RF pulse is applied to a magnetized sample at the Larmor frequency, an initial phase coherence of the individual protons is established and maximum M_{xy} is achieved. Rotating at the Larmor frequency, the transverse magnetic field of the excited sample induces signal in the receiver antenna coil (in the laboratory frame of reference). A damped sinusoidal electronic signal, known as the *free induction decay* (FID), is produced (Fig. 12-15).

The FID amplitude decay is caused by loss of M_{xy} phase coherence due to intrinsic micromagnetic inhomogeneities in the sample's structure, whereby individual protons

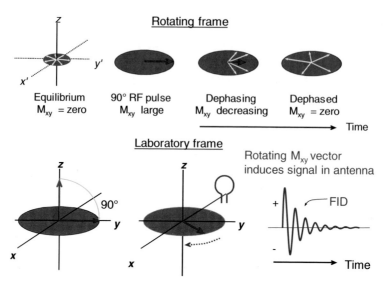

■ **FIGURE 12-15 Top.** Conversion of longitudinal magnetization, M_z, into transverse magnetization, M_{xy}, results in an initial phase coherence of the individual spins of the sample. The magnetic moment vector precesses at the Larmor frequency (stationary in the rotating frame), and dephases with time. **Bottom.** In the laboratory frame, M_{xy} precesses and induces a signal in an antenna receiver sensitive to transverse magnetization. A FID signal is produced with positive and negative variations oscillating at the Larmor frequency, and decaying with time due to the loss of phase coherence.

in the bulk water and hydration layer coupled to macromolecules precess at incrementally different frequencies arising from the slight changes in local magnetic field strength. Phase coherence is lost over time as an exponential decay. Elapsed time between the peak transverse signal (e.g., directly after a 90-degree RF pulse) and 37% of the peak level ($1/e$) is the T2 relaxation time (Fig. 12-16A). Mathematically, this is expressed as

$$M_{xy}(t) = M_0 e^{-t/T2}$$

where $M_{xy}(t)$ is the transverse magnetic moment at time t for a sample that has M_0 transverse magnetization at $t = 0$. When $t = T2$, then $e^{-1} = 0.37$ and $M_{xy} = 0.37\, M_0$.

The molecular structure of the magnetized sample and characteristics of the bound water protons strongly affects its T2 decay value. Amorphous structures (e.g., cerebral spinal fluid [CSF] or highly edematous tissues) contain mobile molecules with fast and rapid molecular motion. Without structural constraint (e.g., lack of a hydration layer), these tissues do not support intrinsic magnetic field inhomogeneities, and thus exhibit long T2 values. As molecular size increases for specific tissues, constrained molecular motion and the presence of the hydration layer produce magnetic field domains within the structure and increase spin dephasing that causes more rapid decay with the result of shorter T2 values. For large, nonmoving structures, stationary magnetic inhomogeneities in the hydration layer result in these types of tissues (e.g., bone) having a very short T2.

Extrinsic magnetic inhomogeneities, such as the imperfect main magnetic field, B_0, or susceptibility agents in the tissues (e.g., MR contrast materials, paramagnetic or ferromagnetic objects), add to the loss of phase coherence from intrinsic inhomogeneities and further reduce the decay constant, known as T2* under these conditions (Fig. 12-16B).

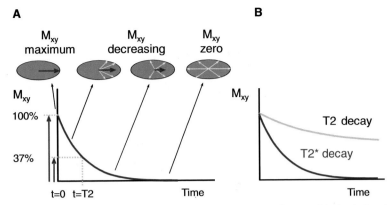

■ **FIGURE 12-16 A.** The loss of M_{xy} phase coherence occurs exponentially caused by intrinsic spin-spin interactions in the tissues and extrinsic magnetic field inhomogeneities. The exponential decay constant, T2, is the time over which the signal decays to 37% of the initial transverse magnetization (e.g., after a 90-degree pulse). **B.** T2 is the decay time resulting from *intrinsic* magnetic properties of the sample. T2* is the decay time resulting from *both intrinsic and extrinsic magnetic field variations.* T2 is always longer than T2*.

Return to Equilibrium: T1 Relaxation

Longitudinal magnetization begins to recover immediately after the B_1 excitation pulse, simultaneous with transverse decay; however, the return to equilibrium conditions occurs over a longer time period. *Spin-lattice relaxation* is the term describing the release of energy back to the *lattice* (the molecular arrangement and structure of the hydration layer), and the regrowth of M_z. This occurs exponentially as

$$M_z(t) = M_0(1 - e^{-t/T1})$$

where $M_z(t)$ is the longitudinal magnetization at time t and $T1$ is the time needed for the recovery of 63% of M_z after a 90-degree pulse (at $t = 0$, $M_z = 0$, and at $t = T1$, $M_z = 0.63\,M_0$), as shown in Figure 12-17. When $t = 3 \times T1$, then $M_z = 0.95\,M_0$, and for $t > 5 \times T1$, then $M_z \approx M_0$, and full longitudinal magnetization equilibrium is established.

Since M_z does not generate an MR signal directly, determination of T1 for a specific tissue requires a specific "sequence," as shown in Figure 12-18. At equilibrium, a 90-degree pulse sets $M_z = 0$. After a delay time, ΔT, the recovered M_z component is converted to M_{xy} by a second 90-degree pulse, and the resulting peak amplitude

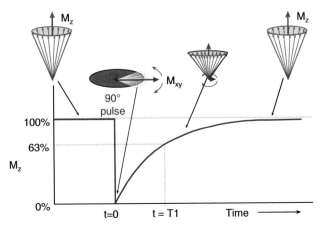

■ **FIGURE 12-17** After a 90-degree pulse, M_z is converted from a maximum value at equilibrium to $M_z = 0$. Return of M_z to equilibrium occurs exponentially and is characterized by the spin-lattice T1 relaxation constant. After an elapsed time equal to T1, 63% of the longitudinal magnetization is recovered. Spin-lattice recovery takes longer than spin-spin decay (T2).

■ FIGURE 12-18 Spin-lattice relaxation for a sample can be measured by using various delay times between two 90-degree RF pulses. After an initial 90-degree pulse, $M_z = 0$, another 90-degree pulse separated by a known delay is applied, and the longitudinal magnetization that has recovered during the delay is converted to transverse magnetization. The maximum amplitude of the resultant FID is recorded as a function of delay times between initial pulse and readout (three different delay time experiments are shown in this example), and the points are fit to an exponential recovery function to determine T1.

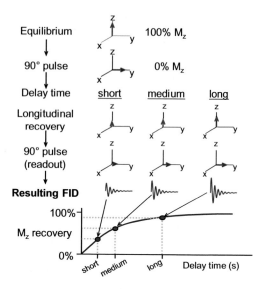

is recorded. By repeating the sequence from equilibrium conditions with different delay times, ΔT between 90-degree pulses, data points that lie on the recovery curve are fit to an exponential equation and T1 is estimated.

The T1 relaxation time depends on the rate of energy dissipation into the surrounding molecular lattice and hydration layer and varies substantially for different tissue structures and pathologies. This can be explained from a classical physics perspective by considering the "tumbling" frequencies of the protons in bulk water and the hydration layers present relative to the Larmor precessional frequency of the protons. Energy transfer is most efficient when a maximal overlap of these frequencies occurs. Small molecules and unbound, bulk water have tumbling frequencies across a broad spectrum, with low-, intermediate-, and high-frequency components. Large, slowly moving molecules have a very tight hydration layer and exhibit low tumbling frequencies that concentrate in the lowest part of the frequency spectrum. Moderately sized molecules (e.g., proteins) and viscous fluids have a moderately bound hydration layer that produce molecular tumbling frequencies more closely matched to the Larmor frequency. This is more fully described in the "Two Compartment Fast Exchange Model" (Fullerton, et.al, 1982; Bottomley, et. al, 1984). The water in the hydration layer and bulk water exchange rapidly (on the order of 100,000 transitions per second) so that a weighted average of the T1 is observed. Therefore, the T1 time is strongly dependent on the physical characteristics of the tissues and their associated hydration layers. Therefore for solid and slowly moving structures, the hydration layer permits only low-frequency molecular tumbling frequencies and consequently, there is almost no spectral overlap with the Larmor frequency. For unstructured tissues and fluids in bulk water, there is also only a small spectral overlap with the tumbling frequencies. In each of these situations, release of energy is constrained and T1 relaxation time is long. For structured and moderately sized proteins and fatty tissues, molecular tumbling frequencies are most conducive to spin-lattice relaxation because of a larger overlap with the Larmor frequency and result in a relatively short T1 relaxation time, as shown in Figure 12-19. Typical T1 values are in the range of 0.1 to 1 s for soft tissues, and 1 to 4 s in aqueous tissues (e.g., CSF).

As the main magnetic field strength increases, a corresponding increase in the Larmor precessional frequency causes a decrease in the overlap with the molecular tumbling frequencies and a longer T1 recovery time. Gadolinium chelated with

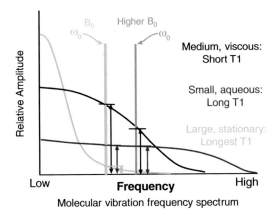

■ **FIGURE 12-19** A classical physics explanation of spin-lattice relaxation is based upon the tumbling frequency of the protons in water molecules of a sample material and its frequency spectrum. Large, stationary structures have water protons with tight hydration layers that exhibit little tumbling motion and a low-frequency spectrum (*aqua* curve). Bulk water and small-sized, aqueous materials have frequencies distributed over a broad range (*purple* curve). Medium-sized, proteinacious materials have a hydration layer that slows down the tumbling frequency of protons sufficiently to allow tumbling at the Larmor frequency (*black* curve). The overlap of the Larmor precessional frequency (vertical bar) with the molecular vibration spectrum indicates the likelihood of spin-lattice relaxation. With higher field strengths, the T1 relaxation becomes *longer* as the tumbling frequency spectrum overlap is decreased.

complex macromolecules are effective in decreasing T1 relaxation time of local tissues by creating a hydration layer that forms a spin-lattice energy sink and results in a rapid return to equilibrium.

Comparison of T1 and T2

T1 is on the order of 5 to 10 times longer than T2. Molecular motion, size, and interactions influence T1 and T2 relaxation (Fig. 12-20). Because most tissues of interest for clinical MR applications are intermediate to small-sized molecules, tissues

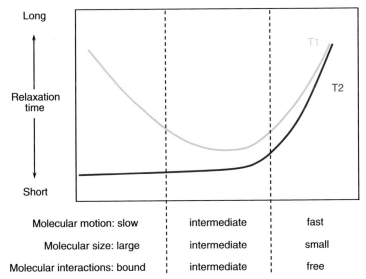

■ **FIGURE 12-20** Factors affecting T1 and T2 relaxation times of different tissues are generally based on molecular motion, size, and interactions that have an impact on the local magnetic field variations (T2 decay) and structure with intrinsic tumbling frequencies coupling to the Larmor frequency (T1 recovery). The relaxation times (vertical axis) are different for T1 and T2.

TABLE 12-4 T1 AND T2 RELAXATION CONSTANTS FOR SEVERAL TISSUES[a]

TISSUE	T1, 0.5 T (ms)	T1, 1.5 T (ms)	T2 (ms)
Fat	210	260	80
Liver	350	500	40
Muscle	550	870	45
White matter	500	780	90
Gray matter	650	900	100
Cerebrospinal fluid	1,800	2,400	160

[a]Estimates only, as reported values for T1 and T2 span a wide range.

with a longer T1 usually have a longer T2, and those with a shorter T1 usually have a shorter T2. In Table 12-4, a comparison of T1 and T2 values for various tissues is listed. Depending on the main magnetic field strength, measurement methods, and biological variation, these relaxation values vary widely. Agents that disrupt the local magnetic field environment, such as paramagnetic blood degradation products, elements with unpaired electron spins (e.g., gadolinium), or any ferromagnetic materials, cause a significant decrease in T2*. In situations where a macromolecule binds free water into a hydration layer, T1 is also significantly decreased.

To summarize, T1 > T2 > T2*, and the specific relaxation times are a characteristic of the tissues. T1 values are longer for higher field strength magnets, while T2 values are unaffected. Thus, the T1, T2, and T2* decay constants, as well as proton density are fundamental properties of tissues, and can be exploited by machine-dependent acquisition techniques in MRI and MRS to aid in the diagnosis of pathologic conditions such as cancer, multiple sclerosis, or hematoma.

12.4 Basic Acquisition Parameters

Emphasizing the differences of T1 and T2, relaxation time constants, and proton density of the tissues is the key to the exquisite contrast sensitivity of MR images, but at the same time, the need to spatially localize the tissues is also required. First, basic machine-based parameters are described.

Time of Repetition

Acquiring an MR image relies on the repetition of a sequence of events in order to sample the volume of interest and periodically build the complete dataset over time. The time of repetition (TR) is the period between B_1 excitation pulses. During the TR interval, T2 decay and T1 recovery occur in the tissues. TR values range from extremely short (millisecond) to extremely long (10,000 ms) time periods, determined by the type of sequence employed.

Time of Echo

Excitation of protons with the B_1 RF pulse creates the M_{xy} FID signal. To separate the RF energy deposition and returning signal, an "echo" is induced to appear at a later time, with the application of a 180-degree RF inversion pulse. This can also be achieved with a gradient field and subsequent polarity reversal. The time of echo (TE) is the time between the excitation pulse and the appearance of the peak amplitude of an induced echo, which is determined by applying a 180-degree RF inversion pulse or gradient polarity reversal at a time equal to TE/2.

Time of Inversion

The TI is the time between an initial inversion/excitation (180 degrees) RF pulse that produces maximum tissue saturation, and a 90-degree readout pulse. During the TI, M_z recovery occurs. The readout pulse converts the recovered M_z into M_{xy}, which is then measured with the formation of an echo at time TE as discussed above.

Partial Saturation

Saturation is a state of tissue magnetization from equilibrium conditions. At equilibrium, the protons in a material are *unsaturated*, with full M_z amplitude. The first excitation (B_1) pulse in the sequence produces the largest transverse magnetization, and recovery of the longitudinal magnetization occurs at the T1 time constant over the TR interval. However, because the TR is less than at least five times the T1 of the sample, M_z recovery is incomplete. Consequently, less M_{xy} amplitude is generated in the second excitation pulse. After the third pulse, a "steady-state" equilibrium is reached, where the amount of M_z recovery and M_{xy} signal amplitude are constant, and the tissues achieve a state of *partial saturation* (Fig. 12-21). Tissues with short T1 have relatively less saturation than tissues with long T1. Partial saturation has an impact on tissue contrast, and explains certain findings such as unsaturated protons in blood outside of the volume moving into the volume and generating a bright vascular signal on entry slices into the volume.

12.5 Basic Pulse Sequences

Three major pulse sequences perform the bulk of data acquisition (DAQ) for imaging: spin echo (SE), inversion recovery (IR), and gradient echo (GE). When used in conjunction with spatial localization methods, "contrast-weighted" images are obtained. In the following sections, the salient points and considerations of generating tissue contrast are discussed.

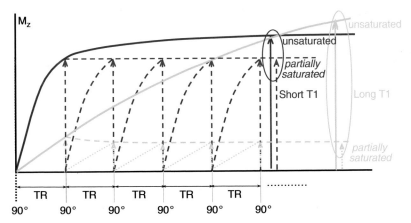

■ **FIGURE 12-21** Partial saturation of tissues occurs because the repetition time between excitation pulses does not allow for full return to equilibrium, and the M_z amplitude for the next RF pulse is reduced. After the third excitation pulse, a steady-state equilibrium is reached, where the amount of longitudinal magnetization is the same from pulse to pulse, as is the transverse magnetization for a tissue with a specific T1 decay constant. Tissues with long T1 experience a greater partial saturation than do tissues with short T1 as shown above. Partial saturation is important in understanding contrast mechanisms and signal from unsaturated and saturated tissues.

Spin Echo

SE describes the excitation of the magnetized protons in a sample with a 90-degree RF pulse and production of a FID, followed by a refocusing 180-degree RF pulse to produce an echo. The 90-degree pulse converts M_z into M_{xy}, and creates the largest phase coherent transverse magnetization that immediately begins to decay at a rate described by T2* relaxation. The 180-degree RF pulse, applied at TE/2, inverts the spin system and induces phase coherence at TE, as depicted in the rotating frame in Figure 12-22. Inversion of the spin system causes the protons to experience external magnetic field variations opposite of that prior to TE/2, resulting in the cancellation of the extrinsic inhomogeneities and associated dephasing effects. In the rotating frame of reference, the echo magnetization vector reforms in the opposite direction from the initial transverse magnetization vector.

Subsequent 180-degree RF pulses during the TR interval (Fig. 12-23) produce corresponding echoes with peak amplitudes that are reduced by intrinsic T2 decay of the tissues, and are immune from extrinsic inhomogeneities. Digital sampling and acquisition of the signal occurs in a time window symmetric about TE, during the evolution and decay of each echo.

Spin Echo Contrast Weighting

Contrast is proportional to the difference in signal intensity between adjacent pixels in an image, corresponding to different voxels in the patient. The details of signal localization and image acquisition in MRI are discussed in Section 12.6. Here, the signal intensity variations for different tissues based upon TR and TE settings are described without consideration of spatial localization.

Ignoring the signal due to moving protons (e.g., blood flow), the signal intensity produced by an MR system for a specific tissue using a SE sequence is

$$S \propto r_H \left[1 - e^{TR/T1}\right] e^{-TE/T2}$$

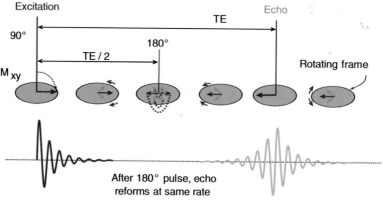

■ FIGURE 12-22 The SE pulse sequence starts with a 90-degree pulse and produces an FID that decays according to T2* relaxation. After a delay time TE/2, a 180-degree RF pulse inverts the spins that re-establishes phase coherence and produces an echo at a time TE. Inhomogeneities of external magnetic fields are canceled, and the peak amplitude of the echo is determined by T2 decay. The rotating frame shows the evolution of the echo vector in the opposite direction of the FID. The sequence is repeated for each repetition period, TR.

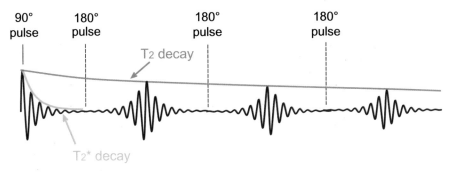

■ **FIGURE 12-23** "True" T2 decay is determined from multiple 180-degree refocusing pulses acquired during the repetition period. While the FID envelope decays with the T2* decay constant, the peak amplitudes of subsequent echoes decay exponentially according to the T2 decay constant, as extrinsic magnetic field inhomogeneities are cancelled.

where ρ_H is the proton density, $T1$ and $T2$ are physical properties of tissue, and TR and TE are pulse sequence timing parameters. For the same pulse sequence, different values of T1, T2, and ρ_H change the signal intensity S, and generate contrast amongst different tissues. Importantly, by changing the pulse sequence parameters TR and TE, the contrast dependence can be weighted toward T1, proton density, or T2 characteristics of the tissues.

T1 Weighting

A "T1-weighted" SE sequence is designed to produce contrast chiefly based on the T1 characteristics of tissues, with de-emphasis of T2 and proton density contributions to the signal. This is achieved by using a relatively short TR to maximize the differences in longitudinal magnetization recovery during the return to equilibrium, and a short TE to minimize T2 decay during signal acquisition. In Figure 12-24, on the left is the graph of longitudinal recovery in steady-state partial saturation after a 90-degree RF excitation at time t = 0, depicting four tissues (CSF, gray matter, white matter, and fat). The next 90-degree RF pulse occurs at the selected TR interval, chosen to create the largest signal difference between the tissues based upon their respective T1 recovery values, which is shown to be about 600 ms (the red vertical line). At this instant in time, all M_z recovered for each tissue is converted to M_{xy}, with respective signal amplitudes projected over to the transverse magnetization graph on the right. Decay immediately occurs, t = 0, at a rate based upon respective T2 values of the tissues. To minimize T2 decay and to maintain the differences in signal amplitude due to T1 recovery, the TE time is kept short (red vertical line). Horizontal projections from the TE intersection with each of the curves graphically illustrate the relative signal amplitudes acquired according to tissue type. Fat, with a short T1, has a large signal, because there is greater recovery of the M_z vector over the TR period. White and gray matter have intermediate T1 values with intermediate signal amplitude, and CSF, with a long T1, has the lowest signal amplitude. A short TE preserves the T1 signal differences by not allowing any significant transverse (T2) decay.

T1-weighted SE contrast therefore requires a short TR and a short TE. A T1-weighted axial image of the brain acquired with TR = 500 ms and TE = 8 ms is illustrated in Figure 12-25. Fat is the most intense signal, followed by white matter, gray matter, and CSF. Typical SE T1-weighting machine parameters are TR = 400 to 600 ms and TE = 3 to 10 ms.

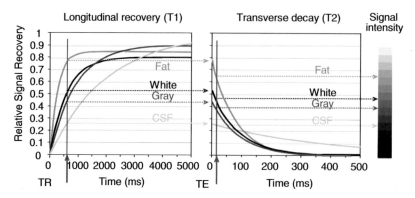

■ **FIGURE 12-24** T1-weighted contrast: Longitudinal recovery (**left**) and transverse decay (**right**) diagrams (note the values of the x-axis time scales) show four brain tissues and T1 and T2 relaxation constants. T1-weighted contrast requires the selection of a TR that emphasizes the differences in the T1 characteristics of the tissues (e.g., TR = ∼ 500 *ms*), and reduces the T2 characteristics by using a short TE so that transverse decay is reduced (e.g., TE ≤ 15 *ms*).

Proton Density Weighting

Proton density contrast weighting relies mainly on differences in the number of magnetized protons per unit volume of tissue. At equilibrium, tissues with a large proton density, such as lipids, fats, and CSF, have a corresponding large M_z compared to other soft tissues. Contrast based on proton density differences is achieved by reducing the contributions of T1 recovery and T2 decay. T1 differences are reduced by selecting a long TR value to allow substantial recovery of M_z. T2 differences of the tissues are reduced by selecting a short TE value. Longitudinal recovery and transverse decay graphs for proton density weighting, using a long TR and a short TE, are illustrated in Figure 12-26. Contrast is generated from variations in proton density (CSF > fat > gray matter > white matter). Figure 12-27 shows a proton

■ **FIGURE 12-25** T1 contrast weighting, TR=500 ms, TE=8 ms. Short TR (400 to 600 ms) generates T1 relaxation-dependent signals. Signals with short T1 have high signal intensity (fat and white matter), while signals with long T1 have low signal intensity (CSF). Short TE (less than 15 ms) preserves the T1 tissue differences by not allowing significant T2 decay to occur.

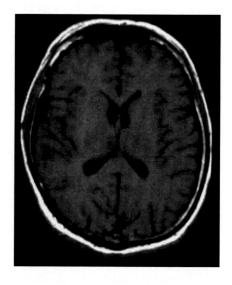

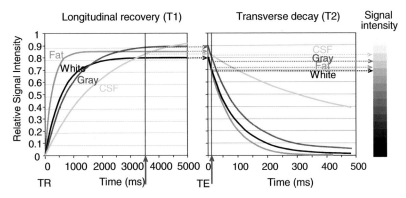

■ FIGURE 12-26 Proton density weighting: Proton (spin) density weighted contrast requires the use of a long TR (e.g., greater than 2,000 *ms*) to reduce T1 effects, and a short TE (e.g., less than 35 *ms*) to reduce T2 influence in the acquired signals. Note that the average overall signal intensity is higher.

density-weighted image with TR = 2,400 ms and TE = 30 ms. Fat and CSF display as a relatively bright signal, and a slight contrast inversion between white and gray matter occurs. A typical proton density-weighted image has a TR between 2,000 and 4,000 ms (see footnote in Table 12.5) and a TE between 3 and 30 ms. The proton density SE sequence achieves the highest overall signal intensity and the largest signal-to-noise ratio (SNR); however, the image contrast is relatively low, and therefore the contrast-to-noise ratio is not necessarily larger than achievable with T1 or T2 contrast weighting.

T2 Weighting

T2 contrast weighting follows directly from the proton density-weighting sequence: reduce T1 differences in tissues with a long TR, and emphasize T2 differences with a *long* TE. The T2-weighted signal is generated from the second echo produced by a

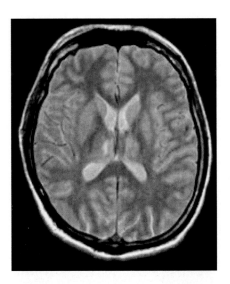

■ FIGURE 12-27 Proton density contrast weighting, TR=2400 ms, TE=30 ms.. Long TR minimizes T1 relaxation differences of the tissues. Signals with large proton density have higher signal intensity (CSF). Short TE preserves the proton density differences without allowing significant T2 decay. This sequence produces a high peak SNR, even though the contrast differences are less than a T2-weighted image.

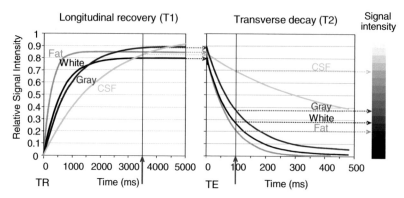

■ FIGURE 12-28 T2 weighted contrast requires the use of a long TR (e.g., greater than 2,000 ms) to reduce T1 influences, and a long TE (e.g., greater than 80 ms) to allow for T2 decay to evolve. Compared to the proton density weighting, the difference is with longer TE.

second 180-degree pulse of a long TR spin echo pulse sequence, where the first echo is proton density weighted, with short TE. T2 contrast differences are manifested by allowing M_{xy} signal decay as shown in Figure 12-28. Compared with a T1-weighted image, inversion of tissue contrast occurs in the image where CSF is bright, and gray and white matter are reversed in intensity.

A T2-weighted image (Fig. 12-29) demonstrates high tissue contrast, compared with either the T1-weighted or proton density-weighted images. As TE is increased, more T2-weighted contrast is achieved, but at the expense of less M_{xy} signal and greater image noise. However, even with low signal amplitudes, image processing with *window width* and *window level* adjustments can remap the signals over the full range of the display, so that the overall average brightness is similar for all images. The typical T2-weighted sequence uses a TR of approximately 2,000 to 4,000 ms and a TE of 80 to 120 ms.

■ FIGURE 12-29 T2 contrast weighting. Long TR minimizes T1 relaxation differences of the tissues. Long TE allows T2 decay differences to be manifested. A second echo provides time for T2 decay to occur, so a T2 W image is typically acquired in concert with a PD W image. While this sequence has high contrast, the signal decay reduces the overall signal and therefore the SNR.

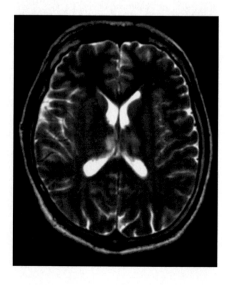

TABLE 12-5   SE PULSE SEQUENCE CONTRAST WEIGHTING PARAMETERS

PARAMETER	T1 CONTRAST	PROTON DENSITY CONTRAST[a]	T2 CONTRAST
TR (ms)	400–600	2,000–4,000	2,000–4,000
TE (ms)	5–30	5–30	60–150

[a]Strictly speaking, SE images with TR less than 3,000 ms are not proton density with respect to the CSF; because of its long T1, only 70% of the CSF magnetization recovery will have occurred and will not appear as bright as for a true PD image. True PD image intensities can be obtained with fast spin echo methods (Chapter 13) with longer TR (e.g., 8,000 ms).
TE, time of echo; TR, time of repetition.

Spin Echo Parameters

Table 12-5 lists typical contrast-weighting values of TR and TE for SE imaging. For conventional SE sequences, both proton density and T2-weighted contrast signals are acquired during each TR by acquiring two echoes with a short TE and a long TE (Fig. 12-30).

Inversion Recovery

IR emphasizes T1 relaxation times of the tissues by extending the amplitude of the longitudinal recovery by a factor of two. An initial 180-degree RF pulse inverts M_z to $-M_z$. After a programmed delay, the time of inversion—TI, a 90-degree RF (readout) pulse rotates the recovered fraction of M_z into the transverse plane to generate the FID. A second 180-degree pulse (or gradient polarity reversal, see next section, GE) at TE/2 produces an echo at TE (Fig. 12-31); in this situation, the sequence is called *inversion recovery spin echo* (IR SE). The TR for IR is the time between 180-degree initiation pulses. Partial saturation of the protons and steady-state equilibrium of the longitudinal magnetization is achieved after the first three excitations in the sequence. The echo amplitude associated with a given tissue depends on TI, TE, TR, and magnitude (positive or negative) of M_z.

The signal intensity at a location (x,y) in the image matrix for an IR SE acquisition with nonmoving anatomy is approximated as

$$S \propto \rho_H \left(1 - 2e^{-TI/T1}\right) \left(1 - e^{-(TR-TD)/T1}\right) \left(e^{-TE/T2}\right)$$

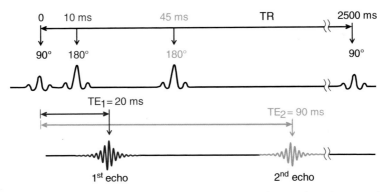

■ **FIGURE 12-30** SE with two 180-degree refocusing pulses after the initial 90-degree excitation pulse. The early echo contains information related to proton density of the tissues, and the longer echo provides T2 weighting. This double echo method is used for providing proton density content and T2 weighted content independently during the same TR interval, and used to fill two separate k-space repositories that are used in producing the final proton density and T2 weighted images.

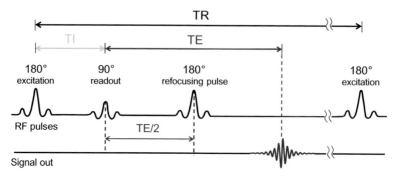

■ **FIGURE 12-31** Inversion-recovery SE sequence is shown. The initial 180-degree excitation pulse inverts the longitudinal magnetization, and thus requires a factor of two times recovery of the longitudinal magnetization over time. The "inversion time" (TI) is the delay between the excitation pulse and conversion to transverse magnetization of the recovered longitudinal magnetization. Subsequently, a second 180-degree pulse is applied at TE/2, which refocuses the transverse magnetization as an echo at time TE. The signal strength is chiefly a function of the T1 characteristics of the tissues, as the TE values are kept short.

where the factor of 2 in the first part of the equation arises from the longitudinal magnetization recovery from $-M_z$ to M_z, and all other parameters are as previously described. For the TI to control contrast between tissues, it follows that TR must be relatively long and TE short. The RF sequence is shown in Figure 12-31.

The IR sequence produces "negative" longitudinal magnetization that results in negative (in phase) or positive (out of phase) transverse magnetization when short TI is used. The actual signals are acquired as magnitude (absolute values) such that M_z values are positive.

Short Tau Inversion Recovery

Short Tau Inversion Recovery, or STIR, is a pulse sequence that uses a very short TI and magnitude signal processing, where M_z signal amplitude is always positive (Fig. 12-32).

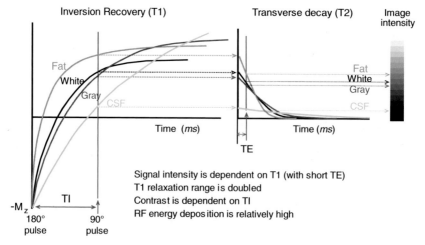

■ **FIGURE 12-32** The IR longitudinal recovery diagram shows the 2 × M_z range provided by the 180-degree excitation pulse. A 90-degree readout pulse at a time TI and a 180-degree refocusing pulse at a time TE/2 from the readout pulse forms the echo at time TE. The time scale is not explicitly indicated on the x-axis. A short TE is used to reduce T2 contrast characteristics.

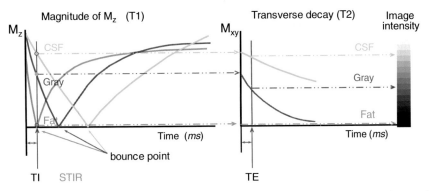

■ **FIGURE 12-33** IR longitudinal magnetization as a function of time, with magnitude signal processing. All tissues go through a null (the bounce point) at a time dependent on T1. The inversion time (TI) is adjusted to select a time to null a certain tissue type. Shown above is the STIR (Short Tau IR) used for suppressing the signal due to fat tissues, achieved with TI = approximately 150 ms (0.693 × 260 ms).

In this situation, materials with short T1 have a lower signal intensity (the reverse of a standard T1-weighted image), and all tissues at some point during recovery have $M_z = 0$. This is known as the *bounce point* or tissue null. Selection of an appropriate TI can thus suppress tissue signals (e.g., fats/lipids, CSF) depending on their T1 relaxation times. The signal null ($M_z = 0$) occurs at TI = $ln(2) \times$ T1, where *ln* is the natural log and $ln(2) = 0.693$. Since T1 for fat at 1.5T is approximately 260 ms, TI is selected as 0.693 × 260 ms = 180 ms. A typical STIR sequence uses TI of 140 to 180 ms and TR of approximately 2,500 ms. Compared with a T1-weighted examination, STIR reduces distracting fat signals (Fig. 12-33) and chemical shift artifacts (explained in Chapter 13) (Fig. 12-34).

Fluid Attenuated Inversion Recovery

The signal levels of CSF and other tissues with long T1 relaxation constants can be overwhelming in the magnitude IR image. Fluid attenuated IR, the *FLAIR* sequence,

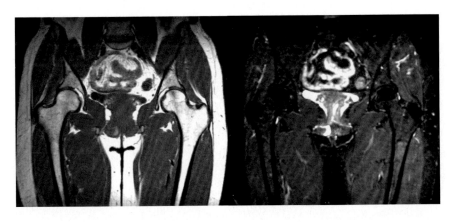

T1   STIR

■ **FIGURE 12-34** SE T1-weighting versus STIR technique. **Left**. T1 W with TR = 750 ms, TE = 13 ms. **Right**. STIR with TR = 5,520 ms, TI = 150 ms, TE = 8 ms. The fat is uniformly suppressed in the STIR image, providing details of nonfat structures otherwise difficult to discern.

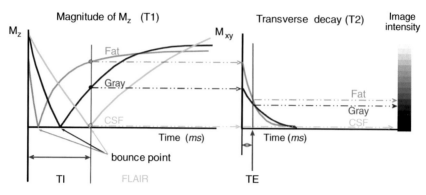

■ **FIGURE 12-35** Shown above is the FLAIR acquisition, with the TI set to the null of CSF, which reduces the large CSF signals and allows the visualization of subtle details otherwise hidden. TE is short to not allow T2 "contamination" of the signals.

reduces CSF signal and other water-bound anatomy in the MR image by using a TI selected at or near the bounce point of CSF to permit better evaluation of the surrounding anatomy as shown in Figure 12-35. Reducing the CSF signal (T1 ≈ 2,500 ms @ 1.5 T) requires TI = 0.693 × 2,500 ms, or ≈ 1,700 ms. A comparison of T1, T2, and FLAIR sequences demonstrates the contrast differences achievable by reducing signals of one tissue to be able to visualize another (see Fig. 12-36).

Summary, Spin Echo Sequences

MR contrast schemes for clinical imaging use the SE or an IR variant of the SE pulse sequences for many examinations. SE and IR SE sequences are less sensitive to magnetic field inhomogeneities, magnetic susceptibilities, and generally give high SNR and CNR. The downsides are the relatively long TR and corresponding long acquisition times.

Gradient Echo

The *GE* technique uses a magnetic field gradient applied in one direction and then reversed to induce the formation of an echo, instead of the 180-degree

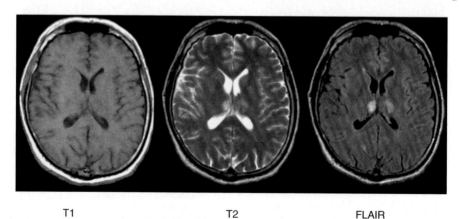

| T1 | T2 | FLAIR |

■ **FIGURE 12-36 Left.** T1-weighted spin-echo axial brain image (TR = 549 ms, TE = 11 ms); Middle: T2 weighted spin-echo image (TR = 2,400 ms, TE = 90 ms); **Right.** FLAIR image (TR = 10,000 ms, TI = 2,400 ms, TE = 150 ms).

inversion pulse. For a FID signal generated under a linear gradient, the transverse magnetization dephases rapidly as the gradient is applied. After a predetermined time, the nearly instantaneous reversal of the GE polarity will rephase the protons and produce a *GE* that occurs when the opposite gradient polarity of equal strength has been applied for the same time as the initial gradient. The induced GE signal is acquired just before and after the peak amplitude, as illustrated in Figure 12-37.

The GE is not a true SE but a purposeful dephasing and rephasing of the FID. Magnetic field (B_0) inhomogeneities and tissue susceptibilities caused by paramagnetic or diamagnetic tissues or contrast agents are emphasized in GE imaging. This is because the dephasing and rephasing of the FID signals occur in the same direction relative to the main magnetic field. In this situation, unlike a 180-degree refocusing RF pulse, the external magnetic field variations are not cancelled. Compare Figures 12-22 and 12-37 and the direction of the M_{xy} vector in the rotating frame. For SE techniques, the FID and echo vectors form in opposite directions, whereas with GE, the FID and echo form in the same direction. Significant sensitivity to field nonuniformity and magnetic susceptibility agents thus occurs, as M_{xy} decay is a strong function of T2*, which is much shorter than the "true" T2 achieved in SE sequences. Timing of the gradient echo is controlled either by inserting a time delay between the negative and positive gradients or by reducing the amplitude of the reversed gradient, thereby extending the time for the rephasing process to occur.

A major variable determining tissue contrast in GE sequences is the flip angle. Depending on the desired image contrast, flip angles of a few degrees to more than 90 degrees are used, a majority of which are small angles much less than 60 degrees. In the realm of very short TR, smaller flip angles require less time and create more transverse magnetization compared to larger flip angles. A plot of M_{xy} signal amplitude versus TR as a function of flip angle (Fig. 12-38) shows that smaller flip angles produce more M_{xy} signal than larger flip angles when TR is less than 200 ms.

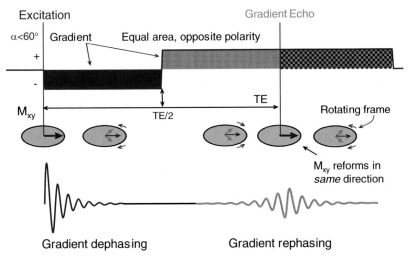

■ **FIGURE 12-37** A magnetic field gradient induces the formation of an "echo" (instead of a 180-degree RF pulse). Transverse magnetization spins are dephased with an applied gradient of one polarity and rephased with the gradient reversed in polarity; this produces a "gradient echo." Note that the rotating frame depicts the magnetic moment vector of the echo in the *same direction* as the FID relative to the main magnetic field, and therefore extrinsic inhomogeneities are not cancelled.

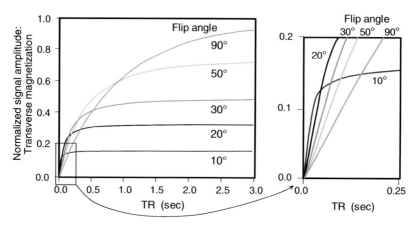

■ **FIGURE 12-38** Transverse magnetization as a function of TR and the flip angle is shown. For small flip angles and very short TR, the transverse magnetization is higher for small flip angles compared to larger flip angles. Detail is shown on the right.

Ultimately, tissue contrast in GE pulse sequences depends on TR, TE, and flip angle along with specialized manipulation of the acquisition sequence.

Gradient Echo Sequences with Long TR

For GE sequences with "long" TR (greater than 200 ms) and flip angles greater than 45 degrees, contrast behavior is similar to that of SE sequences. The major difference is image contrast that is based on T2* rather than T2, because external magnetic field inhomogeneities are not cancelled. As for clinical interpretation, the mechanisms of contrast based on T2* are different from those based on T2, particularly for MRI contrast agents. A relatively long TE tends to emphasize the differences between T2* and T2, rather than improve T2 contrast, as would be expected in an SE sequence. T1 weighting is achieved with a short TE (5 to 10 ms). In most situations, however, GE imaging is not useful with long TR, except when contrast produced by magnetic susceptibility differences is desired.

Gradient Echo Sequences with short TR, less than 50 ms

Reducing the repetition period below 50 ms does not allow for transverse decay (T2*) to fully occur, and a steady-state equilibrium of longitudinal and transverse magnetization from pulse to pulse exists. The persistent transverse magnetization is produced from previous RF excitations, and multiple signals are generated: (1) the FID signal generated at the end of the current RF pulse, and once rephased, contains T2* or T1 information depending on the TE; (2) a stimulated echo generated from the previous RF pulse acting on the persistent transverse magnetization accruing from the RF pulse twice displaced. The stimulated echo contains T2 and T2* weighting. This is schematically shown in Figure 12-39 for a train of RF pulses and the generated signals.

Given the nature of the overlapping signals, there are generic GE acquisitions termed coherent, incoherent, and steady-state free precession (SSFP) that provide differential tissue contrast weighting.

Coherent GE

The coherent GE sequence is shown in Figure 12-40, indicating the timing of the RF pulse with the dephasing and rephasing implemented by reversal of gradient

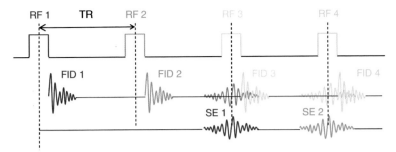

■ **FIGURE 12-39** GE acquisition with short TR less than 50 ms and flip angles upto 45 degrees produces two signals: (1) the FID from the current RF pulse and (2) stimulated echo from the previous RF pulse resulting from persistent transverse magnetization. These signals overlap, but are shown distinct in the illustration for clarity. Resultant image contrast is due to the ratio of T1 to T2 in a tissue because of the mixed signals generated by the combined FID (chiefly T1 and T2* contrast) and SE (chiefly T2 and T2* contrast) in the digitized signal. With the train of RF excitation pulses, RF pulse 2 stimulates the echo formation of the FID produced from RF pulse 1, which appears during RF pulse 3 and superimposes on the current (RF pulse 3) FID. While this is a conceptual illustration, in fact, the actual situation is much more complicated, as there are many higher order stimulated and gradient echoes that contribute to the observed signal.

polarity to generate an echo at a selectable time TE for the frequency encode gradient (FEG), where identification of proton position based upon frequency is performed. (Note: the various encoding gradients used to localize the protons are discussed in the next section of this chapter.) Also involved in this sequence is the phase encode gradient (PEG), which is applied and incrementally changed for each TR to identify proton position in the direction perpendicular to the FEG based upon phase changes of the protons after the PEG is turned off. A "rewinder PEG" of the same strength but opposite polarity is applied after the echo to realign the phase prior to the next RF pulse. The combined FID and simulated echo signals are generated during the GE, and produce tissue contrast dependent on flip angle, TR, and TE. With moderate flip angles of 30 to 60 degrees, the differences in tissue contrast are primarily based upon T2/T1 ratios. Since most tissues with a long

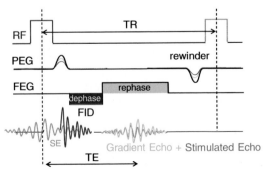

■ **FIGURE 12-40** Coherent GE: Multiple gradients are used for localizing the protons, including the PEG and the FEG. In addition to localizing protons, these gradients are intrinsic to the manipulation of the signals in the coherent GE acquisition. As shown above, the PEG is applied after the RF pulse but prior to the FEG, to determine location in one direction by adding a known phase to the protons based on location per TR interval. Subsequently, a rewinder gradient of the same strength but opposite polarity resets the phase prior to the next TR excitation. The FEG is the gradient that generates the echo from the FID plus the stimulated echo from the previous RF pulse.

TABLE 12-6   GRADIENT RECALLED ECHO WEIGHTING (STEADY-STATE)

PARAMETER	T1	T2/T1	T2	T2*	PROTON DENSITY
Flip angle (degrees)	45–90	30–50	5–15	5–15	5–30
TR (ms)	200–400	10–50	200–400	100–300	100–300
TE (ms)	3–15	3–15	30–50	10–20	5–15

T2 also have a long T1 and vice versa, there is very little tissue contrast generated. In certain applications such as MR angiography, this is a good outcome, so that anatomical contrast differences that would otherwise compete with the bright blood when displayed by image processing techniques (described in Chapter 13) would reduce the image quality.

This acquisition technique is described by the acronyms GRASS (gradient recalled acquisition in the steady state), FISP (fast imaging with steady-state precession), FAST (Fourier acquired steady state), and other acronyms coined by MRI equipment manufacturers. Table 12-6 indicates typical parameter values for contrast desired in steady-state and GE acquisitions. The steady-state sequences with coherent echoes produce T2* and proton density contrast. A GRASS/FISP sequence using TR = 35 ms, TE = 3 ms, and flip angle = 20 degrees shows unremarkable contrast, but blood flow shows up as a bright signal (Fig. 12-41). This technique enhances vascular contrast, from which MR angiography sequences can be reconstructed.

Incoherent, "Spoiled" Gradient Echo Techniques

With very short TR steady-state acquisitions, T1 weighting *cannot* be achieved to any great extent, owing to either a small difference in longitudinal magnetization with small flip angles or dominance of the T2* effects for larger flip angles produced

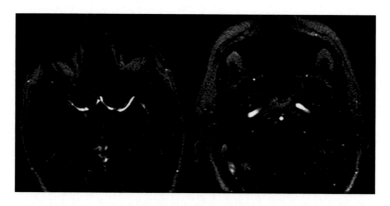

TR=35 *ms*, TE=3 *ms*, flip angle=20

■ **FIGURE 12-41** A *steady-state* gradient recalled echo (GRASS) sequence (TR = 24 *ms*, TE = 4.7 *ms*, flip angle = 50 degrees) of two slices out of a volume acquisition is shown. Contrast is unremarkable for white and gray matter because of a T2-/T1-weighting dependence. Blood flow appears as a relatively bright signal. MR angiography (see Chapter 13) depends on pulse sequences such as these to reduce the contrast of the anatomy relative to the vasculature.

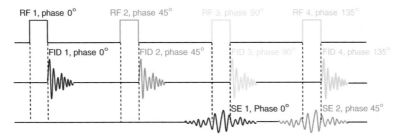

■ **FIGURE 12-42** Incoherent (spoiled) GE acquisition: Persistent transverse magnetization is dephased by each RF pulse; the superposition of the FID from the current RF pulse with a stimulated-echo from the previous RF pulse is separable, because of differences in the phase of the generated signals. In an actual sequence with TR of 5 to 6 ms, several of stimulated echoes will contribute to the signal, along with the FID. Particular angles of phase increment (typically 117 or 123 degrees) have been determined empirically to cause cancellation by destructive interference of the magnetization from the different coherence pathways to eliminate the signal, leaving only the signal from the FID. T1 contrast can be preferentially generated without contamination of the signals due to the T2 characteristics of the tissues.

by persistent residual transverse magnetization created by stimulated echoes. The T2* influence can be reduced by using a long TR (usually not an option), or by "spoiling" the steady-state transverse magnetization by introducing incoherent phase differences from pulse to pulse. The latter is achieved by adding a phase shift to successive RF pulses during the excitation of protons. Both the RF transmitter and RF receiver are phase locked, so that the receiver discriminates the phase of the GE from the SE generated by the previous RF pulse, now out of phase, as shown in Figure 12-42. Mostly, T1-weighted contrast is obtained, with short TR, short TE, and moderate to large flip angle. Spoiled transverse magnetization gradient recalled echo (SPGR) is often used in three-dimensional volume acquisitions because of the extremely short acquisition time allowed by the short TR of the GE sequence and the good contrast rendition of the anatomy provided by T1 weighting (Fig. 12-43).

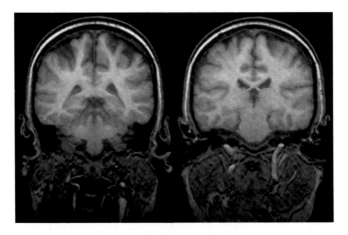

TR=8 *ms*, TE=1.9 *ms*, flip angle=20°
Note T1 contrast and high blood vessel signal

■ **FIGURE 12-43** Incoherent (spoiled) GE images. The ability to achieve T1 contrast weighting is extremely useful for rapid three-dimensional volume imaging. Bright blood (lower portion of each image) and magnetic susceptibility artifacts are characteristic of this sequence. TR = 8 *ms*, TE = 1.9 *ms*, flip angle = 20 degrees.

MR contrast agents (e.g., gadolinium) produce greater contrast with T1-weighted SPGR than with a comparable T1-weighted SE sequence because of the greater sensitivity to magnetic susceptibility. The downsides of spoiled GE techniques are the increased sensitivity to other artifacts such as chemical shift and magnetic field inhomogeneities, as well as lower SNR.

Steady-State Free Precession

In GE sequences with short TR (less than 50 ms), the TE is not long enough to generate any T2 contrast, and GE rephasing is inefficient and dominated by T2* effects. The SSFP sequence emphasizes acquisition of only the stimulated echo, which arises from the previous RF pulse and appears during the next RF pulse at a time equal to 2 × TR (see Fig. 12-39). To reposition the stimulated echo to an earlier time in the TR interval for signal acquisition, a rewinder gradient is applied, which speeds up the rephasing process initiated by the RF pulse, so that it reforms and decays just before the next RF pulse. In the SSFP sequence, there are two TE values: one is the *actual TE*, the time between the peak stimulated echo amplitude and the *next* excitation pulse, and the other is the *effective TE*, the time from the echo and the RF pulse that created its FID. The effective TE is thus longer than the TR and is calculated as: effective TE = 2 × TR-actual TE. So for TR = 50 ms and TE = 5 ms, the effective TE is 95 ms, which means that the stimulated echo has had 95 ms to manifest T2 weighting. SSFP sequences provide true T2 contrast weighting, are useful for brain and joint imaging, and can be used with three-dimensional volumetric acquisitions (as discussed in Chapter 13) (Figs. 12-44 and 12-45). "Balanced" SSFP sequences generate accumulated gradient echo (FID) and stimulated echo signals with the use of symmetrical gradients in 3 spatial directions, which null phase shifts induced by flow. Balanced SSFP provides T2/T1 contrast and high speed acquisitions, particularly useful for cardiac imaging (Chavan, et.al., 2008).

Summary, Gradient Echo contrast

For GE acquisition in the realm of short TR, persistent transverse magnetization produces two signals: (1) the FID produced from the RF pulse just applied and

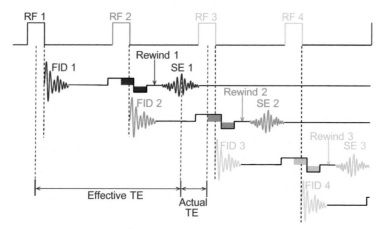

■ **FIGURE 12-44** SSFP uses a rewinder gradient to position each stimulated echo so that it appears just before the next excitation pulse, and is acquired separately from the FID. Since rephasing of the stimulated echo is initiated by an RF pulse rather than a gradient, more T2 rather than T2* weighting occurs. The *actual* TE is the time from the peak echo amplitude to the center of the next RF pulse. The *effective* TE is 2 × TR−actual TE (This is shown in the lower left of the figure).

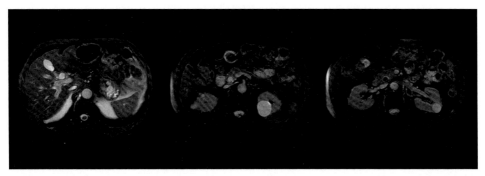

■ **FIGURE 12-45** Three abdominal post gadolinium contrast axial images are part of a breath-hold dataset using a "balanced SSFP" acquisition, which simultaneously accumulates the FID and the stimulated echo with contrast varying according to the T2/T1 ratio (TR: 3.34 ms, TE: 1.2 milliseconds, Flip angle 70 degrees, matrix size 192 × 320). Each image is acquired in approximately 700 milliseconds, making this sequence useful for reducing voluntary and involuntary patient motion in contrast enhanced abdominal and cardiac imaging.

(2) the stimulated echo from the residual transverse magnetization. From these two generated signals, coherent, incoherent, or SSFP sequences are used in order to generate different contrast-weighting schemes. Coherent GE uses the combined FID and SE signals and produces contrast mainly depending on the ratio of T2/T1 or T2*/T1; incoherent (or spoiled) GE produces contrast mainly based on T1, and SSFP samples the SE signal only, thus producing signals that are more T2 weighted. Figure 12-46 shows the signals and the timing of acquisition for these three scenarios. Note that these are generic, not fully inclusive, and do not include specific sequences implemented by the major manufacturers that do not fit into this simplified categorization. Additionally the term SSFP is used differently by the manufacturers. One should consult the specific applications manuals and descriptions of the specific models and pulse sequence implementations for more detailed information (Also see Chapter 13, Table 1 for a brief comparison of GE sequences). Details of GE techniques are reviewed in an article by Chavhan, et.al. (2008).

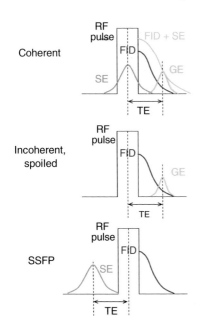

■ **FIGURE 12-46** A schematic summary of the three major GE sequences (RF, RadioFrequency; FID, Free Induction Decay; GE, Gradient Echo; SE, Stimulated or Spin Echo; TE, Time of Echo) are shown. Coherent GE uses signals from the FID and the SE to produce the image, typically with contrast dependent on T2/T1 weighting, and low contrast. Incoherent GE eliminates the detection of the SE, thus, providing a means to generate T1-weighted contrast from the FID signal. SSFP uses the SE signal, which provides mainly T2-weighted contrast. Balanced SSFP uses both the gradient and stimulated echo to produce a T2/T1 weighting with symmetrically applied gradients in three dimensions.

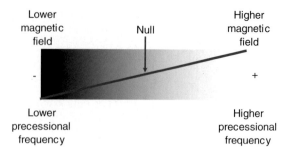

■ **FIGURE 12-47** The gradient magnetic field creates a net positive and negative magnetic environment that adds to and subtracts from the main magnetic field. Associated with the local change in magnetic field is a positionally dependent change in precessional frequencies, per the Larmor equation. The precessional frequencies directly vary across the field in proportion to the applied gradient strength.

 ## MR Signal Localization

Spatial localization is essential for creating MR images and determining the location of discrete sample volumes for MR spectroscopy. This is achieved by superimposing linear magnetic field variations on the main (B_0) field to generate corresponding position-dependent variations in precessional frequency of the protons (Fig. 12-47). Simultaneous application of an RF excitation (B_1 pulse) excites only those protons in resonance within the frequency bandwidth (BW) of the B_1 RF pulse by absorbing energy.

Magnetic Field Gradients

Inside the magnet bore, three sets of gradients reside along the logical coordinate axes—x, y, and z—and produce a magnetic field variation determined by the magnitude of the applied current in each coil set (Fig. 12-48). When independently energized, the three coils (x, y, z) can produce a linearly variable magnetic field in

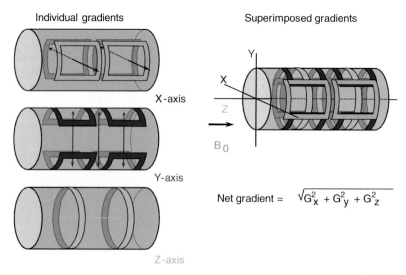

■ **FIGURE 12-48** Within the large stationary magnetic field, field gradients are produced by three separate coil pairs placed within the central core of the magnet, along the x, y, or z directions. In modern systems, the current loops are distributed across the cylinders for the x-, y- and z- gradients, which generates a lower, but more uniform gradient field. Magnetic field gradients of arbitrary direction are produced by the vector addition of the individual gradients turned on simultaneously. Any gradient direction is possible by superimposition of magnetic fields generated by the three-axis gradient system.

any direction, where the net gradient is equal to $\sqrt{G_x^2 + G_y^2 + G_z^2}$. Gradient polarity reversals (positive to negative and negative to positive changes in magnetic field strength) are achieved by reversing the current direction in the gradient coils.

Two important properties of magnetic gradients are: (1) The *gradient field strength* is determined by its peak amplitude and slope (change over distance), and typically ranges from 1 to 50 mT/m. (2) The *slew rate* is the time to achieve the peak magnetic field amplitude. Typical slew rates of gradient fields are from 5 to 250 mT/m/ms. As the gradient field is turned on, *eddy currents* are induced in nearby conductors such as adjacent RF coils and the patient, which produce magnetic fields that oppose the gradient field and limit the achievable slew rate. Actively shielded gradient coils and compensation circuits can reduce problems caused by eddy currents.

In a gradient magnetic field, protons maintain precessional frequencies corresponding to local magnetic field strength. At the middle of the gradient, called the *null*, there is no change in the field strength or precessional frequency. With a linear gradient, the magnetic field increases and decreases linearly from the null, as does the precessional frequency (Fig. 12-47 and Table 12-7). In the rotating frame of reference, incremental changes of frequency occur symmetrically about the null, and the positions of protons are encoded by frequency and phase. The frequency BW is the range of frequencies over the FOV, and the frequency BW per pixel is the BW divided by the number of discrete samples. Gradient amplitude can also be expressed in frequency per distance. For instance, a 10-mT/m gradient can be expressed as 10 mT/m × 42.58 MHz/T × 1 T/1,000 mT = 0.4258 MHz/m, which is equivalent to 425.8 kHz/m or 425.8 Hz/mm. The relationship of gradient strength and frequency BW across the FOV is independent of the main magnet field strength.

Localization of protons in the three-dimensional volume requires the application of three distinct gradients during the pulse sequence: slice select, frequency encode, and phase encode. These gradients are sequenced in a specific order, depending on the pulse sequences employed. Often, the three gradients overlap partially or completely during the scan to achieve a desired spin state, or to leave protons in their original phase state after the application of the gradient(s).

TABLE 12-7   PRECESSIONAL FREQUENCY VARIATION AT 1.5 T ALONG AN APPLIED GRADIENT

Gradient field strength	3 mT/m = 127.74 Hz/mm
Main magnetic field strength	1.5 T
FOV	0.15 m = 150 mm
Linear gradient amplitude over FOV	0.45 mT; from −0.225 mT to +0.225 mT
Maximum magnetic field (frequency)	1.500225 T (63.8795805 MHz)
Unchanged magnetic field at null	1.500000 T (63.8700000 MHz)
Minimum magnetic field	1.499775 T (63.8604195 MHz)
Net frequency range across FOV[a]	0.019161 MHz = 19.2 kHz = 19,161 Hz
Frequency range across FOV (1,278 Hz/cm)[b]	127.74 Hz/mm × 150 mm = 19,161 Hz
Frequency BW per pixel (256 samples)	19,161 Hz/256 = 74.85 Hz/pixel

[a]Calculated using the absolute precessional frequency range: 63.8796–63.8604 MHz.
[b]Calculated using the gradient strength expressed in Hz/mm.

Slice Select Gradient

RF transmitters cannot spatially direct the RF energy to a specific region in the body; rather the RF pulse, when turned on during the application of the slice select gradient (SSG), determines the slice location of protons in the tissues that absorb energy. For axial MR images, the SSG is applied along the long (cranial-caudal) axis of the body. Under the influence of the gradient field, the proton precessional frequencies in the volume are incrementally increased or decreased dependent on their distance from the null. A selective, narrow band RF frequency pulse of a known duration and amplitude delivers energy to the total volume, but only those protons with precessional frequencies matching the RF BW frequencies will absorb energy within a defined slice of tissues as shown in Figure 12-49 (red vertical line indicates energy absorbed due to resonance). If the center frequency of the RF pulse is increased, then a different slab of protons absorbs energy (blue vertical line).

Slice thickness is chiefly determined by the frequency BW of the RF pulse and the gradient strength across the FOV. For a fixed gradient strength, the RF pulse with a narrow BW excites protons within a thin slice, and a wide BW excites a thick slice (Fig. 12-50A). For a fixed RF BW, a high gradient strength produces a large range of frequencies across the FOV and decreases the slice thickness, whereas a low gradient strength produces a small range of frequencies and produces an increase in the slice thickness (Fig. 12-50B).

A combination of a narrow BW and a low gradient strength or a wide BW and a high gradient strength can result in the same slice thickness. Decisions depend chiefly on the SNR and the propensity for "chemical shift" artifacts. SNR is inversely proportional to the receiver BW: $SNR \propto \dfrac{1}{\sqrt{BW}}$; therefore narrow BW and low gradient strength are preferred; however, artifacts due to *chemical shift* (see Chapter 13, Section 13.5, Chemical Shift Artifacts) can be problematic. Consequently, trade-offs in image quality must be considered when determining the optimal RF BW and SSG field strength combinations.

After the SSG is turned off, the protons revert to the precessional frequency of the main magnetic field, but phase coherence is lost. To reestablish the original phase of all stationary protons, a gradient of opposite polarity equal to one-half of the

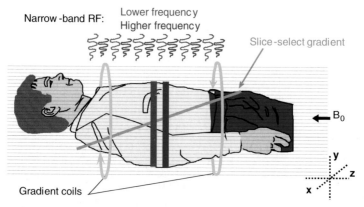

■ **FIGURE 12-49** The *SSG* disperses the precessional frequencies of the protons in a known way along the gradient. A narrow band RF pulse excites only a selected volume (slice) of tissues, determined by frequency, BW, and SSG strength. In the example above, two narrow-band RF pulses with different center frequencies irradiate the whole body during the application of the gradient, and only those protons at the same frequencies as the RF pulses will absorb energy. Note that the higher frequency slice is shifted towards the positive pole of the applied gradient.

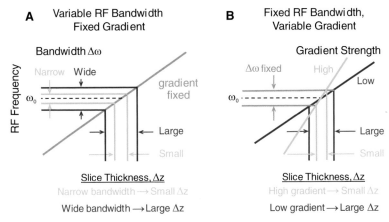

A Variable RF Bandwidth
Fixed Gradient

B Fixed RF Bandwidth,
Variable Gradient

■ **FIGURE 12-50** Slice thickness is dependent on RF BW and gradient strength. **A.** For a fixed gradient strength, the RF BW determines the slice thickness. **B.** For a fixed RF BW, gradient strength determines the slice thickness.

area of the original SSG is applied (Fig. 12-51). For 180-degree RF excitations, the rephasing gradient is not necessary, as all protons maintain their phase relationships because of the symmetry of the RF pulse and spin inversion.

To summarize, the SSG is applied simultaneously with a RF pulse of a known BW to create proton excitation in a single plane with a known slice thickness, and to localize signals orthogonal to the gradient. It is the first of three gradients applied to the volume.

Frequency Encode Gradient

The *FEG*, also known as the *readout gradient*, is applied in a direction perpendicular to the SSG, along the "logical" x-axis, during the evolution and decay of the induced echo. Net changes in precessional frequencies are distributed symmetrically from 0 at the null to $+f_{max}$ and $-f_{max}$ at the edges of the FOV (Fig. 12-52) under the applied FEG. The composite signal is amplified, digitized, and processed by the Fourier transform to convert frequency into spatial position (Fig. 12-53). A spatial "projection" is created by integrating the resultant Fourier transformed signal amplitudes perpendicular to the direction of the applied gradient at corresponding spatial positions.

The SSG in concert with an incremental rotation of the FEG direction about the object can produce data projections through the object as a function of angle, as shown in Figure 12-54. With a sufficient number of projections, filtered back-projection can be used for reconstructing a tomographic image (see Chapter 11 on

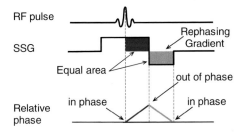

■ **FIGURE 12-51** SSG rephasing. At the peak of the RF pulse, all protons in the slice are in phase, but the SSG causes the spins to become dephased after the gradient is turned off. To reestablish phase coherence, a reverse polarity gradient is applied equal to one-half the area of the original SSG. At the next pulse, the relative phase will be identical.

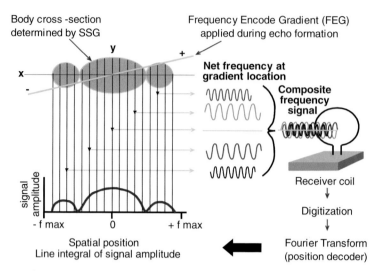

■ **FIGURE 12-52** The *FEG* is applied in an orthogonal direction to the SSG, and confers *a spatially dependent variation* in the precessional frequencies of the protons. Acting only on those protons in a slice determined by the SSG excitation, the composite signal is acquired, digitized, demodulated (Larmor frequency removed), and Fourier transformed into frequency and amplitude information. A one-dimensional array represents a *projection* of the slice of tissue (amplitude and position) at a specific angle. (Demodulation into net frequencies occurs *after* detection by the receiver coil; this is shown in the figure for clarity only.)

CT Reconstruction). In fact, this is how some of the first MR images were reconstructed from individual projections, using a rotating FEG. However, inefficient acquisition and data handling, in addition to motion artifacts, has led to near-universal acquisition with phase encoding techniques.

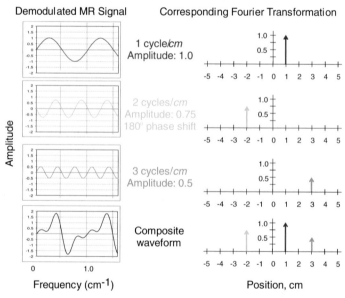

■ **FIGURE 12-53** Spatial frequency signals (cycles/cm) and their Fourier transforms (spatial position) are shown for three simple sinusoidal waveforms with a specific amplitude and phase. The Fourier transform decodes the frequency, phase and amplitude variations in the spatial frequency domain into a corresponding position and amplitude in the spatial domain. A 180-degree phase shift (second from the top) is shifted in the negative direction from the origin. The composite waveform (a summation of all waveforms, lower left) is decoded by Fourier transformation into the corresponding positions and amplitudes (lower right).

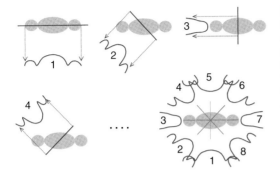

■ **FIGURE 12-54** A rotating FEG in the x-y plane allows the acquisition of individual projections as a function of angle, by repeating the SSG – FEG sequence with incremental change of the FEG direction. This example shows eight projections; to have sampling sufficient for high SNR and resolution would require hundreds of projections about the object.

Phase Encode Gradient

Position of the protons in the third orthogonal dimension is determined with a PEG, which is applied after the SSG but before the FEG, along the third orthogonal axis. Phase in this context represents a linear variation in the starting point of sinusoidal waves that precess at the same frequency. Phase changes are purposefully introduced by the application of a short duration PEG within each data acquisition (DAQ) interval. Prior to the PEG, all protons have the same phase, and turning on the PEG introduces a linear variation in the precessional frequency of the protons according to their position along the gradient. After a brief interval, the PEG is turned off, all protons revert to the Larmor frequency, and linear phase shifts are manifested by a specific gradient strength and polarity. Incremental positive phase change is introduced for protons under the positive pole, negative phase change under the negative pole, and no phase change occurs for protons at the null of the PEG. Throughout the acquisition sequence, the PEG strength and polarity is incrementally changed to introduce specific known phase changes as a function of position across the FOV for each acquisition interval (Fig. 12-55). Spatial encoding is determined by the amount of phase shift that has occurred. Protons located at the center

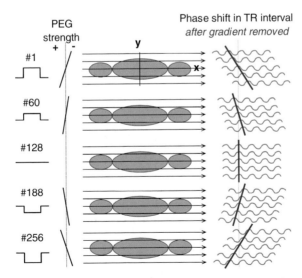

■ **FIGURE 12-55** The PEG is applied *before* the FEG and *after* the SSG. The PEG produces a spatially dependent variation in angular frequency of the excited spins for a brief duration, and generates a spatially dependent variation in phase when the spins return to the Larmor frequency. Incremental changes in the PEG strength for each TR interval spatially encodes the phase variations: protons at the null of the PEG do not experience any phase change, while protons in the periphery experience a large phase change dependent on their distance from the null. The incremental variation of the PEG strength can be thought of as providing specific "views" of the volume because the SSG and FEG remain fixed throughout the acquisition.

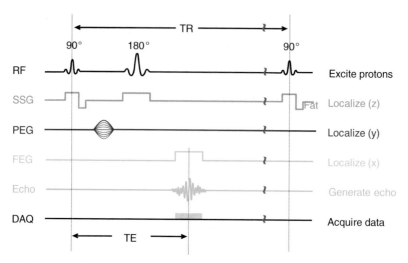

■ **FIGURE 12-56** A typical spin-echo pulse sequence diagram indicates the timing of the SSG, PEG, and FEG during the repetition time (TR) interval, synchronized with the RF pulses and the DAQ when the echo appears. Each TR interval is repeated with a different PEG strength (this appears as multiple lines in the illustration, but only one PEG strength is applied per TR as indicated by the bold line in this figure).

of the FOV, the PEG null, do not exhibit a phase shift. Protons located at the edges of the FOV exhibit the largest positive to negative (or negative to positive) phase shifts. Protons located at intermediate distances from the null experience intermediate phase shifts (positive or negative). Each location along the phase encode axis is spatially encoded by the amount of phase shifts experienced by the protons. For sequential acquisition sequences, each sample in the PEG direction is separated in time by the TR interval.

Gradient Sequencing

An acquisition of an *SE* pulse sequence is illustrated in Figure 12-56, showing the timing of the SSG in conjunction with the 90-degree RF excitation pulse, the application of a short duration PEG at a known strength, followed by a 180-degree refocusing RF pulse at TE/2, and the echo envelope with the peak amplitude occurring at TE. This sequence is repeated with slight incremental changes in the PEG strength to define the three dimensions in the image over the acquisition time.

12.7 "K-Space" Data Acquisition and Image Reconstruction

MR data are initially stored in the k-space matrix, the "frequency domain" repository (Fig. 12-57). K-space describes a two-dimensional matrix of positive and negative spatial frequency values, encoded as complex numbers (e.g., a + bi, $i = \sqrt{-1}$). The matrix is divided into four quadrants, with the origin at the center representing frequency = 0. Frequency domain data are encoded in the k_x direction by the FEG, and in the k_y direction by the PEG in most image sequences. The lowest spatial frequency increment (the fundamental frequency) is the BW across each pixel (see Table 12-7). The maximum useful frequency (the Nyquist frequency) is equal to ½ frequency range across the k_x or k_y directions, as the frequencies are encoded from $-f_{max}$ to $+ f_{max}$. The periodic nature of the frequency domain has a built-in symmetry described by "symmetric" and "antisymmetric" functions (e.g., cosine and sine waves). "Real," "imaginary," and "magnitude" describe specific phase and amplitude characteristics of the composite MR frequency waveforms. Partial acquisitions are

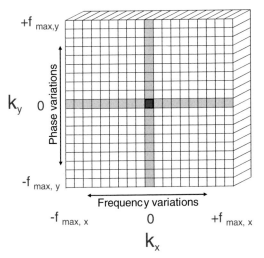

■ **FIGURE 12-57** The k-space matrix is the repository for spatial frequency signals acquired during
the evolution and decay of the echo. The k_x axis
(along the rows) and the k_y axis (along the columns) have units of cycles/unit distance. Each axis
is symmetric about the center of k-space, ranging from $-f_{max}$ to $+f_{max}$ along the rows and the
columns. The matrix is filled one row at a time in
a conventional acquisition with the FEG induced
frequency variations mapped along the k_x axis and
the PEG induced phase variations mapped along
the k_y axis.

possible (e.g., one-half of the k-space matrix plus one line) with complex conjugate
symmetry filling the remainder (See Chapter 13, Section 1, "Data Synthesis").

Two-Dimensional Data Acquisition

MR data are acquired as a complex, composite frequency waveform. With methodical
variations of the PEG during each excitation, the k-space matrix is filled to produce
the desired variations across the frequency and phase encode directions as shown in
Figure 12-58.

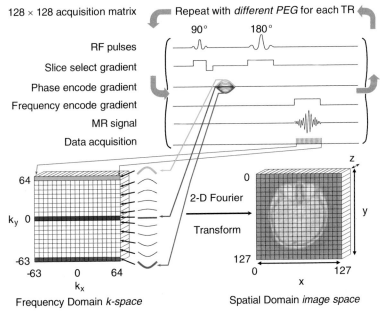

■ **FIGURE 12-58** MR data are acquired into k-space matrix, where each row in k-space represents spatially
dependent frequency variations under a fixed FEG strength, and each column represents spatially dependent
phase shift variations under an incrementally varied PEG strength. Data are placed in a specific row determined
by the PEG strength for each TR interval. The grayscale image is constructed from the two-dimensional Fourier
transformation of the k-space matrix by sequential application of one-dimensional transforms along each row,
and then along each column of the intermediate transformed data. The output image matrix is arranged with
the image coordinate pair, x = 0, y = 0 at the upper left of the image matrix.

A summary description of the two-dimensional spin-echo image acquisition steps follows.

1. A narrow band RF excitation pulse simultaneously applied with the SSG causes a specific slab of tissues with protons at the same frequency to absorb energy. Transverse magnetization, M_{xy}, is produced with amplitude dependent on the saturation of the protons and the angle of excitation. A 90-degree flip angle produces the largest M_{xy}.

2. A PEG is applied for a brief duration, which introduces a phase difference among the protons along the phase encode direction to produce a specific "view" of the data along the k_y axis, corresponding to the strength of the PEG,

3. A refocusing 180-degree RF pulse is delivered at TE/2 to invert and reestablish the phase coherence of the transverse magnetization at time TE.

4. During the evolution and decay of the echo signal, the FEG is applied orthogonal to both the SSG and PEG directions, generating spatially dependent changes in the precessional frequencies of the protons.

5. Data sampling and acquisition of the complex signal occurs simultaneous to the FEG. A one-dimensional inverse Fourier transform converts the digital data into discrete frequency values and corresponding amplitudes to determine position along the k_x (readout) direction.

6. Data are deposited in the k-space matrix at a row location specifically determined by the strength of the PEG. For each TR, an incremental variation of the PEG strength sequentially fills each row. In some sequences, the phase encode data are acquired in nonsequential order to fill portions of k-space more pertinent to the requirements of the exam (e.g., in the low-frequency, central area of k-space). Once filled, the k-space matrix columns contain positionally dependent variations in phase change along the k_y (phase encode) direction.

7. After all rows are filled, an inverse Fourier transform decodes the frequency domain variations in phase for each of the columns of k-space to produce the spatial domain representation.

8. The final image is scaled and adjusted to represent the proton density, T1, T2, and flow characteristics of the tissues using a grayscale range, where each pixel represents a voxel.

The bulk of image information representing the lower spatial frequencies is contained in the center of k-space, whereas the higher spatial frequencies are contained in the periphery, as shown in Figure 12-59, representing a grayscale rendition of k-space for a sagittal slice of a brain MR image acquisition. The innermost areas represent the bulk of the anatomy, while the outer areas of *k-space* contain the detail and resolution components of the anatomy, as shown by reconstructed images.

Two-Dimensional Multiplanar Acquisition

Direct axial, coronal, sagittal, or oblique planes can be obtained by energizing the appropriate gradient coils during the image acquisition, as shown in Figure 12-60. The SSG determines the orientation of the slices: axial uses z-axis coils; coronal uses y-axis coils; and sagittal uses x-axis coils for selection of the slice orientation. Oblique plane acquisition depends on a combination of the x-, y-, and z-axis coils energized simultaneously. SSG, PEG, and FEG applications are perpendicular to each other, and acquisition of data into the k-space matrix remains the same, with the FEG along the k_x axis and the PEG along the k_y axis.

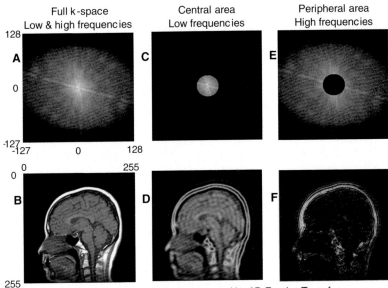

Spatial domain images reconstructed by 2D Fourier Transform

■ **FIGURE 12-59 A.** Image representations of *k-space* segmentation show a concentration of information around the origin (the k-space images are logarithmically amplified for display of the lowest amplitude signals). **B.** Inverse two-dimensional Fourier transformation converts the data into a visible image. **C.** Segmenting a radius of 25 pixels out of 128 in the central area and zeroing out the periphery extracts a majority of the low-frequency information. **D.** The corresponding image demonstrates the majority of the image content is in the center of k-space. **E.** Zeroing out the central portion and leaving the peripheral areas isolates the higher spatial frequency signals. **F.** The resulting image is chiefly comprised of high frequency detail and resolution. Ringing that is visible in the image is due to the sharp masking transition from the image data to zero.

12.8 Summary

The basics of magnetic resonance are covered in this chapter, including the simplest descriptions of magnetism, magnetic characteristics of the elements, and magnetization of tissue samples. Important is the description of the intrinsic decay constants T1, T2, T2*, and proton density in terms of tissue-specific structures and variation in the intrinsic and extrinsic local magnetic fields. Contrast between tissues is determined by pulse sequences including SE, IR, GE, and their associated parameters

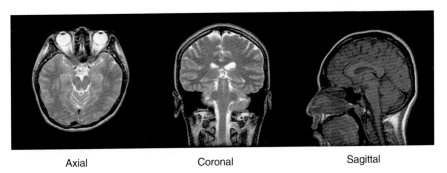

Axial   Coronal   Sagittal

■ **FIGURE 12-60** Direct acquisitions of axial, coronal, and sagittal tomographic images are possible by electronically energizing the magnetic field gradients in a different order without moving the patient. Oblique planes can also be obtained. PEG (k_y axis) and FEG (k_x axis) are perpendicular to the SSG.

TR, TE, TI, and flip angle. In addition to generating contrast, the ability to spatially localize the protons and create a two-dimensional image is as important, so that the differences can be appreciated in a grayscale rendition of the anatomy. The concepts of the frequency domain description of the signals and the k-space acquisition matrix are integral to the discussion, as well as the Fourier transform and the conversion of frequency to spatial domain representations of the data, necessary for visualization. In the next chapter, more details are given for image acquisition time, various pulse sequence designs, how image acquisition time is shortened, and characteristics of the image in terms of SNR, CNR, and artifacts. Unique capabilities for noninvasive "biopsy" of tissues, quality control, equipment, MR safety, and biological effects are also discussed.

REFERENCES AND SUGGESTED READINGS

Bottomley PA, Foster TH, Argersinger RE, Pfeifer LM. A review of normal tissue hydrogen NMR relaxation mechanisms from 1-100 MHz: dependence on tissue type, NMR frequency, temperature, species, excision, and age. *Med Phys* 1984;11:425–448.

Chavhan GB, Babyn PS, Jankharia BG, Cheng HM,Shroff MM. Steady-State MR Imaging Sequences: Physics, Classification, and Clinical Applications. *Radiographics* 2008;28:1147–1160.

Fullerton GD, Potter JL, Dornbluth NC. NMR relaxation of protons in tissues and other macromolecular water solutions. *Magn Reson Imaging* 1982; 1:209–228.

NessAiver M. *All you really need to know about MRI physics*. Baltimore, MD: Simply Physics, 1997.

Pooley RA. AAPM/RSNA physics tutorial for residents: fundamental Physics of MR imaging. *Radiographics* 2005;25:1087–1099.

Westbrook C, Kaut-Roth C, Talbot J. *MRI in practice*. 3rd ed. Malden, MA: Blackwell Publishing, 2005.

CHAPTER 13

Magnetic Resonance Imaging: Advanced Image Acquisition Methods, Artifacts, Spectroscopy, Quality Control, Siting, Bioeffects, and Safety

The essence of magnetic resonance imaging (MRI) in medicine is the acquisition, manipulation, display, and archive of datasets that have clinical relevance in the context of making a diagnosis or performing research for new applications and opportunities. There are many advantages and limitations of MRI and MR spectroscopy (MRS) as a solution to a clinical problem. Certainly, as described previously (note that this chapter assumes a working knowledge of Chapter 12 content), the great advantages of MR are the ability to generate images with outstanding tissue contrast and good resolution, without resorting to ionizing radiation. Capabilities of MR extend far beyond those basics, into fast acquisition sequences, perfusion and diffusion imaging, MR angiography (MRA), tractography, spectroscopy, and a host of other useful or potentially useful clinical applications. Major limitations of MR are also noteworthy, including extended acquisition times, MR artifacts, patient claustrophobia, tissue heating, and acoustic noise to name a few. MR safety, often ignored, is also of huge concern to the safety of the patient.

In this second of two MR chapters, advanced pulse sequences and fast image acquisition methods, dedicated radiofrequency (RF) coils, methods for perfusion, diffusion, and angiography imaging, image quality metrics, common artifacts, spectroscopy, MR equipment and siting, as well as MR safety issues are described and discussed with respect to the underlying physics.

The concepts of image acquisition and timing issues for standard and advanced pulse sequences into k-space is discussed first, with several methods that can be used to reduce acquisition times and many of the trade-offs that must be considered.

13.1 Image Acquisition Time

A defining character of MRI is the tremendous range of acquisition time needed to image a patient volume. Times ranging from as low as 50 ms to tens of minutes are commonly required depending on the study, pulse sequence, number of images in the dataset, and desired image quality. When MR was initially considered to be a potential diagnostic imaging modality in the late 1970s, the prevailing conventional wisdom gave no chance for widespread applicability because of the extremely long times required to generate a single slice from a sequentially acquired dataset, which required several minutes or more per slice. Breakthroughs in technology, equipment design, RF coils, the unique attributes of the k-space matrix, and methods of acquiring data drastically shortened acquisition times (or effective acquisition times) quickly, and propelled the rapid adoption of MRI in the mid-1980s. By the early 1990s, MRI established its clinical value that continues to expand today.

Acquisition Time, Two-Dimensional Fourier Transform Spin Echo Imaging

The time to acquire an image is determined by the data needed to fill the fraction of k-space that allows the image to be reconstructed by Fourier transform methods. For a standard spin echo sequence, the relevant parameters are the TR, number of phase encoding steps, and number of excitations (NEX) used for averaging identical repeat cycles, as

$$\text{Acquisition time} = \text{TR} \times \text{\# PEG Steps} \times \text{NEX}$$

Even though there may be multiple echoes as illustrated in Figure 13-1, there is also the same number of k-space repositories to capture the data in a specific, single row of k-space defined by the strength of the PEG, as shown for the first echo with proton density weighting and second echo with T2 weighting for this double echo acquisition. Thus, effective imaging time can be reduced by producing two (or more) images of the same slice within the TR interval. In addition, the matrix size that defines k-space is often not square (e.g., 256 × 256, 128 × 128), but

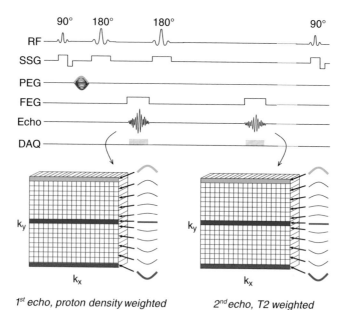

1st echo, proton density weighted   *2nd echo, T2 weighted*

■ **FIGURE 13-1** Standard spin echo pulse sequence is shown with two echoes per TR interval to encode proton density contrast (short TE, first echo), and T2 contrast (long TE, second echo). In this acquisition, two separate images are acquired independently by storing in a designated k-space matrix according to echo time. A single PEG strength is momentarily applied to induce phase variations to encode the row to be filled in each of the matrices (see the *red* PEG encoding for the last row in k-space, for instance). The full k-space matrix requires the sequence to be repeated with incremental variations in the PEG strength until each k-space row is fully populated. If averaging is desired, then an identical sequence (without incrementing the PEG) is repeated and averaged in the same row.

rectangular (e.g., 256 × 192, 256 × 128) where the small matrix dimension is most frequently along the phase encode direction to minimize the number of incremental PEG strength applications during the acquisition. A 256 × 192 image matrix and two averages (NEX) per phase encode step with a TR = 600 ms (for T1 weighting) requires imaging time of 0.6 s × 192 × 2 = 230.4 s = 3.84 min for a single slice! For a proton density and T2-weighted double echo sequence with TR = 2,500 ms (Fig. 13-1), this increases to 16 min, although two images are created in that time. Of course, a simple first-order method would be to eliminate the number of averages (NEX), which reduces the time by a factor of 2; however, the downsides are an increase in the statistical variability of the data, which decreases the image signal-to-noise ratio (SNR) and makes the image appear "noisy." Methods to reduce acquisition time and/or time per slice are crucial to making MR exam times reasonable, as described by various methods below.

Multislice Data Acquisition

The average acquisition time per reconstructed image slice in a single-slice spin echo sequence is clinically unacceptable. However, the average time per slice is significantly reduced using multislice acquisition methods, where several slices within the tissue volume are selectively excited in a sequential timing scheme during the TR interval to fully utilize the dead time waiting for longitudinal recovery in an adjacent slice, as shown in Figure 13-2. This requires cycling all of the gradients and tuning the RF excitation pulse many times during the TR interval. The total number of slices that can be acquired simultaneously is a function of TR, TE, and machine limitations:

$$\text{Total Number of Slices} = TR/(TE + C),$$

where C is a constant dependent on the MR equipment capabilities (computer speed; gradient capabilities; sequence options; additional pulses, e.g., spoiling pulses in standard SE; use of spatial saturation; and chemical shift, among others). Each slice and each echo, if multiecho, requires its own k-space repository to store data as it is acquired. Long TR acquisitions such as proton density and T2-weighted sequences

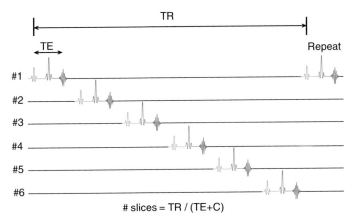

■ FIGURE 13-2 Multislice two-dimensional image acquisition is accomplished by discretely exciting different slabs of tissue during the TR period; appropriate changes of the RF excitation bandwidth, SSG, PEG, and FEG parameters are necessary. Because of diffuse excitation profiles, RF irradiation of adjacent slices leads to partial saturation and loss of contrast. The number of slices (volume) that can be obtained is a function of the TR, TE, and C, the latter representing the capabilities of the MR system and type of pulse sequence.

can produce a greater number of slices over a given volume than T1-weighted sequences with a short TR. The chief trade-off is a loss of tissue contrast due to *cross-excitation* of adjacent slices due to nonsquare excitation profiles, causing undesired proton saturation as explained in Section 13.5 on artifacts.

Data Synthesis

Data "synthesis" takes advantage of the symmetry and redundant characteristics of the frequency domain signals in k-space. The acquisition of as little as one-half the data plus one row of k-space allows the mirroring of "complex conjugate" data to fill the remainder of the matrix (Fig. 13-3). In the phase encode direction, "half Fourier," "½ NEX," or "phase conjugate symmetry" (vendor-specific names) techniques effectively reduce the number of required TR intervals by one-half plus one line, and thus can reduce the acquisition time by nearly one-half. In the frequency encode direction, "fractional echo" or "read conjugate symmetry" refers to reading a fraction of the echo. While there is no scan time reduction when all the phase encode steps are acquired, there is a significant echo time reduction, which can reduce motion-related artifacts, such as dephasing of blood. However, the penalty for either half Fourier or fractional echo techniques is a reduction in the SNR (caused by a reduced NEX or

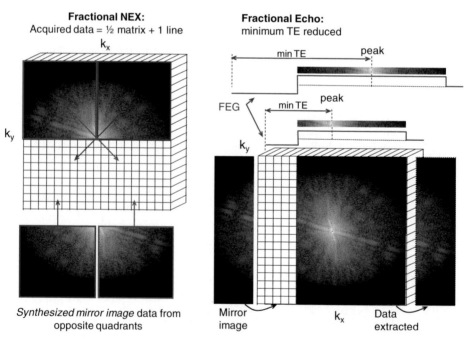

■ **FIGURE 13-3** Fractional NEX and Fractional Echo. **Left**. Data synthesis uses the redundant characteristics of the frequency domain. This is an example of phase conjugate symmetry, in which ½ of the PEG views +1 extra are acquired, and the complex conjugate of the data is reflected in the symmetric quadrants. Acquisition time is thus reduced by approximately $\sqrt{2}$ (~ 40%), although image noise is increased by approximately $\sqrt{2}$. Right: Fractional echo acquisition is performed when only part of the echo is read during the application of the FEG. Usually, the peak of the echo is centered in the middle of the readout gradient, and the echo signals prior to the peak are identical mirror images after the peak. With fractional echo, the echo is no longer centered, and the sampling window is shifted such that only the peak echo and the dephasing part of the echo are sampled. As the peak of the echo is closer to the RF excitation pulse, TE can be reduced, which can improve T1 and proton density weighting contrast. A larger number of slices can also be obtained with a shorter TE in a multislice acquisition (see Fig. 13-2).

data sampling in the volume) and the potential for artifacts if the approximations in the complex conjugation of the signals are not accurate. Other inaccuracies result from inhomogeneities of the magnetic field, imperfect linear gradient fields, and the presence of magnetic susceptibility agents in the volume being imaged.

Fast Pulse Sequences

Fast Spin Echo (FSE) techniques use multiple PEG steps in conjunction with multiple 180-degree refocusing RF pulses to produce an echo train length (ETL) with corresponding digital data acquisitions per TR interval, as illustrated in Figure 13-4. Multiple k-space rows are filled during each TR equal to the ETL, which is also the reduction factor for acquisition time. "Effective echo time" is determined when the central views in k-space are acquired, which are usually the first echoes, and subsequent echoes are usually spaced apart via increased PEG strength with the same echo spacing time. "*Phase re-ordering*" optimizes SNR by acquiring the low-frequency information with the early echoes (lowest amount of T2 decay), and the high-frequency, peripheral information with late echoes, where the impact on overall image SNR is lower. The FSE technique has the advantage of spin echo image acquisition, namely immunity from external magnetic field inhomogeneities, with 4×, 8×, to 16× faster acquisition time. However, each echo experiences different amounts of intrinsic T2 decay, which results in image contrast differences when compared with conventional spin echo images of similar TR and TE. Lower signal levels in the later echoes produce less SNR, and fewer images can be acquired in the image volume during the same acquisition. A T2-weighted spin echo image (TR = 2,000 ms, 256 phase encode steps, one average) requires approximately 8.5 min, while a corresponding FSE with an ETL of 4 (Fig. 13-4) requires about 2.1 min.

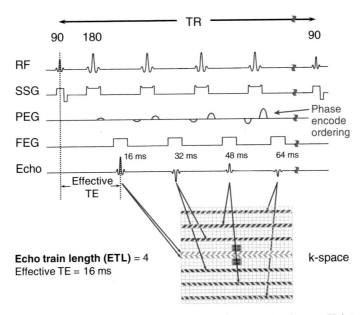

■ **FIGURE 13-4** Conventional FSE uses multiple 180-degree refocusing RF pulses per TR interval with incremental changes in the PEG to fill several views in k-space (the ETL). This example illustrates an ETL of four, with an "effective" TE equal to 16 *ms*. Total time of the acquisition is reduced by the ETL factor. The reversed polarity PEG steps reestablish coherent phase before the next gradient application. Slightly different PEG strengths are applied to fill the center of k-space first, and then the periphery with later echoes, continuing until all views are recorded. As shown, data can be mirrored using conjugate symmetry to reduce the overall time by another factor of two.

Longer TR values allow for a greater ETL, which will offset the longer TR in terms of overall acquisition time, and will also allow more proton density weighting. Specific FSE sequences for T2 weighting and multiecho FSE are employed with variations in phase reordering and data acquisition. FSE is also known as "turbo spin echo" or "RARE" (rapid acquisition with refocused echoes).

A Gradient Echo (GE) Acquisition pulse sequence is similar to a standard spin echo sequence with a readout gradient reversal substituting for the 180-degree pulse (Fig. 13-5). Repetition of the acquisition sequence occurs for each PEG step and with each average. With small flip angles and gradient reversals, a considerable reduction in TR and TE is possible for fast image acquisition; however, the ability to acquire multiple slices is compromised. A PEG rewinder pulse of opposite polarity is applied to maintain phase relationships from pulse to pulse in the coherent image acquisition. Spoiler gradients are used to eliminate persistent transverse magnetization from stimulated echoes for incoherent GE (see Chapter 12, Section 12.5).

Acquisition times are calculated in the same way as spin echo; a GE sequence for a 256 × 192 image matrix, two averages, and a TR = 30 ms, results in an imaging time equal to 192 × 2 × 0.03 s = 15.5 s. A conventional spin echo requires 3.84 min for a TR = 600 ms. Trade-offs for fast acquisition speed include SNR losses, magnetic susceptibility artifacts, and less immunity from magnetic field inhomogeneities. There are several acronyms for GE sequences, including GRASS, FISP, Spoiled GRASS, FLASH, SSFP, etc., depending on the manufacturer of the equipment. Table 13-1 describes a partial list of the different GE sequences and their method of data acquisition.

Echo Planar Image (EPI) Acquisition is a technique that provides extremely fast imaging time. Spin Echo (SE-EPI) and Gradient Echo (GE-EPI) are two methods used for acquiring data, and a third is a hybrid of the two, GRASE (Gradient and Spin Echo). Single-shot (all of the image information is acquired within 1 TR interval) or multishot EPI has been implemented with these methods. For single-shot SE-EPI,

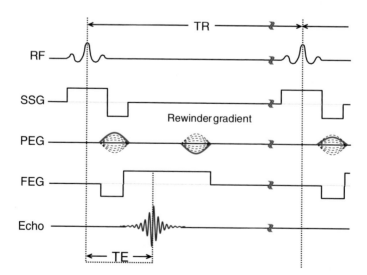

■ **FIGURE 13-5** Coherent GE pulse sequence uses a small flip angle (30 to 40 degrees) RF pulse simultaneous to the SSG. Phase and frequency encode gradients are applied shortly afterward (with a TE of less than 3 *ms* in certain sequences). A PEG "rewinder" (reverse polarity) reestablishes the phase conditions prior to the next pulse, simultaneous with the extended FEG duration.

TABLE 13-1   COMPARISON OF MANUFACTURER-NAMED ACRONYMS FOR GE SEQUENCES

SEQUENCE	GENERAL ELECTRIC	PHILIPS	SIEMENS	TOSHIBA
Coherent GE	GRASS, FGR FMPGR	FFE	FISP	Field echo
Incoherent GE (RF spoiled)	SPGR, FSPGR	T1 FFE		Field echo
Incoherent GE (Gradient spoiled)	MPGR		FLASH	Field echo
Steady-state free precession	SSFP, DE FGR	T2 FFE	PSIF	
SSFP: balanced sequence / true FISP	FIESTA	Balanced FFE	True FISP	True SSFP

Note: Not all manufacturers are listed in this table, nor are all GE sequences. (Blank areas indicate particular sequence is not performed (at time of publication).

image acquisition typically begins with a standard 90-degree flip, then a PEG/FEG gradient application to initiate the acquisition of data in the periphery of the k-space, followed by a 180-degree echo-producing RF pulse. Immediately after, an oscillating readout gradient and phase encode gradient "blips" are continuously applied to stimulate echo formation and rapidly fill k-space in a stepped "zig-zag" pattern (Fig. 13-6). The "effective" echo time occurs at a time TE, when the maximum amplitude of the induced GEs occurs. Acquisition of the data must proceed in a period less than T2* (around 50 ms), placing high demands on the sampling rate, the gradient coils (shielded coils are required, with low induced "eddy currents"), the RF transmitter/receiver, and RF energy deposition limitations. For GE-EPI, a similar acquisition strategy is implemented but without a 180 degrees refocusing RF pulse, allowing for faster acquisition time. SE-EPI is generally longer, but better image quality is achieved; on the other hand, larger RF energy deposition to the patient occurs. EPI acquisition can

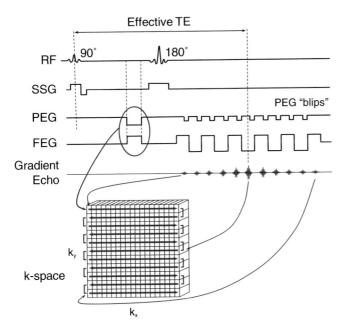

■ **FIGURE 13-6** Single shot Echo Planar Spin Echo image (SE-EPI) acquisition sequence. Data is deposited in k-space, initially positioned by a simultaneous PEG and FEG application to locate the initial row and column position (in this example, the upper left), followed by phase encode gradient "blips" simultaneous to FEG oscillations, to fill *k-space* line by line by introducing 1-row phase changes in a zig-zag pattern. Image matrix sizes of 64 × 64 and 128 × 64 are common.

be preceded with any type of RF pulse, for instance FLAIR (EPI-FLAIR), which will produce images much faster than the corresponding conventional FLAIR sequence.

The GRASE (Gradient and Spin Echo) sequence combines the initial spin echo with a series of GEs, followed by an RF rephasing (180 degrees) pulse, and the pattern is repeated until k-space is filled. This hybrid sequence achieves the benefits of both types of rephasing: the speed of the gradient and the ability of the RF pulse to compensate for $T2^*$ effects, providing significant improvements in image quality compared to the standard EPI methods. A trade-off is a longer acquisition time (e.g., greater than 100 ms) and much greater energy deposition from the multiple 180 degrees RF pulses.

EPI acquisitions typically have poor SNR, low resolution (matrices of 64 × 64 or 128 × 64 are typical), and many artifacts, particularly of chemical shift and magnetic susceptibility origin. Nevertheless, EPI offers real-time "snapshot" image capability with 50 ms total acquisition time. EPI is emerging as a clinical tool for studying time-dependent physiologic processes and functional imaging. Concerns of safety with EPI, chiefly related to the rapid switching of gradients and possible nerve stimulation of the patient, the associated acoustic noise, image artifacts, distortion, and chemical shift are components that will limit use for many imaging procedures.

Other K-Space Filling Methods

Methods to fill k-space in a nonsequential way can enhance signal, contrast, and achieve rapid scan times as shown in Figure 13-7. *Centric k-space filling* has been discussed with FSE imaging (above), where the lower strength phase encode gradi-

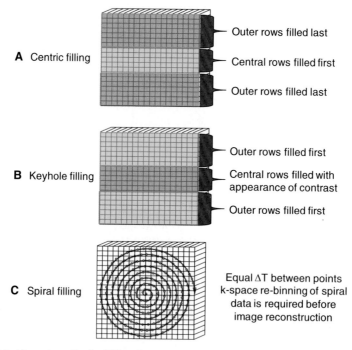

A Centric filling
— Outer rows filled last
— Central rows filled first
— Outer rows filled last

B Keyhole filling
— Outer rows filled first
— Central rows filled with appearance of contrast
— Outer rows filled first

C Spiral filling
Equal ΔT between points k-space re-binning of spiral data is required before image reconstruction

■ **FIGURE 13-7** Alternate methods of filling k-space. **A.** Centric filling applies the lower strength PEG's first to maximize signal and contrast from the earliest echoes of a FSE or GE sequence. **B.** Keyhole filling applies PEG's of higher strength first to fill the outer portions of k-space, and the central lines are filled only during a certain part of the sequence, such as with arrival of contrast signal. **C.** Spiral data acquisition occurs with sinusoidal oscillation of the X and Y gradients 90 degrees out of phase with each other, with samples beginning in the center of k-space and spiraling out to the periphery. Interpolating the data into the k_x, k_y matrix is required in order to apply 2DFT image reconstruction.

ents are applied first, filling the center of k-space when the echoes have their highest amplitude. This type of filling is also important for fast GE techniques, where the image contrast and the SNR fall quickly with time from the initial excitation pulse.

Keyhole filling methods fill k-space similarly to centric filling, except the central lines are filled when important events occur during the sequence, in situations such as contrast-enhanced angiography. Outer areas of k-space are filled first, and when gadolinium appears in the imaging volume, the center areas are filled. At the end of the scan, the outer and central k-space regions are meshed to produce an image with both good contrast and resolution.

Spiral filling is an alternate method of filling k-space radially, which involves the simultaneous oscillation of equivalent encoding gradients to sample data points during echo formation in a spiral, starting at the origin (the center of the k-space) and spiraling outward to the periphery in the prescribed acquisition plane. The same contrast mechanisms are available in spiral sequences (e.g., T1, T2, proton density weighting), and spin or GEs can be obtained. After acquisition of the signals, an additional post-processing step, re-gridding, is necessary to convert the spiral data into the rectilinear matrix for two-dimensional Fourier transform (2DFT). Spiral scanning is an efficient method for acquiring data and sampling information in the center of k-space, where the bulk of image information is contained.

A variant of radial sampling with enhanced filling of the center of k-space is known generically as "blade" imaging, and commonly as **propeller**: Periodically Rotated Overlapping Parallel Lines with Enhanced Reconstruction, where a rectangular block of data is acquired and then rotated about the center of k-space. Redundant information concentrated in the center of k-space is used for improvement of SNR or for the identification of times during the scan in which the patient may have moved, so that those blocks of data can be processed with a phase-shifting algorithm to eliminate the movement effect on the data during the reconstruction process and to mitigate motion artifacts to a great extent. Filling of k-space for this method is shown in Figure 13-8.

Parallel Imaging

Parallel imaging is a technique that fills k-space by using the response of multiple receive RF coils that are coupled together with independent channels, so that data can be acquired simultaneously. Specific hardware and software are necessary for the electronic orchestration of this capability. Typically, 2, 4, 5, 7, 8, 16, 18 (or more) coils are arranged around the area to be imaged; if a 4-coil configuration is used, then during each TR period, each coil acquires a view of the data as the acquisition sequence proceeds. Lines in k-space are defined only after the processing of linear combinations of the signals that are received by all of the coils. Since 4 views of the data are acquired per TR interval, scan time can be decreased by a factor of 4 (known as the *reduction factor*). However, the acquisition of the signals have gaps, and the FOV in the phase direction is reduced to one-quarter of its original size. This results in a known aliasing of the information (a wrapped image—see section on Artifacts), that is rectified by using the measured sensitivity profile of each coil to calculate from where the signal is coming. This sensitivity profile determines the position of the signal based on its amplitude, where the signal near the coil has a higher amplitude than that farthest away. As a result of the process, commonly known as SENSE (SENSitivity Encoding—there are several acronyms coined by the manufacturers), the image can be unwrapped and combined with the unwrapped images from each of the other coils. A simple two-coil example is shown in Figure 13-9 for a breast image application of SENSE, in which improved resolution is desired over reduced scan time.

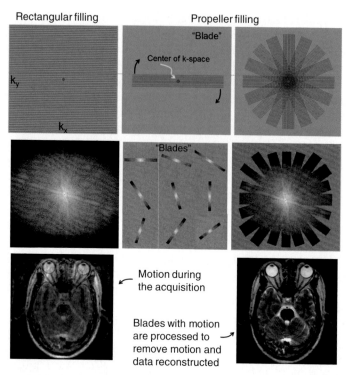

■ **FIGURE 13-8** The propeller data acquisition compared to a rectangular filling of k-space is shown above. Instead of acquiring single lines of information to fill k-space consecutively as shown in the upper left and middle left, a rectangular data acquisition at a specific angle (e.g., 0 degree) is acquired encompassing several lines of k-space, which represents a "blade" of information. The partial acquisition is rotated about the center of k-space at angular increments, which provides a dense sampling of data at the center of k-space and less in the periphery as shown by the schematic (upper right illustration). If the patient moves during a portion of the examination (lower left image), the blades in which the motion occurred can be identified, reprocessed, and the image reconstructed without the motion artifacts (lower right image).

■ **FIGURE 13-9** Parallel imaging with two RF coils. **Top**. A single coil acquisition of a breast MR exam over the full FOV. **Middle**. Individual coils with every-other row of k-space being filled represent ½ FOV, with image overlap caused by aliasing. **Bottom**. After SENSE processing, images are combined to deliver twice the spatial resolution in the left/right (Phase) direction, with the same imaging time.

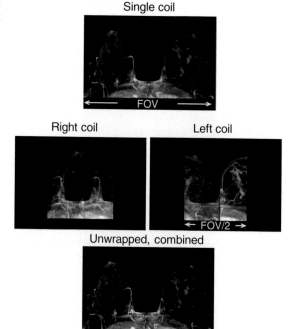

Parallel imaging can be used to either reduce scan times or improve resolution. It also can be used with most pulse sequences. There are obvious benefits in terms of scan times and/or resolution, but there is a slight loss of SNR due to the manipulation of the signals, and chemical shift artifacts (explained in the Artifacts section) may increase. Patient motion can also cause misalignment between the undersampled data and the reference scans of the coils.

Three-Dimensional Fourier Transform Image Acquisition

Three-dimensional image acquisition (volume imaging) requires the use of a broadband, nonselective, or "slab-selective" RF pulse to excite a large volume of protons simultaneously. Two phase gradients are discretely applied in the slice encode and phase encode directions, prior to the frequency encode (readout) gradient (Fig. 13-10). The image acquisition time is equal to

TR × # Phase Encode Steps (z-axis) × # Phase Encode Steps
    (y-axis) × # Signal Averages

A three-dimensional Fourier transform (three one-dimensional Fourier transforms) is applied for each column, row, and depth axis in the image matrix "cube." Volumes obtained can be either isotropic, the same size in all three directions, or anisotropic, where at least one dimension is different in size. The advantage of the former is equal resolution in all directions; reformations of images from the volume do not suffer from degradations of larger sample size from other directions. After the spatial domain data are obtained, individual two-dimensional slices in any arbitrary plane are extracted by interpolation of the cube data.

When using a standard TR of 600 ms with one average for a T1-weighted exam, a 128 × 128 × 128 cube requires 163 min or about 2.7 h! Obviously, this is unacceptable for standard clinical imaging. GE pulse sequences with TR of 50 ms acquire the same image volume in about 15 min. Another shortcut is with anisotropic voxels, where the phase encode steps in one dimension are reduced, albeit with a loss of resolution. A major benefit to isotropic three-dimensional acquisition is the uniform resolution

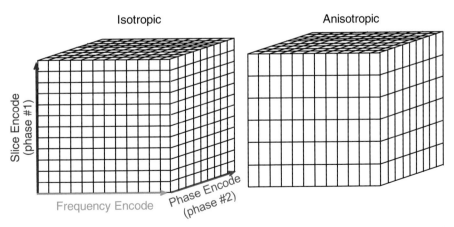

■ FIGURE 13-10 Three-dimensional image acquisition requires the application of a broadband RF pulse to excite all of the protons in the volume simultaneously, followed by a phase encode gradient along the slice encode direction, a phase encode gradient along the phase encode direction, and a frequency encode gradient in the readout direction. Spatial location is decoded sequentially by the Fourier transform along each encode path, storing intermediate results in the three-dimensional k-space matrix.

in all directions when extracting any two-dimensional image from the matrix cube. In addition, high SNR is achieved compared to a similar two-dimensional image, allowing reconstruction of very thin slices with good detail (less partial volume averaging) and high SNR. A downside is the increased probability of motion artifacts and increased computer hardware requirements for data handling and storage.

13.2 MR Image Characteristics

Spatial Resolution and Contrast Sensitivity

Spatial resolution, contrast sensitivity, and SNR parameters form the basis for evaluating the MR image characteristics. The spatial resolution is dependent on the FOV, which determines pixel size, the gradient field strength, which determines the FOV, the receiver coil characteristics (head coil, body coil, and various surface coil designs), the sampling bandwidth, and the image matrix. Common image matrix sizes are 128 × 128, 256 × 128, 256 × 192, and 256 × 256, with 512 × 256, 512 × 512, and 1,024 × 512 becoming prevalent. In general, MR provides spatial resolution approximately equivalent to that of CT, with pixel dimensions on the order of 0.5 to 1.0 mm for a high-contrast object and a reasonably large FOV (greater than 250 mm). A 250 mm FOV and a 256 × 256 matrix will have a pixel size on the order of 1 mm. In small FOV acquisitions with high gradient strengths and with surface coil receivers, the effective pixel size can be smaller than 0.1 to 0.2 mm (of course, with a limited FOV of 25 to 50 mm. Slice thickness in MRI is usually 5 to 10 mm and represents the dimension that produces the most partial volume averaging.

Spatial resolution can be improved with higher field strength magnets due to a larger SNR, which allows thinner slice acquisition, and/or higher sampling rates (smaller pixels) for a given acquisition. However, with higher B_0, increased RF absorption, artifact production, and a lengthening of T1 relaxation occur. The latter decreases T1 contrast sensitivity because of increased saturation of the longitudinal magnetization.

Contrast sensitivity is the major attribute of MR. The spectacular contrast sensitivity of MR enables the exquisite discrimination of soft tissues and contrast due to blood flow. This sensitivity is achieved through differences in the T1, T2, proton density, and flow velocity characteristics. Contrast, which is dependent upon these parameters, is achieved through the proper application of pulse sequences, as discussed previously. MR contrast materials, usually susceptibility agents that disrupt the local magnetic field to enhance T2 decay or provide a relaxation mechanism for shorter T1 recovery time (e.g., bound water in hydration layers), are becoming important enhancement agents for differentiation of normal and diseased tissues. The absolute contrast sensitivity of the MR image is ultimately limited by the SNR and presence of image artifacts.

Signal-to-Noise Ratio, SNR

There are numerous dependencies on the ultimate SNR achievable by the MR system. The intrinsic signal intensity based on T1, T2, and proton density parameters has been discussed; to summarize, the TR, TE, and flip angle will have an impact on the magnitude of the signal generated in the image. While there are many mitigating factors, a long TR increases the longitudinal magnetization recovery and increases the SNR; a long TE increases the transverse magnetization decay and reduces the SNR; a smaller flip angle (reduced from 90 degrees) reduces the SNR. Therefore, spin echo pulse sequences with large flip angle, long TR, short TE, coarse matrix, large FOV, thick slices, and many averages will generate the best SNR; however, the resultant image may not be clinically relevant or desirable. While SNR is important, it's not everything.

For a given pulse sequence (TR, TE, flip angle), the SNR of the MR image is dependent on a number of variables, as shown in the equation below for a two-dimensional image acquisition:

$$\text{SNR} \propto I \times \text{voxel}_{x,y,z} \times \frac{\sqrt{\text{NEX}}}{\sqrt{\text{BW}}} \times f(\text{QF}) \times f(B) \times f(\text{slice gap}) \times f(\text{reconstruction})$$

where I is the intrinsic signal intensity based on pulse sequence, $\text{voxel}_{x,y,z}$ is the voxel volume, determined by FOV, image matrix, and slice thickness, NEX is the number of excitations, determined by the number (or fractional number) of repeated signal acquisitions into the same voxels. BW is the frequency bandwidth of the RF receiver, $f(\text{QF})$ is the function of the coil quality factor parameter (tuning the coil), $f(B)$ is the function of magnetic field strength, B, $f(\text{slice gap})$ is the function of interslice gap effects, and $f(\text{reconstruction})$ is the function of the reconstruction algorithm.

Other factors in the above equation are explained briefly below.

Voxel Volume

The voxel volume is equal to

$$\text{Volume} = \frac{\text{FOV}_x}{\text{No. of pixels, } x} \times \frac{\text{FOV}_y}{\text{No. of pixels, } y} \times \text{Slice thickness, } z$$

SNR is linearly proportional to the voxel volume. Thus, by reducing the image matrix size from 256×256 to 256×128 over the same FOV, the effective voxel size increases by a factor of two, and therefore increases the SNR by a factor of two for the same image acquisition time (e.g., 256 phase encodes with one average versus 128 phase encodes with two averages).

Signal Averages

Signal averaging (also known as number of excitations, NEX) is achieved by averaging sets of data acquired using an identical pulse sequence (same PEG strength). The SNR is proportional to the square root of the number of signal averages. A 2-NEX acquisition requires a doubling (100% increase) of the acquisition time for a 40% increase in the SNR $\left(\sqrt{2} = 1.4\right)$ Doubling the SNR requires 4 NEX. In some cases, less than 1 average (e.g., ½ or ¾ NEX) can be selected. Here, the number of phase encode steps is reduced by ½ or ¼, and the missing data are synthesized in the k-space matrix. Imaging time is therefore reduced by a similar amount; however, a loss of SNR accompanies the shorter imaging times by the same square root factor.

RF Bandwidth

The receiver bandwidth defines the range of frequencies to which the detector is tuned during the application of the readout gradient. A narrow bandwidth (a narrow spread of frequencies around the center frequency) provides a higher SNR, proportional to $\frac{1}{\sqrt{\text{BW}}}$. A twofold reduction in RF bandwidth—from 8 to 4 kHz, for instance—increases the SNR by 1.4 × (40% increase). This is mainly related to the fact that the white noise, which is relatively constant across the bandwidth, does not change, while the signal distribution changes with bandwidth. In the spatial domain, bandwidth is inversely proportional to the sample dwell time, ΔT to sample the signal: $BW = 1/\Delta T$. Therefore, a narrow bandwidth has a longer dwell time, which increases the signal height (Fig. 13-11), compared to the shorter dwell time for the broad bandwidth signal, thus spreading the signal over a larger range of frequencies. The SNR is reduced by the square root of the dwell time. However, any decrease in RF bandwidth must be coupled with a decrease in gradient strength to maintain the sampling across the FOV, which might be unacceptable if chemical shift artifacts are of concern (see Artifacts, below). Narrower bandwidths also require a longer time for sampling, and therefore affect the minimum TE time that is possible for an imaging sequence. Clinical situations that can use narrow bandwidths are with T2-weighted images and long TEs that allow the echo to evolve over an extended period, particularly in situations where fat saturation pulses are used to reduce the effects of chemical shift in the acquired images. Use of broad bandwidth settings is necessary when very short TEs are required, such as in fast GE imaging to reduce the sampling time.

RF Coil Quality Factor

The coil quality factor is an indication of RF coil sensitivity to induced currents in response to signals emanating from the patient. Coil losses that lead to lower SNR are caused by patient "loading" effects and eddy currents, among other factor. Patient loading refers to the electric impedance characteristics of the body, which to a certain extent acts like an antenna. This effect causes a variation in the magnetic field that is different

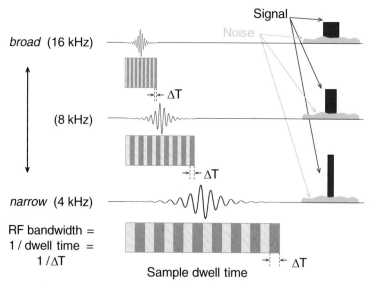

■ **FIGURE 13-11** RF Receiver Bandwidth is determined by the FEG strength, the FOV, and sampling rate. This figure illustrates the spatial domain view of SNR and corresponding sample dwell time. Evolution of the echo in the broad bandwidth situation occurs rapidly with minimal dwell time, which might be needed in situations where very short TE is required, even though the SNR is reduced. On the other hand, in T2 weighted images requiring a long TE, narrow bandwidth can improve SNR.

for each patient, and must be measured and corrected for. Consequently, tuning the receiver coil to the resonance frequency is mandatory before image acquisition. Eddy currents are signals that are opposite of the induced current produced by transverse magnetization in the RF coil, and reduce the overall signal. Quadrature coils increase the SNR as two coils are used in the reception of the signal; phased array coils increase the SNR even more when the data from several coils are added together (see Parallel Imaging, Section 13.1). The proximity of the receiver coil to the volume of interest affects the coil quality factor, but there are trade-offs with image uniformity. Positioning of the coil with respect to the direction of the main magnetic field is also an issue that occurs with air core (horizontal B_0) to solid core (vertical B_0) magnets. Body receiver coils positioned in the bore of the magnet have a moderate quality factor, whereas surface coils have a high quality factor. With the body coil, the signal is relatively uniform across the FOV; however, with surface coils, the signal falls off abruptly near the edges of the field, limiting the useful imaging depth and resulting in nonuniform brightness across the image.

Magnetic Field Strength

Magnetic field strength influences the SNR of the image by a factor of $B^{1.0}$ to $B^{1.5}$. Thus, one would expect a three- to fivefold improvement in SNR with a 1.5 T magnet over a 0.5 T magnet. Although the gains in the SNR are real, other considerations mitigate the SNR improvement in the clinical environment, including longer T1 relaxation times and greater RF absorption, as discussed previously.

Cross-Excitation

Cross-excitation occurs from the nonrectangular RF excitation profiles in the spatial domain and the resultant overlap of adjacent slices in multislice image acquisition sequences. This saturates the protons and reduces contrast and the contrast-to-noise ratio. To avoid cross-excitation, interslice gaps or interleaving procedures are necessary (see Artifacts section, below).

Image Acquisition and Reconstruction Algorithms

Image acquisition and reconstruction algorithms have a profound effect on SNR. The various acquisition/reconstruction methods that have been used in the past and those used today are, in order of increasing SNR, point acquisition methods, line acquisition methods, two-dimensional Fourier transform acquisition methods, and three-dimensional Fourier transform volume acquisition methods. In each of these techniques, the volume of tissue that is excited is the major contributing factor to improving the SNR and image quality. Reconstruction filters and image processing algorithms will also affect the SNR. High-pass filtration methods that increase edge definition will generally decrease the SNR, while low-pass filtration methods that smooth the image data will generally increase the SNR at the cost of reduced resolution.

Summary, Image Quality

The best possible image quality is always desirable, but not always achievable because of the trade-off between SNR, scan speed, and spatial resolution. To increase one of these three components of image quality involves the consideration of reducing one or both of the other two. It is thus a balancing act that is chosen by the operator, the protocol, and the patient in order to acquire images with the best diagnostic yield.

MR parameters that may be changed include TR, TE, TI, ETL, Matrix Size, Slice Thickness, Field of view, and NEX. Working with these parameters in the optimization of acquisition protocols to achieve high image quality is essential.

13.3 Signal from Flow

The appearance of moving fluid (vascular and cerebrospinal fluid [CSF]) in MR images is complicated by many factors, including flow velocity, vessel orientation, laminar versus turbulent flow patterns, pulse sequences, and image acquisition modes. Flow-related mechanisms combine with image acquisition parameters to alter contrast. Signal due to flow covers the entire gray scale of MR signal intensities, from "black blood" to "bright blood" levels, and flow can be a source of artifacts. The signal from flow can also be exploited to produce MR angiographic images.

Low signal intensities (flow voids) are often a result of *high-velocity signal loss* (HVSL), in which protons in the flowing blood move out of the slice during echo reformation, causing a lower signal. *Flow turbulence* can also cause flow voids, by causing a dephasing of protons in the blood with a resulting loss of the tissue magetization in the area of turbulence. With HVSL, the amount of signal loss depends on the velocity of the moving fluid. Pulse sequences to produce "black blood" in images can be very useful in cardiac and vascular imaging. A typical black blood pulse sequence uses a "double inversion recovery" method, whereby a nonselective 180-degree RF pulse is initially applied, inverting all protons in the body, and is followed by a selective 180-degree RF pulse that restores the magnetization in the selected slice. During the inversion time, blood outside of the excited slice with inverted protons flows into the slice, producing no signal; therefore, the blood appears dark.

Flow-Related Enhancement

Flow-related enhancement is a process that causes increased signal intensity due to flowing protons; it occurs during imaging of a volume of tissues. *Even-echo rephasing* is a phenomenon that causes flow to exhibit increased signal on even echoes in a multiple-echo image acquisition. Flowing protons that experience two subsequent 180-degree pulses (even echoes) generate higher signal intensity due to a constructive rephasing of protons during echo formation. This effect is prominent in slow laminar flow (e.g., veins show up as bright structures on even-echo images).

Flow enhancement in GE images is pronounced for both venous and arterial structures, as well as CSF. The high intensity is caused by the wash-in (between subsequent RF excitations) of fully unsaturated protons into a volume of partially saturated protons due to the short TR used with gradient imaging. During the next excitation, the signal amplitude resulting from the moving unsaturated protons is about 10 times greater than that of the nonmoving saturated protons. With GE techniques, the degree of enhancement depends on the velocity of the blood, the slice or volume thickness, and the TR. As blood velocity increases, unsaturated blood exhibits the greatest signal. Similarly, a thinner slice or decreased repetition time results in higher flow enhancement. In arterial imaging of high-velocity flow, it is possible to have bright blood throughout the imaging volume of a three-dimensional acquisition if unsaturated blood can penetrate into the volume prior to experiencing an RF pulse.

Signal from blood is dependent on the relative saturation of the surrounding tissues and the incoming blood flow in the vasculature. In a multislice volume,

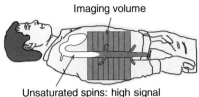

Imaging volume

Unsaturated spins: high signal

Flow-Related Enhancement

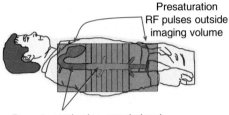

Presaturation
RF pulses outside
imaging volume

Pre-saturated spins: equal signal

Flow presaturation

■ **FIGURE 13-12** The repeated RF excitation within an imaging volume produces partial saturation of the tissue magnetization (**top** figure, **gray** area). Unsaturated protons flowing into the volume generate a large signal difference that is bright relative to the surrounding tissues. Bright blood effects can be reduced by applying pre-saturation RF pulses adjacent to the imaging volume, so that protons in inflowing blood will have a similar partial saturation (**bottom** figure; note no blood signal).

repeated excitation of the tissues and blood causes a partial saturation of the protons, dependent on the T1 characteristics and the TR of the pulse sequence. Blood outside of the imaged volume does not interact with the RF excitations, and therefore these unsaturated protons may enter the imaged volume and produce a large signal compared to the blood within the volume. This is known as flow-related enhancement. As the pulse sequence continues, the unsaturated blood becomes partially saturated and the protons of the blood produce a similar signal to the tissues in the inner slices of the volume (Fig. 13-12). In some situations, flow-related enhancement is undesirable and is eliminated with the use of "presaturation" pulses applied to volumes just above and below the imaging volume. These same saturation pulses are also helpful in reducing motion artifacts caused by adjacent tissues outside the imaging volume.

MR Angiography

Exploitation of blood flow enhancement is the basis for MRA. Two techniques to create images of vascular anatomy include time-of-flight and phase contrast angiography.

Time-of-Flight Angiography

The time-of-flight technique relies on the tagging of blood in one region of the body and detecting it in another. This differentiates moving blood from the surround stationary tissues. Tagging is accomplished by proton saturation, inversion, or relaxation to change the longitudinal magnetization of moving blood. The penetration of the tagged blood into a volume depends on the T1, velocity, and direction of the blood. Since the detectable range is limited by the eventual saturation of the tagged blood, long vessels are difficult to visualize simultaneously in a three-dimensional volume. For these reasons, a two-dimensional stack of slices is typically acquired, where even slowly moving blood can penetrate the region of RF excitation in thin slices (Fig. 13-13). Each slice is acquired separately, and blood moving in one direction (north or south, e.g., arteries versus veins) can be selected by delivering a presaturation pulse on an adjacent slab superior or inferior to the slab of data acquisition. Thin slices are also helpful in preserving resolution of the flow pattern. Often used for the two-dimensional

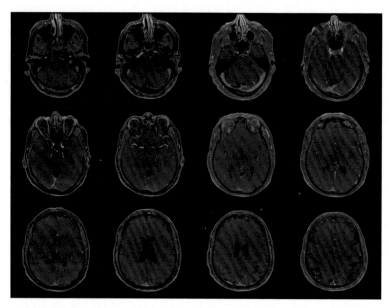

■ **FIGURE 13-13** The *time of flight* MRA acquisition collects each slice separately with a sequence to enhance blood flow. Exploitation of blood flow is achieved by detecting unsaturated protons moving into the volume, producing a bright signal. A coherent GE image acquisition pulse sequence is shown, TR = 24 ms, TE = 3.1 ms, Flip Angle = 20 degrees. Every 10th image in the stack is displayed above, from left to right and top to bottom.

image acquisition is a "GRASS" or "FISP" GE technique that produces relatively poor anatomic contrast, yet provides a high-contrast "bright blood" signal. Magnetization transfer contrast sequences (see below) are also employed to increase the contrast of the signals due to blood by reducing the background anatomic contrast.

Two-dimensional TOF MRA images are obtained by projecting the content of the stack of slices at a specific angle through the volume. A maximum intensity projection (MIP) algorithm detects the largest signal along a given ray through the volume and places this value in the image (Fig. 13-14). The superimposition of residual

■ **FIGURE 13-14** A simple illustration shows how the MIP algorithm extracts the highest (maximum) signals in the two-dimensional stack of images along a specific direction in the volume, and produces projection images with maximum intensity variations as a function of angle.

Projections are cast through the image stack (volume)
The *maximum* signal along each line is projected

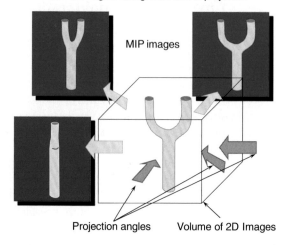

stationary anatomy often requires further data manipulation to suppress undesirable signals. This is achieved in a variety of ways, the simplest of which is setting a window threshold. Another method is to acquire a dataset without contrast, and subtract the noncontrast MIP from the contrast MIP to reduce background signals. Clinical MRA images show the three-dimensional characteristics of the vascular anatomy from several angles around the volume stack (Fig. 13-15) with some residual signals from the stationary anatomy. Time-of-flight angiography often produces variation in vessel intensity dependent on orientation with respect to the image plane, a situation that is less than optimal.

Phase Contrast Angiography

Phase contrast imaging relies on the phase change that occurs in moving protons such as blood. One method of inducing a phase change is dependent on the application of a bipolar gradient (one gradient with positive polarity followed by a second gradient with negative polarity, separated by a delay time ΔT). In a second acquisition of the same view of the data (same PEG), the polarity of the bipolar gradients is reversed, and moving protons are encoded with negative phase, while the stationary protons exhibit no phase change (Fig. 13-16). Subtracting the second excitation from the first cancels the magnetization due to stationary protons but enhances magnetization due to moving protons. Alternating the bipolar gradient polarity for each subsequent excitation during the acquisition provides phase contrast image information. The degree of phase shift is directly related to the velocity encoding (VENC) time, ΔT, between the positive and negative lobes of the bipolar gradients and the velocity of the protons within the excited volume. Proper selection of the VENC time

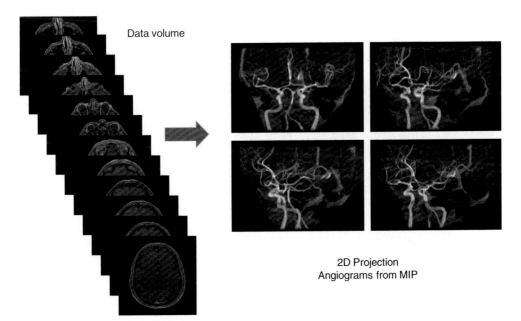

Data volume

2D Projection
Angiograms from MIP

■ **FIGURE 13-15** A volume stack of bright blood images (left) is used with MIP processing to create a series of projection angiograms at regular intervals; the three-dimensional perspective is appreciated in a stack view, with virtual rotation of the vasculature.

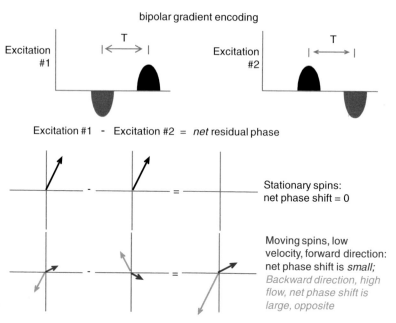

■ **FIGURE 13-16** Phase Contrast Angiography uses consecutive excitations that have a bipolar gradient encoding with the polarity reversed between the first and second excitation, as shown in the top row. Magnetization vectors (lower two rows) illustrate the effect of the bipolar gradients on stationary and moving spins for the first and second excitations. Subtracting the two will cancel stationary tissue magnetization and enhance phase differences caused by the velocity of moving blood.

is necessary to avoid phase wrap error (exceeding 180-degree phase change) and to ensure an optimal phase shift range for the velocities encountered. Intensity variations are dependent on the amount of phase shift, where the brightest pixel values represent the largest forward (or backward) velocity, a mid-scale value represents 0 velocity, and the darkest pixel values represent the largest backward (or forward) velocity. Figure 13-17 shows a representative magnitude and phase contrast image of the cardiac vasculature. Unlike the time-of-flight methods, the phase contrast image

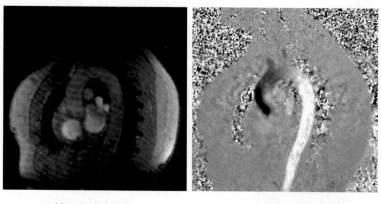

Magnitude Image   Phase Image

■ **FIGURE 13-17** Magnitude (**left**) and phase (**right**) images provide contrast of flowing blood. Magnitude images are sensitive to flow, but not to direction; phase images provide direction and velocity information. The blood flow from the heart shows forward flow in the ascending aorta (*dark* area) and forward flow in the descending aorta at this point in the heart cycle for the phase image. Some bright flow patterns in the ascending aorta represent backward flow to the coronary arteries. Grayscale amplitude is proportional to velocity, where intermediate grayscale is 0 velocity.

is inherently quantitative, and when calibrated carefully, provides an estimate of the mean blood flow velocity and direction. Two- and three-dimensional phase contrast image acquisitions for MRA are possible.

Gradient Moment Nulling

In spin echo and gradient recalled echo imaging, the slice select and readout gradients are balanced, so that the uniform dephasing with the initial gradient application is rephased by an opposite polarity gradient of equal area. However, when moving protons are subjected to the gradients, the amount of phase dispersion is not compensated (Fig. 13-18). This phase dispersal can cause ghosting (faint, displaced copies of the anatomy) in images. It is possible, however, to rephase the protons by a gradient moment nulling technique. With constant velocity flow (first-order motion), all protons can be rephased using the application of a gradient triplet. In this technique, an initial positive gradient of unit area is followed by a negative gradient of twice the area, which creates phase changes that are compensated by a third positive gradient of unit area. The velocity compensated gradient (right graph in Fig. 13-18) depicts the evolution of the proton phase back to zero for both stationary and moving protons. Note that the overall applied gradient has a net area of zero—equal to the sum of the positive and negative areas. Higher order corrections such as second- or third-order moment nulling to correct for acceleration and other motions are possible, but these techniques require more complicated gradient switching. Gradient moment nulling can be applied to both the slice select and readout gradients to correct for problems such as motion ghosting as elicited by CSF pulsatile flow.

13.3 Perfusion and Diffusion Contrast Imaging

Perfusion of tissues via the capillary bed permits the delivery of oxygen and nutrients to the cells and removal of waste (e.g., CO_2) from the cells. Conventional perfusion measurements are based on the uptake and wash-out of radioactive tracers or other exogenous tracers that can be quantified from image sequences using well-characterized imaging equipment and calibration procedures. For MR perfusion images, exogenous

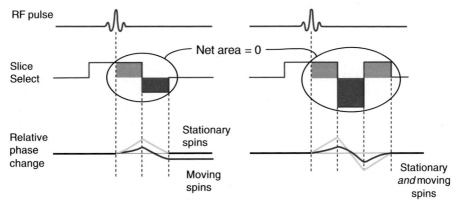

■ **FIGURE 13-18 Left.** Phase dispersion of stationary and moving spins under the influence of an applied gradient (no flow compensation) as the gradient is inverted is shown. The stationary spins return to the original phase state, whereas the moving spins do not. **Right.** *Gradient moment nulling* of first order linear velocity (flow compensation) requires a doubling of the negative gradient amplitude followed by a positive gradient such that the total summed area is equal to zero. This will return both the stationary spins *and* the moving spins back to their original phase state.

and endogenous tracer methods are used. Freely diffusible tracers using nuclei such as ^2H (deuterium), ^3He, ^{17}O, and ^{19}F are employed in experimental procedures to produce differential contrast in the tissues. More clinically relevant are intravascular blood pool agents such as gadolinium–diethylenetriaminepentaacetic acid, which modify the relaxation of protons in the blood in addition to producing a shorter T2*. This produces signal changes that can be visualized in pre and post contrast images (Fig. 13-19). Endogenous tracer methods do not use externally added agents, but instead depend on the ability to generate contrast from specific excitation or diffusion mechanisms. For example, labeling of inflowing protons ("black blood" perfusion) uses protons in the blood as the contrast agent. Tagged (labeled) protons outside of the imaging volume perfuse into the tissues, resulting in a drop in signal intensity, a time course of events that can be monitored by quantitative measurements.

Functional MRI (fMRI) is based on the increase in blood flow to the local vasculature that accompanies neural activity in the specific areas of the brain, resulting in a local reduction of deoxyhemoglobin because the increase in blood flow occurs without an increase in oxygen extraction. As deoxyhemoglobin is a paramagnetic agent, it alters the T2*-weighted MRI image signal. Thus, this endogenous contrast enhancing agent serves as the signal for fMRI. Area voxels (represented by x-y coordinates and z slice thickness) of high metabolic activity resulting from a task-induced stimulus produce a correlated signal for Blood Oxygen Level Dependent (BOLD) acquisition techniques. A BOLD sequence produces multiple T2*-weighted images of the head before the application of the stimulus. The patient is repeatedly subjected to the stimulus and multiple BOLD images are acquired. Because the BOLD sequence produces images that are highly dependent on blood oxygen levels, areas of high metabolic activity will demonstrate a change in signal when the prestimulus image data set is subtracted, voxel by voxel, from post-stimulus image data set. Voxel locations defined by significant

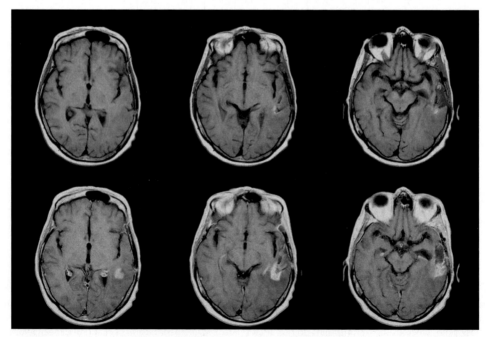

■ FIGURE 13-19 Pre (**top row**) and post (**bottom row**) gadolinium contrast T1-weighted MR axial images of the brain illustrate the signal change that occurs with the appearance of gadolinium by shortening the T1 time of the perfused tissues.

signal changes indicate regions of the brain activated by a specific task. Stimuli in fMRI experiments can be physical (finger movement), sensory (light flashes or sounds), or cognitive (repetition of "good" or "bad" word sequences, complex problem solving), among others. To improve the SNR in the fMRI images, a stimulus is typically applied in a repetitive, periodic sequence, and BOLD images are acquired continuously, tagged with the timing of the stimulus. Regions in the brain that demonstrate time-dependent activity and correlate with the time-dependent application of the stimulus are statistically analyzed, and coded using a color scale, while voxels that do not show a significant intensity change are not colored. The resultant color map is overlaid onto a grayscale image of the brain for anatomic reference, as shown in Figure 13-20.

High-speed imaging and T2* weighting necessary for fMRI is typically achieved with EPI acquisition techniques that can be acquired in as little as 50 ms for a 64 × 64 acquisition matrix. Gradient Recalled Echo acquisitions using standard sequences are also employed with multiple contiguous slices (e.g., 16 slices, slice thickness 5 mm, TR = 3 s, TE = 60 ms, 90-degree flip angle) at 1.5 T, with 25 to 30 complete head acquisitions. The latter acquisition techniques provide better spatial resolution but rely on very cooperative subjects and a much longer exam time.

Diffusion Weighted Imaging

Diffusion relates to the random motion of water molecules in tissues. Interaction of the local cellular structure with the movement of water molecules produces anisotropic, directionally dependent diffusion (e.g., in the white matter of brain tissues).

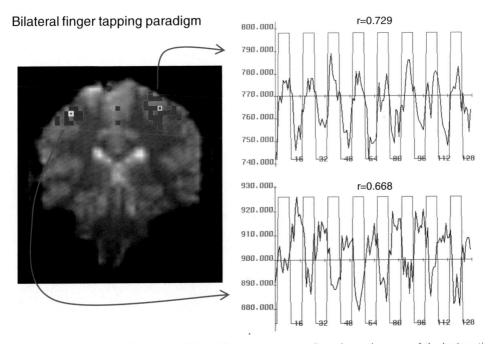

Bilateral finger tapping paradigm

■ **FIGURE 13-20** Functional MR image bilateral finger tapping paradigm shows the areas of the brain activated by this repeated activity. The paradigm was a right finger tap alternated by a left finger tap (time sequence on the right side of the figure) and the correlated BOLD signals (*black traces*) derived from the echo planar image sequence. A voxel-by-voxel correlation of the periodic stimulus and MR signal is performed, and when exceeding a correlation threshold, a color overlay is added to the grayscale image. In this example, *red* indicates the right finger tap that excites the left motor cortex, which appears on the right side of the image, and blue the left finger tap. (Figure compliments of MH Buonocore, MD, PhD University of California Davis.)

■ FIGURE 13-21 The basic elements of a DWI pulse sequence are shown. The diffusion weighting gradients are of amplitude G, duration of the gradients δ and time between gradients is Δ.

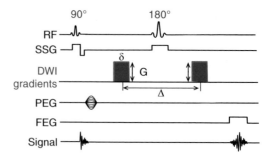

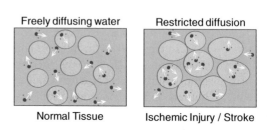

Freely diffusing water   Restricted diffusion

Normal Tissue   Ischemic Injury / Stroke

Diffusion sequences use strong MR gradients applied symmetrically about the refocusing pulse to produce signal differences based on the mobility and directionality of water diffusion, as shown in Figure 13-21. Tissues with more water mobility (normal) have a greater signal loss than those of lesser water mobility (injury) under the influence of the diffusion weighted imaging (DWI) gradients.

The in vivo structural integrity of certain tissues (healthy, diseased, or injured) can be measured by the use of DWI, in which water diffusion characteristics are determined through the generation of apparent diffusion coefficient (ADC) maps. This requires two or more acquisitions with different DWI parameters. A low ADC corresponds to high signal intensity on a calculated image, which represents restricted diffusion (Fig. 13-22). ADC maps of the brain and the spinal cord have shown prom-

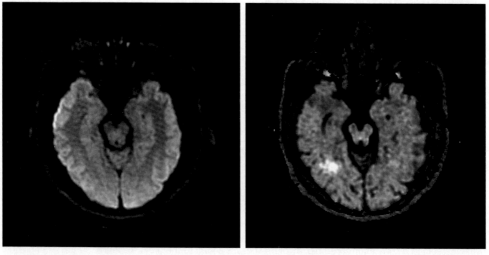

■ FIGURE 13-22 **Left**. Diffusion weighted image. **Right**. Calculated ADC image, showing an area of increased brightness related to restricted mobility of water molecules.

ise in predicting and evaluating pathophysiology before it is visible on conventional T1- or T2-weighted images. DWI is also a sensitive indicator for early detection of ischemic injury. Areas of acute stroke show a drastic reduction in the diffusion coefficient compared with nonischemic tissues. Diagnosis of multiple sclerosis is a potential application, based on the measurements of the diffusion coefficients in three-dimensional space.

Various acquisition techniques are used to generate diffusion-weighted contrast. Standard spin echo and EPI pulse sequences with applied diffusion gradients of high strength are used. Challenges for DWI are the extreme sensitivity to motion of the head and brain, which is chiefly caused by the large pulsed gradients required for the diffusion preparation. Eddy currents are also an issue, which reduce the effectiveness of the gradient fields, so compensated gradient coils are necessary. Several strategies have been devised to overcome the motion sensitivity problem, including common electrocardiographic gating and motion compensation methods.

13.4 Magnetization Transfer Contrast

Magnetization transfer contrast is the result of selective observation of the interaction between protons in free water molecules and protons contained in the macromolecules of a protein. Magnetization exchange occurs between the two proton groups because of coupling or chemical exchange. Because the protons exist in slightly different magnetic environments, the selective saturation of the protons in the macromolecule can be excited separately from the bulk water by using narrow-band RF pulses (because the Larmor frequencies are different). A transfer of the magnetization from the protons in the macromolecule partially saturates the protons in bulk water, even though these protons have not experienced an RF excitation pulse (Fig. 13-23). Reduced signal from the

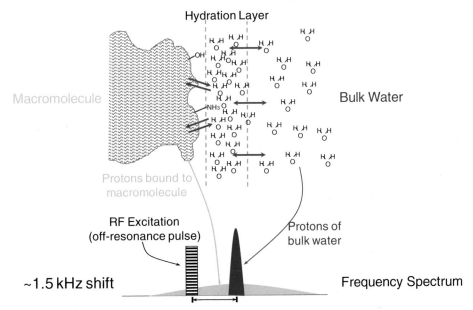

■ **FIGURE 13-23** Magnetization transfer contrast is implemented with an off-resonance RF pulse of about 1,500 Hz from the Larmor frequency. Excitation of hydrogen atoms on macromolecules is transferred via the hydration layer to adjacent "free-water" hydrogen atoms. A partial saturation of the tissues reduces the signals that would otherwise compete with signals from blood flow, making this useful for time-of-flight MRA.

adjacent free water protons by the saturation "label" affects only those protons having a chemical exchange with the macromolecules and improves local image contrast in many situations by decreasing the otherwise large signal generated by the protons in the bulk water. This technique is used for anatomic MRI of the heart, the eye, multiple sclerosis, knee cartilage, and general MRA. Tissue characterization is also possible, because the image contrast in part is caused by the surface chemistry of the macromolecule and the tissue-specific factors that affect the magnetization transfer characteristics.

Magnetization transfer contrast pulse sequences are often used in conjunction with MRA time-of-flight methods. Hydrogen atoms constitute a large fraction of macromolecules in proteins, are tightly bound to these macromolecules, and have a very short T2 decay with a broad range of resonance frequencies compared to protons in free water. Selective excitation of these protons is achieved with an off-resonance RF pulse of approximately 1,500 Hz from the Larmor frequency, causing their saturation. The protons in the hydration layer bound to these molecules are affected by the magnetization and become partially saturated themselves. MR signals from these tissues are suppressed, with an impact of reducing the contrast variation of the anatomy. As a result, the differential contrast of the flow-enhanced signals is increased, with overall better image quality angiographic sequence.

13.5 MR Artifacts

Artifacts manifest as positive or negative signal intensities that do not accurately represent the imaged anatomy. Although some artifacts are relatively insignificant and are easily identified, others can limit the diagnostic potential of the exam by obscuring or mimicking pathologic processes or anatomy. One must realize the impact of MR acquisition protocols and understand the etiology of artifact production to exploit the information they convey.

To minimize the impact of MR artifacts, a working knowledge of MR physics as well as image acquisition techniques is required. On the one hand, there are many variables and options available that complicate the decision-making process for MR image acquisition. On the other, the wealth of choices enhances the goal of achieving diagnostically accurate images. MR artifacts are classified into three broad areas—those based on the machine, on the patient, and on signal processing.

Machine-Dependent Artifacts

Magnetic field inhomogeneities are either global or focal field perturbations that lead to the mismapping of tissues within the image, and cause more rapid T2 relaxation. Distortion or misplacement of anatomy occurs when the magnetic field is not completely homogeneous. Proper site planning, self-shielded magnets, automatic shimming, and preventive maintenance procedures help to reduce inhomogeneities.

Focal field inhomogeneities arise from many causes. Ferromagnetic objects in or on the patient (e.g., makeup, metallic implants, prostheses, surgical clips, dentures) produce field distortions and cause protons to precess at frequencies different from the Larmor frequency in the local area. Incorrect proton mapping, displacement, and appearance as a signal void with a peripherally enhanced rim of increased signal are common findings. Geometric distortion of surrounding tissue is also usually evident. Even nonferromagnetic conducting materials (e.g., aluminum) produce field distortions that disturb the local magnetic environment. Partial compensation by the spin echo (180-degree RF) pulse sequence reduces these artifacts; on the other hand, the gradient-refocused echo sequence accentuates distortions, since the protons always experience the same direction of the focal magnetic inhomogeneities within the patient.

Susceptibility Artifacts

Magnetic susceptibility is the ratio of the induced internal magnetization in a tissue to the external magnetic field. As long as the magnetic susceptibility of the tissues being imaged is relatively unchanged across the field of view, then the magnetic field will remain uniform. Any drastic changes in the magnetic susceptibility will distort the magnetic field. The most common susceptibility changes occur at tissue-air interfaces (e.g., lungs and sinuses), which cause a signal loss due to more rapid dephasing (T2*) at the tissue-air interface (Fig. 13-24). Any metal (ferrous or not) may have a significant effect on the adjacent local tissues due to changes in susceptibility and the resultant magnetic field distortions. Paramagnetic agents exhibit a weak magnetization and increase the local magnetic field causing an artifactual reduction in the surrounding T2* relaxation.

Magnetic susceptibility can be quite helpful in some diagnoses. Most notable is the ability to diagnose the age of a hemorrhage based on the signal characteristics of the blood degradation products, which are different in the acute, subacute, and chronic phases. Some of the iron-containing compounds (deoxyhemoglobin, methemoglobin, hemosiderin, and ferritin) can dramatically shorten T1 and T2 relaxation of nearby protons. The amount of associated free water, the type and structure of the iron-containing molecules, the distribution (intracellular versus extracellular), and the magnetic field strength all influence the degree of relaxation effect that may be seen. For example, in the acute stage, T2 shortening occurs due to the paramagnetic susceptibility of the organized deoxyhemoglobin in the local area, without any large effect on the T1 relaxation time. When red blood cells lyse during the subacute stage, the hemoglobin is altered into methemoglobin, and spin-lattice relaxation is enhanced with the formation of a hydration layer, which shortens T1 relaxation, leading to a much stronger signal

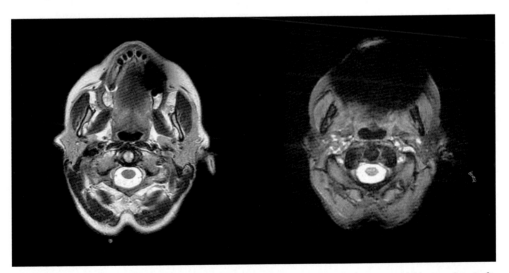

■ **FIGURE 13-24** Susceptibility artifacts due to dental fillings are shown in the same axial image slice. **Left.** Axial T2-weighted fast spin echo image illustrates significant suppression of susceptibility artifacts with 180-degree refocusing pulse. **Right.** Axial T2*-weighted gradient echo image illustrates significant image void exacerbated by the gradient echo, where external inhomogeneities are not canceled in the reformed echo.

on T1-weighted images. Increased signal intensity on T1-weighted images not found in the acute stage of hemorrhage identifies the subacute stage. In the chronic stage, hemosiderin, found in the phagocytic cells in sites of previous hemorrhage, disrupts the local magnetic homogeneity, causes loss of signal intensity, and leads to signal void, producing a characteristic dark rim around the hemorrhage site.

Gadolinium-based contrast agents (paramagnetic characteristics shorten T2 and hydration layer interactions shorten T1) are widely used in MRI. Tissues that uptake gadolinium contrast agents exhibit shortened T1 relaxation and demonstrate increased signal on T1-weighted images. Although focal inhomogeneities are generally considered problematic, there are certain physiologic and anatomic manifestations that can be identified and diagnostic information obtained.

Gradient Field Artifacts

Magnetic field gradients spatially encode the location of the signals emanating from excited protons within the volume being imaged. Proper reconstruction requires linear, matched, and properly sequenced gradients. The slice select gradient defines the volume (slice). Phase and frequency encoding gradients provide the spatial information in the other two dimensions.

Since the reconstruction algorithm assumes ideal, linear gradients, any deviation or temporal instability will be represented as a distortion. Gradient strength has a tendency to fall off at the periphery of the FOV. Consequently, anatomic compression occurs, especially pronounced on coronal and sagittal images having a large FOV, typically greater than 35 cm (Fig. 13-25). Minimizing the spatial distortion entails either reducing the FOV by lowering the gradient field strength or by holding the gradient field strength and number of samples constant while decreasing the frequency bandwidth. Of course, gradient calibration is part of a continuous quality control (QC) checklist, and geometric accuracy must be periodically verified.

Anatomic proportions may simulate abnormalities, so verification of pixel dimensions in the PEG and FEG directions are necessary. If the strength of the FEG and the strength of the largest PEG are different, the height or width of the pixels can become distorted and produce inaccurate measurements. Ideally, the phase and frequency encoding gradients should be assigned to the smaller and larger dimensions of the object, respectively, to preserve spatial resolution while limiting the number of phase encoding steps. In practice, this is not always possible, because motion artifacts or high-intensity

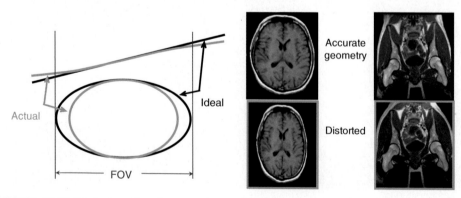

■ **FIGURE 13-25** Gradient nonlinearity causes image distortions by mis-mapping anatomy. In the above examples, the strength of the gradient at the periphery is less than the ideal (*orange line* versus *black line*). This results in a compression of the imaged anatomy, with inaccurate geometry (images with *orange* border). For comparison, images acquired with linear corrections are shown above.

signals that need to be displaced away from important areas of interest after an initial scan might require swapping the frequency and phase encode gradient directions.

RF Coil Artifacts

RF surface coils produce variations in uniformity across the image caused by RF excitation variability, attenuation, mismatching, and sensitivity falloff with distance. Proximal to the surface coil, receive signals are intense, and with distance, signal intensity is attenuated, resulting in grayscale shading and loss of brightness in the image. Nonuniform image intensities are the all-too-frequent result. Also, compensation for the disturbance of the magnetic field by the patient is typically compensated by an automatic shimming calibration. When this is not performed, or performed inadequately, a significant negative impact on image quality occurs. Examples of variable response are shown in Figure 13-26.

Other common artifacts from RF coils occur with RF quadrature coils (coils that simultaneously measure the signal from orthogonal views) that have two separate amplifier and gain controls. If the amplifiers are imbalanced, a bright spot in the center of the image, known as a center point artifact, arises as a "0 frequency" direct current offset. Variations in gain between the quadrature coils can cause ghosting of objects diagonally in the image. The bottom line for all RF coils is the need for continuous measurement and consistent calibration of their response, so that artifacts are minimized.

RF Artifacts

RF pulses and precessional frequencies of MRI instruments occupy the same frequencies of common RF sources, such as TV and radio broadcasts, electric motors, fluorescent lights, and computers. Stray RF signals that propagate to the MRI antenna can produce various artifacts in the image. Narrow-band noise creates noise patterns perpendicular to the frequency encoding direction. The exact position and spatial extent depends on the resonant frequency of the imager, applied gradient field strength, and bandwidth of the noise. A narrow band pattern of black/white

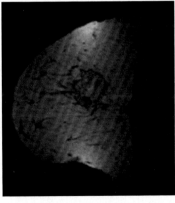
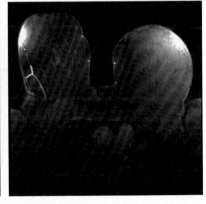

 Coil close to skin   Inadequate shimming for fat saturation

■ **FIGURE 13-26** Signal intensity variations occur when surface RF receive coils are too close to the skin, as exemplified by the MR breast image on the left. With inadequate shimming calibration, saturation pulses for adipose tissue in the breast is uneven, causing a significant variation in the uniformity of the reconstructed image. From Hendrick RE, *Breast MRI: fundamentals and technical aspects*. New York, NY: Springer, 2007. By permission.

alternating noise produces a "zipper" artifact. Broadband RF noise disrupts the image over a much larger area of the reconstructed image with diffuse, contrast-reducing "herringbone" artifacts. Appropriate site planning and the use of properly installed RF shielding materials (e.g., a Faraday cage) reduce stray RF interference to an acceptably low level. An example RF zipper artifact is shown in Figure 13-44.

RF energy received by adjacent slices during a multislice acquisition excite and saturate protons in adjacent slices, chiefly due to RF pulses without sharp off/on/off transitions. This is known as cross-excitation. On T2-weighted images, the slice-to-slice interference degrades the SNR; on T1-weighted images, the extra partial saturation reduces image contrast by reducing longitudinal recovery during the TR interval. A typical truncated "sinc" RF profile and overlap areas in adjacent slices are shown in Figure 13-27. Interslice gaps reduce the overlap of the profile tails, and pseudo-rectangular RF pulse profiles reduce the spatial extent of the tails. Important anatomic findings could exist within the gaps, so *slice interleaving* is a technique to mitigate cross-excitation by reordering slices into two groups with gaps. During the first half of the TR, the first slices are acquired (slices 1 to 5), followed by the second group of slices that are positioned in the gap of the first group (slices 6 to 10). This method reduces cross-excitation by separating the adjacent slice excitations in time. The most effective method is to acquire two independent sets of gapped multislice images, but the image time is doubled. The most appropriate solution is to devise RF pulses that approximate a rectangular profile; however, the additional time necessary for producing such an RF pulse can be prohibitive.

K-Space Errors

Errors in k-space encoding affect all areas of the reconstructed image, and cause the artifactual superimposition of wave patterns across the FOV. Each individual pixel value in k-space contributes to all pixel values in image space as a frequency harmonic with a signal amplitude. One bad pixel introduces a significant artifact, rendering the image suboptimal, as shown in Figure 13-28.

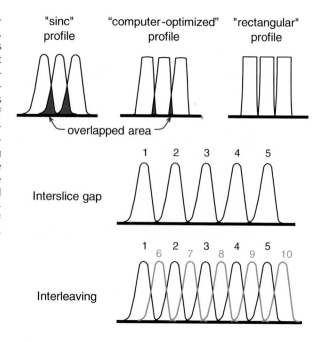

■ FIGURE 13-27 **Top.** Poor pulse profiles are caused by truncated RF pulses, and resulting profile overlap causes unwanted partial saturation in adjacent slices, with a loss of SNR and CNR. Optimized pulses are produced by considering the tradeoff of pulse duration versus excitation profile. **Bottom.** Reduction of cross-excitation is achieved with interslice gaps, but anatomy at the gap location might be missed. An interleaving technique acquires the first half of the images with an interslice gap, and the second half of the images are positioned in the gaps of the first images. The separation in time reduces the amount of contrast reducing saturation of the adjacent slices.

Bad pixel in k-space   Resultant image

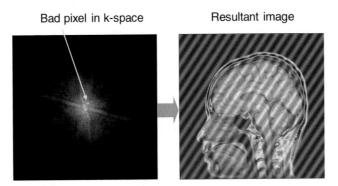

■ **FIGURE 13-28** A single bad pixel in k-space causes a significant artifact in the reconstructed image. The bad pixel is located at $k_x = 2$, $k_y = 3$, which produces a superimposed sinusoidal wave on the spatial domain image as shown above.

Motion Artifacts

The most ubiquitous and noticeable artifacts in MRI arise with patient motion, including voluntary and involuntary movement, and flow (blood, CSF). Although motion artifacts are not unique to MRI, the long acquisition time of certain MRI sequences increases the probability of motion blurring and contrast resolution losses. Motion artifacts occur mostly along the phase encode direction, as adjacent phase encoding measurements in k-space are separated by a TR interval that can last 3,000 ms or longer. Even very slight motion can cause a change in the recorded phase variation across the FOV throughout the MR acquisition sequence. Examples of motion artifacts are shown in Figure 13-29. The frequency encode direction is less affected, especially by periodic motion, since the evolution of the echo signal, frequency encoding, and sampling occur simultaneously over several milliseconds. Ghost images, which are faint copies of the image displaced along the phase encode direction, are the visual result of patient motion.

Several techniques can compensate for motion-related artifacts. The simplest technique transposes the PEG and FEG to relocate the motion artifacts out of the

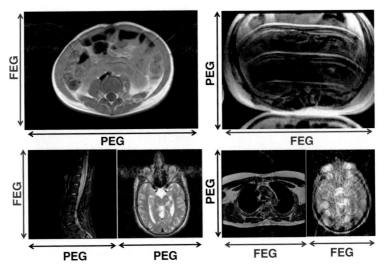

■ **FIGURE 13-29** Motion artifacts, particularly of flow patterns, are most always displayed in the phase encode gradient direction. Slight changes in phase produce multiple ghost images of the anatomy, since the variation in phase caused by motion can be substantial between excitations.

region of diagnostic interest with the same pulse sequences. This does not reduce the magnitude of the artifacts, however, and often there is a mismatch when placing the PEG along the long axis of a rectangular FOV (e.g., an exam of the thoracic spine) in terms of longer examination times or a significant loss of spatial resolution or of SNR.

There are other motion compensation methods:

1. Cardiac and respiratory gating—signal acquisition at a particular cyclic location synchronizes the phase changes applied across the anatomy (Fig. 13-30).
2. Respiratory ordering of the phase encoding projections based on location within the respiratory cycle. Mechanical or video devices provide signals to monitor the cycle.
3. Signal averaging to reduce artifacts of random motion by making displaced signals less conspicuous relative to stationary anatomy.
4. Short TE spin echo sequences (limited to proton density, T1-weighted scans, fractional echo acquisition, Fig. 13-3). Note: Long TE scans (T2 weighting) are more susceptible to motion.
5. Gradient moment nulling (additional gradient pulses for flow compensation) to help rephase protons that are dephased due to motion. Most often, these techniques require a longer TE and are more useful for T2-weighted scans (Fig. 13-18).
6. Presaturation pulses applied outside the imaging region to reduce flow artifacts from inflowing protons, as well as other patient motions that occur in the periphery (Fig. 13-12).
7. Multiple redundant sampling in the center of k-space (e.g., propeller) to identify and remove those sequences contributing to motion, without deleteriously affecting the image (Fig. 13-8).

Chemical Shift Artifacts of the First Kind

There are two types of chemical shift artifacts that affect the display of anatomy due to the precessional frequency differences of protons in fat versus protons in water. Chemical shift refers to the resonance frequency variations resulting from intrinsic

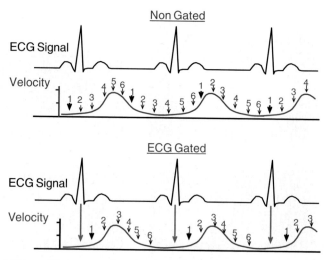

■ **FIGURE 13-30** Motion artifacts occur when data is acquired without consideration of physiologic periodicity. **Top**. The electrocardiogram measures the R-wave at each heartbeat, but data acquisition proceeds in a linear fashion without regard to reproducibility. The result is a set of images degraded with motion artifact, with diagnostic usefulness marginal, at best. **Bottom**. Acquisition of images proceeds with the detection of the R-wave signal and synchronization of the collection of image data in a stepwise fashion over the period between R-waves. A reduced number of images or extended acquisition time is required to collect the data.

magnetic shielding of anatomic structures. Molecular structure and electron orbital characteristics produce fields that shield the main magnetic field and give rise to distinct peaks in the MR spectrum. In the case of proton spectra, peaks correspond to water and fat, and in the case of breast imaging, silicone material is another material to consider. Lower frequencies of about 3.5 parts per million for protons in fat and 5.0 parts per million for protons in silicone occur, compared to the resonance frequency of protons in water (Fig. 13-31). Since resonance frequency increases linearly with field strength, the absolute difference between the fat and water resonance also increases, making high field strength magnets more susceptible to chemical shift artifact.

Data acquisition methods cannot directly discriminate a frequency shift due to the application of a frequency encode gradient or a chemical shift artifact. Water and fat differences therefore cannot be distinguished by the frequency difference induced by the gradient. The protons in fat resonate at a slightly lower frequency than the corresponding protons in water, and cause a shift in the anatomy (misregistration of water and fat moieties) along the frequency encode gradient direction.

A sample calculation in the example below demonstrates frequency variations in fat and water for two different magnetic field and gradient field strengths:

Chemical shift artifact numerical calculation for field strength, with a 3.5-ppm (3.5×10^{-6}) variation in resonance frequency between fat and water results in the following frequency differences:

$$1.5 \text{ T}: 63.8 \times 10^6 \text{Hz} \times 3.5 \times 10^{-6} = 223 \text{ Hz}$$

$$3.0 \text{ T}: 127.7 \times 10^6 \text{Hz} \times 3.5 \times 10^{-6} = 447 \text{ Hz}$$

Thus, the chemical shift is more severe for higher field strength magnets.

Chemical shift artifact numerical calculation for gradient strength results in the following numerical calculations for a 25-cm (0.25 m) FOV, 256 × 256 matrix:

Low gradient strength: 2.5 mT/m × 0.25 m = 0.000625 T variation, gives frequency range of 0.000625 T × 42.58 MHz/T = 26.6 kHz across FOV and 26.6 kHz/256 pixels = 104 Hz/pixel

High gradient strength: 10 mT/m × 0.25 m = 0.0025 T variation, gives frequency range of 0.0025 T × 42.58 MHz/T = 106.5 kHz across FOV and 106.5 kHz/256 pixels = 416 Hz/pixel.

Thus, a chemical shift occurrence is more severe for lower gradient strengths, since displacement will occur over a large number of pixels. With a higher gradient strength, water and fat are more closely contained within the broader pixel boundary bandwidths. Normal and low bandwidth images are illustrated in Figure 13-32.

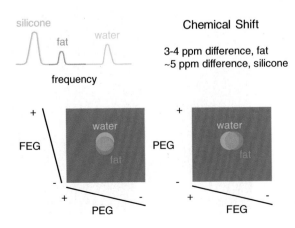

■ FIGURE 13-31 Chemical shift refers to the slightly different precessional frequencies of protons in different materials or tissues. The shifts (in ppm) are referenced to water for fat and silicone. Fat chemical shift artifacts are represented by a shift of water and fat in the images of anatomical structure, mainly in the frequency encode gradient direction. Swapping the PEG and the FEG will cause a shift of the fat and water components of the tissues in the image.

High Bandwidth   Low Bandwidth

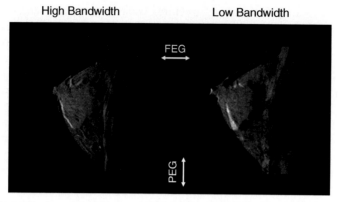

■ **FIGURE 13-32** MR images of the breast, containing glandular and adipose tissue, are acquired under a high bandwidth (32 kHz) and a low bandwidth (4 kHz), illustrating the more severe chemical shift with low readout gradient strength and bandwidth. (Reprinted by permission, Hendrick RE. *Breast MRI: fundamentals and technical aspects.* New York, NY: Springer, 2007.)

RF bandwidth and gradient strength considerations can mitigate chemical shift artifacts. While higher gradient strength can confine the chemical shift of fat within the pixel bandwidth boundaries, a significant SNR penalty occurs with the broad RF bandwidth required to achieve a given slice thickness. A more widely used method is to use lower gradient strengths and narrow bandwidths in combination with off-resonance "chemical presaturation" RF pulses to minimize the fat (or the silicone) signal in the image (Fig. 13-33). Another alternative is to use STIR techniques to eliminate the signals due to fat at the "bounce point." Swapping the phase and frequency gradient directions or changing the polarity of the frequency encode gradient can displace chemical shift artifacts from a specific image region, even though the chemical shift displacement still exists. Identification of fat in a specific anatomic region is easily discerned from the chemical shift artifact displacement caused by changes in FEG/PEG gradient directions.

Chemical Shift Artifacts of the Second Kind

Chemical shift artifacts of the second kind occur with GE images, resulting from the rephasing and dephasing of the echo in the same direction relative to the main magnetic field. Signal appearance is dependent on the selection of TE. This happens because of constructive (in phase) or destructive (out of phase) transverse magnetization events that occur periodically due to the difference in precessional frequencies. At 1.5 T, the chemical shift

■ **FIGURE 13-33** The left image of the lumbar spine is Spin Echo T1 weighted, TR = 450 ms, TE = 14 ms. The right image is T1 weighted with chemical fat saturation pulses, TR = 667 ms, TE = 8 ms. In both images, the FEG is vertically oriented.

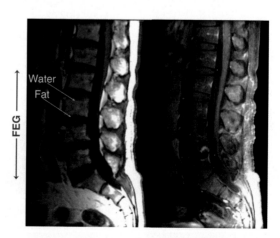

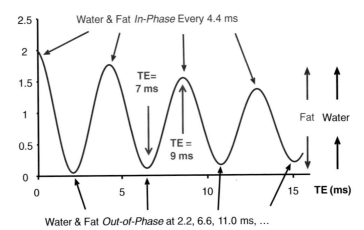

■ **FIGURE 13-34** For GE image sequences, signal intensity of the transverse magnetization vector due to the 220 Hz lower precessional frequency of fat protons, where in-phase magnetization occurs every 4.4 ms $(1/220 s^{-1})$, and out-of-phase magnetization occurs every 4.4 ms shifted by ½ cycle (2.2 ms). Signal intensity is dependent on the selection of TE, as shown above.

is 220 Hz, and the periodicity of each peak (in phase) between water and fat occurs at 0, 4.5, 9.0, 13.5, ... ms, and each valley (out of phase) at 2.25, 6.75, 11.0, ... ms, as shown in Figure 13-34. Thus, selection of TE at 9 ms will lead to a constructive addition of water and fat, and TE at 7 ms will lead to a destructive addition of water and fat. The in-phase timing will lead to a conventional chemical shift image of the first kind, while the out-of-phase timing will lead to a chemical shift image of the second kind, manifesting a dark rim around heterogeneous water and fat anatomical structures, shown in Figure 13-35.

Ringing Artifacts

Ringing artifact (also known as Gibbs phenomenon) occurs near sharp boundaries and high-contrast transitions in the image, and appears as multiple, regularly spaced parallel bands of alternating bright and dark signal that slowly fades with distance.

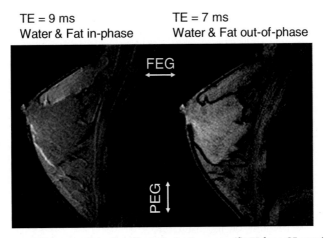

■ **FIGURE 13-35** Breast MRI images show the effect of selecting a specific TE for a GE acquisition. On the left, chemical shift of the "first kind" is shown with TE = 9 ms and water and fat in phase for transverse magnetization, shifted only due to the intrinsic chemical shift differences of fat and water. On the right, chemical shift of the second kind is additionally manifested with TE = 7 ms, due to fat and water being out of phase, creating a lower signal at all fat-water interfaces, and resulting in reduced intensity. (Reprinted by permission, Hendrick RE. *Breast MRI: fundamentals and technical aspects.* New York, NY: Springer, 2007.)

The cause is the insufficient sampling of high frequencies inherent at sharp discontinuities in the signal. Images of objects can be reconstructed from a summation of sinusoidal waveforms of specific amplitudes and frequencies, as shown in Figure 13-36 for a simple rectangular object. In the figure, the summation of frequency harmonics, each with a particular amplitude and phase, approximates the distribution of the object, but initially does very poorly, particularly at the sharp edges. As the number of higher frequency harmonics increase, a better estimate is achieved, although an infinite number of frequencies are theoretically necessary to reconstruct the sharp edge perfectly.

In the MR acquisition, the number of frequency samples is determined by the number of pixels (frequency, k_x, or phase, k_y, increments) across the k-space matrix. For 256 pixels, 128 discrete frequencies are depicted, and for 128 pixels, 64 discrete frequencies are specified (the k-space matrix is symmetric in quadrants and duplicated about its center). A lack of high-frequency signals causes the "ringing" at sharp transitions described as a diminishing hyper- and hypointense signal oscillation from the transition. Ringing artifacts are thus more likely for smaller digital matrix sizes (Fig. 13-37, 256 versus 128 matrix). Ringing artifact commonly occurs at skull/brain interfaces, where there is a large transition in signal amplitude.

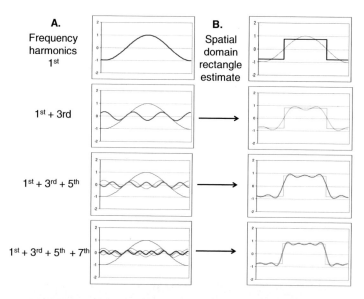

A. Frequency harmonics 1st

B. Spatial domain rectangle estimate

1st + 3rd

1st + 3rd + 5th

1st + 3rd + 5th + 7th

■ **FIGURE 13-36** The synthesis of a spatial object occurs by the summation of frequency harmonics in the MR image. **A. Left column**: frequency harmonics that estimate a rectangle function with progressively higher frequencies and lower amplitudes are shown. **B. Middle column**: As higher frequency harmonics are included, the summed result more faithfully represents the object shape, in this example a rectangle with two vertical edges. The number of frequencies encoded in the MR image is dependent on the matrix size. **C. Right column**: A sharp transition boundary in an MR image is represented with 256 samples better than with 128 samples (frequency harmonics in k-space). The amount of ringing caused by insufficient sampling is reduced with a larger number of samples.

C. Sharp transition in MR image:

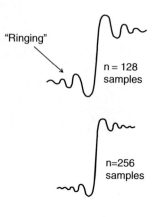

"Ringing"

n = 128 samples

n = 256 samples

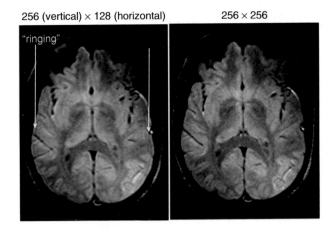

256 (vertical) × 128 (horizontal)   256 × 256

"ringing"

■ **FIGURE 13-37** Example of ringing artifacts caused by a sharp signal transition at the skull in a brain image for a 256 × 128 matrix (left) along the short (horizontal) axis, and the elimination of the artifact in a 256 × 256 matrix (right). The short axis defines the PEG direction.

Wraparound Artifacts

The wraparound artifact is a result of the mismapping of anatomy that lies outside of the FOV but within the slice volume. The anatomy is usually displaced to the opposite side of the image. It is caused by nonlinear gradients or by undersampling of the frequencies contained within the returned signal envelope. For the latter, the sampling rate must be twice the maximal frequency that occurs in the object (the Nyquist sampling limit). Otherwise, the Fourier transform cannot distinguish frequencies that are present in the data above the Nyquist frequency limit, and instead assigns a lower frequency value to them (Fig. 13-38). Frequency signals will "wraparound" to the opposite side of the image, masquerading as low-frequency (aliased) signals.

In the frequency encode direction, a low-pass filter can be applied to the acquired time domain signal to eliminate frequencies beyond the Nyquist frequency. In the phase encode direction, aliasing artifacts can be reduced by increasing the number of phase encode steps (the trade-off is increased image time). Another approach is to move the region of anatomic interest to the center of the imaging volume to avoid the

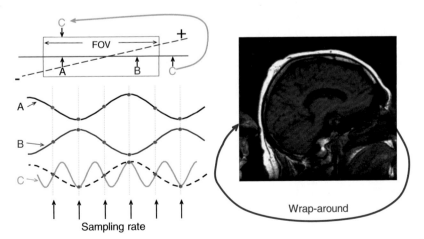

■ **FIGURE 13-38 Left.** Wraparound artifacts are caused by aliasing. Shown is a fixed sampling rate and net precessional frequencies occurring at position *A* and position *B* within the FOV that have identical frequencies but different phase. If signal from position *C* is at *twice* the frequency of *B* and insufficiently sampled, the same frequency and phase will be assigned to *C* as that assigned to *A*, and therefore will appear at that location. **Right.** A wraparound artifact example displaces anatomy from one side of the image (or outside of the FOV) to the other side.

overlapping anatomy, which usually occurs at the periphery of the FOV. An "antialiasing" saturation pulse just outside of the FOV is yet another method of eliminating high-frequency signals that would otherwise be aliased into the lower frequency spectrum. This example of wrap-around artifact is easy to interpret. In some cases, the artifact is not as well delineated (e.g., the top of the skull wrapping into the brain).

Partial Volume Artifacts

Partial volume artifacts arise from the finite size of the voxel over which the signal is averaged. This results in a loss of detail and spatial resolution. Reduction of partial volume artifacts is accomplished by using a smaller pixel size and/or a smaller slice thickness. With a smaller voxel, the SNR is reduced for a similar imaging time, resulting in a noisier signal with less low-contrast sensitivity. Of course, with a greater NEX (averages), the SNR can be maintained, at the cost of longer imaging time.

13.6 Magnetic Resonance Spectroscopy

Magnetic resonance spectroscopy (MRS) is a method to measure tissue chemistry (an "electronic" biopsy) by recording and evaluating signals from metabolites by identifying metabolic peaks caused by frequency shifts (in parts per million, ppm) relative to a frequency standard. In vivo MRS can be performed with ^{1}H (proton), ^{23}Na (sodium), and ^{31}P (phosphorus) nuclei, but proton spectroscopy provides a much higher SNR and can be included in a conventional MRI protocol with about 10 to 15 min extra exam time. Uses of MRS include serial evaluation of biochemical changes in tumors, analyzing metabolic disorders, infections and diseases, as well as evaluation of therapeutic oncology treatments for tumor recurrence versus radiation damage. Early applications were dedicated to brain disorders, but now breast, liver, and prostate MRS are also performed. Correlation of spectroscopy results and MR images are always advised before making a final diagnosis.

In MRS, signals are derived from the amplitude of proton metabolites in targeted tissues. In these metabolites, chemical shifts occur due to electron cloud shielding of the nuclei, causing slightly different resonance frequencies, which exist in a frequency range between water and fat. The very small signal amplitudes of the metabolites require suppression of the extremely large (~10,000 times higher) amplitudes due to bulk water and fat protons, as shown in Figure 13-39. This is achieved by using specific chemical saturation techniques, such as CHESS (Chemical Shift-Selective) or STIR (see Chapter 12). In many cases, the areas evaluated are away from fat structures, and only bulk water signal suppression is necessary; however, in organs such as the liver and the breast, suppression of both fat and water are required. Once the water and fat signals are suppressed, localization of the targeted area volume is achieved by either a single voxel or multivoxel technique.

Single voxel MRS sampling areas, covering a volume of about 1 cm^3 are delineated by a STEAM (Stimulated echo acquisition mode) or a PRESS (Point Resolved Spectroscopy) sequence. The STEAM method uses a 90-degree excitation pulse and 90-degree refocusing pulse to collect the signal in conjunction with gradients to define each dimension of the voxel. The PRESS sequence uses a 90-degree excitation and 180-degree refocusing pulse in each direction. STEAM achieves shorter echo times and superior voxel boundaries, but with lower SNR. After the voxel data are collected, a Fourier transform is applied to separate the composite signal into individual frequencies, which are plotted as a trace for a normal brain spectrum (Fig. 13-40). The resulting line widths are based on homogeneity of the main magnetic field as

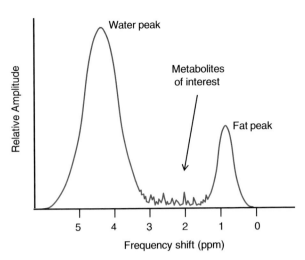

■ **FIGURE 13-39** MRS metabolites of interest in comparison to the water and fat peaks commonly used for imaging. In order to isolate the very small signals, chemical saturation of the water (and fat when present) signal is essential.

well as the magnetic field strength. Higher field strengths (e.g., 3.0 T) will improve resolution of the peaks and corresponding SNR.

Multivoxel MRS uses a CSI (Chemical Shift Imaging) technique to delineate multiple voxels of approximately 1 cm³ volume in 1, 2, or 3 planes over a rectangular block of several centimeters, achievable with more sophisticated equipment and longer scan times. This is followed by MRSI (Magnetic Resonance Spectroscopic Imaging) where the signal intensity of a single metabolite in each voxel is color encoded for each voxel according to concentration and the generated parameter maps superimposed on the anatomical MR image. In practice, the single voxel technique is used to make the initial diagnosis because the SNR is high and all metabolites are represented in the MRS trace. Then, a multivoxel acquisition to assess the distribution of a specific metabolite is performed.

Proton MRS can be performed with short (20 to 40 ms), intermediate (135 to 145 ms), or long (270 to 290 ms) echo times. For short TE, numerous resonances from metabolites of lesser importance (with shorter T2) can make the spectra more difficult to interpret, and with long echo times, SNR losses are too severe. Therefore, most MRS acquisitions use a TE of approximately 135 ms at 1.5 T. Metabolites of interest for brain spectroscopy are listed in Table 13-2.

Applications of MRS are achieved through the interpretation of the spectra that are obtained from the lesion, from its surroundings, and presumably healthy tissue in

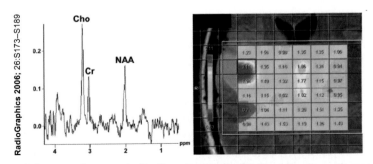

MR Spectrum from anaplastic oligoastrocytoma   Choline / Creatine ratio map

■ **FIGURE 13-40** **Left:** Intermediate echo (TE=135 ms) single voxel spectrum is shown, positioned over an anaplastic oligoastrocytoma brain lesion. Note the elevated Choline peak and lowered Creatine and NAA peaks. **Right:** Multivoxel spectrum is color coded to the Choline / Creatine ratio, illustrating the regional variation of the metabolites corresponding to tumor. From Al-Okaili RN, Krejza J, Wang S, Woo JH, Melhem ER. *Advanced MR Imaging Techniques in the Diagnosis of Intraaxial Brain Tumors in Adults.* Radiographics 2006; 26: S173-S189. By permission.

TABLE 13-2   METABOLITES IN MRS AT 1.5 T

ABBREVIATION	METABOLITE	SHIFT (PPM)	PROPERTIES/SIGNIFICANCE IN THE BRAIN
Cho	Phosphocholine	3.22	Membrane turnover, cell proliferation
Cr	Creatine	3.02 and 3.93	Temporary store for energy-rich phosphates
NAA	N-acetyl-L-aspartate	2.01	Presence of intact glioneural structures
Lactate		1.33 (inverted)	Anaerobic glycolysis
Lipids	Free fatty acids	1.2–1.4	Necrosis

the same scan. Main criteria include the presence or absence of pathologic metabolites (lactate or lipids) and the relationships between the concentrations of choline, creatine, and NAA as ratios. Spectra are usually scaled to the highest peak, and y-axis values will usually differ between measurements, so caution must be observed to avoid potential misdiagnoses.

In a tumor, high cell turnover causes an increase in choline concentration along with a corresponding depression of the NAA peak caused by the loss of healthy glioneural structures. In addition, the creatine peak may also be reduced depending on the energy status of the tumor; it is often used to serve as an internal reference for calculating ratios of metabolites. When a lipid peak is observed, this is a sign of hypoxia and the likelihood of a high-grade malignancy. Table 13-3 lists qualitative findings for MRS spectroscopy in evaluating brain tumors for the ratios of NAA/Cr, NAA/Cho, and Cho/Cr. Examples of single voxel and multivoxel spectra are shown in Figure 13-40, illustrating the use of the spectral peaks for diagnostic interpretation of the ratios, and a MRSI color-encoded graphic display of the spatial distribution of findings. There is certainly much more than determining ratios, and differential diagnoses are often clouded by indistinct peaks, poor SNR, and tumor heterogeneity, among other causes. MRS at 3 T field strength enjoys much better SNR, improved spectral resolution, and faster scans. Because of the higher spectral resolution, familiar single target peaks at 1.5 T become a collection of peaks at 3 T.

13.7 Ancillary Components

Ancillary components are necessary for the proper functioning of the MR system. Shim coils are active or passive magnetic field devices that are used to adjust the main magnetic field and to improve the homogeneity in the sensitive central volume of the

TABLE 13-3   RATIOS OF METABOLITE PEAKS IN MRS INDICATING "NORMAL" AND "ABNORMAL" STATUS

METABOLITE RATIO	NORMAL	ABNORMAL
NAA/Cr	2.0	<1.6
NAA/Cho	1.6	<1.2
Cho/Cr	1.2	>1.5

scanner. Gradient coils, as previously discussed, are wire conductors that produce a linear superimposed gradient magnetic field on the main magnetic field. The gradient coils are located inside the cylinder of the magnet, and are responsible for the banging noise one hears during imaging. This noise is caused by the flexing and torque experienced by the gradient coil from the rapidly changing magnetic fields when energized.

Radiofrequency Coils

A wide variety of transmit and receive coils complement a MR scanner. **RF transmitter coils** create an oscillating secondary magnetic field formed by passing an alternating current through a loop of wire. To accomplish excitation and resonance, the created secondary B_1 field must be arranged at right angles to the main magnetic field, B_0. In an air core design with a horizontal field, the RF coil secondary field should be in the transverse or vertical axes, as the B_1 field is created perpendicular to the transmit coils themselves. RF transmitter coils are therefore oriented above, below, or at the sides of the patient, and are usually cylindrical. In most systems, the body coil contained within the bore of the magnet is most frequently used, but also transmitter coils for the head, extremity, and some breast coils are coupled to a receiver coil.

Very often, transmit and receive functions are separated to handle the variety of imaging situations that arise, and to maximize the SNR for an imaging sequence. All **RF receiver coils** must resonate and efficiently store energy at the Larmor frequency. This is determined by the inductance and capacitance properties of the coil. RF transmit and receive coils need to be tuned prior to each acquisition and matched to accommodate the different magnetic inductance of each patient. Receiver coils must be properly placed to adequately detect the MR signal.

Proximity RF coils include volume or bird-cage coils, the design of choice for brain imaging, the single-turn solenoid for imaging the extremities and the breasts, and the saddle coil. These coils are typically operated as both a transmitter and receiver of RF energy (Fig. 13-41). *Volume coils* encompass the total area of the anatomy of interest and yield uniform excitation and SNR over the entire imaging volume. However, because of their relatively large size, images are produced with lower SNR than other types of coils. Enhanced performance is obtained with a process known as quadrature excitation and detection, which enables the energy to be transmitted and the signals to be received by two pairs of coils oriented at right angles, either electronically or physically. This detector manages two simultaneous channels known as the real (records MR information in phase with a reference signal) and the imaginary (records MR information 90 degree out of phase with the reference signal) channels, and increases the SNR up to a factor of $\sqrt{2}$. If imbalances in the offset or gain of these detectors occur, then artifacts will be manifested, such as a "center point" artifact.

Surface coils are used to achieve high SNR and high resolution when imaging anatomy near the surface of the patient, such as the spine. They are typically receive-only designs, and are usually small and shaped for a specific imaging exam and for patient comfort. The received signal sensitivity, however, is limited to the volume located around the coil at a depth into the patient equal to the radius of the coil, which causes a loss of signal with depth. There are now intracavitary coils for endorectal, endovascular, endovaginal, esophageal, and urethral local imaging, and can be used to receive signals from deep within the patient. In general, a body coil is used to transmit the RF energy and the local coil is used to receive the MR signal.

Phased array coils consisting of multiple coils and receivers are made of several overlapping loops, which extend the imaging FOV in one direction (Fig. 13-41). The

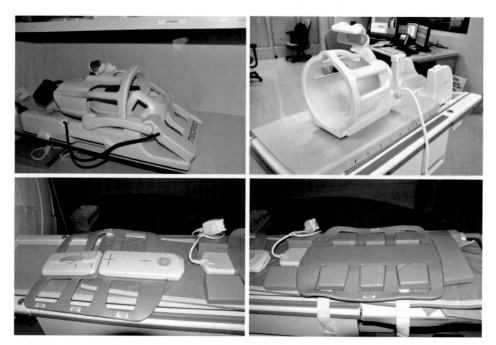

■ **FIGURE 13-41** Radiofrequency surface coils improve image quality and SNR for specific examinations. Upper left is a dedicated head and neck coil. Upper right is a dedicated head coil; the lower left and lower right images illustrate the two components of an 8 channel phased array coil for body imaging.

small FOV of each individual coil provides excellent SNR and resolution, and each is combined to produce a composite image with the advantages of the local surface coil, so that all data can be acquired in a single sequence. Phased array coils for the spine, pelvis, breast, cardiac, and temperomandibular joint applications are commonly purchased with an MR system for optimal image quality.

Multi-channel encoding coils with as many as N = 32 elements allow for detection and encoding based upon the detection of a sensitivity map of the signals near the coil. These coils are used in *parallel imaging* to fill N multiple lines of k-space per TR interval, by assigning certain coil responses to specific regions as the data are acquired simultaneously and using software to link them electronically. By filling k-space quicker, the scan time can be reduced by the number of elements in the coil. However, since each line of k-space is encoded by separate coils, the gap between each line for a specific coil is N times greater than if k-space had been filled normally. Since the FOV dimension in the phase encode direction is inversely proportional to the spacing, the size of the FOV is reduced to 1/N its original size, and as a result, aliasing of signals outside of the FOV in the phase encode direction occurs, and each coil response produces a wrapped image. To overcome the aliasing, the system uses the sensitivity profile of each coil to calculate where the signal is coming from relative to the coil based on its amplitude—the signal generated near the coil has a higher amplitude than the signal furthest away. Using this process (called SENSE, ASSET, GRAPPA, iPAT by the various manufacturers), the image is unwrapped and combined with the unwrapped images from the other coils to form one summed image of the slice, with high SNR and resolution (see Figure 13-9). Parallel imaging can be used to either reduce scan time or improve resolution, in conjunction with most pulse sequences. Downsides include image misalignment when combining images due to patient motion, and increase in chemical shift artifacts, due to a range of frequencies mapped across each coil. Nevertheless, multi-coil parallel imaging techniques are now common and increasing in use.

RF coil safety requires regular inspection of the coil condition, including the conductive wires leading to the coils from the connectors. These wires have the capacity to transmit heat, which may burn the insulating material of the wires or burn the patient. It is important to ensure that the coils are not looped and do not touch the patient or the bore of the magnet. Damage to the insulation requires immediate repair, as this could result in extreme heating, fire, and potential harm to the patient.

MR System Subcomponents

The control interfaces, RF source, detector, and amplifier, analog to digital converter (digitizer), pulse programmer, computer system, gradient power supplies, and image display are crucial components of the MR system. They integrate and synchronize the tasks necessary to produce the MR image (Fig. 13-42).

The operator interface and computer systems vary with the manufacturer, but most consist of a computer system, dedicated processor for Fourier transformation, image processor to form the image, disk drives for storage of raw data and pulse sequence parameters, and a power distribution system to distribute and filter the direct and alternating current. The operator's console is located outside of the scan room, and provides the interface to the hardware and software for data acquisition.

13.8 Magnet Siting, Quality Control

Magnet Siting

Superconductive magnets produce extensive magnetic fringe fields, and create potentially hazardous conditions in adjacent areas. In addition, extremely small signal amplitudes generated by the protons in the body during an imaging procedure have a frequency common to commercial FM broadcasts. Thus, two requirements must

MRI system components

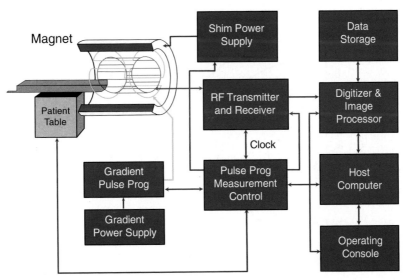

■ **FIGURE 13-42** A block diagram of a typical MRI system shows the components and interfaces between subsystems. Not shown is the **Faraday cage that surrounds the magnet assembly** to eliminate environmental RF noise.

be considered for MR system siting: protect the local environment from the magnet system and protect the magnet from the local environment.

Fringe fields from a high field strength magnet can extend quite far—roughly equal to αB_0, where α is a constant dependent on the magnet bore size and magnet configuration. Fringe fields can potentially cause a disruption of electronic signals and sensitive electronic devices. An unshielded 1.5-T magnet has a 1-mT fringe field at a distance of approximately 9.3 m, a 0.5-mT field at 11.5 m, and a 0.3-mT field at 14.1 m from the center of the magnet. Magnetic shielding is one way to reduce fringe field interactions in adjacent areas. Passive (e.g., thick metal walls close to the magnet) and active (e.g., electromagnet systems strategically placed in the magnet housing) magnetic shielding systems permit a significant reduction in the extent of the fringe fields for high field strength, air core magnets (Fig. 13-43). Patients with pacemakers or ferromagnetic aneurysm clips must avoid fringe fields above 0.5 mT. Magnetically sensitive equipment such as image intensifiers, gamma cameras, and color TVs are severely impacted by fringe fields of less than 0.3 mT, as electromagnetic focusing in these devices is disrupted.

Administrative control for magnetic fringe fields is 0.5 mT, requiring controlled access to areas that exceed this level. Magnetic fields below 0.5 mT are considered safe for the patient population. Disruption of the fringe fields can reduce the homogeneity of the active imaging volume. Any large metallic object (elevator, automobile, etc.) traveling through the fringe field can produce such an effect.

Environmental RF noise must be reduced to protect the extremely sensitive receiver within the magnet from interfering signals. The typical approach for stray RF signal protection is the construction of a Faraday cage, an internal enclosure consisting of RF attenuating copper sheet and/or copper wire mesh. The room containing the MRI system is typically lined with copper sheet (walls) and mesh (windows). This is a costly construction item but provides effective protection from stray RF noise (Fig. 13-44).

Field Uniformity

In addition to magnetic field strength, field uniformity is an important characteristic, expressed in parts per million (ppm) over a given volume, such as 40 cm^3. This is based upon the precessional frequency of the proton, which is determined from the

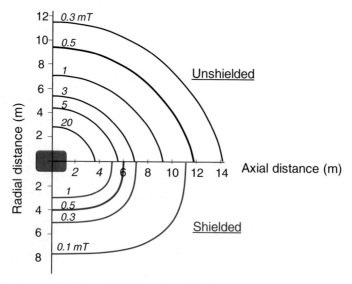

■ **FIGURE 13-43** An unshielded (top half of diagram) and shielded (bottom half of diagram) 1.5 T magnet and the magnetic fringe field strengths plotted with radial distance (vertical axis) and axial distance (horizontal axis).

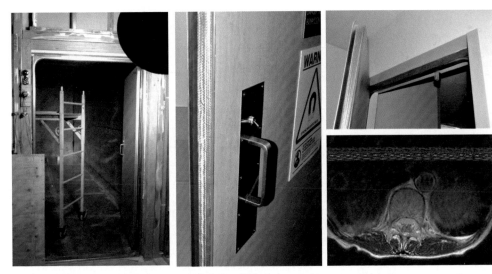

■ **FIGURE 13-44** The MR scanner room requires protection from extraneous radiofrequency signals. This is achieved with the installation of a "Faraday cage" comprised of copper sheet that lines the inner walls of the room (**left**), copper mesh covering the operator viewing window (not shown), and a copper lined door and doorjamb with an inflatable bladder conductor (note switch above the door handle) to seal the door (**middle and upper right**). A leak in the Faraday cage will result in RF artifacts that will occur at specific frequencies as streaks across the image, perpendicular to the FEG direction. (**Lower right**. FEG is vertical, PEG is horizontal.)

proton gyromagnetic ratio. At 1.5 T, the precessional frequency is 1.5 T × 42.58 MHz/T = 63.8 MHz = 63.8 × 10^6 cycles/s, and a specification of 2 ppm homogeneity (2×10^{-6}) gives a frequency uniformity of about 128 cycles/s (Hz) over the volume. Typical homogeneities range from less than 1 ppm for a small FOV (e.g. 150 mm) to greater than 10 ppm for a large FOV (e.g., 400 mm). Field uniformity is achieved by manipulating the main field peripherally with passive and active "shim" coils, which exist in proximity to the main magnetic field. These coils interact with the fringe fields and adjust the variation of the central magnetic field.

Quality Control

Like any imaging system, the MRI scanner is only as good as the weakest link in the imaging chain. The components of the MR system that must be periodically checked include the magnetic field strength, magnetic field homogeneity, system field shimming, gradient linearity, system RF tuning, receiver coil optimization, environmental noise sources, power supplies, peripheral equipment, and control systems among others. A QC program should be designed to assess the basic day-to-day functionality of the scanner. A set of QC tests is listed in Table 13-4. Qualitative and quantitative measurements of system performance should be obtained on a periodic basis, with a test frequency dependent on the likelihood of detecting a change in the baseline values outside of normal operating limits.

The American College of Radiology has an MRI accreditation program that specifies requirements for system operation, QC, and the training requirements of technologists, radiologists, and physicists involved in scanner operation. The accreditation process evaluates the qualifications of personnel, equipment performance, effectiveness of QC procedures, and quality of clinical images—factors that are consistent with the maintenance of a state-of-the-art facility.

TABLE 13-4 RECOMMENDED QC TESTS FOR MRI SYSTEMS

High-contrast spatial resolution
Slice thickness accuracy
Slice position accuracy
RF center frequency tuning
Geometric accuracy and spatial uniformity
Signal uniformity
Low-contrast resolution (sensitivity)
Image artifact evaluation
Operational controls (e.g., table movement control and alignment lighting checks)
Preventive maintenance logging and documentation
Review of system log book and operations

MRI phantoms are composed of materials that produce MR signals with carefully defined relaxation times. Some materials are aqueous paramagnetic solutions; pure gelatin, agar, silicone, or agarose; and organic doped gels, paramagnetic doped gels, and others. Water is most frequently used, but it is necessary to adjust the T1 and T2 relaxation times of (doped) water, so that images can be acquired using pulse sequence timing for patients (e.g., this is achieved by adding nickel, aqueous oxygen, aqueous manganese, or gadolinium). For example, the ACR MR Accreditation phantom (Fig. 13-45) is a cylindrical phantom of 190 mm inside diameter and 148 mm inside length. It is filled with a 10 millimolar solution of nickel chloride and 75 millimolar sodium chloride. Inside the phantom are several structures that are used in a variety of tests for scanner performance. In this phantom, seven quantitative tests are made by scanning the phantom with specific instructions, and include geometric accuracy, high contrast spatial resolution, slice thickness accuracy, slice position accuracy, image intensity uniformity, percent signal ghosting, and low-contrast object detectability. Details

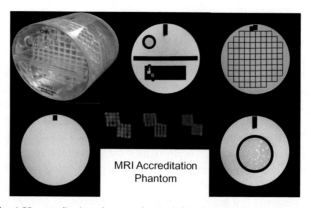

■ **FIGURE 13-45** The ACR accreditation phantom (upper left) and selected images scanned from the phantom are shown above. Upper middle is the spatial resolution module, and just below is a magnification image of the test targets. The upper right shows the geometric distortion module, the lower right is the low contrast sensitivity module, and the lower left is the uniformity module. Not all images are shown; specific details are described in the accreditation documentation available on the ACR website, http://www.acr.org.

on measurement analysis, recommended action criteria, and causes of failure/corrective action are included in the guidance. Some phantoms have standards with known T1, T2, and proton density values to evaluate the quantitative accuracy of the scanner, and to determine the ability to achieve an expected contrast level for a given pulse sequence. Homogeneity phantoms determine the spatial uniformity of transmit and receive RF magnetic fields. Ideal performance is a spatially uniform excitation of the protons and a spatially uniform sensitivity across the imaged object.

13.9 MR Bioeffects and Safety

Although ionizing radiation is not used with MRI and MRS, perception of the general public is that MR is a very safe modality, safety aspects are often an afterthought, particularly in terms of operational activities and training of personnel who work in the area and around the magnet. There are very many important bioeffects and safety issues to be considered for MR. These include the presence of strong magnetic fields, RF energy, time-varying magnetic gradient fields, cryogenic liquids, a confined imaging device (claustrophobia), and noisy operation (gradient coil activation and deactivation, creating acoustic noise). Patients with implants, prostheses, aneurysm clips, pacemakers, heart valves, etc., should be aware of considerable torque on the devices which when placed in the magnetic field, could cause serious adverse effects. Nonmetallic implant materials can also lead to significant heating under rapidly changing gradient fields. Consideration of the distortions and artifacts on the acquired images and possibility of misdiagnosis are also a concern. Ferromagnetic materials inadvertently brought into the imaging room (e.g., an IV pole) are attracted to the magnetic field and can become a deadly projectile to the occupant within the bore of the magnet. Many unfortunate deaths have been attributed to carelessness and lack of a safety culture around an MR scanner. Signage exists in three categories to help identify MR-compatible materials. "MR safe" is a square green sign, and is put on materials and objects that are wholly nonmetallic; "not MR safe" is round red, and is placed on all ferromagnetic and many conducting metals; "MR conditional" signage is triangular yellow, placed on objects that may or may not be safe until further investigation is performed. These signs are shown in Figure 13-46.

In extreme emergencies, the superconducting magnet can be turned off by a manually controlled "quench" procedure. Even under the best circumstances, the quench procedure subjects the magnet to a 260 degrees temperature difference in a short period of time. If performed too quickly, major physical damage to the magnet

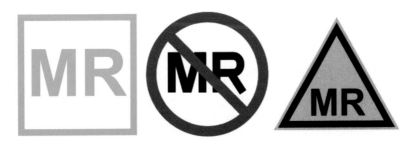

■ FIGURE 13-46 MR labeling includes on the left, MR safe materials that have been found not to interact with the strong MR field or disrupt operation; in the middle, NOT MR safe labels that contraindicate bringing materials with this designation past Zone 2 (see discussion later in this section; on the right, more consideration required before bringing such labeled objects into the scan room).

TABLE 13-5   MRI SAFETY GUIDELINES

ISSUE	PARAMETER	VARIABLES	SPECIFIED VALUE
Static magnetic field	Magnetic field (B_0)	Maximum strength	3.0 T
	Inadvertent exposure	Maximum	0.0005 T
Changing magnetic field (dB/dt)	Axial gradients	$\tau > 120$ µs	<20 T/s
		12 µs $< \tau <$ 120 µs	<2400/τ (µs) T/s
		$\tau < 12$ µs	<200 T/s
	Transverse gradients		<3× axial gradients
	System		<6 T/s
RF power deposition	Temperature	Core of body	<18°C
		Maximum head	<38°C
		Maximum trunk	<39°C
		Maximum extremities	<40°C
	Specific absorption rate (SAR)	Whole body (average)	<4 W/kg
		Head (average)	<3 W/kg
		Head or torso per gram	<8 W/kg
		Extremities per gram	<12 W/kg
Acoustic noise levels		Peak pressure	200 pascals
		Average pressure	105 dBA

τ rise time of gradients.
[a]In some clinical applications, higher field strengths (e.g., 4.0 T) are allowed.

can occur. Because of risks to personnel, equipment, and physical facilities, manual quenches should only be initiated after careful considerations and preparation. Uncontrolled quenching is the result of a sudden loss of superconductivity in the main magnet coils, which can result in the explosive conversion of liquid helium to gas, and jeopardize the safety of those in the room and adjacent areas. In the event of insufficient gas outflow, oxygen can be displaced and build up of pressure in the room can prevent the entry door from being easily opened.

MRI is considered "safe" when used within the regulatory guidelines required of the manufacturers by the Food and Drug Administration (Table 13-5). Serious bioeffects are demonstrated with static and varying magnetic fields at strengths significantly higher (10 to 20 times greater) than those used for typical diagnostic imaging.

Static Magnetic Fields

The long-term biologic effects of high magnetic field strengths are not well known. At lower magnetic field strengths, there have not been any reports of deleterious or nonreversable biologic effects, either acute or chronic. With very high field strength magnets (e.g., 4 T or higher), there has been anecdotal mention of dizziness and disorientation of personnel and patients as they move through the field. With systems in excess of 20 T, enzyme kinetic changes have been documented, increased membrane permeability shown, and altered biopotentials have been measured. These effects have not been demonstrated in magnetic fields below 10 T. Effects on ECG traces have shown an increased amplitude of the *T* wave, presumably due to the magneto-hemodynamic effect, caused by conductive fluid such as blood moving across a magnetic field. When this occurs, sometimes the elevated *T* wave will be mistaken for the desired *R* wave, creating an insufficient gating situation. For this reason, it is recommended that ECG leads are not used for patient monitoring, but rather an alternative such as pulse oximetry be used.

Varying Magnetic Field Effects

The time-varying magnetic fields encountered in the MRI system are due to the gradient switching used for localization of the protons. Magnetic fields that vary their strength with time are generally of greater concern than static fields because oscillating magnetic fields can induce electrical current flow in conductors. The maximum allowed changing gradient fields depend on the rise times of the gradients, as listed in Table 13-5. At extremely high levels of magnetic field variation, effects such as visual phosphenes (the sensation of flashes of light being seen) can result because of induced currents in the nerves or tissues. Other consequences such as bone healing and cardiac fibrillation have been suggested in the literature. The most common bioeffect of MR systems is tissue heating caused by RF energy deposition and/or by rapid switching of high strength gradients. RF coils and antennas can present burn hazards when electrical currents and conductive loops are present, and must have proper insulation—both electrical and thermal.

RF Exposure, Acoustic Noise Limits, Specific Absorption Rate

RF exposure causes heating of tissues. There are obvious effects of overheating, and therefore a power deposition limit is imposed by governmental regulations on the manufacturers for various aspects of MRI and MRS operation. Table 13-5 lists some of the categories and the maximum values permitted for clinical use. The rationale for imposing limits on static and varying magnetic fields is based on the ability of the resting body to dissipate heat buildup caused by the deposition and absorption of thermal energy. Other indicators, such as acoustic noise levels and pressure amplitudes, are determined from limits that are shown to have reversible (unaffected) outcomes for clinically approved sequences. Hearing protection should always be available to the patient. For research sequences and procedures that have not been approved by the FDA, patients or volunteers are to have hearing protection in place.

Pregnancy-related Issues and Pediatric Patient Concerns

Pregnant healthcare staff and physicians are permitted to work in and around the MR environment throughout all stages of pregnancy and assist as needed in setting up the patient and the exam. However, they are not to remain in the magnet scanning room (Zone 4). Regarding the scanning of pregnant patients, current data have not yielded any deleterious effects on the developing fetus with common examinations, and no special considerations are warranted, as long as the benefit-risk-ratio of doing the study is that for any other typical patient. Another consideration is the administration of contrast, which should not be routinely provided. A well-documented consideration to administer contrast based on the overwhelming potential benefit to the patient or fetus relative to the risk of exposing them to gadolinium-based agents and potential deleterious effects of free gadolinium ions, as there are studies that have documented that the agents do pass the placental barrier and do enter the fetus.

For pediatric patients, the largest issues are sedation and monitoring. Special attention to sedation protocols, adherence to standards of care regarding sedation guidelines, and monitoring patients during the scan with MR-safe temperature monitoring and isolation transport units are crucial to maintaining patient safety.

MR Personnel and MR Safety Zones

The American College of Radiology has published a white paper describing the recommendations for MR safety in general, and MR safety "zones" and MR personnel definitions in particular in their 2007 publication (ACR white paper reference). MR safety policies, procedures, and safe practices are suggested in the guidance. In an effort to maintain a buffer zone around the "always on" magnet, MR safety zones are categorized from Zone 1 to Zone 4. Zone 1 is the area freely accessible to the general public, in essence everywhere outside of the MR magnet area and building. Zone 2 represents the interface between Zone 1 and Zone 3—typically the reception area, where patients are registered and MR screening questions take place. Zone 3 is a restricted area comprised of the MR control room and computer room that only specific personnel can access, namely, those specifically trained as MR personnel (described below) and appropriately screened patients and other individuals (nurses,

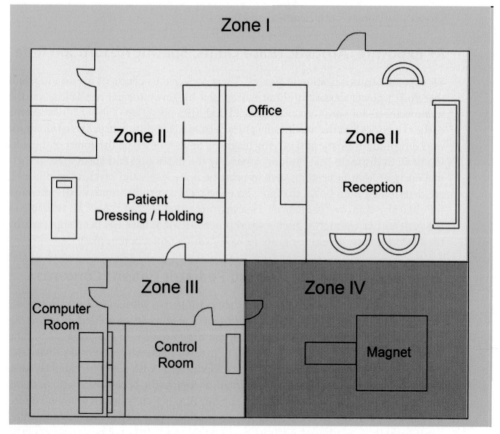

■ FIGURE 13-47 Zoning concept for describing areas in an MR system environment include Zone 1, unrestricted access; Zone 2, interface between unrestricted and restricted areas; Zone 3, restricted area only allowed for MR personnel and screened individuals; Zone 4, the area of the scanner and high magnetic field strength. (Adapted from Kanal E., et.al. Guidance Document for Safe MR Practices: 2007.)

support staff). Zone 4 represents the MR magnet room, and is always located within the confines of Zone 3. Demarcation of these zones should be clearly marked and identified. Figure 13-47 illustrates the zoning concept.

Furthermore, there are personnel definitions describing criteria that must be achieved before access can be granted to Zone 3 and Zone 4 areas. *Non-MR personnel* are patients, visitors, for staff who do not have the appropriate education or training that meet the criteria for Level 1 or Level 2 MR personnel. *Level 1 MR personnel* have passed minimal safety and education training on MR safety issues and have a basic understanding of the effects of MR magnets, dangers of projectiles, effects of strong magnetic fields, etc. These individuals can work in Zone 3 and Zone 4 areas without supervision or oversight; examples are MR office staff, patient aides, and custodial staff. *Level 2 MR personnel* are more extensively trained in the broader aspects of MR safety issues, for example, understanding the potential for thermal loading, burns, neuromuscular excitation, and induced currents from gradients. These individuals are the gatekeepers of access into Zone 4, and take the action and the leadership role in the event of a patient code, ensuring that only properly screened support staff are allowed access. Those responding to a code must be made aware of and comply with MR safety protocols. Examples of personnel designated as Level 2 include MR technologists, MR medical physicists, radiologists, and department nursing staff.

Designated personnel are required to continuously maintain their safety credentials, by acquiring continuous education credits throughout the year on MR safety aspects, and taking an annual test and achieving a minimum passing score.

Summary

Meeting the needs of the MR exam and using the equipment safely and effectively requires the understanding of the basic physics underpinnings described in Chapter 12, and the details of advanced acquisition methods, image characteristics, artifacts/pitfalls, and MR safety/bioeffects covered in this chapter. The reader is encouraged to keep up with the rapid developments of MRI and MRS by referring to recent literature and websites dedicated to MRI education and technological advances.

REFERENCES AND SUGGESTED READINGS

American College of Radiology MRI Accreditation Program, Phantom Test Guidance and other documentation for the MRI accreditation program, available at http://www.acr.org/accreditation/mri/mri_qc_forms.aspx, accessed May 30, 2011.

Hendrick RE. *Breast MRI: fundamentals and technical aspects.* New York, NY: Springer, 2007.

Kanal E, Barkovich AJ, Bell C, et.al. ACR guidance document for safe MR practices: 2007. *AJR Am J Roentgenol.* 2007;188:1–27.

NessAiver M. *All you really need to know about MRI physics.* Baltimore, MD: Simply Physics, 1997.

Al-Okaili RN, Krejza J, Wang S, Woo JH, Melhem ER. *Advanced MR Imaging Techniques in the Diagnosis of Intraaxial Brain Tumors in Adults.* Radiographics 2006; 26: S173-S189.

Westbrook C, Kaut-Roth C, Talbot J. *MRI in practice.* 3rd ed. Malden, MA: Blackwell Publishing, 2005.

CHAPTER 14

Ultrasound

Ultrasound is the term that describes sound waves of frequencies exceeding the range of human hearing and their propagation in a medium. Medical diagnostic ultrasound is a modality that uses ultrasound energy and the acoustic properties of the body to produce an image from stationary and moving tissues. In ultrasound imaging, a short pulse of mechanical energy is delivered to the tissues. The pulse travels at the speed of sound, and with changes in the tissue acoustic properties, a fraction of the pulse is reflected as an echo that returns to the source. Collection of the echoes over time and recording of the echo amplitudes provide information about the tissues along the path of travel. Repeating the process hundreds of times with a small incremental change in the direction of the pulse interrogates a volume, from which a gray-scale tomographic image can be synthesized. Generation of the sound pulses and detection of the echoes are accomplished with a transducer, which also directs the ultrasound pulse along a linear path through the patient. Along a given beam path, the depth of an echo-producing structure is determined from the time between the pulse emission and the echo return, and the amplitude of the echo is encoded as a gray-scale value (Fig. 14-1). In addition to two-dimensional (2D) tomographic imaging, ultrasound provides anatomical distance and volume measurements, motion studies, blood velocity measurements, and 3D imaging.

Historically, medical uses of ultrasound came about shortly after the close of World War II, derived from underwater sonar research. Initial clinical applications monitored changes in the propagation of pulses through the brain to detect intracerebral hematoma and brain tumors based upon the displacement of the midline. Ultrasound rapidly progressed through the 1960s from simple "A-mode" scans to "B-mode" applications and compound "B-scan" images using analog electronics. Advances in equipment design, data acquisition techniques, and data processing capabilities have led to electronic transducer arrays, digital electronics, and real-time image display. This progress is changing the scope of ultrasound and its applications in diagnostic radiology and other areas of medicine. High-resolution, real-time imaging, harmonic imaging, 3D data acquisition, and power Doppler are a few of the innovations introduced into clinical practice. Contrast agents for better delineation of the anatomy, measurement of tissue perfusion, precise drug delivery mechanisms, and determination of elastic properties of the tissues are examples of current research.

The characteristics, properties, and production of ultrasound are described, followed by modes of ultrasound interaction, instrumentation, and image acquisition methods. Signal processing and image display methods show how the ultrasound image is produced, and how evaluation of the blood velocity through Doppler techniques is achieved. Types of image artifacts that can occur, quality control (QC) tests, and potential ultrasound bioeffects complete the overview.

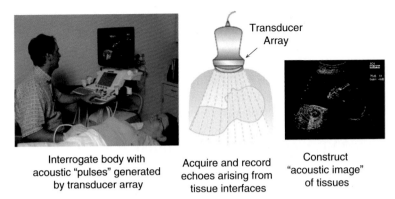

| Interrogate body with acoustic "pulses" generated by transducer array | Acquire and record echoes arising from tissue interfaces | Construct "acoustic image" of tissues |

■ **FIGURE 14-1** A major use of ultrasound is the acquisition and display of the acoustic properties of tissues. A transducer array (transmitter and receiver of ultrasound pulses) directs sound waves into the patient, receives the returning echoes, and converts the echo amplitudes into a 2D tomographic image using the ultrasound acquisition system. Exams requiring a high level of safety such as obstetrics are increasing the use of ultrasound in diagnostic radiology. Photo credit: Emi Manning UC Davis Health System.

 ## Characteristics of Sound

Propagation of Sound

Sound is mechanical energy that propagates through a continuous, elastic medium by the compression and rarefaction of "particles" that comprise it. A simple model of an elastic medium is that of a spring, as shown in Figure 14-2. Compression is caused by a mechanical deformation induced by an external force (such as a plane piston), with a resultant increase in the pressure of the medium. Rarefaction occurs following the compression event—as the backward motion of the piston reverses the force, the compressed particles transfer their energy to adjacent particles with a subsequent reduction in the local pressure amplitude. The section of the spring in contact with the piston then stretches and becomes decompressed (a rarefaction), while the compression continues to travel forward. With continued back-and-forth motion of the piston, a

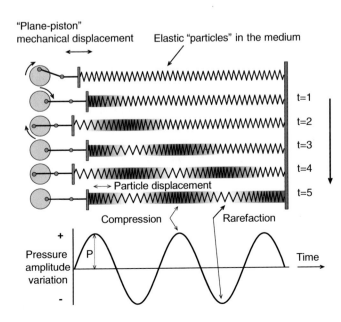

■ **FIGURE 14-2** Ultrasound energy is generated by a mechanical displacement in compressible medium, which is modeled as an elastic spring. Energy propagation is shown as a function of time, resulting in areas of compression and rarefaction with corresponding variations in positive and negative pressure amplitude, *P* (lower diagram). Particles in the medium have only minor displacement as the wave front passes.

series of compressions and rarefactions propagate through the continuous medium (the spring). Any change with respect to position in the elasticity of the spring disturbs the wave train and causes some or all of the energy to be reflected. While the medium itself is necessary for mechanical energy transfer (i.e., sound propagation), the constituent "particles" of the medium act only to transfer mechanical energy; these particles experience only very small back-and-forth displacements. Energy propagation occurs as a wave front in the direction of energy travel, known as a longitudinal wave.

Wavelength, Frequency, and Speed

The *wavelength* (λ) of the ultrasound energy is the distance (usually expressed in units of *mm* or *μm*) between compressions or rarefactions, or between any two points that repeat on the sinusoidal wave of pressure amplitude (see Fig. 14-2). The *frequency* (f) is the number of times the wave oscillates through one cycle each second (s). Sound waves with frequencies less than 15 cycles per second (Hz) are called infrasound, and the range between 15 Hz and 20 kHz comprises the audible acoustic spectrum. Ultrasound represents the frequency range above 20 kHz. Medical ultrasound uses frequencies in the range of 2 to 10 MHz, with specialized ultrasound applications up to 50 MHz. The *period* is the time duration of one wave cycle and is equal to $1/f$, where f is expressed in cycles/s. The *speed of sound* is the distance traveled by the wave per unit time and is equal to the wavelength divided by the period. Since period and frequency are inversely related, the relationship between speed, wavelength, and frequency for sound waves is

$$c = \lambda f$$

where c (*m/s*) is the speed of sound in the medium, λ (*m*) is the wavelength, and f (cycles/s) is the frequency.

The speed of sound is dependent on the propagation medium and varies widely in different materials. The wave speed is determined by the ratio of the bulk modulus (B) (a measure of the stiffness of a medium and its resistance to being compressed) and the density (ρ) of the medium:

$$c = \sqrt{\frac{B}{\rho}}$$

SI units are kg/(m-s^2), kg/m^3, and *m/s* for B, ρ and c, respectively. A highly compressible medium, such as air, has a low speed of sound, while a less compressible medium, such as bone, has a higher speed of sound. A less dense medium has a higher speed of sound than a denser medium (e.g., dry air versus humid air). The speeds of sound in materials encountered in medical ultrasound are listed in Table 14-1. Of major importance is the average speed for "soft tissue" (1,540 *m/s*), fatty tissue (1,450 *m/s*), and air (330 *m/s*). The difference in the speed of sound at tissue boundaries is a fundamental property that generates echoes (and contrast) in an ultrasound image. Medical ultrasound machines use a speed of sound of 1,540 *m/s* when determining localization of reflectors and creating the acoustic image. The speed of sound in soft tissue can be expressed in different units; besides 1,540 *m/s*, most common are 154,000 *cm/s* and 1.54 *mm/μs*, which are often helpful in simplifying conversion factors or estimating values.

The ultrasound frequency is unaffected by changes in sound speed as the acoustic beam propagates through different media. Thus, the ultrasound wavelength is dependent on the medium. Examples of the wavelength change as a function of frequency and propagation medium are given below.

TABLE 14-1   DENSITY AND SPEED OF SOUND IN TISSUES AND MATERIALS FOR MEDICAL ULTRASOUND

MATERIAL	DENSITY (kg/m³)	c (m/s)	c (mm/µs)
Air	1.2	330	0.33
Lung	300	600	0.60
Fat	924	1,450	1.45
Water	1,000	1,480	1.48
"Soft Tissue"	1,050	1,540	1.54
Kidney	1,041	1,565	1.57
Blood	1,058	1,560	1.56
Liver	1,061	1,555	1.55
Muscle	1,068	1,600	1.60
Skull bone	1,912	4,080	4.08
PZT	7,500	4,000	4.00

EXAMPLE: A 2-MHz beam has a wavelength in soft tissue of

$$\lambda = \frac{c}{f} = \frac{1540\ m/s}{2 \times 10^6/s} = 770 \times 10^{-6}\ m = 7.7 \times 10^{-4}\ m \times 1000 \frac{mm}{m} = 0.77\ mm$$

A 10-MHz ultrasound beam has a corresponding wavelength in soft tissue of

$$= \frac{1540\ m/s}{10 \times 10^6/s} = 154 \times 10^{-6}\ m = 1.54 \times 10^{-4}\ m \times 1000 \frac{mm}{m} \cong 0.15\ mm$$

Higher frequency sound has shorter wavelength, as shown in Figure 14-3.

EXAMPLE: A 5-MHz beam travels from soft tissue into fat. Calculate the wavelength in each medium, and determine the percent wavelength change.

In soft tissue,

$$\lambda = \frac{c}{f} = \frac{1540\ m/s}{5 \times 10^6/s} = 3.08 \times 10^{-6}\ m \cong 0.31\ mm$$

In fat,

$$= \frac{1450\ m/s}{5 \times 10^6/s} = 2.9 \times 10^{-6}\ m \cong 0.29\ mm$$

A *decrease* in wavelength of 5.8% occurs in going from soft tissue into fat, due to the differences in the speed of sound. This is depicted in Figure 14-3 for a 5-MHz ultrasound beam.

The wavelength in mm in soft tissue can be calculated directly by dividing the speed of sound in mm/µs (c = 1,540 m/s = 1.54 mm/µs) by the frequency in MHz, as

$$\lambda(mm,\ soft\ tissue) = \frac{c}{f} = \frac{1.54\ mm/\mu s}{f(MHz)} = \frac{1.54\ mm/10^{-6}\ s}{f(10^6/s)} = \frac{1.54\ mm}{f\ (MHz)}$$

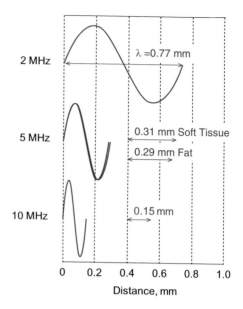

■ **FIGURE 14-3** Ultrasound wavelength is determined by the frequency and the speed of sound in the propagation medium. Wavelengths in soft tissue are calculated for 2-, 5-, and 10-MHz ultrasound sources for soft tissue (**blue**). A comparison of wavelength in fat (**purple**) to soft tissue at 5 MHz is also shown.

Thus, it can quickly be determined that the wavelength of a 10-MHz beam is 0.154 mm, and that of a 1-MHz beam is 1.54 mm by using this simple change in units.

The spatial resolution of the ultrasound image and the attenuation of the ultrasound beam energy depend on the wavelength and frequency, respectively. Ultrasound wavelength affects the spatial resolution achievable along the direction of the beam. A high-frequency ultrasound beam (small wavelength) provides better resolution and image detail than a low-frequency beam; however, the depth of beam penetration is significantly reduced at higher frequency. Ultrasound frequencies used for imaging are therefore selected according to the imaging application. For body parts requiring greater travel distance of the sound waves (e.g., abdominal imaging), lower frequency ultrasound is used (3.5 to 5 MHz) to image structures at significant depths. For small body parts or organs close to the skin surface (e.g., thyroid, breast), higher frequency ultrasound is selected (7.5 to 10 MHz). Most medical imaging applications use ultrasound frequencies in the range of 2 to 10 MHz.

Modern ultrasound equipment consists of multiple sound transmitters aligned in an array that create sound beams independently. Interaction of two or more separate ultrasound beams in a medium can result in *constructive* and/or *destructive wave interference*, as shown in Figure 14-4. The amount of constructive or destructive interference depends on several factors, but the most important are the phase (position of the periodic wave with respect to a reference point) and amplitude of the interacting beams. With phase differences occurring because of the distances between individual transmitters and time of transmitter excitation, all of the individual beams' interactions can generate complex interference patterns, which are very important in shaping and steering the composite ultrasound beam.

Pressure, Intensity, and the *dB* Scale

Sound energy causes particle displacements and variations in local pressure amplitude, P, in the propagation medium. Pressure amplitude is defined as the peak maximum or peak minimum value from the average pressure on the medium in the absence of a sound wave. In the case of a symmetrical waveform, the positive and

Wave interference patterns

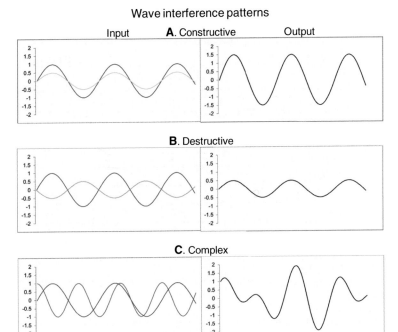

■ **FIGURE 14-4** Interaction of waves in a propagation medium, plotted as amplitude versus time. **A.** Constructive interference occurs with two ultrasound waves of the same frequency and phase, resulting in a higher amplitude output wave. **B.** Destructive interference occurs with the waves 180 degrees out-of-phase, resulting in a lower amplitude output wave. **C.** Complex interference occurs when waves of slightly different frequency interact, resulting in an output waveform of higher and lower amplitude.

negative pressure amplitudes are equal (lower portion of Fig. 14-2); however, in most diagnostic ultrasound applications, the compressional amplitude significantly exceeds the rarefactional amplitude. The SI unit of pressure is the Pascal (Pa), defined as one Newton per square meter (N/m²). The average atmospheric pressure on earth at sea level is approximately equal to 100,000 Pa. Diagnostic ultrasound beams typically deliver peak pressure levels that exceed ten times the earth's atmospheric pressure, or about one MPa (mega Pascal).

Intensity, I, is the amount of power (energy per unit time) per unit area and is proportional to the square of the pressure amplitude, $I \propto P^2$. Medical diagnostic ultrasound intensity levels are described in units of milliwatts/cm^2—the amount of energy per unit time per unit area. The absolute intensity level depends upon the method of ultrasound production (e.g., pulsed or continuous—a discussion of these parameters can be found in Section 14.11 of this chapter). Relative intensity and pressure levels are described as a logarithmic ratio, the *decibel (dB)*. The relative intensity in *dB* for intensity ratios is calculated as

$$\text{relative intensity (dB)} = 10 \log \left(\frac{I_2}{I_1} \right)$$

where I_1 and I_2 are intensity values that are compared as a *relative measure*, and "log" denotes the base 10 logarithm. In diagnostic ultrasound, the ratio of the intensity of the incident pulse to that of the returning echo can span a range of one million times or more. The logarithm function compresses the large and expands the small ratios into a more manageable number range. An intensity ratio of 10^6 (e.g., an incident intensity

TABLE 14-2   INTENSITY RATIO AND CORRESPONDING DECIBEL VALUES

INTENSITY RATIO		DECIBELS (dB)
I_2/I_1	LOG (I_2/I_1)	
1	0	0
2	0.3	3
10	1	10
100	2	20
10,000	4	40
1,000,000	6	60
0.5	−0.3	−3
0.01	−2	−20
0.0001	−4	−40
0.000001	−6	−60

one million times greater than the returning echo intensity) is equal to 60 *dB*, whereas an intensity ratio of 10^2 is equal to 20 *dB*. A change of 10 in the *dB* scale corresponds to an order of magnitude (10 times) change in intensity; a change of 20 corresponds to two orders of magnitude (100 times) change, and so forth. When the intensity ratio is greater than one (e.g., the incident ultrasound intensity to the detected echo intensity), the *dB* values are positive; when less than one, the *dB* values are negative. A loss of 3 *dB* (−3 *dB*) represents a 50% loss of signal intensity. The tissue thickness that reduces the ultrasound intensity by 3 *dB* is considered the "half-value" thickness (HVT). In Table 14-2, intensity ratios, logarithms, and the corresponding intensity dB values are listed.

EXAMPLE: Calculate the remaining intensity of a 100 mW ultrasound pulse that loses 30 dB while traveling through tissue.

$$\text{relative intensity } (dB) = 10 \log \frac{I_2}{I_1} ; \qquad \text{defining equation}$$

$$-30 \ dB = 10 \log \frac{I_2}{100 \text{ mW}} ; \qquad \text{divide each side of the equation by 10:}$$

$$-3 = \log \frac{I_2}{100 \text{ mW}} ; \qquad \text{exponentiate using base 10}$$

$$10^{-3} = \frac{I_2}{100 \text{ mW}} ; \qquad \text{solve for } I_2 :$$

$$I_2 = 0.001 \times 100 \text{ mW} = 0.1 \text{ mW}$$

14.2   Interactions of Ultrasound with Matter

Ultrasound interactions are determined by the acoustic properties of matter. As ultrasound energy propagates through a medium, interactions include reflection, refraction, scattering, and absorption. *Reflection* occurs at tissue boundaries where there is a difference in the *acoustic impedance* of adjacent materials. When the incident beam is perpendicular to the boundary, a fraction of the beam (an echo) returns directly back to the source; the transmitted fraction of the beam continues in the initial direction. For non-normal incidence, the incident angle is that made relative to normal incidence; the reflected angle is equal to the incident angle. *Refraction* describes the change in direction of the transmitted ultrasound energy with nonperpendicular incidence. *Scattering* occurs by reflection or refraction, usually by small particles within the tissue medium, causes the beam to diffuse in many directions, and gives rise to the characteristic texture and gray scale in the acoustic image. *Attenuation* refers to the loss of intensity of the ultrasound beam from absorption and scattering in the medium. *Absorption* is the process whereby acoustic energy is converted to heat energy, whereby, sound energy is lost and cannot be recovered.

Acoustic Impedance

The acoustic impedance (Z) of a material is defined as

$$Z = \rho c$$

where ρ is the density in kg/m^3 and c is the speed of sound in m/s. The SI unit for acoustic impedance is $kg/(m^2 s)$, with the special name the *rayl*, where 1 rayl is equal to $1 \ kg/(m^2 s)$. Table 14-3 lists the acoustic impedances of materials and tissues commonly encountered in medical ultrasonography. In a simplistic way, the acoustic impedance can be likened to the stiffness and flexibility of a compressible medium such as a spring, as mentioned at the beginning of this chapter. When springs with different compressibility are connected together, the energy transfer from one spring to another depends mainly on stiffness. A large difference in the stiffness results in a large reflection of energy, an extreme example of which is a spring attached to a wall. Minor differences in stiffness or compressibility allow the continued propagation of energy, with little reflection at the interface. Sound propagating through a patient behaves similarly. Soft tissue adjacent to air-filled lungs represents a large difference in acoustic impedance; thus, ultrasonic energy incident on the lungs from soft tissue is almost entirely reflected. When adjacent tissues have similar acoustic impedances, only minor reflections of the incident energy occur. Acoustic impedance gives rise to differences in transmission and reflection of ultrasound energy, which is the means for producing an image using pulse-echo techniques.

TABLE 14-3 ACOUSTIC IMPEDANCE, Z = ρc, FOR AIR, WATER, AND SELECTED TISSUES

TISSUE	Z (RAYLS)
Air	0.0004×10^6
Lung	0.18×10^6
Fat	1.34×10^6
Water	1.48×10^6
Kidney	1.63×10^6
Blood	1.65×10^6
Liver	1.65×10^6
Muscle	1.71×10^6
Skull bone	$7.8 \ \times 10^6$

Reflection

The reflection of ultrasound energy at a boundary between two tissues occurs because of the differences in the acoustic impedances of the two tissues. The reflection coefficient describes the fraction of sound intensity incident on an interface that is reflected. For perpendicular incidence (Fig. 14-5A), the *intensity* reflection coefficient, R_I, is expressed as

$$R_I = \frac{I_r}{I_i} = \left(\frac{Z_2 - Z_1}{Z_2 + Z_1}\right)^2$$

The subscripts 1 and 2 represent tissues proximal and distal to the boundary. The intensity transmission coefficient, T_I, is defined as the fraction of the incident intensity that is transmitted across an interface. With conservation of energy, the intensity transmission coefficient is $T_I = 1 - R_I$. For a fat-muscle interface, the intensity reflection and transmission coefficients are calculated as

$$R_{I,\,(Fat \rightarrow Muscle)} = \frac{I_r}{I_i} = \left(\frac{1.71 - 1.34}{1.71 + 1.34}\right)^2 = 0.015; \quad T_{I,\,(Fat \rightarrow Muscle)} = 1 - R_{I,\,(Fat \rightarrow Muscle)} = 0.985$$

The actual intensity reflected or transmitted at a boundary is the product of the incident intensity and the reflection coefficient. For example, an intensity of 40 mW/cm^2 incident on a boundary with $R_I = 0.015$ reflects $40 \times 0.015 = 0.6$ mW/cm^2. The intensity reflection coefficient at a tissue interface is readily calculated from the acoustic impedance of each tissue. Examples of tissue interfaces and respective reflection coefficients are listed in Table 14-4. For a typical muscle-fat interface, approximately 1% of the ultrasound intensity is reflected, and thus almost 99% of the intensity is transmitted to greater depths in the tissues. At a muscle-air interface, nearly 100% of incident intensity is reflected, making anatomy unobservable beyond an air-filled cavity. This is why acoustic coupling gel must be used between the face of the transducer and the skin to eliminate air pockets. A conduit of tissue that allows ultrasound transmission through structures such as the lung is known as an "acoustic window."

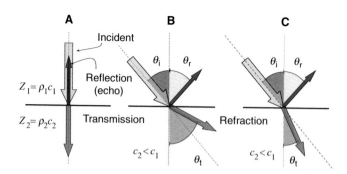

■ FIGURE 14-5 Reflection and refraction of ultrasound occur at tissue boundaries with differences in acoustic impedance, Z. **A.** With perpendicular incidence (90 degrees), a fraction of the beam is transmitted and a fraction of the beam is reflected to the source at a tissue boundary. **B.** With nonperpendicular incidence, (90 degrees), the reflected fraction of the beam is directed away from the transducer at an angle $\theta_r = \theta_i$ and the transmitted fraction of the beam is refracted in the transmission medium at a transmitted refraction angle greater than the incident angle ($\theta_t > \theta_i$) when $c_2 > c_1$. **C.** Refraction angle of the transmitted beam is less than that of the incident angle when $c_1 > c_2$.

TABLE 14-4 PRESSURE AND REFLECTION COEFFICIENTS FOR VARIOUS INTERFACES

TISSUE INTERFACE	PRESSURE REFLECTION	INTENSITY REFLECTION
Liver-Kidney	−0.006	0.00003
Liver-Fat	−0.10	0.011
Fat-Muscle	0.12	0.015
Muscle-Bone	0.64	0.41
Muscle-Lung	−0.81	0.65
Muscle-Air	−0.99	0.99

When the beam is perpendicular to the tissue boundary, the sound is returned back to the transducer as an echo. As sound travels from a medium of lower acoustic impedance into a medium of higher acoustic impedance, the reflected wave experiences a 180-degree phase shift in pressure amplitude, as shown by the negative sign on the pressure amplitude values in Table 14-4. (Note: the reflected pressure amplitude is calculated as the ratio of the difference divided by the sum of the acoustic impedances.)

The above discussion assumes a "smooth" interface between tissues, where the wavelength of the ultrasound beam is much greater than the structural variations of the boundary. With higher frequency ultrasound beams, the wavelength becomes smaller, and the boundary no longer appears smooth. In this case, returning echoes are diffusely scattered throughout the medium, and only a small fraction of the incident intensity returns to the ultrasound transducer.

For nonperpendicular incidence at an angle θ_i (Fig. 14-5B,C), the ultrasound energy is reflected at an angle θ_r equal to the incident angle, $\theta_i = \theta_r$. Echoes are directed away from the source of ultrasound and are thus undetected.

Refraction

Refraction describes the change in direction of the transmitted ultrasound energy at a tissue boundary when the beam is not perpendicular to the boundary. Ultrasound frequency does not change when propagating through various media, but a change in the speed of sound may occur. Angles of incidence, reflection, and transmission are measured relative to the normal incidence on the boundary, as shown in Figure 14-5B,C. The angle of refraction (θ_t) is determined by the speed of sound change that occurs at the boundary and is related to the angle of incidence (θ_i) by Snell's law:

$$\frac{\sin\theta_t}{\sin\theta_i} = \frac{c_2}{c_1}$$

where θ_i and θ_t are the incident and transmitted angles, c_1 and c_2 are the speeds of sound in medium 1 and 2, and medium 2 carries the transmitted ultrasound energy. For small angles of incidence and transmission, Snell's law can be approximated as

$$\frac{\theta_t}{\theta_i} \cong \frac{c_2}{c_1}$$

When $c_2 > c_1$, the angle of transmission is greater than the angle of incidence as shown in Figure 14-5B, and the opposite when $c_2 < c_1$, as shown in Figure 14-5C. No refraction occurs when the speed of sound is the same in the two media, or with perpendicular incidence. This straight-line propagation is assumed in ultrasound signal processing, and when refraction does occur, misplacement of anatomy in the image can result.

A situation called total reflection occurs when $c_2 > c_1$ and the angle of incidence of the sound beam with the boundary between two media exceeds an angle called the critical angle. In this case, the sound beam does not penetrate the second medium at all but travels along the boundary. The critical angle (θ_c) is calculated by setting $\theta_t = 90$ degree in Snell's law (equation above), producing the equation $\sin\theta_c = c_1/c_2$.

Scattering

Acoustic scattering arises from objects and interfaces within a tissue that are about the size of the wavelength or smaller and represent a rough or *nonspecular reflector* surface, as shown in Figure 14-6. Most organs have a characteristic structure that gives rise to a defined scatter "signature" and provides much of the diagnostic information contained in the ultrasound image. A *specular reflector* is a smooth boundary between two media, where the dimensions of the boundary are much larger than the wavelength of the incident ultrasound energy. Because nonspecular reflectors reflect sound in all directions, the amplitudes of the returning echoes are significantly weaker than echoes from tissue boundaries. Fortunately, the dynamic range of the ultrasound receiver is sufficient to detect echo information over a wide range of amplitudes. Intensities of returning echoes from nonspecular reflectors in the tissue parenchyma are not greatly affected by beam direction, unlike the strong directional dependence of specular reflectors. Parenchyma-generated echoes typically have similar echo strengths and gray-scale levels in the image. Differences in scatter amplitude that occur from one region to another cause corresponding brightness changes on the ultrasound display.

In general, the echo signal amplitude from the insonated tissues depends on the number of scatterers per unit volume, the acoustic impedance differences at the scatterer interfaces, the sizes of the scatterers, and the ultrasonic frequency. Hyperechoic (higher scatter amplitude) and hypoechoic (lower scatter amplitude) are terms used for describing the scatter characteristics relative to the average background signal. Hyperechoic areas usually have greater numbers of scatterers, larger acoustic impedance differences, and larger scatterers. Acoustic scattering from nonspecular reflectors increases with frequency, while specular reflection is relatively independent

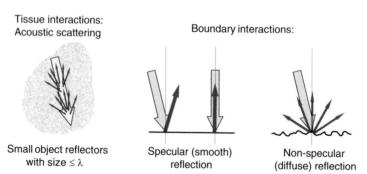

■ FIGURE 14-6 Ultrasound scattering. Small particle reflectors within a tissue or organ cause a diffuse scattering pattern that is characteristic of the particle size, giving rise to specific tissue or organ "signatures." Boundary interactions with ultrasound can also scatter the beam, particularly at higher frequencies. Specular and nonspecular boundary characteristics are partially dependent on the wavelength of the incident ultrasound. As the wavelength becomes smaller, the boundary becomes "rough," resulting in scattering from the surface because of nonperpendicular boundaries.

TABLE 14-5   ATTENUATION COEFFICIENTS FOR SELECTED TISSUES AT 1 MHz

TISSUE COMPOSITION	ATTENUATION COEFFICIENT (1-MHz BEAM, *dB/cm*)
Water	0.0002
Blood	0.18
Soft tissues	0.3–0.8
Brain	0.3–0.5
Liver	0.4–0.7
Fat	0.5–1.8
Smooth muscle	0.2–0.6
Tendon	0.9–1.1
Bone, cortical	13–26
Lung	40

of frequency. It is often possible to enhance the scattered echo signals over the specular echo signals by using higher ultrasound frequencies.

Attenuation

Ultrasound attenuation, the loss of acoustic energy with distance traveled, is caused chiefly by scattering and tissue absorption of the incident beam. Absorbed acoustic energy is converted to heat in the tissue. The *attenuation coefficient, μ,* expressed in units of *dB/cm*, is the relative intensity loss per centimeter of travel for a given medium. Tissues and fluids have widely varying attenuation coefficients, as listed in Table 14-5 for a 1-MHz ultrasound beam. Ultrasound attenuation expressed in *dB* is approximately proportional to frequency. An approximate rule of thumb for "soft tissue" is 0.5 *dB* per *cm* per MHz or 0.5 (*dB/cm*)/MHz. The product of the ultrasound frequency (in MHz) with 0.5 (*dB/cm*)/MHz gives the approximate attenuation coefficient in *dB/cm*. Thus, a 2-MHz ultrasound beam will have approximately twice the attenuation of a 1-MHz beam; a 10-MHz beam will have *ten times* the attenuation per unit distance. Since the *dB* scale progresses logarithmically, the beam intensity is exponentially attenuated with distance (Fig. 14-7). The ultrasound *HVT* is the thickness of tissue necessary to attenuate the incident intensity by 50%, which is equal to a 3 *dB* reduction in intensity. As the frequency increases, the HVT decreases, as demonstrated by the examples below.

EXAMPLE 1: Calculate the approximate intensity HVT in soft tissue for ultrasound beams of 2 and 10 MHz. Determine the number of HVTs the incident beam and the echo travel at a 6-*cm* depth.

Answer: Information needed is (1) the attenuation coefficient approximation 0.5 (*dB/cm*)/MHz and (2) the HVT intensity expressed as a 3 *dB* loss. Given this information, the HVT in soft tissue for a *f* MHz beam is

$$HVT_{f(MHz)} \ (cm) = \frac{3 \ dB}{attenuation\,coefficient\,(dB\,/\,cm)} = \frac{3 \ dB}{\frac{0.5(dB\,/\,cm)}{MHz} \times f(MHz)} = \frac{6}{f}$$

$$HVT_{2\,MHz}\ (cm) = \frac{3\ dB}{\dfrac{0.5\ (dB/cm)}{MHz} \times 2\ MHz} = 3\ cm$$

$$HVT_{10\,MHz}\ (cm) = \frac{6}{10} = 0.6\ cm$$

Number of HVTs:

A 6-cm depth requires a *travel distance* of 12 cm (round-trip).

For a 2-MHz beam, this is 12 $cm/(3\ cm\ /HVT_{2\,MHz}) = 4\ HVT_{2\,MHz}$.

For a 10-MHz beam, this is 12 $cm/(0.6\ cm/HVT_{10\,MHz}) = 20\ HVT_{10\,MHz}$.

EXAMPLE 2: Calculate the approximate intensity loss of a 5-MHz ultrasound wave traveling round-trip to a depth of 4 cm in the liver and reflected from an encapsulated air pocket (100% reflection at the boundary).

Answer: Using 0.5 *dB/*(cm-MHz) for a 5-MHz transducer, the attenuation coefficient is 2.5 *dB/cm*. The total distance traveled by the ultrasound pulse is 8 *cm* (4 *cm* to the depth of interest and 4 *cm* back to the transducer). Thus, the total attenuation is 2.5 *dB/cm* × 8 *cm* = 20 *dB* The incident intensity relative to the returning intensity (100% reflection at the boundary) is

$$20\ dB = 10\ \log(\frac{I_{Incident}}{I_{Echo}})$$

$$2 = \log(\frac{I_{Incident}}{I_{Echo}})$$

$$10^2 = \frac{I_{Incident}}{I_{Echo}}\ \text{Therefore,}\ I_{Incident} = 100\ I_{Echo}$$

The echo intensity is one-hundredth of the incident intensity in this example, or −20 dB. If the boundary reflected 1% of the incident intensity (a typical value), the returning echo intensity would be (100/0.01) or 10,000 times *less* than the incident intensity, or −40 dB. Considering the depth and travel distance of the ultrasound energy, the detector system must have a dynamic range of 120 to 140 dB to be sensitive to acoustic signals generated in the medium. When penetration to deeper structures is important, lower frequency ultrasound transducers must be used. Another

■ **FIGURE 14-7** Ultrasound attenuation occurs exponentially with penetration depth and increases with increased frequency. The plots are estimates of a single frequency ultrasound wave with an attenuation coefficient of (0.5 dB/cm)/MHz of ultrasound intensity versus penetration depth. Note that the total distance traveled by the ultrasound pulse and echo is twice the penetration depth.

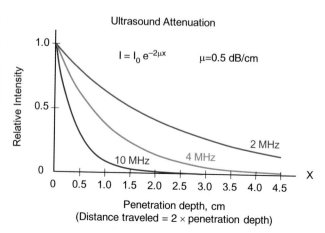

Ultrasound Attenuation

$I = I_0\ e^{-2\mu x}$ $\mu=0.5\ dB/cm$

10 MHz   4 MHz   2 MHz

Relative Intensity

Penetration depth, cm
(Distance traveled = 2 × penetration depth)

consequence of frequency-dependent attenuation is the preferential removal of the highest frequency components in a broadband ultrasound pulse (discussed below in Section 14.3) and a shift to lower frequencies.

14.3 Ultrasound Transducers

Ultrasound is produced and detected with a *transducer*, comprised of one or more ceramic elements with electromechanical properties and peripheral components. The ceramic element converts electrical energy into mechanical energy to produce ultrasound and mechanical energy into electrical energy for ultrasound detection. Over the past several decades, the transducer assembly has evolved considerably in design, function, and capability, from a single-element resonance crystal to a broadband transducer array of hundreds of individual elements. A simple single-element, plane-piston source transducer is illustrated in Figure 14-8. Major components include the piezoelectric material, matching layer, backing block, acoustic absorber, insulating cover, tuning coil, sensor electrodes, and transducer housing.

Piezoelectric Materials

A piezoelectric material (often a crystal or ceramic) is the functional component of the transducer. It converts electrical energy into mechanical (sound) energy by physical deformation of the crystal structure. Conversely, mechanical pressure applied to its surface creates electrical energy. Piezoelectric materials are characterized by a well-defined molecular arrangement of electrical dipoles, as shown in Figure 14-9. Electrical dipoles are molecular entities containing positive and negative electric charges that have an overall neutral charge. When mechanically compressed by an externally applied pressure, the alignment of the dipoles is disturbed from the equilibrium position to cause an imbalance of the charge distribution. A potential difference (voltage) is created across the element with one surface maintaining a net positive charge and one surface a net negative charge. Surface electrodes measure the magnitude of voltage, which is proportional to the incident mechanical pressure amplitude. Conversely, application of an external voltage through conductors attached to the surface electrodes induces the mechanical expansion and contraction of the transducer element.

Piezoelectric materials are available from natural and synthetic materials. An example of a natural piezoelectric material is quartz crystal, commonly used in watches and other timepieces to provide a mechanical vibration source at 32.768 kHz for interval timing. (This is one of several oscillation frequencies of quartz, determined by the

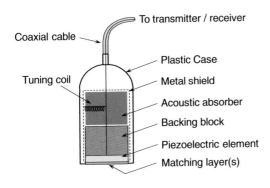

To transmitter / receiver

Coaxial cable

Plastic Case

Tuning coil

Metal shield

Acoustic absorber

Backing block

Piezoelectric element

Matching layer(s)

■ **FIGURE   14-8** A single-element ultrasound transducer assembly is comprised of the piezoelectric ceramic, the backing block, acoustic absorber, tuning coil and metal shield, transducer housing, coaxial cable and voltage source, and the ceramic to tissue matching layer.

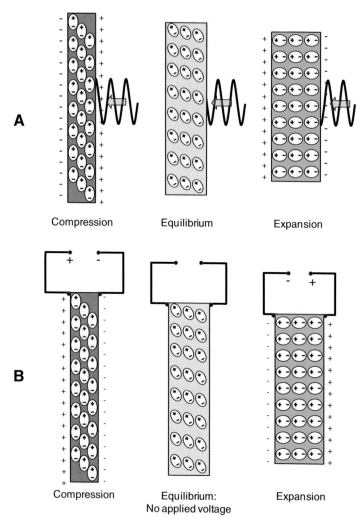

■ **FIGURE 14-9** The piezoelectric element is comprised of aligned molecular dipoles. **A.** Under the influence of mechanical pressure from an adjacent medium (e.g., an ultrasound echo), the element thickness contracts (at the peak pressure amplitude), achieves equilibrium (with no pressure), or expands (at the peak rarefactional pressure) causing realignment of the electrical dipoles to produce positive and negative surface charge. Surface electrodes (not shown) measure the charge variation (voltage) as a function of time **B.** An external voltage source applied to the element surfaces causes compression or expansion from equilibrium by realignment of the dipoles in response to the electrical attraction or repulsion force.

crystal cut and machining properties.) Ultrasound transducers for medical imaging applications employ a synthetic piezoelectric ceramic, most often *lead-zirconate-titanate* (PZT)—a compound with the structure of molecular dipoles. The piezoelectric attributes are attained after a process of molecular synthesis, heating, orientation of internal dipole structures with an applied external voltage, cooling to permanently maintain the dipole orientation, and cutting into a specific shape. For PZT in its natural state, no piezoelectric properties are exhibited; however, heating the material past its "Curie temperature" (e.g., 328°C to 365°C) and applying an external voltage causes the dipoles to align in the ceramic. The external voltage is maintained until the material has cooled to below its Curie temperature. Once the material has cooled, the dipoles retain their alignment. At equilibrium, there is no net charge on ceramic

Reflection

The reflection of ultrasound energy at a boundary between two tissues occurs because of the differences in the acoustic impedances of the two tissues. The reflection coefficient describes the fraction of sound intensity incident on an interface that is reflected. For perpendicular incidence (Fig. 14-5A), the *intensity* reflection coefficient, R_1, is expressed as

$$R_1 = \frac{I_r}{I_i} = \left(\frac{Z_2 - Z_1}{Z_2 + Z_1}\right)^2$$

The subscripts 1 and 2 represent tissues proximal and distal to the boundary. The intensity transmission coefficient, T_1, is defined as the fraction of the incident intensity that is transmitted across an interface. With conservation of energy, the intensity transmission coefficient is $T_1 = 1 - R_1$ For a fat-muscle interface, the intensity reflection and transmission coefficients are calculated as

$$R_{1,\,(Fat\rightarrow Muscle)} = \frac{I_r}{I_i} = \left(\frac{1.71-1.34}{1.71+1.34}\right)^2 = 0.015;\ \ T_{1,\,(Fat\rightarrow Muscle)} = 1 - R_{1,\,(Fat\rightarrow Muscle)} = 0.985$$

The actual intensity reflected or transmitted at a boundary is the product of the incident intensity and the reflection coefficient. For example, an intensity of 40 mW/*cm²* incident on a boundary with $R_1 = 0.015$ reflects 40 × 0.015 = 0.6 mW/*cm²*. The intensity reflection coefficient at a tissue interface is readily calculated from the acoustic impedance of each tissue. Examples of tissue interfaces and respective reflection coefficients are listed in Table 14-4. For a typical muscle-fat interface, approximately 1% of the ultrasound intensity is reflected, and thus almost 99% of the intensity is transmitted to greater depths in the tissues. At a muscle-air interface, nearly 100% of incident intensity is reflected, making anatomy unobservable beyond an air-filled cavity. This is why acoustic coupling gel must be used between the face of the transducer and the skin to eliminate air pockets. A conduit of tissue that allows ultrasound transmission through structures such as the lung is known as an "acoustic window."

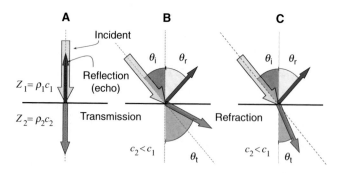

■ **FIGURE 14-5** Reflection and refraction of ultrasound occur at tissue boundaries with differences in acoustic impedance, Z. **A.** With perpendicular incidence (90 degrees), a fraction of the beam is transmitted and a fraction of the beam is reflected to the source at a tissue boundary. **B.** With nonperpendicular incidence, (90 degrees), the reflected fraction of the beam is directed away from the transducer at an angle $\theta_r = \theta_i$ and the transmitted fraction of the beam is refracted in the transmission medium at a transmitted refraction angle greater than the incident angle $(\theta_t > \theta_i)$ when $c_2 > c_1$. **C.** Refraction angle of the transmitted beam is less than that of the incident angle when $c_1 > c_2$.

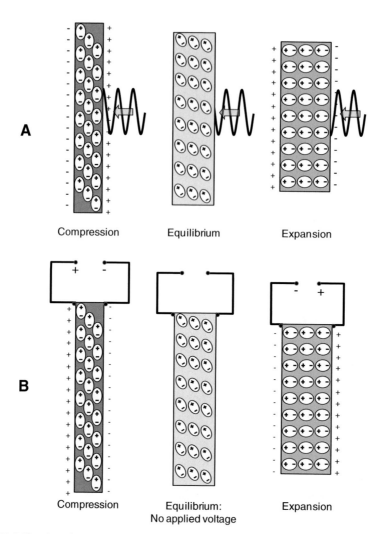

A

Compression   Equilibrium   Expansion

B

Compression   Equilibrium: Expansion
                     No applied voltage

■ **FIGURE 14-9** The piezoelectric element is comprised of aligned molecular dipoles. **A.** Under the influence of mechanical pressure from an adjacent medium (e.g., an ultrasound echo), the element thickness contracts (at the peak pressure amplitude), achieves equilibrium (with no pressure), or expands (at the peak rarefactional pressure) causing realignment of the electrical dipoles to produce positive and negative surface charge. Surface electrodes (not shown) measure the charge variation (voltage) as a function of time **B.** An external voltage source applied to the element surfaces causes compression or expansion from equilibrium by realignment of the dipoles in response to the electrical attraction or repulsion force.

crystal cut and machining properties.) Ultrasound transducers for medical imaging applications employ a synthetic piezoelectric ceramic, most often *lead-zirconate-titanate* (PZT)—a compound with the structure of molecular dipoles. The piezoelectric attributes are attained after a process of molecular synthesis, heating, orientation of internal dipole structures with an applied external voltage, cooling to permanently maintain the dipole orientation, and cutting into a specific shape. For PZT in its natural state, no piezoelectric properties are exhibited; however, heating the material past its "Curie temperature" (e.g., 328°C to 365°C) and applying an external voltage causes the dipoles to align in the ceramic. The external voltage is maintained until the material has cooled to below its Curie temperature. Once the material has cooled, the dipoles retain their alignment. At equilibrium, there is no net charge on ceramic

f_0 is determined by the transducer thickness equal to ½ λ

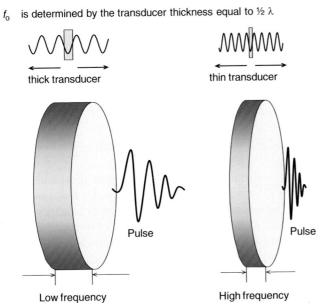

thick transducer

thin transducer

Low frequency

High frequency

Pulse

Pulse

■ **FIGURE 14-10** A short-duration voltage spike causes the resonance piezoelectric element to vibrate at its natural frequency, f_0, which is determined by the thickness of the transducer equal to ½ λ. Low-frequency oscillation is produced with a thicker piezoelectric element. The spatial pulse length (SPL) is a function of the operating frequency and the adjacent damping block.

surfaces. When compressed, an imbalance of charge produces a voltage between the surfaces. Similarly, when a voltage is applied between electrodes attached to both surfaces, mechanical deformation occurs, as illustrated in Figure 14-9A,B.

Resonance Transducers

Resonance transducers for pulse-echo ultrasound imaging operate in a "resonance" mode, whereby a voltage (usually 150 V) of very short duration (a voltage spike of ~1 μs) is applied, causing the piezoelectric material to initially contract and then subsequently vibrate at a natural resonance frequency. This frequency is selected by the "thickness cut" of the PZT, due to the preferential emission of ½-wavelength ultrasound waves in the piezoelectric material as illustrated in Figure 14-10. The operating frequency is determined from the speed of sound in, and the thickness of, the piezoelectric material. For example, a 5-MHz transducer will have a wavelength in PZT (speed of sound in PZT is ~4,000 m/s) of

$$\lambda = \frac{c}{f} = \frac{4{,}000\,m/s}{5\times10^6/s} = 8 \times 10^4\,m = 0.8\,mm$$

To achieve the 5-MHz resonance frequency, a transducer element thickness of ½ × 0.8 mm = 0.4 mm is required. Higher frequencies are achieved with thinner elements, and lower frequencies with thicker elements. Resonance transducers transmit and receive preferentially at a single "center frequency."

Damping Block

The damping block, layered on the back of the piezoelectric element, absorbs the backward directed ultrasound energy and attenuates stray ultrasound signals from the housing. This component also dampens the transducer vibration to create an ultrasound pulse with a short spatial pulse length (SPL), which is necessary to preserve detail along the beam axis (axial resolution). Dampening of the vibration (also known as "ring-down") lessens the purity of the resonance frequency and introduces a broadband frequency spectrum. With ring-down, an increase in the bandwidth (range of frequencies) of the ultrasound pulse occurs by introducing higher and lower frequencies above and below the center (resonance) frequency. The "Q factor" describes the bandwidth of the sound emanating from a transducer as

$$Q = \frac{f_0}{\text{bandwidth}}$$

where f_0 is the center frequency and the bandwidth is the width of the frequency distribution.

A "high Q" transducer has a narrow bandwidth (i.e., very little damping) and a corresponding long SPL. A "low Q" transducer has a wide bandwidth and short SPL. Imaging applications require a broad bandwidth transducer in order to achieve high spatial resolution along the direction of beam travel. Blood velocity measurements by Doppler instrumentation (explained in Section 14.9) require a relatively narrow-band transducer response in order to preserve velocity information encoded by changes in the echo frequency relative to the incident frequency. Continuous-wave ultrasound transducers have a very high Q characteristic. An example of a "high Q" and "low Q" ultrasound pulse illustrates the relationship to SPL in Figure 14-11. While the Q factor is derived from the term "quality factor," a transducer with a low Q does not imply poor quality in the signal.

Matching Layer

The *matching layer* provides the interface between the raw transducer element and the tissue and minimizes the acoustic impedance differences between the transducer and the patient. It consists of layers of materials with acoustic impedances that are intermediate to soft tissue and the transducer material. The thickness of each layer is equal to ¼ wavelength, determined from the center operating frequency of the

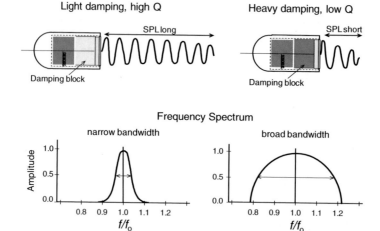

■ **FIGURE 14-11** Effect of damping block on the frequency spectrum. The damping block is adjacent to the backside of the transducer and limits the vibration of the element to a small number of cycles. Light damping allows many cycles to occur (**top left**), which results in an extended SPL (number of cycles times the wavelength) and a narrow frequency bandwidth (range of frequencies contained in the pulse (**bottom left**). Heavy damping reduces the SPL and broadens the frequency bandwidth (**top and bottom right**). The Q factor describes the center frequency divided by the bandwidth.

transducer and speed characteristics of the matching layer. For example, the wavelength of sound in a matching layer with a speed of sound of 2,000 *m/s* for a 5-MHz ultrasound beam is 0.4 *mm*. The optimal matching layer thickness is equal to ¼ λ = ¼ × 0.4 *mm* = 0.1 *mm*. In addition to the matching layer, acoustic coupling gel (with acoustic impedance similar to soft tissue) is used between the transducer and the skin of the patient to eliminate air pockets that could attenuate and reflect the ultrasound beam.

Nonresonance (Broad Bandwidth) "Multifrequency" Transducers

Modern transducer design coupled with digital signal processing enables "multifrequency" or "multihertz" transducer operation, whereby the center frequency can be adjusted in the transmit mode. Unlike the resonance transducer design, the piezoelectric element is intricately machined into a large number of small "rods" and then filled with an epoxy resin to create a smooth surface (Fig. 14-12). The acoustic properties are closer to tissue than a pure PZT material and thus provide a greater transmission efficiency of the ultrasound beam without resorting to multiple matching layers. Broadband multifrequency transducers have bandwidths that exceed 80% of the center frequency (Fig. 14-12B).

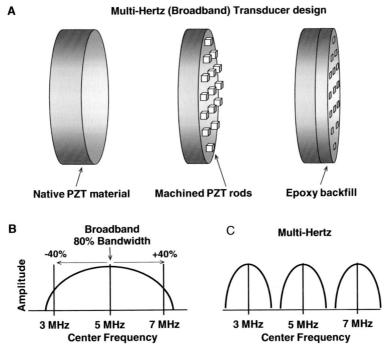

■ **FIGURE 14-12 A.** "Multi-Hertz" broadband transducer elements are created from a native piezoelectric material into multiple small "rods" with epoxy backfill. This creates a ceramic element with acoustic characteristics closer to soft tissue and produces frequencies with very broad bandwidth. **B.** Bandwidth is often described as a percentage of the center frequency. The graph shows an 80% bandwidth (±40%) for a 5-MHz frequency transducer (3- to 7-MHz operational sensitivity). **C.** Multi-Hertz operation depends on the broad bandwidth transducer element to be sensitive to a range of returning frequencies during the reception of echoes with subsequent digital signal processing to select the bandwidth(s) of interest.

Excitation of the multifrequency transducer is accomplished with a short square wave burst of approximately 150 V with one to three cycles, unlike the voltage spike used for resonance transducers. This allows the center frequency to be selected within the limits of the transducer bandwidth. Likewise, the broad bandwidth response permits the reception of echoes within a wide range of frequencies. For instance, ultrasound pulses can be produced at a low frequency, and the echoes received at higher frequency. "Harmonic imaging" is a recently introduced technique that uses this ability—lower frequency ultrasound is transmitted into the patient, and the higher frequency harmonics (e.g., two times the transmitted center frequency), created from the interaction with contrast agents and tissues, are received as echoes. Native tissue harmonic imaging has certain advantages including greater depth of penetration, noise and clutter removal, and improved lateral spatial resolution. Operational characteristics of multihertz transducers and harmonic imaging are explained in Section 14.7.

Transducer Arrays

The majority of ultrasound systems employ transducers with many individual rectangular piezoelectric elements arranged in linear or curvilinear arrays. Typically, 128 to 512 individual rectangular elements comprise the transducer assembly. Each element has a width typically less than ½ wavelength and a length of several millimeters. Two modes of activation are used to produce a beam. These are the "linear" (sequential) and "phased" activation/receive modes as illustrated in Figure 14-13.

Linear Arrays

Linear array transducers typically contain 256 to 512 elements; physically these are the largest transducer assemblies. In operation, the simultaneous firing of a small group of approximately 20 adjacent elements produces the ultrasound beam. The simultaneous activation produces a synthetic aperture (effective transducer width) defined by the number of active elements. Echoes are detected in the receive mode by acquiring signals from most of the transducer elements. Subsequent "A-line" (see Section 14.5) acquisition occurs by firing another group of transducer elements displaced by one or two elements. A rectangular field of view (FOV) is produced with this transducer arrangement. For a curvilinear array, a trapezoidal FOV is produced.

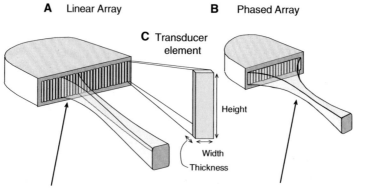

■ **FIGURE 14-13** Multielement transducer arrays. **A.** A linear (or curvilinear) array produces a beam by firing a subset of the total number of transducer elements as a group. **B.** A phased array produces a beam from all of the transducer elements fired with fractional time delays in order to steer and focus the beam. **C.** The transducer element in an array has a thickness, width, and height; the width is typically on the order of ½ wavelength; and the height depends on the transducer design and slice-thickness requirements.

Phased Arrays

A phased-array transducer is usually comprised of 64 to 128 individual elements in a smaller package than a linear array transducer. All transducer elements are activated nearly simultaneously to produce a single ultrasound beam. By using time delays in the electrical activation of the discrete elements across the face of the transducer, the ultrasound beam can be steered and focused electronically without physically moving the transducer on the patient. During ultrasound signal reception, all of the transducer elements detect the returning echoes from the beam path, and sophisticated detection algorithms synthesize the data to form the image.

Capacitive Micromachined Ultrasonic Transducers

Another method of producing high-frequency ultrasound is with the use of capacitive micromachined ultrasound transducers (CMUT), which bring the fabrication technology of integrated circuits into the field of medical ultrasound. These devices, first investigated in the early 1990s, are silicon-based electrostatic transducers, recently shown to be competitive with the lead-zirconate-titanate for producing and receiving ultrasonic data for patient imaging. The basic element of a CMUT is a capacitor cell with a fixed electrode (backplate) and a free electrode (membrane). The principle of operation is electrostatic transduction, whereby an alternating voltage is applied between the membrane and the backplate, and the modulation of the electrostatic force results in membrane vibration with the generation of ultrasound. Conversely, when the membrane is subject to an incident ultrasound wave, the capacitance change can be detected as a current or a voltage signal. For signal detection, a direct current bias voltage must be used in the reception for signal detection and for transmission for linear operation of the array. Fabrication of these transducers with precisely controlled geometric and mechanical properties is possible with microfabrication technologies in the megahertz range; lateral dimensions of the membranes are on the order of 10 microns and a thickness of about 1 to 2 μm. Because of precise micromachining, the electrode separation is made small, which enables high electric fields inside the gap and an ability to have high transduction efficiency.

The main advantages of CMUT arrays compared to PZT are better acoustic matching with the propagation medium, which allows wider bandwidth capabilities, improved resolution, potentially lower costs with easier fabrication, and the ability to have integrated circuits on the same "wafer." CMUT arrays feature improved axial resolution; however, further improvements in both sensitivity and resolution are needed to fully compete with piezoelectric arrays, especially in areas where high depth of penetration is required. Future 2D arrays show much promise in leading ultrasound to improvements in efficiency, speed, multibandwidth operation, and volumetric imaging. These transducers will certainly have an impact on the ultrasound imaging systems of the future.

 ## Ultrasound Beam Properties

The ultrasound beam propagates as a longitudinal wave from the transducer surface into the propagation medium, and exhibits two distinct beam patterns: a slightly converging beam out to a distance determined by the geometry and frequency of the transducer (the near field), and a diverging beam beyond that point (the far field). For an unfocused, single-element transducer, the distance of the near field is determined by the transducer diameter and the frequency of the transmitted sound

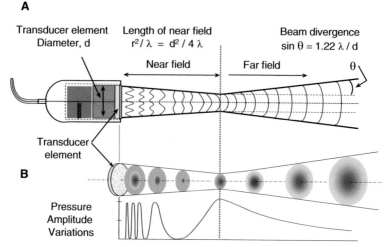

A

Transducer element Length of near field Beam divergence
Diameter, d $r^2 / \lambda = d^2 / 4\lambda$ $\sin \theta = 1.22 \, \lambda / d$

Near field Far field

Transducer element

B

Pressure Amplitude Variations

■ **FIGURE 14-14 A.** The ultrasound beam from a single, circular transducer element is characterized by the near field as a converging beam and far field as a diverging beam. **B.** Pressure amplitude variations in the near field are quite complex and rapidly changing, while in the far field are monotonically decreasing.

(Fig. 14-14). For multiple transducer element arrays, an "effective" transducer diameter is determined by the excitation of a group of transducer elements. Because of the interactions of each of the individual beams and the ability to focus and steer the overall beam, the formulas for a single-element, unfocused transducer are not directly applicable.

The Near Field

The near field, also known as the Fresnel zone, is adjacent to the transducer face and has a converging beam profile. Beam convergence in the near field occurs because of multiple constructive and destructive interference patterns of the ultrasound waves from the transducer surface. "Huygens' principle" describes a large transducer surface as an infinite number of point sources of sound energy where each point is characterized as a radial emitter. As individual wave patterns interact, the peaks and troughs from adjacent sources constructively and destructively interfere causing the beam profile to be tightly collimated in the near field. The ultrasound beam path is thus largely confined to the dimensions of the active portion of the transducer surface, with the beam diameter converging to approximately half the transducer diameter at the end of the near field. The near field length is dependent on the transducer diameter and propagation wavelength:

$$\text{Near Field Length} = \frac{d^2}{4\lambda} = \frac{r^2}{\lambda};$$

where d is the transducer diameter, r is the transducer radius, and λ is the wavelength of ultrasound in the propagation medium. In soft tissue, $\lambda = \dfrac{1.54 \; mm}{f \; (\text{MHz})}$, and the near field length can be expressed as a function of diameter and frequency:

$$\text{Near Field Length (soft tissue)} = \frac{d^2 (mm^2) \; f(\text{MHz})}{4 \times 1.54 \; mm}$$

This equation indicates that the near field distance is increased as the physical diameter and the operation frequency of the transducer are increased. Lateral resolution (the ability of the system to resolve objects in a direction perpendicular to the beam direction) is dependent on the beam diameter and is best at the end of the near field for a single-element transducer. Lateral resolution is poor in areas close to and far from the transducer surface.

Pressure amplitude characteristics in the near field are very complex, caused by the constructive and destructive interference wave patterns of the ultrasound beam. Peak ultrasound pressure occurs at the end of the near field, corresponding to the minimum beam diameter for a single-element transducer. Pressures vary rapidly from peak compression to peak rarefaction several times during transit through the near field. Only when the far field is reached do the ultrasound pressure variations decrease continuously (Fig. 14-14B).

The Far Field

The far field is also known as the Fraunhofer zone and is where the beam diverges. For a large-area single-element transducer, the angle of ultrasound beam divergence, θ, for the far field is given by

$$\sin \theta = 1.22 \frac{\lambda}{d}$$

where d is the effective diameter of the transducer and λ is the wavelength. Less beam divergence occurs with high-frequency, large-diameter transducers. Unlike the near field, where beam intensity varies from maximum to minimum to maximum in a converging beam, ultrasound intensity in the far field decreases monotonically with distance.

Transducer Array Beam Formation and Focusing

In a transducer array, the narrow piezoelectric element width (typically between one-half to one wavelength) produces a diverging beam at a distance very close to the transducer face. Formation and convergence of the ultrasound beam occur with the operation of several or all of the transducer elements at the same time. Transducer elements in a linear array that are fired simultaneously produce an effective transducer width equal to the sum of the widths of the individual elements. Individual beams interact via "constructive" and "destructive" interference to produce a collimated beam that has properties similar to the properties of a single transducer of the same size. With a phased-array transducer, the beam is formed by interaction of the individual wave fronts from each transducer, each with a slight difference in excitation time. Minor phase differences of adjacent beams form constructive and destructive wave summations that "steer" or "focus" the beam profile.

Transmit Focus

For a single transducer or group of simultaneously fired transducers in a linear array, the focal distance is a function of the transducer diameter, the center operating frequency, and the presence of any acoustic lenses attached to the element surface. This focal depth is unchangeable. Phased array transducers and many linear array transducers allow a selectable focal distance by applying specific timing delays between transducer elements that cause the beam to converge at a specified distance. A shallow focal zone (close to the transducer surface) is produced by firing outer transducers in the array before the inner transducers in a symmetrical pattern, as shown in Figure 14-15. Greater focal distances are achieved by reducing the delay time differences amongst the transducer elements, resulting in more distal beam convergence. Multiple

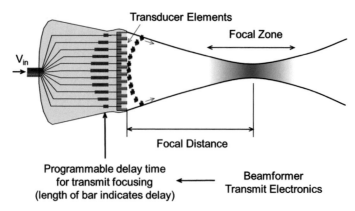

■ **FIGURE 14-15** A phased-array transducer assembly uses all elements to produce the ultrasound beam. Focusing is achieved by implementing a programmable delay time (beam former electronics) for the excitation of the individual transducer elements (focusing requires the outer elements in the array be energized first). Phase differences of the individual ultrasound pulses result in a minimum beam diameter (the focal distance) at a predictable depth in tissue.

transmit focal zones are created by repeatedly acquiring data over the same volume, but with different phase timing of the transducer array elements.

Receive Focus

In a phased-array transducer, the echoes received by all of the individual transducer elements are summed together to create the ultrasound signal from a given depth. Echoes received at the edge of the element array travel a slightly longer distance than those received at the center of the array, particularly at shallow depths. Signals from individual transducer elements therefore must be rephased to avoid a loss of resolution when the individual signals are synthesized to make an image. *Dynamic receive focusing* is a method to rephase the signals by dynamically introducing electronic delays as function of depth (time). At shallow depths, rephasing delays between adjacent transducer elements are greatest. With greater depth, there is less difference, so the phase delay circuitry for the receiver varies as a function of echo listening time, as shown in Figure 14-16. In addition to phased-array transducers, many linear array transducers permit dynamic receive focusing amongst the active element group.

■ **FIGURE 14-16** Dynamic receive focusing. All transducer elements in the phased array are active during the receive mode, and to maintain focus, the receive focus timing must be continuously adjusted in order to compensate for differences in arrival time across the array as a function of time (depth of the echo). Depicted are an early time (top illustration) of proximal echo arrival and a later time of distal echo arrival. To achieve phase alignment of the echo responses by all elements, variable timing is implemented as a function of element position after the transmit pulse in the beam former. The output of all phase-aligned echoes is summed.

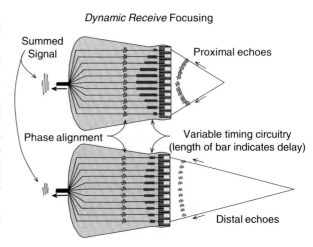

A

Transducer crystal

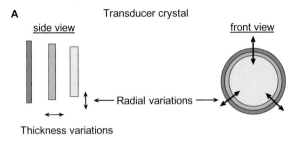

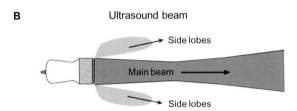

side view

front view

← Radial variations →

Thickness variations

Thickness variations

B

Ultrasound beam

Side lobes

Main beam

Side lobes

■ **FIGURE 14-17** **A.** A single transducer of a multielement array produces the main ultrasound beam in "thickness mode" vibration; however, radial expansion and contraction also occur. **B.** Side lobe energy in a multielement transducer array is created from the radial transducer vibration, which is directed away from the main beam. Echoes received from the side lobe energy are mapped into the main beam, creating unwanted artifacts.

Dynamic Aperture

The lateral spatial resolution of the linear array beam varies with depth, dependent on the linear dimension of the transducer width (aperture). A process termed *dynamic aperture* increases the number of active *receiving* elements in the array with reflector depth, so that the lateral resolution does not degrade with depth of propagation.

Side Lobes and Grating Lobes

Side lobes are unwanted emissions of ultrasound energy directed away from the main pulse, caused by the radial expansion and contraction of the transducer element during thickness contraction and expansion (Fig. 14-17). In the receive mode of transducer operation, echoes generated from the side lobes are unavoidably remapped along the main beam, which can introduce artifacts in the image. In continuous mode operation, the narrow frequency bandwidth of the transducer (high Q) causes the side lobe energy to be a significant fraction of the total beam. In pulsed mode operation, the low Q, broadband ultrasound beam produces a spectrum of acoustic wavelengths that reduce the emission of side lobe energy.

For multielement arrays, side lobe emission occurs in a forward direction along the main beam. By keeping the individual transducer element widths small (less than ½ wavelength), the side lobe emissions are reduced. Another method to minimize side lobes with array transducers is to reduce the amplitude of the peripheral transducer element excitations relative to the central element excitations.

Grating lobes result when ultrasound energy is emitted far off-axis by multielement arrays and are a consequence of the noncontinuous transducer surface of the discrete elements. The grating lobe effect is equivalent to placing a grating in front of a continuous transducer element, producing coherent waves directed at a large angle away from the main beam (Fig. 14-18). This misdirected energy of relatively low amplitude can result in the appearance of highly reflective objects in the main beam.

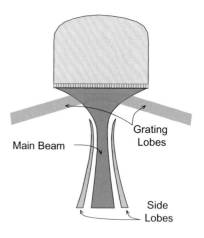

■ **FIGURE 14-18** Side and grating lobes are off-axis energy emissions produced by linear and phased-array transducers. Side lobes are forward directed; grating lobes are emitted from the array surface at very large angles.

Spatial Resolution

In ultrasound, the major factor that limits the spatial resolution and visibility of detail is the volume of the acoustic pulse. The axial, lateral, and elevational (slice-thickness) dimensions determine the minimal volume element (Fig. 14-19). Each dimension has an effect on the resolvability of objects in the image.

Axial Resolution

Axial resolution (also known as linear, range, longitudinal, or depth resolution) refers to the ability to discern two closely spaced objects in the direction of the beam. Achieving good axial resolution requires that the returning echoes be distinct without overlap. The minimal required separation distance between two reflectors is

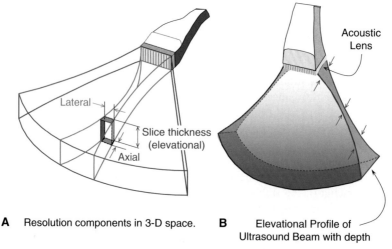

A   Resolution components in 3-D space.   **B**   Elevational Profile of Ultrasound Beam with depth

■ **FIGURE 14-19 A.** The axial, lateral, and elevational (slice-thickness) contributions in three dimensions are shown for a phased-array transducer ultrasound beam. Axial resolution, along the direction of the beam, is independent of depth; lateral resolution and elevational resolution are strongly depth dependent. Lateral resolution is determined by transmit and receive focus electronics; elevational resolution is determined by the height of the transducer elements. At the focal distance, axial is better than lateral and lateral is better than elevational resolution. **B.** Elevational resolution profile with an acoustic lens across the transducer array produces a focal zone in the slice-thickness direction.

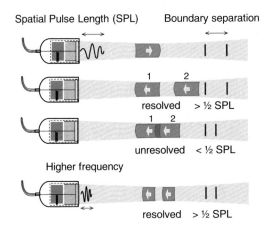

Spatial Pulse Length (SPL)   Boundary separation

resolved   > ½ SPL

unresolved   < ½ SPL

Higher frequency

resolved   > ½ SPL

■ **FIGURE 14-20** Axial resolution is equal to ½ SPL. Tissue boundaries that are separated by a distance greater than ½ SPL produce echoes from the first boundary that are completely distinct from echoes reflected from the second boundary, whereas boundaries with less than ½ SPL result in overlap of the returning echoes. Higher frequencies reduce the SPL and thus improve the axial resolution, as shown in the lower diagram.

one-half of the SPL to avoid the overlap of returning echoes, as the distance traveled between two reflectors is twice the separation distance. Objects spaced closer than ½ SPL will not be resolved (Fig. 14-20).

The SPL is the number of cycles emitted per pulse by the transducer multiplied by the wavelength. Shorter pulses, producing better axial resolution, can be achieved with greater damping of the transducer element (to reduce the pulse duration and number of cycles) or with higher frequency (to reduce wavelength). For imaging applications, the ultrasound pulse typically consists of three cycles. At 5 MHz (wavelength of 0.31 *mm*), the SPL is about 3 × 0.31 = 0.93 *mm,* which provides an axial resolution of ½ (0.93 *mm*) = 0.47 *mm.* At a given frequency, shorter pulse lengths require heavy damping and low Q, broad bandwidth operation. For a constant damping factor, higher frequencies (shorter wavelengths) give better axial resolution, but the imaging depth is reduced. Axial resolution remains constant with depth.

Lateral Resolution

Lateral resolution, also known as azimuthal resolution, refers to the ability to discern as separate two closely spaced objects perpendicular to the beam direction. For both single-element transducers and multielement array transducers, the beam diameter determines the lateral resolution (see Fig. 14-21). Since the beam diameter varies with distance from the transducer in the near and far field, the lateral resolution is depth dependent. The best lateral resolution occurs at the near field–far field interface. At this depth, the effective beam diameter is approximately equal to ½ the transducer diameter. In the far field, the beam diverges and substantially reduces the lateral resolution.

The lateral resolution of linear and curvilinear array transducers can be varied. The number of elements simultaneously activated in a group defines an "effective" transducer width that has similar behavior to a single-transducer element of the same width. Transmit and receive focusing along a single line is possible to produce focal zones with depth along each line.

For the phased-array transducer, focusing to a specific depth is achieved by both beam steering and transmit/receive focusing to reduce the effective beam width and improve lateral resolution, especially in the near field. Multiple transmit/receive focal zones can be implemented to maintain lateral resolution as a function of depth (Fig. 14-22). Each focal zone requires separate pulse-echo sequences to acquire data. One way to accomplish this is to acquire data along one beam direction multiple

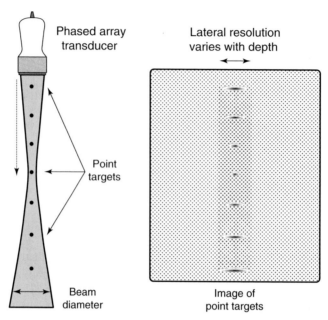

■ **FIGURE 14-21** Lateral resolution indicates the ability to discern objects perpendicular to the direction of beam travel and is determined by the beam diameter. Point objects in the beam are averaged over the effective beam diameter in the ultrasound image as a function of depth. Best lateral resolution occurs at the focal distance; good resolution occurs over the focal zone.

times (depending on the number of transmit focal zones) and to accept only the echoes within each focal zone, building up a single line of in-focus zones by meshing the information together. Increasing the number of focal zones improves overall in-focus lateral resolution with depth, but the amount of time required to produce an image increases, with a consequent reduction in frame rate and/or number of scan lines per image (see section on image quality).

■ **FIGURE 14-22** Phased-array transducers have multiple user selectable transmit and receive focal zones implemented by the beam former electronics. Each focal zone requires the excitation of the entire array for a given focal distance. Subsequent processing meshes the independently acquired data to enhance the lateral focal zone over a greater distance. Good lateral resolution over an extended depth is achieved, but the image frame rate is reduced.

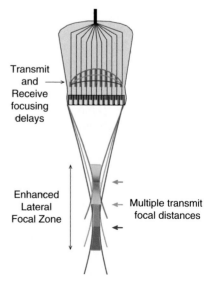

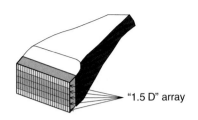

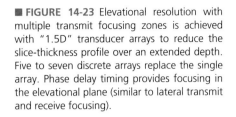

■ **FIGURE 14-23** Elevational resolution with multiple transmit focusing zones is achieved with "1.5D" transducer arrays to reduce the slice-thickness profile over an extended depth. Five to seven discrete arrays replace the single array. Phase delay timing provides focusing in the elevational plane (similar to lateral transmit and receive focusing).

"1.5 D" array

Multiple transmit focal zones: elevational plane

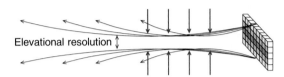

Elevational resolution

Elevational Resolution

The elevational or slice-thickness dimension of the ultrasound beam is perpendicular to the image plane. Slice thickness plays a significant part in image resolution, particularly with respect to volume averaging of acoustic details in the regions close to the transducer and in the far field beyond the focal zone. Elevational resolution is dependent on the transducer element height in much the same way that the lateral resolution is dependent on the transducer element width (Fig. 14-19B). Slice thickness is typically the weakest measure of resolution for array transducers. Use of a fixed focal length lens across the entire surface of the array provides improved elevational resolution at a fixed focal distance. Unfortunately, this compromises resolution due to partial volume averaging before and after the elevational focal zone.

Multiple linear array transducers with five to seven rows, known as *1.5D transducer arrays*, have the ability to steer and focus the beam in the elevational dimension. Elevational focusing is implemented with phased excitation of the outer to inner arrays to minimize the slice-thickness dimension at a given depth (Fig. 14-23). By using subsequent excitations with different focusing distances, multiple transmit focusing can produce smaller slice thickness over a range of tissue depths. A disadvantage of elevational focusing is a frame rate reduction penalty required for multiple excitations to build one image. The increased width of the transducer array also limits positioning flexibility. Extension to future full 2D transducer arrays with enhancements in computational power will allow 3D imaging with uniform resolution throughout the image volume.

14.5 Image Data Acquisition

Understanding ultrasonic image formation requires knowledge of ultrasound production, propagation, and interactions. Images are created using a *pulse-echo* mode format of ultrasound production and detection. Each pulse is directionally transmitted into the patient and experiences partial reflections from tissue interfaces that create echoes, which return to the transducer. Image formation using the pulse-echo approach requires a number of hardware components: the beam former, pulser, receiver, amplifier, scan converter/image memory, and display system (Fig. 14-24). The detection and processing of the echo signals is the subject of this section.

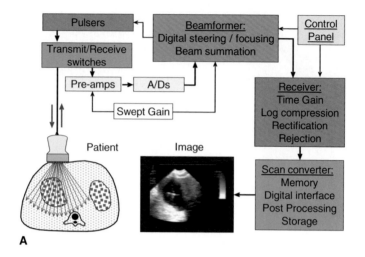

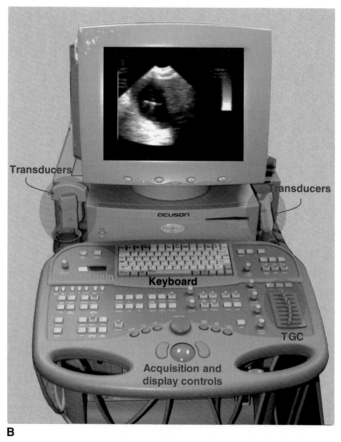

■ **FIGURE 14-24 A.** Components of the ultrasound imager. This schematic depicts the design of a *digital acquisition/digital beam former system*, where *each* of the transducer elements in the array has a pulser, transmit-receive switch, preamplifier, and ADC (e.g., for a 128-element phased array, there are 128 components as shaded boxes). Swept gain reduces the dynamic range of the signals prior to digitization. The beam former provides focusing, steering, and summation of the beam; the receiver processes the data for optimal display, and the scan converter produces the output image rendered on the monitor. Thick lines indicate the path of ultrasound data through the system. **B.** A commercial ultrasound scanner system is comprised of a keyboard, various acquisition and processing controls including transmit gain and TGC, several transducer selections, an image display monitor, and other components/interfaces not shown.

Ultrasound equipment has digital electronics and processing, and current state-of-the-art systems use various combinations of mostly digital and some analog electronics. The discussion below assumes a hybrid analog and digital processing capability for image data acquisition and refers to the modules illustrated in Figure 14-24A.

Beam Former

The beam former is responsible for generating the electronic delays for individual transducer elements in an array to achieve transmit and receive focusing and, in phased arrays, beam steering. Most modern, high-end ultrasound equipment incorporates a *digital beam former* and digital electronics for both transmit and receive functions. A digital beam former controls application-specific integrated circuits that provide transmit/receive switches, digital-to-analog and analog-to-digital converters (ADCs), and preamplification and time gain compensation (TGC) circuitry for each of the transducer elements in the array. Each of these components is explained below. Major advantages of digital acquisition and processing include the flexibility to introduce new ultrasound capabilities by programmable software algorithms and enhanced control of the acoustic beam.

Pulser

The pulser (also known as the transmitter) provides the electrical voltage for exciting the piezoelectric transducer elements and controls the output transmit power by adjustment of the applied voltage. In digital beam former systems, a digital-to-analog converter (DAC) determines the amplitude of the voltage. An increase in transmit amplitude creates higher intensity sound and improves echo detection from weaker reflectors. A direct consequence is higher signal-to-noise ratio in the images but also higher power deposition to the patient. User controls of the output power are labeled "output," "power," "*dB*," or "transmit" by the manufacturer. In some systems, a low power setting for obstetric imaging is available to reduce power deposition to the fetus. A method for indicating output power in terms of a thermal index (TI) and mechanical index (MI) is provided by ultrasound equipment manufacturers (see Section 14.11).

Transmit/Receive Switch

The transmit/receive switch, synchronized with the pulser, isolates the high voltage associated with pulsing (~150 V) from the sensitive amplification stages during receive mode, with induced voltages ranging from approximately 1 V to 2 µV from the returning echoes. After the *ring-down* time, when vibration of the piezoelectric material has stopped, the transducer electronics are switched to sensing surface charge variations of mechanical deflection caused by the returning echoes, over a period up to about 1,000 µs (1 *ms*).

Pulse-Echo Operation

In the *pulse-echo* mode of transducer operation, the ultrasound beam is intermittently transmitted, with a majority of the time occupied by listening for echoes. The ultrasound pulse is created with a short voltage waveform provided by the *pulser* of the ultrasound system. This event is sometimes known as the *main bang*. The generated pulse is typically two to three cycles long, dependent on the damping characteristics of the transducer elements. With a speed of sound of 1,540 *m/s* (0.154 *cm/μs*), the time delay between the transmission pulse and the detection of the echo is directly related to the depth of the interface as

$$\text{Time }(\mu s) = \frac{2D(cm)}{c\,(cm/\mu s)} = \frac{2D(cm)}{0.154\,cm/\mu s} = 13\mu s\,/\,cm \times D(cm)$$

$$\text{Distance }(cm) = \frac{c\,(cm/\mu s) \times \text{Time }(\mu s)}{2} = 0.077 \times \text{Time}(\mu s)$$

where *c*, the speed of sound, is expressed in *cm/μs*; distance from the transducer to the reflector, *D*, is expressed in *cm*; the constant 2 represents the round-trip distance; and time is expressed in μs. One pulse-echo sequence produces one amplitude-modulated (A-line) of image data. The timing of the data excitation and echo acquisition relates to distance (Fig. 14-25). Many repetitions of the pulse-echo sequence are necessary to construct an image from the individual A-lines.

The number of times the transducer is pulsed per second is known as the *pulse repetition frequency* (PRF). For imaging, the PRF typically ranges from 2,000 to 4,000 pulses per second (2 to 4 kHz). The time between pulses is the *pulse repetition period* (PRP), equal to the inverse of the PRF. An increase in PRF results in a decrease in echo listening time. The maximum PRF is determined by the time required for echoes from the most distant structures to reach the transducer. If a second pulse occurs before the detection of the most distant echoes, these more distant echoes can be confused with prompt echoes from the second pulse, and artifacts can occur. The *maximal range* is determined from the product of the speed of sound and the PRP divided by 2 (the factor of 2 accounts for round-trip distance):

$$\text{Maximal range }(cm) = 154{,}000\,cm/s \times \text{PRP}(s) \times \tfrac{1}{2}$$
$$= 77{,}000 \times \text{PRP}(s) = 77{,}000\,/\,\text{PRF}(s^{-1}).$$

A 500 μs PRP corresponds to a PRF of 2 kHz and a maximal range of 38.5 *cm*. For a PRP of 250 μs (PRF of 4 kHz), the maximum depth is halved to 19.3 *cm*. Higher ultrasound frequency operation has limited penetration depth, allowing high PRFs.

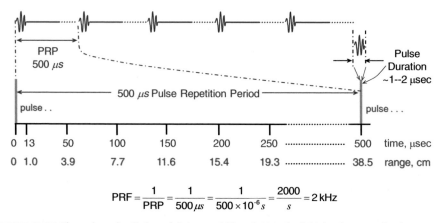

$$\text{PRF} = \frac{1}{\text{PRP}} = \frac{1}{500\,\mu s} = \frac{1}{500 \times 10^{-6}\,s} = \frac{2000}{s} = 2\,\text{kHz}$$

■ **FIGURE 14-25** The pulse-echo timing of data acquisition depicts the initial pulse occurring in a very short time span, the pulse duration = 1 to 2 μs and the time between pulses, the PRP = 500 μs in this example. The number of pulses per second is 2,000/s, or 2 kHz. Range (one-half the round-trip distance) is calculated assuming a speed of sound = 1,540 *m/s*.

Conversely, lower frequency operation requires lower PRFs because echoes can return from greater depths. Ultrasound transducer frequency should not be confused with PRF, and the period of the sound wave $(1/f)$ should not be confused with the PRP $(1/PRF)$. The ultrasound frequency is calibrated in MHz, whereas PRF is in kHz, and the ultrasound period is measured in *microseconds* compared to *milliseconds* for the PRP.

Pulse duration is the ratio of the number of cycles in the pulse to the transducer frequency and is equal to the instantaneous "on" time. A pulse consisting of two cycles with a center frequency of 2 MHz has a duration of 1 µs. *Duty cycle*, the fraction of "on" time, is equal to the pulse duration divided by the PRP. For real-time imaging applications, the duty cycle is typically 0.2% to 0.4%, indicating that greater than 99.5% of the scan time is spent "listening" to echoes as opposed to producing acoustic energy. Intensity levels in medical ultrasonography are very low when averaged over time, as is the intensity when averaged over space due to the collimation of the beam.

For clinical data acquisition, a typical range of PRF, PRP, and duty cycle values are listed in Table 14-6.

Preamplification and Analog-to-Digital Conversion

In multielement array transducers, all preprocessing steps are performed in parallel. Each transducer element produces a small voltage proportional to the pressure amplitude of the returning echoes. An initial preamplification increases the detected voltages to useful signal levels. This is combined with a *fixed* swept gain (Fig.14-26), to compensate for the exponential attenuation occurring with distance (time) traveled. Large variations in echo amplitude (voltage produced in the piezo-electric element) with time are reduced from approximately 1,000,000:1 or 120 dB to about 1,000:1 or 60 dB.

Early ultrasound units used analog electronic circuits for all functions, which were susceptible to drift and instability. Even today, the initial stages of the receiver often use analog electronic circuits. Digital electronics were first introduced in ultrasound for functions such as image formation and display. Since then, there has been a tendency to implement more and more of the signal preprocessing functions in digital circuitry, particularly in high-end ultrasound systems.

In state-of-the-art ultrasound units, each piezoelectric element has its own pre-amplifier and ADC. A typical sampling rate of 20 to 40 MHz with 8 to 12 bits of precision is used (ADCs were discussed in Chapter 5). ADCs with larger bit depths and sampling rates are necessary for systems that digitize the signals directly from the preamplification stage. In systems where digitization of the signal occurs after analog beam formation and summing, a single ADC with less demanding requirements is typically employed.

TABLE 14-6   TYPICAL PRF, PRP, AND DUTY CYCLE VALUES FOR ULTRASOUND OPERATION MODES

OPERATION MODE	PRF (Hz)	PRP (µs)	DUTY CYCLE (%)
M-mode	500	2000	0.05
Real-time	2000 – 4000	500 – 250	0.2 – 0.4
Pulsed Doppler	4000 – 12000	250 – 83	0.4 – 1.2

Adapted from Zagzebski, J. *Essentials of ultrasound physics.* St. Louis, MO: Mosby-Year Book, 1996.

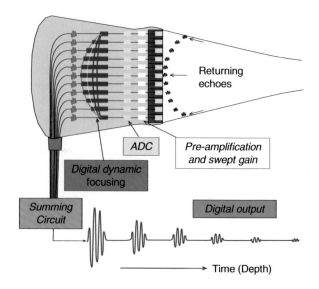

■ **FIGURE 14-26** A phased-array transducer produces a pulsed beam that is focused at a programmable depth and receives echoes during the PRP. This figure shows a digital beam former system, with the analog to digital converter (ADC) converting the signals before the beam focus and steering manipulation. Timed electronic delays phase align the echoes, with the output summed to form the ultrasound echo train along a specific beam direction.

Beam Steering, Dynamic Focusing, and Signal Summation

Echo reception includes electronic delays to adjust for beam direction and dynamic receive focusing to align the phase of detected echoes from the individual elements in the array as a function of echo depth. In digital beam former systems, this is accomplished with digital processing algorithms. Following phase alignment, the preprocessed signals from all of the active transducer elements are summed as shown in Figure 14-26. The output signal represents the acoustic information gathered during the PRP along a single beam direction. This information is sent to the receiver for further processing before rendering into a 2D image.

Receiver

The receiver accepts data from the beam former during the PRP, which represents echo information as a function of time (depth). Subsequent signal processing occurs in the following sequence (Fig. 14-27):

1. **Gain adjustments and dynamic frequency tuning.**
   TGC is a user-adjustable amplification of the returning echo signals as a function of time, to further compensate for beam attenuation. TGC (also known as time varied gain, depth gain compensation, and swept gain) can be changed to meet the needs of a specific imaging application. The ideal TGC curve makes all equally reflective boundaries equal in signal amplitude, regardless of the depth of the boundary (Fig. 14-28). Variations in the output signals are thus indicative of the acoustic impedance differences between tissue boundaries. User adjustment is typically achieved by multiple slider potentiometers, where each slider represents a given depth in the image, or by a 3-knob TGC control, which controls the initial gain, slope, and far gain of the echo signals. For multielement transducers, TGC is applied simultaneously to the signal from each of the individual elements. The TGC amplification effectively reduces the maximum to minimum range of the echo voltages as a function of time to approximately 50 dB (300:1).
   Dynamic frequency tuning is a feature of some broadband receivers that changes the sensitivity of the tuner bandwidth with time, so that echoes from shallow depths are tuned to a higher frequency range, while echoes from deeper

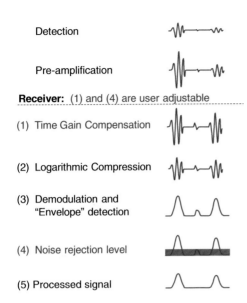

Detection

Pre-amplification

Receiver: (1) and (4) are user adjustable

(1) Time Gain Compensation

(2) Logarithmic Compression

(3) Demodulation and "Envelope" detection

(4) Noise rejection level

(5) Processed signal

■ FIGURE 14-27 The receiver processes the data streaming from the beam former. Steps include TGC, dynamic range compression, rectification, demodulation, and noise rejection. The user has the ability to adjust the TGC and the noise rejection level.

structures are tuned to lower frequencies. The purpose of this is to accommodate for beam softening, where increased attenuation of higher frequencies in a broad bandwidth pulse occurs as a function of depth. Dynamic frequency tuning allows the receiver to make the most efficient use of the ultrasound frequencies incident on the transducer.

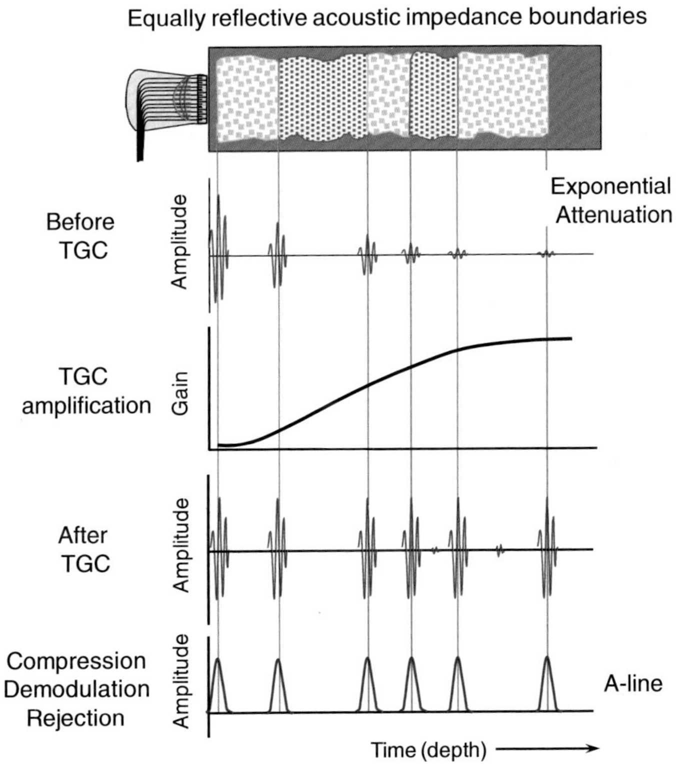

Equally reflective acoustic impedance boundaries

Before TGC — Amplitude

Exponential Attenuation

TGC amplification — Gain

After TGC — Amplitude

Compression Demodulation Rejection — Amplitude

A-line

Time (depth) ⟶

■ FIGURE 14-28 TGC amplifies the acquired signals with respect to time after the initial pulse by operator adjustments (usually a set of five to six slide potentiometers; see Fig. 14-24B). Processed A-line data with appropriate TGC demonstrate that equally reflective interfaces have equal amplitude.

2. **Dynamic range (logarithmic) compression.** *Dynamic range* defines the effective operational range of an electronic device from the threshold signal level to the saturation level. Key components in the ultrasound detection and display that are most affected by a wide dynamic range include the ADC and the display. For receiver systems with an 8-bit ADC, the dynamic range is 20 log (256) = 48 dB, certainly not enough to accurately digitize a 50-dB signal. Video monitors and film have a dynamic range of about 100:1 to 150:1 and therefore require a reduced range of input signals to accurately render the display output. Thus, after TGC, the signals must be reduced to 20 to 30 dB, which is accomplished by compression using *logarithmic amplification* to increase the smallest echo amplitudes and to decrease the largest amplitudes. Logarithmic amplification produces an output signal proportional to the logarithm of the input signal. Logarithmic amplification is performed by an analog signal processor in less costly ultrasound systems and digitally in high-end digital systems having ADCs with a large bit depth. In any case, an appropriate range of signals is achieved for display of the amplitude variations as gray scale on the monitor or for printing on film.
3. **Rectification, demodulation, and envelope detection.** *Rectification* inverts the negative amplitude signals of the echo to positive values. *Demodulation and envelope detection* convert the rectified amplitudes of the echo into a smoothed, single pulse.
4. **Rejection** level adjustment sets the threshold of signal amplitudes allowed to pass to the digitization and display subsystems. This removes a significant amount of undesirable low-level noise and clutter generated from scattered sound or by the electronics.
5. **Processed images** are optimized for gray-scale range and viewing on the limited dynamic range monitors, so that subsequent adjustments to the images are unnecessary.

In the above listed steps, the operator has the ability to control the TGC and noise/clutter rejection. The amount of amplification (overall gain) necessary is dependent on the initial power (transmit gain) settings of the ultrasound system. Higher intensities are achieved by exciting the transducer elements with larger voltages. This increases the amplitude of the returning echoes and reduces the need for electronic amplification gain but also deposits more energy into the patient, where heating or mechanical interactions can be significant. Conversely, lower ultrasound power settings, such as those used in obstetrical ultrasound, require a greater overall electronic gain to amplify weaker echo signals into the appropriate range for TGC. TGC allows the operator to manipulate depth-dependent gain to improve image uniformity and compensate for unusual imaging situations. Inappropriate adjustment of TGC can lead to artifactual enhancement of tissue boundaries and tissue texture as well as nonuniform response versus depth. The noise rejection level sets a threshold to clean up low-level signals in the electronic signal. It is usually adjusted in conjunction with the transmit power level setting of the ultrasound instrument.

Echo Display Modes

A-mode

A-mode (A for amplitude) is the display of the *processed* information from the receiver versus time (after the receiver processing steps shown in Fig. 14-27). As echoes return from tissue boundaries and scatterers (a function of the acoustic impedance differences in the tissues), a digital signal proportional to echo amplitude is produced as a function of time. One "A-line" of data per PRP is the result. As the speed of sound equates to depth (round-trip time), the tissue interfaces along the path of the ultrasound beam are localized by distance from the transducer. The earliest uses of ultrasound in medicine used A-mode information to determine the midline position of the brain for revealing possible mass effect of brain tumors. A-mode and A-line information is currently used in ophthalmology applications for precise distance measurements of the eye. Otherwise, A-mode display by itself is seldom used.

B-mode

B-mode (B for brightness) is the electronic conversion of the A-mode and A-line information into brightness-modulated dots along the A-line trajectory. In general, the brightness of the dot is proportional to the echo signal amplitude (depending upon signal processing parameters). The B-mode display is used for M-mode and 2D gray-scale imaging.

M-mode

M-mode (M for motion) is a technique that uses B-mode information to display the echoes from a moving organ, such as the myocardium and valve leaflets, from a fixed transducer position and beam direction on the patient (Fig. 14-29). The echo data from a single ultrasound beam passing through moving anatomy are acquired and displayed as a function of time, represented by reflector depth on the vertical axis (beam path direction) and time on the horizontal axis. M-mode can provide excellent temporal resolution of motion patterns, allowing the evaluation of the function of heart valves and other cardiac anatomy. Only one anatomical dimension is represented by the M-mode technique, and with advances in real-time 2D echocardiography, Doppler, and color flow imaging, this display mode is of much less importance than in the past.

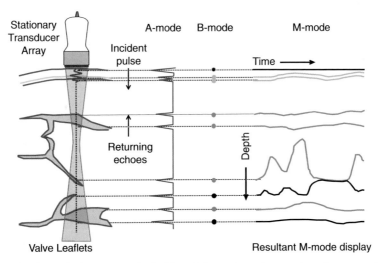

■ **FIGURE 14-29** Ultrasonic data are acquired with a stationary transducer or transducer array. The A-mode data (vertical *blue* trace) represent echo amplitudes during one pulse-echo period. The amplitudes are encoded to brightness (B-mode) as a series of variable intensity dots. The A-mode line and corresponding B-mode dots change position as the valve leaflets move within the stationary beam. By deflecting the dots horizontally in time on a storage display, motion graphs (M-mode) are created, depicting the periodic (or lack of periodic) motion.

Scan Converter

The function of the scan converter is to create 2D images from echo information from distinct beam directions and to perform *scan conversion* to enable image data to be viewed on video display monitors. Scan conversion is necessary because the image acquisition and display occur in different formats. Early scan converters were of an analog design, using storage cathode ray tubes to capture data. These devices drifted easily and were unstable over time. Current scan converters use digital technology for storage and manipulation of data. Digital scan converters are extremely stable and allow subsequent image processing by the application of a variety of mathematical functions.

Digital information streams to the scan converter memory, configured as a matrix of small picture elements (pixels) that represent a rectangular coordinate display. Most ultrasound instruments have an approximately 500×500 pixel matrix (variations between manufacturers exist). Each pixel has a memory address that uniquely defines its location within the matrix. During image acquisition, the digital signals are inserted into the matrix at memory addresses that correspond as close as possible to the relative reflector positions in the body. Transducer beam, orientation, and echo delay times determine the correct pixel addresses (matrix coordinates) in which to deposit the digital information. Misalignment between the digital image matrix and the beam trajectory, particularly for sector-scan formats at larger depths, requires data interpolation to fill in empty or partially filled pixels. The final image is most often recorded with $512 \times 512 \times 8$ bits per pixel, representing about ¼ Mbytes of data. For color display, the bit depth is often as much as 24 bits (1 byte per primary color).

14.6 Two-Dimensional Image Display and Storage

A 2D ultrasound image is acquired by sweeping a pulsed ultrasound beam over the volume of interest and displaying echo signals using B-mode conversion of the A-mode signals. Echo position is based upon the delay time between the pulse initiation and the reception of the echo, using the speed of sound in soft tissue (1,540 *m/s*). The 2D image is progressively built up or continuously updated as the beam is swept through the object.

Early B-mode Scanners—Manual Articulating Arm with Static Display

Early B-mode scanners were made with a single-element transducer mounted on an articulating arm with angular position encoders to determine the location of the ultrasound beam path. This information was necessary to place echo signals at proper positions in the image. The mechanical arm constrained the transducer to a plane, so that the resultant image depicted a tomographic slice. An image was built up on an analog scan converter and storage display by repeated pulsing and positional changes of the transducer (Fig. 14-30), requiring several seconds per image. Linear, sector, or "compound" scans could be performed. Compound scans used a combination of linear and sector transducer motions to improve the probability of perpendicular pulse incidence to organ boundaries so that echoes would return to the transducer. Image quality with these systems was highly dependent on the skill of the sonographer.

Articulating Arm Single Transducer System

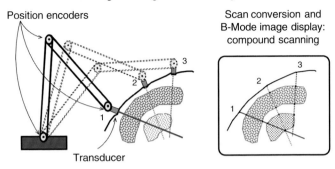

■ FIGURE 14-30 Articulating arm B-mode scanning produces an acoustic tomographic slice of the body. Position encoders track the 3D position of the transducer to allow the scan converter to place the gray-scale–encoded A-line data in the 2D image plane. Shown is a compound scan (multiple compound directions of the single-element transducer) along a plane of the body and the corresponding image lines. Compounding was performed manually, building an image over several seconds, to ensure that the ultrasound beam was perpendicular to the boundary at some point during the scan.

Mechanical Scanning and Real-Time Display

The next step in the evolution of medical ultrasound imaging was dynamic scanning with "real-time" display. This was achieved by implementing periodic mechanical motion of the transducer. Early scanners used a single-element transducer to produce a real-time sector scan image by wobbling the transducer. Enhanced performance was obtained with rotation of a number of transducers on a wheel within the transducer housing. The update of the screen display was determined by the PRF, the oscillation or rotation frequency of the transducer, and the positional information provided by an encoder attached to the rocking or rotating transducer. The number of A-lines that comprised the image was determined by the penetration depth and the image update rate.

Electronic Scanning and Real-Time Display

State-of-the-art ultrasound scanners employ array transducers with multiple piezo-electric elements to electronically sweep an ultrasound beam across the volume of interest for dynamic ultrasound imaging. Array transducers are available as linear/curvilinear arrays and phased arrays. They are distinguished by the way in which the beam is produced and by the FOV coverage that is possible.

Linear and curvilinear array transducers produce rectangular and trapezoidal images, respectively (Fig. 14-31). They are typically composed of 256 to 512 discrete transducer elements of ½ to 1 wavelength width each in an enclosure from about 6 to 8 *cm* wide. A small group of adjacent elements (~15 to 20) is simultaneously activated to create an active transducer area defined by the width (sum of the individual element widths in the group) and the height of the elements. This beam propagates perpendicular to the surface of the transducer, with a single line of echo information acquired during the PRP. A shift of one or more transducer elements and repeating the simultaneous excitation of the group produce the next A-line of data. The ultrasound beam sweeps across the volume of interest in a sequential fashion, with the number of A-lines approximately equal to the number of transducer elements. Advantages of the linear array are the wide FOV for regions close to the transducer and uniform, rectangular sampling across the image. Electronic delays within the

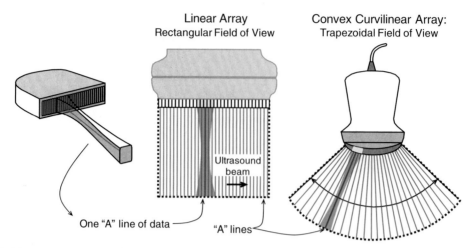

Linear Array
Rectangular Field of View

Convex Curvilinear Array:
Trapezoidal Field of View

Ultrasound beam

One "A" line of data

"A" lines

■ **FIGURE 14-31** Linear and curvilinear array transducers produce an image by activating a subgroup of the transducer elements that form one A-line of data in the scanned object and shifting the active elements by one to acquire the next line of data. Linear arrays produce rectangular image formats; curvilinear arrays produce a trapezoidal format with a wide FOV.

subgroup of transducer elements allow transmit and dynamic receive focusing for improved lateral resolution with depth.

Phased-array transducers are typically comprised of a tightly grouped array of 64, 128, or 256 transducer elements in a 3- to 5-*cm*-wide enclosure. All transducer elements are involved in producing the ultrasound beam and recording the returning echoes. The ultrasound beam is steered by adjusting the delays applied to the individual transducer elements by the beam former. This time delay sequence is varied from one transmit pulse to the next in order to change the sweep angle across the FOV in a sector scan. (Fig. 14-32 shows three separate beams during the sweep.)

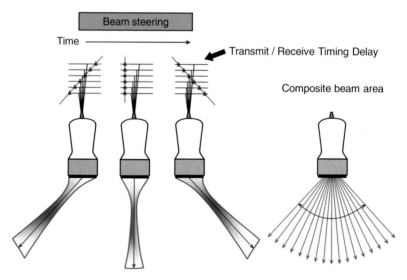

Beam steering

Time

Transmit / Receive Timing Delay

Composite beam area

■ **FIGURE 14-32** The phased-array transducer electronically steers the ultrasound beam by introducing phase delays during the transmit *and* receive timing of the beam former. Lateral focusing also occurs along the beam direction. A sector format composite image is produced (**right**), with the number of A-lines dependent on several imaging factors discussed in the text.

A similar time-delay strategy (dynamic receive focusing) is used to spatially synchronize the returning ultrasound echoes as they strike each transducer element (see Fig. 14-26). In addition to the beam steering capabilities, lateral focusing, multiple transmit focal zones, and dynamic receive focusing are used in phased arrays.

The small overall size of the phased-array transducer entrance window allows flexibility in positioning, particularly through the intercostal space—a small ultrasound conduit in front of the lungs—to allow cardiac imaging. In addition, it is possible to use the phased-array transducer in conjunction with external triggers, such as EKG, to produce M-mode scans at the same time as 2D images, and to allow duplex Doppler/color flow imaging.

Spatial compounding is a method in which ultrasound information is obtained from several different angles of insonation and combined to produce a single image. In fact, the idea of spatial compound scans existed from the earliest implementations of static ultrasound B-scan imaging, as depicted in Figure 14-30. In linear array transducer systems, electronic beam steering allows the insonation of tissues from multiple angles as shown in Figure 14-33, and by averaging the data, the resultant compound image improves image quality in a variety of applications including breast imaging, thyroid, atherosclerotic plaque, and musculoskeletal ultrasound imaging. As each image is produced from multiple angles of insonation, the likelihood that one of these angles will be perpendicular to a specular reflector is increased, and in turn higher echo amplitudes are generated for better definition in the image. In addition, curved surfaces appear more continuous. Speckle noise, a random source of image variation, is reduced by the averaging process of forming the compound image, with a corresponding increase in signal-to-noise ratio. One downside to spatial compounding is the persistence effect of frame averaging, the loss of temporal resolution, and the increase in spatial blurring of moving objects, so it is not particularly useful in situations with voluntary and involuntary patient motion. Spatial compounding is also implemented on phased-array transducers.

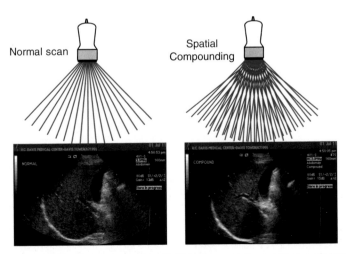

■ FIGURE 14-33 A vector phased array transducer (**left**) in the normal acquisition mode insonates tissues to yield a sector image. Compound scanning (**right**) uses ultrasound beams produced at several angles achieved by electronic steering (three are shown above) to acquire directional acoustic image data subsequently averaged to produce a single image. Note the oversampling patterns in this mode, and since the scan lines are acquired sequentially, the frame rate is reduced by the number of insonation angles used to produce the compound image.

Real-Time Ultrasound Imaging: Frame Rate, FOV, Depth, and Spatial Sampling Trade-Offs

The 2D image (a single *frame*) is created from a number of A-lines, N (typically 100 or more), acquired across the FOV. A larger number of lines will produce a higher quality image; however, the finite time for pulse-echo propagation places an upper limit on N that also impacts the desired temporal resolution. The acquisition time for each line, T_{line} = 13 $\mu s/cm$ × D (cm), is required for the echo data to be unambiguously collected from a depth, D (see Fig. 14-25, which illustrates time and depth relationships). Thus, the time necessary per frame, T_{frame}, is given by N × T_{line} = N × 13 $\mu s/cm$ × D (cm). The *frame rate per second* is the reciprocal of the time required per frame:

$$\text{Frame rate} = \frac{1}{T_{frame}} = \frac{1}{N \times 13\ \mu s \times D(cm)} = \frac{0.077/\mu s}{N \times D(cm)} = \frac{77000\ /\ s}{N \times D(cm)}$$

This equation describes the maximum frame rate possible in terms of N and D. If either N or D increases without a corresponding decrease of the other variable, then the maximum frame rate will decrease. For a given procedure, the sonographer must consider the compromises among frame rate, imaging depth, and number of lines/frame. A secondary consideration is the line density (LD) (spacing between lines), determined by N and the FOV. Higher frame rates can be achieved by reducing the imaging depth, number of lines, or FOV as illustrated in Figure 14-34. The spatial sampling (LD) of the ultrasound beam decreases with depth for sector and trapezoidal scan formats and remains constant with depth for the rectangular format (linear array).

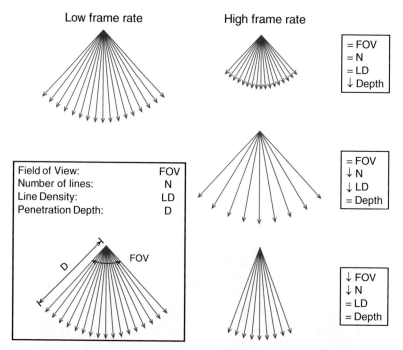

■ FIGURE 14-34 Ultrasound image quality depends on several factors. The number of lines per image, frame rate, field of view (FOV), line density (LD), and penetration depth (*D*) are interrelated (see *inset* figure). For a low frame rate image acquisition with a large penetration depth, a large number of A-lines and a high LD, depicted on the right, are options that can be made with a high frame rate acquisition. Reducing the penetration depth allows an equal LD, equal number of lines, and equal FOV (**top right**). Maintaining equal penetration depth and equal FOV reduces the number of lines and the LD (**middle right**). Keeping the LD and penetration depth equal reduces the FOV and number of lines (**bottom right**).

Another factor that affects frame rate is transmit focusing, whereby the ultrasound beam (each A-line) is focused at multiple depths for improved lateral resolution (see Fig. 14-22). The frame rate will be decreased by a factor approximately equal to the number of transmit focal zones placed on the image, since the beam former electronics must transmit an independent set of pulses for each focal zone.

Scan LD is an important component of image quality. Insufficient LD can cause the image to appear pixelated from the interpolation of several pixels to fill unscanned volumes and can cause the loss of image resolution, particularly at a depth. This might happen when one achieves high temporal resolution (high frame rates) at the expense of LD.

Image Display

For digital flat-panel displays, digital information from the scan converter can be directly converted into a viewable image. For analog monitor displays, the digital scan converter memory requires a DAC and electronics to produce a compatible video signal. The DAC converts the digital pixel data, in a raster pattern, into a corresponding analog video signal compatible with specific video monitors (refer to Chapter 5 for detailed explanation). Window and level adjustments of the digital data, to modify the brightness and contrast of the displayed image, are applied to the output signals without changing the digital memory values (only the look-up-transformation table), before digital-to-analog conversion.

The displayed pixel density can limit the quality and resolution of the image. Employing a "zoom" feature on many ultrasound instruments can enhance the image information to improve and delineate details within the image that are otherwise blurred. Two types of methods, "read" zoom and "write" zoom, are usually available. "Read" zoom enlarges a user-defined region of the stored image and expands the information over a larger number of pixels in the displayed image. Even though the displayed region becomes larger, the resolution of the image itself does not change. Using "write" zoom requires the operator to rescan the area of the patient that corresponds to the user-selectable area. When enabled, the transducer scans the selected area and only the echo data within the limited region are acquired. Figure 14-35 demonstrates the large FOV image and a write zoom resampling of the image content. The latter allows a greater LD, and higher sampling across the FOV provides improved resolution and image quality.

Besides the B-mode data used for the 2D image, other information from M-mode and Doppler signal processing can also be displayed. During operation of the ultrasound scanner, information in the memory is continuously updated in real time. When ultrasound scanning is stopped, the last image acquired is displayed on the screen until ultrasound scanning resumes.

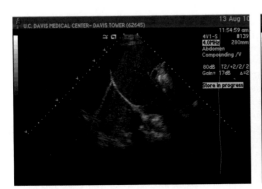 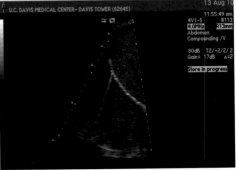

■ **FIGURE 14-35** Large FOV sector scan image (**left**) and corresponding write zoom image (**right**).

Image Storage

Ultrasound images are typically comprised of 640 × 480 or 512 × 512 pixels. Each pixel has a depth of 8 bits (1 byte) of digital data, providing up to 256 levels of gray scale. Image storage (without compression) is approximately ¼ MB per image. For real-time imaging (10 to 30 frames per second), this can amount to hundreds of megabytes of data for video clip acquisitions, depending on the complexity of the examination. Color images used for Doppler studies (Section 14.7) increase the storage requirements further because of larger numbers of bits needed for color resolution (full fidelity color requires 24 bits/pixel, one byte each for the red, green, and blue primary colors).

14.7   Doppler Ultrasound

Doppler ultrasound is based on the shift of frequency in an ultrasound wave caused by a moving reflector, such as blood cells in the vasculature (Fig. 14-36). This is the same effect that causes a siren on a fire truck to sound high pitched as the truck approaches the listener (the wavelength is compressed) and a shift to a lower pitch sound as it passes by and continues on (the wavelength is expanded). The moving reflectors in the body are the blood cells. By comparing the incident ultrasound frequency with the reflected ultrasound frequency from the blood cells, it is possible to discern the velocity of the blood. Not only can blood velocity (and indirectly blood flow) be measured, but the information provided by the Doppler techniques can also be used to create color blood flow maps of the vasculature. The interpretation of Doppler signals in clinical practice, however, requires the extraction of information about the blood flow from the potential confounding aspects related to the technique itself. Therefore, an understanding of the physical principles of Doppler ultrasound is an absolute prerequisite for the interpretation of the acquired information.

Doppler Frequency Shift

The *Doppler shift* is the difference between the incident frequency and reflected frequency. When the reflector is moving directly away from or toward the source of sound, the Doppler frequency shift (f_d) is calculated as

$$f_d = f_r - f_i = \frac{\text{reflector speed}}{\text{reflector speed} + \text{speed of sound}} \times 2 \times f_i$$

■ **FIGURE 14-36** Doppler ultrasound exploits changes in frequency from interaction with moving objects. Sound waves reflected from a moving object are compressed (higher frequency) when moving toward the transducer and expanded (lower frequency) when moving away from the transducer compared to the incident sound wave frequency. The difference between the incident and returning frequencies is called the Doppler shift frequency.

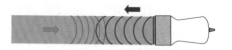

Blood moving towards transducer
produces higher frequency echoes.

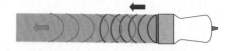

Blood moving away from transducer
produces lower frequency echoes.

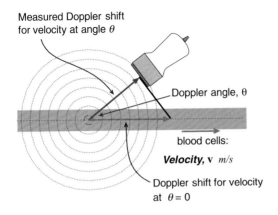

Measured Doppler shift for velocity at angle θ

Doppler angle, θ

blood cells:

Velocity, v *m/s*

Doppler shift for velocity at $\theta = 0$

■ **FIGURE 14-37** Geometry of Doppler ultrasound data acquisition. The Doppler shift varies as a function of the angle (θ) of the incident ultrasound pulse and the axis of the blood vessel for a fixed blood velocity, v. The maximum Doppler shift occurs at an angle $\theta = 0$ For a larger Doppler angle (θ), the measured Doppler shift is less by a factor of cos(θ), and velocity estimates are compensated by 1/cos (θ).

where f_i is the frequency of the sound incident on the reflector and f_r is the frequency of the reflected sound. Thus, the Doppler shift is proportional to the velocity of the blood cells.

When the sound waves and blood cells are not moving in parallel directions, the equation must be modified to account for less Doppler shift. The angle between the direction of blood flow and the direction of the sound is called the Doppler angle (Fig. 14-37). The component of the velocity vector directed toward the transducer is less than the velocity vector along the vessel axis by the cosine of the angle, cos (θ). Without correction for this discrepancy, the Doppler shift will be less and an underestimate of the actual blood velocity will occur. The Doppler angle joins the adjacent side and hypotenuse of a right triangle; therefore, the component of the blood velocity in the direction of the sound (adjacent side) is equal to the actual blood velocity (hypotenuse) multiplied by the cosine of the angle (θ). (Note: In physics, the term *velocity* refers to a vector quantity, describing both the distance traveled per unit time (*speed*) and the direction of movement such as blood flow.) As the velocity of blood cells (peak of ~200 *cm/s*) is significantly less than the speed of sound (154,000 *cm/s*), the denominator can be simplified with an extremely small error by neglecting the velocity of the blood. This results in the generalized Doppler shift equation:

$$f_d = \frac{2\, f_i\, \text{v}\, \cos(\boldsymbol{\theta})}{c}$$

where **v** is the velocity of blood, c is the speed of sound in soft tissue, and θ is the Doppler angle.

Calculation of the blood velocity is straightforward by rearranging the Doppler equation:

$$\text{v} = \frac{f_d c}{2\, f_i\, \cos(\boldsymbol{\theta})}$$

Thus, the measured Doppler shift at a Doppler angle θ is adjusted by 1/cos(θ) in order to achieve accurate velocity estimates. Selected cosine values are cos $0° = 1$, cos $30° = 0.87$, cos $45° = 0.707$, cos $60° = 0.5$, and cos $90° = 0$. At a 60-degree Doppler angle, the measured Doppler frequency is ½ the actual Doppler frequency, and at 90 degrees, the measured frequency is 0. The *preferred* Doppler angle ranges from 30 to 60 degrees. At too large an angle (greater than 60 degrees), the apparent

TABLE 14-7   DOPPLER ANGLE AND ERROR ESTIMATES OF BLOOD VELOCITY FOR A A +3-DEGREE ANGLE ACCURACY ERROR

ANGLE (DEGREES)	SET ANGLE (DEGREES)	ACTUAL VELOCITY (cm/s)	ESTIMATED VELOCITY (cm/s)	PERCENT ERROR (%)
0	3	100	100.1	0.14
25	28	100	102.6	2.65
45	48	100	105.7	5.68
60	63	100	110.1	10.1
80	83	100	142.5	42.5

Doppler shift is small, and minor errors in angle accuracy can result in large errors in velocity (Table 14-7). At too small an angle (e.g., less than 20 degrees), refraction and critical angle interactions can cause problems, as can aliasing of the signal in pulsed Doppler studies.

The Doppler frequency shifts for moving blood occur in the audible range. It is both customary and convenient to convert these frequency shifts into an audible signal through a loudspeaker that can be heard by the sonographer to aid in positioning and to assist in diagnosis.

EXAMPLE   Given: f_i = 5 MHz, v = 35 cm/s, and θ = 45 degrees, calculate the Doppler shift frequency.

$$f_d = \frac{2 \times 5\times10^6 /s \times 35cm/s \times 0.707}{154,000\ cm/s} = 1.6\times10^3 /s = 1.6\,kHz$$

The frequency shift of 1.6 kHz is in the audible range (15 Hz to 20 kHz). With an increased Doppler angle, the measured Doppler shift is *decreased* according to cos (θ) since the projection of the velocity vector toward the transducer decreases (and thus the audible frequencies decrease to lower pitch).

Continuous Doppler Operation

The continuous wave Doppler system is the simplest and least expensive device for measuring blood velocity. Two transducers are required, with one transmitting the incident ultrasound and the other detecting the resultant continuous echoes (Fig. 14-38). An oscillator produces a resonant frequency to drive the transmit transducer and provides the same frequency signal to the demodulator, which compares the returning frequency to the incident frequency. The receiver amplifies the returning signal and extracts the residual information containing the Doppler shift frequency by using a "low-pass" filter, which removes the superimposed high-frequency oscillations. The Doppler signal contains very low-frequency signals from vessel walls and other moving specular reflectors that a *wall filter* selectively removes. An audio amplifier amplifies the Doppler signal to an audible sound level, and a recorder tracks spectrum changes as a function of time for analysis of transient pulsatile flow.

Continuous wave Doppler suffers from depth selectivity with accuracy affected by object motion within the beam path. Multiple overlying vessels will result in superimposition, making it difficult to distinguish a specific Doppler signal. Spectral

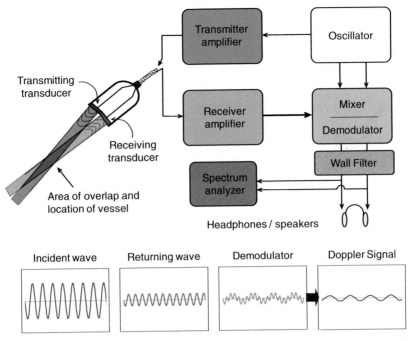

■ **FIGURE 14-38** Block diagram of a continuous wave Doppler system. Two transducers are required: one as a transmitter and the other as a receiver. The area of overlap determines the position of blood velocity measurement. Signals from the receiver are mixed with the original frequency to extract the Doppler signal. A low-pass filter removes the highest frequencies in the demodulated signals, and a high-pass filter (Wall filter) removes the lowest frequencies due to tissue and transducer motion to extract the desired Doppler shift.

broadening of the frequencies occurs with a large sample area across the vessel profile (composed of high velocity in the center and slower velocities at the edge of the vessels). Advantages of continuous mode include high accuracy of the Doppler shift measurement because a narrow frequency bandwidth is used and no aliasing when high velocities are measured, as occurs with pulsed Doppler operation (see below).

Quadrature Detection

The demodulation technique measures the magnitude of the Doppler shift but does not reveal the direction of the Doppler shift, that is, whether the flow is toward or away from the transducers. A method of signal processing called quadrature detection is phase sensitive and can indicate the direction of flow either toward or away from the transducers.

Pulsed Doppler Operation

Pulsed Doppler ultrasound combines the velocity determination of continuous wave Doppler systems and the range discrimination of pulse-echo imaging. A transducer tuned for pulsed Doppler operation is used in a pulse-echo format, similar to imaging. The SPL is longer (a minimum of 5 cycles per pulse up to 25 cycles per pulse) to provide a higher Q factor and improve the measurement accuracy of the frequency shift (although at the expense of axial resolution). Depth selection is achieved with an electronic time gate circuit to reject all echo signals except those falling within the gate window, as determined by the operator. In some systems, multiple gates provide profile patterns of velocity

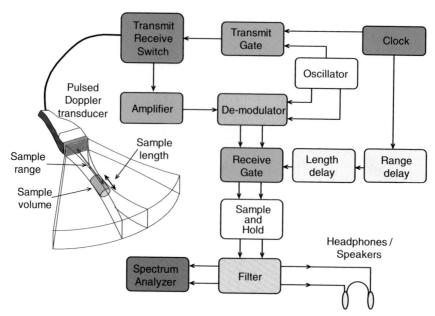

■ **FIGURE 14-39** Block diagram of a pulsed Doppler system. Isolation of a selected area is achieved by gating the time of echo return and analyzing only those echoes that fall within the time window of the gate. In the pulsed mode, the Doppler signal is discretely sampled in time to estimate the frequency shifts occurring in the Doppler gate. Because axial resolution isn't as important as narrow bandwidths to better estimate the Doppler shift, a long spatial pulse width (high Q factor) is employed.

values across a vessel. Figure 14-39 illustrates a simple block diagram of the pulsed Doppler system and the system subcomponents necessary for data processing.

Each Doppler pulse does not contain enough information to completely determine the Doppler shift, but only a *sample* of the shifted frequencies measured as a phase change. Stationary objects within the sample volume do not generate a phase change in the returning echo when compared to the oscillator phase, but a moving object does. Repeated echoes from the active gate are analyzed in the sample/hold circuit, and a Doppler signal is gradually built up (Fig. 14-40A). The discrete measurements acquired at the *PRF* produce the synthesized Doppler signal. According to sampling theory, a signal can be reconstructed unambiguously as long as the true frequency (e.g., the Doppler shift) is less than half the sampling rate. Thus, the *PRF must be at least twice the maximal Doppler frequency shift* encountered in the measurement.

The maximum Doppler shift Δf_{max} that is unambiguously determined in the pulsed Doppler acquisition follows directly from the Doppler equation by substituting V_{max} for V:

$$\Delta f_{max} = \frac{PRF}{2} = \frac{2 f_0 V_{max} \cos(\boldsymbol{\theta})}{c}$$

Rearranging the equation and solving for V_{max}:

$$V_{max} = \frac{c \times PRF}{4 \times f_0 \times \cos(\boldsymbol{\theta})}$$

shows that the maximum blood velocity that is *accurately* determined is increased with larger PRF, lower operating frequency, and larger angle (the cosine of the angle gets smaller with larger angles from 0 to 90 degrees).

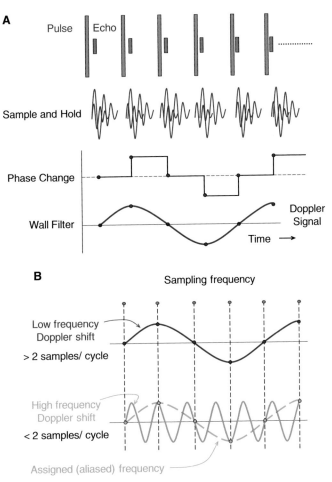

■ **FIGURE 14-40 A.** The returning ultrasound pulses from the Doppler gate are sampled over several pulse-echo cycles (in this example, six times), in order to estimate Doppler shifts (if any) caused by moving blood cells. A sample and hold circuit measures a variation of signal with time (note that the echo [*purple line*] and the pulse [*blue line*] vary in phase, which are recorded and analyzed by Fourier transform methods to determine the Doppler shift frequencies). The wall filter removes the low-frequency degradations caused by transducer and patient motion. **B.** Aliasing occurs when the frequencies in the sampled signal are greater than ½ the PRF (sampling frequency). In this example, a signal of twice the frequency is analyzed as if it were the lower frequency and thus mimics (aliases) the lower frequency.

For Doppler shift frequencies exceeding one-half the PRF, aliasing will occur, causing a potentially significant error in the velocity estimation of the blood (Fig. 14-40B). Thus, a 1.6-kHz Doppler shift requires a minimum PRF of 2×1.6 kHz = 3.2 kHz. One cannot simply increase the PRF to arbitrarily high values, because of echo transit time and possible echo ambiguity. Use of a larger angle between the ultrasound beam direction and the blood flow direction (e.g., 60 degrees) reduces the Doppler shift. Thus, higher velocities can be unambiguously determined for a given PRF at larger Doppler angles. However, at larger angles (e.g., 60 to 90 degrees), small errors in angle estimation cause significant errors in the estimation of blood velocity (see Table 14-7).

A 180-degree phase shift in the Doppler frequency represents blood that is moving away from the transducer. Often, higher frequency signals in the spectrum will be interpreted as lower frequency signals with a 180-degree phase shift, such that the highest blood velocities in the center of a vessel are measured as having reverse flow. This is another manifestation of aliasing.

Duplex Scanning

Duplex scanning refers to the combination of 2D B-mode imaging and pulsed Doppler data acquisition. Without visual guidance to the vessel of interest, pulsed Doppler systems would be of little use. A duplex scanner operates in the imaging mode and creates a real-time image. The Doppler gate is positioned over the vessel of interest with size (length and width) appropriate for evaluation of blood velocity, and at an orientation (angle with respect to the interrogating US beam) that represents the Doppler angle. When switched to Doppler mode, the scanner electronics determines the proper timing to extract data only from within the user-defined gate.

Instrumentation for duplex scanning is available in several configurations. Most often, electronic array transducers switch between a group of transducers used to create a B-mode image and one or more transducers used for the Doppler information.

The duplex system allows estimation of the blood velocity directly from the Doppler shift frequency, since the velocity of sound and the transducer frequency are known, while the Doppler angle can be estimated from the B-mode image and input into the scanner computer for calculation. Once the velocity is known, flow (in units of cm^3/s) is estimated as the product of the vessel's cross-sectional area (cm^2) times the velocity (cm/s).

Errors in the flow volume may occur. The vessel axis might not lie totally within the scanned plane, the vessel might be curved, or flow might be altered from the perceived direction. The beam-vessel angle (Doppler angle) could be in error, which is much more problematic for very large angles, particularly those greater than 60 degrees, as explained previously. The Doppler gate (sample area) could be mispositioned or of inappropriate size, such that the velocities are an overestimate (gate area too small) or underestimate (gate area too large) of the average velocity. Noncircular cross sections will cause errors in the area estimate, and therefore errors in the flow volume.

Multigate pulsed Doppler systems operate with several parallel channels closely spaced across the lumen of a single large vessel. The outputs from all of the gates can be combined to estimate the *velocity profile* across the vessel, which represents the variation of flow velocity within the vessel lumen. Velocities mapped with a color scale visually separate the flow information from the gray-scale image, and a real-time color flow Doppler ultrasound image indicates the direction of flow through color coding. However, time is insufficient to complete the computations necessary for determining the Doppler shifts from a large number of gates to get real-time image update rates, particularly for those located at depth.

Color Flow Imaging

Color flow imaging provides a 2D visual display of moving blood in the vasculature, superimposed upon the conventional gray-scale image as shown in Figure 14-41. Velocities and directions are determined for multiple positions within a subarea of the image and then color encoded (e.g., shades of red for blood moving toward the transducer, and shades of blue for blood moving away from the transducer). Two-dimensional color flow systems do not use the full Doppler shift information because of a lack of time and/or a lack of parallel channels necessary for real-time imaging. Instead, phase-shift autocorrelation or time domain correlation techniques are used.

Phase-shift autocorrelation is a technique to measure the similarity of one scan line measurement to another when the maximum correlation (overlap) occurs. The autocorrelation processor compares the entire echo pulse of one A-line with that of a previous echo pulse separated by a time equal to the PRP. This "self-scanning" algorithm detects changes in phase between two A-lines of data due to any Doppler shift over the time Δt (Fig. 14-41A). The output correlation varies proportionately with the phase change, which in turn varies proportionately with the velocity at the point along the echo pulse trace. In addition, the direction of the moving object (toward or away from the transducer) is preserved through phase detection of the echo amplitudes. Generally, four to eight traces are used to determine the presence of motion along one A-line of the scanned region. Therefore, the beam must remain stationary for short periods of time before insonating another area in the imaging volume. Additionally, because a gray-scale B-mode image must be acquired at the

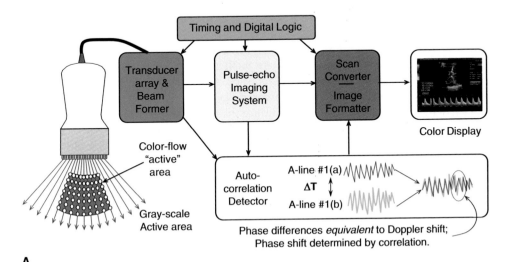

A

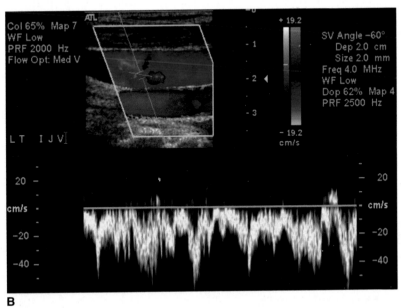

B

■ **FIGURE 14-41 A.** The color flow acquisition produces dynamic gray-scale B-mode images with color-encoded velocity maps in a user-defined "active area" of multiple "gates." **Inset.** Autocorrelation detection is a technique to rapidly determine phase changes (equivalent to Doppler shift) in areas of motion deduced from two (or more) consecutive A-lines of data along the same direction. **B.** Patient data showing arterial and venous flow, with color assignments (red towards and blue away from the transducer) depicting the direction of blood flow. Within the image, the Doppler gate and Doppler angle are shown within the **blue** area, and the bottom graph depicts the Spectral Doppler information extracted from the gate.

same time, the flow information must be interleaved with the image information. The motion data are mapped with a color scale and superimposed on the gray-scale image. FOV determines the processing time necessary to evaluate the color flow data. A smaller FOV delivers a faster frame rate but, of course, sacrifices the area evaluated for flow. One important consideration is keeping the beam at an angle to the vessel axis to avoid a 90-degree angle. This can be achieved by electronic steering of the color flow ultrasound beams or by angling the array transducer relative to the vessel axis (Fig. 14-41B).

Time domain correlation is an alternate method for color flow imaging. It is based upon the measurement that a reflector has moved over a time Δt between consecutive pulse-echo acquisitions (Fig. 14-42). Correlation mathematically determines the degree of similarity between two quantities. From echo train one, a series of templates are formed, which are mathematically manipulated over echo train two to determine the time shifts that result in the best correlation. Stationary reflectors need no time shift for high correlation; moving reflectors require a time Δt (either positive or negative) to produce the maximal correlation. The displacement of the reflector (Δx) is determined by the range equation as $\Delta x = (c\ \Delta t)/2$, where c is the speed of sound. Measured velocity ($\mathbf{V_m}$) is calculated as the displacement divided by the time between pulses (the PRP): $\mathbf{V_m} = \Delta x/\text{PRP}$. Finally, correction for the angle (θ) between the beam axis and the direction of motion (like the standard Doppler correction) is $\mathbf{V} = \mathbf{V_m}/\cos(\theta)$. The velocity determines assignment of color, and the images appear essentially the same as Doppler-processed images. Multiple pulse-echo sequences are typically acquired to provide a good estimate of reflector displacements; frame update rates are reduced corresponding to the number of repeated measurements per line. With time domain correlation methods, short transmit pulses can be used, unlike the longer transmit pulses required for Doppler acquisitions where longer pulses are necessary to achieve narrow bandwidth pulses. This permits better axial resolution. Also, time domain correlation is less prone to aliasing effects compared to Doppler methods because greater time shifts can be tolerated in the returning echo signals from one pulse to the next, which means that higher velocities can be measured.

There are several limitations with color flow imaging. Noise and clutter of slowly moving, solid structures can overwhelm smaller echoes returning from moving blood cells in color flow image. The spatial resolution of the color display is much poorer than the gray-scale image, and variations in velocity are not well resolved in a large vessel. Velocity calculation accuracy by the autocorrelation technique can be limited. Since the color flow map does not fully describe the Doppler frequency spectrum,

■ FIGURE 14-42 Time domain correlation uses a short SPL and an echo "template" to determine positional change of moving reflectors from subsequent echoes. The template scans the echo train to find maximum correlation in each A-line; the displacement between the maximum correlations of each A-line divided by the PRP is the measured velocity.

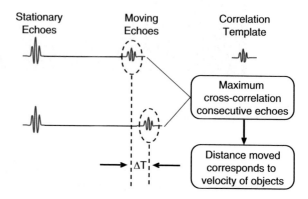

many color 2D units also provide a duplex scanning capability to provide a spectral analysis of specific questionable areas indicated by the color flow examination. Aliasing artifacts due to insufficient sampling of the phase shifts are also a problem that affects the color flow image, causing apparent reversed flow in areas of high velocity (e.g., stenosis).

Doppler Spectral Interpretation

The Doppler signal is typically represented by a spectrum of frequencies resulting from a range of velocities contained within the sampling gate at a specific point in time. Blood flow can exhibit laminar, blunt, or turbulent flow patterns, depending upon the vessel wall characteristics, the size and shape of the vessel, and the flow rate. Fast, laminar flow exists in the center of large, smooth wall vessels, while slower blood flow occurs near the vessel walls, due to frictional forces. Turbulent flow occurs at disruptions in the vessel wall caused by plaque buildup and stenosis. A large Doppler gate that is positioned to encompass the entire lumen of the vessel will contain a large range of blood velocities, while a smaller gate positioned in the center of the vessel will have a smaller, faster range of velocities. A Doppler gate positioned near a stenosis in the turbulent flow pattern will measure the largest range of velocities.

With the pulsatile nature of blood flow, the spectral characteristics vary with time. Interpretation of the frequency shifts and direction of blood flow is accomplished with the fast Fourier transform, which mathematically analyzes the detected signals and generates amplitude versus frequency distribution profile known as the *Doppler spectrum*. In a clinical instrument, the Doppler spectrum is continuously updated in a real-time *spectral Doppler display* (Fig. 14-43). This information is displayed on the video monitor, typically below the 2D B-mode image, as a moving trace, with the blood velocity (proportional to Doppler frequency) as the vertical axis (from $-V_{max}$ to $+ V_{max}$) and time as the horizontal axis. The intensity of the Doppler signal at a particular frequency and moment in time is displayed as the brightness at that point on the display. Velocities in one direction are displayed as positive values along the vertical axis and velocities in the other direction are displayed as negative values. As new data arrive, the information is updated and scrolled from left to right. Pulsatile blood takes on the appearance of a choppy sinusoidal wave through the periodic cycle of the heartbeat.

Interpretation of the spectral display provides the ability to determine the presence of flow, the direction of flow, and characteristics of the flow. It is more difficult to determine a lack of flow, since it is also necessary to ensure that the lack of signal is not due to other acoustical or electrical system parameters or problems. The direction of flow (positive or negative Doppler shift) is best determined with a small Doppler angle (about 30 degrees). Normal flow is typically characterized by a specific spectral Doppler display waveform, which is a consequence of the hemodynamic features of particular vessels. Disturbed and turbulent flow produce Doppler spectra that are correlated with disease processes. In these latter situations, the spectral curve is "filled in" with a wide distribution of frequencies representing a wide range of velocities, as might occur with a vascular stenosis. Vascular impedance and pulsatile velocity changes concurrent with the circulation can be tracked by Doppler spectrum techniques. Pertinent quantitative measures, such as pulsatility index: PI = (max − min)/average and resistive index: RI = (max − min)/max, are dependent on the characteristics of the Doppler spectral display (see Fig. 14-44 for description of max, min, and average values extracted from the display).

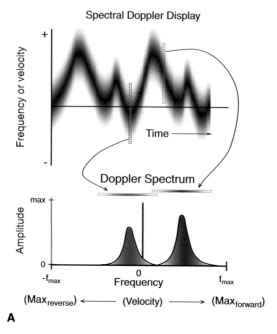

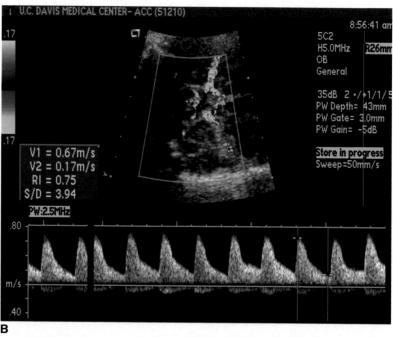

■ **FIGURE 14-43 A.** The spectral Doppler display is a plot of the Doppler shift frequency spectrum displayed vertically, versus time, displayed horizontally. The amplitude of the shift frequency is encoded as gray-scale or color intensity variations. Bottom graph: Two Doppler spectra are shown from the spectral display at two discrete points in time, with amplitude (gray-scale variations) plotted versus frequency (velocity). A broad spectrum (bandwidth) represents turbulent flow, while a narrow spectrum represents laminar flow within the Doppler gate. **B.** Color flow image showing the active color area and the corresponding spectral Doppler display (below) determined from a gate volume positioned over a specific location in the vasculature. The resistive index is calculated from the color intensity spectral display and indicated on the image as RI (note the electronic calipers on the spectrum). The color scale values and velocities in this acquisition are calibrated in m/s.

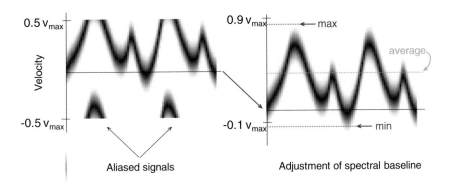

■ FIGURE 14-44 Left. Aliasing of the spectral Doppler display is characterized by "wrap-around" of the highest velocities to the opposite direction when the sampling (PRF) is inadequate. **Right.** Without changing the overall velocity range, the spectral baseline is shifted to incorporate higher forward velocity and less reverse velocity to avoid aliasing. The maximum, average, and minimum spectral Doppler display values allow quantitative determination of clinically relevant information such as pulsatility index and resistive index.

Velocity Aliasing

Aliasing, as described earlier, is an error caused by an insufficient sampling rate (PRF) relative to the high-frequency Doppler signals generated by fast-moving blood. A minimum of two samples per cycle of Doppler shift frequency is required to unambiguously determine the corresponding velocity. In a spectral Doppler display, the aliased signals wrap around to negative amplitude, masquerading as reversed flow (Fig. 14-44, left). The most straightforward method to reduce or eliminate the aliasing error is for the user to adjust the velocity scale to a wider range, as most instruments have the PRF of the Doppler unit linked to the scale setting (a wide range delivers a high PRF). If the scale is already at the maximum PRF, the *spectral baseline*, which represents 0 velocity (0 Doppler shift), can be readjusted to allocate a greater sampling (frequency range) for reflectors moving toward the transducer (Fig. 14-42, right). However, the minimum to the maximum Doppler shift still cannot exceed $\pm PRF/2$. In such a case, the baseline might be adjusted to $-0.1\ V_{max}$ to $+0.9\ V_{max}$, to allow most of the frequency sampling to be assigned to the positive velocities (positive frequency shifts). From the adjusted spectral Doppler display, the maximum, minimum, and average velocities of the blood flow can be determined, and the resistive index as well as other pertinent vascular values can be calculated.

Power Doppler

Doppler analysis places a constraint on the sensitivity to motion, because the signals generated by motion must be extracted to determine velocity and direction from the Doppler and phase shifts in the returning echoes within each gated region. In color flow imaging, the frequency shift encodes the pixel value and assigns a color, which is further divided into positive and negative directions. *Power Doppler* is a signal processing method that relies on the total strength of the Doppler signal (amplitude) and ignores directional (phase) information. The power (also known as energy) mode of signal acquisition is dependent on the amplitude of all Doppler

Color Flow   Power

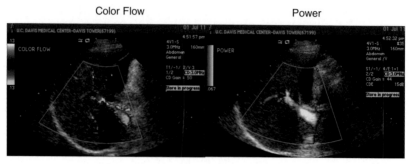

■ **FIGURE 14-45** A comparison of color Doppler (**left**) and power Doppler (**right**) studies shows the enhanced sensitivity of the power Doppler acquisition, particularly in areas perpendicular to the beam direction, where the signal is lost in the color Doppler image. Flow directionality, however, is not available in the power Doppler image.

signals, regardless of the frequency shift. This dramatically improves the sensitivity to motion (e.g., slow blood flow) at the expense of directional and quantitative flow information. Compared to conventional color flow imaging, power Doppler produces images that have more sensitivity to motion and are not affected as much by the Doppler angle (largely nondirectional). Aliasing is not a problem as only the strength of the frequency shifted signals are analyzed, and not the phase. Greater sensitivity allows detection and interpretation of very subtle and slow blood flow. On the other hand, frame rates tend to be slower for the power Doppler imaging mode, and a significant amount of "flash artifacts" occur, which are related to color signals arising from moving tissues, patient motion, or transducer motion. The name "power Doppler" is sometimes mistakenly understood as implying the use of increased transmit power to the patient, but, in fact, the power levels are typically the same as in a standard color flow procedure. The difference is in the processing of the returning signals, where sensitivity is achieved at the expense of direction and quantitation. Images acquired with color flow and power Doppler are illustrated in Figure 14-45.

14.8   Miscellaneous Ultrasound Capabilities

Distance, Area, and Volume Measurements

Measurements of distance, area, and volume are performed routinely in diagnostic ultrasound examinations. This is possible because the speed of sound in soft tissue is known to within about $\pm 1\%$ accuracy ($1,540 \pm 15$ m/s), and calibration of the instrument can be easily performed based on round-trip time of the pulse and the echo. A notable example of common distance evaluations is for fetal age determination by measuring fetal head diameter (Fig. 14-46). Measurement accuracy is achieved by careful selection of reference positions, such as the leading edge to the leading edge of the reflector echo signals along the axis of the beam, as these points are less affected by variations in echo signal amplitude. Measurements between points along the direction of the ultrasound beam are usually more reliable, because of the better axial spatial resolution. Points measured along the lateral plane have a tendency to be smeared out over a larger area due to the poorer lateral resolution of the system. Thus, horizontal and oblique measurements will likely be less accurate. The circumference of a circular object can easily

A   Fetal gestational age (GA) measurements

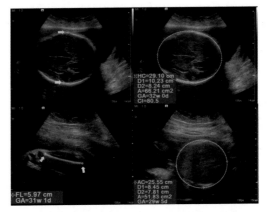

BPD: Biparietal diameter   HC: Head circumference
FL: Femur Length   AC: Abdominal circumference

B   Structured report with composite data

Composite Data

LMP		10/28/2010	
Clinical Age		31w 1d	EDC 8/4/2011
US Age	Average	31w 1d	US EDC 8/4/2011
EFW	Hadlock (BPD, HC, AC, FL)	1604g +/- 237g (3 lb 9oz +/- 8oz)	
EFW%	Jeanty 26		

OB 2D-Mode Ratio Measurements

	Ratio	Range Low	Range High	Growth Author	%
CI	80.5	74.0	83.0		
HC/AC	1.14	0.96	1.17	Campbell	89
FL/BPD	76.7	71.2	87.2		
FL/HC	20.6	17.3	23.3		
FL/AC	23.4	20.0	24.0		

OB Gestational Age Measurements

	Author	w	d	2SD (d)	Mean			Growth Author	%
BPD	Hadlock	31	3	22	7.82	7.82	cm	Hadlock	47
HC	Hadlock	32	0	21	29.10	29.10	cm	Hadlock	38
AC	Hadlock	29	6	15	25.63	25.49	cm	Hadlock	13
						25.84	cm		

■ **FIGURE 14-46 A.** Ultrasound provides accurate distance measurements. Fetal age is often determined by biparietal diameter, circumference measurements (**top**), and femur length, abdominal circumference measurements (**bottom**). Based upon known correlation methods, the gestational age can be calculated for each of the measurements. **B.** The structured report captures and summarizes the data in a tabular format as part of the reporting mechanism.

be calculated from the measured diameter (d) or radius (r), using the relationship circumference = $2\pi r = \pi d$. Distance measurements extend to two dimensions (area) in a straightforward way by assuming a specific geometric shape. Similarly, area measurements in a given image plane extend to 3D volumes by estimating the slice thickness (elevational resolution).

Ultrasound Contrast Agents

Ultrasound contrast agents for vascular and perfusion imaging are becoming extremely important from the clinical perspective. Most agents are comprised of encapsulated microbubbles of 3 to 5 μm diameter containing air, nitrogen, or insoluble gaseous compounds such as perfluorocarbons. Encapsulation materials, such as human albumin, provide a container for the gas to maintain stability for a reasonable time in the vasculature after injection. The natural tendency is for the gas to diffuse rapidly into the bloodstream (e.g., within seconds) even when encapsulated; successful contrast agents maintain stability over a period of time that allows propagation to specific anatomical vascular areas that are targeted for imaging. Because of the small size of the encapsulated bubbles, perfusion of tissues is also possible, but the bubbles must remain extremely stable during the time required for tissue uptake.

The basis for generating an ultrasound signal is the large difference in acoustic impedance between the gas and the fluids and tissues, as well as the compressibility of the bubbles compared to the incompressible materials that are displaced. The bubbles are small compared with the wavelength of the ultrasound beam and thus become a point source of sound, producing reflections in all directions. In addition, the compressibility produces shifts in the returning frequency of the echoes, called frequency harmonics (described in the next section), which are typically higher than the original ultrasound frequency. To fully use the properties of contrast agents, imaging techniques apart from standard B-mode scans are necessary and are based upon the nonlinear compressibility of the gas bubbles and the frequency harmonics that are generated (see below, e.g., pulse inversion harmonic imaging). Destruction of the microbubbles occurs with the incident ultrasound pulse and therefore requires temporal delays between images to allow circulating contrast agent to appear.

Harmonic Imaging

Harmonic frequencies are integral multiples of the frequencies contained in an ultrasound pulse. A pulse with center frequency of f_0 MHz, upon interaction with a medium, will contain high-frequency harmonics of $2 f_0$, $3 f_0$, $4 f_0$, etc. These higher frequencies arise through the vibration of encapsulated gas bubbles used as ultrasound contrast agents or with the *nonlinear propagation* of the ultrasound as it travels through tissues. For contrast agents, the vibration modes of the encapsulated gas reemit higher order harmonics due to the small size of the microbubbles (~3- to 6-μm diameter) and the resultant contraction/expansion from the acoustic pressure variations. *Harmonic imaging* enhances contrast agent imaging by using a low-frequency incident pulse and tuning the receiver (using a multifrequency transducer) to higher frequency harmonics. This approach allows removal of "echo clutter" from fundamental frequency reflections in the near field to improve the sensitivity to the ultrasound contrast agent. Even though the returning harmonic signals have higher attenuation (e.g., the first harmonic will have approximately twice the attenuation coefficient compared to the fundamental frequency), the echoes have to only travel half the distance as the originating ultrasound pulse and thus have a relatively large signal. For harmonic imaging, longer pulse lengths are often used to achieve a higher transducer Q factor. This allows an easier separation of the frequency harmonics from the fundamental frequency. Although the longer SPL degrades axial resolution, the benefits of harmonic imaging overcome the slight degradation in axial resolution.

Based on the harmonic imaging work with microbubble contrast agents, "native tissue" harmonic imaging (imaging higher frequency harmonics produced by tissues when using lower frequency incident sound waves) is now possible and in common use. Harmonic frequencies are generated by the nonlinear distortion of the wave as the high-pressure component (compression) travels faster than the low-pressure component (rarefaction) of the acoustic wave in tissue. This wave distortion, illustrated in Figure 14-47A, increases with depth and localizes in the central area of the beam. The returning echoes comprising the harmonics travel

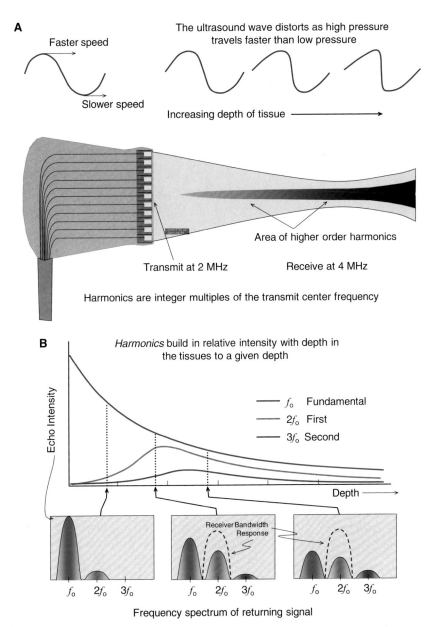

A. Faster speed

Slower speed

The ultrasound wave distorts as high pressure travels faster than low pressure

Increasing depth of tissue

Area of higher order harmonics

Transmit at 2 MHz   Receive at 4 MHz

Harmonics are integer multiples of the transmit center frequency

B. *Harmonics* build in relative intensity with depth in the tissues to a given depth

Echo Intensity

f_o Fundamental
$2f_o$ First
$3f_o$ Second

Depth

Receiver Bandwidth Response

f_o $2f_o$ $3f_o$ f_o $2f_o$ $3f_o$ f_o $2f_o$ $3f_o$

Frequency spectrum of returning signal

■ **FIGURE 14-47 A.** Harmonic frequencies, integer multiples of the fundamental frequency, are produced by the nonlinear propagation of the ultrasound beam, where the high-pressure component travels faster than the low-pressure component of the wave. The wave distortion occurs in the central area of the beam. **B.** Ultrasound harmonic frequencies ($2f_o$, $3f_o$) build with depth and attenuate at a higher, frequency-dependent rate. The frequency spectrum and harmonic amplitudes continuously change with depth (lower figure, displaying three points in time). The transducer bandwidth response must encompass the higher harmonics.

only slightly greater than one-half the distance to the transducer and, despite the higher attenuation, have less but substantial amplitude compared to the fundamental frequency (Fig. 14-47B). The first harmonic (twice the fundamental frequency) is commonly used because it suffers less attenuation than higher order harmonics and because higher order harmonics are likely to exceed the transducer's bandwidth.

C

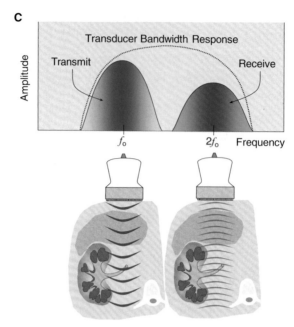

■ FIGURE 14-47 (*Continued*) **C.** Native tissue harmonic imaging uses a lower center frequency spectrum (e.g., 2-MHz spectrum) and receives echoes from the higher harmonics (e.g., 4-MHz spectrum).

Tuning the broadband receiver to the first harmonic spectrum filters out the lower frequency echoes (to the extent that the spectra do not overlap) and eliminates ultrasound reflections and scattering from tissues and objects adjacent to the transducer (Fig. 14-47C). Improved lateral spatial resolution (a majority of the echoes are produced in the central area of the beam), reduced side lobe artifacts, and removal of multiple reverberation artifacts caused by anatomy adjacent to the transducer are some advantages of tissue harmonic imaging. Comparison of conventional and harmonic right kidney images demonstrates improved image quality (Fig. 14-48), typical of many examinations. While not always advantageous, native tissue harmonic imaging

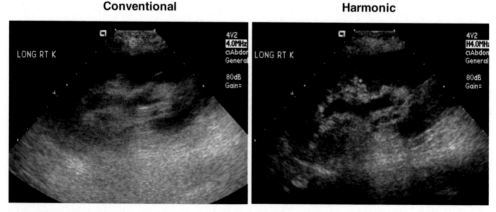

■ FIGURE 14-48 Conventional (**left**) and harmonic image (**right**) of the kidney demonstrate the improved image quality of the harmonic image from reduced echo clutter, increased contrast, and resolution. (Images provided by Dr. Kiran Jain, MD, University of California Davis Health System).

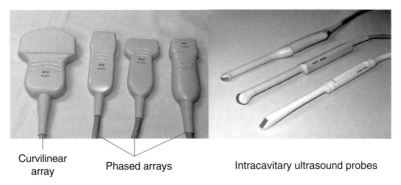

Curvilinear array   Phased arrays   Intracavitary ultrasound probes

■ **FIGURE 14-49** Transducer assemblies come in a variety of shapes and sizes. Each transducer (size, format, frequency) is selected for specific examinations. External (**left**) and intracavitary (**right**) transducers are shown. Intracavitary probes provide an inside out acoustic mapping of soft tissue anatomy.

is best applied in situations such as abdominal imaging that require a lower frequency to achieve adequate penetration to begin with and then switched to the higher frequency harmonic for better quality and less "clutter" adjacent to the transducer.

Transducer Assemblies

Most general-purpose ultrasound units are equipped with at least a linear array abdominal transducer of relatively low frequency (good penetration), and a separate small-parts phased-array transducer of high frequency (high spatial resolution). Special-purpose transducers come in a wide variety of sizes, shapes, and operational frequencies, usually designed for a specific application. Intracavitary transducers for transrectal, transurethral, transvaginal, and transesophageal examinations provide high-resolution, high-frequency imaging of anatomic structures that are in proximity to the cavity walls. For example, transducers for transrectal scanning with linear array or mechanical rotating designs are used routinely to image the bladder or the prostate gland. External and intracavitary transducer probes are shown in Figure 14-49.

Intravascular ultrasound (IVUS) devices are catheter-mounted, typically with a rotating single transducer or phased-array transducer (up to 64 acoustic elements) design, and commonly used in interventional radiology and cardiology procedures. Operating frequencies from about 10 MHz up to 60 MHz are typical, with PRF operation from 15 to 80 kHz create high-resolution (80 to 100 μm detail) acoustic images inside the vessel. The high attenuation and minimal range of the ultrasound allow high PRF sampling. A stack of cylindrical images can be created as the catheter is pulled back through the vasculature of interest, and the vessel volume rendered. Intravascular transducers can be used to assess vessel wall morphology, to differentiate plaque types (fibrous, fibrofatty, necrotic core, dense calcium), to estimate stenosis, and to determine the efficacy of vascular intervention. Figure 14-50 shows IVUS transducer types, depiction of the ultrasound beam, and cylindrical images demonstrating a normal and a diseased vessel lumen.

Ultrasound Biopsy Guidance

Ultrasound is extremely useful for the guidance of biopsy procedures of suspicious solid masses or signs of abnormal tissue change. A fine needle or a core needle is used in many areas of the body, such as the breast, prostate, thyroid, abdominal and

■ FIGURE 14-50 Intravascular ultrasound: devices and images. Catheter-mounted transducer arrays provide an acoustic analysis of the vessel lumen and wall from the inside out. Mechanical (rotating shaft and acoustic mirror with a single transducer) and electronic phased-array transducer assemblies are used. Images show a normal vessel lumen (**lower left**) and reduced luminal stenosis and plaque buildup (**lower right**).

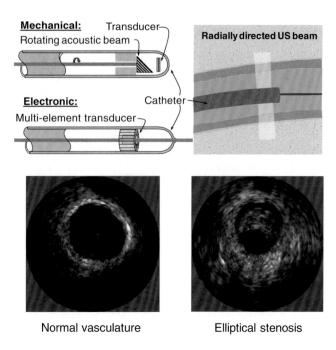

Normal vasculature   Elliptical stenosis

pelvic areas. This is made possible with the excellent needle visibility due to the reflection and scattering of ultrasound under real-time image acquisition.

Three-Dimensional Imaging

3D ultrasound imaging acquires 2D tomographic image data in a series of individual B-scans of a volume of tissue. Forming the 3D dataset requires location of each individual 2D image using known acquisition geometries. Volume sampling can be achieved in several ways with a transducer array: (1) linear translation, (2) freeform motion with external localizers to a reference position, (3) rocking motion, and (4) rotation of the scan (Fig. 14-51A). Three-dimensional image acquisition as a function of time (4D) allows visualization of motion during the scan and rendering of the 3D data. With the volume dataset acquisition geometry known, rendering into a surface display (Fig. 14-51B) by maximal intensity projection processing or volume surface rendering is achieved with data reordering. Applications of various 3D imaging protocols are being actively pursued, particularly in obstetric imaging. Features such as organ boundaries are identified in each image, and the computer calculates the 3D surface, complete with shading effects or false color for the delineation of anatomy.

14.9 Ultrasound Image Quality and Artifacts

Image quality is dependent on the design characteristics of the ultrasound equipment, the numerous equipment variables selected, and positioning skills of the operator. The equipment variables controlled by the operator include transducer frequency, PRF, ultrasound intensity, and TGC curves, among others. Measures of ultrasound image quality include spatial resolution, contrast resolution, image uniformity, and noise characteristics. Image artifacts are common phenomena that can enhance or degrade the diagnostic value of the ultrasound image.

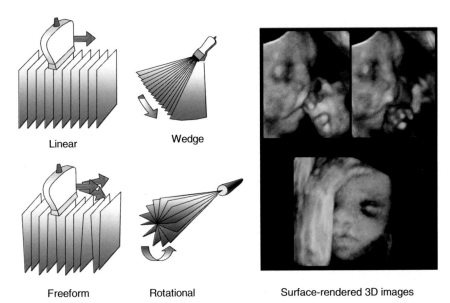

Linear   Wedge

Freeform   Rotational   Surface-rendered 3D images

■ **FIGURE 14-51** 3D ultrasound acquisitions can be accomplished in several ways as depicted on the left in the figure and include linear, wedge, freeform, and circular formats. Reconstruction of the dataset provides 3D surface-shaded and/or wire mesh renditions of the anatomy. The top images on the right are from a 4D acquisition of a fetus at two different points in time. The bottom image shows the 3D surface evaluation of a fetus with a cleft lip.

Spatial Resolution

Ultrasound spatial resolution has components in three directions—axial, lateral, and elevational. Axial resolution is determined by the frequency of the ultrasound and the damping factor of the transducer, which together determine the spatial pulse length. Lateral and elevational resolutions are determined by the dimensions (width and height, respectively) of the transducer aperture, the depth of the object, and mechanical and electronic focusing (see Figs. 14-19 to 14-23). Increasing the depth of lateral resolution focus involves a trade-off of temporal resolution for real-time imaging. Axial and lateral resolutions are in the plane of the image and plainly discernable, while elevational (slice-thickness) resolution is perpendicular to the plane of the image and not as easy to understand or to interpret. Resolution in the axial direction (along the beam) is equal to ½ SPL and independent of depth. Lateral and elevational resolutions are strongly dependent on depth. The minimum resolution in the lateral/elevational directions is typically three to five times greater than axial resolution.

Elevational resolution is a function of the height of the transducer array and is depth dependent as dictated by the near field/far field beam characteristics of the fixed transducer height. Poor elevational resolution occurs adjacent to the transducer array and beyond the near/far field interface. Elevational focusing is possible with an acoustic lens shaped along the height of the elements, which can produce an elevational focal zone closer to the array surface. Alternatively, "1.5D" array transducers have several rows (typically five to seven) of independent elements in the elevational direction ("1.5-D" indicates that the number of elements in the elevational direction is much less than in the lateral direction [over 100 to 200 elements]). Elevational focusing is achieved by introducing phase delays among the elements in different rows to electronically focus the beam in the slice-thickness dimension at a given depth (Fig. 14-23). Multiple elevational transmit focal zones incur a time penalty similar to that required for the multiple lateral focal zones.

Contrast Resolution and Noise

Contrast resolution depends on several interrelated factors. Acoustic impedance differences (Table 14-3) give rise to reflections that delineate tissue boundaries and internal architectures. The density and size of scatterers within tissues or organs produce a specific "texture" (or lack of texture) that provides recognition and detection capabilities over the FOV. Ultrasound scattering introduces additive signals from areas other than from echoes generated by specular reflectors and degrades image contrast. With proper signal processing, attenuation differences (Table 14-5) result in gray-scale differences among the tissues. Areas of low and high attenuation often produce distal signal enhancement or signal loss (e.g., fluid-filled cysts [hypoechoic], gallstones) that allows detection and identification of tissues in the image. Introduction of microbubble contrast agents improves the visualization of the vasculature and tissue perfusion. Spatial compounding provides multiple beam angles to better depict tissue boundaries, as well as provide averaging to reduce stochastic speckle and electronic noise. Harmonic imaging improves image contrast by eliminating unimportant or degrading signals from lower frequency echoes. In addition, Doppler imaging techniques use moving anatomy and sophisticated processing techniques to generate contrast.

Contrast resolution also depends upon spatial resolution. Details within the image are often distributed over the volume element represented in the tomographic slice (e.g., Fig. 14-19), which varies in the lateral and elevational dimensions as a function of depth. In areas where the slice thickness is relatively wide (close to the transducer array surface and at great depth), the returning echoes generated by a small object are averaged over the minimum volume, resulting in a lower signal and possible loss of detection. On the other hand, objects larger than the minimum volume element can actually achieve better contrast relative to the background because the random noise components are reduced by averaging over the volume.

Detection of subtle anatomy in the patient is dependent on the contrast-to-noise ratio. The contrast is generated by differences in signal amplitude as discussed above. Electronic noise is mainly generated by the electronic amplifiers of the system but is occasionally induced by environmental sources such as electrical power fluctuations and equipment malfunction such as a dead or poorly functioning transducer element. A low-noise, high-gain amplifier is crucial for optimal low-contrast resolution. Exponential attenuation of the ultrasound beam, which reduces contrast and increases noise with depth, requires TGC to improve depth uniformity. Image processing that specifically reduces noise, such as temporal or spatial averaging, can increase the contrast-to-noise ratio; however, trade-offs include lower frame rates and/or poorer spatial resolution. Low-power operation (e.g., an obstetrics power setting with low transmit gain) requires higher electronic signal amplification to increase the weak echo amplitudes to useful levels and results in a higher noise level and lower contrast-to-noise ratio. Increasing the transmit power and/or the PRF can improve contrast resolution, but there is a limit with respect to transducer capabilities, and, furthermore, the intensity must be restricted to levels unlikely to cause biological damage.

Artifacts

Artifacts arise from the incorrect display of anatomy or noise during imaging. The causes are machine and operator related, as well as intrinsic to the characteristics and interaction of ultrasound with the tissues. Understanding how artifacts are generated in ultrasound is crucial, which places high demands on the knowledge and experience of the sonographer.

Artifacts can be caused by a variety of mechanisms. For instance, sound travels at different speeds, not just the 1,540 *m/s* average value for soft tissue that is used in the "range equation" for placing echo information in the image matrix. This speed variation results in some echoes being displaced from the expected location in the image display. Sound is refracted when the beam is not perpendicular to a tissue boundary; echoes are deflected to the receiver from areas outside of the main beam and can be mismapped into the image. Improper use of TGC causes suboptimal image quality with nonuniform appearance of tissues within a given band of the image.

Fortunately, most ultrasound artifacts are discernible to the experienced sonographer because of transient appearance and/or obvious effects on the image. Some artifacts are used to advantage as a diagnostic aid in characterization of tissue structures and their composition. Besides aliasing in Doppler and color flow acquisitions discussed in Section 14.7, many common artifacts in B-mode imaging are discussed below.

Refraction

Refraction is a change in the transmitted ultrasound pulse direction at a boundary with nonperpendicular incidence, when the two tissues support a different speed of sound ($C_1 \neq C_2$). Misplaced anatomy often occurs in the image during the scan (Fig. 14-52A). The ultrasonographer must be aware of objects appearing and disappearing with slight differences in orientation of the beam. Anatomical displacement due to refraction artifacts will change with the position of the transducer and angle of incidence with the tissue boundaries.

Shadowing and Enhancement

Shadowing is a hypointense signal area distal to an object or interface and is caused by objects with high attenuation or reflection of the incident beam without the return of echoes. Highly attenuating objects such as bones or kidney stones reduce the intensity of the transmitted beam and can induce low-intensity streaks in the image. Reflection of the incident beam from curved surfaces eliminates the distal propagation of ultrasound and causes streaks or shadowing. Enhancement occurs distal to objects having very low ultrasound attenuation, such as fluid-filled cavities (e.g., a filled bladder or cysts). Hyperintense signals ("through transmission") arise from increased transmission of sound by these structures (Fig. 14-52B).

Reverberation

Reverberation artifacts arise from multiple echoes generated between two closely spaced interfaces reflecting ultrasound energy back and forth during the acquisition of the signal and before the next pulse. These artifacts are often caused by reflections between a highly reflective interface and the transducer or between reflective interfaces such as metallic objects (e.g., bullet fragments), calcified tissues, or air pocket/partial liquid areas of the anatomy. Reverberation echoes are typically manifested as multiple, equally spaced boundaries with decreasing amplitude along a straight line from the transducer (Fig. 14-52C). Comet tail artifact is a form of reverberation. Ring-down artifacts arise from resonant vibrations within fluid trapped between a tetrahedron of air bubbles, which creates a continuous sound wave that is transmitted back to the transducer and displayed as a series of parallel bands extending posterior to a collection of gas.

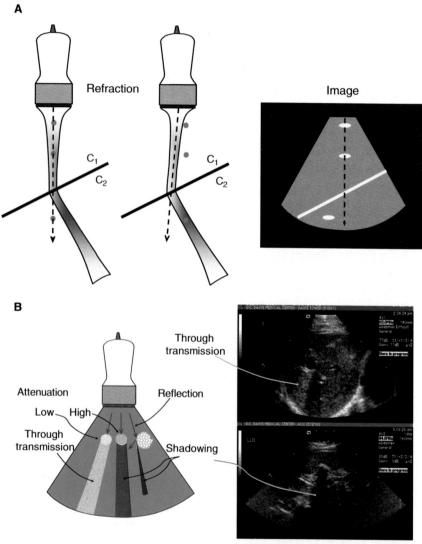

■ **FIGURE 14-52 A.** Refraction is a change in the direction of the ultrasound beam that results from non-perpendicular incidence at a boundary where the two tissues do not have the same speed of sound. During a scan, anatomy can be missed and/or dislocated from the true position. **B.** Attenuation and reflection of the ultrasound beam cause intensity changes. Enhancement occurs distal to objects of low attenuation, manifested by a hyperintense signal, while shadowing occurs distal to objects of high attenuation, resulting in a hypointense signal. At the curved edges of an organ boundary or mass, nonperpendicular reflection can cause distal hypointense streaks and shadowing. Clinical images show through transmission (top) of a low attenuation cyst and shadowing (bottom), caused by high attenuation gallstones. **C.** Reverberation commonly occurs between to strong reflectors, such as an air pocket and the transducer array (left diagram) or with calcium deposits and internal reflections (right image). The echoes bounce back and forth between the two boundaries and produce equally spaced signals of diminishing amplitude in the image. This is often called a "comet-tail" artifact.

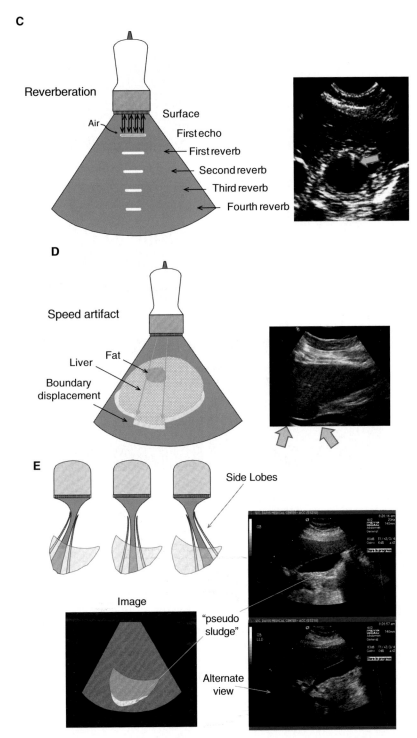

■ **FIGURE 14-52** (*Continued*) **D.** Speed of sound variation in the tissues can cause a mismapping of anatomy. In the case of fatty tissues, the slower speed of sound in fat (1,450 m/s) results in a displacement of the returning echoes from distal anatomy by about 6% of the distance traveled through the mass. **E.** Side lobe energy emissions in transducer arrays can cause anatomy outside of the main beam to be mapped into the main beam. For a curved boundary, such as the gallbladder, side lobe interactions can be remapped and produce findings such as "pseudo" sludge that is not apparent with other scanning angles. Clinical images (top) show pseudosludge, which is not evident after repositioning the transducer assembly (bottom).

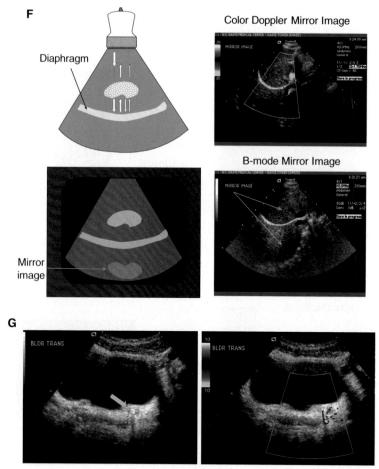

■ FIGURE 14-52 (*Continued*) **F.** A mirror image artifact arises from multiple beam reflections between a mass and a strong reflector, such as the diaphragm. Multiple echoes result in the creation of a mirror image of the mass beyond the diaphragm. Clinical images show mirror artifacts for color Doppler (**top**) and B-mode scan (**bottom**), where the lower arrow points to the artifact mirrored by the diaphragm. **G.** Twinkling artifact occurs with color flow imaging, caused by strong reflectors such as calcified stones, resulting in a changing mixture of colors indicating flow. On the left is a B-mode image of the bladder and the corresponding color flow image (*inset* trapezoidal area) demonstrating the twinkling artifact.

Speed Displacement

The speed displacement artifact is caused by the variability of speed of sound in different tissues. In particular, the lower speed of sound in fat (1,450 m/s) causes edge discontinuities of organ borders distal to fatty tissue (Fig. 14-52D). Edges are mapped outward relative to the nondisplaced tissue borders by about 6% of the distance traveled through the fat (e.g., $(1,540 - 1,450)/1,540 \times 100 = 5.8\%$). Range and distance uncertainty result from the speed artifact, and this also reduces the accuracy of spatial measurements made with ultrasound.

Side Lobes and Grating Lobes

Side lobes are emissions of the ultrasound energy that occur in a direction slightly off-axis from the main beam (see Figs. 14-17 and 14-18) and arise from the expansion of the piezoelectric elements orthogonal to the main beam. Echoes returning from tissues along the propagation direction of the side lobes are positioned in the image as if they occurred along the main beam. One type of side lobe artifact occurs near a highly reflective surface just out of the main beam. Sometimes, side lobes redirect diffuse echoes from adjacent soft tissues into an organ that is normally hypoechoic. This occurs, for instance, in imaging of the gall bladder, where the side lobes produce artifactual "pseudosludge" in an otherwise echo-free organ (Fig. 14-52E). Compared to grating lobes, side lobes are more forward directed and are present with all types of single-element and multielement transducer assemblies.

Grating lobes occur with multielement array transducers and result from the division of a smooth transducer surface into a large number of small elements. Ultrasound energy is produced at a large angle relative to the main beam. This misdirected energy can create ghost images of off-axis high-contrast objects. Grating lobe artifacts are reduced by using very closely spaced elements in the array (less than one-half wavelength apart). Linear array transducers are more prone to grating lobe artifacts than phased-array transducers, chiefly due to the larger width and spacing of the individual elements.

Multipath Reflection and Mirror Image

Near highly reflective surfaces, multiple beam reflections and refractions can find their way back to the transducer. The anatomy involved in these reflections is misplaced on the beam axis more distal to the actual position caused by delays of the echoes returning from the reflector(s). A common example is the interface of the liver and the diaphragm in abdominal imaging. The pulse from the transducer generates echoes from a mass in the liver and continues to the diaphragm, where a very strong echo is produced. This echo travels from the diaphragm back to the mass, producing another set of echoes now directed back to the diaphragm. These echoes are re-reflected from the diaphragm to the transducer. The back and forth travel distance of the second echo set from the mass produces an artifact in the image that resembles a mirror image of the mass, placed beyond the diaphragm (Fig. 14-52F).

Ambiguity

Ambiguity artifacts are created when a high PRF limits the amount of time spent listening for echoes during the PRP. As the PRF *increases*, the PRP *decreases*, with returning echoes still arriving from a greater depth after the next pulse is initiated. Mismapping of very deep echoes to shallow positions can occur in the image.

Twinkling Artifact

Doppler mode detects motion, particularly blood flow, and displays moving blood as red or blue (or selectable color) on the monitor, depending on direction and velocity. The twinkling artifact is represented as a rapidly changing mixture of colors, is typically seen distal to a strong reflector such as a calculus, and is often mistaken for an aneurysm when evaluating vessels. This artifactual appearance is possibly due to echoes from the strong reflector with frequency changes due to the wide bandwidth of the initial pulse and the narrow band "ringing" caused by the structure. Twinkling artifact may be used to identify small renal stones, as shown in Figure 14-52G, and differentiate echogenic foci from calcifications within kidney, gall bladder, and liver.

Slice Thickness

Slice thickness is determined by the beam width of the transducer array perpendicular to the image plane and is greater than the beam width in the image plane. The thickness of the slice profile varies with depth, being broad close to the transducer, narrowing at the elevational focal zone, and widening with distance beyond the focal zone. Consequences of this slice-thickness shape are loss of signal from objects that are much smaller than the volume element due to partial volume averaging and inclusion of signals from highly reflective objects that are not in the imaging plane. These artifacts are most significant at distances close and far from the transducer (see, e.g., Fig. 14-53B).

 ## Ultrasound System Performance and Quality Assurance

The system performance of a diagnostic ultrasound unit is described by several parameters, including sensitivity and dynamic range, spatial resolution, contrast sensitivity, range/distance accuracy, dead zone thickness, and TGC operation. For Doppler studies, PRF, transducer angle estimates, and range gate stability are key issues. To ensure the performance, accuracy, and safety of ultrasound equipment, periodic QC measurements are recommended. The American College of Radiology (ACR) has implemented an accreditation program that specifies recommended periodic QC procedures for ultrasound equipment. The periodic QC testing frequency of ultrasound components should be adjusted to the probability of finding instabilities or maladjustment. This can be assessed by initially performing tests frequently, reviewing logbooks over an extended period, and, with documented stability, reducing the testing rate.

Ultrasound Quality Control

Equipment QC is essentially performed every day during routine scanning by the sonographer, who should and can recognize major problems with the images and the equipment. Ensuring ultrasound image quality, however, requires implementation of a QC program with periodic measurement of system performance to identify problems before serious malfunctions occur. Required are tissue-mimicking phantoms with acoustic targets of various sizes and echogenic features embedded in a medium of uniform attenuation and speed of sound characteristic of soft tissues. Various multipurpose phantoms are available to evaluate the clinical capabilities of the ultrasound system.

A generic phantom comprised of three modules is illustrated in Figure 14-53A–C. The phantom gel filler has tissue-like attenuation of 0.5 to 0.7 (dB/cm)/MHz (higher attenuation provides a more challenging test) and low-contrast targets within a matrix of small scatterers to mimic tissue background. Small, high-contrast reflectors are positioned at known depths for measuring the axial and lateral spatial resolution, for assessing the accuracy of horizontal and vertical distance measurements, and for measuring the depth of the dead zone (the nonimaged area immediately adjacent to the transducer). Another module contains low-contrast, small-diameter spheres (or cylinders) of 2 and 4 mm diameter uniformly spaced with depth, to measure elevational resolution (slice-thickness) variation with depth. The third module is composed of a uniformly distributed scattering material for testing image uniformity and penetration depth.

Spatial resolution, contrast resolution, and distance accuracy are evaluated with one module (Fig. 14-53A). Axial resolution is evaluated by the ability to resolve high-contrast targets separated by 2, 1, 0.5, and 0.25 mm at three different depths. In an optimally functioning system, the axial resolution should be consistent with depth and improve with higher operational frequency. Lateral resolution is evaluated by measuring the lateral spread of the high-contrast targets as a function of depth and transmit focus. Contrast resolution is evaluated with "gray-scale" objects of lower and higher attenuation than the tissue-mimicking gel; more sophisticated phantoms have contrast resolution targets of varying contrast and size. Contrast resolution should improve with increased transmit power. Dead zone depth is determined with the first high-contrast target (positioned at several depths from 0 to ~1 cm) visible in the image. Horizontal and vertical distance measurement accuracy uses the small

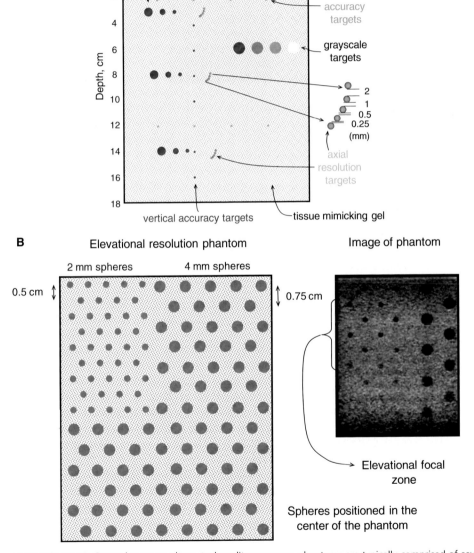

FIGURE 14-53 General-purpose ultrasound quality assurance phantoms are typically comprised of several scanning modules. **A.** System resolution targets (axial and lateral), dead zone depth, vertical and horizontal distance accuracy targets, contrast resolution (gray-scale targets), and low-scatter targets positioned at several depths (to determine penetration depths) are placed in a tissue-mimicking (acoustic scattering) gel. **B.** Elevational resolution is determined with spheres equally distributed along a plane in tissue-mimicking gel. An image of the phantom shows the effects of partial volume averaging and variations in elevational resolution with depth. (Image reprinted by permission of Gammex, Inc., Madison, WI).

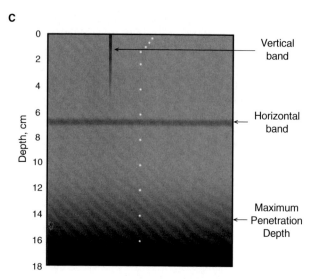

C

■ **FIGURE 14-53** *(Continued)* **C.** The system uniformity module elucidates possible problems with image uniformity. Shown in this figure is a simulation of a transducer malfunction (vertical dropout) and horizontal transition mismatch that occurs with multiple lateral focusing zone image stitching. Penetration depth for uniform response can also be determined.

high-contrast targets. Vertical targets (along the axial beam direction) should have higher precision and accuracy than the corresponding horizontal targets (lateral resolution), and all measurements should be within 5% of the known distance.

Elevational resolution and partial volume effects are evaluated with the "sphere" module (Fig. 14-53B). The ultrasound image of the spherical targets illustrates the effects of slice-thickness variation with depth and the dependence of resolvability on object size. With the introduction of 1.5D transducer arrays as well as 3D imaging capabilities, multiple transmit focal zones to reduce slice thickness at various depths is becoming important, as is the need to verify elevational resolution performance.

Uniformity and penetration depth are measured with the uniformity module (Fig. 14-53C). With a properly adjusted and operating ultrasound system, a uniform response is expected up to the penetration depth capabilities of the transducer array. Higher operational frequencies will display a lower penetration depth. Evidence of vertical-directed shadowing for linear arrays or angular-directed shadowing for phased arrays is an indication of malfunction of a particular transducer element or its associated circuitry. Horizontal variations indicate inadequate handling of transitions between focal zones when in the multifocal mode. These two problems are simulated in the figure of the uniformity module.

During acceptance testing of a new unit, all transducers should be evaluated, and baseline performance measured against manufacturer specifications. The maximum depth of visualization is determined by identifying the deepest low-contrast scatterers in a uniformity phantom that can be perceived in the image. This depth is dependent on the type of transducer and its operating frequency and should be measured to verify that the transducer and instrument components are operating at their designed sensitivity levels. In a 0.7-*dB*/cm-MHz attenuation medium, a depth of 18 cm for abdominal and 8 cm for small-parts transducers is the goal for visualization when a single-transmit focal zone is placed as deeply as possible with maximum transmit power level and optimal TGC adjustments. For a multifrequency transducer, the mid frequency setting should be used. With the same settings, the uniformity section of

TABLE 14-8   RECOMMENDED QC TESTS FOR ACR ACCREDITATION PROGRAM

TEST (GRAY SCALE IMAGING MODE) FOR EACH SCANNER	MINIMUM FREQUENCY
System sensitivity and/or penetration capability	Semiannually
Image uniformity	Semiannually
Photography and other hard copy	Semiannually
Low contrast detectability (optional)	Semiannually
Assurance of electrical and mechanical safety	Semiannually
Horizontal and vertical distance accuracy	At acceptance
Transducers (of different scan format)	Ongoing basis

the phantom without targets assesses gray level and image uniformity. Power and gain settings of the machine can have a significant effect on the apparent size of point-like targets (e.g., high receive gain reveals only large-size targets and has poorer resolution). One method to improve test reproducibility is to set the instrument to the threshold detectability of the targets and to rescan with an increased transmit gain of 20 dB.

Recommended QC procedures for ACR accreditation are listed in Table 14-8. Routine QC testing must occur regularly. The same tests must be performed during each testing period, so that changes can be monitored over time and effective corrective action can be taken. Testing results, corrective action, and the effects of corrective action must be documented and maintained on site. Other equipment-related issues involve cleaning air filters, checking for loose or frayed cables, and checking handles, wheels, and wheel locks as part of the QC tests.

The most frequently reported source of performance instability of an ultrasound system is related to the display on maladjusted video monitors. Drift of the ultrasound instrument settings and/or poor viewing conditions (for instance, portable ultrasound performed in a very bright patient room, potentially causing inappropriately gain-adjusted images) can lead to suboptimal images on the softcopy monitor. The analog contrast and brightness settings for the monitor should be properly established during installation; monitor calibration should be performed according to the DICOM Grayscale Standard Display Function at least semiannually (see Chapter 5) and verified with image test patterns (e.g., the SMPTE pattern).

Doppler Performance Measurements

Doppler techniques are becoming more common in the day-to-day use of medical ultrasound equipment. Reliance on flow measurements to make diagnoses requires demonstration of accurate data acquisition and processing. QC phantoms to assess velocity and flow contain one or more tubes in tissue-mimicking materials at various depths. A blood-mimicking fluid is pushed through the tubes with carefully calibrated pumps to provide a known velocity for assessing the accuracy of the Doppler velocity measurement. Several tests can be performed, including maximum penetration depth at which flow waveforms can be detected, alignment of the sample volume with the duplex B-mode image, accuracy of velocity measurements, and volume flow. For color-flow systems, sensitivity and alignment of the color flow image with the B-scan gray-scale image are assessed.

14.11 Acoustic Power and Bioeffects

Power is the rate of energy production, absorption, or flow. The SI unit of power is the watt (W), defined as one joule of energy per second. Acoustic intensity is the rate at which sound energy flows through a unit area and is usually expressed in units of watts per square centimeter (W/cm²) or milliwatts per square centimeter (mW/cm²).

Ultrasound acoustic power levels are strongly dependent on the operational characteristics of the system, including the transmit power, PRF, transducer frequency, and operation mode. Biological effects (bioeffects) are predominately related to the heating of tissues caused by high intensity levels of ultrasound used to enhance image quality and functionality. For diagnostic imaging, the intensity levels are kept below the threshold for documented bioeffects.

Acoustic Power and Intensity of Pulsed Ultrasound

Measurement Methods

Measurement of ultrasound pressure amplitude within a beam is performed with a hydrophone, a device containing a small (e.g., 0.5-mm-diameter) piezoelectric element coupled to external conductors and mounted in a protective housing. When placed in an ultrasound beam, the hydrophone produces a voltage that is proportional to the variations in pressure amplitude at that point in the beam as a function of time, permitting determination of peak compression and rarefaction amplitude as well as pulse duration and PRP (Fig. 14-54A). Calibrated hydrophones provide absolute measures of pressure, from which the acoustic intensity can be calculated if the acoustic impedance of the medium is accurately known.

Intensity Measures of Pulsed Ultrasound

In the pulsed mode of ultrasound operation, the instantaneous intensity varies greatly with time and position. At a particular location in tissue, the instantaneous intensity is quite large while the ultrasound pulse passes through the tissue, but the pulse duration is only about a microsecond or less, and for the remainder of the PRP, the intensity is nearly zero.

The temporal peak, I_{TP}, is the highest instantaneous intensity in the beam, the temporal average, I_{TA}, is the time-averaged intensity over the PRP, and the pulse average, I_{PA}, is the average intensity of the pulse (Fig. 14-54B). The spatial peak, I_{SP}, is the highest intensity spatially in the beam, and the spatial average, I_{SA}, is the average intensity over the beam area, usually taken to be the area of the transducer (Fig. 14-54C).

The acoustic power contained in the ultrasound beam (watts), averaged over at least one PRP and divided by the beam area (usually the area of the transducer face), is the spatial average–temporal average intensity I_{SATA}. Other meaningful measures for pulsed ultrasound intensity are determined from I_{SATA}, including

1. The spatial average–pulse average intensity, $I_{SAPA} = I_{SATA}/$duty cycle, where $I_{PA} = I_{TA}/$duty cycle
2. The spatial peak–temporal average intensity, $I_{SPTA} = I_{SATA} \times [I_{SP}/I_{SA}]$, which is a good indicator of thermal ultrasound effects
3. The spatial peak–pulse average intensity, $I_{SPPA} = I_{SATA} \times [I_{SP}/I_{SA}]/$duty cycle, an indicator of potential mechanical bioeffects and cavitation

For acoustic ultrasound intensity levels, $I_{SPPA} > I_{SPTA} > I_{SAPA} > I_{SATA}$. Typical acoustical power outputs are listed in Table 14-9. The two most relevant measures are the I_{SPPA} and the I_{SPTA}.

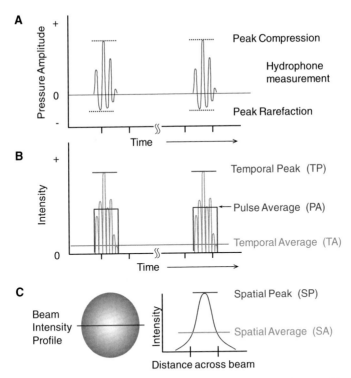

■ **FIGURE 14-54** **A.** Pressure amplitude variations are measured with a hydrophone and include peak compression and peak rarefaction variations with time. **B.** Temporal intensity variations of pulsed ultrasound vary widely, from the temporal peak and temporal average values; pulse average intensity represents the average intensity measured over the pulse duration. **C.** Spatial intensity variations of pulsed ultrasound are described by the spatial peak value and the spatial average value, measured over the beam profile.

Both measurements are required by the US Food and Drug Administration (FDA) for certification of instrumentation. Values of I_{SPTA} for diagnostic imaging are usually below 100 mW/cm^2 for imaging, but for certain Doppler applications, I_{SPTA} can exceed 1,000 mW/cm^2. I_{SPPA} can be several orders of magnitude greater than I_{SPTA}, as shown in Table 14.9. For real-time scanners, the combined intensity descriptors must be modified to consider dwell time (the time the ultrasound beam is directed at a particular region) and the acquisition geometry and spatial sampling. These variations help explain the measured differences between the I_{SPTA} and I_{SPPA} values indicated, which are much less than the duty cycle values that are predicted by the equations above.

TABLE 14-9 TYPICAL INTENSITY MEASURES FOR ULTRASOUND DATA COLLECTION MODES

MODE	PRESSURE AMPLITUDE (MPa)	I_{SPTA} (mW/cm^2)	I_{SPPA} (W/cm^2)	POWER (mW)
B-scan	1.68	19	174	18
M-mode	1.68	73	174	4
Pulsed Doppler	2.48	1,140	288	31
Color flow	2.59	234	325	81

Adapted from compilation of data presented by the American Institute of Ultrasound in Medicine. Note the difference in units for I_{SPTA} (mW/cm^2) versus I_{SPPA} (W/cm^2).

Thermal and mechanical indices of ultrasound operation are now the accepted method of determining power levels for real-time instruments that provide the operator with quantitative estimates of power deposition in the patient. These indices are selected for their relevance to risks from biological effects and are displayed on the monitor during real-time scanning. The sonographer can use these indices to minimize power deposition to the patient (and fetus) consistent with obtaining useful clinical images in the spirit of the ALARA (As Low As Reasonably Achievable) concept.

Thermal Index

The *thermal index*, TI, is the ratio of the acoustical power produced by the transducer to the power required to raise tissue in the beam area by 1°C. This is estimated by the ultrasound system using algorithms that take into account the ultrasonic frequency, beam area, and the acoustic output power of the transducer. Assumptions are made for attenuation and thermal properties of the tissues with long, steady exposure times. An indicated TI value of 2 signifies a possible 2°C increase in the temperature of the tissues when the transducer is stationary. TI values are associated with the I_{SPTA} measure of intensity.

On some scanners, other thermal indices that might be encountered are TIS (S for soft tissue), TIB (B for bone), and TIC (C for cranial bone). These quantities are useful because of the increased heat buildup that can occur at a bone–soft tissue interface when present in the beam, particularly for obstetric scanning of late-term pregnancies, and with the use of Doppler ultrasound (where power levels can be substantially higher).

Mechanical Index

Cavitation is a consequence of the negative pressures (rarefaction of the mechanical wave) that induce bubble formation from the extraction of dissolved gases in the medium. The *mechanical index,* MI is a value that estimates the likelihood of cavitation by the ultrasound beam. The MI is directly proportional to the peak rarefactional (negative) pressure and inversely proportional to the square root of the ultrasound frequency (in MHz). An attenuation of 0.3 (*dB/cm*)/MHz is assumed for the algorithm that estimates the MI. As the ultrasound output power (transmit pulse amplitude) is increased, the MI increases linearly, while an increase in the transducer frequency (say from 2 to 8 MHz) decreases the MI by the square root of 4 or by a factor of two. MI values are associated with the I_{SPPA} measure of intensity.

Biological Mechanisms and Effects

Diagnostic ultrasound has established a remarkable safety record. Significant deleterious bioeffects on either patients or operators of diagnostic ultrasound imaging procedures have not been reported in the literature. Despite the lack of evidence that any harm can be caused by diagnostic intensities of ultrasound, it is prudent and indeed an obligation of the physician to consider issues of benefit versus risk when performing an ultrasound exam and to take all precautions to ensure maximal benefit with minimal risk. The American Institute of Ultrasound in Medicine recommends adherence to the ALARA principles. US FDA requirements for new ultrasound equipment include the display of acoustic output indices (MI and TI) to give the user feedback regarding the power deposition to the patient.

At high intensities, ultrasound can cause biological effects by thermal and mechanical mechanisms. Biological tissues absorb ultrasound energy, which is converted into heat; thus, heat will be generated at all parts of the ultrasonic field in the tissue. Thermal effects are dependent not only on the rate of heat deposition in a particular volume of the body but also on how fast the heat is removed by blood flow and other means of heat conduction. The best indicator of heat deposition is the I_{SPTA} measure of intensity and the calculated TI value. Heat deposition is determined by the average ultrasound intensity in the focal zone and the absorption coefficient of the tissue. Absorption increases with the frequency of the ultrasound and varies with tissue type. Bone has a much higher attenuation (absorption) coefficient than soft tissue, which can cause significant heat deposition at a tissue-bone interface. In diagnostic ultrasound applications, the heating effect is typically well below a temperature rise (e.g., 1°C to 2°C) that would be considered potentially damaging, although some Doppler instruments can approach these levels with high pulse repetition frequencies and longer pulse duration.

Nonthermal mechanisms include mechanical movement of the particles of the medium due to radiation pressure (which can cause force or torque on tissue structures) and acoustic streaming, which can give rise to a steady circulatory flow. With higher energy deposition over a short period, *cavitation* can occur, broadly defined as sonically generated activity of highly compressible bodies composed of gas and/or vapor. Cavitation can be subtle or readily observable and is typically unpredictable and sometimes violent. *Stable cavitation* generally refers to the pulsation (expansion and contraction) of persistent bubbles in the tissue that occur at low and intermediate ultrasound intensities (as used clinically). Chiefly related to the peak rarefactional pressure, the MI is an estimate for producing cavitation. At higher ultrasound intensity levels, *transient cavitation* can occur, whereby the bubbles respond nonlinearly to the driving force, causing a collapse approaching the speed of sound. At this point, the bubbles might dissolve, disintegrate, or rebound. In the minimum volume state, conditions exist that can dissociate the water vapor into free radicals such as H• and OH•, which can cause chemical damage to biologically important molecules such as DNA. Short, high amplitude pulses such as those used in imaging are good candidates for transient cavitation; however, the intensities used in diagnostic imaging are far below the transient cavitation threshold (e.g., 1 kW/cm^2 peak pulse power is necessary for transient cavitation to be evoked).

Although biological effects have been demonstrated at much higher ultrasound power levels and longer durations, the levels and durations for typical imaging and Doppler studies are below the threshold for known undesirable effects. At higher output power, outcomes include macroscopic damage (e.g., rupturing of blood vessels, breaking up cells—indeed, the whole point of shock wave lithotripsy— the breakup of kidney stones) and microscopic damage (e.g., breaking of chromosomes, changes in cell mitotic index). No bioeffects have been shown below I_{SPTA} of 100 mW/cm^2 (Fig. 14-55). Even though ultrasound is considered safe when used properly, prudence dictates that ultrasound exposure be limited to only those patients for whom a definite benefit will be obtained.

14.12 Summary

Ultrasound uses mechanical energy to generate acoustic maps of the body, which can be extremely useful in providing valuable diagnostic information that can be acquired in a very safe and efficient manner. Quality of the exam is extremely operator dependent, and of all medical imaging modalities, ultrasound can be considered an "art" and the operator must have extensive knowledge and understanding of the underlying basic physics to be considered a true "artist." This is also true of

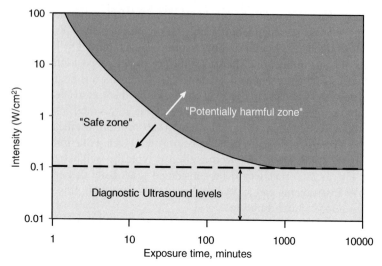

■ **FIGURE 14-55** A diagram of potential bioeffects from ultrasound delineates *safe* and potentially *harmful* regions according to ultrasound intensity levels and exposure time. The dashed line shows the upper limit of intensities typically encountered in diagnostic imaging applications.

the radiologist who must use this physics knowledge to understand the ultrasound interactions, generation of the image, limitations, potential artifacts, and possible pitfalls that are present in order to make a confident diagnosis. Despite the purported safety of ultrasound, precautions must be taken to ensure the appropriateness of the examination and the potential misdiagnoses and deleterious bioeffects that can occur with misuse.

REFERENCES AND SUGGESTED READINGS

American Institute of Ultrasound in Medicine, Official Statements and Reports, available at the AIUM web site: http://www.aium.org

Feldman MK. US Artifacts. Radiographics 29:1179–1189, 2009.

Hangiandreou N. AAPM/RSNA Physics Tutorial for Residents: Topics in US – B-mode US: Basic Concepts and New Technology. Radiographics 23:1019–1033, 2003.

Hedrick WR, Hykes DL, Starchman DE. *Ultrasound Physics and Instrumentation,* Fourth Edition. St. Louis, MO: Mosby, 2005.

Kremkau FW. *Sonography, principles and instruments.* 8th ed. St. Louis, MO: Elsevier Saunders, 2011.

Zagzebski JA. *Essentials of ultrasound physics.* St. Louis, MO: Mosby, Inc., 1996.

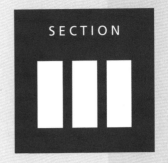

SECTION

III

Nuclear Medicine

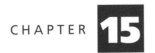
Radioactivity and Nuclear Transformation

Activity

The quantity of radioactive material, expressed as the number of radioactive atoms undergoing nuclear transformation per unit time (t), is called *activity* (A). Described mathematically, activity is equal to the change (dN) in the total number of radioactive atoms (N) in a given period of time (dt), or

$$A = -dN/dt \qquad [15\text{-}1]$$

The minus sign indicates that the number of radioactive atoms decreases with time. Activity has traditionally been expressed in units of curies (Ci). The curie is named after Marie Curie, a Polish-born French chemist and physicist, who won two Nobel prizes for her work with radioactive materials. One for physics in 1903 (with her husband Pierre Curie and Henri Becquerel) for research on radioactivity and another for chemistry in 1911 for her discovery of the elements radium and polonium, the latter named after her native Poland. The term *radioactivity* was coined by Marie Curie reflecting the intense radiation emissions from radium. One Ci is defined as 3.70×10^{10} disintegrations per second (dps), which is roughly equal to the rate of disintegrations from 1 g of radium-226 (Ra-226). A curie is a large amount of radioactivity. In nuclear medicine, activities from 0.1 to 30 mCi of a variety of radionuclides are typically used for imaging studies, and up to 300 mCi of iodine-131 is used for therapy. Although the curie is still the most common unit of radioactivity in the United States, the majority of the world's scientific literature uses the Systeme International (SI) units. The SI unit for radioactivity is the becquerel (Bq), named after Henri Becquerel, who discovered radioactivity in 1896. The becquerel is defined as 1 dps. One millicurie (mCi) is equal to 37 megabecquerels (1 mCi = 37 MBq). Table 15-1 lists the units and prefixes describing various amounts of radioactivity.

Decay Constant

Radioactive decay is a random process. From moment to moment, it is not possible to predict which radioactive atoms in a sample will decay. However, observation of a larger number of radioactive atoms over a period of time allows the average rate of nuclear transformation (decay) to be established. The number of atoms decaying per unit time (dN/dt) is proportional to the number of unstable atoms (N) that are present at any given time:

$$dN/dt \propto N \qquad [15\text{-}2]$$

579

TABLE 15-1   UNITS AND PREFIXES ASSOCIATED WITH VARIOUS QUANTITIES OF RADIOACTIVITY

QUANTITY	SYMBOL	DPS	DPM
Gigabecquerel	GBq	1×10^9	6×10^{10}
Megabecquerel	MBq	1×10^6	6×10^7
Kilobecquerel	kBq	1×10^3	6×10^4
Curie	Ci	3.7×10^{10}	2.22×10^{12}
Millicurie	mCi (10^{-3} Ci)	3.7×10^7	2.22×10^9
Microcurie	μCi (10^{-6} Ci)	3.7×10^4	2.22×10^6
Nanocurie	nCi (10^{-9} Ci)	3.7×10^1	2.22×10^3
Picocurie	pCi (10^{-12} Ci)	3.7×10^{-2}	2.22

Multiply mCi by 37 to obtain MBq or divide MBq by 37 to obtain mCi (e.g., 1 mCi = 37 MBq).

A proportionality can be transformed into an equality by introducing a constant. This constant is called the *decay constant* (λ).

$$-dN/dt = \lambda N \qquad [15\text{-}3]$$

The minus sign indicates that the number of radioactive atoms decaying per unit time (the decay rate or activity of the sample) decreases with time. The decay constant is equal to fraction of the number of radioactive atoms remaining in a sample that decay per unit time. The relationship between activity and λ can be seen by considering Equation 15-1 and substituting A for $-dN/dt$ in Equation 15-3:

$$A = \lambda N \qquad [15\text{-}4]$$

The decay constant is characteristic of each radionuclide. For example, the decay constants for technetium-99m (Tc-99m) and molybdenum-99 (Mo-99) are 0.1151 h^{-1} and 0.252 day^{-1}, respectively.

Physical Half-Life

A useful parameter related to the decay constant is the physical half-life (T½ or T_p½). The half-life is defined as the time required for the number of radioactive atoms in a sample to decrease by one half. The number of radioactive atoms remaining in a sample and the number of elapsed half-lives are related by the following equation:

$$N = N_0/2^n \qquad [15\text{-}5]$$

where N is number of radioactive atoms remaining, N_0 is the initial number of radioactive atoms, and n is the number of half-lives that have elapsed. The relationship between time and the number of radioactive atoms remaining in a sample is demonstrated with Tc-99m (T_p½ ≈ 6 h) in Table 15-2.

After 10 half-lives, the number of radioactive atoms in a sample is reduced by approximately a factor of a thousand. After 20 half-lives, the number of radioactive atoms is reduced to approximately one millionth of the initial number.

The decay constant and the physical half-life are related as follows:

$$\lambda = \ln2 / T_p\text{½} = 0.693 / T_p\text{½} \qquad [15\text{-}6]$$

TABLE 15-2   RADIOACTIVE DECAY[a]

TIME (D)	NO. OF PHYSICAL HALF-LIVES	EXPRESSION	N	$(N/N_0) \times 100$ = % REMAINING
0	0	$N_0/2^0$	10^6	100%
0.25	1	$N_0/2^1$	5×10^5	50%
0.5	2	$N_0/2^2$	2.5×10^5	25%
0.75	3	$N_0/2^3$	1.25×10^5	12.5%
1	4	$N_0/2^4$	6.25×10^4	6.25%
2.5	10	$N_0/2^{10}$	$\approx 10^3$	$\approx 0.1\%$ $(1/1,000)N_0$
5	20	$N_0/2^{20}$	≈ 1	$\approx 0.000001\%$ $(1/1,000,000)N_0$

[a]The influence of radioactive decay on the number of radioactive atoms in a sample is illustrated with technetium-99m, which has a physical half-life of 6 h (0.25 days). The sample initially contains one million (10^6) radioactive atoms (N).

where *ln* 2 denotes the natural logarithm of 2. Note that the derivation of this relationship is identical to that between the half value layer (HVL) and the linear attenuation coefficient (μ) in Chapter 3 (Equation 3-9).

The physical half-life and the decay constant are physical quantities that are inversely related and unique for each radionuclide. Half-lives of radioactive materials range from billions of years to a fraction of a second. Radionuclides used in nuclear medicine typically have half-lives on the order of hours or days. Examples of $T_p\frac{1}{2}$ and λ for radionuclides commonly used in nuclear medicine are listed in Table 15-3.

TABLE 15-3   PHYSICAL HALF-LIFE ($T_p\frac{1}{2}$) AND DECAY CONSTANT (λ) FOR RADIONUCLIDES USED IN NUCLEAR MEDICINE

RADIONUCLIDE	$T_p\frac{1}{2}$	λ
Rubidium-82 (^{82}Rb)	75 s	0.0092 s^{-1}
Fluorine-18 (^{18}F)	110 min	0.0063 min^{-1}
Technetium-99m (^{99m}Tc)	6.02 h	0.1151 h^{-1}
Iodine-123 (^{123}I)	13.27 h	0.0522 h^{-1}
Samarium-153 (^{153}Sm)	1.93 d	0.3591 d^{-1}
Yttrium-90 (^{90}Y)	2.69 d	0.2575 d^{-1}
Molybdenum-99 (^{99}Mo)	2.75 d	0.2522 d^{-1}
Indium-111 (^{111}In)	2.81 d	0.2466 d^{-1}
Thallium-201 (^{201}Tl)	3.04 d	0.2281 d^{-1}
Gallium-67 (^{67}Ga)	3.26 d	0.2126 d^{-1}
Xenon-133 (^{133}Xe)	5.24 d	0.1323 d^{-1}
Iodine-131 (^{131}I)	8.02 d	0.0864 d^{-1}
Phosphorus-32 (^{32}P)	14.26 d	0.0486 d^{-1}
Strontium-82 (^{82}Sr)	25.60 d	0.0271 d^{-1}
Chromium-51 (^{51}Cr)	27.70 d	0.0250 d^{-1}
Strontium-89 (^{89}Sr)	50.53 d	0.0137 d^{-1}
Iodine-125 (^{125}I)	59.41 d	0.0117 d^{-1}
Cobalt-57 (^{57}Co)	271.79 d	0.0025 d^{-1}

Fundamental Decay Equation

By applying the integral calculus to Equation 15-3, a useful relationship is established between the number of radioactive atoms remaining in a sample and time—the fundamental decay equation:

$$N_t = N_0 e^{-\lambda t} \text{ or } A_t = A_0 e^{-\lambda t} \qquad [15\text{-}7]$$

where N_t is the number of radioactive atoms at time t, A_t is the activity at time t, N_0 is the initial number of radioactive atoms, A_0 is the initial activity, e is the base of natural logarithm $= 2.718...$, λ is the decay constant $= \ln 2/T_p\tfrac{1}{2} = 0.693/T_p\tfrac{1}{2}$, and t is the time.

Problem: A nuclear medicine technologist injects a patient with 400 μCi of indium-111–labeled autologous leukocytes ($T_p\tfrac{1}{2}$ 2.81 days). Twenty-four hours later, the patient is imaged. Assuming that none of the activity was excreted, how much activity remains at the time of imaging?

   Solution:
   $A = A_0 e^{-\lambda t}$
   Given:
   $A_0 = 400 \ \mu$Ci
   $\lambda = 0.693/2.81 \text{ days} = 0.247 \text{ days}^{-1}$
   $t = 1$ day
   Note: t and $T_p\tfrac{1}{2}$ must be in the same units of time.
   $A_t = 400 \ \mu$Ci $e^{-(0.247 \text{ days}^{-1})(1 \text{ day})}$
   $A_t = 400 \ \mu$Ci $e^{-0.247}$
   $A_t = (400 \ \mu$Ci$)(0.781)$
   $A_t = 312 \ \mu$Ci

A plot of activity as a function of time on a linear scale results in a curvilinear exponential relationship in which the total activity asymptotically approaches zero (Fig. 15-1). If the logarithm of the activity is plotted versus time (semilog plot), this exponential relationship appears as a straight line (Fig. 15-2).

15.2 Nuclear Transformation

As mentioned previously, when an unstable (i.e., radioactive) atomic nucleus undergoes the spontaneous transformation, called *radioactive decay,* radiation is emitted. If the daughter nucleus is stable, this spontaneous transformation ends. If the daughter is also

■ FIGURE 15-1 Percentage of initial activity as a function of time (linear scale).

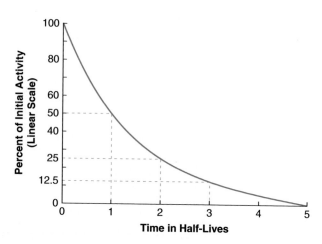

Time in Half-Lives

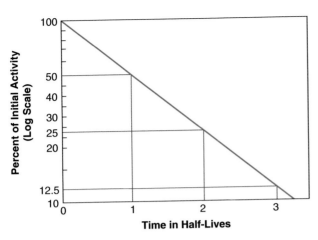

■ **FIGURE 15-2** Percentage of initial activity as a function of time (semilog plot).

unstable, the process continues until a stable nuclide is reached. Most radionuclides decay in one or more of the following ways: (1) alpha decay, (2) beta-minus emission, (3) beta-plus (positron) emission, (4) electron capture, or (5) isomeric transition.

Alpha Decay

Alpha (α) decay is the spontaneous emission of an alpha particle (identical to a helium nucleus consisting of two protons and two neutrons) from the nucleus (Fig. 15-3). Alpha decay typically occurs with heavy nuclides (A > 150) and is often followed by gamma and characteristic x-ray emission. These photon emissions are often accompanied by the competing processes of internal conversion and Auger electron emission. Alpha particles are the heaviest and least penetrating form of radiation considered in this chapter. They are emitted from the atomic nucleus with discrete energies in the range of 2 to 10 MeV. An alpha particle is approximately four times heavier than a proton or neutron and carries an electronic charge twice that of the proton. Alpha decay can be described by the following equation:

$$\underset{Z}{\overset{A}{}}X \rightarrow \underset{Z-2}{\overset{A-4}{}}Y + \underset{2}{\overset{4}{}}He^{2+} + \text{transition energy} \qquad [15-8]$$
$$\left(\underset{\text{particle}}{\overset{\text{alpha}}{}}\right)$$

EXAMPLE:

$$\underset{86}{\overset{220}{}}Rn \rightarrow \underset{84}{\overset{216}{}}Po + \underset{2}{\overset{4}{}}He^{2+} + 6.4 \text{ MeV transition energy}$$

Alpha decay results in a large energy transition and a slight increase in the ratio of neutrons to protons (N/Z ratio):

$$\underset{86}{\overset{220}{}}Rn \qquad \xrightarrow{\quad \alpha^{+2} \quad} \qquad \underset{84}{\overset{216}{}}Po$$

N/Z = 134/86 = 1.56   N/Z = 132/84 = 1.57

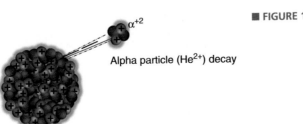

Alpha particle (He²⁺) decay

■ **FIGURE 15-3** Alpha decay.

Alpha particles are not used in medical imaging because their ranges are limited to approximately 1 cm/MeV in air and typically less than 100 μm in tissue. Even the most energetic alpha particles cannot penetrate the dead layer of the skin. However, the intense ionization tracks produced by this high LET radiation (e.g., mean LET of alpha particles is ~100 keV/μm compared to ~3 keV/μm for energetic electrons set in motion by the interaction of diagnostic x-rays in tissue) make them a potentially serious health hazard should alpha-emitting radionuclides enter the body via ingestion, inhalation, or a wound. Research continues to assess the potential therapeutic effectiveness of alpha-emitting radionuclides such as astatine-212, bismuth-212, and bismuth-213 (At-211, Bi-212, and Bi-213) chelated to monoclonal antibodies to produce stable radioimmunoconjugates directed against various tumors as radioimmunotherapeutic agents.

Beta-Minus (Negatron) Decay

Beta-minus (β^-) decay, or negatron decay, characteristically occurs with radionuclides that have an excess number of neutrons compared with the number of protons (i.e., a high N/Z ratio). Beta-minus decay can be described by the following equation:

$$_Z^A X \rightarrow \, _{Z+1}^A Y + \underset{\text{(negatron)}}{\beta^-} + \underset{\text{(antineutrino)}}{\bar{\nu}} + \text{energy} \qquad [15\text{-}9]$$

This mode of decay results in the conversion of a neutron into a proton with the simultaneous ejection of a negatively charged beta particle (β^-) and an antineutrino ($\bar{\nu}$), (Fig. 15-4). With the exception of their origin (the nucleus), beta particles are identical to ordinary electrons. The antineutrino is an electrically neutral subatomic particle whose mass is much smaller than that of an electron. The absence of charge and the infinitesimal mass of antineutrinos make them very difficult to detect because they rarely interact with matter. Beta decay increases the number of protons by 1 and thus transforms the atom into a different element with an atomic number Z + 1. However, the concomitant decrease in the neutron number means that the mass number remains unchanged. Decay modes in which the mass number remains constant are called *isobaric transitions*. Radionuclides produced by nuclear fission are "neutron rich," and therefore most decay by β^- emission. Beta-minus decay decreases the N/Z ratio, bringing the daughter closer to the line of stability (see Chapter 2):

■ FIGURE 15-4 Beta-minus decay.

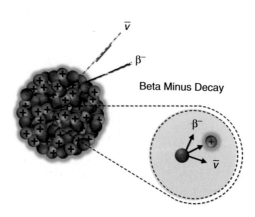

Beta Minus Decay

EXAMPLE:

$$^{32}_{15}P \xrightarrow{\quad \beta^- \quad} ^{32}_{16}S$$

$$N/Z = 17/15 = 1.13 \qquad\qquad N/Z = 16/16 = 1.00$$

Although the β^- particles emitted by a particular radionuclide have a discrete maximal energy (E_{max}), almost all are emitted with energies lower than the maximum. The average energy of the β^- particles is approximately 1/3 E_{max}. The balance of the energy is given to the antineutrino (i.e., $E_{max} = E_{\beta^-} + E_{\bar{v}}$). Thus, beta-minus decay results in a polyenergetic spectrum of β^- energies ranging from zero to E_{max} (Fig. 15-5). Any excess energy in the nucleus after beta decay is emitted as gamma rays, internal conversion electrons, and other associated radiations.

Beta-Plus Decay (Positron Emission)

Just as beta-minus decay is driven by the nuclear instability caused by excess neutrons, "neutron-poor" radionuclides (i.e., those with a low N/Z ratio) are also unstable. Many of these radionuclides decay by beta-plus (positron) emission, which increases the neutron number by one. Beta-plus decay can be described by the following equation:

$$^A_Z X \rightarrow \,^A_{Z-1} Y + \underset{(\text{positron})}{\beta^+} + \underset{(\text{neutrino})}{v} + \text{energy} \qquad\qquad [15\text{-}10]$$

The net result is the conversion of a proton into a neutron with the simultaneous ejection of the positron (β^+) and a neutrino (v). Positron decay decreases the number of protons (atomic number) by 1 and thereby transforms the atom into a different element with an atomic number of $Z-1$ (Fig. 15-6). The daughter atom, with one less proton in the nucleus, initially has one too many orbital electrons and thus is a negative ion. However, the daughter quickly releases the extra orbital electron to the surrounding

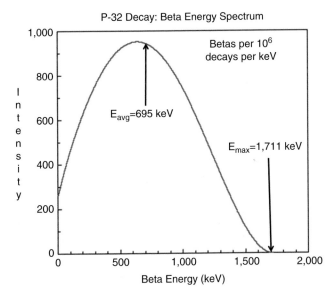

P-32 Decay: Beta Energy Spectrum

E_{avg}=695 keV

E_{max}=1,711 keV

Betas per 10^6 decays per keV

Beta Energy (keV)

■ **FIGURE 15-5** P-32 example. Distribution of beta-minus particle kinetic energy. Number of beta-minus particles emitted per 10^6 decays of P-32 as a function of energy.

■ FIGURE 15-6 Beta-plus decay.

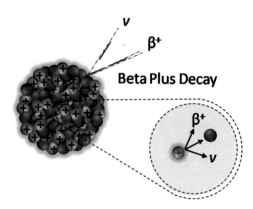

Beta Plus Decay

medium and becomes a neutral atom. Position decay can only occur if the mass of the parent atom exceeds that of the daughter atom by at least the masses of the two electrons (positron and orbital electron). According to Einstein's mass-energy equivalence formula, $E = mc^2$, 511 keV is the energy equivalent of the rest mass of an electron (positively or negatively charged). Therefore, there is an inherent threshold for positron decay equal to the sum of the rest mass energy equivalent of two electrons (i.e., 2×511 keV, or 1.02 MeV).

The number of neutrons is increased by 1; therefore, the transformation is isobaric because the total number of nucleons is unchanged. Accelerator-produced radionuclides, which are typically neutron deficient, often decay by positron emission. Positron decay increases the N/Z ratio, resulting in a daughter closer to the line of stability.

EXAMPLE:

$$ {}^{18}_{9}\text{F} \xrightarrow{\quad \beta^+ \quad} {}^{18}_{8}\text{O} $$

$$ \text{N/Z} = 9/9 = 1 \qquad\qquad \text{N/Z} = 10/8 = 1.25 $$

The energy distribution between the positron and the neutrino is similar to that between the negatron and the antineutrino in beta-minus decay; thus positrons are polyenergetic with an average energy equal to approximately $1/3$ E_{max}. As with β^- decay, excess energy following positron decay is released as gamma rays and other associated radiation.

Although β^+ decay has similarities to β^- decay, there are also important differences. The neutrino and antineutrino are *antiparticles,* as are the positron and negatron. The prefix *anti-* before the name of an elementary particle denotes another particle with certain symmetry characteristics. In the case of charged particles such as the positron, the antiparticle (i.e., the negatron) has a charge equal but opposite to that of the positron and a magnetic moment that is oppositely directed with respect to spin. In the case of neutral particles such as the neutrino and antineutrino, there is no charge; therefore, differentiation between the particles is made solely on the basis of differences in magnetic moment. Other important differences between the particle and antiparticle are their lifetimes and their eventual fates. As mentioned earlier, negatrons are physically identical to ordinary electrons and as such lose their kinetic energy as they traverse matter via excitation and ionization. When they lose all (or almost all) of their kinetic energy, they may be captured by an atom or absorbed into the free electron pool. Positrons undergo a similar process of energy deposition via excitation and ionization; however, when they come to rest, they react violently with their antiparticles (electrons). This process results in the entire rest mass of both particles being instantaneously converted to energy and emitted as two oppositely directed (i.e., ~180 degrees apart) 511-keV *annihilation photons* (Fig. 15-7). Medical imaging of annihilation radiation from positron-emitting radiopharmaceuticals, called positron emission tomography (PET), is discussed in Chapter 19.

Electron Capture Decay

Electron capture (ε) is an alternative to positron decay for neutron-deficient radionuclides. In this decay mode, the nucleus captures an orbital (usually a K- or L-shell) electron, with the conversion of a proton into a neutron and the simultaneous ejection of a neutrino (Fig. 15-8). Electron capture can be described by the following equation:

$$_Z^A X + e^- \rightarrow {}_{Z-1}^A Y + \underset{\text{(neutrino)}}{\nu} + \text{energy}.$$ [15-11]

The net effect of electron capture is the same as positron emission: the atomic number is decreased by 1, creating a different element, and the mass number remains unchanged. Therefore, electron capture is isobaric and results in an increase in the N/Z ratio.

EXAMPLE:

$$_{81}^{201}\text{Tl} \xrightarrow{\ \varepsilon\ } {}_{80}^{201}\text{Hg} + \text{energy}$$

$$N/Z = 120/81 = 1.48 \qquad N/Z = 121/80 = 1.51$$

The capture of an orbital electron creates a vacancy in the electron shell, which is filled by an electron from a higher energy shell. As discussed in Chapter 2, this electron transition results in the emission of characteristic x-rays and/or Auger electrons. For example, thallium-201, (Tl-201) decays to mercury-201 (Hg-201) by electron capture, resulting in the emission of characteristic x-rays. It is these

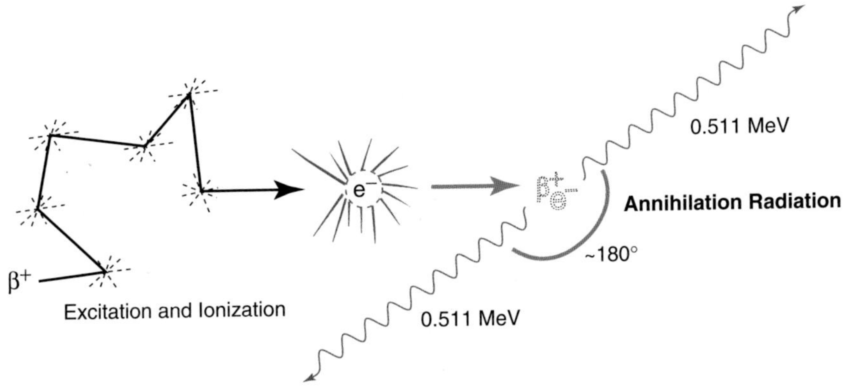

■ **FIGURE 15-7** Annihilation radiation.

■ **FIGURE 15-8** Electron capture decay.

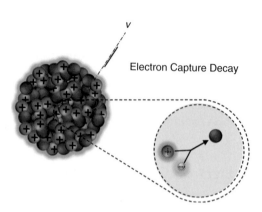

x-rays that are primarily used to create the images in Tl-201 myocardial perfusion studies. As with other modes of decay, if the nucleus is left in an excited state following electron capture, the excess energy will be emitted as gamma rays and other radiations.

As previously mentioned, positron emission requires a mass energy difference between the parent and daughter atoms of at least 1.02 MeV. Neutron-poor radionuclides below this threshold energy decay exclusively by electron capture. Nuclides for which the energy difference between the parent and daughter exceed 1.02 MeV may decay by electron capture or positron emission, or both. Heavier proton-rich nuclides are more likely to decay by electron capture, whereas lighter proton-rich nuclides are more likely to decay by positron emission. This is a result of the closer proximity of the K- or L-shell electrons to the nucleus and the greater magnitude of the coulombic attraction from the positive charges. Although capture of a K- or L-shell electron is the most probable, electron capture can occur with higher energy shell electrons.

The quantum mechanical description of the atom is essential for understanding electron capture. The Bohr model describes electrons in fixed orbits at discrete distances from the nucleus. This model does not permit electrons to be close enough to the nucleus to be captured. However, the quantum mechanical model describes orbital electron locations as probability density functions in which there is a finite probability that an electron will pass close to or even through the nucleus.

Electron capture radionuclides used in medical imaging decay to atoms in excited states that subsequently emit externally detectable x-rays, gamma rays, or both.

Isomeric Transition

Often during radioactive decay, a daughter is formed in an excited (i.e., unstable) state. Gamma rays are emitted as the daughter nucleus undergoes an internal rearrangement and transitions from the excited state to a lower energy state. Once created, most excited states transition almost instantaneously (on the order of 10^{-12} s) to lower energy states with the emission of gamma radiation. However, some excited states persist for longer periods, with half-lives ranging from nanoseconds (10^{-9} s) to more than 30 years. These excited states are called metastable or isomeric states and those with half-lives exceeding a millisecond (10^{-3} s) are denoted by the letter "m" after the mass number (e.g., Tc-99m). Isomeric transition is a decay process that yields gamma radiation without the emission or capture of a particle by the nucleus. There is no change in atomic number, mass number, or neutron number. Thus, this decay mode is isobaric and isotonic, and it occurs between two nuclear energy states with no change in the N/Z ratio.

Isomeric transition can be described by the following equation:

$$^{Am}_{Z}X \rightarrow {}^{A}_{Z}X + (energy) \tag{15-12}$$

The energy is released in the form of gamma rays, internal conversion electrons, or both.

Decay Schemes

Each radionuclide's decay process is a unique characteristic of that radionuclide. The majority of the pertinent information about the decay process and its associated radiation can be summarized in a line diagram called a *decay scheme* (Fig. 15-9). Decay schemes identify the parent, daughter, mode of decay, energy levels including those of excited and metastable states, radiation emissions, and sometimes physical half-life and other characteristics of the decay sequence. The top horizontal line represents the parent, and the bottom horizontal line represents the daughter. Horizontal lines between those two represent intermediate excited or metastable states. By convention, a diagonal arrow to the right indicates an increase in Z, which occurs with beta-minus decay. A diagonal arrow to the left indicates a decrease in Z such as decay by electron capture. A vertical line followed by a diagonal arrow to the left is used to indicate alpha decay and in some cases to indicate positron emission when a radionuclide decays by both electron capture and positron emission (e.g., F-18). Vertical down pointing arrows indicate gamma ray emission, including those emitted during isomeric transition. These diagrams are often accompanied by decay data tables, which provide information on all the significant ionizing radiations emitted from the atom as a result of the nuclear transformation. Examples of these decay schemes and data tables are presented in this section.

Figure 15-10 shows the alpha decay scheme of radon-220 (Rn-220). Rn-220 has a physical half-life of 55 s and decays by one of two possible alpha transitions. Alpha 1 (α_1) at 5.747 MeV occurs 0.07% of the time and is followed immediately by a 0.55-MeV gamma ray (γ_1) to the ground state. The emission of alpha 2 (α_2) with an energy of 6.287 MeV, occurs 99.9% of the time and leads directly to the ground state. The decay data table lists these radiations together with the daughter atom, which has a -2 charge and a small amount of kinetic energy as a result of recoil from the alpha particle emission.

Phosphorus-32 (P-32) is used in nuclear medicine as a therapeutic agent in the treatment of a several diseases, including polycythemia vera, and serous effusions. P-32 has a half-life of 14.3 days and decays directly to its ground state by emitting a beta-minus particle with an E_{max} of 1.71 MeV (Fig. 15-11). The average (mean) energy of the beta-minus particle is approximately 1/3 E_{max} (0.6948 MeV), with the

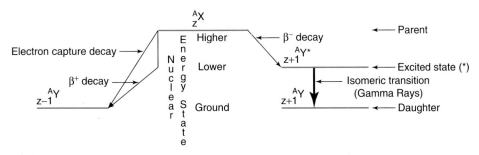

■ FIGURE 15-9 Elements of the generalized decay scheme.

■ **FIGURE 15-10** Principal decay scheme of radon-220.

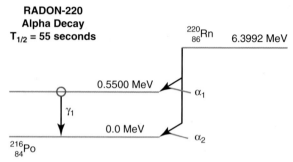

RADON-220
Alpha Decay
$T_{1/2}$ = 55 seconds

$^{220}_{86}$Rn   6.3992 MeV

0.5500 MeV α_1

γ_1

0.0 MeV α_2

$^{216}_{84}$Po

Decay Data Table

Radiation		Mean Number per Disintegration	Mean Energy per Particle (MeV)
Alpha	1	0.0007	5.7470
Recoil Atom		0.0007	0.1064
Alpha	2	0.9993	6.2870
Recoil Atom		0.9993	0.1164
Gamma	1	0.0006	0.5500

antineutrino carrying off the balance of the transition energy. There are no excited energy states or other radiation emitted during this decay; therefore, P-32 is referred to as a *"pure beta emitter."*

A somewhat more complicated decay scheme is associated with the beta-minus decay of Mo-99 to Tc-99 (Fig. 15-12). Eight of the ten possible beta-minus decay transitions are shown with probabilities ranging from 0.822 for beta-minus 8 (i.e., 82.2% of all decays of Mo-99 are by β_8^- transition) to 0.0004 (0.04%) for β_6^-. The sum of all transition probabilities (β_1^- to β_{10}^-) is equal to 1. The average energy of beta particles from the transition is 0.4519 MeV. The β_8^- transition leads directly to a metastable state of technetium 99, Tc-99m, which is 0.1427 MeV above the ground state and decays with a half-life of 6.02 h. Tc-99m is the most widely used radionuclide in nuclear medicine.

After beta decay, there are a number of excited states created that transition to lower energy levels via the emission of gamma rays and/or internal conversion

■ **FIGURE 15-11** Principal decay scheme of phosphorus-32.

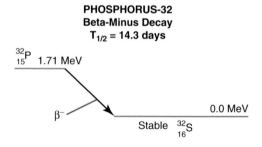

PHOSPHORUS-32
Beta-Minus Decay
$T_{1/2}$ = 14.3 days

$^{32}_{15}$P   1.71 MeV

β^-

0.0 MeV

Stable $^{32}_{16}$S

Decay Data Table

Radiation	Mean Number per Disintegration	Mean Energy per Particle (MeV)
Beta Minus	1.000	0.6948

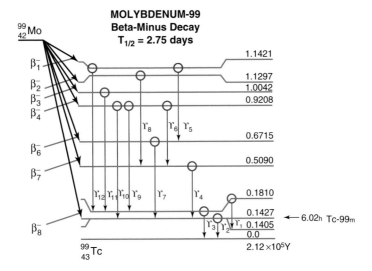

Decay Data Table

Radiation		Mean Number per Disintegration	Mean Energy per Particle (MeV)	Radiation		Mean Number per Disintegration	Mean Energy per Particle (MeV)
Beta Minus	1	0.0010	0.0658	Gamma	4	0.0119	0.3664
Beta Minus	3	0.0014	0.1112	Gamma	5	0.0001	0.4706
Beta Minus	4	0.1640	0.1331	Gamma	6	0.0002	0.4115
Beta Minus	6	0.0004	0.2541	Gamma	7	0.0006	0.5288
Beta Minus	7	0.0114	0.2897	Gamma	8	0.0002	0.6207
Beta Minus	8	0.8220	0.4428	Gamma	9	0.1367	0.7397
Gamma	1	0.0105	0.0406	K Int Con Elect		0.0002	0.7186
K Int Con Elect		0.0428	0.0195	Gamma	10	0.0426	0.7779
L Int Con Elect		0.0053	0.0377	K Int Con Elect		0.0000	0.7571
M Int Con Elect		0.0017	0.0401	Gamma	11	0.0013	0.8230
Gamma	2	0.0452	0.1405	Gamma	12	0.0010	0.9608
K Int Con Elect		0.0058	0.1194	K Alpha-1 X-Ray		0.0253	0.0183
L Int Con Elect		0.0007	0.1377	K Alpha-2 X-Ray		0.0127	0.0182
Gamma	3	0.0600	0.1811	K Beta-1 X-Ray		0.0060	0.0206
K Int Con Elect		0.0085	0.1600	KLL Auger Elect		0.0087	0.0154
L Int Con Elect		0.0012	0.1782	KLX Auger Elect		0.0032	0.0178
M Int Con Elect		0.0004	0.1806	LMM Auger Elect		0.0615	0.0019
				MXY Auger Elect		0.1403	0.0004

■ **FIGURE 15-12** Principal decay scheme of molybdenum-99. Auger electron nomenclature: KXY Auger Elect is an auger electron emitted from the "Y" shell as a result of a transition of an electron of the "X" shell to a vacancy in the K shell. "X" and "Y" are shells higher than the K shell. For example, KLL Auger Elect is an auger electron emitted from the L shell as a result of a transition of another L shell electron to a vacancy in the K shell.

electrons. As previously described, the ejection of an electron by internal conversion of the gamma ray results in the emission of characteristic x-rays, Auger electrons, or both. All of these radiations, their mean energies, and their associated probabilities are included in the decay data table.

The process of gamma ray emission by isomeric transition is of primary importance to nuclear medicine, because most procedures performed depend on the emission and detection of gamma radiation. Figure 15-13 shows the decay scheme for Tc-99m. There are three gamma ray transitions as Tc-99m decays to Tc-99. The gamma 1 (γ_1) transition occurs very infrequently because 99.2% of the time this energy is internally converted resulting in the emission of either an M-shell internal conversion electron (86.2%) with a mean energy of 1.8 keV or an N-shell internal conversion electron (13.0%) with a mean energy of 2.2 keV. After internal conversion, the nucleus is left in an excited state, which is followed almost instantaneously by gamma 2 (γ_2) transition at 140.5 keV to ground state. The γ_2 transition occurs 89.1% of the time with the balance of the transitions from 140.5 keV to ground state

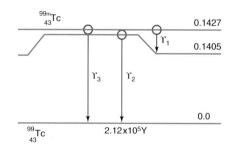

TECHNETIUM 99m
Isomeric Transition
$T_{1/2}$ = 6.02 hrs.

$^{99m}_{43}$Tc ... 0.1427

... 0.1405 Υ_1

Υ_3 Υ_2

0.0

$^{99}_{43}$Tc 2.12×10^5Y

Decay Data Table

Radiation		Mean Number per Disintegration	Mean Energy per Particle (MeV)
Gamma	1	0.0000	0.0021
M Int Con Elect		0.8620	0.0018
N Int Con Elect		0.1300	0.0022
Gamma	2	0.8910	0.1405
K Int Con Elect		0.0892	0.1194
L Int Con Elect		0.0109	0.1375
M Int Con Elect		0.0020	0.1377
Gamma	3	0.0003	0.1426
K Int Con Elect		0.0088	0.1215
L Int Con Elect		0.0035	0.1398
M Int Con Elect		0.0011	0.1422
K Alpha-1 X-Ray		0.0441	0.0183
K Alpha-2 X-Ray		0.0221	0.0182
K Beta-1 X-Ray		0.0105	0.0206
KLL Auger Elect		0.0152	0.0154
KLX Auger Elect		0.0055	0.0178
LMM Auger Elect		0.1093	0.0019
MXY Auger Elect		1.2359	0.0004

■ **FIGURE 15-13** Principal decay scheme of technetium-99m. Auger electron nomenclature: KXY Auger Elect is an auger electron emitted from the "Y" shell as a result of a transition of an electron of the "X" shell to a vacancy in the K shell. "X" and "Y" are shells higher than the K shell. For example, KLL Auger Elect is an auger electron emitted from the L shell as a result of a transition of another L shell electron to a vacancy in the K shell.

occurring primarily via internal conversion. Gamma 2 is the principal photon imaged in nuclear medicine. Like gamma 1, the gamma 3 transition at 142.7 keV occurs very infrequently relative to the probability of internal conversion electron emission. Here again, the vacancies created in orbital electron shells following internal conversion result in the production of characteristic x-rays and Auger electrons.

■ **FIGURE 15-14** Principal decay scheme of fluorine-18.

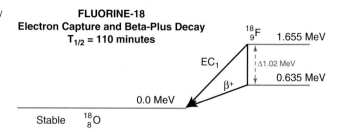

FLUORINE-18
Electron Capture and Beta-Plus Decay
$T_{1/2}$ = 110 minutes

$^{18}_{9}$F   1.655 MeV

EC_1 Δ1.02 MeV

0.635 MeV

β^+

0.0 MeV

Stable $^{18}_{8}$O

Decay Data Table

Radiation	Mean Number per Disintegration	Mean Energy Particle (MeV)
Beta Plus	0.9700	0.2496
Annih. Radiation	1.9400	0.5110

TABLE 15-4   SUMMARY OF RADIONUCLIDE DECAY

TYPE OF DECAY	PRIMARY RADIATION EMITTED	OTHER RADIATION EMITTED	NUCLEAR TRANSFORMATION	CHANGE IN Z	CHANGE IN A	NUCLEAR CONDITION PRIOR TO TRANSFORMATION
Alpha	$^4_2\text{He}^{+2}(\alpha)$	γ-rays C x-rays AE, ICE	$^A_Z X \rightarrow ^{A-4}_{Z-2}X^{-2} + ^4_2\text{He}^{2+} + \text{energy}$	-2	-4	$Z > 83$
Beta minus	β^{-1}	γ-rays C x-rays AE, ICE, $\bar{\nu}$	$^A_Z X \rightarrow ^A_{Z+1}Y + \beta^- + \bar{\nu} + \text{energy}$	$+1$	0	N/Z too large
Beta plus	β^{+1}	γ-rays C x-rays AE, ICE, ν	$^A_Z X \rightarrow ^A_{Z-1}Y + \beta^+ + \nu + \text{energy}$	-1	0	N/Z too small
Electron capture	C x-rays	γ-rays AE,ICE, ν	$^A_Z X + e^- \rightarrow ^A_{Z-1}Y + \nu + \text{energy}$	-1	0	N/Z too small
Isomeric transition	γ-rays	C x-rays AE, ICE	$^{Am}_Z X \rightarrow ^A_Z X + \text{energy}$	0	0	Excited or meta-stable nucleus

ICE, internal conversion e⁻; AE, auger e⁻; C x-rays, Characteristic x-rays; γ-rays, Gamma rays; $\bar{\nu}$, antineutrino; ν, neutrino.

As discussed previously, positron emission and electron capture are competing decay processes for neutron-deficient radionuclides. As shown in Figure 15-14, fluorine-18 (F-18) decays by both modes. F-18 decays by positron emission (represented by a solid vertical line followed by a diagonal arrow to the left) 97% of the time. The length of the vertical part of the line in the diagram represents the sum of the rest mass energy equivalent of the positron and electron (i.e., 1.02 MeV). Electron capture (represented by a diagonal arrow to the left) occurs 3% of the time. The dual mode of decay results in an "effective" decay constant (λ_e) that is the sum of the positron (λ_1) and electron capture (λ_2) decay constants: $\lambda_e = \lambda_1 + \lambda_2$. The decay data table shows that positrons are emitted 97% of the time with an average energy of 0.2496 MeV (~1/3 of 0.635 MeV, which is E_{max}). Furthermore, the interaction of the positron with an electron results in the production of two 511-keV annihilation radiation photons. Because two photons are produced for each positron, their abundance is $2 \times 97\%$, or 194%. ^{18}F is the most widely used radionuclide for PET imaging.

A summary of the characteristics of radionuclide decay modes previously discussed is provided in table 15.4

SUGGESTED READINGS

Cherry SR, et al. *Physics in nuclear medicine*. 4th ed. Philadelphia, PA: Saunders, 2011.
Friedlander G, Kennedy JW, Miller JM. *Nuclear and radiochemistry*. 3rd ed. New York, NY: Wiley, 1981.
Patton JA. Introduction to nuclear physics. *Radiographics* 1998;18:995–1007.

CHAPTER 16

Radionuclide Production, Radiopharmaceuticals, and Internal Dosimetry

16.1 Radionuclide Production

Although many naturally occurring radioactive nuclides exist, all of those commonly administered to patients in nuclear medicine are artificially produced. Artificial radioactivity was discovered in 1934 by Irene Curie (daughter of Marie and Pierre Curie) and Frederic Joliot, who induced radioactivity in boron and aluminum targets by bombarding them with alpha (α) particles from polonium. Positrons continued to be emitted from the targets after the alpha source was removed. Today, more than 2,500 artificial radionuclides have been produced by a variety of methods. Most radionuclides used in nuclear medicine are produced by particle accelerators (e.g., cyclotrons), nuclear reactors, or radionuclide generators.

Cyclotron-Produced Radionuclides

Cyclotrons and other charged-particle accelerators produce radionuclides by bombarding stable nuclei with high-energy charged particles. Positively charged ions such as protons (H^+), deuterons ($^2H^+$), and alpha particles ($^4He^{2+}$) as well as negatively charged hydrogen ions (H^-) are commonly used to produce radionuclides used in medicine. Charged particles must be accelerated to high kinetic energies to overcome and penetrate the repulsive coulombic barrier of the target atoms' nuclei.

In 1930, Cockcroft and Walton applied a clever scheme of cascading a series of transformers, each capable of stepping up the voltage by several hundred thousand volts. The large potentials generated were used to produce artificial radioactivity by accelerating particles to high energies and bombarding stable nuclei with them.

In Berkeley, California, in 1931, E.O. Lawrence capitalized on this development but added a unique dimension in his design of the cyclotron (Fig. 16-1). A cyclotron has a vacuum chamber between the poles of an electromagnet. Inside the vacuum chamber is a pair of hollow, semicircular electrodes, each shaped like the letter D and referred to as "dees." The two dees are separated by a small gap. An alternating high voltage is applied between the two dees. When positive ions are injected into the center of the cyclotron they are attracted to and accelerated toward the negatively charged dee. The static magnetic field constrains the ions to travel in a circular path, whereby the radius of the circle increases as the ions gain kinetic energy (Fig. 16-2). Half way around the circle, the ions approach the gap between the dees; at this time, the polarity of the electrical field between the two dees is reversed, causing the ions to be accelerated toward the negative dee. This cycle is repeated again and again,

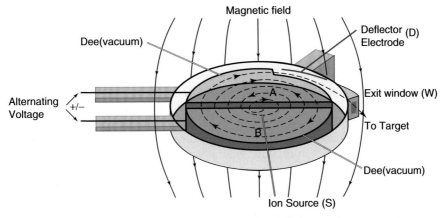

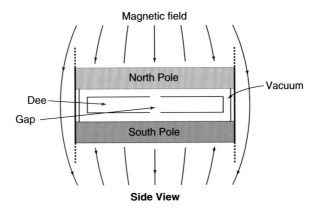

Top and bottom magnet removed

Side View

■ FIGURE 16-1 Schematic view of a cyclotron. Two "dees" (A and B) are seperated by a small gap.

with the particles accelerated each time they cross the gap, acquiring kinetic energy and sweeping out larger and larger circles. As the length of the path between successive accelerations increases, the speed of the particle also increases; hence, the time interval between accelerations remains constant. The cyclic nature of these events led

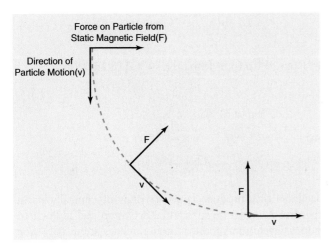

Force on Particle from Static Magnetic Field(F)

Direction of Particle Motion(v)

■ FIGURE 16-2 A constant magnetic field imposes a force (**F**) on a moving charged particle that is perpendicular to the direction of the particle's velocity (**v**). This causes an ion in a cyclotron to move in a circular path. The diameter of the circular path is proportional to the speed of the ion.

to the name "cyclotron." The final kinetic energy achieved by the accelerated particles depends on the type of particle (e.g., protons or deuterons), diameter of the dees,
and the strength of the static magnetic field. Finally, as the ions reach the periphery of
the dees, they are removed from their circular path by a negatively charged deflector
plate (if positive ions are accelerated) or electron stripping foil (if H^- ions are accelerated), emerge through the window, and strike the target. Depending on the design of
the cyclotron, particle energies can range from a few million electron volts (MeV) to
several hundred MeV.

The accelerated ions collide with the target nuclei, causing nuclear reactions.
An incident particle may leave the target nucleus after interacting, transferring
some of its energy to it, or it may be completely absorbed. The specific reaction
depends on the type and energy of the bombarding particle as well as the composition of the target. In either case, target nuclei are left in excited states, and this excitation energy is disposed of by the emission of particulate (protons and neutrons)
and electromagnetic (gamma rays) radiations. Gallium-67 (Ga-67) is an example
of a cyclotron-produced radionuclide. The production reaction is written as
follows:

$$^{68}Zn\ (p,2n)\ ^{67}Ga \qquad\qquad [16\text{-}1]$$

where the target material is zinc-68 (Zn-68), the bombarding particle is a proton (p) accelerated to approximately 20 MeV, two neutrons (2n) are emitted, and
Ga-67 is the product radionuclide. In some cases, the nuclear reaction produces
a radionuclide that decays to the clinically useful radionuclide (see iodine-123
and thallium-201 production below). Most cyclotron-produced radionuclides
are neutron poor and therefore decay by positron emission or electron capture.
The production methods of several cyclotron-produced radionuclides important
to nuclear medicine are shown below, (EC = electron capture, T½ = physical
half-life).

Iodine-123 production:

$$^{127}I\ (p,5n)\ ^{123}Xe \xrightarrow[T_{1/2}\ 2\ hr]{EC} {}^{123}I\ \text{or}$$

$$^{124}Xe(p,2n)\ ^{123}Cs \xrightarrow[T_{1/2}\ 1\,sec]{EC\,or\,\beta^+} {}^{123}Xe \xrightarrow[T_{1/2}\ 2hr]{EC} {}^{123}I \qquad [16\text{-}2]$$

Indium-111 production:

$$^{109}Ag\ (\alpha,2n)\ ^{111}In \quad \text{or} \quad {}^{111}Cd\ (p,n)\ ^{111}In \quad \text{or} \quad {}^{112}Cd\ (p,2n)\ ^{111}In$$

Cobalt-57 production:

$$^{56}Fe\ (d,n)\ ^{57}Co$$

Thallium-201 production:

$$^{203}Tl\ (p,3n)\ ^{201}Pb \xrightarrow[T_{1/2}\ 9.4\ hr]{EC\,or\,\beta^+} {}^{201}Tl$$

Industrial cyclotron facilities that produce large activities of clinically useful
radionuclides are very expensive and require substantial cyclotron and radiochemistry support staff and facilities. Cyclotron-produced radionuclides are usually more
expensive than those produced by other technologies.

Much smaller, specialized cyclotrons, installed in commercial radiopharmacies serving metropolitan areas or in hospitals, have been developed to produce positron-emitting radionuclides for positron emission tomography (PET) (Fig. 16-3). These cyclotrons operate at lower energies (10 to 30 MeV) than industrial cyclotrons and commonly accelerate H⁻ ions. (An H⁻ ion is a proton with two orbital electrons.) In such a cyclotron, the beam is extracted by passing it through a carbon stripping foil, which removes the electrons thus creating an H⁺ ion (proton) beam.

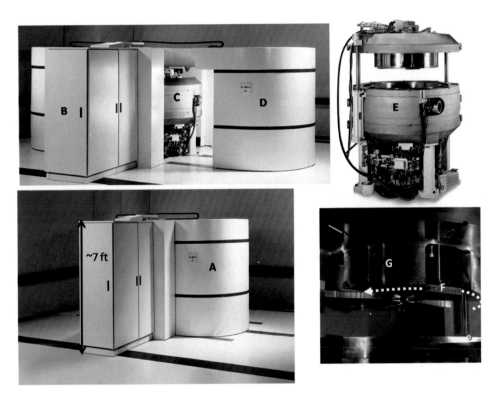

■ **FIGURE 16-3** Commercial self-shielded cyclotron for radionuclide production capable of producing a 60 µA beam of protons accelerated to ~11 MeV is shown with the radiation shields closed (**A**). Designed with a small footprint to fit into a relatively small room (24' × 23' × 14' height) (**B**) Power supply and control cabinet (**C**) Cyclotron assembly approximately 10,000 kg (22,000 lb) (**D**) Retractable radiation shielding (open) approximately 14,500 kg (32,000 lb) of borated concrete and polyethylene. Neutrons and gamma radiation are an unavoidable byproduct of the nuclear reactions which are used to produce the desired radioactive isotopes. Boron and polyethylene are added to the radiation shield to absorb neutrons. The shielding is designed so that radiation exposure rates are reduced to the point where technologists and other radiation workers can occupy the room while the accelerator is in operation (less than 20 uSv/h at 24 ft from the center of the cyclotron). (**E**) Cyclotron assembly open. Hydrogen gas line at the top of the cyclotron assembly provides the source of hydrogen ions to be accelerated. (**F**) One of four cyclotron dees. The acceleration potential is supplied by high frequency voltage. In this system, four dees provide eight accelerations per orbit, thus reducing acceleration path length and beam loss. (**G**) Beam shaping magnets act as powerful lenses to confine ions to the midplane. The *dotted white arrow* shows the beam path through one of the dees.

The radiochemicals produced (in gas or liquid) are sent through tubing in a shielded channel running under the floor to the automated radiochemistry unit located in a shielded enclosure in a room next to the cyclotron. A typical production run from a cyclotron in a commercial radiopharmacy serving a metropolitan area will produce approximately 131 GBq (3.5 Ci) of F-18 during a 2 h irradiation. The radiopharmacy may have three to four production runs a day depending on the clinical demand in the area. (Photos courtesy of Siemens Medical Solutions, Inc.)

Because of the change in the polarity of the charge on each particle, the direction of the forces on the moving particles from the magnetic field is reversed and the beam is diverted out of the cyclotron and onto a target. These commercially available specialized medical cyclotrons have a number of advantages, including automated cyclotron operation and radiochemistry modules, allowing a technologist with proper training to operate the unit. Radiation shielding of cyclotrons is always an important consideration; however, the use of negative ions avoids the creation of unwanted radioactivity in the cyclotron housing and thus reduces the amount of radiation shielding necessary. This substantially reduces the size and weight of the cyclotron facility allowing it to be placed within the hospital close to the PET imaging facilities. Production methods of clinically useful positron-emitting radionuclides are listed below.

Fluorine-18 production: ^{18}O (p,n) ^{18}F $(T_{1/2} = 110$ min$)$
Nitrogen-13 production: ^{16}O(p,α) ^{13}N $(T_{1/2} = 10$ min$)$

Oxygen-15 production: ^{14}N (d,n) ^{15}O or ^{15}N (p,n)^{15}O $(T_{1/2} = 2.0$ min$)$ [16-3]
Carbon-11 production: ^{14}N (p,α) ^{11}C $(T_{1/2} = 20.4$ min$)$

In the interests of design simplicity and cost, some medical cyclotrons accelerate only protons. These advantages may be offset for particular productions such as ^{15}O when an expensive rare isotope ^{15}N that requires proton bombardment must be used in place of the cheap and abundant ^{14}N isotope that requires deuteron bombardment. The medical cyclotrons are usually located near the PET imaging system because of the short half-lives of the radionuclides produced. Fluorine-18 (F-18) is an exception to this generalization because of its longer half-life (110 min).

Nuclear Reactor–Produced Radionuclides

Nuclear reactors are another major source of clinically used radionuclides. Neutrons, being uncharged, have an advantage in that they can penetrate the nucleus without being accelerated to high energies. There are two principal methods by which radionuclides are produced in a reactor: nuclear fission and neutron activation.

Nuclear Fission

Fission is the splitting of an atomic nucleus into two smaller nuclei. Whereas some unstable nuclei fission spontaneously, others require the input of energy to overcome the nuclear binding forces. This energy is often provided by the absorption of neutrons. Neutrons can induce fission only in certain very heavy nuclei. Whereas high-energy neutrons can induce fission in several such nuclei, there are only three nuclei of reasonably long half-life that are fissionable by neutrons of all energies; these are called fissile nuclides.

The most widely used fissile nuclide is uranium-235 (U-235). Elemental uranium exists in nature primarily as U-238 (99.3%) with a small fraction of U-235 (0.7%). U-235 has a high fission cross section (i.e., high fission probability); therefore, its concentration is usually enriched (typically to 3% to 5%) to make the fuel used in nuclear reactors.

When a U-235 nucleus absorbs a neutron, the resulting nucleus (U-236) is in an extremely unstable excited energy state that usually promptly fissions into two smaller nuclei called *fission fragments*. The fission fragments fly apart with very high kinetic energies, with the simultaneous emission of gamma radiation and the ejection of two to five neutrons per fission (Equation 16-4).

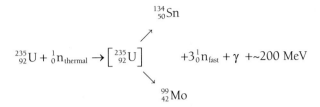

$$^{235}_{92}U + ^{1}_{0}n_{thermal} \rightarrow \left[^{235}_{92}U\right] \qquad +3^{1}_{0}n_{fast} + \gamma + {\sim}200 \text{ MeV}$$

The fission of uranium creates fission fragment nuclei having a wide range of mass numbers. More than 200 radionuclides with mass numbers between 70 and 160 are produced by the fission process (Fig. 16-4). These fission products are neutron rich and therefore almost all of them decay by beta-minus (β^-) particle emission.

Nuclear Reactors and Chain Reactions

The energy released by the nuclear fission of a uranium atom is more than 200 MeV. Under the right conditions, this reaction can be perpetuated if the fission neutrons interact with other U-235 atoms, causing additional fissions and leading to a self-sustaining nuclear chain reaction (Fig. 16-5). The probability of fission with U-235 is greatly enhanced as neutrons slow down or *thermalize*. The neutrons emitted from fission are very energetic (called *fast neutrons*), and are slowed (*moderated*) to thermal energies (~0.025 eV) as they scatter in water in the reactor core. Good moderators are low-Z materials that slow the neutrons without absorbing a significant fraction of them. Water is the most commonly used moderator, although other materials, such as graphite (used in the reactors at the Chernobyl plant in the Ukraine) and heavy water (^2H_2O), are also used.

Some neutrons are absorbed by nonfissionable material in the reactor, while others are moderated and absorbed by U-235 atoms and induce additional fissions. The ratio of the number of fissions in one generation to the number in the previous

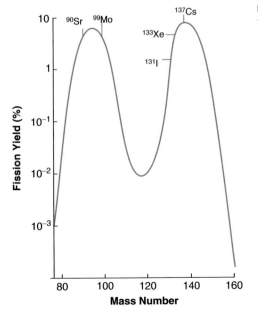

■ FIGURE 16-4 Fission yield as a percentage of total fission products from uranium 235.

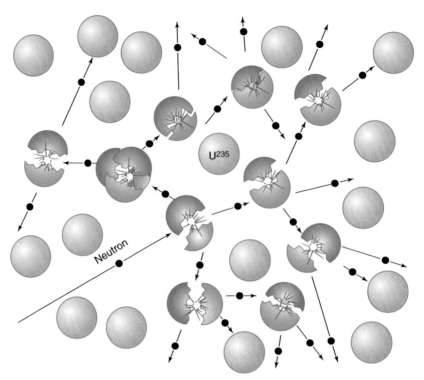

■ **FIGURE 16-5** Schematic of a nuclear chain reaction. The neutrons (shown as small *blackened circles*) are not drawn to scale with respect to the uranium atoms.

generation is called the *multiplication factor*. When the number of fissions per generation is constant, the multiplication factor is 1 and the reactor is said to be *critical*. When the multiplication factor is greater than 1, the rate of the chain reaction increases, at which time the reactor is said to be *supercritical*. If the multiplication factor is less than 1 (i.e., more neutrons being absorbed than produced), the reactor is said to be *subcritical* and the chain reaction will eventually cease.

This chain reaction process is analogous to a room whose floor is filled with mousetraps, each one having a ping-pong ball placed on the trap. Without any form of control, a self-sustaining chain reaction will be initiated when a single ping-pong ball is tossed into the room and springs one of the traps. The nuclear chain reaction is maintained at a desired level by limiting the number of available neutrons through the use of neutron-absorbing *control rods* (containing boron, cadmium, indium, or a mixture of these elements), which are placed in the reactor core between the fuel elements. Inserting the control rods deeper into the core absorbs more neutrons, reducing the reactivity (i.e., causing the neutron flux and power output to decrease with time). Removing the control rods has the opposite effect. If a nuclear reactor accident results in loss of the coolant, the fuel can overheat and melt (so-called *meltdown*). However, because of the design characteristics of the reactor and its fuel, an atomic explosion, like those from nuclear weapons, is impossible.

Figure 16-6 is a diagram of a typical radionuclide production reactor. The fuel is processed into rods of uranium-aluminum alloy approximately 6 cm in diameter and 2.5 m long. These *fuel rods* are encased in zirconium or aluminum, which have favorable neutron and heat transport properties. There may be as many as 1,000 fuel rods in the reactor, depending on the design and the neutron flux requirements. Water

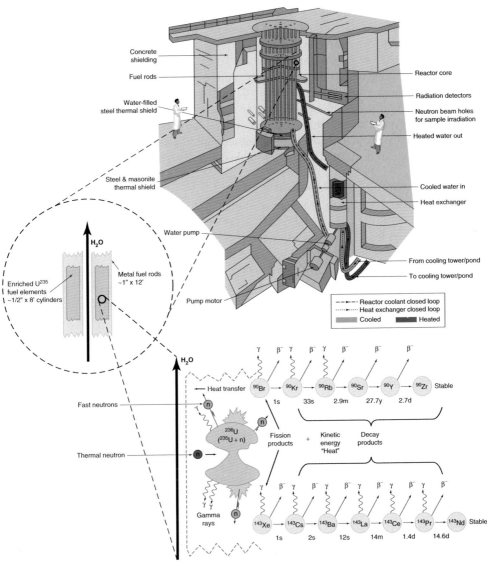

■ **FIGURE 16-6** NRU Radionuclide research/production reactor (adapted from diagram provided courtesy of Atomic Energy of Canada and Chalk River Laboratories, Chalk River, Ontario). Fuel rod assemblies and the fission process are illustrated to show some of the detail and the relationships associated with fission-produced radionuclides.

circulates between the encased fuel rods in a closed loop, whereby the heat generated from the fission process is transferred to cooler water in the heat exchanger. The water in the reactor and in the heat exchanger is in closed loops that do not come into direct physical contact with the fuel. The heat transferred to the cooling water is released to the environment through cooling towers, evaporation ponds, or heat exchangers that transfer the heat to a large body of water. The cooled water is pumped back toward the fuel rods, where it is reheated and the process is repeated.

In commercial nuclear power electric generation stations, the heat generated from the fission process produces high pressure steam that is directed through a steam turbine, which powers an electrical generator. The steam is then condensed to water by the condenser.

Nuclear reactor safety design principles dictate numerous barriers between the radioactivity in the core and the environment. For example, in commercial power reactors, the fuel is encased in metal fuel rods that are surrounded by water and enclosed in a sealed, pressurized, approximately 30-cm-thick steel reactor vessel. These components, together with other highly radioactive reactor systems, are enclosed in a large steel-reinforced concrete shell (~1 to 2 m thick), called the *containment structure*. In addition to serving as a moderator and coolant, the water in the reactor acts as a radiation shield, reducing the radiation levels adjacent to the reactor vessel. Specialized nuclear reactors are used to produce clinically useful radionuclides from fission products or neutron activation of stable target material.

Fission-Produced Radionuclides

The fission products most often used in nuclear medicine are molybdenum-99 (Mo-99), iodine-131 (I-131), and xenon-133 (Xe-133). These products can be chemically separated from other fission products with essentially no stable isotopes (*carrier*) of the radionuclide present. Thus, the concentration or specific activity (measured in MBq or Ci per gram) of these "carrier-free" fission-produced radionuclides is very high. High-specific-activity, carrier-free nuclides are preferred in radiopharmaceutical preparations to increase the labeling efficiency of the preparations and minimize the mass and volume of the injected material.

Neutron Activation–Produced Radionuclides

Neutrons produced by the fission of uranium in a nuclear reactor can be used to create radionuclides by bombarding stable target material placed in the reactor. Ports exist in the reactor core between the fuel elements where samples to be irradiated are inserted. This process, called *neutron activation*, involves the capture of neutrons by stable nuclei, which results in the production of radioactive nuclei. The most common neutron capture reaction for thermal (slow) neutrons is the (n,γ) reaction, in which the capture of the neutron by a nucleus is immediately followed by the emission of a gamma ray. Other thermal neutron capture reactions include the (n,p) and (n,α) reactions, in which the neutron capture is followed by the emission of a proton or an alpha particle, respectively. However, because thermal neutrons can induce these reactions only in a few, low-atomic-mass target nuclides, most neutron activation uses the (n,γ) reaction. Almost all radionuclides produced by neutron activation decay by beta-minus particle emission. Examples of radionuclides produced by neutron activation useful to nuclear medicine are listed below.

Phosphorus-32 production: $^{31}P(n,\gamma)\,^{32}P$ $(T_{1/2} = 14.3\ \text{days})$

[16-5]

Chromium-51 production: $^{50}Cr(n,\gamma)\,^{51}Cr$ $(T_{1/2} = 27.8\ \text{days})$

A radionuclide produced by an (n,γ) reaction is an isotope of the target element. As such, its chemistry is identical to that of the target material, making chemical separation techniques useless. Furthermore, no matter how long the target material is irradiated by neutrons, only a small fraction of the target atoms will undergo neutron capture and become activated. Therefore, the material removed from the reactor will not be carrier free because it will always contain stable isotopes of the radionuclide. In addition, impurities in the target material will cause the production of other radionuclides. The presence of carrier in the mixture limits the ability to concentrate the radionuclide of interest and therefore lowers the specific activity. For this reason, many of the clinically used radionuclides that could be produced by neutron activation (e.g., ^{131}I, ^{99}Mo) are instead produced by nuclear fission to

TABLE 16-1   COMPARISON OF RADIONUCLIDE PRODUCTION METHODS

	PRODUCTION METHOD			
CHARACTERISTIC	LINEAR ACCELERATOR/ CYCLOTRON	NUCLEAR REACTOR (FISSION)	NUCLEAR REACTOR (NEUTRON ACTIVATION)	RADIONUCLIDE GENERATOR
Bombarding particle	Proton, alpha	Neutron	Neutron	Production by decay of parent
Product	Neutron poor	Neutron excess	Neutron excess	Neutron poor or excess
Typical decay pathway	Positron emission, electron capture	Beta-minus	Beta-minus	Several modes
Typically carrier free	Yes	Yes	No	Yes
High specific activity	Yes	Yes	No	Yes
Relative cost	High	Low	Low	Low (^{99m}Tc) High (^{82}Rb)
Radionuclides for nuclear medicine applications	^{11}C, ^{13}N, ^{15}O, ^{18}F, ^{57}Co, ^{67}Ga, ^{68}Ge, ^{111}In, ^{123}I, ^{201}Tl	^{99}Mo, ^{131}I, ^{133}Xe	^{32}P, ^{51}Cr, ^{89}Sr, ^{125}I, ^{153}Sm	^{68}Ga, ^{81m}Kr, ^{82}Rb, ^{90}Y, ^{99m}Tc

maximize specific activity. An exception to the limitations of neutron activation is the production of ^{125}I, in which neutron activation of the target material, ^{124}Xe, produces a radioisotope, ^{125}Xe, that decays to form the desired radioisotope (Equation 16-6). In this case, the product radioisotope can be chemically or physically separated from the target material. Various characteristics of radionuclide production are compared in Table 16-1.

^{125}I production:

$$^{124}Xe\,(n,\gamma)^{125}Xe \xrightarrow[T_{1/2}\ 17\ hr]{EC\ or\ \beta^+} {}^{125}I \qquad [16\text{-}6]$$

Radionuclide Generators

Since the mid-1960s, technetium-99m (Tc-99m) has been the most important radionuclide used in nuclear medicine for a wide variety of radiopharmaceutical applications. However, its relatively short half-life (6 h) makes it impractical to store even a weekly supply. This supply problem is overcome by obtaining the parent Mo-99, which has a longer half-life (67 h) and continually produces Tc-99m. The Tc-99m is collected periodically in sufficient quantities for clinical operations. A system for holding the parent in such a way that the daughter can be easily separated for clinical use is called a *radionuclide generator*.

Molybdenum-99/Technetium-99m Radionuclide Generator

In a molybdenum-99/technetium-99m radionuclide generator, Mo-99 (produced by nuclear fission of U-235 to yield a high-specific-activity, carrier-free parent) is loaded, in the form of ammonium molybdenate $(NH_4^+)(MoO_4^-)$, onto a porous column containing 5 to 10 g of an alumina (Al_2O_3) resin. The ammonium molybdenate becomes attached to the surface of the alumina molecules (a process called *adsorption*). The porous nature of the alumina provides a large surface area for adsorption of the parent.

As with all radionuclide generators, the chemical properties of the parent and daughter are different. In the Mo-99/Tc-99m or "moly" generator, the Tc-99m is much less tightly bound than the Mo-99. The daughter is removed (*eluted*) by the flow of isotonic (normal, 0.9%) saline (the "eluant") through the column. When the saline solution is passed through the column, the chloride ions easily exchange with the TcO_4^- (but not the MoO_4^-) ions, producing sodium pertechnetate, Na^+ ($^{99m}TcO_4^-$). Technetium-99m pertechnetate ($^{99m}TcO_4^-$) is produced in a sterile, pyrogen-free form with high specific activity and a pH (~5.5) that is ideally suited for radiopharmaceutical preparations.

Commercially moly generators have a large reservoir of oxygenated saline (the eluant) connected by tubing to one end of the column and a vacuum extraction vial to the other. On insertion of the vacuum collection vial (contained in a shielded elution tool), saline is drawn through the column and the eluate is collected during elution which takes about 1 to 2 min. Figure 16-7 is a picture and cross-sectional diagram of a moly generator together with an insert that shows details of the generator column. Sterility is achieved by a millipore filter connected to the end of the column, by the use of a bacteriostatic agent in the eluant, or by autoclave sterilization of the loaded column by the manufacturer.

Moly generators are typically delivered with approximately 37 to 740 GBq (1 to 20 Ci) of Mo-99, depending on the workload of the department. The larger activity generators are typically used by commercial radiopharmacies supplying radiopharmaceuticals to multiple nuclear medicine departments. The generators are shielded by the manufacture with lead, tungsten or in the case of higher activity generators depleted uranium. Additional shielding is typically placed around the generator to reduce the exposure of staff during elution. The activity of the daughter at the time of elution depends on the following:

1. The activity of the parent
2. The rate of formation of the daughter, which is equal to the rate of decay of the parent (i.e., $A_o e^{-\lambda_p t}$)
3. The decay rate of the daughter
4. The time since the last elution
5. The elution efficiency (typically 80% to 90%)

Transient Equilibrium

Between elutions, the daughter (Tc-99m) builds up or "grows in" as the parent (Mo-99) continues to decay. After approximately 23 h, the Tc-99m activity reaches a maximum, at which time the production rate and the decay rate are equal and the parent and daughter are said to be in *transient equilibrium*. Once transient equilibrium has been achieved, the daughter activity decreases, with an apparent half-life equal to the half-life of the parent. Transient equilibrium occurs when the half-life of the parent is greater than that of the daughter by a factor of approximately 10. In the general case of transient equilibrium, the daughter activity will exceed the parent at equilibrium. If all of the (Mo-99) decayed to Tc-99m, the Tc-99m activity would slightly exceed (~10% higher) that of the parent at equilibrium. However, approximately 12% of Mo-99 decays directly to Tc-99 without first producing Tc-99m, Figure 16-8. Therefore, at equilibrium, the Tc-99m activity will be only approximately 97% (1.1 × 0.88) that of the parent (Mo-99) activity.

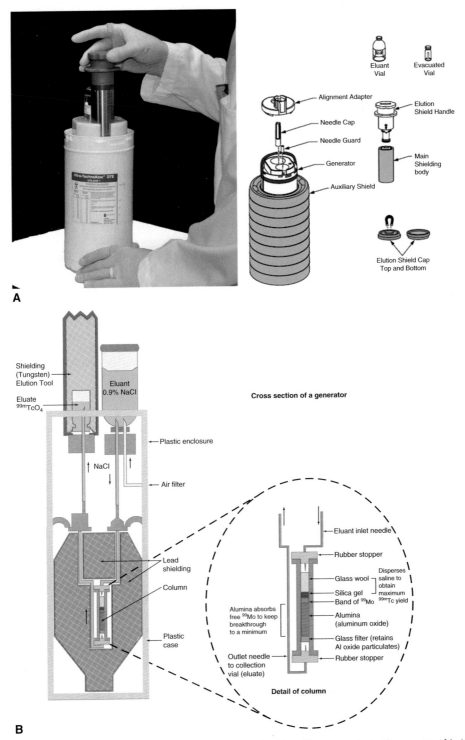

Eluant
Vial

Evacuated
Vial

Alignment Adapter

Needle Cap

Needle Guard

Generator

Auxiliary Shield

Elution
Shield Handle

Main
Shielding
body

Elution Shield Cap
Top and Bottom

A

Shielding
(Tungsten)
Elution Tool

Eluant
0.9% NaCl

Eluate
^{99m}TcO$_4$

Cross section of a generator

Plastic enclosure

↑ NaCl ↓

Air filter

Eluant inlet needle

Rubber stopper

Glass wool ⎤ Disperses
⎟ saline to
Silica gel ⎦ obtain
maximum
Band of ^{99}Mo ^{99m}Tc yield

Lead
shielding

Column

Alumina absorbs
free ^{99}Mo to keep
breakthrough
to a minimum

Alumina
(aluminum oxide)

Glass filter (retains
Al oxide particulates)

Plastic
case

Outlet needle
to collection
vial (eluate)

Rubber stopper

Detail of column

B

■ **FIGURE 16-7** (**A**) Picture of a "wet" molybdenum 99/technetium 99m generator in the process of being eluted (**left**). A spent generator which is no longer radioactive was used in order to minimize dose. For picture clarity, the shielding normally surrounding the generator (illustrated in the accompanying diagram (**right**) is not shown. However correct radiation safety principles (discussed further in chapter 21) are shown including the use of disposable gloves, finger ring and body dosimeters and disposable plastic backed absorbent paper on the bench top to minimize the spread of any contamination. An explosion diagram depicting the generator components, and auxiliary radiation shielding is shown on the right. (**B**) A cross-sectional diagram of the generator interior and column detail. Consult the text for additional information on the elution process. (Adapted from photo and diagrams provided courtesy of Covidien Radiopharmaceuticals St. Louis, MO.)

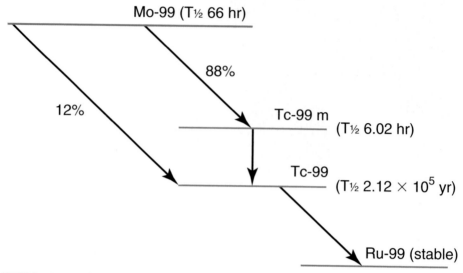

■ **FIGURE 16-8** Simplified decay scheme of Mo-99. Mo-99 decays to Tc 99m approximately 88% of the time. Thus is due to the β_8 transition directly to Tc-99m (~82.2%) along with several other beta transitions to excited states that emit gamma rays (principally the β_4 γ_{10} and β_7 γ_4) to yield Tc-99m. The balance (12%) of Mo-99 decays occurs by other beta transitions to excited states that ultimately yield Tc-99 bypassing the metastable form of Tc (Tc-99m).

Moly generators (sometimes called "cows") are usually delivered weekly and eluted (called "milking the cow") each morning, allowing maximal yield of the daughter. The elution process is approximately 90% efficient. This fact, together with the limitations on Tc-99m yield in the Mo-99 decay scheme, results in a maximum elution yield of approximately 85% of the Mo-99 activity at the time of elution. Therefore, a typical elution on Monday morning from a moly generator with 55.5 GBq (1.5 Ci) of Mo-99 yields approximately 47.2 GBq (1.28 Ci) of Tc-99m in 10 mL of normal saline (a common elution volume). By Friday morning of that week, the same generator would be capable of delivering only about 17.2 GBq (0.47 Ci). The moly generator can be eluted more frequently than every 23 h; however, the Tc-99m yield will be less. Approximately half of the maximal yield will be available 6 h after the last elution. Figure 16-9 shows a typical time-activity curve for a moly generator.

Secular Equilibrium

Although the moly generator is by far the most widely used in nuclear medicine, other generator systems produce clinically useful radionuclides. When the half-life of the parent is much longer than that of the daughter (i.e., more than about 100 times longer), *secular equilibrium* occurs after approximately five to six half-lives of the daughter. In secular equilibrium, the activity of the parent and the daughter are the same if all of the parent atoms decay directly to the daughter. Once secular equilibrium is achieved, the daughter will have an apparent half-life equal to that of the parent. The strontium-82/rubidium-82 (Sr-82/Rb-82) generator, with parent and daughter half-lives of 25.5 d and 75 s, respectively, reaches secular equilibrium within approximately 7.5 min after elution. Figure 16-10 shows a time-activity curve demonstrating secular equilibrium. The characteristics of radionuclide generator systems are compared in Table 16-2.

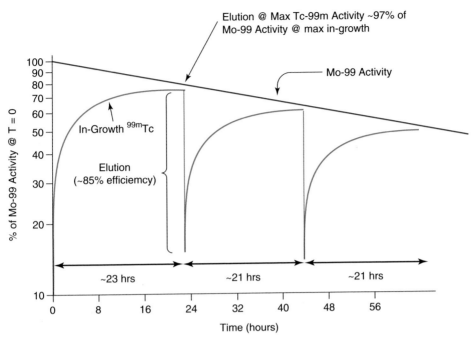

■ FIGURE 16-9 Time-activity curve of a molybdenum 99/technetium 99m radionuclide generator system demonstrating the ingrowth of Tc-99m and subsequent elution. The time to maximum Tc-99m activity, approximately 23 h, assumes there is no residual Tc-99m from a previous elution of the column. Typical elution efficiency is approximately 85% (~15% residual Tc-99m), thus time to maximum Tc-99m activity following the first elution is approximately 21 h. Approximately 50% of the maximum Tc-99m activity is obtained in 6 h. The maximum Tc-99m activity in the eluate is typically 80% to 90% of Mo-99 activity.

Quality Control

The users of moly generators are required to perform molybdenum and alumina breakthrough tests. Mo-99 contamination in the Tc-99m eluate is called *molybdenum breakthrough*. Mo-99 is an undesirable contaminant because its long half-life

TABLE 16-2 CLINICALLY USED RADIONUCLIDE GENERATOR SYSTEMS IN NUCLEAR MEDICINE

PARENT	DECAY MODE AND (HALF-LIFE)	DAUGHTER	TIME OF MAXIMAL INGROWTH (EQUILIBRIUM)	DECAY MODE AND (HALF-LIFE)	DECAY PRODUCT
^{68}Ge	EC (271 d)	^{68}Ga	~6.5 h (S)	β^+ EC (68 min)	^{68}Zn (stable)
^{90}Sr	β^- (28.8 y)	^{90}Y	~1 mo (S)	β^- (2.67 d)	^{90}Zr (stable)
^{81}Rb	β^+ EC (4.6 h)	^{81m}Kr	~80 s (S)	IT (13.5 s)	^{81}Kr[a]
^{82}Sr	EC (25.5 d)	^{82}Rb	~7.5 min (S)	β^+ (75 s)	^{82}Kr (stable)
^{99}Mo	β^- (67 h)	^{99m}Tc	~24 h (T)	IT (6 h)	^{99}Tc[a]

Note: Decay modes: EC, electron capture; β^+, positron emission; β^-, beta-minus; IT, isometric transition (i.e., gamma ray emission). Radionuclide equilibrium; T, transient; S, secular.
[a]These nuclides have half-lives greater than 10^5 y and for medical applications can be considered to be essentially stable.

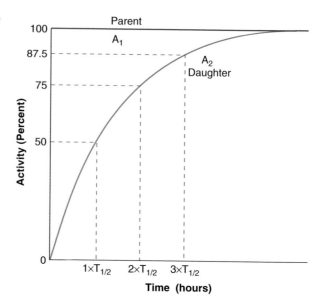

■ **FIGURE 16-10** Time-activity curve demonstrating secular equilibrium.

and highly energetic betas increase the radiation dose to the patient without providing any clinical information. The high-energy gamma rays (~740 and 780 keV) are very penetrating and cannot be efficiently detected by scintillation cameras. The *U.S. Pharmacopeia* (USP) and the U.S. Nuclear Regulatory Commission (NRC) limit the Mo-99 contamination to 0.15 μCi of Mo-99 per mCi of Tc-99m at the time of administration. The Mo-99 contamination is evaluated by placing the Tc-99m eluate in a thick (~6 mm) lead container (provided by the dose calibrator manufacturer), which is placed in the dose calibrator. The high-energy photons of Mo-99 can be detected, whereas virtually all of the Tc-99m 140-keV photons are attenuated by the lead container. Eluates from moly generators rarely exceed permissible Mo-99 contamination limits. The quality control procedures to evaluate breakthrough of radionuclidic contaminates in the eluates from Mo-99/Tc-99m and Sr-82/Rb-82 generators are discussed further in chapter 17 in the context of dose calibrator operations and quality control. It is also possible (although rare) for some of the alumina from the column to contaminate the Tc-99m eluate. Alumina interferes with the preparation of some radiopharmaceuticals (especially sulfur colloid and Tc-99m-labeled red blood cell preparations). The USP limits the amount of alumina to no more than 10 μg alumina per mL of Tc-99m eluate. Commercially available paper test strips and test standards are used to assay for alumina concentrations.

16.2 Radiopharmaceuticals

Characteristics, Applications, Quality Control, and Regulatory Issues in Medical Imaging

The vast majority of radiopharmaceuticals in nuclear medicine today use Tc-99m as the radionuclide. Most Tc-99m radiopharmaceuticals are easily prepared by aseptically injecting a known quantity of Tc-99m pertechnetate into a sterile vial containing the lyophilized (freeze-dried) pharmaceutical. The radiopharmaceutical complex is, in most cases, formed instantaneously and can be used for multiple doses over a period of several hours. Radiopharmaceuticals can be prepared in this fashion (called "kits") as needed in the nuclear medicine department, or they may be delivered to the department by a centralized commercial radiopharmacy that serves several hospitals in the area. Although most Tc-99m radiopharmaceuticals can be prepared rapidly and easily at room temperature, several products (e.g., Tc-99m macroaggregated albumin [MAA]), require multiple steps such as boiling the Tc-99m reagent complex for several minutes. In almost all cases, however, the procedures are simple and the labeling efficiencies are very high (typically greater than 95%).

Other radionuclides common to diagnostic nuclear medicine imaging include ^{123}I, ^{67}Ga, ^{111}In, ^{133}Xe, and ^{201}Tl. Positron-emitting radionuclides are used for PET. ^{18}F, as fluorodeoxyglucose (FDG), is used in approximately 85% of all clinical PET applications. Rubidium 82 (^{82}Rb) is used to assess myocardial perfusion using PET/CT imaging systems, in place of Tl-201 and Tc-99m based myocardial perfusion agents that are imaged using scintillation cameras. A wide variety of other positron-emitting radionuclides are currently being evaluated for their clinical utility, including carbon-11 (^{11}C), nitrogen-13 (^{13}N), oxygen-15 (^{15}O), and gallium-68 (^{68}Ga). The physical characteristics, most common modes of production, decay characteristics, and primary imaging photons (where applicable) of the radionuclides used in nuclear medicine are summarized in Table 16-3.

Ideal Diagnostic Radiopharmaceuticals

Although there are no truly "ideal" diagnostic radiopharmaceuticals, it is helpful to think of currently used agents in light of the ideal characteristics.

Low Radiation Dose

It is important to minimize the radiation exposure to patients while preserving the diagnostic quality of the image. Radionuclides can be selected that have few particulate emissions and a high abundance of clinically useful photons. Most modern scintillation cameras are optimized for photon energies close to 140 keV, which is a compromise among patient attenuation, spatial resolution, and detection efficiency. Photons whose energies are too low are largely attenuated by the body, increasing the patient dose without contributing to image formation. High-energy photons are more likely to escape the body but have poor detection efficiency and easily penetrate collimator septa of scintillation cameras (see Chapter 18). A radiopharmaceutical should have an effective half-life long enough to complete the study with an adequate concentration in the tissues of interest but short enough to minimize the patient dose.

High Target/Nontarget Activity

The ability to detect and evaluate lesions depends largely on the concentration of the radiopharmaceutical in the organ, tissue or, lesion of interest or on a clinically useful uptake and clearance pattern. Maximum concentration of the radiopharmaceutical in the target tissues of interest while minimizing the uptake in surrounding (nontarget) tissues and organs improves contrast and the ability to detect subtle abnormalities in the radiopharmaceutical's distribution. Maximizing this target/nontarget ratio is characteristic of all clinically useful radiopharmaceuticals and is improved by observing the recommended interval between injection and imaging for the specific agent. This interval is a compromise between the uptake of the activity in target tissue, washout of the activity in the background (nontarget) tissues and practical considerations of clinic operations. With some radiopharmaceuticals such as the bone scanning agent Tc-99m labeled methylene-diphosphonate (^{99m}Tc-MDP)

TABLE 16-3 PHYSICAL CHARACTERISTICS OF CLINICALLY USED RADIONUCLIDES

RADIONUCLIDE	METHOD OF PRODUCTION	MODE OF DECAY (%)	PRINCIPAL PHOTONS keV (% ABUNDANCE)	PHYSICAL HALF-LIFE	COMMENTS
Chromium-51 (^{51}Cr)	Neutron activation	EC (100)	320 (9)	27.8 d	Used for in vivo red cell mass determinations (not used for imaging; samples counted in a NaI(Tl) well counter).
Cobalt-57 (^{57}Co)	Cyclotron produced	EC (100)	122 (86) 136 (11)	271 d	Principally used as a uniform flood field source for scintillation camera quality control.
Gallium-67 (^{67}Ga)	Cyclotron produced	EC (100)	93 (40) 184 (20) 300 (17) 393 (4)	78 h	Typically use the 93, 184, and 300 keV photons for imaging.
Indium-111 (^{111}In)	Cyclotron produced	EC (100)	171 (90) 245 (94)	2.8 d	Typically used when the kinetics require imaging more than 24 h after injection. Both photons are used in imaging.
Iodine-123 (^{123}I)	Cyclotron produced	EC (100)	159 (83)	13.2 h	Has replaced ^{131}I for diagnostic imaging to reduce patient radiation dose.
Iodine-125 (^{125}I)	Neutron activation	EC (100)	35 (6) 27 (39) XR 28 (76) XR 31 (20) XR	60.2 d	Typically used as ^{125}I albumin for in vivo blood/plasma volume determinations (not used for imaging; samples counted in a NaI(Tl) well counter).
Krypton-81m (^{81m}Kr)	Generator product	IT (100)	190 (67) 181 (6) 740 (12)	13 s	This ultrashort-lived generator-produced radionuclide is a gas and can be used to perform serial lung ventilation studies with very little radiation exposure to patient or staff. The expense and short $T_{1/2}$ of the parent (^{81}Rb, 4.6 h) limits its use.
Molybdenum-99 (^{99}Mo)	Nuclear fission (^{235}U)	β^- (100)	740 (12) 780 (4)	67 h	Parent material for Mo/Tc generator. Not used directly as a radiopharmaceutical; 740- and 780-keV photons used to identify "moly breakthrough."
Technetium-99m (^{99m}Tc)	Generator product	IT (100)	140 (88)	6.02 h	This radionuclide accounts for more than 70% of all imaging studies.

Radionuclide	Production	Decay mode (%)	Emissions keV (%)	Half-life	Comments
Xenon-133 (^{133}Xe)	Nuclear fission (^{235}U)	β^- (100)	81 (37)	5.3 d	^{133}Xe is a heavier-than-air gas. Low abundance and low energy of photon reduces image resolution.
Thallium (^{201}Tl)	Cyclotron produced	EC (100)	69–80 (94) XR	73.1 h	The majority of clinically useful photons are low-energy x-rays (69–80 keV) from mercury 201 (^{201}Hg), the daughter of ^{201}Tl. Although these photons are in high abundance (94%), their low energy results in significant patient attenuation, which is particularly difficult with female patients, in whom breast artifacts in myocardial imaging often makes interpretation more difficult.
Positron-emitting radionuclides					
Carbon-11 (^{11}C)	Cyclotron produced	β^+ (99.8)	511 AR (200)	20.4 min	Carbon-11 production: ^{14}N (p,α) ^{11}C Short half life requires on-site cyclotron for imaging. Primarily clinical research applications.
Fluorine-18 (^{18}F)	Cyclotron produced	β^+ (97) EC (3)	511 AR (193)	110 min	This radionuclide accounts for more than 70–80% of all clinical PET studies; typically formulated as FDG. Cyclotron produced via ^{18}O (p,n) ^{18}F reaction.
Nitrogen-13 (^{13}N)	Cyclotron produced	β^+ (99.8)	511 AR (200)	10 min	Cyclotron produced via ^{16}O (p,α) ^{13}N reaction. Short half life requires on-site cyclotron for imaging. Primarily clinical research applications.
Oxygen-15 (^{15}O)	Cyclotron produced	β^+ (99.9)	511 AR (200)	122 s	Cyclotron produced via ^{14}N (d,n) ^{15}O or ^{15}N (p,n) ^{15}O. Short half life requires on-site cyclotron for imaging. Primarily clinical research applications.
Gallium-68 (^{68}Ga)	Generator product	β^+ (89) EC (11)	511 AR (184)	68 min	Ga-68 is a generator decay product of Ge-68, which is linear accelerator produced via a Ga-69 (p,2n) Ge-68 reaction.
Rubidium-82 (^{82}Rb)	Generator product	β^+ (95) EC (5)	511 AR (190) 776 (13)	75 s	Rb-82 is a generator decay product of Sr-82, which is cyclotron produced via a Rb-85 (p,4n) Sr-82 reaction. The half-life of Sr-82 is 25 d (600 h) and is in secular equilibrium with Rb-82 within ~8 min after elution.

(continued)

TABLE 16-3 PHYSICAL CHARACTERISTICS OF CLINICALLY USED RADIONUCLIDES (continued)

RADIONUCLIDE	METHOD OF PRODUCTION	MODE OF DECAY (%)	PRINCIPAL PHOTONS keV (% ABUNDANCE)	PHYSICAL HALF-LIFE	COMMENTS
Therapeutic radionuclides					
Iodine-131 (^{131}I)	Nuclear fission (^{235}U)	β^- (100)	284 (6) 364 (81) 637 (7)	8.0 d	Used for treatment of hyperthyroidism and thyroid cancer: 364-keV photon used for imaging. Resolution and detection efficiency are poor due to high energy of photons. High patient dose, mostly from β^- particles.
Iodine-125 (^{125}I)	Neutron activation	EC (100)	35 (6) 27 (39) XR 28 (76) XR 31 (20) XR	60.2d	Recent use as ^{125}I Iotrex™ liquid brachytherapy source in Proxima GliaSite® radiation therapy system for treatment of recurrent gliomas and metastatic brain tumors.
Phosphorus-32 (^{32}P)	Neutron activation	β^- (100)	None	14.26 d	Prepared as either sodium phosphate for treatment of myeloproliferative disorders such as polycythemia vera and thrombocytosis or colloidal chromic phosphate for intracavitary therapy of malignant ascites, malignant pleural effusions, malignant pericardial effusions, and malignant brain cysts.
Samarium-153 (^{153}Sm)	Neutron activation	β^- (100)	103 (29)	1.93 d	As ^{153}Sm lexidronam ethylene diamine tetra methylene phosphonic acid (EDTMPA) used for pain relief from metastatic bone lesions. Advantage compared to ^{89}Sr is that the ^{153}Sm distribution can be imaged.
Strontium-89 (^{89}Sr)	Neutron activation	β^- (100)	None	50.53 d	As strontium chloride for pain relief from metastatic bone lesions.
Yttrium-90 (^{90}Y)	Generator product daughter of Sr-90	β^- (100)	None Bremsstrahlung x-ray imaging is possible to confirm delivery to treatment region	2.67 d	Bound to murine monoclonal antibodies, used to treat certain non-Hodgkin's lymphomas. Also used bound to microspheres (glass or resin) for intrahepatic arterial delivery of the Y-90 microspheres for the treatment of unresectable metastatic liver tumors. Y-90 is a generator decay product of Sr-90, which is a fission product.

Note: β^-, Beta-minus decay; β^+, beta-plus (positron) decay; AR, annihilation radiation; EC, electron capture; IT, isomeric transition (i.e., gamma ray emission), XR, x-ray.

instructions to the patient to be well hydrated and void prior to imaging improves image quality, lesion detectability and reduces patient dose. Abnormalities can be identified as localized areas of increased radiopharmaceutical concentration, called "hot spots" (e.g., a stress fracture in a bone scan), or as "cold spots" in which the radiopharmaceutical's normal localization in a tissue is altered by a disease process (e.g., perfusion defect in a lung scan with ^{99m}Tc-MAA). Disassociation of the radionuclide from the radiopharmaceutical alters the desired biodistribution, thus degrading image quality. Good quality control over radiopharmaceutical preparation helps to ensure that the radionuclide is bound to the pharmaceutical.

Safety, Convenience, and Cost-Effectiveness

Low chemical toxicity is enhanced by the use of high-specific-activity, carrier-free radionuclides that also facilitate radiopharmaceutical preparation and minimize the required amount of the isotope. For example, 3.7 GBq (100 mCi) of I-131 contains only 0.833 μg of iodine. Radionuclides should also have a chemical form, pH, concentration, and other characteristics that facilitate rapid complexing with the pharmaceutical under normal laboratory conditions. The compounded radiopharmaceutical should be stable, with a shelf life compatible with clinical use, and should be readily available from several manufacturers to minimize cost.

Therapeutic Radiopharmaceuticals

Radiopharmaceuticals are also used for the treatment of a number of diseases. The goal of radiopharmaceutical therapy is to deliver a sufficiently large dose to the target organ, tissue, or cell type while limiting the dose to nontarget tissue to minimize deterministic effects such as bone marrow suppression and to minimize the risk of cancer.

All currently approved therapeutic radiopharmaceuticals emit beta particles, but research continues with radiopharmaceuticals containing short-lived alpha particle–emitting radionuclides such as astatine-211(At-211) and Auger electron–emitting radionuclides such as I-125 and In-111.

Commonly used therapeutic radiopharmaceuticals include I-131 NaI for hyperthyroidism and thyroid cancer, Sr-89 chloride and Sm-153 lexidronam for relief of pain from cancer metastatic to bone, I-131 and Y-90 labeled monoclonal antibodies for treatment of certain non-Hodgkin's lymphomas, and P-32 as sodium phosphate for bone marrow disorders such as polycythemia vera. Radionuclides used for radiopharmaceutical therapy are listed in Table 16-3.

Radiopharmaceutical Mechanisms of Localization

Radiopharmaceutical concentration in tissue is driven by one or more of the following mechanisms: (1) compartmental localization and leakage, (2) cell sequestration, (3) phagocytosis, (4) passive diffusion, (5) active transport, (6) capillary blockade, (7) perfusion, (8) chemotaxis, (9) antibody-antigen complexation, (10) receptor binding, and (11) physiochemical adsorption.

Compartmental Localization and Leakage

Compartmental localization refers to the introduction of the radiopharmaceutical into a well-defined anatomic compartment. Examples include Xe-133 gas inhalation into the lung, intraperitoneal instillation of P-32 chromic phosphate, and Tc-99m-labeled RBCs injected into the circulatory system. Compartmental leakage is used to identify an abnormal opening in an otherwise closed compartment, as when labeled RBCs are used to detect gastrointestinal bleeding.

Cell Sequestration

To evaluate splenic morphology and function, RBCs are withdrawn from the patient, labeled with Tc-99m, and slightly damaged by *in vitro* heating in a boiling water bath for approximately 30 min. After they have been reinjected, the spleen's ability to recognize and remove (i.e., sequester) the damaged RBCs is evaluated.

Phagocytosis

The cells of the reticuloendothelial system are distributed in the liver (~85%), spleen (~10%), and bone marrow (~5%). These cells recognize small foreign substances in the blood and remove them by phagocytosis. In a liver scan, for example, Tc-99m-labeled sulfur colloid particles (~100 nm) are recognized, being substantially smaller than circulating cellular elements, and are rapidly removed from circulation.

Passive Diffusion

Passive diffusion is simply the free movement of a substance from a region of high concentration to one of lower concentration. Anatomic and physiologic mechanisms exist in the brain tissue and surrounding vasculature that allow essential nutrients, metabolites, and lipid-soluble compounds to pass freely between the plasma and brain tissue while many water-soluble substances (including most radiopharmaceuticals) are prevented from entering healthy brain tissue. This system, called the blood-brain barrier, protects and regulates access to the brain. Disruptions of the blood-brain barrier can be produced by trauma, neoplasms, and inflammation. The disruption permits radiopharmaceuticals such as Tc-99m diethylenetriaminepentaacetic acid (DTPA), which is normally excluded by the blood-brain barrier, to follow the concentration gradient and enter the affected brain tissue.

Active Transport

Active transport involves cellular metabolic processes that expend energy to concentrate the radiopharmaceutical into a tissue against a concentration gradient and above plasma levels. The classic example in nuclear medicine is the trapping and organification of radioactive iodide. Trapping of iodide in the thyroid gland occurs by transport against a concentration gradient into follicular cells, where it is oxidized to a highly reactive iodine by a peroxidase enzyme system. Organification follows, resulting in the production of radiolabeled triiodothyronine (T_3) and thyroxine (T_4). Another example is the localization of thallium (a potassium analog) in muscle tissue. The concentration of Tl-201 is mediated by the energy-dependent Na^+/K^+ ionic pump. Nonuniform distribution of Tl-201 in the myocardium indicates a myocardial perfusion deficit. F-18 FDG is a glucose analog that concentrates in cells that rely upon glucose as an energy source, or in cells whose dependence on glucose increases under pathophysiological conditions. FDG is actively transported into the cell where it is phosphorylated and trapped for several hours as FDG-6-phosphate. The retention and clearance of FDG reflects glucose metabolism in a given tissue. FDG is used to assist in the evaluation of malignancy in patients with known or suspected diagnoses of cancer. In addition, FDG is used to assess regional cardiac glucose metabolism for the evaluation of hibernating myocardium (i.e., the reversible loss of systolic function) in patients with coronary artery disease.

Capillary Blockade

When particles slightly larger than RBCs are injected intravenously, they become trapped in the capillary beds. A common example in nuclear medicine is in the assessment of pulmonary perfusion by the injection of Tc-99m-MAA, which is trapped in the pulmonary capillary bed. Imaging the distribution of Tc-99m-MAA provides a representative assessment of pulmonary perfusion. The "microemboli" created by this radiopharmaceutical do not pose a significant clinical risk because only a very small percentage of the pulmonary capillaries are blocked and the MAA is eventually removed by biodegradation.

Perfusion

Relative perfusion of a tissue or organ system is an important diagnostic element in many nuclear medical procedures. For example, the perfusion phase of a three-phase bone scan helps to distinguish between an acute process (e.g., osteomyelitis) and remote fracture. Perfusion is also an important diagnostic element in examinations such as renograms, cerebral and hepatic blood flow studies and myocardial perfusion studies.

Chemotaxis

Chemotaxis describes the movement of a cell such as a leukocyte in response to a chemical stimulus. ^{111}In- and ^{99m}Tc-labeled leukocytes respond to products formed in immunologic reactions by migrating and accumulating at the site of the reaction as part of an overall inflammatory response.

Antibody-Antigen Complexation

An antigen is a biomolecule (typically a protein) that is capable of inducing the production of, and binding to, an antibody in the body. The antibody has a strong and specific affinity for the antigen. An *in vitro* test called radioimmunoassay (RIA) makes use of the competition between a radiolabeled antigen and the same antigen in the patient's serum for antibody binding sites. RIA, developed by Berson and Yalow in the late 1950s (Berson and Yalow 1960), led to a Nobel Prize in Medicine for Yalow in 1977, five years after the untimely death of Berson. RIA techniques have been employed to measure minute quantities of various enzymes, antigens, drugs, and hormones; however, many of these tests have been replaced by immunoassays using nonradioactive labels. At equilibrium, the more unlabeled serum antigen that is present, the less radiolabeled antigen (free antigen) will become bound to the antibody (bound antigen). The serum level is measured by comparing the ratio between bound and free antigen in the sample to a known standard for that particular assay.

Antigen-antibody complexation is also used in diagnostic imaging with such agents as In-111-labeled monoclonal antibodies for the detection of colorectal carcinoma. This class of immunospecific radiopharmaceuticals promises to provide an exciting new approach to diagnostic imaging. In addition, a variety of radiolabeled (typically with I-131 or Y-90) monoclonal antibodies directed toward tumors are being used in an attempt to deliver tumoricidal radiation doses. This procedure, called radioimmunotherapy, has proven effective in the treatment of some non-Hodgkin's lymphomas and is under clinical investigation for other malignancies.

Receptor Binding

This class of radiopharmaceuticals is characterized by their high affinity to bind to specific receptor sites. For example, the uptake of In-111-octreotide, used for the localization of neuroendocrine and other tumors, is based on the binding of a somatostatin analog to receptor sites in tumors.

Physiochemical Adsorption

The localization of methylenediphosphonate (MDP) occurs primarily by adsorption in the mineral phase of the bone. MDP concentrations are significantly higher in amorphous calcium than in mature hydroxyapatite crystalline structures, which helps to explain its concentration in areas of increased osteogenic activity.

A summary of the characteristics and clinical utility of commonly used radiopharmaceuticals is provided in Appendix F-1.

Radiopharmaceutical Quality Control

Aside from the radionuclidic purity quality control performed on the ^{99m}Tc-pertechnetate generator eluate, the most common radiopharmaceutical quality control procedure is the test for radiochemical purity. The radiochemical purity assay identifies the fraction of the total radioactivity that is in the desired chemical form. Radiochemical impurity can occur as the result of temperature changes, presence of unwanted oxidizing or reducing agents, pH changes, or radiation damage to the radiopharmaceutical (called autoradiolysis). The presence of radiochemical impurities compromises the diagnostic utility of the radiopharmaceutical by reducing uptake in the organ of interest and increasing background activity, thereby degrading image quality. In addition to lowering the diagnostic quality of the examination, radiochemical impurities unnecessarily increase patient dose.

The most common method to determine the amount of radiochemical impurity in a radiopharmaceutical preparation is thin-layer chromatography. This test is performed by placing a small aliquot ($\sim$1 drop) of the radiopharmaceutical preparation approximately 1 cm from one end of a small rectangular paper (e.g., Whatman filter paper) or a silica-coated plastic strip. This strip is called the "stationary phase." The end of the strip with the spot of radiopharmaceutical is then lowered into a glass vial containing an appropriate solvent (e.g., saline, acetone, or 85% methanol), such that the solvent front begins just below the spot. The depth of the solvent in the vial must be low enough, so that the spot of radiopharmaceutical on the strip is above the solvent. The solvent will slowly move up the strip and the various radiochemicals will partition themselves at specific locations identified by their reference values (R_f), which ranges from 0 to 1 along the strip, according to their relative solubilities. The reference value number is the fraction of the total distance on the strip, (from the origin, where the spot of the radiopharmaceutical is placed to a predetermined line near the top of the strip where the solvent front ends), traveled by a particular radiochemical. Once the solvent front has reached the top, the strip is removed and dried. The strip is cut into sections, and the percentage of the total radioactivity on each section of the strip is assayed and recorded. The movements of radiopharmaceuticals and their contaminants have been characterized for several solvents. Comparison of the results with these reference values allows the identities and percentages of the radiochemical impurities to be determined.

The two principal radiochemical impurities in technetium-labeled radiopharmaceuticals are free (i.e., unbound) Tc-99m-pertechnetate and hydrolyzed Tc-99m. The Tc-99m radiopharmaceutical complex and its associated impurities will, depending upon the solvent, either remain at the origin ($R_f = 0$) or move with the solvent front to a location near the end of the strip. For example, with Whatman 31 ET chromatography paper as the stationary phase in an acetone solvent, Tc-99m-MAA remains at the origin and any free pertechnetate or hydrolyzed Tc-99m migrates close to the solvent front ($R_f = 0.9$). On the other hand, I-131 (as bound NaI) moves with the solvent front ($R_f = 1$) in an 85% methanol solvent, while the impurity (unbound iodide) moves approximately 20% of the distance from the origin ($R_f = 0.2$). These assays are easy to perform and should be used as part of a routine radiopharmacy quality control program and whenever there is a question about the radiochemical integrity of a radiopharmaceutical preparation.

Internal Dosimetry

The radiation doses to patients from diagnostic imaging procedures are an important issue and, in the absence of a medical physicist at an institution (e.g., private practice radiology), radiologists and nuclear medicine physicians are often consulted as the local experts. Radiation dosimetry is primarily of interest because radiation dose quantities serve as indices of the risk from diagnostic imaging procedures using ionizing radiation. Dosimetry also plays an important role in radiopharmaceutical therapy where estimates of activity necessary to produce tumoricidal doses must be weighed against potential radiotoxicity to healthy tissue. In nuclear medicine procedures, the chemical form of the radiopharmaceutical, its route of administration (e.g., intravenous injection, ingestion, inhalation), the administered activity, the radionuclide, and patient-specific disease states and pharmacokinetics determine the patient dose.

Radiopharmaceutical Dosimetry: Methodology

Several formalized methodologies have been proposed for calculation of internal dose. The Medical Internal Radiation Dosimetry (MIRD) and Radiation Dose Assessment Resource (RADAR) task groups of the Society of Nuclear Medicine have developed formalisms for calculating the radiation dose to selected organs and the whole body from internally administered radionuclides. These formalisms take into account variables related to the physics of energy deposition by ionizing radiation as well as those associated with the biologic system for which the dose is being calculated. Although some of the variables are known with a high degree of accuracy, others are based on estimates or simplifying assumptions that, taken together, provide an approximation of the dose to the average (reference) adult, adolescent, child, and the fetus. Prior to the widespread availability of microcomputers, basic standardized computational anthropomorphic phantoms were developed by utilizing a combination of simple geometric shapes (e.g., cones, spheres, cylinders) to represent the human body (Fig. 16-11A). Over the years, greater computer processing power and more complex calculational techniques allowed for much more sophisticated and anatomically accurate phantoms to be developed. Today, these newer phantoms are available for adult males and females, children of different ages, and the pregnant female (Fig. 16-11B).

The internal dosimetry formalism has two main elements: (1) estimation of the number of nuclear transformations occurring in various "source" organs containing radioactive material and (2) estimation of the energy absorbed in selected "target" organs for which the dose is being calculated from the radiation emitted in source organs (Fig. 16-12).

MIRD Formalism

The MIRD formalism designates a source organ in which activity is located as r_S, and a target organ for which the dose is being calculated as r_T. Following the administration of the radiopharmaceutical, the mean dose to a particular target organ or tissue over a defined dose integration period (T_D) is calculated from the following equation (Bolch 2009)

$$D(r_T, T_D) = \sum_{r_S} \int_0^{T_D} A(r_S, t) \frac{1}{M(r_T, t)} \sum_i E_i Y_i \phi(r_T \leftarrow r_S, E_i, t) \qquad [16\text{-}7]$$

where $A(r_S, t)$ is the activity for each source organ (r_S) at time (t); $M(r_T, t)$ is the target organ mass at time t; E_i is the mean energy of a given radiation emission i; and Y_i

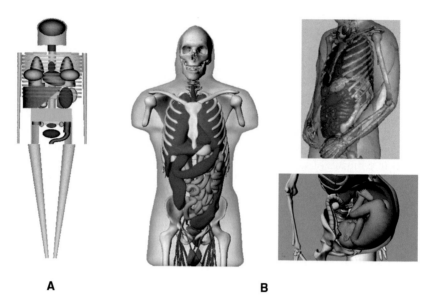

A   **B**

■ **FIGURE 16-11 (A)** First-generation computational anthropomorphic phantoms (referred to as the Fisher-Snyder phantoms) were developed utilizing simplified geometric shapes. Monte Carlo computer programs were used simulate the creation and transport of radiation from the decay of radionuclides inside the body. **(B)** More sophisticated and anatomically correct phantoms are currently available for adult males and females, children of different ages and the pregnant female. (Adapted from Stabin MG, Emmons-Keenan MA, Segars WP, Fernald MJ. *The Vanderbilt University Reference Adult and Pediatric Phantom Series*, and Xu XG, Shi C, Stabin MG, Taranenko V. Pregnant female/fetus computational phantoms and the latest RPI-P series representing 3, 6, and 9 months gestational periods. In: *Handbook of Anatomical Models for Radiation Dosimetry*. Boca Raton, FL: CRC Press, 2009.)

is its yield (i.e., number emitted per nuclear transformation) and $\phi(r_T\leftarrow r_S,E_i,t)$, the absorbed fraction, is the fraction of the energy emitted in the source organ r_S that is absorbed in the target r_T for a given radiation emission i at time t. All of the terms after the activity term have also been consolidated into *S factors*, which gives the absorbed dose in the target, r_T, per disintegration in each source organ r_S (rad/μCi-hr). The MIRD committee has not published S factors in SI units (Gy/Bq-s).

If the dose to a patient is being calculated from the administration of a diagnostic radiopharmaceuticals during which there would be no significant change in the mass of the source or target organs over time (a situation more relevant to therapy where the mass of a tumor may change over time), the calculation simplifies to this time-independent form:

$$D(r_T,T_D) = \sum_{r_S} \tilde{A}\ (r_S,T_D)S(r_T \leftarrow r_S) \qquad [16\text{-}8]$$

where term $\tilde{A}(r_S,T_D)$ represents the *time-integrated activity* (i.e., total number of disintegrations) in the source organ or tissue during the specified dose integration period T_D. The factors that influence the time-integrated activity in a source organ are discussed below.

RADAR Formalism

The last publication of complete tables of S-values for an anthropomorphic phantom was in 1975. Since that time, the RADAR group published a method for

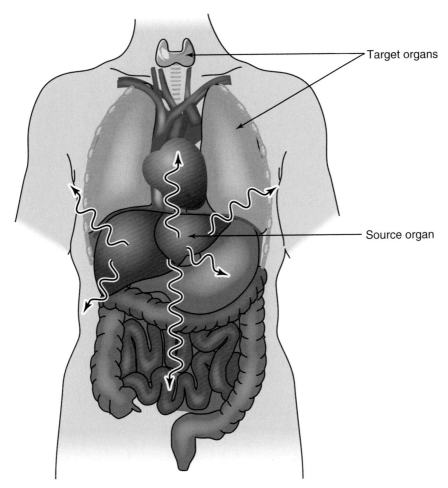

■ **FIGURE 16-12** Illustration of source and target organ concept for calculation of the dose to the lungs and thyroid gland (target organs) from a radiopharmaceutical (e.g., technetium-99m sulfur colloid) primarily located in the liver (source organ). Note that the relative geometry and mass of the source and target organs together with the physical decay characteristic of the radionuclide and its associated radiopharmaceutical kinetics all play a part in determining the dose to any particular organ.

calculation of internal dose for which the numerous variables and complexities inherent in such a calculation are represented by simplified terms and symbols (Stabin, 2003).

$$D_T = N_s \times DF \qquad\qquad [16\text{-}9]$$

Here D_T is the dose in target organ T; N_s is the number of disintegrations that occur in any source region (i.e., the time integrated activity); and DF is the *dose factor*, representing the absorbed dose in the target (T) per disintegration in each source organ, incorporating the same variables as in the MIRD S factors. This method has been implemented in software (OLINDA/EXM) designed to run on a desktop computer (Stabin, 2005). The software can perform dose calculation for over 800 radionuclides in six reference adult and child models (Cristy, 1987), and three models of the pregnant female (representing the end of each trimester) using absorbed fractions calculated by Oak Ridge National Laboratory (Stabin, 1995). Version 2 of this software will perform calculations using these historical phantoms as well as the new, more mathematically sophisticated and anatomically correct image-based models that have been developed over the last decade for adults, children, and pregnant females.

Time-Integrated Activity

The MIRD committee used the term *cumulated activity* for many years to represent the time-integral of activity in Equation 16-7. The integral of any time-activity curve is the total number of nuclear transformations from the radionuclide located in a particular source organ. The RADAR method uses the term N_s, to represent the number of disintegrations occurring in a source organ. The units of Bq-s (Becquerel seconds) express the total number of disintegrations (i.e., disintegrations per unit time $\times$ time = disintegrations).

Calculating the number of disintegrations in the various organs requires fitting time-activity data to mathematical functions (typically one or more exponentials) or creation and solution of a theoretical compartmental model describing the kinetics of the radiopharmaceutical in the body. A compartment may be a physical space (e.g., blood in the vasculature) or a physiological compartment (e.g., iodine as thyroxine). Such a model is typically created from a knowledge of anatomy, physiology and the rates of transfer among compartments based on studies of the *in-vivo* behavior of the radiopharmaceutical in animals and humans. Figure 16-13 shows a compartmental model for radioactive ionic or elemental iodine.

However, for some radiopharmaceuticals, a simplified single compartment model may provide a reasonable approximation. In this case, activity is accumulated by an organ and gradually eliminated. The total number of disintegrations in a source organ depends on (1) the administered activity, (2) the fraction of the administered activity "taken up" by the source organ, and (3) the rate of elimination from the source organ.

Figure 16-14 shows a simple kinetic model representing the accumulation and elimination of radioactivity in a source organ (liver). The activity localized in the source organ (A_f) is a fraction (f) of the injected activity (A_0), (i.e., $A_f = A_0 \times f$). If we assume there is exponential biological excretion, two processes will act to reduce the total activity in the source organ: (1) physical decay of the radionuclide, as represented by its physical half-life T_p, and (2) biologic elimination, as represented by the biologic half-life T_b. Taken together, the reduction of activity in a source organ with time can be expressed as an *effective half-life* (T_e) that is calculated as follows:

$$T_e = \frac{T_p \times T_b}{T_p + T_b}$$ [16-10]

In a manner analogous to radioactive decay, the activity remaining in a source organ after a time (t) is

$$A(r_S,t) = fA_0\, e^{-\lambda_e t}$$ [16-11]

where λ_e is the effective decay constant, equal to $0.693/T_e$.

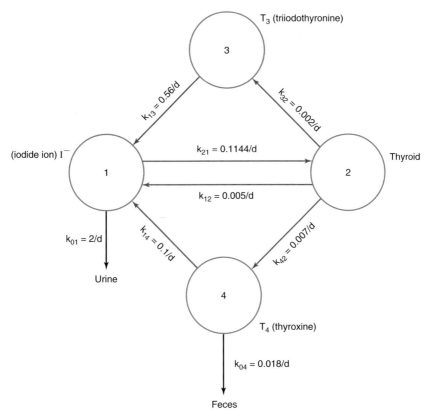

■ **FIGURE 16-13** A simplified compartmental model of iodine kinetics in humans. Compartment 1 is extra thyroidal iodide, compartment 2 is thyroidal iodine, compartment 3 is extrathyroidal T_3 (triiodothyronine), and compartment 4 is extrathyroidal T_4 (thyroxine). The compartmental transfer coefficient or *rate constant* k_{xy} describes the relative rate at which iodine is transferred from compartment y to compartment x. For example k_{21} is the rate constant for the transfer of extrathyroidal iodide (compartment 1) to the thyroid gland (compartment 2). Iodine also leaves the thyroid gland in the form of T_3 and T_4 (k_{32}, k_{42}) as well as some release of free iodine back into the extrathyroidal space (k_{12}). The relative values of the rate constants for the elimination of iodine into the urine and feces (k_{01}, k_{04}) indicate that the vast majority of the iodine is eliminated in the urine. These rate constants can be greatly altered by pathology (e.g., hyperthyroidism) or other conditions (e.g., low iodine diet). Reference: Mones Berman, Kinetic Models for Absorbed Dose Calculations, MIRD Pamphlet No. 12, Society of Nuclear Medicine, 1977.

Just as one cannot predict the range of a single photon before it interacts, it is not possible to know when any particular radioactive atom will decay. However, one can describe the *mean life* (τ) or average time to decay for atoms of a specific radionuclide in a manner analogous to the mean free path (MFP) for photons discussed in Chapter 3. Just as the "average" distance traveled by the photons before interacting can be described in terms of its linear attenuation coefficient (μ) or half-value layer (HVL), ($1/\mu$ or 1.44 HVL), the mean life of a nuclide is equal to $1/\lambda$ or 1.44 $T_p\frac{1}{2}$. For the purpose of radiation dosimetry where the removal of radioactive atoms from a source organ is more completely described by the effective half-life (T_e), mean life in the organ becomes $1/\lambda_e$ or 1.44 T_e. The total number of nuclear transformations is equal to the area under the time-activity curve. The area under this curve (Fig. 16-15) can be shown to be equal to the product of the initial amount of activity in the source

■ **FIGURE 16-14** Simplified kinetics model of the accumulation and elimination of radioactivity in a source organ (e.g., liver). A fraction (*f*) of the injected activity (A_0) is localized in the source organ in which the initial activity (A_f) is reduced by physical decay and biologic excretion of the radiopharmaceutical.

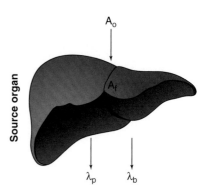

organ ($A_0 \times f$) and the mean life (1.44 T_e). Therefore the total number of nuclear transformations (*N*) can be expressed as

$$N = 1.44\ T_e A_0 f \qquad\qquad [16\text{-}12]$$

As discussed in the RADAR dosimetry model, the dose factor (*DF*) is the absorbed dose in the target (T) per disintegration in a specified source organ. The DF is expressed in units of mGy/MBq-s, and like the S factor, it is determined by the mass of the target organ; the quantity, type, and mean energy of the ionizing radiation emitted per disintegration (i.e., decay scheme); and finally the fraction of the emitted radiation energy that reaches and is absorbed by the target organ.

Each dose factor is specific to a particular source organ—target organ pair and a specific radionuclide. Dose factors are provided in tabular form or incorporated into computer programs for many common diagnostic and therapeutic radionuclides. Table 16-4 lists some dose factors from the OLINDA/EXM program for Tc-99m. This computer program can be used for calculating organ and effective doses from a wide variety of radiopharmaceuticals used in nuclear medicine.

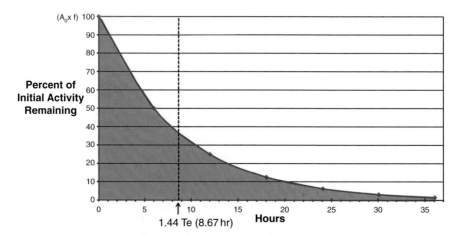

■ **FIGURE 16-15** Time activity curve for a hypothetical Tc-99m labeled radiopharmaceutical that has a very long biological half-life (T_b) compared to the 6.02 h physical half-life (T_p) of Tc-99m, thus $T_e = T_p$. The cumulated activity is equal to the area under the curve which is numerically equal to ($A_0 \cdot f$) (1.44 T_e) representing the total number of nuclear transformations (disintegrations) in the specified source organ.

Example Dose Calculations

The simplest example of an internal dose calculation would be a situation in which the radiopharmaceutical instantly localizes in a single organ and remains there with an infinite T_b. Although most radiopharmaceuticals do not meet both of these assumptions, this hypothetical example is considered for the purpose of demonstrating the calculational technique in its simplest possible application.

EXAMPLE: A patient is injected with 100 MBq of Tc-99m-sulfur colloid. Estimate the absorbed dose to the (1) liver, (2) testes, and (3) red bone marrow.

Assumptions:
1. All of the injected activity is uniformly distributed in the liver.
2. The uptake of Tc-99m-sulfur colloid in the liver from the blood is instantaneous.
3. There is no biologic removal of Tc-99m-sulfur colloid from the liver.

In this case, the testes and red bone marrow are target organs, whereas the liver is both a source and a target organ. The average dose to any target organ can be estimated by applying the RADAR formalism in Equation 16-9:

$$D_T = N_s \times DF$$

STEP 1. Calculate the number of disintegrations (N_s) in the source organ (i.e., liver) by inserting the appropriate values into Equation 16-12 (Note that because T_b is infinite, $T_e = T_p$):

$$N_s = 1.44 \times 6 \, hr \times 1 \times 100 \, MBq = 980 \, MBq - hr \left(\frac{3600 \, s}{hr} \right)$$

$$N_s = 3.1 \times 10^6 \, MBq\text{-s or } 3.1 \times 10^{12} \text{ disintegrations}$$

STEP 2. Find the appropriate dose factors for each target/source organ pair and the radionuclide of interest (i.e., Tc-99m) from Table 16-4. The appropriate dose factors found at the intersection of the source organ's column (i.e., liver) and the individual target organ's row (i.e., liver, testes, or red bone marrow).

TARGET (r_T)	SOURCE (r_S)	DOSE FACTOR (mGy/MBq-s)
Liver	Liver	3.16×10^{-6}
Red bone marrow	Liver	8.32×10^{-8}
Testes	Liver	1.57×10^{-9}

STEP 3. Organize the assembled information in a table of organ doses:

TARGET ORGAN (r_T)	N_s (MBq-s)	×	DOSE FACTOR (mGy/MBq-s)	=	D_T (mGy)
Liver	3.1×10^6		3.16×10^{-6}		9.8
Red bone marrow	3.1×10^6		8.32×10^{-8}		0.26
Testes	3.1×10^6		1.57×10^{-9}		0.0049

Compared to the dose to the liver the relatively low dose to the testes and red bone marrow is largely due to the fact that only a small fraction of the isotropically emitted penetrating radiation (i.e., gamma rays and x-rays) is directed toward, and absorbed by, these tissues.

TABLE 16-4 Tc-99m DOSE FACTORS (mGy/MBq-s) FOR SOME SOURCE/TARGET ORGAN COMBINATIONS*

TARGET ORGANS	SOURCE ORGANS										
	ADRENALS	BRAIN	LLI CONTENTS	SI CONTENT	STOMACH CONTENTS	ULI CONTENTS	HEART CONTENTS	HEART WALL	KIDNEYS	LIVER	LUNGS
Adrenals	1.80E-04	4.18E-10	2.25E-08	7.46E-08	2.73E-07	9.58E-08	2.53E-07	2.85E-07	7.24E-07	4.35E-07	2.33E-07
Brain	4.18E-10	4.23E-06	1.57E-11	3.91E-11	4.27E-10	4.68E-11	3.14E-09	2.54E-09	1.58E-10	8.16E-10	7.63E-09
Breasts	5.05E-08	3.17E-09	2.28E-09	7.35E-09	5.73E-08	8.00E-09	2.41E-07	2.61E-07	1.99E-08	6.82E-08	2.33E-07
Gallbladder Wall	3.57E-07	1.54E-10	6.49E-08	4.38E-07	3.05E-07	7.53E-07	1.03E-07	1.22E-07	4.09E-07	8.70E-07	7.46E-08
LLI Wall	1.98E-08	1.32E-11	1.23E-05	5.92E-07	9.10E-08	2.14E-07	4.06E-09	4.90E-09	5.50E-08	1.44E-08	3.29E-09
Small Intestine	7.46E-08	3.91E-11	7.16E-07	4.22E-06	2.08E-07	1.25E-06	1.57E-08	2.06E-08	2.13E-07	1.16E-07	1.35E-08
Stomach Wall	2.85E-07	2.52E-10	1.24E-07	2.13E-07	8.53E-06	2.86E-07	1.66E-07	2.65E-07	2.53E-07	1.48E-07	1.19E-07
ULI Wall	9.41E-08	4.76E-11	3.10E-07	1.36E-06	2.65E-07	8.37E-06	2.12E-08	2.65E-08	2.12E-07	1.88E-07	1.81E-08
Heart Wall	2.85E-07	2.54E-09	5.42E-09	2.06E-08	2.33E-07	2.97E-08	5.48E-06	1.19E-05	8.22E-08	2.33E-07	4.40E-07
Kidneys	7.24E-07	1.58E-10	7.10E-08	2.13E-07	2.73E-07	2.12E-07	6.45E-08	8.22E-08	1.32E-05	2.93E-07	6.66E-08
Liver	4.35E-07	8.16E-10	1.80E-08	1.16E-07	1.47E-07	1.87E-07	2.13E-07	2.33E-07	2.93E-07	*3.16E-06*	1.97E-07
Lungs	2.33E-07	7.63E-09	4.50E-09	1.35E-08	1.10E-07	1.77E-08	4.59E-07	4.40E-07	6.66E-08	2.09E-07	3.57E-06
Muscle	1.12E-07	2.21E-08	1.23E-07	1.12E-07	9.96E-08	1.07E-07	8.83E-08	9.20E-08	9.79E-08	7.52E-08	9.34E-08
Ovaries	3.14E-08	1.52E-08	1.26E-06	9.23E-08	5.85E-08	7.71E-07	4.55E-09	6.15E-09	7.02E-08	3.81E-08	5.39E-09
Pancreas	1.09E-06	4.15E-10	5.21E-08	1.42E-07	1.23E-06	1.62E-07	2.65E-07	3.57E-07	4.97E-07	3.86E-07	1.74E-07
Red Marrow	2.53E-07	1.01E-07	2.01E-07	1.79E-07	7.50E-08	1.43E-07	1.11E-07	1.11E-07	1.71E-07	*8.32E-08*	1.11E-07
Osteogenic Cells	2.67E-07	2.99E-07	1.82E-07	1.49E-07	1.03E-07	1.27E-07	1.60E-07	1.60E-07	1.62E-07	1.24E-07	1.66E-07
Skin	3.41E-08	3.97E-08	3.62E-08	3.01E-08	3.41E-08	3.09E-08	3.41E-08	3.70E-08	3.79E-08	3.62E-08	4.02E-08

Spleen	4.58E-07	5.19E-10	6.53E-08	1.01E-07	7.83E-07	1.05E-07	1.24E-07	1.67E-07	6.63E-07	7.22E-08	1.64E-07
Testes	1.54E-09	1.46E-12	1.40E-07	2.61E-08	2.90E-09	1.92E-08	5.16E-10	6.16E-10	3.10E-09	*1.57E-09*	3.67E-10
Thymus	5.66E-08	6.88E-09	2.04E-09	4.66E-09	3.65E-08	5.43E-09	8.87E-07	7.35E-07	1.73E-08	5.93E-08	2.85E-07
Thyroid	8.11E-09	1.35E-07	2.48E-10	4.87E-10	2.62E-09	7.69E-10	5.17E-08	4.33E-08	2.95E-09	8.64E-09	8.82E-08
Urinary Bladder Wall	7.55E-09	6.02E-12	4.98E-07	2.12E-07	1.73E-08	1.61E-07	2.22E-09	2.17E-09	1.87E-08	1.16E-08	1.33E-09
Uterus	1.89E-08	1.31E-11	5.17E-07	8.37E-07	5.05E-08	3.97E-07	4.87E-09	5.47E-09	6.42E-08	3.29E-08	4.10E-09
Total Body	1.72E-07	1.25E-07	1.49E-07	1.59E-07	1.17E-07	1.41E-07	1.17E-07	1.65E-07	1.58E-07	1.59E-07	1.44E-07

*OLINDA/EXM v1.0.

Note: GI, gastrointestinal; SI, small intestine; ULI, upper large intestine; LLI, lower large intestine; Bold italicized correspond to values in MIRD example problem. E, exponential (e.g., 4.6E-05 $=4.6 \times 10^{-5}$).

Whole Body Dose and Effective Dose

Dose factor tables always include entries for the *whole body* of the reference adult, child, or pregnant woman. As is the case for individual organs, all energy absorbed from all emissions are summed and then divided by the mass, in this case, of the whole body. Researchers and regulators usually note this quantity, but in nuclear medicine, it is of questionable utility. If the whole body is fairly uniformly irradiated, this quantity may be useful in risk assessment, but this is rarely the case with radiopharmaceuticals, as they are specifically designed to target specific tissues. Averaging all of the energy absorbed in particular organs over the mass of the whole body may give a misleading result. As an example, imagine that we have I-131 activity only in the thyroid of an adult male. Let's say there were 100 MBq-hr in the thyroid, whose mass is about 20 g. The dose to the thyroid is

$$D = 100\text{MBq-hr} \times \left(\frac{3600s}{hr}\right) 1.59 \times 10^{-3} \frac{mGy}{MBq\text{-}s} = 570mGy$$

One can use the dose factor for thyroid to total body and calculate a "total body dose" of 0.27 mGy but it is of very little value. The dose to the thyroid, on the other hand, can be useful in evaluating the potential risk by using the ICRP 103 methodology to calculate an effective dose (see Chapter 3) or to calculate the relative or absolute thyroid cancer risk from the dose based on organ-specific risk estimates (see discussion of risk calculations in Chapter 20). However, in the RADAR or MIRD dosimetry systems, the "whole body dose" is calculated by taking all of the beta energy that was absorbed in the 20 g of thyroid and averaging it over 73,000 g of body tissue (mass of the reference person) and adding the photon energy that was fairly uniformly received by tissues outside of the thyroid. There is little one can do with a dose calculated in this manner that would have any relevence to the assessment of potential health risks.

Recall (from Chapter 3) that in the effective dose model, tissue weighting factors (w_T) are used to account for the differences among individual organs and tissues to harm (i.e., detriment) from radiation-induced cancer, genetic, and other stochastic effects. The w_T values were chosen on the basis of age and gender averaged estimates of relative radiation induced detriment for each of organs and tissues listed. To reflect the combined detriment from stochastic effects due to the equivalent doses in all the organs and tissues of the body, the equivalent dose in each organ and tissue is multiplied by its corresponding w_T, and the results are added to give the effective dose.

$$E = \sum_T H_T \times w_T$$

If one were to recalculate the effective dose for the Tc-99m-sulfur colloid dosimetry example illustrated above, this time including all the source and target organs, more realistic kinetics, and a more typical administered activity for an adult liver/spleen scan of 200 MBq, the effective dose would be approximately 1.9 mSv. This value could be used to compare the relative risk of the Tc-99m-sulfur colloid liver scan to an alternative diagnostic imaging procedure using ionizing radiation such as an abdominal CT scan for which the effective dose (~8 mSv), and thus the risk, may be approximately four times higher.

It is important to remember that the effective dose concept was developed for the purpose of radiation protection where the reference population for which the w_T values were developed included a distribution of both genders and all ages. Effective dose was not intended, nor is it correct to assume that it can be used, to provide individual risk estimates to a particular patient from medical imaging procedures. This is a consequence of the fact that the magnitude of risk for stochastic effects are dependent on variables beyond just organ/tissue doses such as age at time of exposure and gender. For example, as discussed in Chapter 20, radiation exposure in children carriers a greater cancer risk than the same dose in adult patients. Thus, calculating risk on the basis of effective doses for a pediatric patient population would likely underestimate the actual cancer risk and such calculations are inappropriate anytime there are significant dissimilarities between the age and gender of a particular patient or patient population and the ICRP reference population. The effective dose methodology was not developed to assess radiation-induced health risks in patients receiving radiopharmaceutical therapy, even if the patient populations are similar to the age and gender distributions of the ICRP reference population.

Accuracy of Dose Calculations

Although the methods shown here provide reasonable estimates of organ doses, the typical application of this technique usually includes several significant assumptions, limitations, and simplifications that, taken together, could result in significant differences between the true and calculated doses. These include the following:

1. The radioactivity is assumed to be uniformly distributed in each source organ. This is rarely the case and, in fact, significant pathology (e.g., cirrhosis of the liver) or characteristics of the radiopharmaceutical may result in a highly nonuniform activity distribution.
2. The dose factors derived from early computational models were based on organ sizes and geometries that were idealized into simplified shapes to reduce the computational complexity. Significant improvements have been made over the last few decades and more detailed and anatomically correct anthropomorphic phantoms are now available.
3. Each organ is assumed to be homogeneous in density and composition.
4. Even the newer more detailed "reference" adult, adolescent, and child phantoms are just approximations of the physical dimensions of any given individual.
5. Although the radiobiologic effect of the dose occurs at the molecular level, the energy deposition is averaged over the entire mass of the target organs and therefore does not reflect the actual microdosimetry on a molecular or cellular level.
6. Dose contributions from bremsstrahlung and other minor radiation sources are ignored.
7. With a few exceptions, low-energy photons and all particulate radiations are assumed to be absorbed locally (i.e., nonpenetrating).

Taken together, radiopharmaceutical dose estimate may be different (higher or lower) by a factor of two or more than the actual dose in any given individual. This is particularly true in patients with significant disease states that alter the kinetics of the normal radiopharmaceutical distribution. However, for patients who have had individualized dosimetry performed prior to receiving radionuclide therapy, the total uncertainty in an individual dose estimate can be reduced to a value of perhaps ~10% to 20% (Stabin 2008). In addition, the time-activity curves used for each initial organ dose estimate during the developmental phase of a radiopharmaceutical is usually based on laboratory animal data. This information is only slowly adjusted by data aquired in human subjects and quantitative evaluation of biodistributions and kinetics. The FDA does not currently require manufacturers to update their package inserts as better radiopharmaceutical dosimetry becomes available. Therefore, organ doses listed in package inserts (especially those of older agents) are often not the best source of dosimetry information (Appendix H, Fig. H-3). The ICRP, utilizing similar methodology, reference data on biokinetics, and new ORNL phantoms discussed above, have compiled the most comprehensive collection of dose estimates for radiopharmaceuticals in their publications 53, 80, and 106 (ICRP 1987, ICRP 1998, ICRP 2009).

In addition to the development of child and fetal dosimetry models, advances in the use of radioimmunotherapeutic pharmaceuticals have increased the need for patient-specific dosimetry that takes advantage of individual kinetics and anatomic information. A good overview of these issues and models can be found in several recent reviews (see suggested reading).

For the most commonly used diagnostic and therapeutic radiopharmaceutical agents, Appendix F-2 summarizes the typically administered adult dose, the organ receiving the highest radiation dose and its dose, the gonadal dose, and the adult effective dose. For most of these same radiopharmaceuticals, Appendix F-3A provides a table of effective doses per unit activity administered in 15-, 10-, 5-, and 1-year-old patients, Appendix F-3B provides the North American consensus guidelines for administered radiopharmaceutical activities in children and adolescents, Appendix F4-A provides a table of absorbed doses to the embryo or fetus at early, 3, 6, and 9 months gestation per unit activity of commonly used radiopharmaceuticals administered to the mother, Appendix F4-B provides a table of effective doses to the newborn and infant per unit activity of specific radiopharmaceuticals administered from the mother's breast milk and Appendix F4-C provides a table of breast dose from radiopharmaceuticals excreted in breast milk.

Regulatory Issues

Investigational Radiopharmaceuticals

All pharmaceuticals for human use, whether radioactive or not, are regulated by the U.S. Food and Drug Administration (FDA). A request to evaluate a new radiopharmaceutical for human use is submitted to the FDA in an application called a "Notice of Claimed Investigational Exemption for a New Drug" (IND). The IND can be sponsored by either an individual physician or a radiopharmaceutical manufacturer who will work with a group of clinical investigators to collect the necessary data. The IND application includes the names and credentials of the investigators, the clinical protocol, details of the research project, details of the manufacturing of the drug, and animal toxicology data. The clinical investigation of the new radio pharmaceutical occurs in three stages. Phase I focuses on a limited number of patients and is designed to provide information on the pharmacologic distribution, metabolism, dosimetry, toxicity, optimal dose schedule, and adverse reactions. Phase II studies include a limited number of patients with specific diseases to begin the assessment of the drug's efficacy, refine the dose schedule, and collect more information on safety. Phase III clinical trials involve a much larger number of patients (and are typically conducted by several institutions) to provide more extensive (i.e., statistically significant) information on efficacy, safety, and dose administration. To obtain approval to market a new radiopharmaceutical, a "New Drug Application" (NDA) must be submitted to and approved by the FDA. Approval of a new radiopharmaceutical typically requires 5 to 10 years from laboratory work to NDA. The package insert of an approved radiopharmaceutical describes the intended purpose of the radiopharmaceutical, the suggested dose, dosimetry, adverse reactions, clinical pharmacology, and contraindications.

Any research involving human subjects conducted, supported, or otherwise regulated by a federal department or agency must be conducted in accordance with the

Federal Policy for the Protection of Human Subjects, (Federal Register, 1991); this policy is codified in the regulations of 15 federal departments and agencies. This policy requires that all research involving human subjects be reviewed and approved by an institutional review board (IRB) and that informed consent be obtained from each research subject. Most academic medical institutions have IRBs. An IRB comprises clinical, scientific, legal, and other experts and must include at least one member who is not otherwise affiliated with the institution. Informed consent must be sought in a manner that minimizes the possibility of coercion and provides the subject sufficient opportunity to decide whether or not to participate. The information presented must be in language understandable to the subject. It must include a statement that the study involves research, the purposes of the research, a description of the procedures, and identification of any procedures that are experimental; a description of any reasonably foreseeable risks or discomforts; a description of any likely benefits to the subject or to others; a disclosure of alternative treatments; and a statement that participation is voluntary, that refusal will involve no penalty or loss of benefits, and that the subject may discontinue participation at any time.

Byproduct Material, Authorized Users, Written Directives, and Medical Events

Medical use of Byproduct Material

Although the production of radiopharmaceuticals is regulated by the FDA, the medical use of radioactive material is regulated under the terms of a license issued to a specific legal entity (such as a clinic or hospital which is the *licensee*) by the U.S. Nuclear Regulatory Commission (NRC) or, a comparable state agency (i.e., an agreement state, which is discussed further in Chapter 21). The NRC's regulations apply to the use of *byproduct material*. Until recently, the regulatory definition of byproduct material included radionuclides that were the byproducts of nuclear fission or nuclear activation but excluded others such as accelerator-produced radionuclides. The current NRC's definition of byproduct material, however, has been broadened to include virtually all radioactive material used in medicine. The regulations regarding the medical use of radioactive material are contained in Title 10, Part 35, of the *Code of Federal Regulations* (10 CFR 35).

Authorized User

An *authorized user* (AU), in the context of the practice of nuclear medicine, is a physician who is responsible for the medical use of radioactive material and is designated by name on a license for the medical use of radioactive material or is approved by the radiation safety committee of a medical institution whose license authorizes such actions. Such a physician may be certified by a medical specialty board, such as the American Board of Radiology, whose certification process includes all of the requirements identified in Part 35 for the medical use of unsealed sources of radioactive materials for diagnosis and therapy. Alternatively a physician can apply to the NRC or comparable state agency for AU status by providing documentation of the specific education, training and experience requirements contained in 10 CFR 35.

Written Directive

The NRC requires that, before the administration of a dosage of I-131 sodium iodide greater than 1.11 MBq (30 μCi) or any therapeutic dosage of unsealed byproduct material, a *written directive* must be signed and dated by an authorized user. The written directive must contain the patient or human research subject's name and must describe the radioactive drug, the activity, and (for radionuclides other than I-131) the route of administration. In addition, the NRC requires the implementation of written procedures to provide, for each administration requiring a written directive, high confidence that the patient or human research subject's identity is verified before the administration and that each administration is performed in accordance with the written directive.

Medical Events

The NRC defines certain errors in the administration of radiopharmaceuticals as *medical events*, and requires specific actions to be taken within specified time periods following the recognition of the error. The initial report to the NRC, (or, in an agreement state, the comparable state agency) must be made by telephone no later than the next calendar day after the discovery of the event and must be followed by a written report within 15 days. This report must include specific information such as a description of the incident, the cause of the medical event, the effect (if any) on the individual or individuals involved, and proposed corrective actions. The referring physician must be notified of the medical event, and the patient must also be notified, unless the referring physician states that he or she will inform the patient or that, based on medical judgment, notification of the patient would be harmful. Additional details regarding these reporting requirements can be found in 10 CFR 35.

The NRC defines a medical event as:

A. The administration of NRC-licensed radioactive materials that results in one of the following conditions (1, 2 or 3 below) unless its occurrence was as the direct result of patient intervention (e.g., an I-131 therapy patient takes only one-half of the prescribed treatment and then refuses to take the balance of the prescribed dosage):

1. A dose that differs from the prescribed dose or dose that would have resulted from the prescribed *dosage* (i.e., administered activity) by more than 0.05 Sv (5 rem) effective dose equivalent, 0.5 Sv (50 rem) to an organ or tissue, or 0.5 Sv (50 rem) shallow dose equivalent to the skin; and one of the following conditions (i or ii) has also occurred.
   (i) The total dose delivered differs from the prescribed dose by 20% or more;
   (ii) The total dosage delivered differs from the prescribed dosage by 20% or more or falls outside the prescribed dosage range. Falling outside the prescribed dosage range means the administration of activity that is greater or less than a predetermined range of activity for a given procedure that has been established by the licensee.

2. A dose that exceeds 0.05 Sv (5 rem) effective dose equivalent, 0.5 Sv (50 rem) to an organ or tissue, or 0.5 Sv (50 rem) shallow dose equivalent to the skin from any of the following
   (i) An administration of a wrong radioactive drug containing byproduct material;
   (ii) An administration of a radioactive drug containing byproduct material through the wrong route of administration;
   (iii) An administration of a dose or dosage to the wrong individual or human research subject.

3. A dose to the skin or an organ or tissue other than the treatment site that exceeds by 0.5 Sv (50 rem) and 50% or more of the dose expected from the administration defined in the written directive.

B. Any event resulting from intervention of a patient or human research subject in which the administration of byproduct material or radiation from byproduct material results or will result in unintended permanent functional damage to an organ or a physiological system, as determined by a physician.

This definition of a medical event was summarized from NRC regulations. It applies only to the use of unsealed byproduct material and omits the definition of a medical event involving the use of sealed sources of byproduct material to treat patients (e.g., conventional brachytherapy treatment of prostate cancer with I-125 seeds by radiation oncologists). The complete regulations regarding written directives, authorized users and medical events can be found in 10 CFR 35. State regulatory requirements should be consulted, because they may differ from federal regulations.

SUGGESTED READING

Dillehay G, Ellerbroek Balon H, et al. Practice guideline for the performance of therapy with unsealed radiopharmaceutical sources. *Int J Radiat Oncol Biol Phys* 2006;64(5,1):1299–1307.

Hung JC, Ponto JA, Hammes RJ. Radiopharmaceutical-related pitfalls and artifacts. *Semin Nucl Med* 1996;26:208–255.

Macey DJ, Williams LE, Breitz HB, et al. *AAPM report no.71, A primer for radioimmunotherapy and radionuclide therapy.* Madison, WI: Medical Physics Publishing; 2001.

Medley CM, Vivian GC. Radionuclide developments. *Br J Radiol* 1997;70:133–144.

Ponto JA. The AAPM/RSNA physics tutorial for residents: radiopharmaceuticals. *Radiographics* 1998;18:1395–1404.

Rhodes BA, Hladik WB, Norenberg JP. Clinical radiopharmacy: principles and practices. *Semin Nud Med* 1996;26:77–84.

Saha GB. *Fundamentals of nuclear pharmacy.* 5th ed. New York, NY: Springer-Verlag, 2004.

Sampson CB, ed. *Textbook of radiopharmacy: theory and practice.* 2nd ed. New York, NY: Gordon and Breach Publishers, 1995.

Loevinger R, Budinger T, Watson E. MIRD primer for absorbed dose calculations. New York, NY: Society of Nuclear Medicine, 1991.

Stabin M. Nuclear medicine dosimetry. *Phys Med Biol* 2006:51.

Toohey RE, Stabin MG, Watson EE. The AAPM/RSNA physics tutorial for residents. Internal radiation dosimetry: principles and applications. *Radiographics* 2000;20:533–546.

Zanzonico PB. Internal radionuclide radiation dosimetry: a review of basic concepts and recent developments. *J Nuclear Med* 2000;41:297–308.

SELECTED REFERENCES

Bolch WE, Eckerman KF, Sgouros G, Thomas SR. MIRD Pamphlet No. 21: A Generalized Schema for Radiopharmaceutical Dosimetry—Standardization of nomenclature. *J Nucl Med* 2009;50: 477–484.

Cristy M, Eckerman K. Specific absorbed fractions of energy at various ages from internal photons sources. ORNL/TM-8381 V1-V7. Oak Ridge, TN: Oak Ridge National Laboratory, 1987.

Federal Register 1991: Federal Register. *Federal Policy for the Protection of Human Subjects.* June 18, 1991: 28003–28032.

ICRP 1987: Publication 53: Biokinetics and Dosimetry: General Considerations. *Ann ICRP* 1987; 18(1–4).

ICRP 1998: ICRP Publication 80: Radiation Dose to Patients from Radiopharmaceuticals: Addendum 2 to ICRP Publication 53. *Ann ICRP* 1998;28(3).

ICRP 2008: ICRP Publication 106: Radiation Dose to Patients from Radiopharmaceuticals A Third Addendum to ICRP Publication 53 ICRP. *Ann ICRP.* 2008 38(1–2).

Robbins RJ. *Chromatography of Technetium-99m Radiopharmaceuticals – A Practical Guide.* Society of Nuclear Medicine, Reston, VA, 1985.

Stabin M, Watson E, Cristy M, Ryman J, Eckerman K, Davis J, Marshall D, Gehlen K. mathematical models and specific absorbed fractions of photon energy in the nonpregnant adult female and at the end of each trimester of pregnancy. *ORNL Report ORNL/TM* 1995;12907.

Stabin MG. MIRDOSE: personal computer software for internal dose assessment in nuclear medicine. *J Nucl Med* 1996;37(3):538–546.

Stabin MG. Uncertainties in internal dose calculations for radiopharmaceuticals. *J Nucl Med* 2008;49: 853–860.

Stabin MG, Siegel JA. Physical models and dose factors for use in internal dose assessment. *Health Physics* 2003;85(3):294–310.

Stabin MG, Sparks RB, Crowe E. OLINDA/EXM: the second-generation personal computer software for internal dose assessment in nuclear medicine. *J Nucl Med* 2005;46.

Yalow, RS, Berson, SA. Immunoassay of endogenous plasma insulin in main. *J clin invest* 1960;39: 1157–1175.

CHAPTER 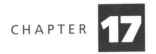 **17**

Radiation Detection and Measurement

The detection and measurement of ionizing radiation are the basis for the majority of diagnostic imaging. In this chapter, the basic concepts of radiation detection and measurement are introduced, followed by a discussion of the characteristics of specific types of detectors. The electronic systems used for pulse height spectroscopy and the use of sodium iodide (NaI) scintillators to perform gamma-ray spectroscopy are described, followed by a discussion of detector applications. The use of radiation detectors in imaging devices is covered in other chapters.

All detectors of ionizing radiation require the interaction of the radiation with matter. Ionizing radiation deposits energy in matter by ionization and excitation. *Ionization* is the removal of electrons from atoms or molecules. (An atom or molecule stripped of an electron has a net positive charge and is called a *cation*. In many gases, the free electrons become attached to uncharged atoms or molecules, forming negatively charged *anions*. An ion pair consists of a cation and its associated free electron or anion.) *Excitation* is the elevation of electrons to excited states in atoms, molecules, or a crystal. Excitation and ionization may produce chemical changes or the emission of visible light or ultraviolet (UV) radiation. Most energy deposited by ionizing radiation is ultimately converted into thermal energy.

The amount of energy deposited in matter by a single interaction is very small. For example, a 140-keV gamma ray deposits 2.24×10^{-14} Joules if completely absorbed. To raise the temperature of 1 g of water by 1°C (i.e., 1 calorie) would require the complete absorption of 187 trillion (187×10^{12}) of these photons. For this reason, most radiation detectors provide signal amplification. In detectors that produce an electrical signal, the amplification is electronic. In photographic film, the amplification is achieved chemically.

17.1 Types of Detectors and Basic Principles

Radiation detectors may be classified by their detection method. A *gas-filled detector* consists of a volume of gas between two electrodes. Ions produced in the gas by the radiation are collected by the electrodes, resulting in an electrical signal.

The interaction of ionizing radiation with certain materials produces ultraviolet radiation and/or visible light. These materials are called *scintillators*. They are commonly attached to or incorporated in devices that convert the UV radiation and light into an electrical signal. For other applications, photographic film is used to record the light emitted by the scintillators. Many years ago, in physics research and medical fluoroscopy, the light from scintillators was viewed directly with dark-adapted eyes.

Semiconductor detectors are especially pure crystals of silicon, germanium, or other semiconductor materials to which trace amounts of impurity atoms have been added so that they act as diodes. A diode is an electronic device with two terminals that permits a large electrical current to flow when a voltage is applied in one direction,

633

but very little current when the voltage is applied in the opposite direction. When used to detect radiation, a voltage is applied in the direction in which little current flows. When an interaction occurs in the crystal, electrons are raised to an excited state, allowing a momentary pulse of electrical current to flow through the device.

Detectors may also be classified by the type of information produced. Detectors, such as Geiger-Mueller (GM) detectors, that indicate the number of interactions occurring in the detector are called *counters*. Detectors that yield information about the energy distribution of the incident radiation, such as NaI scintillation detectors, are called *spectrometers*. Detectors that indicate the net amount of energy deposited in the detector by multiple interactions are called *dosimeters*.

Pulse and Current Modes of Operation

Many radiation detectors produce an electrical signal after each interaction of a particle or photon. The signal generated by the detector passes through a series of electronic circuits, each of which performs a function such as signal amplification, signal processing, or data storage. A detector and its associated electronic circuitry form a *detection system*. There are two fundamental ways that the circuitry may process the signal—pulse mode and current mode. In *pulse mode*, the signal from each interaction is processed individually. In *current mode*, the electrical signals from individual interactions are averaged together, forming a net current signal.

There are advantages and disadvantages to each method of handling the signal. GM detectors are operated in pulse mode, whereas most ionization chambers, including ion chamber survey meters and the dose calibrators used in nuclear medicine, are operated in current mode. Scintillation detectors are operated in pulse mode in nuclear medicine applications, but in current mode in direct digital radiography, fluoroscopy, and x-ray computed tomography (CT).

In this chapter, the term *interaction* typically refers to the interaction of a single photon or charged particle, such as the interaction of a gamma ray by the photoelectric effect or Compton scattering. The term *event* may refer to a single interaction, or it may refer to something more complex, such as two nearly simultaneous interactions in a detector. In instruments which process the signals from individual interactions or events in pulse mode, an interaction or event that is registered is referred to as a *count*.

Effect of Interaction Rate on Detectors Operated in Pulse Mode

The main problem with using a radiation detector or detection system in pulse mode is that two interactions must be separated by a finite amount of time if they are to produce distinct signals. This interval is called the *dead time* of the system. If a second interaction occurs during this time interval, its signal will be lost; furthermore, if it is close enough in time to the first interaction, it may even distort the signal from the first interaction. The fraction of counts lost from dead-time effects is smallest at low interaction rates and increases with increasing interaction rate.

The dead time of a detection system is largely determined by the component in the series with the longest dead time. For example, the detector usually has the longest dead time in GM counter systems, whereas in multichannel analyzer (MCA) systems (see later discussion), the analog-to-digital converter (ADC) generally has the longest dead time.

The dead times of different types of systems vary widely. GM counters have dead times ranging from tens to hundreds of microseconds, whereas most other systems have dead times of less than a few microseconds. It is important to know the count-rate behavior of a detection system; if a detection system is operated at too high an interaction rate, an artificially low count rate will be obtained.

There are two mathematical models describing the behavior of detector systems operated in pulse mode—paralyzable and nonparalyzable. Although these models

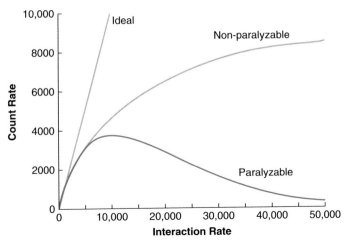

■ **FIGURE 17-1** Effect of interaction rate on measured count rate of paralyzable and nonparalyzable detectors. The "ideal" line represents the response of a hypothetical detector that does not suffer from dead-time count losses (i.e., the count rate is equal to the interaction rate). Note that the y-axis scale is expanded with respect to that of the x-axis; the "ideal" line would be at a 45-degree angle if the scales were equal.

are simplifications of the behavior of real detection systems, real systems may behave like one or the other model. In a *paralyzable* system, an interaction that occurs during the dead time after a previous interaction extends the dead time; in a *nonparalyzable* system, it does not. Figure 17-1 shows the count rates of paralyzable and nonparalyzable detector systems as a function of the rate of interactions in the detector. At very high interaction rates, a paralyzable system will be unable to detect any interactions after the first, because subsequent interactions will extend the dead time, causing the system to indicate a count rate of zero!

Current Mode Operation

When a detector is operated in current mode, all information regarding individual interactions is lost. For example, neither the interaction rate nor the energies deposited by individual interactions can be determined. However, if the amount of electrical charge collected from each interaction is proportional to the energy deposited by that interaction, then the net electrical current is proportional to the dose rate in the detector material. Detectors subject to very high interaction rates are often operated in current mode to avoid dead-time information losses. Image-intensifier tubes and flat panel image receptors in fluoroscopy, detectors in x-ray CT machines, direct digital radiographic image receptors, ion chambers used in phototimed radiography, and most nuclear medicine dose calibrators are operated in current mode.

Spectroscopy

The term *spectroscopy*, literally the viewing of a spectrum, is commonly used to refer to measurements of the energy distributions of radiation fields, and a *spectrometer* is a detection system that yields information about the energy distribution of the incident radiation. Most spectrometers are operated in pulse mode, and the amplitude of each pulse is proportional to the energy deposited in the detector by the interaction causing that pulse. *The energy deposited by an interaction, however, is not always the total energy of the incident particle or photon.* For example, a gamma ray may interact with the detector by Compton scattering, with the scattered photon escaping the detector. In this case, the deposited energy is the difference between the energies of the incident and scattered photons. A *pulse height spectrum* is usually depicted as a

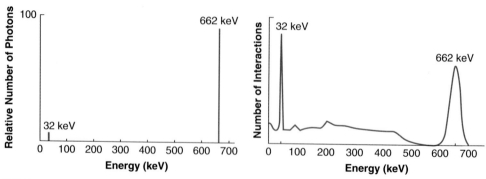

■ **FIGURE 17-2** Energy spectrum of cesium-137 (**left**) and resultant pulse height spectrum from a detector (**right**).

graph of the number of interactions depositing a particular amount of energy in the spectrometer as a function of energy (Fig. 17-2). Because the energy deposited by an interaction may be less than the total energy of the incident particle or photon and also because of random variations in the detection process, *the pulse height spectrum produced by a spectrometer is not identical to the actual energy spectrum of the incident radiation.* The energy resolution of a spectrometer is a measure of its ability to differentiate between particles or photons of different energies. Pulse height spectroscopy is discussed later in this chapter.

Detection Efficiency

The *efficiency (sensitivity)* of a detector is a measure of its ability to detect radiation. The efficiency of a detection system operated in pulse mode is defined as the probability that a particle or photon emitted by a source will be detected. It is measured by placing a source of radiation in the vicinity of the detector and dividing the number of particles or photons detected by the number emitted:

$$\text{Efficiency} = \frac{\text{Number detected}}{\text{Number emitted}} \qquad [17\text{-}1]$$

This equation can be written as follows:

$$\text{Efficiency} = \frac{\text{Number reaching detector}}{\text{Number emitted}} \times \frac{\text{Number detected}}{\text{Number reaching detector}}$$

Therefore, the detection efficiency is the product of two terms, the geometric efficiency and the intrinsic efficiency:

$$\text{Efficiency} = \text{Geometric efficiency} \times \text{Intrinsic efficiency} \qquad [17\text{-}2]$$

where the *geometric efficiency* of a detector is the fraction of emitted particles or photons that reach the detector and the *intrinsic efficiency* is the fraction of those particles or photons reaching the detector that are detected. Because the total, geometric, and intrinsic efficiencies are all probabilities, each ranges from 0 to 1.

The geometric efficiency is determined by the geometric relationship between the source and the detector (Fig. 17-3). It increases as the source is moved toward the detector and approaches 0.5 when a point source is placed against a flat surface of the detector, because in that position one half of the photons or particles are emitted into the detector. For a source inside a well-type detector, the geometric efficiency approaches 1, because most of the particles or photons are intercepted by the detector. (A well-type detector is a detector containing a cavity for the insertion of samples.)

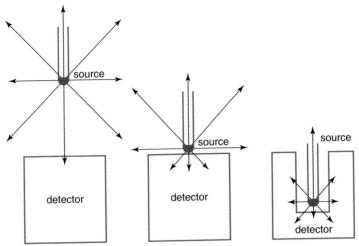

■ **FIGURE 17-3** Geometric efficiency. With a source far from the detector (**left**), the geometric efficiency is less than 50%. With a source against the detector (**center**), the geometric efficiency is approximately 50%. With a source in a well detector (**right**), the geometric efficiency is greater than 50%.

The intrinsic efficiency of a detector in detecting photons, also called the *quantum detection efficiency* (QDE), is determined by the energy of the photons and the atomic number, density, and thickness of the detector. If a parallel beam of monoenergetic photons is incident upon a detector of uniform thickness, the intrinsic efficiency of the detector is given by the following equation:

$$\text{Intrinsic efficiency} = 1 - e^{-\mu x} = 1 - e^{-(\mu/\rho)\rho x} \qquad [17\text{-}3]$$

where μ is the linear attenuation coefficient of the detector material, ρ is the density of the material, μ/ρ is the mass attenuation coefficient of the material, and x is the thickness of the detector. This equation shows that the intrinsic efficiency for detecting x-rays and gamma rays increases with the thickness of the detector and the density and the mass attenuation coefficient of the detector material. The mass attenuation coefficient increases with the atomic number of the material and, within the range of photon energies used in diagnostic imaging, decreases with increasing photon energy, with the exception of absorption edges (Chapter 3).

17.2 Gas-Filled Detectors

Basic Principles

A gas-filled detector (Fig. 17-4) consists of a volume of gas between two electrodes, with an electric potential difference (voltage) applied between the electrodes. Ionizing radiation forms ion pairs in the gas. The positive ions (cations) are attracted to the negative electrode (cathode), and the electrons or anions are attracted to the positive electrode (anode). In most detectors, the cathode is the wall of the container that holds the gas or a conductive coating on the inside of the wall, and the anode is a wire inside the container. After reaching the anode, the electrons travel through the circuit to the cathode, where they recombine with the cations. This electrical current can be measured with a sensitive ammeter or other electrical circuitry.

There are three types of gas-filled detectors in common use—ionization chambers, proportional counters, and GM counters. The type of detector is determined

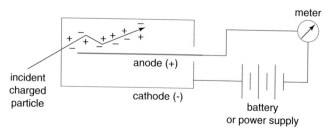

■ **FIGURE 17-4** Gas-filled detector. A charged particle, such as a beta particle, is shown entering the detector from outside and creating ion pairs in the gas inside the detector. This can occur only if the detector has a sufficiently thin wall. When a thick-wall gas-filled detector is used to detect x-rays and gamma rays, the charged particles causing the ionization are mostly electrons generated by Compton and photoelectric interactions of the incident x-rays or gamma rays in the detector wall or in the gas in the detector.

primarily by the voltage applied between the two electrodes. In an ionization chamber, the two electrodes can have almost any configuration: they may be two parallel plates, two concentric cylinders, or a wire within a cylinder. In proportional counters and GM counters, the anode must be a thin wire. Figure 17-5 shows the amount of electrical charge collected after a single interaction as a function of the electrical potential difference (voltage) applied between the two electrodes.

Ionizing radiation produces ion pairs in the gas of the detector. If no voltage is applied between the electrodes, no current flows through the circuit because there is no electric field to attract the charged particles to the electrodes; the ion pairs merely recombine in the gas. When a small voltage is applied, some of the cations

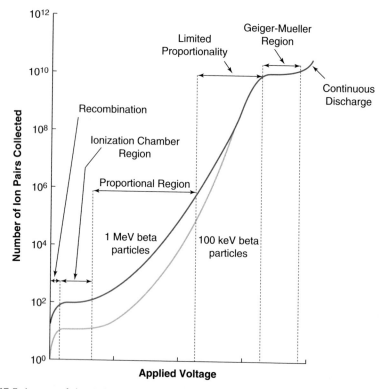

■ **FIGURE 17-5** Amount of electrical charge collected after a single interaction as a function of the electrical potential difference (voltage) applied between the two electrodes of a gas-filled detector. The lower curve shows the charge collected when a 100-keV electron interacts, and the upper curve shows the result from a 1-MeV electron.

are attracted to the cathode and some of the electrons or anions are attracted to the anode before they can recombine. As the voltage is increased, more ions are collected and fewer recombine. This region, in which the current increases as the voltage is raised, is called the *recombination region* of the curve.

As the voltage is increased further, a plateau is reached in the curve. In this region, called the *ionization chamber region*, the applied electric field is sufficiently strong to collect almost all ion pairs; additional increases in the applied voltage do not significantly increase the current. Ionization chambers are operated in this region.

Beyond the ionization region, the collected current again increases as the applied voltage is raised. In this region, called the *proportional region*, electrons approaching the anode are accelerated to such high kinetic energies that they cause additional ionization. This phenomenon, called *gas multiplication*, amplifies the collected current; the amount of amplification increases as the applied voltage is raised.

At any voltage through the ionization chamber region and the proportional region, the amount of electrical charge collected from each interaction is *proportional* to the amount of energy deposited in the gas of the detector by the interaction. For example, the amount of charge collected after an interaction depositing 100 keV is one tenth of that collected from an interaction depositing 1 MeV.

Beyond the proportional region is a region in which the amount of charge collected from each event is the same, regardless of the amount of energy deposited by the interaction. In this region, called the *Geiger-Mueller region* (GM region), the gas multiplication spreads the entire length of the anode. The size of a pulse in the GM region tells us nothing about the energy deposited in the detector by the interaction causing the pulse. Gas-filled detectors cannot be operated at voltages beyond the GM region because they continuously discharge.

Ionization Chambers (Ion Chambers)

Because gas multiplication does not occur at the relatively low voltages applied to ionization chambers, the amount of electrical charge collected from a single interaction is very small and would require huge amplification to be detected. For this reason, ionization chambers are seldom used in pulse mode. The advantage to operating them in current mode is the almost complete freedom from dead-time effects, even in very intense radiation fields. In addition, as shown in Figure 17-5, the voltage applied to an ion chamber can vary significantly without appreciably changing the amount of charge collected.

Almost any gas can be used to fill the chamber. If the gas is air and the walls of the chamber are of a material whose effective atomic number is similar to air, the amount of current produced is proportional to the *exposure rate* (exposure is the amount of electrical charge produced per mass of air). Air-filled ion chambers are used in portable survey meters and can accurately indicate exposure rates from less than 1 mR/h to tens or hundreds of roentgens per hour (Fig. 17-6). Air-filled ion chambers are also used for performing quality-assurance testing of diagnostic and therapeutic x-ray machines, and they are the detectors in most x-ray machine phototimers. Measurements using an air-filled ion chamber that is open to the atmosphere are affected by the density of the air in the chamber, which is determined by ambient air pressure and temperature. Measurements using such chambers that require great accuracy must be corrected for these factors.

In very intense radiation fields, there can be signal loss due to recombination of ions before they are collected at the electrodes, causing the current from an ion chamber to deviate from proportionality to the intensity of the radiation. An ion chamber intended for use in such fields may have a small gas volume, a low gas density, and/or a high applied voltage to reduce this effect.

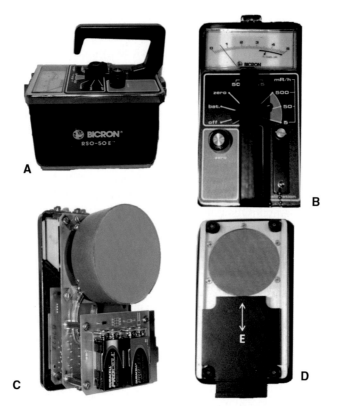

■ FIGURE 17-6 Portable air-filled ionization chamber survey meter (**A**). This particular instrument measures exposure rates ranging from about 0.1 mR/h to 50 R/h. The exposure rate is indicated by the position of the red needle on the scale. The scale is selected using the range knob located below the scale (**B**). In this case, the needle is pointing to a value of 0.6 on the scale, and the range selector is set at 50 mR/h. Thus, the exposure rate being shown is 6 mR/h. The interior of the instrument is shown (**C**) and the ion chamber, covered with a thin Mylar membrane, is easily seen. On the bottom of the meter case (**D**) is a slide (**E**) that can cover or expose the thin Mylar window of the ion chamber. This slide should be opened when measuring low-energy x-ray and gamma-ray radiation. The slide can also be used to determine if there is a significant beta radiation component in the radiation being measured. If there is no substantial change in the measured exposure rate with the slide open (where beta radiation can penetrate the thin membrane and enter the ion chamber) or closed (where the ion chamber is shielded from beta radiation), the radiation can be considered to be comprised primarily of x-rays or gamma rays.

Gas-filled detectors tend to have low intrinsic efficiencies for detecting x-rays and gamma rays because of the low densities of gases and the low atomic numbers of most common gases. The sensitivity of ion chambers to x-rays and gamma rays can be enhanced by filling them with a gas that has a high atomic number, such as argon ($Z = 18$) or xenon ($Z = 54$), and pressurizing the gas to increase its density. Well-type ion chambers called dose calibrators are used in nuclear medicine to assay the activities of dosages of radiopharmaceuticals to be administered to patients; many are filled with pressurized argon. Xenon-filled pressurized ion chambers were formerly used as detectors in some CT machines.

Air filled ion chambers are commonly used to measure the related quantities air kerma and exposure rate. These quantities were defined in Chapter 3. Air kerma is the initial kinetic energy transferred to charged particles, in this case electrons liberated in air by the radiation, per mass air and exposure is the amount of electrical charge created in air by ionization caused by these electrons, per mass air. There is a problem measuring the ionization in the small volume of air in an ionization chamber of reasonable size. The energetic electrons released by interactions in the air have long ranges in air and many of them would escape the air in the chamber and cause much of their ionization elsewhere. This problem can be partially solved by building the ion chamber with thick walls of a material whose effective atomic number is similar to that of air. In this case, the number of electrons escaping the volume of air is approximately matched by a similar number of electrons released in the chamber wall entering the air in the ion chamber. This situation, if achieved, is called *electronic equilibrium*. For this reason, most ion chambers for measuring exposure or air kerma have thick air-equivalent walls, or are equipped with removable air-equivalent buildup caps to establish electronic equilibrium. The thickness of material needed to establish electronic equilibrium increases with the energy of the x- or gamma rays. However, thick walls or buildup caps may significantly attenuate low energy x- and gamma rays. Many ion chamber survey meters have windows that may be opened in the thick material around the ion chamber to permit more accurate measurement of low energy x- and gamma rays.Electronic equilibrium, also called charged particle equilibrium, is discussed in detail in more advanced texts (Attix, 1986; Knoll, 2010).

Proportional Counters

Unlike ion chambers, which can function with almost any gas, including air, a proportional counter must contain a gas with low electron affinity, so that few free electrons become attached to gas molecules. Because gas multiplication can produce a charge-per-interaction that is hundreds or thousands of times larger than that produced by an ion chamber, proportional counters can be operated in pulse mode as counters or spectrometers. They are commonly used in standards laboratories, in health physics laboratories, and for physics research. They are seldom used in medical centers.

Multiwire proportional counters, which indicate the position of an interaction in the detector, have been studied for use in nuclear medicine imaging devices. They have not achieved acceptance because of their low efficiencies for detecting x-rays and gamma rays from the radionuclides commonly used in nuclear medicine.

Geiger-Mueller Counters

GM counters must also contain gases with specific properties, discussed in more advanced texts. Because gas multiplication produces billions of ion pairs after an interaction, the signal from a GM detector requires little additional amplification. For this reason, GM detectors are often used for inexpensive survey meters.

GM detectors have high efficiencies for detecting charged particles that penetrate the walls of the detectors; almost every such particle reaching the interior of a detector is counted. Many GM detectors are equipped with thin windows to allow beta particles and conversion electrons to reach the gas and be detected. Very weak charged particles, such as the beta particles emitted by tritium (^{3}H, E_{max} = 18 keV), which is extensively used in biomedical research, cannot penetrate the windows; therefore, contamination by ^{3}H cannot be detected with a GM survey meter. Flat, thin-window GM detectors, called "pancake"-type detectors, are very useful for finding radioactive contamination (Fig. 17-7).

In general, GM survey meters are very inefficient detectors of x-rays and gamma rays, which tend to pass through the gas without interaction. Most of those that are detected have interacted with the walls of the detectors, with the resultant electrons scattered into the gas inside the detectors.

The size of the voltage pulse from a GM tube is independent of the energy deposited in the detector by the interaction causing the pulse: an interaction that deposits 1 keV causes a voltage pulse of the same size as one caused by an interaction that deposits 1 MeV. Therefore, GM detectors cannot be used as spectrometers or precise dose-rate meters. Many portable GM survey meters display measurements in units

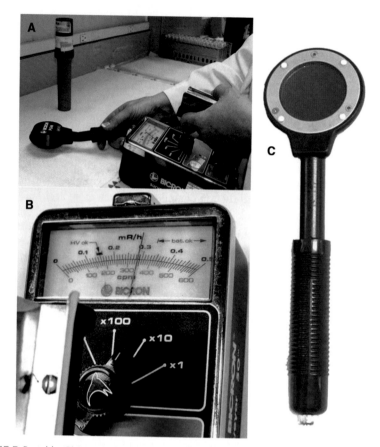

■ **FIGURE 17-7** Portable GM survey meter with a thin-window "pancake" probe. In the upper left (**A**), a survey for radioactive contamination is being performed. In the lower left (**B**), the range knob below the display is set to X10 and so the red needle on the meter indicates a count rate of about 3,500 counts per minute (cpm). The thin window of the GM probe (**C**) is designed to permit beta particles and conversion electrons whose energies exceed about 45 keV to reach the sensitive volume inside the tube, and the large surface area of the detector reduces the time needed to survey a surface.

of milliroentgens per hour. However, the GM counter cannot truly measure exposure rates, and so its reading must be considered only an approximation. If a GM survey meter is calibrated to indicate exposure rate for 662-keV gamma rays from ^{137}Cs (commonly used for calibrations), it may overrespond by as much as a factor of 5 for photons of lower energies, such as 80 keV. If an accurate measurement of exposure rate is required, an air-filled ionization chamber survey meter should be used.

This overresponse of a GM tube to low-energy x-rays and gamma rays can be partially corrected by placing a thin layer of a material with a moderately high atomic number (e.g., tin) around the detector. The increasing attenuation coefficient of the material (due to the photoelectric effect) with decreasing photon energy significantly flattens the energy response of the detector. Such GM tubes are called *energy-compensated detectors*. The disadvantage of an energy-compensated detector is that its sensitivity to lower energy photons is substantially reduced and its energy threshold, below which photons cannot be detected at all, is increased. Energy-compensated GM detectors commonly have windows that can be opened to expose the thin tube walls so that high-energy beta particles and low-energy photons can be detected.

GM detectors suffer from extremely long dead times, ranging from tens to hundreds of microseconds. For this reason, GM counters are seldom used when accurate measurements are required of count rates greater than a few hundred counts per second. A portable GM survey meter may become paralyzed in a very high radiation field and yield a reading of zero. Ionization chamber instruments should always be used to measure high intensity x-ray and gamma ray fields.

17.3 Scintillation Detectors

Basic Principles

Scintillators are materials that emit visible light or ultraviolet radiation after the interaction of ionizing radiation with the material. Scintillators are the oldest type of radiation detectors; Roentgen discovered x-radiation and the fact that x-rays induce scintillation in barium platinocyanide in the same fortuitous experiment. Scintillators are used in conventional film-screen radiography, many direct digital radiographic image receptors, fluoroscopy, scintillation cameras, CT scanners, and positron emission tomography (PET) scanners.

Although the light emitted from a single interaction can be seen if the viewer's eyes are dark adapted, most scintillation detectors incorporate a means of signal amplification. In conventional film-screen radiography, photographic film is used to amplify and record the signal. In other applications, electronic devices such as photomultiplier tubes (PMTs), photodiodes, or image-intensifier tubes convert the light into electrical signals. PMTs and image-intensifier tubes amplify the signal as well. However, most photodiodes do not provide amplification; if amplification of the signal is required, it must be provided by an electronic amplifier. A *scintillation detector* consists of a scintillator and a device, such as a PMT, that converts the light into an electrical signal.

When ionizing radiation interacts with a scintillator, electrons are raised to an excited energy level. Ultimately, these electrons fall back to a lower energy state, with the emission of visible light or ultraviolet radiation. Most scintillators have more than one mode for the emission of visible light or ultraviolet radiation, and each mode has its characteristic decay constant. *Luminescence* is the emission of light after excitation. *Fluorescence* is the prompt emission of light, whereas *phosphorescence* (also called *afterglow*) is the delayed emission of light. When scintillation detectors are operated in current mode, the prompt signal from an interaction cannot be separated from the phosphorescence caused by previous interactions. When a scintillation detector is operated in pulse mode, afterglow is less important because electronic circuits can separate the rapidly rising and falling components of the prompt signal from the slowly decaying delayed signal resulting from previous interactions.

It is useful, before discussing actual scintillation materials, to consider properties that are desirable in a scintillator.

1. The *conversion efficiency*, the fraction of deposited energy that is converted into light or ultraviolet (UV) radiation, should be high. (Conversion efficiency should not be confused with detection efficiency.)
2. For many applications, the decay times of excited states should be short. (Light or UV radiation is emitted promptly after an interaction.)
3. The material should be transparent to its own emissions. (Most emitted light or UV radiation escapes reabsorption.)
4. The frequency spectrum (color) of emitted light or UV radiation should match the spectral sensitivity of the light receptor (PMT, photodiode, or film).
5. If used for x-ray and gamma-ray detection, the attenuation coefficient (μ) should be large, so that detectors made of the scintillator have high detection efficiencies.

Materials with large atomic numbers and high densities have large attenuation coefficients.

6. The material should be rugged, unaffected by moisture, and inexpensive to manufacture.

In all scintillators, the amount of light emitted after an interaction increases with the energy deposited by the interaction. Therefore, scintillators may be operated in pulse mode as spectrometers. When a scintillator is used for spectroscopy, its energy resolution (ability to distinguish between interactions depositing different energies) is primarily determined by its conversion efficiency. A high conversion efficiency is required for superior energy resolution.

There are several categories of materials that scintillate. Many organic compounds exhibit scintillation. In these materials, the scintillation is a property of the molecular structure. Solid organic scintillators are used for timing experiments in particle physics because of their extremely prompt light emission. Organic scintillators include the liquid scintillation fluids that are used extensively in biomedical research. Samples containing radioactive tracers such as ^{3}H, ^{14}C, and ^{32}P are mixed in vials with liquid scintillators, and the light flashes are detected and counted by PMTs and associated electronic circuits. Organic scintillators are not used for medical imaging because the low atomic numbers of their constituent elements and their low densities make them poor x-ray and gamma-ray detectors. When photons in the diagnostic energy range do interact with organic scintillators, it is primarily by Compton scattering.

There are also many inorganic crystalline materials that exhibit scintillation. In these materials, the scintillation is a property of the crystalline structure: if the crystal is dissolved, the scintillation ceases. Many of these materials have much larger average atomic numbers and higher densities than organic scintillators and therefore are excellent photon detectors. They are widely used for radiation measurements and imaging in radiology.

Most inorganic scintillation crystals are deliberately grown with trace amounts of impurity elements called *activators*. The atoms of these activators form preferred sites in the crystals for the excited electrons to return to the ground state. The activators modify the frequency (color) of the emitted light, the promptness of the light emission, and the proportion of the emitted light that escapes reabsorption in the crystal.

Inorganic Crystalline Scintillators in Radiology

No one scintillation material is best for all applications in radiology. Sodium iodide activated with thallium [NaI(Tl)] is used for most nuclear medicine applications. It is coupled to PMTs and operated in pulse mode in scintillation cameras, thyroid probes, and gamma well counters. Its high content of iodine (Z = 53) and high density provide a high photoelectric absorption probability for x-rays and gamma rays emitted by common nuclear medicine radiopharmaceuticals (70 to 365 keV). It has a very high conversion efficiency; approximately 13% of deposited energy is converted into light. Because a light photon has an energy of about 3 eV, approximately one light photon is emitted for every 23 eV absorbed by the crystal. This high conversion efficiency gives it a very good energy resolution. It emits light very promptly (decay constant, 250 ns), permitting it to be used in pulse mode at interaction rates greater than 100,000/s. Very large crystals can be manufactured; for example, the rectangular crystals of one modern scintillation camera are 59 cm (23 inches) long, 44.5 cm (17.5 inches) wide, and 0.95 cm thick. Unfortunately, NaI(Tl) crystals are fragile; they crack easily if struck or subjected to rapid temperature change. Also, they are hygroscopic (i.e., they absorb water from the atmosphere) and therefore must be hermetically sealed.

Positron emission tomography (PET), discussed in Chapter 19, requires high detection efficiency for 511-keV annihilation photons and a prompt signal from each interaction because the signals must be processed in pulse mode at high interaction rates. PET detectors are thick crystals of high-density, high atomic number scintillators optically coupled to PMTs. For many years, bismuth germanate ($Bi_4Ge_3O_{12}$, often abbreviated as "BGO") was the preferred scintillator. The high atomic number of bismuth ($Z = 83$) and the high density of the crystal yield a high intrinsic efficiency for the 511-keV positron annihilation photons. The primary component of the light emission is sufficiently prompt (decay constant, 300 ns) for PET. NaI(Tl) was used in early and some less-expensive PET scanners. Today, lutetium oxyorthosilicate (Lu_2SiO_4O, abbreviated LSO), lutetium yttrium oxyorthosilicate ($Lu_xY_{2-x}SiO_4O$, abbreviated LYSO), and gadolinium oxyorthosilicate (Gd_2SiO_4O, abbreviated GSO), all activated with cerium, are used in newer PET scanners. Their densities and effective atomic numbers are similar to those of BGO, but their conversion efficiencies are much larger and they emit light much more promptly.

Calcium tungstate ($CaWO_4$) was used for many years in intensifying screens in film-screen radiography. It was largely replaced by rare-earth phosphors, such as gadolinium oxysulfide activated with terbium. The intensifying screen is an application of scintillators that does not require very prompt light emission, because the film usually remains in contact with the screen for at least several seconds after exposure. Cesium iodide activated with thallium is used as the phosphor layer of many indirect-detection thin-film transistor radiographic and fluoroscopic image receptors, described in Chapters 7 and 9. Cesium iodide activated with sodium is used as the input phosphor and zinc cadmium sulfide activated with silver is used as the output phosphor of image-intensifier tubes in fluoroscopes.

Scintillators coupled to photodiodes are used as the detectors in CT scanners, as described in Chapter 10. The extremely high x-ray flux experienced by the detectors necessitates current mode operation to avoid dead-time effects. With the rotational speed of CT scanners as high as three rotations per second, the scintillators used in CT must have very little afterglow. Cadmium tungstate and gadolinium ceramics are scintillators used in CT. Table 17-1 lists the properties of several inorganic crystalline scintillators of importance in radiology and nuclear medicine.

Conversion of Light into an Electrical Signal

Photomultiplier Tubes

PMTs perform two functions—conversion of ultraviolet and visible light photons into an electrical signal and signal amplification, on the order of millions to billions. As shown in Figure 17-8, a PMT consists of an evacuated glass tube containing a *photocathode*, typically 10 to 12 electrodes called *dynodes*, and an *anode*. The photocathode is a very thin electrode, located just inside the glass entrance window of the PMT, which emits electrons when struck by visible light. Photocathodes are inefficient; approximately one electron is emitted from the photocathode for every five UV or light photons incident upon it. A high-voltage power supply provides a voltage of approximately 1,000 V, and a series of resistors divides the voltage into equal increments. The first dynode is given a voltage of about +100 V with respect to the photocathode; successive dynodes have voltages that increase by approximately 100 V per dynode. The electrons emitted by the photocathode are attracted to the first dynode and are accelerated to kinetic energies equal to the potential difference between the photocathode and the first dynode. (If the potential difference is 100 V, the kinetic energy of each electron is 100 eV.) When these electrons strike the first dynode, about five electrons are ejected from the dynode for each electron hitting it. These electrons are then attracted to the second dynode, reaching kinetic energies equal to the potential difference between the first and second dynodes, and causing

TABLE 17-1 INORGANIC SCINTILLATORS USED IN MEDICAL IMAGING

MATERIAL	ATOMIC NUMBERS	DENSITY (g/cm³)	WAVELENGTH OF MAXIMAL EMISSION (nm)	CONVERSION EFFICIENCY[a] (%)	DECAY CONSTANT (μS)	AFTERGLOW (%)	USES
NaI(Tl)	11, 53	3.67	415	100	0.25	0.3–5 @ 6 ms	Scintillation cameras
$Bi_4Ge_3O_{12}$	83, 32, 8	7.13	480	12–14	0.3	0.005 @ 3 ms	PET scanners
Lu_2SiO_4O(Ce)	71, 14, 8	7.4	420	75	40	—	PET scanners
CsI(Na)	55, 53	4.51	420	85	0.63	—	Input phosphor of image-intensifier tubes
CsI(Tl)	55, 53	4.51	550	45[b]	1.0	0.5–5 @ 6 ms	Thin-film transistor radiographic and fluoroscopic image receptors
ZnCdS(Ag)	30, 48, 16	—	—	—	—	—	Output phosphor of image-intensifier tubes
$CdWO_4$	48, 74, 8	7.90	475	40	14	0.1 @ 3 ms	Computed tomographic (CT) scanners
$CaWO_4$	20, 74, 8	6.12	—	14–18	0.9–20	—	Radiographic screens
Gd_2O_2S(Tb)	64, 8, 16	7.34	—	—	560	—	Radiographic screens

[a]Relative to NaI(Tl), using a PMT to measure light.

[b]The light emitted by CsI(Tl) does not match the spectral sensitivity of PMTs very well; its conversion efficiency is much larger if measured with a photodiode.

Source: Data on NaI(Tl), BGO, CsI(Na), CsI(Tl), and $CdWO_4$ courtesy of Saint-Gobain Crystals, Hiram, OH. Data on LSO from Ficke DC, Hood JT, Ter-Pogossian MM. A spheroid positron emission tomograph for brain imaging: a feasibility study. JNM 1996: 37:1222.

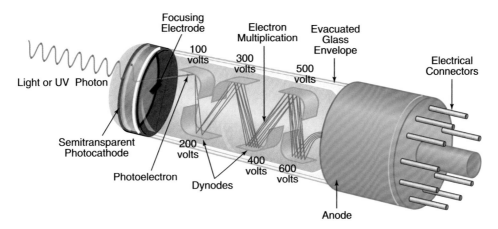

■ FIGURE 17-8 Diagram of a PMT showing the main components (photocathode, focusing electrode, dynodes, and anode) and illustrating the process of electron multiplication. Actual PMTs typically have 10 to 12 dynodes.

about five electrons to be ejected from the second dynode for each electron hitting it. This process continues down the chain of dynodes, with the number of electrons being multiplied by a factor of 5 at each stage. The total amplification of the PMT is the product of the individual multiplications at each dynode. If a PMT has ten dynodes and the amplification at each stage is 5, the total amplification will be

$$5 \times 5 \times 5 \times 5 \times 5 \times 5 \times 5 \times 5 \times 5 \times 5 = 5^{10} \approx 10,000,000$$

The amplification can be adjusted by changing the voltage applied to the PMT.

When a scintillator is coupled to a PMT, an optical coupling material is placed between the two components to minimize reflection losses. The scintillator is usually surrounded on all other sides by a highly reflective material, often magnesium oxide powder.

Photodiodes

Photodiodes are semiconductor diodes that convert light into electrical signals. (The principles of operation of semiconductor diodes are discussed later in this chapter.) In use, photodiodes are reverse biased. *Reverse bias* means that the voltage is applied with the polarity such that essentially no electrical current flows. When the photodiode is exposed to light, an electrical current is generated that is proportional to the intensity of the light. Photodiodes are sometimes used with scintillators instead of PMTs. Photodiodes produce more electrical noise than PMTs do, but they are smaller and less expensive. Most photodiodes, unlike PMTs, do not amplify the signal. However, a type of photodiode called an avalanche photodiode does provide signal amplification, although not as much as a PMT. Photodiodes coupled to $CdWO_4$ or other scintillators are used in current mode in CT scanners. Photodiodes are also essential components of indirect-detection thin-film transistor radiographic and fluoroscopic image receptors, which use scintillators to convert x-ray energy into light.

Scintillators with Trapping of Excited Electrons

In most applications of scintillators, the prompt emission of light after an interaction is desirable. However, there are inorganic scintillators in which electrons become trapped in excited states after interactions with ionizing radiation. These trapped electrons can be released by heating or exposure to light; the electrons then fall to their ground state with the emission of light, which can be detected by a PMT or other sensor. These trapped electrons, in effect, store information about the radiation exposure. Such scintillators can be used for dosimetry or for radiographic imaging.

Thermoluminescent Dosimeters and Optically Stimulated Luminescent Dosimeters

As mentioned above, scintillators with electron trapping can be used for dosimetry. In the case of *thermoluminescent dosimeters* (TLDs), to read the signal after exposure to ionizing radiation, a sample of TLD material is heated, the light is detected and converted into an electrical signal by a PMT, and the resultant signal is integrated and displayed. The amount of light emitted by the TLD increases with the amount of energy absorbed by the TLD, but may deviate from proportionality, particularly at higher doses. After the TLD has been read, it may be baked in an oven to release the remaining trapped electrons and reused.

Lithium fluoride (LiF) is one of the most useful TLD materials. It is commercially available in forms with different trace impurities (Mg and Ti or Mg, Cu, and P), giving differences in properties such as sensitivity and linearity of response with dose. LiF has trapping centers that exhibit almost negligible release of trapped electrons at room temperature, so there is little loss of information with time from exposure to the reading of the TLD. The effective atomic number of LiF is close to that of tissue, so the amount of light emission is almost proportional to the tissue dose over a wide range of x-ray and gamma-ray energies. It is commonly used instead of photographic film for personnel dosimetry.

In optically stimulated luminescense (OSL), the trapped excited electrons are released by exposure to light, commonly produced by a laser, of a frequency optimal for releasing the trapped electrons. The most commonly used OSL material is aluminum oxide (Al_2O_3) activated with a small amount of carbon. The effective atomic number of aluminum oxide is significantly higher than that of soft tissue, and so dose to this material is not proportional to dose to soft tissue over the full range of energies used in medical imaging. Methods for compensating for this effect are discussed in Chapter 21.

Photostimulable Phosphors

Photostimulable phosphors (PSPs), like TLDs, are scintillators in which a fraction of the excited electrons become trapped. PSP plates are used in radiography as image receptors, instead of film-screen cassettes. Although the trapped electrons could be released by heating, a laser is used to scan the plate and release them. The electrons then fall to the ground state, with the emission of light. Barium fluorohalide activated with europium is commonly used for PSP imaging plates. In this material, the wavelength that is most efficient in stimulating luminescence is in the red portion of the spectrum, whereas the stimulated luminescence itself is in the blue-violet portion of the spectrum. The stimulated emissions are converted into an electrical signal by PMTs. After the plate is read by the laser, it may be exposed to light to release the remaining trapped electrons that can be reused. The use of PSPs in radiography has been discussed further in Chapter 7.

17.4 Semiconductor Detectors

Semiconductors are crystalline materials whose electrical conductivities are less than those of metals but more than those of crystalline insulators. Silicon and germanium are common semiconductor materials.

In crystalline materials, electrons exist in energy bands, separated by forbidden gaps. In metals (e.g., copper), the least tightly bound electrons exist in a partially occupied band, called the conduction band. The conduction-band electrons are mobile, providing high electrical conductivity. In an insulator or a semiconductor,

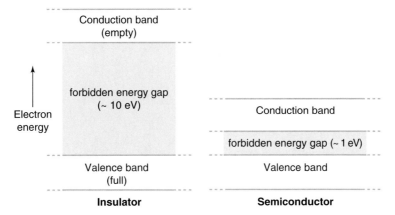

Electron energy

Conduction band
(empty)

forbidden energy gap
(~ 10 eV)

Valence band
(full)

Insulator

Conduction band

forbidden energy gap (~ 1 eV)

Valence band

Semiconductor

■ **FIGURE 17-9** Energy band structure of a crystalline insulator and a semiconductor material.

the valence electrons exist in a filled valence band. In semiconductors, these valence-band electrons participate in covalent bonds and so are immobile. The next higher energy band, the conduction band, is empty of electrons. However, if an electron is placed in the conduction band, it is mobile, as are the upper band electrons in metals. The difference between insulators and semiconductors is the magnitude of the energy gap between the valence and conduction bands. In insulators, the band gap is greater than 5 eV, whereas in semiconductors, it is about 1 eV or less (Fig. 17-9). In semiconductors, valence-band electrons can be raised to the conduction band by ionizing radiation, visible light or ultraviolet radiation, or thermal energy.

When a valence-band electron is raised to the conduction band, it leaves behind a vacancy in the valence band. This vacancy is called a *hole*. Because a hole is the absence of an electron, it is considered to have a net positive charge, equal but opposite to that of an electron. When another valence-band electron fills the hole, a hole is created at that electron's former location. Thus, holes behave as mobile positive charges in the valence band even though positively charged particles do not physically move in the material. The hole-electron pairs formed in a semiconductor material by ionizing radiation are analogous to the ion pairs formed in a gas by ionizing radiation.

A crystal of a semiconductor material can be used as a radiation detector. A voltage is placed between two terminals on opposite sides of the crystal. When ionizing radiation interacts with the detector, electrons in the crystal are raised to an excited state, permitting an electrical current to flow, similar to a gas-filled ionization chamber. Unfortunately, the radiation-induced current, unless it is very large, is masked by a larger current induced by the applied voltage.

To reduce the magnitude of the voltage-induced current so that the signal from radiation interactions can be detected, the semiconductor crystal is "doped" with a trace amount of impurities so that it acts as a diode (see earlier discussion of types of detectors). The impurity atoms fill sites in the crystal lattice that would otherwise be occupied by atoms of the semiconductor material. If atoms of the impurity material have more valence electrons than those of the semiconductor material, the impurity atoms provide mobile electrons in the conduction band. A semiconductor material containing an electron-donor impurity is called an *n-type material* (Fig. 17-10). N-type material has mobile electrons in the conduction band. On the other hand, an impurity with fewer valence electrons than the semiconductor material provides sites in the valence band that can accept electrons. When a valence-band electron fills one of these sites, it creates a hole at its former location. Semiconductor material doped with a hole-forming impurity is called *p-type material*. P-type material has mobile holes in the valence band.

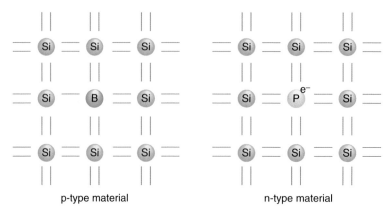

■ **FIGURE 17-10** P-type and n-type impurities in a crystal of a semiconductor material, silicon in this example. N-type impurities provide mobile electrons in the conduction band, whereas p-type impurities provide acceptor sites in the valence band. When filled by electrons, these acceptor sites create holes that act as mobile positive charges. (Si, silicon; B, boron; P, phosphorus.)

A semiconductor diode consists of a crystal of semiconductor material with a region of n-type material that forms a junction with a region of p-type material (Fig. 17-11). If an external voltage is applied with the positive polarity on the p-type side of the diode and the negative polarity on the n-type side, the holes in the p-type material and the mobile conduction-band electrons of the n-type material are drawn to the junction. There, the mobile electrons fall into the valence band to fill holes. Applying an external voltage in this manner is referred to as *forward bias*. Forward bias permits a current to flow with little resistance.

On the other hand, if an external voltage is applied with the opposite polarity—that is, with the negative polarity on the p-type side of the diode and the positive polarity on the n-type side—the holes in the p-type material and the mobile conduction-band electrons of the n-type material are drawn away from the junction. Applying the external voltage in this polarity is referred to as *reverse bias*. Reverse bias draws the charge carriers away from the n-p junction, forming a region depleted of current carriers. Very little electrical current flows when a diode is reverse biased.

■ **FIGURE 17-11** Semiconductor diode. When no bias is applied, a few holes migrate into the n-type material and a few conduction-band electrons migrate into the p-type material. With forward bias, the external voltage is applied with the positive polarity on the p-side of the junction and negative polarity on the n-side, causing the charge carriers to be swept into the junction and a large current to flow. With negative bias, the charge carriers are drawn away from the junction, creating a region depleted of charge carriers that acts as a solid-state ion chamber.

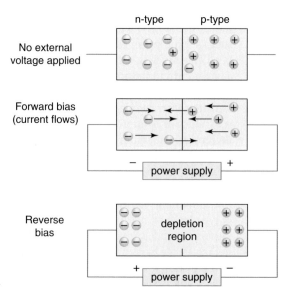

A reverse-biased semiconductor diode can be used to detect visible light and UV radiation or ionizing radiation. The photons of light or ionization and excitation produced by ionizing radiation can excite lower energy electrons in the depletion region of the diode to higher energy bands, producing hole-electron pairs. The electrical field in the depletion region sweeps the holes toward the p-type side and the conduction-band electrons toward the n-type side, causing a momentary pulse of current to flow after the interaction.

Photodiodes are semiconductor diodes that convert light into an electrical current. As mentioned previously, they are used in conjunction with scintillators as detectors in CT scanners. Scintillation-based thin-film transistor radiographic and fluoroscopic image receptors, discussed in Chapter 7, incorporate a photodiode in each detector element.

Semiconductor detectors are semiconductor diodes designed for the detection of ionizing radiation. The amount of charge generated by an interaction is proportional to the energy deposited in the detector by the interaction; therefore, semiconductor detectors are spectrometers. Because thermal energy can also raise electrons to the conduction band, many types of semiconductor detectors used for x-ray and gamma-ray spectroscopy must be cooled with liquid nitrogen.

The energy resolution of germanium semiconductor detectors is greatly superior to that of NaI(Tl) scintillation detectors. Liquid nitrogen–cooled germanium detectors are widely used for the identification of individual gamma ray–emitting radionuclides in mixed radionuclide samples because of their superb energy resolution.

Semiconductor detectors are seldom used for medical imaging devices because of high expense, because of low quantum detection efficiencies in comparison to scintillators such as NaI(Tl) (Z of iodine = 53, Z of germanium = 32, Z of silicon = 14), because they can be manufactured only in limited sizes, and because many such devices require cooling.

Efforts are being made to develop semiconductor detectors of higher atomic number than germanium that can be operated at room temperature. A leading candidate to date is cadmium zinc telluride (CZT). A small-field-of-view nuclear medicine camera using CZT detectors has been developed.

A layer of a semiconductor material, amorphous selenium (Z = 34), is used in some radiographic image receptors, including those in some mammography systems. The selenium is commonly referred to as a "photoconductor." In these image receptors, the selenium layer is electrically coupled to a rectangular array of thin film transistor detector elements which collect and store the mobile electrical charges produced in the selenium by x-ray interactions during image acquisition. These image receptors are discussed in Chapters 7 and 8.

17.5 Pulse Height Spectroscopy

Many radiation detectors, such as scintillation detectors, semiconductor detectors, and proportional counters, produce electrical pulses whose amplitudes are proportional to the energies deposited in the detectors by individual interactions. *Pulse height analyzers* (PHAs) are electronic systems that may be used with these detectors to perform pulse height spectroscopy and energy-selective counting. In energy-selective counting, only interactions that deposit energies within a certain energy range are counted. Energy-selective counting can be used to reduce the effects of background radiation, to reduce the effects of scatter, or to separate events caused by different radionuclides in a sample containing multiple radionuclides. Two types of PHAs are *single-channel analyzers* (SCAs) and *multichannel analyzers* (MCAs). MCAs determine spectra much more efficiently than do SCA systems, but they are more expensive. Pulse height discrimination circuits are incorporated in scintillation cameras and other nuclear medicine imaging devices to reduce the effects of scatter on the images.

Single-Channel Analyzer Systems

Function of a Single-Channel Analyzer System

Figure 17-12 depicts an SCA system. Although the system is shown with an NaI(Tl) crystal and PMT, it could be used with any pulse-mode spectrometer. The high-voltage power supply typically provides 800 to 1,200 V to the PMT. The series of resistors divides the total voltage into increments that are applied to the dynodes and anode of the PMT. Raising the voltage increases the magnitude of the voltage pulses from the PMT.

The detector is often located some distance from the majority of the electronic components. The pulses from the PMT are usually routed to a preamplifier (pre-amp), which is connected to the PMT by as short a cable as possible. The function of the preamp is to amplify the voltage pulses further, so as to minimize distortion and attenuation of the signal during transmission to the remainder of the system. The pulses from the preamp are routed to the amplifier, which further amplifies the pulses and modifies their shapes. The gains of most amplifiers are adjustable.

The pulses from the amplifier then proceed to the SCA. The user is allowed to set two voltage levels, a lower level and an upper level. If a voltage pulse whose amplitude is less than the lower level or greater than the upper level is received from the amplifier, the SCA does nothing. If a voltage pulse whose amplitude is greater than the lower level but less than the upper level is received from the amplifier, the SCA produces a single logic pulse. A logic pulse is a voltage pulse of fixed amplitude and duration. Figure 17-13 illustrates the operation of an SCA. The counter counts the logic pulses from the SCA for a time interval set by the timer.

Many SCAs permit the user to select the mode by which the two knobs set the lower and upper levels. In one mode, usually called *LL/UL mode,* one knob directly sets the lower level and the other sets the upper level. In another mode, called *window mode,* one knob (often labeled E or energy) sets the midpoint of the range of accept-able pulse heights and the other knob (often labeled ΔE or window) sets the range of voltages around this value. In this mode, the lower level voltage is $E - \Delta E/2$ and the upper level voltage is $E + \Delta E/2$. (In some SCAs, the range of acceptable pulse heights is from E to $E + \Delta E$.) Window mode is convenient for plotting a spectrum.

■ FIGURE 17-12 SCA system with NaI(Tl) detector and PMT.

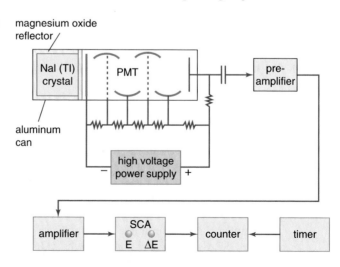

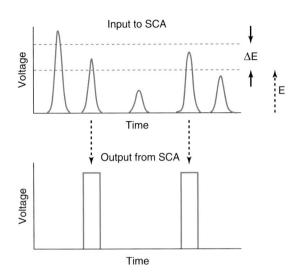

Plotting a Spectrum Using a Single-Channel Analyzer

To obtain the pulse height spectrum of a sample of radioactive material using an SCA system, the SCA is placed in window mode, the E setting is set to zero, and a small window (ΔE) setting is selected. A series of counts is taken for a fixed length of time per count, with the E setting increased before each count but without changing the window setting. Each count is plotted on graph paper as a function of baseline (E) setting.

Energy Calibration of a Single-Channel Analyzer System

On most SCAs, each of the two knobs permits values from 0 to 1,000 to be selected. By adjusting the amplification of the pulses reaching the SCA—either by changing the voltage produced by the high-voltage power supply or by changing the amplifier gain—the system can be calibrated so that these knob settings directly indicate keV.

A ^{137}Cs source, which emits 662-keV gamma rays, is usually used. A narrow window is set, centered about a setting of 662. For example, the SCA may be placed into LL/UL mode with lower level value of 655 and an upper level value of 669 selected. Then the voltage produced by the high-voltage power supply is increased in steps, with a count taken after each step. The counts first increase and then decrease. When the voltage that produces the largest count is selected, the two knobs on the SCA directly indicate keV. This procedure is called *peaking* the SCA system.

Multichannel Analyzer Systems

An MCA system permits an energy spectrum to be automatically acquired much more quickly and easily than does an SCA system. Figure 17-14 is a diagram of a counting system using an MCA. The detector, high-voltage power supply, preamp, and amplifier are the same as were those described for SCA systems. The MCA consists of an analog-to-digital converter (ADC), a memory containing many storage locations called *channels,* control circuitry, and a timer. The memory of an MCA typically ranges from 256 to 8,192 channels, each of which can store a single integer. When the acquisition of a spectrum begins, all of the channels are set to zero. When each voltage pulse from the amplifier is received, it is converted into a binary digital signal, the value of which is proportional to the amplitude of the analog voltage pulse. (ADCs are discussed in Chapter 5.) This digital signal designates a particular channel in the MCA's memory. The number stored in that channel is then incremented by 1.

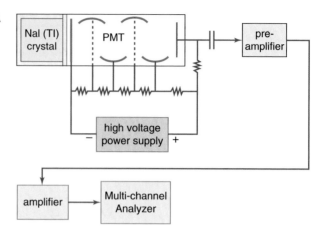

As many pulses are processed, a spectrum is generated in the memory of the MCA. Figure 17-15 illustrates the operation of an MCA. Today, most MCAs are interfaced to digital computers that store, process, and display the resultant spectra.

X-ray and Gamma-Ray Spectroscopy with Sodium Iodide Detectors

X-ray and gamma-ray spectroscopy is best performed with semiconductor detectors because of their superior energy resolution. However, high detection efficiency

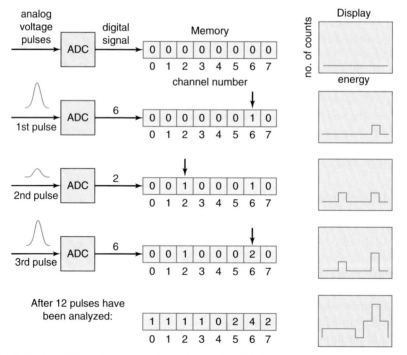

■ **FIGURE 17-15** Acquisition of a spectrum by an MCA. The digital signal produced by the ADC is a binary signal, as described in Chapter 5. After the analog pulses are digitized by the ADC, they are sorted into bins (channels) by height, forming an energy spectrum. Although this figure depicts an MCA with 8 channels, actual MCAs have as many as 8,192 channels.

is more important than ultrahigh energy resolution for most nuclear medicine applications, so most spectroscopy systems in nuclear medicine use NaI(Tl) crystals coupled to PMTs.

Interactions of Photons with a Spectrometer

There are a number of mechanisms by which an x-ray or gamma ray can deposit energy in the detector, several of which deposit only a fraction of the incident photon energy. As illustrated in Figure 17-16, an incident photon can deposit its full energy by a photoelectric interaction (A) or by one or more Compton scatters followed by a photoelectric interaction (B). However, a photon will deposit only a fraction of its energy if it interacts by Compton scattering and the scattered photon escapes the detector (C). In that case, the energy deposited depends on the scattering angle, with larger angle scatters depositing larger energies. Even if the incident photon interacts by the photoelectric effect, less than its total energy will be deposited if the inner-shell electron vacancy created by the interaction results in the emission of a characteristic x-ray that escapes the detector (D).

Most detectors are shielded to reduce the effects of natural background radiation and nearby radiation sources. Figure 17-16 shows two ways by which an x-ray or gamma-ray interaction in the shield of the detector can deposit energy in the detector. The photon may Compton scatter in the shield, with the scattered photon striking the detector (E), or a characteristic x-ray from the shield may interact with the detector (F).

Most interactions of x-rays and gamma rays with an NaI(Tl) detector are with iodine atoms, because iodine has a much larger atomic number than sodium does. Although thallium has an even larger atomic number, it is only a trace impurity.

Spectrum of Cesium-137

The spectrum of ^{137}Cs is often used to introduce pulse height spectroscopy because of the simple decay scheme of this radionuclide. As shown at the top of Figure 17-17, ^{137}Cs decays by beta particle emission to ^{137m}Ba, whose nucleus is in an excited state. The ^{137m}Ba nucleus attains its ground state by the emission of a 662-keV gamma ray 90% of the time. In 10% of the decays, a conversion electron is emitted instead of a gamma ray. The conversion electron is usually followed by the emission of an approximately 32-keV K-shell characteristic x-ray as an outer-shell electron fills the inner-shell vacancy.

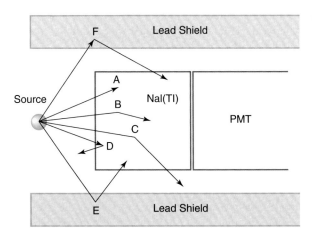

■ **FIGURE 17-16** Interactions of x-rays and gamma rays with an NaI(Tl) detector. See text for description.

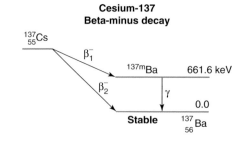

**Cesium-137
Beta-minus decay**

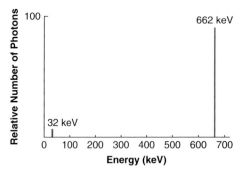
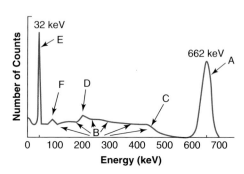

■ **FIGURE 17-17** Decay scheme of ^{137}Cs (**top**), actual energy spectrum (**left**), and pulse height spectrum obtained using an NaI(Tl) scintillation detector (**right**). See text for description of pulse height spectrum. (*A*) photopeak, due to complete absorption of 662-keV gamma rays in the crystal; (*B*) Compton continuum; (*C*) Compton edge; (*D*) backscatter peak; (*E*) barium x-ray photopeak; and (*F*) photopeak caused by absorption of lead *K*-shell x-rays (72 to 88 keV) from the shield.

In the left in Figure 17-17 is the actual energy spectrum of ^{137}Cs, and on the right is its pulse height spectrum obtained with the use of an NaI(Tl) detector. There are two reasons for the differences between the spectra. First, there are a number of mechanisms by which an x-ray or gamma ray can deposit energy in the detector, several of which deposit only a fraction of the incident photon energy. Second, there are random variations in the processes by which the energy deposited in the detector is converted into an electrical signal. In the case of an NaI(Tl) crystal coupled to a PMT, there are random variations in the fraction of deposited energy converted into light, the fraction of the light that reaches the photocathode of the PMT, and the number of electrons ejected from the back of the photocathode per unit energy deposited by the light. These factors cause random variations in the size of the voltage pulses produced by the detector, even when the incident x-rays or gamma rays deposit exactly the same energy. The energy resolution of a spectrometer is a measure of the effect of these random variations on the resultant spectrum.

In the pulse height spectrum of ^{137}Cs, on the right in Figure 17-17, the photopeak (A) is caused by interactions in which the energy of an incident 662-keV photon is entirely absorbed in the crystal. This may occur by a single photoelectric interaction or by one or more Compton scattering interactions followed by a photoelectric interaction. The Compton continuum (B) is caused by 662-keV photons that scatter in the crystal, with the scattered photons escaping the crystal. Each portion of the continuum corresponds to a particular scattering angle. The Compton edge (C) is the upper limit of the Compton continuum. The backscatter peak (D) is caused by 662-keV photons that scatter from the shielding around the detector into the detector. The barium x-ray photopeak (E) is a second photopeak caused by the absorption of barium *K*-shell x-rays (31 to 37 keV), which are emitted after the emission of conversion electrons. Another photopeak (F) is caused by lead *K*-shell x-rays (72 to 88 keV) from the shield.

Spectrum of Technetium-99m

The decay scheme of ^{99m}Tc is shown at the top in Figure 17-18. ^{99m}Tc is an isomer of ^{99}Tc that decays by isomeric transition to its ground state, with the emission of a 140.5-keV gamma ray. In 11% of the transitions, a conversion electron is emitted instead of a gamma ray.

The pulse height spectrum of ^{99m}Tc is shown at the bottom of Figure 17-18. The photopeak (A) is caused by the total absorption of the 140-keV gamma rays. The escape peak (B) is caused by 140-keV gamma rays that interact with the crystal by the photoelectric effect but with the resultant iodine *K*-shell x-rays (28 to 33 keV) escaping the crystal. There is also a photopeak (C) caused by the absorption of lead *K*-shell x-rays from the shield. The Compton continuum is quite small, unlike the continuum in the spectrum of ^{137}Cs, because the photoelectric effect predominates in iodine at 140 keV.

Spectrum of Iodine-125

^{125}I decays by electron capture followed by the emission of a 35.5-keV gamma ray (6.7% of decays) or a conversion electron. The electron capture usually leaves the

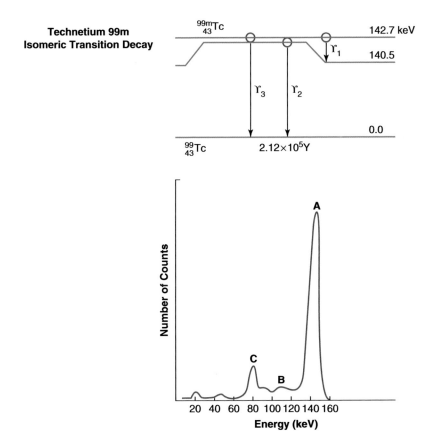

■ **FIGURE 17-18** Decay scheme of ^{99m}Tc (**top**) and its pulse height spectrum on an NaI(Tl) scintillation detector (**bottom**). See text for details.

daughter nucleus with a vacancy in the *K*-shell. The emission of a conversion electron usually also results in a *K*-shell vacancy. Each transformation of an ¹²⁵I atom therefore results in the emission, on the average, of 1.47 x-rays or gamma rays with energies between 27 and 36 keV.

Figure 17-19 shows two pulse height spectra from ¹²⁵I. The spectrum on the left was acquired with the source located 7.5 cm from an NaI(Tl) detector, and the one on the right was collected with the source in an NaI(Tl) well detector. The spectrum on the left shows a large photopeak at about 30 keV, whereas the spectrum on the right shows a peak at about 30 keV and a smaller peak at about 60 keV. The 60-keV peak in the spectrum from the well detector is a *sum peak* caused by two photons simultaneously striking the detector. The sum peak is not apparent in the spectrum with the source 7.5 cm from the detector because the much lower detection efficiency renders unlikely the simultaneous interaction of two photons with the detector.

Performance Characteristics

Energy Resolution

The energy resolution of a spectrometer is a measure of its ability to differentiate between particles or photons of different energies. It can be determined by irradiating the detector with monoenergetic particles or photons and measuring the width of the resultant peak in the pulse height spectrum. Statistical effects in the detection process cause the amplitudes of the pulses from the detector to randomly vary about the mean pulse height, giving the peak a gaussian shape. (These statistical effects are one reason why the pulse height spectrum produced by a spectrometer is not identical to the actual energy spectrum of the radiation.) A wider peak implies a poorer energy resolution.

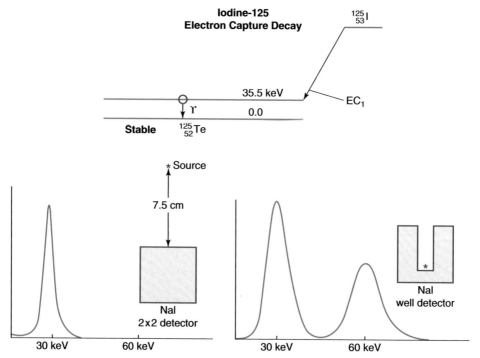

■ **FIGURE 17-19** Decay scheme and spectrum of ¹²⁵I source located 7.5 cm from solid NaI(Tl) crystal (**left**) and in NaI(Tl) well counter (**right**).

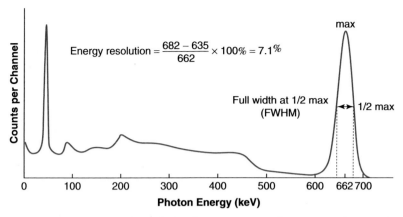

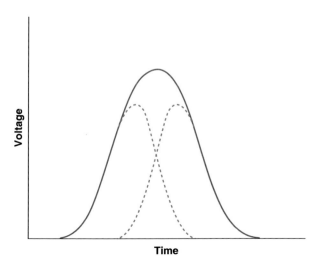

■ **FIGURE 17-20** Energy resolution of a pulse height spectrometer. The spectrum shown is that of ^{137}Cs, obtained by an NaI(Tl) scintillator coupled to a PMT.

The width is usually measured at half the maximal height of the peak, as illustrated in Figure 17-20. This is called the full width at half maximum (FWHM). The FWHM is then divided by the pulse amplitude corresponding to the maximum of the peak:

$$\text{Energy resolution} = \frac{\text{FWHM}}{\text{Pulse amplitude at center of peak}} \times 100\% \qquad [17\text{-}4]$$

For example, the energy resolution of a 5-cm-diameter and 5-cm-thick cylindrical NaI(Tl) crystal, coupled to a PMT and exposed to the 662-keV gamma rays of ^{137}Cs, is typically about 7% to 8%.

Count-Rate Effects in Spectrometers

In pulse height spectroscopy, count-rate effects are best understood as pulse pileup. Figure 17-21 depicts the signal from a detector in which two interactions occur, separated by a very short time interval. The detector produces a single pulse, which is the sum of the individual signals from the two interactions, having a higher amplitude than the signal from either individual interaction. Because of this effect, operating a pulse height spectrometer at a high count rate causes loss of counts and misplacement of counts in the spectrum.

■ **FIGURE 17-21** Pulse pileup. The dashed lines represent the signals produced by two individual interactions in the detector that occur at almost the same time. The *solid line* depicts the actual pulse produced by the detector. This single pulse is the sum of the signals from the two interactions.

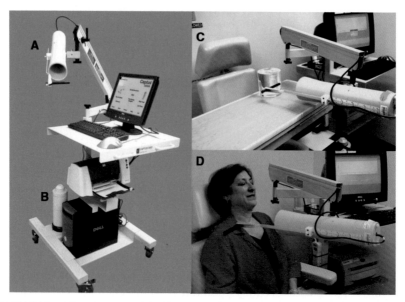

■ **FIGURE 17-22** Thyroid probe system (**A**). (Photograph courtesy Capintec, Inc., Ramsey, New Jersey.) The personal computer has added circuitry and software so that it functions as an MCA. An NaI(Tl) well detector (**B**), discussed later in this chapter, for counting samples for radioactivity is part of this system. For thyroid uptake tests, the radioiodine capsules are placed in a Lucite neck phantom before patient administration and counted individually (**C**). At 4 to 6 h and again at about 24 h after administration, the radioactivity in the patient's neck is counted at the same distance from the probe as was the neck phantom (**D**).

17.6 Nonimaging Detector Applications

Sodium Iodide Thyroid Probe and Well Counter

Thyroid Probe

A nuclear medicine department typically has a thyroid probe for measuring the uptake of ^{123}I or ^{131}I by the thyroid glands of patients and for monitoring the activities of ^{131}I in the thyroid glands of staff members who handle large activities of ^{131}I. A thyroid probe, as shown in Figures 17-22 and 17-23, usually consists of a 5.1-cm (2-inch)-diameter and 5.1-cm-thick cylindrical NaI(Tl) crystal coupled to a PMT, which in turn is connected to a preamplifier. The probe is shielded on the sides and back with lead and is equipped with a collimator so that it detects photons only from a limited portion of the patient. The thyroid probe is connected to a high-voltage power supply and either an SCA or an MCA system.

■ **FIGURE 17-23** Diagram of a thyroid probe.

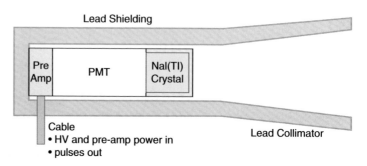

Thyroid Uptake Measurements

Thyroid uptake measurements may be performed using one or two capsules of ^{123}I or ^{131}I sodium iodide. A neck phantom, consisting of a Lucite cylinder of diameter similar to the neck and containing a hole parallel to its axis for a radioiodine capsule, is required. In the two-capsule method, the capsules should have almost identical activities. Each capsule is placed in the neck phantom and counted separately. Then, one capsule is swallowed by the patient. The other capsule is called the "standard." Next, the emissions from the patient's neck are counted, typically at 4 to 6 h after administration, and again at 24 h after administration. Each time that the patient's thyroid is counted, the patient's distal thigh is also counted for the same length of time, to approximate nonthyroidal activity in the neck, and a background count is obtained. All counts are performed with the NaI crystal at the same distance, typically 20 to 30 cm, from the thyroid phantom or the patient's neck or thigh. (This distance reduces the effects of small differences in distance between the detector and the objects being counted.) Furthermore, each time that the patient's thyroid is counted, the remaining capsule is placed in the neck phantom and counted. Finally, the uptake is calculated for each neck measurement:

$$\text{Uptake} = \frac{(\text{Thyroid count} - \text{Thigh count})}{(\text{Count of standard in phantom} - \text{Background count})}$$

$$\times \frac{\text{Initial count of standard in phantom}}{\text{Initial count of patient capsule in phantom}}$$

Some nuclear medicine laboratories instead use a method that requires only one capsule. In this method, a single capsule is obtained, counted in the neck phantom, and swallowed by the patient. As in the previous method, the patient's neck and distal thigh are counted, typically at 4 to 6 h and again at 24 h after administration. The times of the capsule administration and the neck counts are recorded. Finally, the uptake is calculated for each neck measurement:

$$\frac{(\text{Thyroid count} - \text{Thigh count})}{(\text{Count of capsule in phantom} - \text{Background count})} \times e^{0.693t/T_{1/2}}$$

where $T_{1/2}$ is the physical half-life of the radionuclide and t is the time elapsed between the count of the capsule in the phantom and the thyroid count. The single-capsule method avoids the cost of the second capsule and requires fewer measurements, but it is more susceptible to instability of the equipment, technologist error, and dead-time effects.

Sodium Iodide Well Counter

A nuclear medicine department also usually has an NaI(Tl) well counter, shown in Figures 17-22B and 17-24. The NaI(Tl) well counter may be used for clinical tests such as Schilling tests (a test of vitamin B_{12} absorption), plasma or red blood cell volume determinations, and radioimmunoassays, although radioimmunoassays have been largely replaced by immunoassays that do not use radioactivity. The well counter is also commonly used to assay wipe test samples to detect radioactive contamination. The well counter usually consists of a cylindrical NaI(Tl) crystal, either 5.1 cm (2 inches) in diameter and 5.1 cm thick or 7.6 cm (3 inches) in diameter and 7.6 cm thick, with a hole in the crystal for the insertion of samples. This configuration gives the counter an extremely high efficiency, permitting it to assay samples containing activities of less than 1 nCi (10^{-3} μCi). The crystal is

■ **FIGURE 17-24** Diagram of an NaI(Tl) well counter.

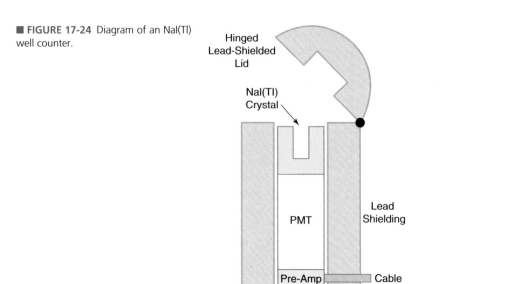

■ **FIGURE 17-24** Diagram of an NaI(Tl) well counter.

coupled to a PMT, which in turn is connected to a preamplifier. A well counter in a nuclear medicine department should have a thick lead shield, because it is used to count samples containing nanocurie activities in the vicinity of millicurie activities of high-energy gamma-ray emitters such as ^{67}Ga, ^{111}In, and ^{131}I. The well counter is connected to a high-voltage power supply and either an SCA or an MCA system. Departments that perform large numbers of radioimmunoassays often use automatic well counters, such as the one shown in Figure 17-25, to count large numbers of samples.

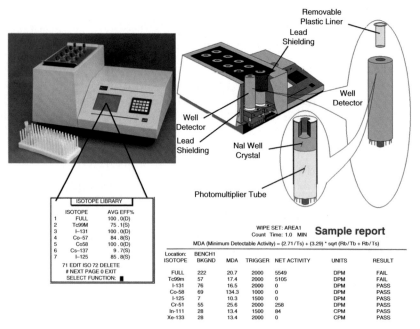

■ **FIGURE 17-25** Automatic gamma well counter. (Photograph courtesy Laboratory Technologies, Inc.)

Sample Volume and Dead-Time Effects in Sodium Iodide Well Counters

The position of a sample in a sodium iodide well counter has a dramatic effect on the detection efficiency. When liquid samples in vials of a particular shape and size are counted, the detection efficiency falls as the volume increases. Most nuclear medicine *in vitro* tests require the comparison of a liquid sample from the patient with a reference sample. It is crucial that both samples be in identical containers and have identical volumes.

In addition, the high efficiency of the NaI well counter can cause unacceptable dead-time count losses, even with sample activities in the microcurie range. It is important to ensure that the activity placed in the well counter is sufficiently small so that dead-time effects do not cause a falsely low count. In general, well counters should not be used at apparent count rates exceeding about 5,000 cps, which limits samples of ^{125}I and ^{57}Co to activities less than about 0.2 μCi. However, larger activities of some radionuclides may be counted without significant losses; for example, activities of ^{51}Cr as large as 5 μCi may be counted, because only about one out of every ten decays yields a gamma ray.

Quality Assurance for the Sodium Iodide Thyroid Probe and Well Counter

Both of these instruments should have energy calibrations (as discussed earlier for an SCA system) performed daily, with the results recorded. A background count and a constancy test, using a source with a long half-life such as ^{137}Cs, also should be performed daily for both the well counter and the thyroid probe to test for radioactive contamination or instrument malfunction. On the day the constancy test is begun, a counting window is set to tightly encompass the photopeak, and a count is taken and corrected for background. Limits called "action levels" are established which, if exceeded, cause the person performing the test to notify the chief technologist, physicist, or physician. On each subsequent day, a count is taken using the same source, window setting, and counting time; corrected for background; recorded; and compared with the action levels. If each day's count were mistakenly compared with the previous day's count instead of the first day's count, slow changes in the instrument would not be discovered. Periodically, a new first day count and action levels should be established, accounting for decay of the radioactive source. This will prevent the constancy test count from exceeding an action level because of decreasing source activity. Also, spectra should be plotted annually for commonly measured radionuclides, usually ^{123}I and ^{131}I for the thyroid probe and perhaps ^{57}Co (Schilling tests), ^{125}I (radioimmunoassays), and ^{51}Cr (red cell volumes and survival studies) for the well counter, to verify that the SCA windows fit the photopeaks. This testing is greatly simplified if the department has an MCA.

Dose Calibrator

A dose calibrator, shown in Figure 17-26, is used to measure the activities of dosages of radiopharmaceuticals to be administered to patients. The U.S. Nuclear Regulatory Commission (NRC) and state regulatory agencies require that dosages of x-ray– and gamma ray–emitting radiopharmaceuticals be determined before administration to patients. NRC allows administration of a "unit dosage" (an individual patient dosage prepared by a commercial radiopharmacy, without any further manipulation of its activity by the nuclear medicine department that administers it) without measurement. It also permits determination of activities of non-unit dosages by volumetric measurements and mathematical calculations. Most dose calibrators are well-type

■ **FIGURE 17-26** Dose calibrator. The detector is a well-geometry ion chamber filled with pressurized argon. The syringe and vial holder (**A**) is used to place radioactive material, in this case in a syringe, into the detector. This reduces exposure to the hands and permits the activity to be measured in a reproducible geometry. The removable plastic insert (**B**) prevents contamination of the well.

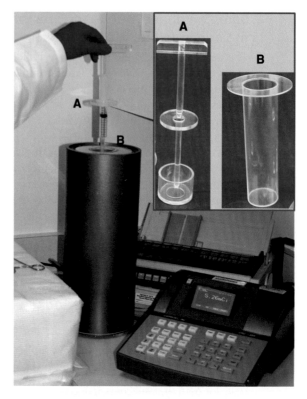

ionization chambers that are filled with argon ($Z = 18$) and pressurized to maximize sensitivity. Most dose calibrators have shielding around their chambers to protect users from the radioactive material being assayed and to prevent nearby sources of radiation from affecting the measurements.

A dose calibrator cannot directly measure activity. Instead, it measures the intensity of the radiation emitted by a dosage of a radiopharmaceutical. The manufacturer of a dose calibrator determines calibration factors relating the magnitude of the signal from the detector to activity for specific radionuclides commonly used in nuclear medicine. The user pushes a button or turns a dial on the dose calibrator to designate the radionuclide being measured, thereby specifying a calibration factor, and the dose calibrator displays the measured activity.

Operating Characteristics

Dose calibrators using ionization chambers are operated in current mode, thereby avoiding dead-time effects. They can accurately assay activities as large as 2 Ci. For the same reasons, they are relatively insensitive and cannot accurately assay activities less than about 1 μCi. In general, the identification and measurement of activities of radionuclides in samples containing multiple radionuclides is not possible. The measurement accuracy is affected by the position in the well of the dosages being measured, so it is important that all measurements be made with the dosages at the same position. Most dose calibrators have large wells, which reduce the effect of position on the measurements.

Dose calibrators using large well-type ionization chambers are in general not significantly affected by changes in the sample volume or container for most radionuclides. However, the measured activities of certain radionuclides, especially those such as ^{111}I, ^{123}I, ^{125}I, and ^{133}Xe that emit weak x-rays or gamma rays, are highly dependent on factors such as whether the containers (e.g., syringe or vial) are glass or plastic and the thicknesses of the containers' walls. There is currently no generally accepted solution to this problem. Some radiopharmaceutical manufacturers provide correction factors for these radionuclides; these correction factors are specific to the radionuclide, the container, and the model of dose calibrator.

There are even greater problems with attenuation effects when assaying the dosages of pure beta-emitting radionuclides, such as ^{32}P and ^{89}Sr. For this reason, the NRC does not require unit dosages of these radionuclides to be assayed in a dose calibrator before administration. However, most nuclear medicine departments assay these, but only to verify that the activities as assayed by the vendor are not in error by a large amount.

Dose Calibrator Quality Assurance

Because the assay of activity using the dose calibrator is often the only assurance that the patient is receiving the prescribed activity, quality assurance testing of the dose calibrator is required by the NRC and state regulatory agencies. The NRC requires the testing to be in accordance with nationally recognized standards or the manufacturer's instructions. The following set of tests is commonly performed to satisfy this requirement.

The device should be tested for *accuracy* upon installation and annually thereafter. Two or more sealed radioactive sources (often ^{57}Co and ^{137}Cs) whose activities are known within 5% are assayed. The measured activities must be within 10% of the actual activities.

The device should also be tested for *linearity* (a measure of the effect that the amount of activity has on the accuracy) upon installation and quarterly thereafter. The most common method requires a vial of ^{99m}Tc containing the maximal activity that would be administered to a patient. The vial is measured two or three times daily until it decays to less than 30 μCi; the measured activities and times of the measurements are recorded. One measurement is assumed to be correct and, from this measurement, activities are calculated for the times of the other measurements. No measurement may differ from the corresponding calculated activity by more than 10%. An alternative to the decay method for testing linearity is the use of commercially available lead cylindrical sleeves of different thickness that simulate radioactive decay via attenuation (Figure 17-27). These devices must be calibrated prior to first use by comparing their simulated decay with the decay method described above.

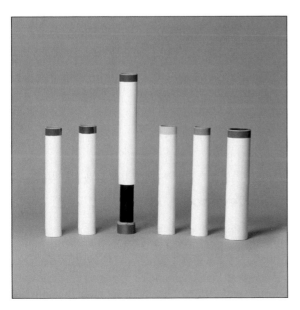

■ **FIGURE 17-27** Set of cylindrical lead sleeves used to test dose calibrator linearity. These color-coded sleeves of different thicknesses use attenuation to simulate radioactive decay over periods of 6, 12, 20, 30, 40, and 50 h for ^{99m}Tc. Additional sleeves are available that can extend the simulated decay interval up to 350 h. Photo courtesy of Fluke Biomedical Radiation Management Services, Cleveland, Ohio.

The device should be tested for *constancy* before its first use each day. At least one sealed source (usually ^{57}Co) is assayed, and its measured activity, corrected for decay, must not differ from its measured activity on the date of the last accuracy test by more than 10%. (Most laboratories perform a daily accuracy test, which is more rigorous, in lieu of a daily constancy test.)

Finally, the dose calibrator should be tested for geometry dependence on installation. This is usually done by placing a small volume of a radiochemical, often ^{99m}Tc pertechnetate, in a vial or syringe and assaying its activity after each of several dilutions. If volume effects are found to affect measurements by more than 10%, correction factors must be determined. The geometry test must be performed for syringe and vial sizes commonly used. Dose calibrators should also be appropriately tested after repair or adjustment.

The calibration factors of individual radionuclide settings should be verified for radionuclides assayed for clinical purposes. This can be performed by placing a source of any radionuclide in the dose calibrator, recording the indicated activity using a clinical radionuclide setting (e.g., ^{131}I), recording the indicated activity using the setting of a radionuclide used for accuracy determination (e.g., ^{57}Co or ^{137}Cs), and verifying that the ratio of the two indicated activities is that specified by the manufacturer of the dose calibrator.

Molybdenum-99 Concentration Testing

When a ^{99}Mo/^{99m}Tc generator is eluted, it is possible to obtain an abnormally large amount of ^{99}Mo in the eluate. (Radionuclide generators are discussed in Chapter 16.) If a radiopharmaceutical contaminated with ^{99}Mo is administered to a patient, the patient will receive an increased radiation dose (^{99}Mo emits high-energy beta particles and has a 66-h half-life) and the quality of the resultant images may be degraded by the high-energy ^{99}Mo gamma rays. The NRC requires that any ^{99m}Tc to be administered to a human must not contain more than 0.15 kBq of ^{99}Mo per MBq of ^{99m}Tc (0.15 μCi of ^{99}Mo per mCi of ^{99m}Tc) at the time of administration and that the first elution of a generator must be assayed for ^{99}Mo concentration.

The concentration of ^{99}Mo is most commonly measured with a dose calibrator and a special lead container that is supplied by the manufacturer. The walls of the lead container are sufficiently thick to stop almost all of the gamma rays from ^{99m}Tc (140 keV) but thin enough to be penetrated by many of the higher energy gamma rays from ^{99}Mo (740 and 778 keV). To perform the measurement, the empty lead container is first assayed in the dose calibrator. Next, the vial of ^{99m}Tc is placed in the lead container and assayed. Finally, the vial of ^{99m}Tc alone is assayed. The ^{99}Mo concentration is then obtained using the following equation:

$$\text{Concentration} = K \cdot \frac{A_{vial-in-container} - A_{empty-container}}{A_{vial}} \qquad [17\text{-}5]$$

where K is a correction factor supplied by the manufacturer of the dose calibrator that accounts for the attenuation of the ^{99}Mo gamma rays by the lead container.

^{82}Sr and ^{85}Sr Concentration Testing

Myocardial perfusion can by assessed by PET using the radiopharmaceutical ^{82}Rb chloride. In clinical practice, ^{82}Rb chloride is obtained from an ^{82}Sr/^{82}Rb generator. (These generators are discussed in Chapter 16.) When an ^{82}Sr/^{82}Rb generator is eluted, it is possible to obtain an abnormally large amount of ^{82}Sr or ^{85}Sr, a radioactive contaminant in the production of ^{82}Sr, in the eluate. The NRC requires that any ^{82}Rb chloride to be administered to a human not contain more than 0.02 kBq of ^{82}Sr or

0.2 kBq of ^{85}Sr per MBq of ^{82}Rb at the time of administration and that the concentrations of these radionuclides be measured before the first patient use each day. A dose calibrator is generally used to assay the concentration of the unwanted contaminants ^{82}Sr and ^{85}Sr in the eluate. The measurement procedures are contained in the package insert provided by the manufacturer of the generators. The eluate is allowed to decay for an hour so that only ^{82}Sr and ^{85}Sr remain. The sample is then assayed in the dose calibrator, and the amounts of ^{82}Sr and ^{85}Sr are estimated from an assumed ratio.

17.7 Counting Statistics

Introduction

Sources of Error

There are three types of errors in measurements. The first is *systematic error*. Systematic error occurs when measurements differ from the correct values in a systematic fashion. For example, systematic error occurs in radiation measurements if a detector is used in pulse mode at too high an interaction rate; dead-time count losses cause the measured count rate to be lower than the actual interaction rate. The second type of error is *random error*. Random error is caused by random fluctuations in whatever is being measured or in the measurement process itself. The third type of error is the *blunder* (e.g., setting the single-channel analyzer window incorrectly for a single measurement).

Random Error in Radiation Detection

The processes by which radiation is emitted and interacts with matter are random in nature. Whether a particular radioactive nucleus decays within a specified time interval, the direction of an x-ray emitted by an electron striking the target of an x-ray tube, whether a particular x ray passes through a patient to reach the film cassette of an x-ray machine, and whether a gamma ray incident upon a scintillation camera crystal is detected are all random phenomena. Therefore, all radiation measurements, including medical imaging, are subject to random error. Counting statistics enable judgments of the validity of measurements that are subject to random error.

Characterization of Data

Accuracy and Precision

If a measurement is close to the correct value, it is said to be *accurate*. If measurements are reproducible, they are said to be *precise*. Precision does not imply accuracy; a set of measurements may be very close together (precise) but not close to the correct value (i.e., inaccurate). If a set of measurements differs from the correct value in a systematic fashion (systematic error), the data are said to be *biased*.

Measures of Central Tendency—Mean and Median

Two measures of central tendency of a set of measurements are the *mean* (average) and the median. The mean ($\bar{x}$) of a set of measurements is defined as follows:

$$\bar{x} = \frac{x_1 + x_2 + \ldots + x_N}{N} \qquad [17\text{-}6]$$

where N is the number of measurements.

To obtain the *median* of a set of measurements, they must first be put in order by size. The median is the middle measurement if the number of measurements is odd, and it is the average of the two midmost measurements if the number of measurements is even. For example, to obtain the median of the five measurements 8, 14, 5, 9, and 12, they are first sorted by size: 5, 8, 9, 12, and 14. The median is 9. The advantage of the median over the mean is that the median is less affected by outliers. An outlier is a measurement that is much greater or much less than the others.

Measures of Variability—Variance and Standard Deviation

The variance and standard deviation are measures of the variability (spread) of a set of measurements. The variance (σ^2) is determined from a set of measurements by subtracting the mean from each measurement, squaring the differences, summing the squares, and dividing by one less than the number of measurements:

$$\sigma^2 = \frac{(x_1 - \bar{x})^2 + (x_2 - \bar{x})^2 + \ldots + (x_N - \bar{x})^2}{N - 1} \qquad [17\text{-}7]$$

where N is the total number of measurements and $\bar{x}$ is the sample mean.

The *standard deviation* (σ) is the square root of the variance:

$$\sigma = \sqrt{\sigma^2} \qquad [17\text{-}8]$$

The *fractional standard deviation* (also referred to as the *fractional error* or *coefficient of variation*) is the standard deviation divided by the mean:

$$\text{Fractional standard deviation} = \sigma / \bar{x} \qquad [17\text{-}9]$$

Probability Distribution Functions for Binary Processes

Binary Processes

A *trial* is an event that may have more than one outcome. A *binary process* is a process in which a trial can only have two outcomes, one of which is arbitrarily called a *success*. A toss of a coin is a binary process. The toss of a die can be considered a binary process if, for example, a "two" is selected as a success and any other outcome is considered to be a failure. Whether a particular radioactive nucleus decays during a specified time interval is a binary process. Whether a particular x-ray or gamma ray is detected by a radiation detector is a binary process. Table 17-2 lists examples of binary processes.

A measurement consists of counting the number of successes from a specified number of trials. Tossing ten coins and counting the number of "heads" is a measurement. Placing a radioactive sample on a detector and recording the number of events detected is a measurement.

TABLE 17-2 BINARY PROCESSES

TRIAL	DEFINITION OF A SUCCESS	PROBABILITY OF A SUCCESS
Toss of a coin	"Heads"	1/2
Toss of a die	"A four"	1/6
Observation of a radioactive nucleus for a time "t"	It decays	$1 - e^{-\lambda t}$
Observation of a detector of efficiency E placed near a radioactive nucleus for a time "t"	A count	$E(1 - e^{-\lambda t})$

Source: Adapted from Knoll GF. *Radiation detection and measurement*, 4th ed. New York, NY: John Wiley, 2010.

Probability Distribution Functions—Binomial, Poisson, and Gaussian

A probability distribution function (pdf) describes the probability of obtaining each outcome from a measurement—for example, the probability of obtaining six "heads" in a throw of ten coins. There are three probability distribution functions relevant to binary processes—the binomial, the Poisson, and the Gaussian (normal). The binomial distribution exactly describes the probability of each outcome from a measurement of a binary process:

$$P(x) = \frac{N!}{x!(N-x)!} p^x (1-p)^{N-x} \qquad [17\text{-}10]$$

where N is the total number of trials in a measurement, p is the probability of success in a single trial, and x is the number of successes. The mathematical notation $N!$, called *factorial notation*, is simply shorthand for the product

$$N! = N \cdot (N-1) \cdot (N-2) \cdots 3 \cdot 2 \cdot 1 \qquad [17\text{-}11]$$

For example, $5! = 5\cdot4\cdot3\cdot2\cdot1 = 120$. If we wish to know the probability of obtaining two heads in a toss of four coins, $x = 2$, $N = 4$, and $p = 0.5$. The probability of obtaining two heads is

$$P(two\text{-}heads) = \frac{4!}{2!(4-2)!}(0.5)^2(1-0.5)^{4-2} = 0.375$$

Figure 17-28 is a graph of the binomial distribution. It can be shown that the sum of the probabilities of all outcomes for the binomial distribution is 1.0 and that the mean ($\bar{x}$) and standard deviation (σ) of the binomial distribution are as follows:

$$\bar{x} = pN \quad \text{and} \quad \sigma = \sqrt{pN(1-p)} \qquad [17\text{-}12]$$

If the probability of a success in a trial is much less than 1 (not true for a toss of a coin, but true for most radiation measurements), the standard deviation is approximated by the following:

$$\sigma = \sqrt{pN(1-p)} \approx \sqrt{pN} = \sqrt{\bar{x}} \qquad [17\text{-}13]$$

Because of the factorials in Equation 17-10, it is difficult to use if either x or N is large. The Poisson and Gaussian distributions are approximations to the binomial pdf that are often used when x or N is large. Figure 17-29 shows a Gaussian distribution.

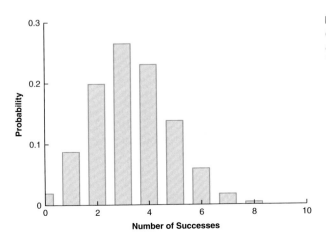

■ **FIGURE 17-28** Binomial probability distribution function when the probability of a success in a single trial (*p*) is 1/3 and the number of trials (*N*) is 10.

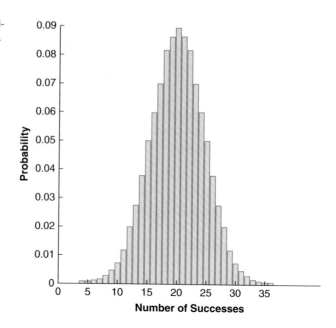

■ **FIGURE 17-29** Gaussian probability distribution function for pN = 20.

Estimating the Uncertainty of a Single Measurement

Estimated Standard Deviation

The standard deviation can be estimated, as previously described, by making several measurements and applying Equations 17-7 and 17-8. Nevertheless, if the process being measured is a binary process, the standard deviation can be estimated from a single measurement. The single measurement is probably close to the mean. Because the standard deviation is approximately the square root of the mean, it is also approximately the square root of the single measurement:

$$\sigma \approx \sqrt{x} \qquad [17\text{-}14]$$

where x is the single measurement. The fractional standard deviation of a single measurement may also be estimated as:

$$\text{Fractional error} = \frac{\sigma}{x} \approx \frac{\sqrt{x}}{x} = \frac{1}{\sqrt{x}} \qquad [17\text{-}15]$$

For example, a single measurement of a radioactive source yields 1,256 counts. The estimated standard deviation is

$$\sigma \approx \sqrt{1,256 \text{ cts}} = 35.4 \text{ cts}$$

The fractional standard deviation is estimated as

$$\text{Fractional error} = 35.4 \text{ cts}/1,256 \text{ cts} = 0.028 = 2.8\%$$

Table 17-3 lists the estimated fractional errors for various numbers of counts. The fractional error decreases with the number of counts.

Confidence Intervals

Table 17-4 lists intervals about a measurement, called *confidence intervals*, for which the probability of containing the true mean is specified. There is a 68.3% probability than the true mean is within one standard deviation (1 σ) of a measurement, a 95% probability

TABLE 17-3 FRACTIONAL ERRORS (PERCENT STANDARD DEVIATIONS) FOR SEVERAL NUMBERS OF COUNTS

COUNT	FRACTIONAL ERROR (%)
100	10.0
1,000	3.2
10,000	1.0
100,000	0.32

that it is within 2 σ of a measurement, and a 99.7% probability that it is within 3 σ of a measurement, assuming that the measurements follow a gaussian distribution.

For example, a count of 853 is obtained. Determine the interval about this count in which there is a 95% probability of finding the true mean.

First, the standard deviation is estimated as

$$\sigma \approx \sqrt{853 \text{ cts}} = 29.2 \text{ cts}$$

From Table 17-4, the 95% confidence interval is determined as follows:

$$853 \text{ cts} \pm 1.96 \ \sigma = 853 \text{ cts} \pm 1.96 \ (29.2 \text{ cts}) = 853 \text{ cts} \pm 57.2 \text{ cts}$$

So, the 95% confidence interval ranges from 796 to 910 counts.

Propagation of Error

In nuclear medicine, calculations are frequently performed using numbers that incorporate random error. It is often necessary to estimate the uncertainty in the results of these calculations. Although the standard deviation of a count may be estimated by simply taking its square root, it is incorrect to calculate the standard deviation of the result of a calculation by taking its square root. Instead, the standard deviations of the actual counts must first be calculated and entered into propagation of error equations to obtain the standard deviation of the result.

Multiplication or Division of a Number with Error by a Number without Error

It is often necessary to multiply or divide a number containing random error by a number that does not contain random error. For example, to calculate a count rate, a

TABLE 17-4 CONFIDENCE INTERVALS

INTERVAL ABOUT MEASUREMENT	PROBABILITY THAT MEAN IS WITHIN INTERVAL (%)
$\pm 0.674\sigma$	50.0
$\pm 1\sigma$	68.3
$\pm 1.64\sigma$	90.0
$\pm 1.96\sigma$	95.0
$\pm 2.58\sigma$	99.0
$\pm 3\sigma$	99.7

Source: Adapted from Knoll GF. *Radiation detection and measurement,* 4th ed. New York, NY: John Wiley, 2010.

count (which incorporates random error) is divided by a counting time (which does not involve significant random error). If a number x has a standard deviation σ and is multiplied by a number c without random error, the standard deviation of the product cx is $c\sigma$. If a number x has a standard deviation σ and is divided by a number c without random error, the standard deviation of the quotient x/c is σ/c.

For example, a 5-min count of a radioactive sample yields 952 counts. The count rate is 952 cts/5 min = 190 cts/min. The standard deviation and percent standard deviation of the count are

$$\sigma \approx \sqrt{952 \text{ cts}} = 30.8 \text{ cts}$$

$$\text{Fractional error} = 30.8 \text{ cts}/952 \text{ cts} = 0.032 = 3.2\%$$

The standard deviation of the count rate is

$$\sigma = 30.8 \text{ cts}/5 \text{ min} = 6.16 \text{ cts/min}$$

$$\text{Fractional error} = 6.16 \text{ cts}/190 \text{ cts} = 3.2\%$$

Notice that the percent standard deviation is not affected when a number is multiplied or divided by a number without random error.

Addition or Subtraction of Numbers with Error

It is often necessary to add or subtract numbers with random error. For example, a background count may be subtracted from a count of a radioactive sample. Whether two numbers are added or subtracted, the same equation is used to calculate the standard deviation of the result, as shown in Table 17-5.

For example, a count of a radioactive sample yields 1,952 counts, and a background count with the sample removed from the detector yields 1,451 counts.

The count of the sample, corrected for background, is

$$1,952 \text{ cts} -1,451 \text{ cts} = 501 \text{ cts}$$

The standard deviation and percent standard deviation of the original sample count are

$$\sigma_{s+b} \approx \sqrt{1,952 \text{ cts}} = 44.2 \text{ cts}$$

$$\text{Fractional error} = 44.2 \text{ cts}/1,952 \text{ cts} = 2.3\%$$

TABLE 17-5   PROPAGATION OF ERROR EQUATIONS

DESCRIPTION	OPERATION	STANDARD DEVIATION
Multiplication of a number with random error by a number without random error	cx	$c\sigma$
Division of a number with random error by a number without random error	x/c	σ/c
Addition of two numbers containing random errors	$x_1 + x_2$	$\sqrt{\sigma_1^2 + \sigma_2^2}$
Subtraction of two numbers containing random errors	$x_1 - x_2$	$\sqrt{\sigma_1^2 + \sigma_2^2}$

Note: c is a number without random error, σ is the standard deviation of x, σ_1 is the standard deviation of x_1, and σ_2 is the standard deviation of x_2.

The standard deviation and percent standard deviation of the background count are

$$\sigma_b \approx \sqrt{1,451 \text{ cts}} = 38.1 \text{ cts}$$

$$\text{Fractional error} = 38.1 \text{ cts}/1,451 \text{ cts} = 2.6\%$$

The standard deviation and percent standard deviation of the sample count corrected for background are

$$\sigma_s \approx \sqrt{(44.2 \text{ cts})^2 + (38.3 \text{cts})^2} = 58.3 \text{ cts}$$

$$\text{Fractional error} = 58.1 \text{ cts}/501 \text{ cts} = 11.6\%$$

Note that the fractional error of the difference is much larger than the fractional error of either count. The fractional error of the difference of two numbers of similar magnitude can be much larger than the fractional errors of the two numbers.

Combination Problems

It is sometimes necessary to perform mathematical operations in series, for example, to subtract two numbers and then to divide the difference by another number. The standard deviation is calculated for each intermediate result in the series by entering the standard deviations from the previous step into the appropriate propagation of error equation in Table 17-5.

For example, a 5-min count of a radioactive sample yields 1,290 counts and a 5-min background count yields 451 counts. What is the count rate due to the sample alone and its standard deviation?

First, the count is corrected for background:

$$\text{Count} = 1,290 \text{ cts} - 451 \text{ cts} = 839 \text{ cts}$$

The estimated standard deviation of each count and the difference are calculated:

$$\sigma_{s+b} \approx \sqrt{1,290 \text{ cts}} = 35.9 \text{ cts and } \sigma_b \approx \sqrt{451 \text{ cts}} = 21.2 \text{ cts}$$

$$\sigma_s \approx \sqrt{(35.9 \text{ cts})^2 + (21.2 \text{ cts})^2} = 41.7 \text{ cts}$$

Finally, the count rate due to the source alone and its standard deviation are calculated:

$$\text{Count rate} = 839 \text{ cts}/5 \text{ min} = 168 \text{ cts/min}$$

$$\sigma_s/c = 41.7 \text{ cts}/5 \text{ min} = 8.3 \text{ cts/min}$$

SUGGESTED READING

Attix FH. *Introduction to radiological physics and radiation dosimetry*, New York, NY: John Wiley, 1986

Cherry, R., Simon et.al. *Physics in Nuclear Medicine*. 4th ed., Philadelphia: Saunders, 2011.

Knoll GF. *Radiation detection and measurement*, 4th ed. New York, NY: John Wiley, 2010.

Patton JA, Harris CC. Gamma well counter. In: Sandler MP, et al., eds. *Diagnostic nuclear medicine*, 3rd ed. Baltimore, MD: Williams & Wilkins, 1996:59–65.

Ranger NT. The AAPM/RSNA physics tutorial for residents: radiation detectors in nuclear medicine. *Radiographics* 1999;19:481–502.

Rzeszotarski MS. The AAPM/RSNA physics tutorial for residents: counting statistics. *Radiographics* 1999;19:765–782.

CHAPTER 18

Nuclear Imaging—The Scintillation Camera

Nuclear imaging produces images of the distributions of radionuclides in patients. Because charged particles from radioactivity in a patient are almost entirely absorbed within the patient, nuclear imaging uses gamma rays, characteristic x-rays (usually from radionuclides that decay by electron capture), or annihilation photons (from positron-emitting radionuclides) to form images.

To form a projection image, an imaging system must determine not only the photon flux density (number of x- or gamma rays per unit area) at each point in the image plane but also the directions of the detected photons. In x-ray transmission imaging, the primary photons travel known paths diverging radially from a point (the focal spot of the x-ray tube). In contrast, the x- or gamma rays from the radionuclide in each volume element of a patient are emitted isotropically (equally in all directions). Nuclear medicine instruments designed to image gamma- and x-ray–emitting radionuclides use *collimators* that permit photons following certain trajectories to reach the detector but absorb most of the rest. A heavy price is paid for using collimation—the vast majority (typically well over 99.95%) of emitted photons is wasted. Thus, collimation, although necessary for the formation of projection images, severely limits the performance of these devices. Instruments for imaging positron (β^+)-emitting radionuclides can avoid collimation by exploiting the unique properties of annihilation radiation to determine the directions of the photons.

The earliest widely successful nuclear medicine imaging device, the rectilinear scanner, which dominated nuclear imaging from the early 1950s through the late 1960s, used a moving radiation detector to sample the photon fluence at a small region of the image plane at a time[1]. This was improved upon by the use of a large-area position-sensitive detector (a detector indicating the location of each interaction) to sample simultaneously the photon fluence over the entire image plane. The Anger scintillation camera, which currently dominates nuclear imaging, is an example of the latter method. The scanning detector system is less expensive, but the position-sensitive detector system permits more rapid image acquisition and has replaced single scanning detector systems.

Nuclear imaging devices using gas-filled detectors (such as multiwire proportional counters) have been developed. Unfortunately, the low densities of gases, even when pressurized, yield low detection efficiencies for the x- and gamma-ray energies commonly used in nuclear imaging. To obtain a sufficient number of interactions to form statistically valid images without imparting an excessive radiation dose to the patient, nearly all nuclear imaging devices in routine clinical use utilize solid inorganic scintillators as detectors because of their superior detection efficiency. Efforts are being made to develop nuclear imaging devices using semiconductor detectors. This will require the development of a high atomic number, high-density

---

[1]Cassen B, Curtis L, Reed A, Libby RL. Instrumentation for 1-131 use in medical studies. Nucleonics 1951: 9: 46–9.

semiconductor detector of sufficient thickness for absorbing the x- and gamma rays commonly used in nuclear imaging and that can be operated at room temperature. The leading detector material to date is cadmium zinc telluride (CZT). A small field of view (FOV) camera using CZT semiconductor detectors has been developed.

The attenuation of x-rays in the patient is useful in radiography, fluoroscopy, and x-ray computed tomography and, in fact, is necessary for image formation. However, in nuclear imaging, attenuation is usually a hindrance; it causes a loss of information and, especially when it is very nonuniform, it is a source of artifacts.

The quality of a nuclear medicine image is determined not only by the performance of the nuclear imaging device but also by the properties of the radiopharmaceutical used. For example, the ability of a radiopharmaceutical to preferentially accumulate in a lesion of interest largely determines the smallest such lesion that can be detected. Furthermore, the dosimetric properties of a radiopharmaceutical determine the maximal activity that can be administered to a patient, which in turn affects the amount of statistical noise (quantum mottle) in the image and the spatial resolution. For example, in the 1950s and 1960s, radiopharmaceuticals labeled with I-131 and Hg-203 were commonly used. The long half-lives of these radionuclides and their beta particle emissions limited administered activities to approximately 150 microcuries (μCi). These low administered activities and the high-energy gamma rays of these radionuclides required the use of collimators providing poor spatial resolution. Many modern radiopharmaceuticals are labeled with technetium-99m (Tc-99m), whose short half-life (6.01 h) and isomeric transition decay (~88% of the energy is emitted as 140-keV gamma rays; only ~12% is given to conversion electrons and other emissions unlikely to escape the patient) permit activities of up to about 35 millicuries (mCi) to be administered. The high gamma-ray flux from such an activity permits the use of high-resolution (low-efficiency) collimators. Radiopharmaceuticals are discussed in Chapter 16.

18.1 Planar Nuclear Imaging: The Anger Scintillation Camera

The Anger gamma scintillation camera, developed by Hal O. Anger at the Donner Laboratory in Berkeley, California, in the 1950s, is by far the most common nuclear medicine imaging device.[2] However, it did not begin to replace the rectilinear scanner significantly until the late 1960s, when its spatial resolution became comparable to that of the rectilinear scanner and Tc-99m-labeled radiopharmaceuticals, for which it is ideally suited, became commonly used in nuclear medicine. Most of the advantages of the scintillation camera over the rectilinear scanner stem from its ability simultaneously to collect data over a large area of the patient, rather than one small area at a time. This permits the more rapid acquisition of images and enables dynamic studies that depict the redistribution of radionuclides to be performed. Because the scintillation camera wastes fewer x- or gamma rays than earlier imaging devices, its images have less quantum mottle (statistical noise) and it can be used with higher resolution collimators, thereby producing images of better spatial resolution. The scintillation camera is also more flexible in its positioning, permitting images to be obtained from almost any angle. Although it can produce satisfactory images using x- or gamma rays ranging in energy from about 70 keV (Tl-201) to 364 keV (I-131) or perhaps even 511 keV (F-18), the scintillation camera is best suited for imaging photons with energies in the range of 100 to 200 keV. Figure 18-1 shows a modern scintillation camera.

---

[2]Hal O. Anger, Scintillation Camera, Review of Scientific Instruments, 29, 1958, 27–33.

■ **FIGURE 18-1** Modern dual rectangular head scintillation camera. The two heads are in a 90 degree orientation for cardiac SPECT imaging (discussed in Chapter 19). (Courtesy of Siemens Medical Solutions.)

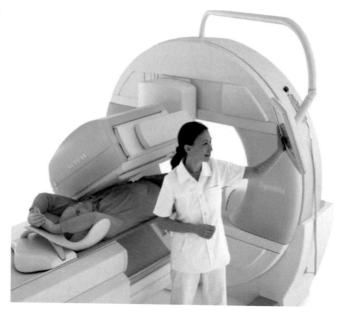

Scintillation cameras of other designs have been devised, and one, the multicrystal scintillation camera (briefly described later in this chapter), achieved limited commercial success. However, the superior performance of the Anger camera for most applications has caused it to dominate nuclear imaging. The term *scintillation camera* will refer exclusively to the Anger scintillation camera throughout this chapter.

Design and Principles of Operation

Detector and Electronic Circuits

A scintillation camera head (Fig. 18-2) contains a disk-shaped (mostly on older cameras) or rectangular thallium-activated sodium iodide [NaI(Tl)] crystal, typically 0.95 cm (⅜ inch) thick, optically coupled to a large number (typically 37 to 91) of 5.1- to 7.6-cm (2- to 3-inch) diameter photomultiplier tubes (PMTs). PMTs and NaI(Tl) scintillation crystals were described in Chapter 17. The NaI(Tl) crystals of modern cameras have large areas; the rectangular crystals of one manufacturer are 59 x 44.5 cm (23 x 17.4 in.), with a field-of-view of about 53 by 39 cm. Some

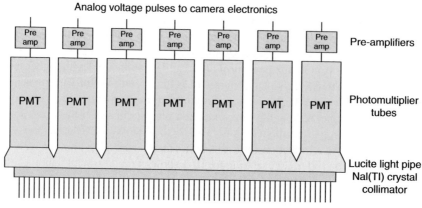

■ **FIGURE 18-2** Scintillation camera detector.

camera designs incorporate a Lucite light pipe between the glass cover of the crystal and PMTs; in others, the PMTs are directly coupled to the glass cover. In most cameras, a preamplifier is connected to the output of each PMT. Between the patient and the crystal is a collimator, usually made of lead, that only allows x- or gamma rays approaching from certain directions to reach the crystal. The collimator is essential; a scintillation camera without a collimator does not generate meaningful images. Figure 18-2 shows a parallel-hole collimator.

The lead walls, called *septa*, between the holes in the collimator absorb most photons approaching the collimator from directions that are not aligned with the holes. Most photons approaching the collimator from a nearly perpendicular direction pass through the holes; many of these are absorbed in the sodium iodide crystal, causing the emission of visible light and ultraviolet (UV) radiation. The light and UV photons are converted into electrical signals and amplified by the PMTs. These signals are further amplified by the preamplifiers (preamps). The amplitude of the electrical pulse produced by each PMT is proportional to the amount of light it received following an x- or gamma-ray interaction in the crystal.

Because the collimator septa intercept most photons approaching the camera along paths not aligned with the collimator holes, the pattern of photon interactions in the crystal forms a two-dimensional projection of the three-dimensional activity distribution in the patient. The PMTs closest to each photon interaction in the crystal receive more light than those that are more distant, causing them to produce larger voltage pulses. The relative amplitudes of the pulses from the PMTs following each interaction contain sufficient information to determine the location of the interaction in the plane of the crystal within a few mm.

Early scintillation cameras formed images on photographic film using only analog electronic circuitry. In the late 1970s, digital circuitry began to be used for some functions. Modern scintillation cameras have an analog-to-digital converter (ADC) for the signal from the preamplifier (preamp) following each PMT (Fig. 18-3). ADCs are described in Chapter 5. The remaining circuits used for signal processing and image formation are digital. The digitized signals from the preamps are sent to two circuits. The position circuit receives the signals from the individual preamps after each x- or gamma-ray interaction in the crystal and, by determining the centroid of these signals, produced an X-position signal and a Y-position signal that together specify the position of the interaction in the plane of the crystal. The summing circuit adds the signals from the individual preamps to produce an energy (Z) signal proportional in amplitude to the total energy deposited in the crystal by the interaction. These digital signals are then sent to correction circuits, described later in this chapter, to correct position-dependent systematic errors in event position assignment and energy determination (see Spatial Linearity and Uniformity, below). These correction circuits greatly improve the spatial linearity and uniformity of the images. The corrected energy (Z) signal is sent to an energy discrimination circuit. An interaction in the camera's crystal is recorded as a count in the image only if the energy (Z) signal is within a preset energy window. Scintillation cameras permit as many as four energy windows to be set for imaging radionuclides, such as Ga-67 and In-111, which emit useful photons of more than one energy. Following energy discrimination, the X- and Y-position signals are sent to a digital computer, where they are formed into a digital projection image, as described in Section 18.2 below, that can be displayed on a monitor.

Collimators

The collimator of a scintillation camera forms the projection image by permitting x- or gamma-ray photons approaching the camera from certain directions to reach the

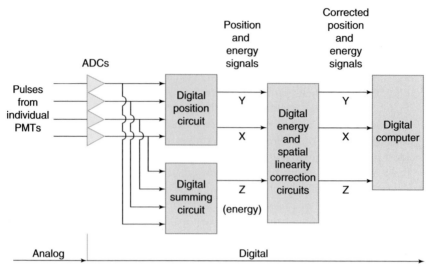

■ **FIGURE 18-3** Electronic circuits of a modern digital scintillation camera. An actual scintillation camera has many more than four PMTs and ADCs.

crystal while absorbing most of the other photons. Collimators are made of high atomic number, high-density materials, usually lead. The most commonly used collimator is the *parallel-hole collimator*, which contains thousands of parallel holes (Fig. 18-4). The holes may be round, square, or triangular; however, most state-of-the-art collimators have hexagonal holes and are usually made from lead foil, although some are cast. The partitions between the holes are called *septa*. The septa must be thick enough to absorb most of the photons incident upon them. For this reason, collimators designed

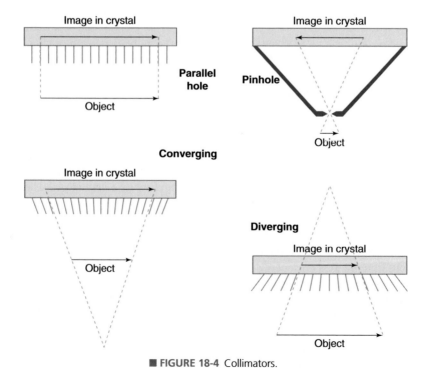

■ **FIGURE 18-4** Collimators.

for use with radionuclides that emit higher energy photons have thicker septa. There is an inherent compromise between the spatial resolution and efficiency (sensitivity) of collimators. Modifying a collimator to improve its spatial resolution (e.g., by reducing the size of the holes or lengthening the collimator) reduces its efficiency. Most scintillation cameras are provided with a selection of parallel-hole collimators. These may include "low-energy, high-sensitivity"; "low-energy, all-purpose" (LEAP); "low-energy, high-resolution"; "medium-energy" (suitable for Ga-67 and In-111), "high-energy" (for I-131); and "ultra–high-energy" (for F 18) collimators. The size of the image produced by a parallel-hole collimator is not affected by the distance of the object from the collimator. However, its spatial resolution degrades rapidly with increasing collimator-to-object distance. The field-of-view (FOV) of a parallel-hole collimator does not change with distance from the collimator.

A *pinhole collimator* (Fig. 18-4) is commonly used to produce magnified views of small objects, such as the thyroid gland or a hip joint. It consists of a small (typically 3- to 5-mm diameter) hole in a piece of lead or tungsten mounted at the apex of a leaded cone. Its function is identical to the pinhole in a pinhole photographic camera. As shown in the figure, the pinhole collimator produces a magnified image whose orientation is reversed. The magnification of the pinhole collimator decreases as an object is moved away from the pinhole. If an object is as far from the pinhole as the pinhole is from the crystal of the camera, the object is not magnified and, if the object is moved yet farther from the pinhole, it is minified. (Clinical imaging is not performed at these distances.) There are pitfalls in the use of pinhole collimators due to the decreasing magnification with distance. For example, a thyroid nodule deep in the mediastinum can appear to be in the thyroid itself. Pinhole collimators are used extensively in pediatric nuclear medicine. On some pinhole collimators, the part containing the hole can be removed and replaced with a part with a hole of another diameter; this allows the hole size to be varied for different clinical applications.

A *converging collimator* (Fig. 18-4) has many holes, all aimed at a focal point in front of the camera. As shown in the figure, the converging collimator magnifies the image. The magnification increases as the object is moved away from the collimator. A disadvantage of a converging collimator is that its FOV decreases with distance from the collimator. A *diverging collimator* (Fig. 18-4) has many holes aimed at a focal point behind the camera. It produces a minified image in which the amount of minification increases as the object is moved away from the camera. A diverging collimator may be used to image a part of a patient using a camera whose FOV, if a parallel-hole collimator were used, would be smaller than the body part to be imaged. For example, a diverging collimator could enable a mobile scintillation camera with a 25- or 30-cm diameter crystal to perform a lung study of a patient in the intensive care unit. If a diverging collimator is reversed on a camera, it becomes a converging collimator. The diverging collimator is seldom used today, because it has inferior imaging characteristics to the parallel-hole collimator and the large rectangular crystals of most modern cameras render it unnecessary. The converging collimator is also seldom used; its imaging characteristics are superior, in theory, to the parallel-hole collimator, but its decreasing FOV with distance and varying magnification with distance have discouraged its use. However, a hybrid of the parallel-hole and converging collimator, called a *fan-beam collimator*, may be used in single photon emission computed tomography (SPECT) to take advantage of the favorable imaging properties of the converging collimator (see Chapter 19).

Many special-purpose collimators, such as the seven-pinhole collimator, have been developed. However, most of them have not enjoyed wide acceptance. The performance characteristics of parallel-hole, pinhole, and fan-beam collimators are discussed below (see Performance).

Principles of Image Formation

In nuclear imaging, which can also be called emission imaging, the photons from each point in the patient are emitted isotropically. Figure 18-5 shows the fates of the x- and gamma rays emitted in a patient being imaged. Some photons escape the patient without interaction, some scatter within the patient before escaping, and some are absorbed within the patient. Many of the photons escaping the patient are not detected because they are emitted in directions away from the image receptor. The collimator absorbs the vast majority of those photons that reach it. As a result, only a tiny fraction of the emitted photons (about 1 to 2 in 10,000 for typical low-energy parallel-hole collimators) has trajectories permitting passage through the collimator holes; thus, well over 99.9% of the photons emitted during imaging are wasted. Some photons penetrate the septa of the collimator without interaction. Of those reaching the crystal, some are absorbed in the crystal, some scatter from the crystal, and some pass through the crystal without interaction. The relative probabilities of these events depend on the energies of the photons and the thickness of the crystal. Of those photons absorbed in the crystal, some are absorbed by a single photoelectric absorption, whereas others undergo one or more Compton scatters before a photoelectric absorption. It is also possible for two photons to interact simultaneously with the crystal; if the energy (Z) signal from the coincident interactions is within the energy window of the energy discrimination circuit, the result will be a single count mispositioned in the image. The fraction of simultaneous interactions increases with the interaction rate of the camera.

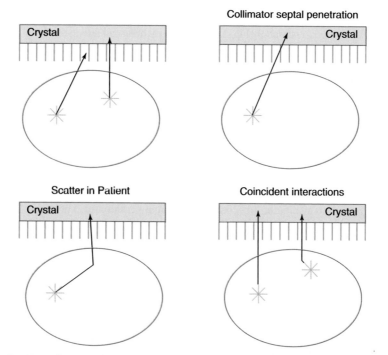

■ FIGURE 18-5 Ways that x- and gamma rays interact with a scintillation camera. All of these, other than the ones depicted in the upper left, cause a loss of contrast and spatial resolution and add statistical noise. However, interactions by photons that have scattered though large angles and many coincident interactions are rejected by pulse height discrimination circuits.

Interactions in the crystal of photons that have been scattered in the patient, photons that have penetrated the collimator septa, photons that undergo one or more scatters in the crystal, and coincident interactions reduce the spatial resolution and image contrast and increase random noise. The function of the camera's energy discrimination circuits (also known as pulse height analyzers) is to reduce this loss of resolution and contrast by rejecting photons that scatter in the patient or result in coincident interactions. Unfortunately, the limited energy resolution of the camera causes a wide photopeak, and low-energy photons can scatter through large angles with only a small energy loss. For example, a 140-keV photon scattering 45 degrees will only lose 7.4% of its energy. An energy window that encompasses most of the photopeak will unfortunately still accept a significant fraction of the scattered photons and coincident interactions.

It is instructive to compare single photon emission imaging with x-ray transmission imaging (Table 18-1). In x-ray transmission imaging, including radiography and fluoroscopy, an image is projected on the image receptor because the x-rays originate from a very small source that approximates a point. In comparison, the photons in nuclear imaging are emitted isotropically throughout the patient and therefore collimation is necessary to form a projection image. Furthermore, in x-ray transmission imaging, x-rays that have scattered in the patient can be distinguished from primary x-rays by their directions and thus can be largely removed by grids. In emission imaging, primary photons cannot be distinguished from scattered photons by their directions. The collimator removes about the same fraction of scattered photons as it does primary photons and, unlike the grid in x-ray transmission imaging, does not reduce the fraction of counts in the resultant image due to scatter. Scattered photons in nuclear imaging can only be differentiated from primary photons by energy, because scattering reduces photon energy. In emission imaging, energy discrimination is used to reduce the fraction of counts in the image caused by scattered radiation. Finally, nuclear imaging devices must use pulse mode (the signal from each interaction is processed separately) for event localization and so that interaction-by-interaction energy discrimination can be employed; x-ray transmission imaging systems have photon fluxes that are too high to allow a radiation detector to detect, discriminate, and record on a photon-by-photon basis.

Alternative Camera Design—the Multielement Camera

An alternative to the Anger scintillation camera for nuclear medicine imaging is the multi-detector element camera. An image receptor of such a camera is a two-dimensional array of many small independent detector elements. Such cameras are used with collimators for image formation, as are Anger scintillation cameras.

TABLE 18-1 COMPARISON OF SINGLE-PHOTON NUCLEAR IMAGING WITH X-RAY TRANSMISSION IMAGING

	PRINCIPLE OF IMAGE FORMATION	SCATTER REJECTION	PULSE OR CURRENT MODE
X-ray transmission imaging	Point source	Grid or air gap	Current
Scintillation camera	Collimation	Pulse height discrimination	Pulse

One such camera, the Baird Atomic System 77, achieved limited clinical acceptance in the 1970s and early 1980s. It consisted of 294 NaI(Tl) scintillation crystals arranged in an array of 14 rows and 21 columns. A clever arrangement of light pipes was used to route the light from the crystals to 35 PMTs, with all crystals in a row connected to one PMT and all crystals in a column being connected to another PMT. Light signals being simultaneously received by the PMT for a column and another PMT for a row identified the crystal in which a gamma ray or x-ray interaction occurred. Since that time, other multielement cameras have been developed. Each detector element of one design is a CsI(Tl) scintillation crystal optically coupled to a single photodiode and, in another design, each detector element is a CZT semiconductor detector.

The intrinsic spatial resolution of a multi-element detector camera is determined by the physical dimensions of the independent detector elements. An advantage to the multielement camera design is that very high interaction rates can be tolerated with only limited dead-time losses because of the independent detectors in the image receptor. A disadvantage is the complexity of the electronics needed to process the signals from such a large number of independent detectors.

Performance

Measures of Performance

Measures of the performance of a scintillation camera with the collimator attached are called *system* or *extrinsic* measurements. Measures of camera performance with the collimator removed are called *intrinsic* measurements. System measurements give the best indication of clinical performance, but intrinsic measurements are often more useful for comparing the performance of different cameras, because they isolate camera performance from collimator performance.

Uniformity is a measure of a camera's response to uniform irradiation of the detector surface. The ideal response is a perfectly uniform image. Intrinsic uniformity is usually measured by placing a point radionuclide source (typically 150 µCi of Tc-99m) in front of the uncollimated camera. The source should be placed at least four times the largest dimension of the crystal away to ensure uniform irradiation of the camera surface and at least five times away, if the uniformity image is to be analyzed quantitatively using a computer. System uniformity, which reveals collimator as well as camera defects, is assessed by placing a uniform planar radionuclide source in front of the collimated camera. Solid planar sealed sources of Co-57 (typically 5 to 10 mCi when new) and planar sources that may be filled with a Tc-99m solution are commercially available. A planar source should be large enough to cover the crystal of the camera. The uniformity of the resultant images may be analyzed by a computer or evaluated visually.

Spatial resolution is a measure of a camera's ability to accurately portray spatial variations in activity concentration and to distinguish as separate radioactive objects in close proximity. The *system spatial resolution* is evaluated by acquiring an image of a line source, such as a capillary tube filled with Tc-99m, using a computer interfaced to the collimated camera and determining the line spread function (LSF). The LSF, described in Chapter 4, is a cross-sectional profile of the image of a line source. The full-width-at-half-maximum (FWHM), the full-width-at-tenth-maximum, and the modulation transfer function (described in Chapter 4) may all be derived from the LSF.

The system spatial resolution, if measured in air so that scatter is not present, is determined by the collimator resolution and the intrinsic resolution of the camera.

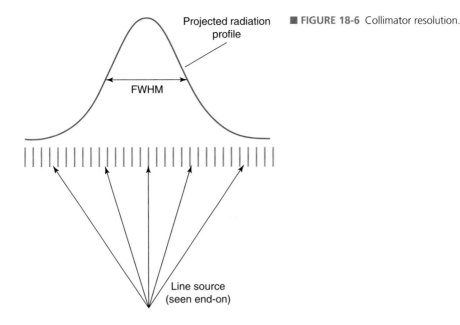

■ **FIGURE** 18-6 Collimator resolution.

The *collimator resolution* is defined as the FWHM of the radiation transmitted through the collimator from a line source (Fig. 18-6). It is not directly measured, but calculated from the system and intrinsic resolutions. The *intrinsic resolution* is determined quantitatively by acquiring an image with a sheet of lead containing one or more thin slits placed against the uncollimated camera using a point source. The point source should be positioned at least five times the largest dimension of the camera's crystal away. The system (R_S), collimator (R_C), and intrinsic (R_I) resolutions, as indicated by the FWHMs of the LSFs, are related by the following equation:

$$R_S = \sqrt{R_C^2 + R_I^2}$$ [18-1]

Some types of collimators magnify (converging, pinhole) or minify (diverging) the image. For these collimators, the system and collimator resolutions should be corrected for the collimator magnification, so that they refer to distances in the object rather than distances in the camera crystal:

$$R_S' = \sqrt{R_C'^2 + (R_I / m)^2}$$ [18-2]

where $R_S' = R_S/m$ is the system resolution corrected for magnification, $R_C' = R_C/m$ is the collimator resolution corrected for magnification, and m is the collimator magnification (image size in crystal/object size). The collimator magnification is determined as follows:

$m = 1.0$ for parallel-hole collimators
$m = $ (pinhole-to-crystal distance)/(object-to-pinhole distance) for pinhole collimators
$m = f/(f - x)$ for converging collimators
$m = f/(f + x)$ for diverging collimators

where f is the distance from the crystal to the focal point of the collimator and x is the distance of the object from the crystal. It will be seen later in this section that the collimator and system resolutions degrade (FWHM of the LSF, corrected for collimator magnification, increases) with increasing distance between the line source and collimator.

As can be seen from Equation 18-2, collimator magnification reduces the deleterious effect of intrinsic spatial resolution on the overall system resolution. Geometric magnification in x-ray transmission imaging reduces the effect of image receptor blur for the same reason.

In routine practice, the intrinsic spatial resolution is semiquantitatively evaluated by imaging a parallel line or a four-quadrant bar phantom (Fig. 18-7) in contact with the camera face, using a planar radionuclide source if the camera is collimated or a distant point source if the collimator is removed, and visually noting the smallest bars that are resolved. By convention, the widths of the bars are the same as the widths of the spaces between the bars. The size of the smallest bars that are resolved is approximately related to the FWHM of the LSF:

$$(\text{FWHM of the LSF}) \approx 1.7 \times (\text{Size of smallest bars resolved}) \qquad [18\text{-}3]$$

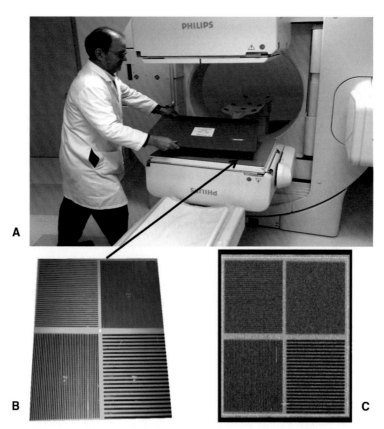

A

B

C

■ **FIGURE 18-7** Use of a bar phantom for evaluating spatial resolution. A plastic rectangular flood source containing up to10 mCi (370 MBq) of uniformly distributed Co-57 (**A**) is placed on top of the bar phantom (**B**), which is resting on top of the camera head collimator. The bar phantom has four quadrants, each consisting of parallel lead bars with a specific width and spacing between the bars. An image (**C**) is acquired with approximately 10 million counts and the lines are visually inspected for linearity and determination of closest spacing between the bars that can be seen resolved as separate lines. A typical four-quadrant bar phantom for a modern scintillation camera might have 2.0-, 2.5-, 3.0-, and 3.5-mm wide lead bars, with the widths of the spaces equal to the widths of the bars. This extrinsic resolution test (performed with the collimator attached to the camera) evaluates the system resolution. An intrinsic resolution test is performed with the collimator removed from the camera head. In this case, the bar phantom is placed against the crystal of the uncollimated camera head and irradiated by a point source containing 100 to 200 μCi (3.7 to 7.4 MBq) of Tc-99m in a syringe placed at least four camera crystal diameters away.

Spatial linearity (lack of spatial distortion) is a measure of the camera's ability to portray the shapes of objects accurately. It is determined from the images of a bar phantom, line source, or other phantom by assessing the straightness of the lines in the image. Spatial nonlinearities can significantly degrade the uniformity, as will be discussed later in this chapter.

Multienergy spatial registration, commonly called *multiple window spatial registration*, is a measure of the camera's ability to maintain the same image magnification, regardless of the energies deposited in the crystal by the incident x- or gamma rays. (Image magnification is defined as the distance between two points in the image divided by the actual distance between the two points in the object being imaged.) Higher energy x- and gamma-ray photons produce larger signals from the individual PMTs than do lower energy photons. The position circuit of the scintillation camera normalizes the X- and Y-position signals by the energy signal, so that the position signals are independent of the deposited energy. If a radionuclide emitting useful photons of several energies, such as Ga-67 (93-, 185-, and 300-keV gamma rays), is imaged and the normalization is not properly performed, the resultant image will be a superposition of images of different magnifications (Fig. 18-8). The multienergy spatial registration can be tested by imaging several point sources of Ga-67, offset from the center of the camera, using only one major gamma ray at a time. The centroid of the count distribution of each source should be at the same position in the image for all three gamma-ray energies.

The *system efficiency* (sensitivity) of a scintillation camera is the fraction of x- or gamma rays emitted by a source that produces counts in the image. The system efficiency is important because it, in conjunction with imaging time, determines the amount of quantum mottle (graininess) in the images. The system efficiency (E_s) is the product of three factors: the collimator efficiency (E_c), the intrinsic efficiency of the crystal (E_i), and the fraction (f) of interacting photons accepted by the energy discrimination circuits:

$$E_s = E_c \times E_i \times f \qquad \text{[18-4]}$$

The *collimator efficiency* is the fraction of photons emitted by a source that penetrate the collimator holes. In general, it is a function of the distance between the source and the collimator and the design of the collimator. The *intrinsic efficiency*, the fraction

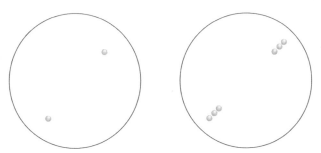

■ **FIGURE 18-8** Multienergy spatial registration. **Left.** A simulated image of two point sources of a radionuclide emitting gamma rays of three different energies, illustrating proper normalization of the X- and Y-position signals for deposited energy. **Right.** A simulated image of the same two point sources, showing improper adjustment of the energy normalization circuit. The maladjustment causes higher energy photons to produce larger X and Y values than lower energy photons interacting at the same position in the camera's crystal, resulting in multiple images of each point source. A less severe maladjustment would cause each point source to appear as an ellipse, rather than three discrete dots.

of photons penetrating the collimator that interact with the NaI(Tl) crystal, is determined by the thickness of the crystal and the energy of the photons:

$$E_i = 1 - e^{-\mu x} \qquad [18\text{-}5]$$

where μ is the linear attenuation coefficient of sodium iodide and x is the thickness of the crystal. The last two factors in Equation 18-4 can be combined to form the *photopeak efficiency*, defined as the fraction of photons reaching the crystal that produce counts in the photopeak of the energy spectrum:

$$E_p = E_i \times f \qquad [18\text{-}6]$$

This equation assumes that the window of the energy discrimination circuit has been adjusted to encompass the photopeak exactly. In theory, the system efficiency and each of its components range from zero to one. In reality, low-energy all-purpose parallel-hole collimators have efficiencies of about 2×10^{-4} and low-energy high-resolution parallel-hole collimators have efficiencies of about 1×10^{-4}.

The *energy resolution* of a scintillation camera is a measure of its ability to distinguish between interactions depositing different energies in its crystal. A camera with superior energy resolution is able to reject a larger fraction of photons that have scattered in the patient or have undergone coincident interactions, thereby producing images of better contrast and less relative random noise. The energy resolution is measured by exposing the camera to a point source of a radionuclide, usually Tc-99m, emitting monoenergetic photons and acquiring a spectrum of the energy (Z) pulses, using either the nuclear medicine computer interfaced to the camera, if it has the capability, or a multichannel analyzer. The energy resolution is calculated from the FWHM of the photopeak (see Pulse Height Spectroscopy in Chapter 17). The FWHM is divided by the energy of the photon (140 keV for Tc-99m) and is expressed as a percentage. A wider FWHM implies poorer energy resolution.

Scintillation cameras are operated in pulse mode (see Design and Principles of Operation, above) and therefore suffer from dead-time count losses at high interaction rates. They behave as paralyzable systems (see Chapter 17); the indicated count rate initially increases as the imaged activity increases, but ultimately reaches a maximum and decreases thereafter. The count-rate performance of a camera is usually specified by (1) the observed count rate at 20% count loss and (2) the maximal count rate. These count rates may be measured with or without scatter. Both are reduced when measured with scatter. Table 18-2 lists typical values for modern cameras. These high count rates are usually achieved by implementing a high count-rate mode that degrades the spatial and energy resolutions.

Some scintillation cameras can correctly process the PMT signals when two or more interactions occur simultaneously in the crystal, provided that the interactions are separated by sufficient distance. This significantly increases the number of interactions that are correctly registered at high interaction rates.

Design Factors Determining Performance

Intrinsic Spatial Resolution and Intrinsic Efficiency

The intrinsic spatial resolution of a scintillation camera is determined by the types of interactions by which the x- or gamma rays deposit energy in the camera's crystal and the statistics of the detection of the visible light photons emitted following these interactions. The most important of these is the random error associated

TABLE 18-2   TYPICAL INTRINSIC PERFORMANCE CHARACTERISTICS OF A MODERN SCINTILLATION CAMERA, MEASURED BY NEMA PROTOCOL

Intrinsic spatial resolution (FWHM of LSF for 140 keV)[a]	2.7–4.2 mm
Energy resolution (FWHM of photopeak for 140 keV photons)	9.2%–11%
Integral uniformity (max. pixel – min. pixel)/(max. pixel + min. pixel)	2%–5%
Absolute spatial linearity	Less than 1.5 mm
Observed count rate at 20% count loss (measured without scatter)	110,000–260,000 counts/s
Observed maximal count rate (measured without scatter)	170,000–500,000 counts/s

[a]Intrinsic spatial resolution is for a 0.95-cm (3/8-inch) thick crystal; thicker crystals cause slightly worse spatial resolution.
FWHM, full width at half maximum; LSF, line spread function; NEMA, National Electrical Manufacturers Association.

with the collection of ultraviolet (UV) and visible light photons and subsequent production of electrical signals by the PMTs. Approximately one UV or visible light photon is emitted in the NaI crystal for every 25 eV deposited by an x- or gamma ray. For example, when a 140-keV gamma ray is absorbed by the crystal, approximately 140,000/25 = 5,600 UV or visible light photons are produced. About two-thirds of these, approximately 3,700 photons, reach the photocathodes of the PMTs. Only about one out of every five of these causes an electron to escape a photocathode, giving rise to about 750 electrons. These electrons are divided among the PMTs, with the most being produced in the PMTs closest to the interaction. Thus, only a small number of photoelectrons is generated in any one PMT after an interaction. Because the processes by which the absorption of a gamma ray causes the release of electrons from a photocathode are random, the pulses from the PMTs after an interaction contain significant random errors that, in turn, cause errors in the X and Y signals produced by the position circuit of the camera and the energy (Z) signal. These random errors limit both the intrinsic spatial resolution and the energy resolution of the camera. The energy of the incident x- or gamma rays determines the amount of random error in the event localization process; higher energy photons provide lower relative random errors and therefore superior intrinsic spatial resolution. For example, the gamma rays from Tc-99m (140 keV) produce better spatial resolution than do the x-rays from Tl-201 (69 to 80 keV), because each Tc-99m gamma ray produces about twice as many light photons when absorbed. There is relatively little improvement in intrinsic spatial resolution for gamma-ray energies above 250 keV because the improvement in spatial resolution due to more visible light photons is largely offset by the increased likelihood of scattering in the crystal before photoelectric absorption (discussed below).

The quantum detection efficiency of the PMTs in detecting the UV and visible light photons produced in the crystal is the most significant factor limiting the intrinsic spatial resolution (typically only 20% to 25% of the UV and visible light photons incident on a photocathode contribute to the signal from the PMT). The size of the PMTs also affects the spatial resolution slightly; using PMTs of smaller diameter improves the spatial resolution by providing better sampling of the light emitted following each interaction in the crystal.

A thinner NaI crystal provides better intrinsic spatial resolution than a thicker crystal. A thinner crystal permits less spreading of the light before it reaches the PMTs. Furthermore, a thinner crystal reduces the likelihood of an incident x- or gamma ray undergoing one or more Compton scatters in the crystal followed by photoelectric absorption. Compton scattering in the crystal can cause the centroid of the energy deposition to be significantly offset from the site of the initial interaction in the crystal. The likelihood of one or more scatters in the crystal preceding the photoelectric absorption increases with the energy of the x- or gamma ray.

The intrinsic efficiency of a scintillation camera is determined by the thickness of the crystal and the energy of the incident x- or gamma rays. Figure 18-9 is a graph of photopeak efficiency (fraction of incident x- or gamma rays producing counts in the photopeak) as a function of photon energy for NaI(Tl) crystals 0.635 cm (¼ inch), 1.27 cm (½ inch), and 2.54 cm (1 inch) thick. Most modern cameras have 0.95-cm (⅜ inch) thick crystals. The photopeak efficiency of these crystals is greater than 80% for the 140-keV gamma rays from Tc-99m, but less than 30% for the 364-keV gamma rays from I-131. Some cameras, designed primarily for imaging radionuclides such as Tl-201 and Tc-99m, which emit low-energy photons, have 0.635-cm (¼ inch) thick crystals. Other cameras, designed to provide greater intrinsic efficiency for imaging radionuclides such as I-131 which emit high-energy gamma rays, have 1.27- to 2.5-cm (½ to 1 inch) thick crystals.

There is a design compromise between the intrinsic efficiency of the camera, which increases with crystal thickness, and intrinsic spatial resolution, which degrades with crystal thickness. This design compromise is similar to the design compromise between the spatial resolution of scintillator-based image receptors used in radiography and fluoroscopy, which deteriorates with increasing phosphor layer thickness, and detection efficiency, which improves with increasing thickness.

Collimator Resolution and Collimator Efficiency

The collimator spatial resolution, as defined above, of multihole collimators (parallel-hole, converging, and diverging) is determined by the geometry of the holes. The spatial resolution improves (narrower FWHM of the LSF) as the diameters of the holes are reduced and the lengths of the holes (thickness of the collimator) are increased. Unfortunately, changing the hole geometry to improve the spatial resolution in general reduces the collimator's efficiency. *The resultant compromise between collimator efficiency and collimator resolution is the single most significant limitation on scintillation camera performance.*

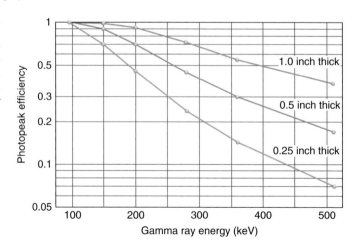

■ FIGURE 18-9 Calculated photopeak efficiency as a function of x- or gamma-ray energy for NaI(Tl) crystals. (Data from Anger HO, Davis DH. Gamma-ray detection efficiency and image resolution in sodium iodide. *Rev Sci Instr* 1964;35:693.)

The spatial resolution of a parallel-hole collimator decreases (i.e., FWHM of the LSF increases) linearly as the collimator-to-object distance increases. This degradation of collimator spatial resolution with increasing collimator-to-object distance is also one of the most important factors limiting scintillation camera performance. However, the efficiency of a parallel-hole collimator is nearly constant over the collimator-to-object distances used for clinical imaging. Although the number of photons passing through a particular collimator hole decreases as the square of the distance, the number of holes through which photons can pass increases as the square of the distance. The efficiency of a parallel-hole collimator, neglecting septal penetration, is approximately

$$E_C \approx \frac{A}{4\pi l^2} g \qquad\qquad [18\text{-}7]$$

where A is the cross-sectional area of a single collimator hole, l is the length of a hole (i.e., the thickness of the collimator), and g is the fraction of the frontal area of the collimator that is not blocked by the collimator septa (g = total area of holes in collimator face/area of collimator face).

Figure 18-10 depicts the line spread function (LSF) of a parallel-hole collimator as a function of source-to-collimator distance. The width of the LSF increases with distance. Nevertheless, the area under the LSF (total number of counts) does not significantly decrease with distance.

The spatial resolution of a pinhole collimator, along its central axis, corrected for collimator magnification, is approximately equal to

$$R'_C \approx d\,\frac{f + x}{f} \qquad\qquad [18\text{-}8]$$

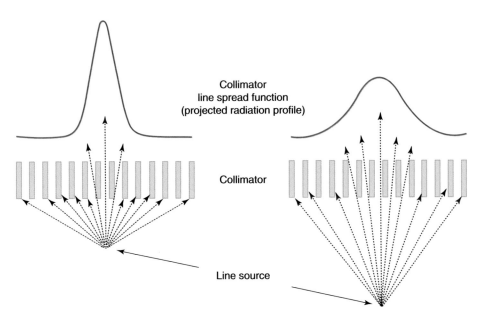

■ **FIGURE 18-10** Line spread function (LSF) of a parallel-hole collimator as a function of source-to-collimator distance. The full-width-at-half-maximum (FWHM) of the LSF increases linearly with distance from the source to the collimator; however, the total area under the LSF (photon fluence through the collimator) decreases very little with source to collimator distance. (In both figures, the line source is seen "end-on.")

TABLE 18-3   THE EFFECT OF INCREASING COLLIMATOR-TO-OBJECT DISTANCE ON COLLIMATOR PERFORMANCE PARAMETERS

COLLIMATOR	SPATIAL RESOLUTION[a]	EFFICIENCY	FIELD SIZE	MAGNIFICATION
Parallel hole	Decreases	Approximately constant	Constant	Constant ($m = 1.0$)
Converging	Decreases	Increases	Decreases	Increases ($m >1$ at collimator surface)
Diverging	Decreases	Decreases	Increases	Decreases ($m <1$ at collimator surface)
Pinhole	Decreases	Decreases	Increases	Decreases (m largest near pinhole)

[a]Spatial resolution corrected for magnification.

where d is the diameter of the pinhole, f is the distance from the crystal to the pinhole, and x is the distance from the pinhole to the object. The efficiency of a pinhole collimator, along its central axis, neglecting penetration around the pinhole, is

$$E_C = d^2/16x^2 \qquad [18\text{-}9]$$

Thus, the spatial resolution of the collimator improves (i.e., R'_C decreases) as the diameter of the pinhole is reduced, but the collimator efficiency decreases as the square of the pinhole diameter. Both the collimator spatial resolution and the efficiency are best for objects close to the pinhole (small x). The efficiency decreases rapidly with increasing pinhole-to-object distance.

The spatial resolution of all collimators decreases with increasing gamma-ray energy because of increasing collimator septal penetration or, in the case of pinhole collimators, penetration around the pinhole. Table 18-3 compares the characteristics of different types of collimators.

System Spatial Resolution and Efficiency

The system spatial resolution and efficiency are determined by the intrinsic and collimator resolutions and efficiencies, as described by Equations 18-2 and 18-4. Figure 18-11 (top) shows the effect of object-to collimator distance on system spatial resolution. The system resolutions shown in this figure are corrected for magnification. *The system spatial resolution, when corrected for magnification, is degraded (i.e., FWHM of the LSF increases) as the collimator-to-object distance increases for all types of collimators.* This degradation of resolution with increasing patient-to-collimator distance is among the most important factors in image acquisition. Technologists should make every effort to minimize this distance during clinical imaging.

Figure 18-11 (bottom) shows the effect of object-to-collimator distance on system efficiency. The system efficiency with a parallel-hole collimator is nearly constant with distance. The system efficiency with a pinhole collimator decreases significantly with distance. The system efficiency of a fan-beam collimator (described in the following chapter) increases with collimator-to-object distance.

Modern scintillation cameras with 0.95-cm (⅜ inch) thick crystals typically have intrinsic spatial resolutions slightly less than 4.0 mm FWHM for the 140-key gamma rays of Tc-99m. One manufacturer's low-energy high-resolution parallel-hole collimator has a resolution of 1.5 mm FWHM at the face of the collimator and 6.4 mm at

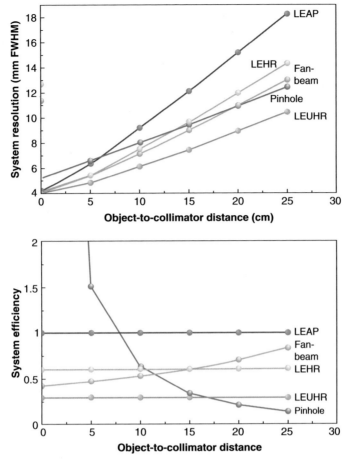

■ **FIGURE 18-11** System spatial resolution (**top**) and efficiency (**bottom**) as a function of object-to-collimator distance (in cm). System resolutions for pinhole and fan-beam collimators are corrected for magnification. System efficiencies are relative to a low-energy, all-purpose (LEAP) parallel-hole collimator (system efficiency 340 cpm/μCi Tc-99m for a 0.95-cm- thick crystal). LEHR, low-energy, high-resolution parallel-hole collimator; LEUHR, low-energy, ultra-high-resolution parallel-hole collimator. (Data courtesy of the late William Guth of Siemens Medical Systems, Nuclear Medicine Group.)

10 cm from the collimator. The system resolutions, calculated from Equation 18-1, are as follows:

$$R_S = \sqrt{(1.5 \text{ mm})^2 + (4.0 \text{ mm})^2} = 4.3 \text{ mm at 0 cm} \qquad [18\text{-}9a]$$

and

$$R_S = \sqrt{(6.4 \text{ mm})^2 + (4.0 \text{ mm})^2} = 7.5 \text{ mm at 10 cm} \qquad [18\text{-}9b]$$

Thus, the system resolution is only slightly worse than the intrinsic resolution at the collimator face, but is largely determined by the collimator resolution at typical imaging distances for internal organs.

Spatial Linearity and Uniformity

Fully analog scintillation cameras, now obsolete, suffered from significant spatial nonlinearity and nonuniformity. These distortions were caused by systematic (non-random) effects, which vary with position on the face of the camera, in the detection

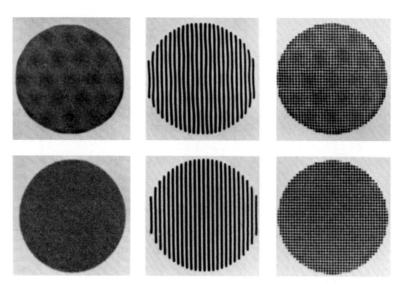

■ **FIGURE 18-12** Pairs of uniformity images, lead slit-mask (lead sheet with thin slits) images, and orthogonal hole phantom (lead sheet with a rectangular array of holes) images, with scintillation camera's digital correction circuitry disabled (**top**) to demonstrate nonuniformities and spatial nonlinearities inherent to a scintillation camera and with correction circuitry functioning (**bottom**), demonstrating effectiveness of linearity and energy (Z) signal correction circuitry. (Photographs courtesy of Everett W. Stoub, Ph.D., formerly of Siemens Gammasonics, Inc.)

and collection of signals from individual x- or gamma rays. Because these position-dependent effects are not random, corrections for them can be made. Modern digital cameras use tables of position-specific correction factors for this function.

Spatial nonlinearity (Fig. 18-12 top center and top right) is caused by the non-random (i.e., systematic) mispositioning of events. It is mainly due to the calculated locations of the interactions being shifted in the resultant image toward the center of the nearest PMT by the position circuit of the camera. Modern cameras have digital circuits that use tables of correction factors to correct each pair of X- and Y-position signals for spatial nonlinearities (Fig. 18-13). One lookup table contains an X-position correction for each portion of the crystal and another table contains corrections for the Y direction. Each pair of digital position signals is used to "look up" a pair of X and Y corrections in the tables. The corrections are added to the uncorrected X and Y values. The corrected X and Y values (X′ and Y′ in Fig. 18-13) are sent to a computer or other device that accepts them in digital form for image formation.

■ **FIGURE 18-13** Spatial linearity correction circuitry of a scintillation camera.

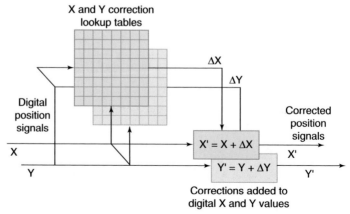

X and Y correction lookup tables

ΔX

ΔY

Digital position signals

Corrected position signals

X

$X' = X + \Delta X$

X′

Y

$Y' = Y + \Delta Y$

Y′

Corrections added to digital X and Y values

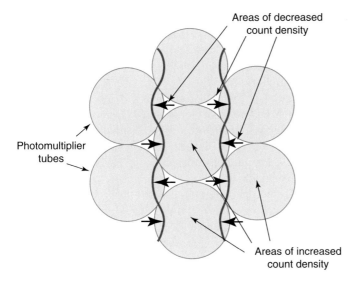

Areas of decreased
count density

Photomultiplier
tubes

Areas of increased
count density

■ **FIGURE 18-14** Spatial non-linearities cause nonuniformities. The two vertical wavy lines represent straight lines in the object that have been distorted. The scintillation camera's position circuit causes the locations of individual counts to be shifted toward the center of the nearest photomultiplier tube (PMT), causing an enhanced count density toward the center of the PMT and a decreased count density between the PMTs, as seen in the *top left image* in Figure 18-12.

There are three major causes of nonuniformity. The first is spatial nonlinearities. As shown in Figure 18-14, the systematic mispositioning of events imposes local variations in the count density. Spatial nonlinearities that are almost imperceptible can cause significant nonuniformities. The linearity correction circuitry previously described effectively corrects this source of nonuniformity.

The second major cause of nonuniformity is that the position of the interaction in the crystal affects the magnitude of the energy (Z) signal. It may be caused by local variations in the crystal in the light generation and light transmission to the PMTs and by variations in the light detection and gains of the PMTs. If these regional variations in energy signal are not corrected, the fraction of interactions rejected by the energy discrimination circuits will vary with position in the crystal. These positional variations in the magnitude of the energy signal are corrected by digital electronic circuitry in modern cameras (Fig. 18-15).

The third major cause of nonuniformity is local variations in the efficiency of the camera in absorbing x- or gamma rays, such as manufacturing defects or damage

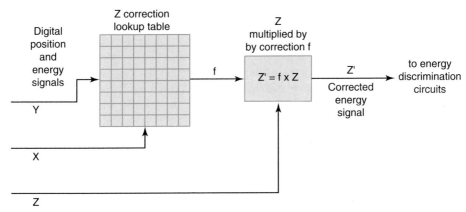

■ **FIGURE 18-15** Energy (Z) signal correction circuitry of a scintillation camera. The digital X- and Y-position signals are used to "look up" a position-dependent correction factor. The uncorrected Z value is multiplied by the correction factor. Finally, the corrected Z value is transmitted to the energy discrimination circuits.

to the collimator. These may be corrected by acquiring an image of an extremely uniform planar source using a computer interfaced to the camera. A correction factor is determined for each pixel in the image by dividing the average pixel count by that pixel count. Each pixel in a clinical image is multiplied by its correction factor to compensate for this cause of nonuniformity.

The digital spatial linearity and energy correction circuits of a modern scintillation camera do not directly affect its intrinsic spatial resolution. However, the obsolete fully analog cameras, which lacked these corrections, used means such as thick light pipes and light absorbers between the crystal and PMTs to improve spatial linearity and uniformity. These reduced the amount of light reaching the PMTs. As mentioned previously, the intrinsic spatial resolution and the energy resolution are largely determined by the statistics of the detection of light photons from the crystal. The loss of signal from light photons in fully analog cameras significantly limited their intrinsic spatial and energy resolutions. The use of digital linearity and energy correction permits camera designs that maximize light collection, thereby providing much better intrinsic spatial resolution and energy resolution than fully analog cameras.

NEMA Specifications for Performance Measurements of Scintillation Cameras

The National Electrical Manufacturers Association (NEMA) publishes a document that specifies standard methods for measuring camera performance.[3] All manufacturers of scintillation cameras publish NEMA performance measurements of their cameras, which are used by prospective purchasers in comparing cameras and for writing purchase specifications. Before the advent of NEMA standards, manufacturers measured the performance of scintillation cameras in a variety of ways, making it difficult to compare the manufacturers' specifications for different cameras objectively. The measurement methods specified by NEMA require specialized equipment and are not intended to be performed by the nuclear medicine department. However, it is possible to perform simplified versions of the NEMA tests to determine whether a newly purchased camera meets the published specifications. Unfortunately, the NEMA protocols omit testing of a number of important camera performance parameters.

Effects of Scatter, Collimator Spatial Resolution, and Attenuation on Projection Images

Ideally, a nuclear medicine projection image would be a two-dimensional projection of the three-dimensional activity distribution in the patient. If this were the case, the number of counts in each point in the image would be proportional to the average activity concentration along a straight line through the corresponding anatomy of the patient. There are three main reasons why nuclear medicine images are not ideal projection images—attenuation of photons in the patient, inclusion of Compton scattered photons in the image, and the degradation of spatial resolution with distance from the collimator. Furthermore, because most nuclear medicine images are acquired over periods of many seconds or even minutes, patient motion, particularly respiratory motion, is a source of image blurring.

Attenuation in the patient by Compton scattering and the photoelectric effect prevents some photons that would otherwise pass through the collimator holes from contributing to the image. The amount of attenuation is mainly determined

[3]Performance Measures of Gamma Cameras, NEMA NU 1-2007.

by the path length through tissue and the densities of the tissues between a location in the patient and the corresponding point on the camera face. Thus, photons from structures deeper in the patient are much more heavily attenuated than photons from structures closer to the camera face. Attenuation is more severe for lower energy photons, such as the 68- to 80-keV characteristic x-rays emitted by Tl-201 ($\mu \approx 0.19$ cm^{-1}), than for higher energy photons, such as the 140-keV gamma rays from Tc-99m ($\mu = 0.15$ cm^{-1}) Nonuniform attenuation, especially in thoracic and cardiac nuclear imaging, presents a particular problem in image interpretation.

The vast majority of the interactions with soft tissue by x- and gamma rays of the energies used for nuclear medicine imaging are by Compton scattering. Some photons that have scattered in the patient pass through the collimator holes and are detected. As in x-ray transmission imaging such as radiography and CT, the relative number of scattered photons is greater when imaging thicker parts of the patient, such as the abdomen, and the main effects of counts in the image from scattered photons are a loss of contrast and an increase in random noise. As was mentioned earlier in this chapter, the number of scattered photons contributing to the image is reduced by pulse height discrimination. However, setting an energy window of sufficient width to encompass most of the photopeak permits a considerable amount of the scatter to contribute to image formation.

Operation and Routine Quality Control

Peaking a scintillation camera means to adjust its energy discrimination windows to center them on the photopeak or photopeaks of the desired radionuclide. Modern cameras display the spectrum as a histogram of the number of interactions as a function of pulse height (Fig. 18-16), like the display produced by a multichannel analyzer (see Chapter 17). On this display, the energy window limits are shown as vertical lines. A narrower energy window provides better scatter rejection, but also reduces the number of unscattered photons recorded in the image.

Peaking may be performed manually by adjusting the energy window settings while viewing the spectrum or automatically by the camera. Older scintillation cameras with mostly analog electronics required adjustment of the energy windows before the first use each day and again before imaging another radionuclide. In modern scintillation cameras, the energy calibration and energy window settings are very stable. For such cameras, peaking is typically adjusted and assessed only at the beginning of each day of use with a single radionuclide, commonly using the Tc-99m or Co-57 source that is used for uniformity assessment. If other radionuclides are imaged during the day, preset energy windows for these radionuclides are used without adjusting them for the actual energy spectra. Adjustment of the energy discrimination windows for the photopeaks of other radionuclides (e.g., In-111, I-123, I-131, Xe-133, and Tl-201) that might be imaged is performed infrequently, such as after major calibrations of the camera. A nearly scatter-free source should be used to assess or adjust the energy windows; using the radiation emitted by a patient to assess or adjust the energy windows would constitute poor practice because of its large scatter component.

The uniformity of the camera should be assessed daily and after each repair. The assessment may be made intrinsically by using a Tc-99m point source, or the system uniformity may be evaluated by using a Co-57 planar source or a fillable flood source. Uniformity images must contain sufficient counts so that quantum mottle does not mask uniformity defects. The number of counts needed increases with the useful area of the camera. As many as 5 to 15 million counts should be obtained for the daily test of a modern large area, rectangular head camera. Uniformity images can be evaluated visually or can be analyzed by a computer program, avoiding the

■ **FIGURE 18-16** Displays of a pulse-height spectrum used for "peaking" the scintillation camera (centering the pulse height analyzer window on the photopeak). The radionuclide is ^{99m}Tc. The energy window is shown by the two vertical lines around the photopeak. **A.** A properly adjusted 20% window. **B.** An improperly adjusted 20% window. **C.** A properly adjusted 15% window.

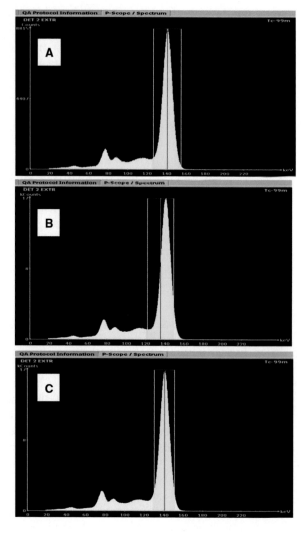

subjectivity of visual evaluation. The uniformity test will reveal most malfunctions of a scintillation camera. Figure 18-17 shows uniformity images from a modern scintillation camera. Multi-hole collimators are easily damaged by careless handling, such as by striking them with an imaging table or dropping heavy objects on them. Technologists should inspect the collimators on each camera daily and whenever changing collimators. Old damage should be marked. The uniformity of each collimator should be evaluated periodically, by using a Co-57 planar source or a fillable flood source and whenever damage is suspected. The frequency of this testing depends on the care taken by the technologists to avoid damaging the collimators and their reliability in visually inspecting the collimators and reporting new damage.

The spatial resolution and spatial linearity are typically assessed at least weekly. If a four-quadrant bar phantom (Fig. 18-7) is used, it should be imaged four times with a 90-degree rotation between images to ensure all quadrants of the camera are evaluated. If a parallel-line phantom is used, it should be imaged twice with a 90-degree rotation between images.

The efficiency of each camera head should be measured periodically. It can be monitored during uniformity tests by always performing the test with the source at

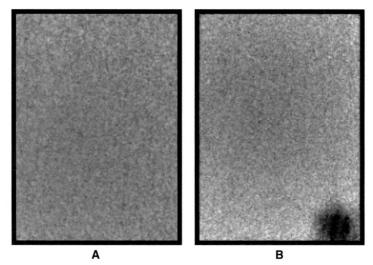

A   **B**

■ **FIGURE 18-17** Uniformity images. **A.** Image from a modern high-performance camera with digital spatial linearity and energy signal correction circuitry. **B.** The other head of the same camera, with an optically decoupled photomultiplier tube. (Images courtesy Carol Moll, CNMT)

the same distance, determining the activity of the source, recording the number of counts and counting time, and calculating the count rate per unit activity.

Each camera should also have a complete evaluation at least annually, which includes not only the items listed above, but also multienergy spatial registration and count-rate performance. Table 19-1 in Chapter 19 contains a recommended schedule for quality control testing of scintillation cameras. Relevant tests should also be performed after each repair or adjustment of a scintillation camera.

New cameras should receive acceptance testing by an experienced medical physicist to determine if the camera's performance meets the purchase specifications and to establish baseline values for routine quality control testing.

Computers, Whole Body Scanning, and SPECT

Almost all scintillation cameras are connected to digital computers. The computer is used for the acquisition, processing, and display of digital images and for control of the movement of the camera heads. Computers used with scintillation cameras are discussed later in this chapter.

Many large-FOV scintillation cameras can perform whole-body scanning. Some systems move the camera past a stationary patient, whereas others move the patient table past a stationary scintillation camera. Moving camera systems require less floor space. In either case, the system must sense the position of the camera relative to the patient table and must add values that specify the position of the camera relative to the table to the X- and Y-position signals. Older systems with round or hexagonal crystals usually had to make two passes over each side of the patient. Modern large-area rectangular head cameras can scan each side of all but extremely obese patients with a single pass, saving considerable time and producing superior image statistics.

Many modern computer-equipped scintillation cameras have heads that can rotate automatically around the patient and acquire images from different views. The computer mathematically manipulates these images to produce cross-sectional images of the activity distribution in the patient. This is called single photon emission computed tomography (SPECT) and is discussed in detail in Chapter 19.

Obtaining High-Quality Images

Attention must be paid to many technical factors to obtain high-quality images. Imaging procedures should be optimized for each type of study. Sufficient counts must be acquired so that quantum mottle in the image does not mask lesions. Imaging times must be as long as possible consistent with patient throughput and lack of patient motion. The camera or table scan speed should be sufficiently slow during whole-body scans to obtain adequate image statistics. The use of a higher resolution collimator may improve spatial resolution and the use of a narrower energy window to reduce scatter may improve image contrast.

Because the spatial resolution of a scintillation camera is degraded significantly as the collimator-to-patient distance is increased, the camera heads should always be as close to the patient as possible. In particular, thick pillows and mattresses on imaging tables should be discouraged when images are acquired with the camera head below the table.

Significant nonuniformities can be caused by careless treatment of the collimators. Collimators are easily damaged by collisions with imaging tables or by placing them on top of other objects when they are removed from the camera.

Patient motion and metal objects worn by patients or in the patients' clothing are common sources of artifacts. Efforts should be made to identify metal objects and to remove them from the patient or from the field of view. The technologist should remain in the room during imaging to minimize patient motion. Furthermore, for safety, a patient should never be left unattended under a moving camera, either in whole-body or SPECT mode.

18.2 Computers in Nuclear Imaging

Most nuclear medicine computer systems consist of commercially available computers with additional components to enable them to acquire, process, and display images from scintillation cameras. A manufacturer may incorporate a computer for image acquisition and camera control in the camera itself and provide a separate computer for image processing and display, or provide a single computer for both purposes.

Modern scintillation cameras create the pairs of X- and Y-position signals using digital circuitry and transfer them to the computer in digital form. The formation of a digital image is described in the following section.

Digital Image Formats in Scintillation Camera Imaging

As discussed in Chapter 5, a digital image consists of a rectangular array of numbers, and an element of the image represented by a single number is called a pixel. In nuclear medicine, each pixel represents the number of counts detected from activity in a specific location within the patient. Common image formats are 64^2 and 128^2 pixels, reflecting the low spatial resolution of scintillation cameras. Whole-body images are stored in larger formats, such as 256 by 1,024 pixels. If one byte (8 bits) is used for each pixel, the image is said to be in *byte mode*; if two bytes are used for each pixel, the image is said to be in *word mode*. A single pixel can store as many as 255 counts in byte mode and 65,535 counts in word mode. Modern nuclear medicine computers may allow only word-mode images.

Image Acquisition

Frame-Mode Acquisition

Image data in nuclear medicine are acquired in either frame or list mode. Figure 18-18 illustrates frame-mode acquisition. Before acquisition begins, a portion of the computer's memory is designated to contain the image. All pixels within this image are set to zero. After acquisition begins, pairs of X- and Y-position signals are received from the camera, each pair corresponding to the detection of a single x- or gamma ray. Each pair of numbers designates a single pixel in the image. One count is added to the counts in that pixel. As many pairs of position signals are received, the image is formed.

There are three types of frame-mode acquisition: *static, dynamic,* and *gated.* In a static acquisition, a single image is acquired for either a preset time interval or until the total number of counts in the image reaches a preset number. In a dynamic acquisition, a series of images is acquired one after another, for a preset time per image. Dynamic image acquisition is used to study dynamic processes, such as the first transit of a bolus of a radiopharmaceutical through the heart or the extraction and excretion of a radiopharmaceutical by the kidneys.

Some dynamic processes occur too rapidly for them to be effectively portrayed by dynamic image acquisition; each image in the sequence would have too few counts to be statistically valid. However, if the dynamic process is repetitive, gated image acquisition may permit the acquisition of an image sequence that accurately

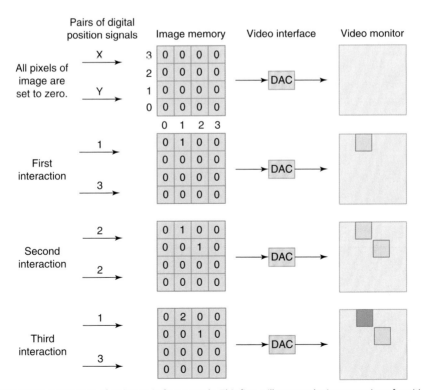

■ FIGURE 18-18 Acquisition of an image in frame mode. This figure illustrates the incorporation of position data from the first three interactions into an image. This example shows a 4 by 4 pixel image for the purpose of illustration. Actual nuclear medicine projection images are typically acquired in formats of 64 x 64 or 128 x 128 pixels.

depicts the dynamic process. Gated acquisition is most commonly used for evaluating cardiac mechanical performance in cardiac blood pool studies and, sometimes, in myocardial perfusion studies. Gated acquisition requires a physiologic monitor that provides a trigger pulse to the computer at the beginning of each cycle of the process being studied. In gated cardiac studies, an electrocardiogram (ECG) monitor provides a trigger pulse to the computer whenever the monitor detects a QRS complex.

Figure 18-19 depicts the acquisition of a gated cardiac image sequence. First, space for the desired number of images (usually 16 to 24 for gated cardiac blood pool imaging) is reserved in the computer's memory. Next, several cardiac cycles are timed and the average time per cycle is determined. The time per cycle is divided by the number of images in the sequence to obtain the time T per image. Then the acquisition begins. When the first trigger pulse is received, the acquisition interface sends the data to the first image in the sequence for a time T. Then it is stored in the second image in the sequence for a time T, after which it is stored in the third image for a time T. This process proceeds until the next trigger pulse is received. Then the process begins anew, with the data being added to that in the first image for a time T, then the second image for a time T, etc. This process is continued until a preset time interval, typically 10 min, has elapsed, enabling sufficient counts to be collected for the image sequence to form a statistically valid depiction of an average cardiac cycle.

List-Mode Acquisition

In *list-mode acquisition*, the pairs of X- and Y-position values are stored in a list (Fig. 18-20), instead of being immediately formed into an image. Periodic timing marks are included in the list. If a physiologic monitor is being used, as in gated cardiac imaging, trigger marks are also included in the list. After acquisition is complete, the list-mode data are reformatted into conventional images for display. The advantage of list-mode acquisition is that it allows great flexibility in how the X and Y values are combined to form images. The disadvantages of list-mode acquisition are that it generates large amounts of data, requiring more memory to acquire and

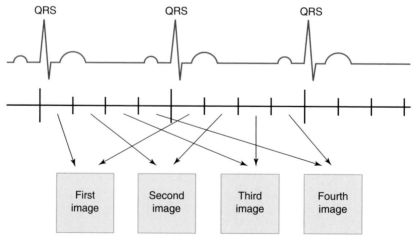

■ **FIGURE 18-19** Acquisition of a gated cardiac image sequence. Only four images are shown here. Sixteen to twenty-four images are typically acquired.

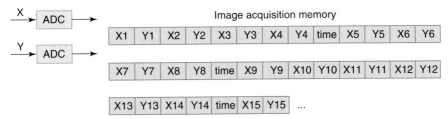

■ FIGURE 18-20 Acquisition of image data in list mode. The digital X- and Y-position signals are stored as a list. Periodically, a timing signal is also stored. The image or images cannot be viewed until the list-mode data are formed into an image matrix or matrices.

disk space to store than frame-mode images, and that the data must be subsequently processed into standard images for viewing.

Image Processing in Nuclear Medicine

A major reason for the use of computers in nuclear medicine is that they provide the ability to present the data in the unprocessed images in ways that are of greater use to the clinician. Although it is not within the scope of this section to provide a comprehensive survey of image processing in nuclear medicine, the following are common examples.

Image Subtraction

When one image is subtracted from another, each pixel count in one image is subtracted from the corresponding pixel count in the other. Negative numbers resulting from these subtractions are set to zero. The resultant image depicts the change in activity that occurs in the patient during the time interval between the acquisitions of the two images.

Regions of Interest and Time-Activity Curves

A *region of interest* (ROI) is a closed boundary that is superimposed on the image. It may be drawn manually or it may be drawn automatically by the computer. The sum of the counts in all pixels in the ROI is an indication of the activity in the corresponding portion of the patient.

To create a *time-activity curve* (TAC), a ROI must first be drawn on one image of a dynamic or gated image sequence. The same ROI is then superimposed on each image in the sequence by the computer and the total number of counts within the ROI is determined for each image. Finally, the counts within the ROI are plotted as a function of image number. The resultant curve is an indication of the activity in the corresponding portion of the patient as a function of time. Figure 18-21 shows ROIs over both kidneys of a patient and TACs describing the uptake and excretion of the radiopharmaceutical Tc-99m MAG-3 by the kidneys.

Spatial Filtering

Nuclear medicine images have a grainy appearance because of the statistical nature of the acquisition process. This quantum mottle can be reduced by a type of spatial filtering called *smoothing*. Unfortunately, smoothing also reduces the spatial resolution of the image. Images should not be smoothed to the extent that clinically significant detail is lost. Smoothing is a type of convolution filtering, which is described in detail in Chapter 4 and Appendix G.

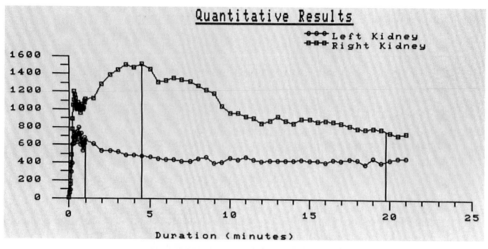

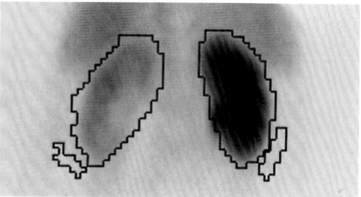

■ FIGURE 18-21 Regions of interest (**bottom**) and time-activity curves (**top**).

Left Ventricular Ejection Fraction

The left ventricular ejection fraction (LVEF) is a measure of the mechanical performance of the left ventricle of the heart. It is defined as the fraction of the end-diastolic volume ejected during a cardiac cycle:

$$LVEF = (V_{ED} - V_{ES})/V_{ED} \qquad [18\text{-}10]$$

where V_{ED} is the end-diastolic volume and V_{ES} is the end-systolic volume of the ventricle. In nuclear medicine, it is can be determined from an equilibrium-gated blood pool image sequence, using Tc-99m–labeled red blood cells. The image sequence is acquired from a left anterior oblique (LAO) projection, with the camera positioned at the angle demonstrating the best separation of the two ventricles, after sufficient time has elapsed for the administered activity to reach a uniform concentration in the blood.

The calculation of the LVEF is based on the assumption that the counts from left ventricular activity are approximately proportional to the ventricular volume throughout the cardiac cycle. A ROI is first drawn around the left ventricular cavity, and a TAC is obtained by superimposing this ROI over all images in the sequence. The first image in the sequence depicts end diastole, and the image containing the least counts in the ROI depicts end systole. The total left ventricular

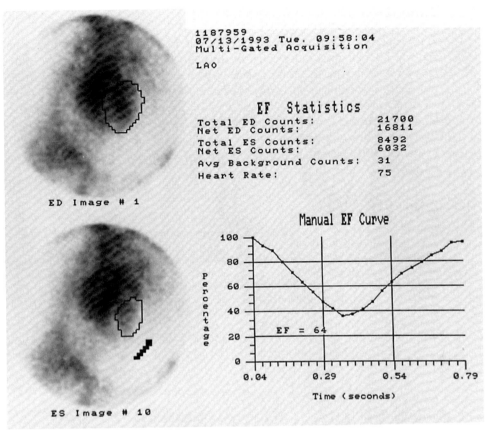

Within the figure:

1187959
07/13/1993 Tue. 09:58:04
Multi-Gated Acquisition

LAO

EF Statistics

Total ED Counts:	21700
Net ED Counts:	16811
Total ES Counts:	8492
Net ES Counts:	6032
Avg Background Counts:	31
Heart Rate:	75

ED Image # 1

Manual EF Curve

Percentage

EF = 64

100, 80, 60, 40, 20, 0

Time (seconds)

0.04   0.29   0.54   0.79

ES Image # 10

■ **FIGURE 18-22** End-diastolic (**top**) and end-systolic (**bottom**) images from a gated cardiac blood-pool study, showing ROIs used to determine the left ventricular ejection fraction (LVEF). The small dark ROI below and to the right of the LV ROI in the end-systolic image is used to determine and correct for the extracardiac ("background") counts.

counts in the end-diastolic and end-systolic images are determined. Some programs use the same ROI around the left ventricle for both images, whereas, in other programs, the ROI is drawn separately in each image to better fit the varying shape of the ventricle. Unfortunately, each of these counts is due not only to activity in the left ventricular cavity but also to activity in surrounding tissues, chambers, and great vessels. To compensate for this "crosstalk" (commonly called "background activity"), another ROI is drawn just beyond the wall of the left ventricle, avoiding active structures such as the spleen, cardiac chambers, and great vessels. The number of counts in the left ventricular ROI due to crosstalk is estimated as follows:

$$\text{Counts crosstalk} = \frac{(\text{Counts in crosstalk ROI})\ (\text{Pixels in LV ROI})}{(\text{Pixels in crosstalk ROI})} \quad [18\text{-}11]$$

Figure 18-22 shows end-diastolic and end-systolic images of the heart from the LAO projection and the ROIs used to determine the LVEF. The LVEF is then calculated using the following equation:

$$\text{LVEF} = \frac{(\text{Counts ED}) - (\text{Counts ES})}{(\text{Counts ED}) - (\text{Counts crosstalk})} \quad [18\text{-}12]$$

Summary

This chapter described the principles of operation of the Anger scintillation camera, which forms images, depicting the distribution of x- and gamma-ray–emitting radionuclides in patients, using a planar crystal of the scintillator NaI(Tl) optically coupled to a two-dimensional array of photomultiplier tubes. The collimator, necessary for formation of projection images, imposes a compromise between spatial resolution and sensitivity in detecting x- and gamma rays. Because of the collimator, the spatial resolution of the images degrades with distance from the face of the camera. In Chapter 19, the use of the scintillation camera to perform computed tomography, called *SPECT*, is described.

SUGGESTED READINGS

Anger HO. Radioisotope cameras. In: Hine GJ, ed. *Instrumentation in nuclear medicine, vol.* 1. New York, NY: Academic Press, 1967:485–552.

Gelfand MJ, Thomas SR. *Effective use of computers in nuclear medicine.* New York, NY: McGraw-Hill, 1988.

Graham LS, Levin CS, Muehllehner G. Anger scintillation camera. In: Sandler MP, et al., eds. *Diagnostic nuclear medicine.* 4th ed. Baltimore, MD: Lippincott Williams & Wilkins, 2003:31–42.

Groch MW. Cardiac function: gated cardiac blood pool and first pass imaging. In: Henkin RE, et al., eds. *Nuclear medicine,* vol. 1. St. Louis, MO: Mosby, 1996:626–643.

Simmons GH, ed. *The scintillation camera.* New York, NY: Society of Nuclear Medicine, 1988.

Yester MV, Graham LS, eds. *Advances in nuclear medicine: the medical physicist's perspective.* Proceedings of the 1998 Nuclear Medicine Mini Summer School, American Association of Physicists in Medicine, June 21–23,1998, Madison, WI.

CHAPTER 19

Nuclear Imaging—Emission Tomography

The formation of projection images in nuclear medicine was discussed in the previous chapter. A nuclear medicine projection image depicts a two-dimensional projection of the three-dimensional activity distribution in the patient. The disadvantage of a projection image is that the contributions to the image from structures at different depths overlap, hindering the ability to discern the image of a structure at a particular depth. Tomographic imaging is fundamentally different—it attempts to depict the activity distribution in a single cross section of the patient.

There are two fundamentally different types of tomography: conventional tomography, also called geometric or focal plane tomography, and computed tomography. In conventional tomography, structures out of a focal plane are not removed from the resultant image; instead, they are blurred by an amount proportional to their distances from the focal plane. Those close to the focal plane suffer little blurring and remain apparent in the image. Even those farther away, although significantly blurred, contribute to the image, thereby reducing contrast and adding noise. In distinction, computed tomography uses mathematical methods to remove overlying structures completely. Computed tomography requires the acquisition of a set of projection images from at least a 180-degree arc about the patient. The projection image information is then mathematically processed by a computer to form images depicting cross sections of the patient. Just as in x-ray transmission imaging, both conventional and computed tomography are possible in nuclear medicine imaging. Both single photon emission computed tomography (SPECT) and positron emission tomography (PET) are forms of computed tomography.

19.1 Focal Plane Tomography in Nuclear Medicine

Focal plane tomography once had a significant role in nuclear medicine, but is seldom used today. The rectilinear scanner, when used with focused collimators, is an example of conventional tomography. A number of other devices have been developed to exploit conventional tomography in nuclear medicine. The Anger tomoscanner used two small scintillation cameras with converging collimators, one above and one below the patient table, to scan the patient in a raster pattern; a single scan produced multiple whole-body images, each showing structures at a different depth in the patient in focus. The seven-pinhole collimator was used with a conventional scintillation camera and computer to produce short-axis images of the heart, each showing structures at a different depth in focus. The rectilinear scanner and the Anger tomoscanner are no longer produced. The seven-pinhole collimator, which never enjoyed wide acceptance, has been almost entirely displaced by SPECT.

The scintillation camera itself, when used for planar imaging with a parallel-hole collimator, produces a weak tomographic effect. The system spatial resolution decreases with distance, causing structures farther from the camera to be more blurred than closer structures. Furthermore, attenuation of photons increases with depth in the patient, also enhancing the visibility of structures closer to the camera. This effect is perhaps most clearly evident in planar skeletal imaging of the body. In the anterior images, for example, the sternum and anterior portions of the ribs are clearly shown, whereas the spine and posterior ribs are barely evident.

19.2   Single Photon Emission Computed Tomography

Design and Principles of Operation

Single photon emission computed tomography (SPECT) generates transverse images depicting the distribution of x- or gamma-ray–emitting nuclides in patients. Standard planar projection images are acquired from an arc of 180 degrees (most cardiac SPECT) or 360 degrees (most noncardiac SPECT) about the patient. Although these images could be obtained by any collimated imaging device, the vast majority of SPECT systems use one or more scintillation camera heads that revolve about the patient. The SPECT system's digital computer then reconstructs the transverse images using either filtered backprojection or an iterative reconstruction method, which are described later in this chapter, as does the computer in an x-ray CT system. Figure 19-1 shows a variety of SPECT systems.

SPECT was invented by David Kuhl and others in the early 1960s, about 10 years before the invention of x-ray CT by Hounsfield (Kuhl and Edwards, 1963). However, in contrast to x-ray CT, most features of interest in SPECT images were also visible in planar nuclear medicine images and SPECT did not come into routine clinical use until the late 1980s.

Image Acquisition

The camera head or heads of a SPECT system revolve about the patient, acquiring projection images. The head or heads may acquire the images while moving (continuous acquisition) or may stop at predefined evenly spaced angles to acquire the images ("step and shoot" acquisition). If the camera heads of a SPECT system produced ideal projection images (i.e., no attenuation by the patient and no degradation of spatial resolution with distance from the camera), projection images from opposite sides of the patient would be mirror images and projection images over a 180-degree arc would be sufficient for transverse image reconstruction. However, in SPECT, attenuation greatly reduces the number of photons from activity in the half of the patient opposite the camera head and this information is greatly blurred by the distance from the collimator. Therefore, for most noncardiac studies, such as bone SPECT, the projection images are acquired over a complete revolution (360 degrees) about the patient. However, most nuclear medicine laboratories acquire cardiac SPECT studies, such as myocardial perfusion studies, over a 180-degree arc symmetric about the heart, typically from the 45-degree right anterior oblique view to the 45-degree left posterior oblique view (Fig. 19-2). The 180-degree acquisition produces reconstructed images of superior contrast and resolution, because the projection images of the heart from the opposite 180 degrees have poor spatial resolution and contrast due to greater distance and attenuation. Although studies have shown that the 180-degree acquisition can introduce artifacts (Liu et al., 2002), the 180-degree acquisition is more commonly used than the 360-degree acquisition for cardiac studies.

SPECT projection images are usually acquired in either a 64^2 or a 128^2 pixel format. Using too small a pixel format reduces the spatial resolution of the projection images and of the resultant reconstructed transverse images. When the 64^2 format is used, typically 60 or 64 projection images are acquired and, when a 128^2 format is chosen, 120 or 128 projection images are acquired. Using too few projections creates radial streak artifacts in the reconstructed transverse images.

The camera heads on older SPECT systems followed circular orbits around the patient while acquiring images. Circular orbits are satisfactory for SPECT imaging of the brain, but cause a loss of spatial resolution in body imaging because the circular

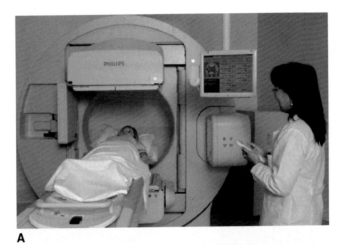

A

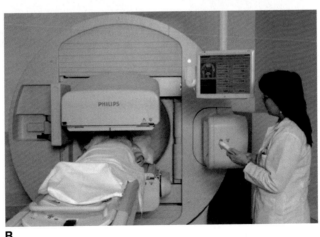

B

■ **FIGURE 19-1 A.** SPECT/CT system with two scintillation camera heads in a fixed 180-degree orientation and a non-diagnostic x-ray CT system for attenuation correction and anatomic correlation. The x-ray source is on the right side of the gantry and a flat-panel x-ray image receptor is on the left. **B.** Technologist moving the upper camera head closer to the patient for SPECT imaging. Photo credit: Emi Manning UC Davis Health System

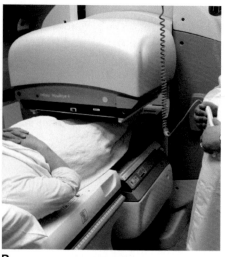

C

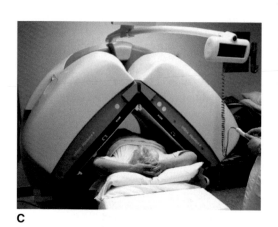

D

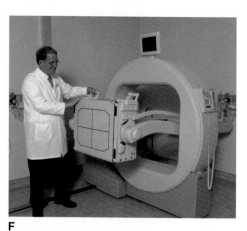

E

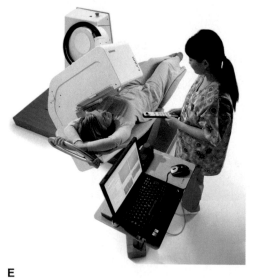

F

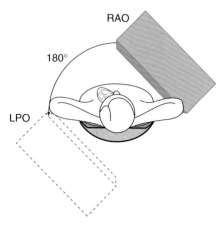

■ **FIGURE 19-1** (*Continued*) **C.** Dual head, variable angle SPECT/CT camera with heads in the 90-degree orientation for cardiac SPECT and in the 180-degree orientation (**D**) for other SPECT or whole body planar imaging. **E.** Dual head, fixed 90-degree SPECT camera for cardiac imaging (Image courtesy Siemens Medical Solutions). **F.** Single head SPECT camera, with head in a position for planar imaging (Image courtesy Emi Manning UC Davis Health System).

■ **FIGURE 19-2** 180-degree cardiac orbit.

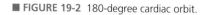

RAO

180°

LPO

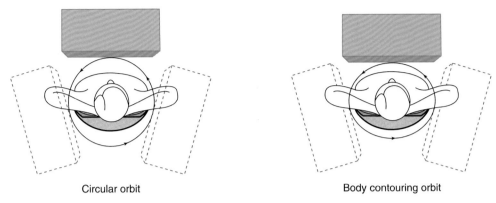

Circular orbit   Body contouring orbit

■ **FIGURE 19-3** Circular (**A**) and body-contouring (**B**) orbits.

orbit causes the camera head to be many centimeters away from the surface of the body during the anterior and perhaps the posterior portions of its orbit (Fig. 19-3). Modern SPECT systems provide noncircular orbits (also called "body contouring") that keep the camera heads in close proximity to the surface of the body throughout the orbit. For some systems, the technologist specifies the noncircular orbit by placing the camera head as close as possible to the patient at several angles, from which the camera's computer determines the orbit. Other systems perform automatic body contouring, using sensors on the camera heads to determine their proximity to the patient at each angle.

In brain SPECT, it is usually possible for the camera head to orbit with a much smaller radius than in body SPECT, thereby producing images of much higher spatial resolution. In many older cameras, a large distance from the physical edge of the camera head to the useful portion of the detector often made it impossible to orbit at a radius within the patient's shoulders while including the base of the brain in the images. These older systems were therefore forced to image the brain with an orbit outside the patient's shoulders, causing a significant loss of resolution. Most modern SPECT systems permit brain imaging with orbits within the patient's shoulders, although a patient's head holder extending beyond the patient table is generally necessary.

Transverse Image Reconstruction

After the projection images are acquired, they are usually corrected for nonuniformities and for center-of-rotation (COR) misalignments. (These corrections are discussed below, "Quality Control in SPECT.") Following these corrections, transverse image reconstruction is performed using either filtered backprojection or iterative methods.

As described in Chapter 10, filtered backprojection consists of two steps. First, the projection images are mathematically filtered. Then, to form a particular transverse image, simple backprojection is performed of the row, corresponding to that transverse image, of each projection image. For example, the fifth row of each projection image is backprojected to form the fifth transverse image. A SPECT study produces transverse images covering the entire field of view of the camera in the axial direction from each revolution of the camera head or heads.

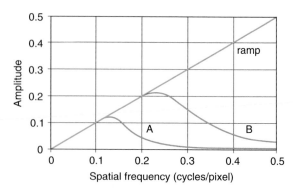

■ **FIGURE** 19-4 Typical filter kernels used for filtered backprojection. The kernels are shown in frequency space. Filter Kernel A is a Butterworth filter of fifth order with a critical frequency of 0.15 Nyquist and Filter Kernel B is a Butterworth filter of fifth order with a critical frequency of 0.27 Nyquist. Filter Kernel A provides more smoothing than Filter Kernel B. A ramp filter, which provides no smoothing, is also shown.

Mathematical theory specifies that the ideal filter kernel, when displayed in the spatial frequency domain, is the ramp filter (Fig. 19-4). (The spatial frequency domain is discussed in Appendix G, Convolution and Fourier Transforms.) However, the actual projection images contain considerable statistical noise, from the random nature of radioactive decay and photon interactions, due to the relatively small number of counts in each pixel. If the images were filtered using a ramp filter kernel and then backprojected, the resultant transverse images would contain an unacceptable amount of statistical noise.

In the spatial frequency domain, statistical noise predominates in the high-frequency portion. Furthermore, the spatial resolution characteristics of the scintillation camera cause a reduction of higher spatial frequency information that increases with distance of the structure being imaged from the camera. To smooth the projection images before backprojection, the ramp filter kernel is modified to "roll off" at higher spatial frequencies. Unfortunately, this reduces the spatial resolution of the projection images and thus of the reconstructed transverse images. A compromise must therefore be made between spatial resolution and statistical noise of the transverse images.

Typically, a different filter kernel is selected for each type of SPECT study; for example, a different kernel would be used for HMPAO brain SPECT than would be used for Tl-201 myocardial perfusion SPECT. The choice of filter kernel for a particular type of study is determined by the amount of statistical noise in the projection images (mainly determined by the injected activity, collimator, and acquisition time per image) and their spatial resolution (determined by the collimator and distances of the camera head(s) from the organ being imaged). The preference of the interpreting physician regarding the appearance of the images also plays a role. Projection images of better spatial resolution and less quantum mottle require a filter with a higher spatial frequency cutoff to avoid unnecessary loss of spatial resolution in the reconstructed transverse images, whereas projection images of poorer spatial resolution and greater quantum mottle require a filter with a lower spatial frequency cutoff to avoid excessive quantum mottle in the reconstructed transverse images. Although the SPECT camera's manufacturer may suggest filters for specific imaging procedures, the filters are usually empirically optimized in each nuclear medicine laboratory. Figure 19-5 shows a SPECT image created using three different filter kernels, illustrating too much smoothing, proper smoothing, and no smoothing.

Filtered backprojection is computationally efficient. However, it is based upon the assumption that the projection images are perfect projections of a three-dimensional

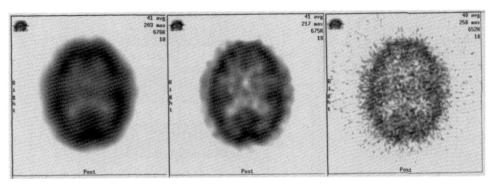

■ **FIGURE 19-5** SPECT images created by filtered backprojection. The projection images were filtered using the filter kernels shown in Figure 19-4. The image on the left, produced using Filter Kernel A, exhibits a significant loss of spatial resolution. The image in the center was produced using Filter Kernel B, which provides a proper amount of smoothing. The image on the right, produced using the ramp filter, shows good spatial resolution, but excessive statistical noise.

object. As discussed in the previous chapter, this is far from true in scintillation camera imaging, mainly because of attenuation of photons in the patient, inclusion of Compton scattered photons in the image, and the degradation of spatial resolution with distance from the collimator.

In SPECT, iterative reconstruction methods are increasingly being used instead of filtered backprojection. In iterative methods, an initial activity distribution in the patient is assumed. Then, projection images are calculated from the assumed activity distribution, using a model of the imaging characteristics of the scintillation camera and the patient. The calculated projection images are compared with the actual projection images and, based upon this comparison, the assumed activity distribution is adjusted. This process is repeated several times, with successive adjustments to the assumed activity distribution, until the calculated projection images approximate the actual projection images (Fig. 19-6).

As was stated above, in each iteration, projection images are calculated from the assumed activity distribution. The calculation of projection images can use the point spread function of the scintillation camera, which takes into account the decreasing spatial resolution with distance from the camera face. The point spread function can be modified to incorporate the effect of photon scattering in the patient. Furthermore, if a map of the attenuation characteristics of the patient is available, the calculation of the projection images can include the effects of attenuation. If this is done, iterative methods will partially compensate for the effects of decreasing spatial resolution with distance, photon scattering in the patient, and attenuation in the patient. Iterative reconstruction can be used to produce higher quality tomographic images than filtered backprojection, or it can be used to produce images of similar quality to those produced by filtered backprojection, but with less administered activity or shorter acquisition times.

Iterative methods are computationally less efficient than filtered backprojection. However, the increasing speed of computers, the small image matrix sizes used in nuclear imaging, and development of computationally efficient algorithms, such as the ordered-subset expectation maximization method (Hudson and Larkin, 1994), have made iterative reconstruction feasible for SPECT. Three-dimensional spatial filtering is commonly performed after iterative reconstruction to reduce image noise.

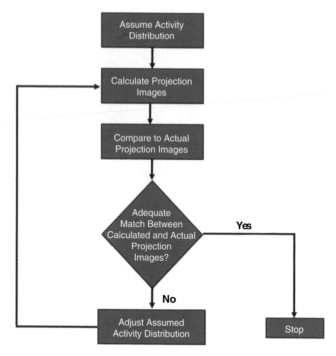

■ **FIGURE 19-6** Flowchart for iterative reconstruction. In some implementations, iterative reconstruction is performed for a specified number of iterations, instead of being terminated when a sufficiently good approximation is achieved.

Attenuation Correction in SPECT

Radioactivity whose x- or gamma rays must traverse long paths through the patient produces fewer counts, due to attenuation, than does activity closer to the surface of the patient adjacent to the camera. For this reason, transverse image slices of a phantom with a uniform activity distribution, such as a cylinder filled with a well-mixed solution of radionuclide, will show a gradual decrease in activity toward the center (Fig. 19-7, on the left). Attenuation effects are more severe in body SPECT than in brain SPECT.

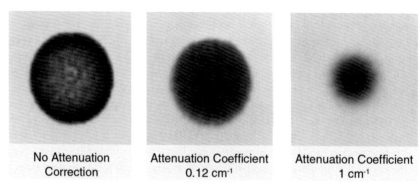

■ **FIGURE 19-7** Attenuation correction. On the left is a reconstructed transverse image slice of a cylindrical phantom containing a well-mixed radionuclide solution. This image shows a decrease in activity toward the center due to attenuation. (A small ring artifact, unrelated to the attenuation, is also visible in the center of the image.) In the center is the same image corrected by the Chang method, using a linear attenuation coefficient of 0.12 cm^{-1}, demonstrating proper attenuation correction. On the right is the same image, corrected by the Chang method using an excessively large attenuation coefficient.

Approximate methods are available for attenuation correction. One of the most common, the Chang method, presumes a constant attenuation coefficient throughout the patient (Chang, 1978). Approximate attenuation corrections can overcompensate or undercompensate for attenuation. If such a method is to be used, its proper functioning should be verified using phantoms before its use in clinical studies.

However, attenuation is not uniform in the patient, particularly in the thorax. These approximate methods cannot compensate for nonuniform attenuation.

Several manufacturers provide SPECT cameras with sealed radioactive sources (commonly containing Gd-153, which emits 97 and 103-keV gamma rays) to measure the attenuation through the patient. The sources are used to acquire transmission data from projections around the patient. After acquisition, the transmission projection data are reconstructed to provide maps of tissue attenuation characteristics across transverse sections of the patient, similar to x-ray CT images. Finally, these attenuation maps are used during an iterative SPECT image reconstruction process to provide attenuation-corrected SPECT images.

The transmission sources are available in several configurations. These include scanning collimated line sources that are used with parallel-hole collimators, arrays of fixed line sources used with parallel-hole collimators, and a fixed line source located at the focal point of a fan-beam collimator.

The transmission data are usually acquired simultaneously with the acquisition of the emission projection data, because performing the two separately can pose significant problems in the spatial alignment of the two data sets and greatly increases the total imaging time. The radionuclide used for the transmission measurements is chosen to have primary gamma ray emissions that differ significantly in energy from those of the radiopharmaceutical. Separate energy windows are used to differentiate the photons emitted by the transmission source from those emitted by the radiopharmaceutical. However, scattering of the higher energy photons in the patient and in the detector causes some cross-talk in the lower energy window.

Major manufacturers of nuclear medicine imaging systems provide systems combining two scintillation camera heads capable of planar imaging and SPECT and an x-ray CT scanner, with a single patient bed. These are referred to as SPECT/CT systems. In SPECT/CT systems, the x-ray CT attenuation image data can be used to correct the radionuclide emission data for attenuation by the patient. This is discussed in more detail later in this chapter.

Attenuation correction using radioactive transmission sources and x-ray CT-derived attenuation maps has been extensively studied in myocardial perfusion SPECT, where attenuation artifacts can mimic perfusion defects. These studies have shown that attenuation correction reduces attenuation artifacts and produces modest improvement in diagnostic performance when the studies are read by experienced clinicians (Hendel et al., 2002; Masood et al., 2005). However, other studies have shown that attenuation correction can cause artifacts, particularly when there is spatial misalignment of the emission data with respect to the attenuation maps determined from the transmission information. It remains common for SPECT myocardial perfusion imaging to be performed without attenuation correction, although that may change with the increasing implementation of SPECT/CT.

Generation of Coronal, Sagittal, and Oblique Images

The pixels from the transverse image slices may be reordered to produce coronal and sagittal images. For cardiac imaging, it is desirable to produce oblique images oriented either parallel (vertical and horizontal long-axis images) or perpendicular (short-axis images) to the long axis of the left ventricle. Because there is considerable anatomic variation among patients regarding the orientation of the long axis of the left ventricle, the long axis of the heart must be determined before the computer can create the oblique images. This task is commonly performed manually by a technologist.

Collimators for SPECT

Most SPECT is performed using parallel-hole collimators. However, specialized collimators have been developed for SPECT. The fan-beam collimator, shown in Figure 19-8, is a hybrid of the converging and parallel-hole collimator. Because it is a parallel-hole collimator in the y-direction, each row of pixels in a projection image corresponds to a single transaxial slice of the subject. In the x-direction, it is a converging collimator, with spatial resolution and efficiency characteristics superior to those of a parallel-hole collimator (see Fig. 18-11). Because a fan-beam collimator is a converging collimator in the cross-axial direction, its field-of-view (FOV) decreases with distance from the collimator. For this reason, the fan-beam collimator is mainly used for brain SPECT; if the collimator is used for body SPECT, portions of the body are excluded from the FOV, which can cause artifacts, called "truncation artifacts," in the reconstructed images.

Multihead SPECT Cameras

To reduce the limitations imposed on SPECT by collimation and limited time per view, camera manufacturers provide SPECT systems with two scintillation camera heads that revolve about the patient (Fig. 19-1) and, in the past, SPECT systems with three heads were commercially available from at least two manufacturers. The use of multiple camera heads permits the use of higher resolution collimators, for a given level of quantum mottle in the tomographic images, than would a single head system. However, the use of multiple camera heads poses considerable technical challenges for the manufacturer. It places severe requirements upon the electrical

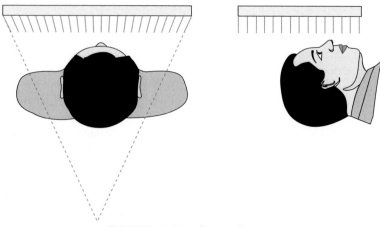

■ **FIGURE 19-8** Fan-beam collimator.

and mechanical stability of the camera heads. In particular, the X and Y offsets and X and Y magnification factors of all the heads must be precisely matched throughout the rotation about the patient. Today's multihead systems are very stable and provide high-quality tomographic images for a variety of clinical applications.

Multihead scintillation cameras are available in several configurations. Double-head cameras with opposed heads (180 degrees head configuration) are good for head and body SPECT and whole-body planar scans (Figure 19-1 A and B). Triple-head, fixed-angle cameras are good for head and body SPECT, but less suitable for whole-body planar scans because of the limited width of the crystals. Double-head, variable-angle cameras are highly versatile, capable of head and body SPECT and whole-body planar scans with the heads in the 180-degree configuration and cardiac SPECT in the 90-degree configuration (Figure 19-1, C and D). (The useful portion of the NaI crystal does not extend all the way to the edge of a camera head. If the two camera heads are placed at an angle of exactly 90 degrees to each other, both heads cannot be close to the patient without parts of the patient being outside of the fields of view. For this reason, one manufacturer provides the option of SPECT acquisitions with the heads at a 76-degree angle to each other.)

Performance

Spatial Resolution

The spatial resolution of a SPECT system can be measured by acquiring a SPECT study of a line source, such as a capillary tube filled with a solution of Tc-99m, placed parallel to the axis of rotation. The National Electrical Manufacturers Association (NEMA) has a protocol for measuring spatial resolution in SPECT. This protocol specifies a cylindrical plastic water-filled phantom, 22 cm in diameter, containing three line sources (Fig. 19-9, on the left) for measuring spatial resolution. The full widths at half maximum (FWHMs) of the line sources are measured from the reconstructed transverse images, as shown on the right in Figure 19-9. A ramp filter is used in the filtered backprojection, so that the filtering does not reduce the spatial resolution. The NEMA spatial resolution measurements are primarily determined by the collimator used. The tangential resolution for the peripheral sources (typically 7 to 8 mm FWHM for low-energy high-resolution parallel-hole collimators) is superior to both the central resolution (typically 9.5 to 12 mm) and the radial resolution for the peripheral sources (typically 9.4 to 12 mm).

These FWHMs measured using the NEMA protocol, while providing a useful index of ultimate system performance, are not necessarily representative of clinical performance, because these spatial resolution studies can be acquired using longer imaging times and closer orbits than would be possible in a patient. Patient studies may require the use of lower resolution (higher efficiency) collimators than the one used in the NEMA measurement to obtain adequate image statistics. In addition, the filters used before backprojection for clinical studies cause more blurring than do the ramp filters used in NEMA spatial resolution measurements. The NEMA spatial resolution measurements fail to show the advantage of SPECT systems with two or three camera heads; double and triple head cameras will permit the use of higher resolution collimators for clinical studies than will single head cameras.

Spatial resolution deteriorates as the radius of the camera orbit increases. For this reason, brain SPECT produces images of much higher spatial resolution than does body SPECT. For optimal spatial resolution, the SPECT camera heads should orbit the patient as closely as possible. Body-contouring orbits (see above, "Design and Operation") provide better resolution than circular orbits.

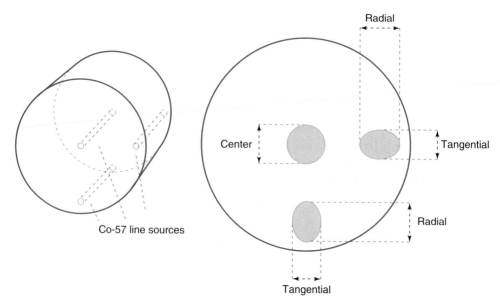

■ **FIGURE 19-9** NEMA phantom for evaluating the spatial resolution of a SPECT camera (**left**). The phantom is a 22-cm diameter plastic cylinder, filled with water and containing three Co-57 line sources. One line source lies along the central axis and the other two are parallel to the central line source, 7.5 cm away. A SPECT study is acquired with a camera radius of rotation (distance from collimator to AOR) of 15 cm. The spatial resolution is measured from reconstructed transverse images, as shown on the right. Horizontal and vertical profiles are taken through the line sources and the FWHMs of these LSFs are determined. The average central resolution (FWHM of the central LSF) and the average tangential and radial resolutions (determined from the FWHMs of the two peripheral sources as shown) are determined. (Adapted from Performance Measurements of Scintillation Cameras, National Electrical Manufacturers Association, 2001.)

Comparison of SPECT to Conventional Planar Scintillation Camera Imaging

In theory, SPECT should produce spatial resolution similar to that of planar scintillation camera imaging. In clinical imaging, its resolution is usually slightly worse. The camera head is usually closer to the patient in conventional planar imaging than in SPECT. The spatial filtering used in SPECT to reduce statistical noise also reduces spatial resolution. The short time per view of SPECT may mandate the use of a lower resolution collimator to obtain adequate numbers of counts.

In planar nuclear imaging, radioactivity in tissues in front of and behind an organ or tissue of interest causes a reduction in contrast. Furthermore, if the activity in these overlapping structures is not uniform, the pattern of this activity distribution is superimposed on the activity distribution in the organ or tissue of interest. As such, it is a source of structural noise that impedes the ability to discern the activity distribution in the organ or tissue of interest. The main advantage of SPECT over conventional planar nuclear imaging is improved contrast and reduced structural noise produced by eliminating counts from the activity in overlapping structures. SPECT using iterative reconstruction can also partially compensate for the effects of the scattering of photons in the patient and collimator effects such as the decreasing spatial resolution with distance from the camera and collimator septal penetration. When attenuation is measured using sealed radioactive transmission sources or an x-ray CT scanner, SPECT can partially compensate for the effects of photon attenuation in the patient.

Quality Control in SPECT

Even though a technical quality control program is important in planar nuclear imaging, it is critical to SPECT. Equipment malfunctions or maladjustments that would not noticeably affect planar images can markedly degrade the spatial resolution of SPECT images and produce significant artifacts, some of which may mimic pathology. Upon installation, a SPECT camera should be tested by a medical physicist. Following acceptance testing, a quality control program should be established to ensure that the system's performance remains comparable to its initial performance.

X and Y Magnification Factors and Multienergy Spatial Registration

The X and Y magnification factors, often called X and Y gains, relate distances in the object being imaged, in the x and y directions, to the numbers of pixels between the corresponding points in the resultant image. The X magnification factor is determined from an image of two point sources placed against the camera's collimator a known distance apart along a line parallel to the x-axis:

$$X_{mag} = \frac{\text{actual distance between centers of point sources}}{\text{number of pixels between centers of point sources}}$$

The Y magnification factor is determined similarly but with the sources parallel to the y-axis. The X and Y magnification factors should be equal. If they are not, the projection images will be distorted in shape, as will be coronal, sagittal, and oblique images. (The transverse images, however, will not be distorted.)

The multienergy spatial registration, described in the previous chapter, is a measure of the camera's ability to maintain the same image magnification, regardless of the energy of the x- or gamma rays forming the image. The multienergy spatial registration is not only important in SPECT when imaging radionuclides such as Ga-67 and In-111, which emit useful photons of more than one energy, but also because uniformity and axis of rotation corrections, to be discussed shortly, determined with one radionuclide will only be valid for others if the multienergy spatial registration is correct.

Alignment of Projection Images to the Axis of Rotation (COR Calibration)

The axis of rotation (AOR) is an imaginary reference line about which the head or heads of a SPECT camera rotate. If a radioactive line source were placed on the AOR, each projection image would depict it as a vertical straight line near the center of the image; this projection of the AOR into the image is called the center-of-rotation (COR). The location of the COR in each projection image must be known to correctly calculate the three-dimensional activity distribution from the projection images. Ideally, the COR is aligned with the center, in the x-direction, of each projection image. However, there may be misalignment of the COR with the centers of the projection images. This misalignment may be mechanical; for example, the camera head may not be exactly centered in the gantry. It can also be electronic. The misalignment may be the same amount in all projection images from a single camera head, or it may vary with the angle of the projection image.

If a COR misalignment is not corrected, it causes a loss of spatial resolution in the resultant transverse images. If the misalignment is large, it can cause a point source to appear as a tiny "doughnut" (Fig. 19-10). (These "doughnut" artifacts are not seen in clinical images; they are visible only in reconstructed images of point or line sources. The "doughnut" artifacts caused by COR misalignment are not centered in the image

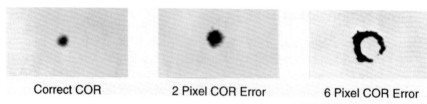

Correct COR   2 Pixel COR Error   6 Pixel COR Error

■ **FIGURE 19-10** Center-of-rotation (COR) misalignment in SPECT. Small misalignments cause blurring (**center**), whereas large misalignments cause point sources to appear as "tiny doughnut" artifacts (**right**). Such "tiny doughnut" artifacts would only be visible in phantom studies and are unlikely to be seen in clinical images.

and so can be distinguished from the ring artifacts caused by nonuniformities.) Scintillation camera manufacturers provide software to assess and correct the effects of COR misalignment. The COR alignment is assessed by placing a point source, several point sources, or a line source in the camera's field of view, acquiring a set of projection images, and analyzing these images using the SPECT system's computer. If a line source is used, it is placed parallel to the AOR.

The SPECT system's computer corrects the COR misalignment by shifting each clinical projection image in the x-direction by the proper number of pixels prior to filtered backprojection or iterative reconstruction. When a line source is used, the COR correction can be performed separately for each transverse slice. If the COR misalignment varies with camera head angle, instead of being constant for all projection images, it can only be corrected if the computer permits angle-by-angle corrections. Separate assessments of the COR correction must be made for different collimators and, on some systems, for different camera zoom factors and image formats (e.g., 64^2 versus 128^2). The COR correction determined using one radionuclide will only be valid for other radionuclides if the multienergy spatial registration is correct.

Uniformity

The uniformity of the camera head or heads is important; nonuniformities that are not apparent in low count daily uniformity studies can cause significant artifacts in SPECT. The artifact caused by a nonuniformity appears in transverse images as a ring centered about the AOR (Fig. 19-11).

■ **FIGURE 19-11** Image of a cylinder filled with a uniform radionuclide solution, showing a ring artifact due to a nonuniformity. The artifact is the dark ring toward the center.

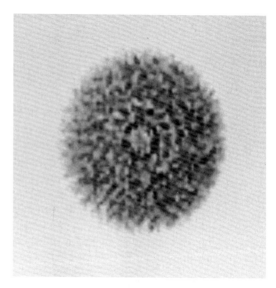

Multihead SPECT systems can produce partial ring artifacts when projection images are not acquired by all heads over a 360-degree arc. Clinically, ring artifacts are most apparent in high-count density studies, such as liver images. However, ring artifacts may be most harmful in studies such as myocardial perfusion images in which, due to poor counting statistics and large variations in count density, they may not be recognized and thus lead to misinterpretation.

The causes of nonuniformities were discussed in the previous chapter. As mentioned in that chapter, modern scintillation cameras have digital circuits using lookup tables to correct the X and Y position signals from each interaction for systematic position-specific errors in event location assignment and the Z (energy) signal for systematic position-specific variations in light collection efficiency. However, these correction circuits cannot correct nonuniformity due to local variations in detection efficiency, such as dents or manufacturing defects in the collimators.

If not too severe, nonuniformities of this latter type can be largely corrected. A very high-count uniformity image is acquired. The ratio of the average pixel count to the count in a specific pixel in this image serves as a correction factor for that pixel. Following the acquisition of a projection image during a SPECT study, each pixel of the projection image is multiplied by the appropriate correction factor before COR correction and filtered backprojection or iterative reconstruction. For the high-count uniformity image, at least 30 million counts should be collected for 64^2 pixel images and 120 million counts for a 128^2 pixel format. These high-count uniformity images are typically acquired weekly to monthly. Correction images must be acquired for each camera head and collimator. For cameras from some manufacturers, separate correction images must be acquired for each radionuclide. The effectiveness of a camera's correction circuitry and of the use of high-count flood correction images can be tested by acquiring a SPECT study of a large plastic container or a SPECT performance phantom filled with a well-mixed solution of Tc-99m and examining the transverse images for ring artifacts. However, this testing will not assess parts of the collimator or camera face outside the projected image of the container or phantom.

Camera Head Tilt

The camera head or heads must be aligned with the axis of rotation (AOR); for most types of collimators, this requires that faces of the heads be exactly parallel to the AOR. If they are not, a loss of spatial resolution and contrast will result from out-of-slice activity being backprojected into each transverse image slice, as shown in Figure 19-12.

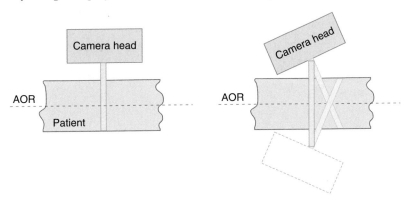

■ **FIGURE 19-12** Head tilt. The camera head on the left is parallel to the axis of rotation (AOR), causing the counts collected in a pixel of the projection image to be backprojected into the corresponding transverse image slice of the patient. The camera head on the right is tilted, causing counts from activity outside of a transverse slice (*along the grey diagonal lines of response*) to be backprojected into the transverse image slice (*orange colored vertical slice*).

The loss of resolution and contrast in each transverse image slice will be less toward the center of the slice and greatest toward the edges of the image. If the AOR of the camera is aligned to be level when the camera is installed and there is a flat surface on the camera head that is parallel to the collimator face, a bubble level may be used to test for head tilt. Some SPECT cameras require the head tilt to be manually adjusted for each acquisition, whereas other systems set it automatically. The accuracy of the automatic systems should be periodically tested. A more reliable method than the bubble level is to place a point source in the camera FOV, centered in the axial (y) direction, but near the edge of the field in the transverse (x) direction. A series of projection images is then acquired. If there is head tilt, the position of the point source will vary in the y-direction from image to image. Proper head tilt can be evaluated from cine viewing of the projection images.

SPECT Quality Control Phantoms

There are commercially available phantoms (Fig. 19-13) that may be filled with a solution of Tc-99m or other radionuclide and used to evaluate system performance. These phantoms are very useful for the semiquantitative assessment of spatial resolution, image contrast, and uniformity, although the small sizes of most such phantoms allow uniformity to be assessed only over a relatively small portion of the camera's face. They are used for acceptance testing of new systems and periodic testing, typically quarterly, thereafter. Table 19-1 provides a suggested schedule for a SPECT quality control program.

19.3   Positron Emission Tomography

Positron emission tomography (PET) generates images depicting the distribution of positron-emitting nuclides in patients. Nearly all PET systems manufactured today are coupled to x-ray CT systems, with a single patient bed passing through the bores of both systems, and are referred to as "PET/CT" systems. Figure 19-14 shows a

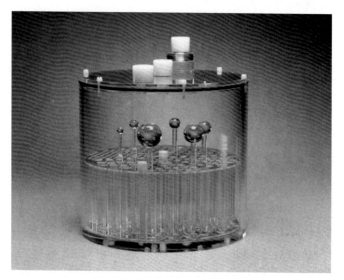

■ FIGURE 19-13 "Jaszczak" phantom for testing SPECT systems, a product of Data Spectrum Corporation. (Photograph courtesy Data Spectrum Corporation.) A soluble radioactive material, typically labeled with Tc-99m, is introduced into the phantom and mixed in the water until it is uniformly distributed. The acrylic plastic spheres and rods are not radioactive and are "cold" objects in the radioactive solution.

TABLE 19-1 RECOMMENDED SCHEDULE FOR ROUTINE QUALITY CONTROL TESTING OF A SCINTILLATION CAMERA

TEST	FREQUENCY	NOTES
Set and check energy discrimination window(s)	Before first use daily	Point (intrinsic) or planar (extrinsic) source of radionuclide
Extrinsic or intrinsic low-count uniformity images of all camera heads	Before first use daily	5–10 million counts, depending upon effective area of camera head
Cine review of projection images and/or review of sinogram[a] (S)	After each clinical SPECT study	Check for patient motion
Visual inspection of collimators for damage	Daily and when changing collimators	If new damage found, acquire a new high-count uniformity calibration image
High count-density extrinsic or intrinsic uniformity images of all camera heads (S)	Weekly to monthly	30 million counts for 64^2 images and 120 million counts for 128^2
Spatial resolution check with bar or hole pattern	Weekly	
Center of rotation (S)	Weekly to monthly	Point or line source(s), as recommended by manufacturer
Efficiency of each camera head	Quarterly	
Reconstructed cylindrical phantom uniformity (S)	Monthly to quarterly	Cylindrical phantom filled with Tc-99m solution
Point source reconstructed spatial resolution (S)	Quarterly, semiannually, or annually	Point source
Reconstructed SPECT phantom (S)	Quarterly	Using a phantom such as the one shown in Figure19-13
Pixel size check	Quarterly	Two point sources
Head tilt angle check (S)	Quarterly	Bubble level or point source
Extrinsic uniformity images of all collimators not tested above	Quarterly or semiannually	Planar source. High-count density images of all collimators used for SPECT
Multienergy spatial registration	Quarterly, semiannually, or annually	Ga-67 point source
Count rate performance	Annually	Tc-99m source

The results of these tests are to be compared with baseline values, typically determined during acceptance testing. If the manufacturer recommends or an accrediting body specifies additional tests or more frequent testing, these recommendations or specifications should take precedence. For tests with multiple frequencies listed, it is recommended that the tests be performed initially at the higher frequency, but the frequency be reduced if the measured parameters prove stable. Tests labeled (S) need not be performed for cameras used only for planar imaging.
[a]A sinogram is an image containing projection data corresponding to a single transaxial image of the patient. Each row of pixels in the sinogram is the row, corresponding to that transaxial image, of one projection image.

PET/CT system. This section discusses PET imaging systems; their use in PET/CT systems is discussed later in this chapter.

In a typical PET system, several rings of detectors surround the patient. PET scanners use *annihilation coincidence detection* (ACD) instead of collimation to obtain projections of the activity distribution in the subject. The PET system's computer then reconstructs the transverse images from the projection data, as does the computer of an x-ray CT or SPECT system. Modern PET scanners are multislice devices,

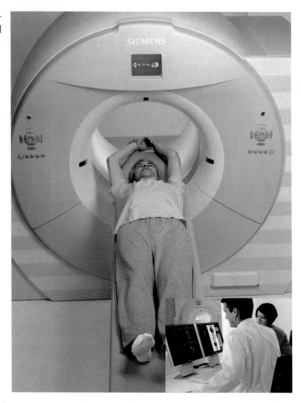

permitting the simultaneous acquisition of as many as 109 transverse images over 21.6 cm of axial distance. The clinical importance of PET today is largely due to its ability to image the radiopharmaceutical fluorine-18 fluorodeoxyglucose (FDG), a glucose analog used for differentiating malignant neoplasms from benign lesions, staging patients with malignant neoplasms, monitoring the response to therapy for neoplasms, differentiating severely hypoperfused but viable myocardium from scar, and other applications. A few other positron-emitting radiopharmaceuticals have been approved for use and many are under development or clinical investigation.

Design and Principles of Operation

Annihilation Coincidence Detection

Positron emission is a mode of radioactive transformation and was discussed in Chapter 15. Positrons emitted in matter lose most of their kinetic energy by causing ionization and excitation. When a positron has lost most of its kinetic energy, it interacts with an electron by *annihilation*, as shown on the left in Figure 19-15. The entire mass of the electron-positron pair is converted into two 511-keV photons, which are emitted in nearly opposite directions. In solids and liquids, positrons travel only very short distances (see Table 19-3) before annihilation.

If both photons from an annihilation interact with detectors and neither photon is scattered in the patient, the annihilation occurred near the line connecting the two interactions, as shown on the right in Figure 19-15. Circuitry within the scanner identifies pairs of interactions occurring at nearly the same time, a process called annihilation coincidence detection (ACD). The circuitry of the scanner then determines the line in space connecting the locations of the two interactions. Thus, ACD establishes the trajectories of detected photons, a function performed by collimation in

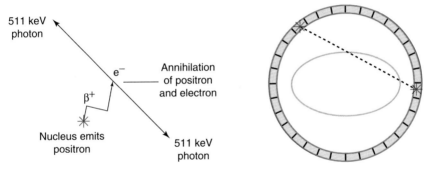

■ **FIGURE 19-15** Annihilation coincidence detection (ACD). When a positron is emitted by a nuclear transforma-tion, it scatters through matter losing energy. After it loses most of its energy, it annihilates with an electron, result-ing in two 511-keV photons that are emitted in nearly opposite directions (**left**). When two interactions are nearly simultaneously detected within a ring of detectors surrounding the patient (**right**), it is presumed that an annihilation occurred on the line connecting the interactions (i.e., line of response). Thus, ACD, by determining the path of the detected photons, performs the same function for a PET scanner as does the collimator of a scintillation camera.

SPECT systems. However, the ACD method is much less wasteful of photons than collimation. Additionally, ACD avoids the degradation of spatial resolution with distance from the detector that occurs when collimation is used to form projection images.

True, Random, and Scatter Coincidences

A *true coincidence* is the nearly simultaneous interaction with the detectors of emis-sions resulting from a single nuclear transformation. A *random coincidence* (also called an *accidental* or *chance coincidence*), which mimics a true coincidence, occurs when emissions from different nuclear transformations interact nearly simultaneously with the detectors (Fig. 19-16). A *scatter coincidence* occurs when one or both of the pho-tons from a single annihilation are scattered, and both are detected (Fig. 19-16). A scatter coincidence is a true coincidence, because both interactions result from a single positron annihilation. Random coincidences and scatter coincidences result in misplaced coincidences, because they are assigned to lines of response (LORs) that do not intersect the actual locations of the annihilations. They are therefore sources of noise, whose main effects are to reduce image contrast and increase statistical noise.

Detection of Interactions

Scintillation crystals coupled to photomultiplier tubes (PMTs) are used as detectors in all commercial PET systems today; the low intrinsic efficiencies of gas-filled and semi-conductor detectors for detecting 511-keV photons make them impractical for use

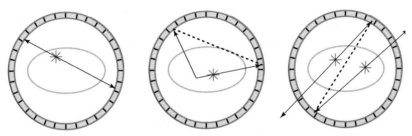

■ **FIGURE 19-16** True coincidence (**left**), scatter coincidence (**center**), and random (accidental) coincidence (**right**). A scatter coincidence is a true coincidence, because it is caused by a single nuclear transformation, but results in a count attributed to the wrong LOR (*dashed line*). The random coincidence is also attributed to the wrong LOR.

in PET. The signals from the PMTs are processed using pulse mode (the signals from each interaction are processed separately from those of other interactions) to create signals identifying the position in the detector, deposited energy, and time of each interaction. The energy signal is used for energy discrimination to reduce mispositioned events due to scatter and the time signal is used for coincidence detection and, in some PET systems, time-of-flight determination (discussed later in this chapter).

In early PET scanners, each scintillation crystal was coupled to a single PMT. In this design, the size of the individual crystal largely determined the spatial resolution of the system; reducing the size (and therefore increasing the number of crystals) improved the resolution. It became increasingly costly and impractical to pack more and more smaller PMTs into each detector ring. Modern designs couple larger crystals to more than one PMT; one such design is shown in Figure 19-17. The relative magnitudes of the signals from the PMTs coupled to a single crystal are used to determine the position of the interaction in the crystal, as in a scintillation camera. In such a system, the crystal and four PMTs comprise a detector. However, an interaction is localized to one of the portions of the crystal separated by the slits and thus each such segment of the crystal can be considered to be a detector element from the perspective of image formation.

The scintillation material must emit light very promptly to permit true coincident interactions to be distinguished from random coincidences and to minimize dead-time count losses at high interaction rates. Also, to maximize the counting efficiency, the material must have a high linear attenuation coefficient for 511-keV photons. A high conversion efficiency (fraction of deposited energy emitted as light or UV radiation) is also important; it permits more precise event localization in the detectors and better energy discrimination. Until recently, most PET systems used crystals of bismuth germanate ($Bi_4Ge_3O_{12}$, abbreviated BGO). The light output of BGO is only 12% to 14% of that of NaI(Tl), but its greater density and average atomic number give it a much higher efficiency in detecting 511-keV annihilation photons. Light is emitted rather slowly from BGO (decay constant of 300 ns), which contributes to dead-time count losses and random coincidences at high interaction rates. Several inorganic scintillators that emit light more quickly are replacing BGO. These include lutetium

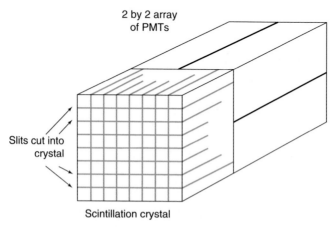

■ FIGURE 19-17 A technique for coupling scintillation crystals to photomultiplier tubes (PMTs). The relative heights of the pulses from the four PMTs are used to determine the position of each interaction in the crystal. The thick (2 to 3 cm) crystal is necessary to provide a reasonable detection efficiency for the 511-keV annihilation photons. The slits cut in the scintillation crystal form light pipes, limiting the spread of light from interactions in the front portion of the crystal, which otherwise would reduce the spatial resolution. This design permits four PMTs to serve 64 detector elements.

oxyorthosilicate (Lu$_2$SiO$_4$O, abbreviated LSO), lutetium yttrium oxyorthosilicate (Lu$_x$Y$_{2-x}$SiO$_4$O, abbreviated LYSO), and gadolinium oxyorthosilicate (Gd$_2$SiO$_4$O, abbreviated GSO), all activated with cerium. Their attenuation properties are nearly as favorable as those of BGO and their much faster light emission produces better performance at high interaction rates, especially in reducing dead-time effects and in discriminating between true and random coincidences. A disadvantage of LSO and LYSO is that they are slightly radioactive; about 2.6% of naturally occurring lutetium is radioactive Lu-176, which has a half-life of 38 billion years, producing about 295 nuclear transformations per second in each cubic centimeter of LSO. NaI(Tl) was used as the scintillator in some less-expensive PET systems. The properties of BGO, LSO, LYSO, and GSO are contrasted with those of NaI(Tl) in Table 19-2.

The energy signals from the detectors are sent to energy discrimination circuits, which can reject events in which the deposited energy differs significantly from 511 keV to reduce the effect of photon scattering in the patient. However, some annihilation photons that have escaped the patient without scattering interact with the detectors by Compton scattering, depositing less than 511 keV. An energy discrimination window that encompasses only the photopeak rejects these valid interactions as well as photons that have scattered in the patient. The energy window can be set to encompass only the photopeak, with maximal rejection of scatter, but also reducing the number of valid interactions detected, or the window can include part of the Compton continuum, increasing the sensitivity, but also increasing the number of scattered photons detected.

The time signals of interactions not rejected by the energy discrimination circuits are used for coincidence detection. When a coincidence is detected, the circuitry or a computer in the scanner determines a line in space connecting the two interactions, as shown in Figure 19-15. This is called a *line of response*. The number of coincidences detected along each LOR is stored in the memory of the computer. Figure 19-18 compares the acquisition of projection data by SPECT and PET systems. Once data acquisition is complete, the computer uses the projection data to produce transverse images of the radionuclide distribution in the patient, as in x-ray CT or SPECT.

TABLE 19-2   PROPERTIES OF SEVERAL INORGANIC SCINTILLATORS OF INTEREST IN PET

SCINTILLATOR	DECAY CONSTANT (ns)	PEAK WAVELENGTH (nm)	ATOMIC NUMBERS	DENSITY (g/cm³)	ATTENUATION COEFFICIENT 511 keV (cm⁻¹)	CONVERSION EFFICIENCY RELATIVE TO NaI
NaI(Tl)	250	415	11,53	3.67	0.343	100%
BGO	300	460	83,32,8	7.17	0.964	12%–14%
GSO(Ce)	56	430	64,14,8	6.71	0.704	41%
LSO(Ce)	40	420	71,14,8	7.4	0.870	75%

Decay constants, peak wavelengths, densities, and conversion efficiencies of BGO, GSO, and LSO (From Ficke DC, Hood JT, Ter-Pogossian MM. A spheroid positron emission tomograph for brain imaging: a feasibility study. *J Nucl Med* 1996;37:1222.)
LYSO(Ce) has a decay constant, peak emission wavelength, and relative conversion efficiency similar to those of LSO (Ce), but its density and attenuation coefficient are less. Its density and attenuation coefficient vary with the proportion of yttrium to lutetium. (Information on LYSO from Chen J, Zhang L, Zhu RY. Large size LYSO crystals for future high energy physics experiments. *IEEE Trans Nucl Sci* 2005;52(6):3133–3140.)

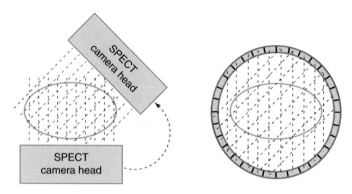

■ **FIGURE** 19-18 Acquisition of projection data by a SPECT system (**left**) and a PET system (**right**), showing how each system collects data for two projections. However, the PET system collects data for all projections simultaneously, whereas the scintillation camera head of the SPECT system must move to collect data from each projection angle.

Timing of Interactions and Detection of Coincidences

To detect coincidences, the times of individual interactions in the detectors must be compared. However, interactions themselves cannot be directly detected; instead, the signals caused by interactions are detected. In scintillators, the emission of light after an interaction is characterized by a relatively rapid increase in intensity followed by a more gradual decrease. A timing circuit connected to each detector must designate one moment that follows each interaction by a constant time interval. The time signal is determined from the leading edge of the electrical signal from the PMTs connected to a detector crystal because the leading edge is steeper than the trailing edge. When the time signals from two detectors occur within a selected time interval called the *time window*, a coincidence is recorded. A typical time window for a system with BGO detectors is 12 ns. A typical time window for a system with LSO detectors, which emit light more promptly, is 4.5 ns.

True versus Random Coincidences

The rate of random coincidences between any pair of detectors is:

$$R_{random} = \tau S_1 S_2 \qquad [19\text{-}1]$$

where τ is the coincidence time window and S_1 and S_2 are the actual count-rates of the detectors, often called *singles rates*. The time window is the designated time interval during which a pair of interactions in different detectors is considered to be a coincidence. The ratio of random to true coincidences increases with increasing activity in the subject and decreases as the time window is shortened. However, there is a limit to how small the time window can be. The time window must accommodate the difference in arrival times of true coincidence photons from annihilations occurring in locations up to the edge of the device's FOV. For example, if the longest path for an unscattered annihilation photon crossing the FOV is 70 cm, the time window can be no shorter than

$$\Delta t = 0.7 \text{ m}/(3.0 \times 10^8 \text{ m/s}) = 2.33 \text{ ns}$$

where 3.0×10^8 m/s is the speed of light. Furthermore, the time window must also be sufficiently long to accommodate the imprecision in the measured times of interactions. Scintillation materials that emit light promptly permit the use of shorter time windows and thus better discrimination between true and random coincidences.

Because the singles rates in individual detectors, ignoring dead-time count losses, are approximately proportional to the activity in the patient, Equation 19-1 shows that the rate of random coincidences is approximately proportional to the square of the activity in the patient. The true coincidence rate, ignoring dead-time count losses, is approximately proportional to the activity in the patient and so the ratio of random coincidences to true coincidences is approximately proportional to the administered activity.

Although individual random coincidences cannot be distinguished from true coincidences, methods of correction are available. The number of random coincidences along each LOR can be measured by adding a time delay to one of the two timing signals used for coincidence detection, so that no true coincidences are detected. Alternatively, the number of random coincidences may be calculated from the single event count-rates of the detectors, using Equation 19-1. The number of random coincidences is then subtracted from the number of true plus random coincidences for each LOR. This method corrects for the magnitude of signal from random coincidences, but not for the statistical noise that they introduce.

Scatter Coincidences

As previously mentioned, a scatter coincidence occurs when one or both of the photons from an annihilation are scattered in the patient and both are detected (Fig. 19-16). The fraction of scatter coincidences is dependent upon the amount of scattering material and thus is less in head than in body imaging. Because scatter coincidences are true coincidences, reducing the activity administered to the patient, reducing the time window, or using a scintillator with faster light emission does not significantly reduce the scatter coincidence fraction. Furthermore, the corrections for random coincidences do not compensate for scatter coincidences. The energy discrimination circuits of the PET scanner can be used to reject some scatter coincidences. As was mentioned previously, energy discrimination to reduce scatter is less effective in PET than in SPECT, because many of the 511-keV annihilation photons interact with the detectors by Compton scattering, depositing less than their entire energies in the detectors. Using an energy window closely enveloping the photopeak will reject many annihilation photons that have not scattered in the patient. The fraction of scatter coincidences can also be reduced by two-dimensional data acquisition and axial septa, as described in the following section. Approximation methods are available for scatter correction. These methods correct for the magnitude of the signal from scatter coincidences, but not for the statistical noise introduced by scatter coincidences.

Two- and Three-Dimensional Data Acquisition

In two-dimensional (slice) data acquisition, coincidences are detected and recorded only within each ring of detector elements or within a few adjacent rings of detector elements. PET scanners designed for two-dimensional acquisition have axial septa, thin annular collimators, typically made of tungsten, to prevent most radiation emitted by activity outside a transaxial slice from reaching the detector ring for that slice (Fig. 19-19). The fraction of scatter coincidences is greatly reduced in PET systems using two-dimensional data acquisition and axial collimation because of the geometry. Consider an annihilation occurring within a particular detector ring with the initial trajectories of the annihilation photons toward the detectors. If either of the photons scatters, it is likely that the new trajectory of the photon will cause it to miss the detector ring, thereby preventing a scatter coincidence. Furthermore, most photons from out-of-slice activity are absorbed by the axial septa.

In two-dimensional data acquisition, coincidences within one or more pairs of adjacent detector rings may be added to improve the sensitivity, as shown in Figure 19-20. The data from each pair of detector rings are added to that of the slice midway between the two rings. For example, if N is the number of a particular ring of detector elements, coincidences between rings $N-1$ and $N+1$ are

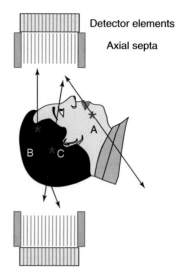

■ FIGURE 19-19 Side view of PET scanner illustrating two-dimensional data acquisition. The axial septa prevent photons from activity outside the field-of-view (**A**) and most scattered photons (**B**) from causing counts in the detectors. However, many valid photon pairs (**C**) are also absorbed.

Detector elements

Axial septa

added to the projection data for ring N. For further sensitivity, coincidences between rings N – 2 and N+2 can also be added to those of ring N. After the data from these pairs of detector rings are added, a standard two-dimensional reconstruction is performed to create a transverse image for this slice. Similarly, coincidences between two immediately adjacent detector rings, that is, between rings N and N+1, can be used to generate a transverse image halfway between these rings. For greater sensitivity, coincidences between rings N – 1 and N+2 can be added to these data. However, increasing the number of pairs of adjacent rings used in two-dimensional acquisition reduces the axial spatial resolution.

In three-dimensional (volume) data acquisition, axial septa are not used and coincidences are detected between many or all detector rings (Fig. 19-21). Three-dimensional acquisition greatly increases the number of true coincidences detected and may permit smaller activities to be administered to patients, compared to two-dimensional image acquisition. There are disadvantages to three-dimensional data

■ FIGURE 19-20 Side view of PET scanner performing two-dimensional data acquisition, showing LORs for a single transverse image. Cross-ring coincidences have been added to those occurring within the ring of detector elements. This increases the number of coincidences detected, but causes a loss of axial spatial resolution that increases with distance from the axis of the scanner.

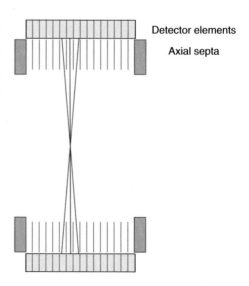

Detector elements

Axial septa

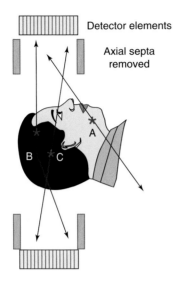

Detector elements

Axial septa removed

■ **FIGURE 19-21** Side view of PET scanner illustrating three-dimensional data acquisition. Without axial septa, interactions from activity outside the FOV (**A**) and scattered photons (**B**) are greatly increased, increasing the dead time, random coincidence fraction, and scatter coincidence fraction. However, the number of true coincidences (**C**) detected is also greatly increased.

acquisition. For the same administered activity, the greatly increased interaction rate increases the random coincidence fraction and the dead-time count losses. Furthermore, the scatter coincidence fraction is much larger and the number of interactions from activity outside the FOV is greatly increased. (Activity outside the FOV causes few true coincidences, but increases the rate of random coincidences detected and dead-time count losses.) Some PET systems are equipped with retractable axial septa, permitting them to perform two- or three-dimensional acquisition.

Figure 19-22 shows the efficiency of coincidence detection when two- or three-dimensional acquisition is used. In two-dimensional acquisition, the efficiency is nearly constant along the axial length of the detector rings. In three-dimensional

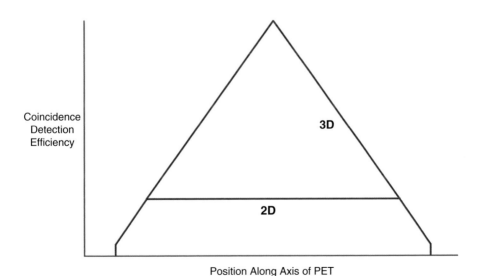

Coincidence Detection Efficiency

3D

2D

Position Along Axis of PET

■ **FIGURE 19-22** Efficiency of coincidence detection along axis of detector rings for two- and three-dimensional data acquisition. The three-dimensional acquisition example presumes that coincidences are detected among all rings of detector elements. The coincidence detection efficiency in two-dimensional acquisition is least if coincidences are detected only within individual rings of detector elements; it substantially increases when coincidences are also detected among adjacent rings, as shown in Figure 19-20.

acquisition, if coincidences are detected among all rings of detector elements, the coincidence detection efficiency increases linearly from the ends of the rings to the center. PET scans of extended lengths of patients are commonly accomplished by a discontinuous motion of the patient table through the system, with the table stopping for individual bed positions. Because of the greatly varying coincidence detection efficiency, much greater overlap of bed positions is necessary when using three-dimensional acquisitions.

Transverse Image Reconstruction

After the projection data are acquired, the data for each LOR are corrected for random coincidences, scatter coincidences, dead-time count losses, and attenuation (described below). Following these corrections, transverse image reconstruction is performed. For two-dimensional data acquisition, image reconstruction methods are similar to those used in SPECT. As in SPECT, either filtered backprojection or iterative reconstruction methods can be used. For three-dimensional data acquisition, special three-dimensional analytical or iterative reconstruction methods are required. These are beyond the scope of this chapter, but are discussed in the suggested readings listed at the end of the chapter.

An advantage of PET over SPECT is that, in PET, the correction for nonuniform attenuation can be applied to the projection data before reconstruction. In SPECT, the correction for nonuniform attenuation is intertwined with and complicates the reconstruction process.

Time of Flight Determination

In theory, measurement of the difference between the times of the interactions in the detectors of a pair of annihilation photons would determine the point on a line between the two interactions where an annihilation occurred. If this were possible, PET would be inherently tomographic and the reconstruction of transverse images from projection data would not be necessary.

The speed of light is 3.0×10^8 m/s. To determine the location of an annihilation within 1 cm would require being able to measure a difference in interaction times of $\Delta t = 1 \text{ cm} / 3.0 \times 10^{10} \text{ cm/s} = 0.033$ ns. Such precision in timing is not possible with current PET scintillators. Fast scintillators such as LSO and LYSO permit determination of the location of an annihilation within several cm. This information can be used in the tomographic reconstruction process to improve the signal-to-noise ratio in the images.

Performance

Spatial Resolution

Modern whole-body PET systems achieve a spatial resolution slightly better than 5-mm FWHM of the LSF in the center of the detector ring when measured by the NEMA standard, *Performance Measurements of Positron Emission Tomographs* (National Electrical Manufacturers Association, NEMA NU 2-2007, Performance Measurements of Positron Emission Tomographs). There are three factors that primarily limit the spatial resolution of PET scanners: (1) the intrinsic spatial resolution of the detectors, (2) the distances traveled by the positrons before annihilation, and (3) the fact that the annihilation photons are not emitted in exactly opposite directions from each other. The intrinsic resolution of the detectors is the major factor determining the spatial resolution in current scanners. In older systems in which the detectors consisted of separate crystals each attached to a single PMT, the size of the crystals

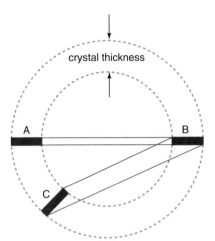

■ **FIGURE 19-23** Cause of reduced spatial resolution with distance from center of PET scanner. Only three crystal segments in the detector ring are shown. For coincident interactions in detectors *A* and *B*, there is little uncertainty in the LOR. When coincidences occur in detectors *B* and *C*, there is greater uncertainty in the LOR. Using thinner crystals would reduce this effect, but would also reduce their intrinsic detection efficiency and thus the number of coincidences detected.

determined the resolution. In clinical imaging, spatial resolution is also reduced by organ motion, most commonly due to respiration.

The spatial resolution of a PET system is best in the center of the detector ring and decreases slightly (FWHM increases) with distance from the center. This occurs because of the considerable thickness of the detectors. Uncertainty in the depth of interaction causes uncertainty in the LOR for annihilation photons that strike the detectors obliquely. Photons emitted from the center of the detector ring can only strike the detectors "head-on," but many of the photons emitted from activity away from the center strike the detectors from oblique angles (Fig. 19-23). Some newer PET systems can estimate the depths of interactions in the detectors and have more uniform spatial resolution across a transverse image.

The distance traveled by the positron before annihilation also slightly degrades the spatial resolution. This distance is determined by the maximal positron energy of the radionuclide and the density of the tissue. A radionuclide that emits lower energy positrons yields better resolution. Table 19-3 lists the maximal energies of positrons emitted by radionuclides commonly used in PET. Activity in denser tissue yields higher resolution than activity in less dense tissue such as lung tissue.

TABLE 19-3   PROPERTIES OF POSITRON-EMITTING RADIONUCLIDES COMMONLY USED IN PET

NUCLIDE	HALF-LIFE (min)	POSITRONS PER TRANSFORMATION	MAXIMAL POSITRON ENERGY (keV)	MAXIMAL POSITRON RANGE (mm)[a]	NOTES
C-11	20.4	1.00	960	4.2	
N-13	10.0	1.00	1198	5.4	
O-15	2.0	1.00	1732	8.4	
F-18	110	0.97	634	2.4	Most common use is F-18 fluorodeoxyglucose.
Rb-82	1.3	0.95	3356	17	Produced by a Sr-82/Rb-82 generator.

The average positron range is much less than the maximal range, because positrons are emitted with a continuum of energies and because the paths of positrons in matter are not straight.
[a]In water from ICRU Report 37.

Although positrons lose nearly all of their momentum before annihilation, the positron and electron possess some residual momentum when they annihilate. Conservation of momentum predicts that the resultant photons will not be emitted in exactly opposite directions. This causes a small loss of resolution, which increases with the diameter of the detector ring.

Efficiency in Annihilation Coincidence Detection

Consider a point source of a positron-emitting radionuclide in air midway between two identical detectors (Fig. 19-24) and assume that all positrons annihilate within the source. The true coincidence rate of the pair of detectors is

$$R_T = 2AG\varepsilon^2 \qquad\qquad [19\text{-}2]$$

where A is the rate of positron emission by the source, G is the geometric efficiency of either detector, and ε is the intrinsic efficiency of either detector. (Geometric and intrinsic efficiency were defined in Chapter 17.) Because the rate of true coincidences detected is proportional to the square of the intrinsic efficiency, maximizing the intrinsic efficiency is very important in PET. For example, if the intrinsic efficiency of a single detector for a 511-keV photon is 0.9, 81% of the annihilation photon pairs emitted toward the detectors will have coincident interactions. However, if the intrinsic efficiency of a single detector is 0.1, only 1% of pairs emitted toward the detectors will have coincident interactions.

As mentioned previously, most PET systems today use crystals of high density, high atomic number scintillators such as BGO, LSO, LYSO, or GSO. These crystals are typically about two to three cm thick. For example, a 2-cm thick crystal of LSO has an intrinsic efficiency of 82%, although energy discrimination reduces the fraction of detected photons used for coincidence detection below this value.

As mentioned above in "Two- and Three-Dimensional Data Acquisition," increasing the axial acceptance angle of annihilation photons greatly increases the efficiency. In PET systems with three-dimensional data acquisition, this can be augmented by adding additional rings of detectors.

Attenuation and Attenuation Correction in PET

Attenuation in PET differs from attenuation in SPECT, because both annihilation photons must escape the patient to cause a coincident event to be registered. The probability of both photons escaping the patient without interaction is the product of the probabilities of each escaping:

$$(e^{-\mu x}) \cdot (e^{-\mu(d-x)}) = e^{-\mu d} \qquad\qquad [19\text{-}3]$$

where d is the total path length through the patient, x is the distance one photon must travel to escape, and $(d-x)$ is the distance the other must travel to escape (Fig. 19-25). Thus, the probability of both escaping the patient without interaction is independent of where on the line the annihilation occurred and is the same as the probability of

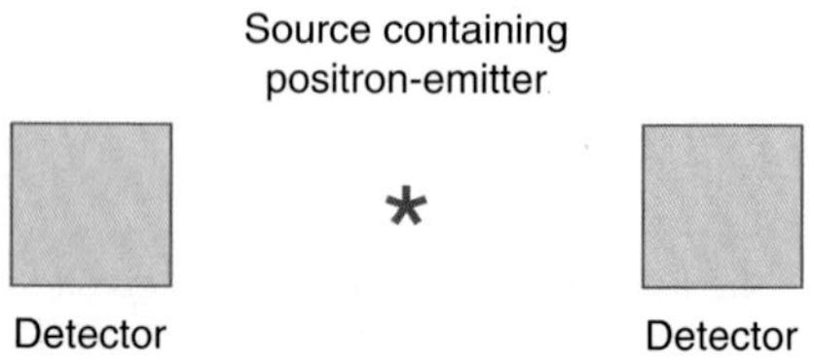

■ FIGURE 19-24 Point source of a positron-emitting radionuclide, in air, midway between two identical detectors.

Source containing positron-emitter

Detector   Detector

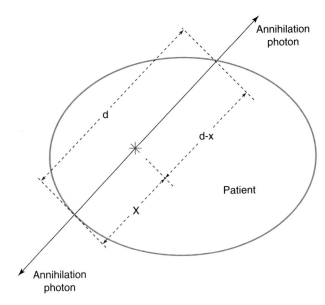

■ **FIGURE 19-25** Attenuation in PET. The probability that both annihilation photons emitted along a particular LOR escape interaction in the patient is independent of the position on the LOR where the annihilation occurred.

a single 511-keV photon passing entirely through the patient along the same path. (Equation 19-3 was derived for the case of uniform attenuation, but this principle is also valid for nonuniform attenuation.)

Even though the attenuation coefficient for 511-keV annihilation photons in soft tissue ($\mu/\rho = 0.095$ cm²/g) is lower than those of photons emitted by most radionuclides used in SPECT ($\mu/\rho = 0.15$ cm²/g for 140 keV gamma rays), the average path length for both to escape is much longer. For a 20-cm path in soft tissue, the chance of both annihilation photons of a pair escaping the tissue without interaction is only about 15%. Thus, attenuation is more severe in PET than in SPECT. The vast majority of the interactions with tissue are Compton scattering. Attenuation causes a loss of information and, because the loss is not the same for all LORs, causes artifacts in the reconstructed tomographic images. The loss of information also contributes to the statistical noise in the images.

As in SPECT, both approximate methods and methods using radioactive sources to measure the attenuation have been used for attenuation correction in PET. Most of the approximate methods used a profile of the patient and presume a uniform attenuation coefficient within the profile.

Many older PET systems provided one or more retractable positron-emitting sources inside the detector ring between the detectors and the patient to measure the transmission of annihilation photons from the sources through the patient. As mentioned above, the probability that a single annihilation photon from a source will pass through the patient without interaction is the same as the probability that both photons from an annihilation in the patient traveling along the same path through the patient will escape interaction. These sources were usually configured as rods and were parallel to the axis of the scanner (Fig. 19-26). The sources revolved around the patient, so that attenuation was measured along all LORs through the patient. These sources usually contained Ge-68, which has a half-life of 271 days and decays to Ga-68, which primarily decays by positron emission. Alternatively, a source containing a gamma ray-emitting radionuclide, such as Cs-137 (662-keV gamma ray), has been used for attenuation measurements instead of a positron-emitting radionuclide source. When a gamma ray-emitting radionuclide is used to measure the attenuation, the known position of the source

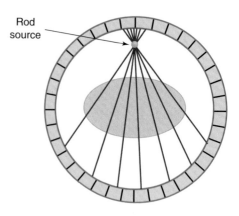

■ **FIGURE 19-26** Rod source for attenuation correction in a dedicated PET system.

and the location where a gamma ray is detected together determine a LOR for that interaction. In either case, the transmission data acquired using the external sources were used to correct the emission data for attenuation prior to transverse image reconstruction.

There are the advantages and disadvantages to attenuation correction from transmission measurements using radioactive sources. The transmission measurements increased the imaging time; slightly increased the radiation dose to the patient; and increased the statistical noise in the images. Also, spatial misregistration between the attenuation map and the emission data, most often caused by patient motion, can cause significant artifacts if the transmission data are not acquired simultaneously with the emission data.

Today, nearly every PET system manufactured is coupled to an x-ray CT system. These are called PET/CT systems. On such systems, the x-ray transmission information is used to correct the PET information for attenuation and so they are not provided with radioactive transmission sources for attenuation correction. PET/CT systems are discussed in detail later in this chapter.

Alternatives to Dedicated PET Systems—Multihead SPECT Cameras with Coincidence Detection Capability and SPECT with High Energy Collimators

Double and triple head SPECT cameras with coincidence detection capability have been commercially available. These cameras had planar NaI(Tl) crystals coupled to PMTs. With standard nuclear medicine collimators mounted, they functioned as conventional scintillation cameras and could perform planar nuclear medicine imaging and SPECT. With the collimators removed or replaced by slit collimators which reduce the rate of interactions by photons from out-of-field activity, they could perform coincidence imaging of positron-emitting radiopharmaceuticals. When used for coincidence imaging, these cameras provided spatial resolution similar to that of dedicated PET systems. The smaller attenuation coefficient of sodium iodide with respect to common PET scintillators and the thin crystal of a typical scintillation camera limited the intrinsic efficiency of each detector in detecting annihilation photons. For this reason, many cameras intended for coincidence imaging had thicker NaI crystals than standard scintillation cameras, with thicknesses ranging from 1.27 to 2.5 cm (1/2 to 1 inch). These thicker crystals significantly increased the number of true coincidences detected. However, even with thicker crystals, they detected much smaller numbers of true coincidences than dedicated PET systems. The lower coincidence detection sensitivity caused more statistical noise in the images than in images from a dedicated

PET system. Many studies were performed comparing multihead scintillation cameras capable of coincidence detection with dedicated PET systems for the task of detecting lesions with concentrations of F-18 FDG; these studies showed that the coincidence scintillation cameras had comparable performance for the detection of large lesions, but significantly worse performance in detecting small lesions in the patients, in comparison to dedicated PET systems (Boren et al., 1999; Delbeke et al., 1999; Oturai et al., 2004; Tiepolt et al., 2000; Yutani et al., 1999; Zhang et al., 2002; Zimny et al., 1999).

Some scintillation cameras can perform planar imaging and SPECT of positron emitters using collimators designed for 511-keV photons. These collimators have very thick septa and have very low collimator efficiencies. Despite the thick septa, the images produced suffer from considerable septal penetration. Also, the thick septa produce collimator pattern artifacts in the images. However, attenuation by the patient is less significant than in coincidence imaging. The gantries of such cameras must be able to support very heavy camera heads, because of the weight of 511-keV collimators and because the camera heads must contain adequate shielding for 511-keV photons from outside the FOV. F-18 FDG imaging with high-energy collimators does not appear to be acceptable for the evaluation and staging of neoplasms (Macfarlane et al., 1995), because of its limited detection efficiency and spatial resolution.

Quality Control in PET

Daily, typically before the first patient imaging, a scan is performed of a uniform positron-emitting source. This may be a line source or a cylindrical source. Ge-68 is a radionuclide commonly used in these sources; its daughter Ga-68, with which it is in secular equilibrium, emits positrons. This scan, typically displayed as detector maps or sinograms, will reveal poorly performing or inoperative detectors, detectors requiring normalization, and detectors with improperly set energy windows. Tomographic uniformity is periodically assessed using a cylindrical phantom with the uniform distribution of a positron-emitting radionuclide. If the daily or periodic uniformity scans reveal changes in detector efficiencies, a detector normalization calibration is performed to measure the efficiencies of all the detector LORs in the system and update the stored normalization factors. Periodically, an absolute activity calibration should also be performed if clinical measurements of activity concentration are to be performed. A medical physicist should perform a complete systems test and review the quality control program at least annually. This systems test assesses many parameters, including spatial resolution, statistical noise, count-rate performance, sensitivity, and image quality.

19.4 Dual Modality Imaging—SPECT/CT, PET/CT, and PET/MRI

Nuclear medicine tomographic imaging, whether SPECT or PET, of cancer, infections, and inflammatory diseases often reveals lesions with greater radionuclide concentrations than surrounding tissue, but often provides little information regarding their exact locations in the organs of the patients. Spatial coregistration of the SPECT or PET images with images from another modality, such as x-ray CT or MRI, that provides good depiction of anatomy can be very useful. This can be accomplished by imaging the patient using separate SPECT or PET and CT or MRI systems and aligning the resultant images using multimodality image registration software. However, it is difficult to align the patient on the bed of the second imaging system exactly the same as on the first system, which in turn makes it very difficult to accurately align the SPECT or PET data with the CT or MRI data.

As mentioned earlier in this chapter, another problem common to both SPECT and PET is attenuation of the gamma rays, x-rays, or annihilation photons by the patient, causing a reduction in apparent activity toward the centers of transverse images and attenuation artifacts, particularly when attenuation is nonuniform. In both SPECT and PET, manufacturers have provided the capability to perform attenuation correction using sealed radioactive sources to measure the transmission through the patient from the various projection angles. As mentioned earlier, the use of radioactive sources for attenuation correction in SPECT was not met with universal acceptance, whereas the use of external sources for attenuation correction in PET was generally accepted. However, in PET, the use of radioactive sources for attenuation correction increased imaging times, reducing patient throughput.

To solve these problems, systems have been developed that incorporate a PET or SPECT system and a conventional x-ray CT system in a single gantry or in coupled gantries (Fig. 19-14 and Fig. 19-1A,B). The patient lies on a bed that passes through the bores of both systems. X-ray CT imaging is performed of the same length of the patient as the PET or SPECT imaging, either before or after the PET or SPECT image acquisition. Because the patient's position on the bed is the same during CT and PET or SPECT image acquisition, accurate coregistration of the CT and PET or SPECT information is usually possible. In the coregistered images, the PET or SPECT information is usually superimposed in color on grayscale CT images (Fig. 19-27).

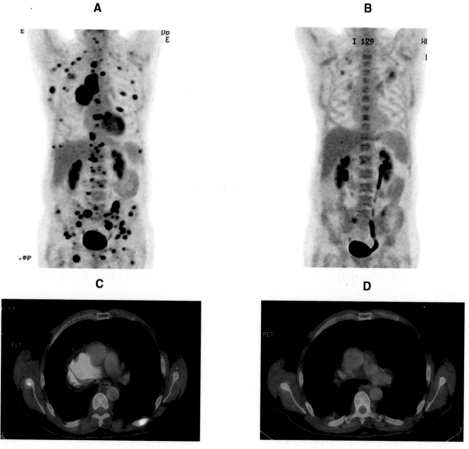

■ **FIGURE 19-27** Coregistered PET and CT images. (Images courtesy of D. K. Shelton, M.D., UC Davis Medical Center.)

Advantages of using x-ray CT systems instead of radioactive sources for attenuation correction are much quicker attenuation scans, permitting increased patient throughput and reducing the likelihood of patient motion; less statistical noise in the attenuation data due to the high x-ray flux from the CT; and higher spatial resolution attenuation data. However, there are disadvantages as well, which are discussed below.

Manufacturers have provided SPECT/CT and PET/CT systems with x-ray CT subsystems that are capable of producing diagnostic quality CT images and with less-expensive CT systems that are not capable of producing diagnostic quality CT images. If the x-ray CT subsystem is capable of diagnostic quality imaging, it may be used with low tube current, providing low dose but nondiagnostic CT information for attenuation correction and anatomic localization only, or with high tube current, providing diagnostic quality CT images.

Nearly all PET systems sold today are integrated PET/x-ray CT systems, because of their ability to provide attenuation-corrected PET images coregistered to x-ray CT images with high patient throughput. Efforts are underway to develop combined PET/MRI systems. These are discussed later in this chapter.

Attenuation Correction in PET/CT

As mentioned above, the x-ray CT provides information that can be used for attenuation correction of the PET information, replacing the positron-emitting rod sources formerly used for attenuation correction by PET systems. A modern x-ray CT system can provide the attenuation information, with very little statistical noise, in a fraction of a minute, in comparison with the many minutes required when positron-emitting rod sources were used.

An x-ray CT system measures the average linear attenuation coefficients, averaged over the x-ray energy spectrum, for individual volume elements (voxels) of the patient. However, linear attenuation coefficients for 511-keV annihilation photons are necessary for attenuation correction of PET information. Linear attenuation coefficients, measured using the x-rays from x-ray CT systems, are very different from those for 511-keV photons, and the ratio between the coefficients depends upon the material in the individual voxel. If the x-ray CT information is to be used for correction of the PET emission information, the linear attenuation coefficient for each voxel for 511-keV photons must be estimated from the linear attenuation coefficient (or, equivalently, the CT number) for that voxel for x-rays from the CT system.

The linear attenuation coefficient is the product of the density of a material and its mass attenuation coefficient. Table 19-4 lists the mass attenuation coefficients for 70-keV x-rays and 511-keV annihilation photons for several materials. The mass attenuation coefficients in the CT energy range vary greatly with the atomic number (Z) of the material because of the photoelectric effect. Although the interactions of the x-rays from an x-ray CT system with soft tissue and bodily fluids are mainly by Compton scattering, their interactions with higher atomic number materials such as bone mineral, x-ray contrast material, and metal objects in the body, are by both the photoelectric effect and Compton scattering. However, 511-keV annihilation photons almost entirely interact with all these materials by Compton scattering. As discussed in Chapter 3, the Compton scattering component of the linear attenuation coefficient for photons of a specific energy is determined by the number of electrons per volume, which in turn is largely determined by the density of the material.

The commonly used methods for estimating the linear attenuation coefficients for 511-keV photons from the CT numbers (defined in Chapter 10) are based upon making assumptions about the composition of the material in individual voxels using

TABLE 19-4   COMPARISON OF MASS ATTENUATION COEFFICIENTS FOR SOME TISSUES AND MATERIALS

PHOTON ENERGY (keV)	MASS ATTENUATION COEFFICIENTS (cm²/g)			
	SKELETAL MUSCLE	CORTICAL BONE	TITANIUM	IODINE
70	0.192	0.263	0.545	5.02
511	0.0951	0.0894	0.0811	0.0952

Hubbell JH, Seltzer SM. Tables of X-Ray Mass Attenuation Coefficients and Mass Energy-Absorption Coefficients 1 keV to 20 MeV for Elements Z=1 to 92 and 48 Additional Substances of Dosimetric Interest, NISTIR 5632, US Department of Commerce, May 1995.
For x-rays of a typical energy (70 keV) produced by a CT scanner, the likelihood of the photoelectric effect has a large effect on mass attenuation coefficients and so they vary greatly with the atomic numbers of the material. However, for 511-keV annihilation photons, Compton scattering is by far the most likely interaction in these materials and the mass attenuation coefficient varies little with atomic number. Note that attenuation is determined by the linear attenuation coefficient, which is the product of the mass attenuation coefficient and the density of the material.

their CT numbers. One method for estimating the linear attenuation coefficients for 511-keV photons from the CT numbers is to divide the voxels into two groups: those with CT numbers less than a value such as 50 and those with CT numbers greater than this value (Carney et al., 2006). Voxels with CT numbers less than this value are assumed to contain only soft tissue, body fluids, gas, or a mixture of them, whereas voxels with CT numbers greater than this value are assumed to contain bone mineral and soft tissue. For each of these two groups, the linear attenuation coefficient for 511-keV photons is calculated from a linear equation relating these linear attenuation coefficients to the CT number. For voxels in the low CT number group:

$$\mu_{511keV} = (9.6 \times 10^{-5} cm^{-1}) \cdot (CTnumber + 1,000)$$

This equation will yield the correct linear attenuation coefficients for air (CT number $= -1000$, $\mu_{511\,keV} = 0$) and water (CT number $= 0$, $\mu_{511\,keV} = 0.096$ cm⁻¹) and approximately correct linear attenuation coefficients for most soft tissues. For voxels in the high CT number group, the linear attenuation coefficient for 511-keV photons is calculated from

$$\mu_{511keV} = m \cdot (CTnumber) + b$$

where m and b are empirically determined constants that differ with the kV used by the x-ray CT system. In effect, the linear equation for the lower CT number voxels uses the CT number to determine the density of the soft tissue in a voxel, whereas the linear equation for the high CT number voxels uses the CT number to determine the ratio of mass of bone mineral to mass of soft tissue in a voxel. These methods for estimating the linear attenuation coefficients for 511-keV photons from CT numbers are successful when the assumptions about the composition of material in a voxel are valid, but can fail badly when these assumptions are not correct.

Incorrect estimation of the linear attenuation coefficients for 511-keV photons can cause artifacts in the attenuation-corrected images. This commonly occurs when there is a material, such as metal or concentrated x-ray contrast material, that does not conform to the assumptions implicit in the method used to estimate attenuation coefficients for 511-keV photons from the x-ray CT data. If the attenuation coefficient for 511-keV photons is significantly overestimated, the artifact typically appears as a falsely elevated radionuclide concentration. Such artifacts are discussed below.

Artifacts in PET/CT Imaging

Most things that cause artifacts in CT imaging, such as implanted metal objects that cause star artifacts and patient motion, can in turn cause artifacts in attenuation-corrected PET/CT images. However, there are also artifacts, discussed below, that are not artifacts in the PET images or the CT images themselves, but are caused by the interactions of the two image sets.

Spatial Misregistration Artifacts

Despite the fact that the patient lies in the same position for both the PET and x-ray CT scans, spatial misregistration of image information can still occur because the PET and x-ray CT image information are not acquired simultaneously. Misregistration most commonly occurs due to organ motion, particularly in or near the thorax due to respiration. The x-ray CT imaging is commonly performed during a single breath-hold to produce images without the effects of respiratory motion, whereas the PET imaging occurs during normal resting respiration. In particular, if the CT imaging is performed with breath-holding after full inspiration and the PET imaging is acquired during shallow breathing, F-18 FDG avid lesions located in the liver close to the diaphragm or in the chest wall may appear to be in the lungs in the fused PET/CT images. Figure 19-28 shows a case of misregistration due to respiratory motion.

A partial solution to this problem is to acquire low-dose x-ray CT information for image coregistration and attenuation correction during normal resting breathing and, if needed, to acquire separate high-dose diagnostic quality CT images during breath holding at maximal inspiration. Another partial solution is to acquire the CT images with breath holding at midinspiration or midexpiration. Some systems allow respiratory gating to be performed during the PET acquisition. Respiratory gating can reduce respiratory motion artifacts and permit more accurate determination of tissue volumes and activity concentrations, but increases the acquisition time.

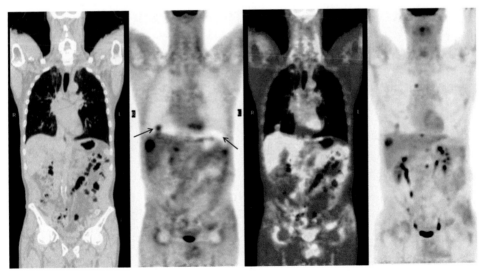

■ FIGURE 19- 28 PET/CT study showing diaphragmatic misregistration with superimposition of a hypermetabolic liver nodule over the right lung base on the fused PET-CT. **Left to right:** coronal CT, attenuation-corrected PET, fused attenuation corrected PET-CT, and attenuation-corrected PET maximum intensity projection images. CT shows no nodule in the right lung base, and attenuation-corrected PET and fused PET-CT images show a clear band above the diaphragm due to misregistration. (Images and interpretation courtesy of George M. Segall , M.D., VA Palo Alto Health Care System.)

Attenuation Correction Artifacts

When x-ray CT information is used for attenuation correction of the PET information, incorrect estimation of linear attenuation coefficients for 511-keV photons can cause artifacts. As mentioned above under Attenuation Correction in PET/CT, material in the patient that does not meet the assumptions inherent in the method to estimate attenuation coefficients for 511-keV photons from x-ray CT data can cause significant errors in attenuation correction. If the attenuation coefficient for 511-keV photons is significantly overestimated, the artifact typically appears as a falsely elevated radionuclide concentration. This can occur where there are metallic objects in the body, such as pacemakers, orthopedic devices, or body piercings, or concentrations of x-ray contrast material. Such an artifact is shown in Figure 19-29.

Voluminous metal objects, such as hip implants, in the patient may not cause such attenuation artifacts displaying falsely elevated radionuclide concentration. Although the attenuation coefficient for 511-keV photons is greatly overestimated, there is no positron-emitting radionuclide in the metal object and so the attenuation correction and image reconstruction process has no signal to incorrectly overamplify.

As mentioned above, x-ray contrast material, commonly containing iodine (intravascular contrast material) or barium (contrast material for GI studies) can also cause errors in attenuation correction (Mawlawi et al., 2006; Otero et al., 2009). It appears that such material, unless concentrated in a particular location, is not likely to have clinically significant effects.

A focus of apparent enhanced uptake in the attenuation-corrected images can be confirmed or refuted by a review of the corresponding uncorrected images. Spatial misregistrations of CT and PET data can also cause errors in attenuation correction (Goerres et al., 2003). Such an artifact appears at the level of the diaphragm (band of falsely-low pixel values) in the middle two images in Figure 19-28.

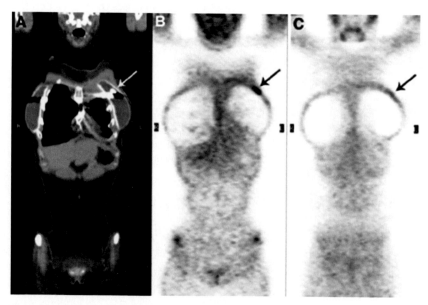

■ FIGURE 19-29 Attenuation correction artifact caused by overestimation of attenuation by a metal object, in this case a body piercing. CT image (**A**) shows a streaking artifact at the location of the metal object on the left breast. Overestimation of attenuation causes the attenuation-corrected PET image (**B**) to display a falsely elevated concentration of F-18 FDG at the location of the metal object. Notice that that concentration of F-18 FDG is not elevated in the PET image (**C**) that is not attenuation corrected. (Images courtesy of Sureshbabu W, Mawlawi O. PET/CT imaging artifacts. *J Nucl Med Technol* 2005;33:156–161.)

Truncation Artifacts

The radial FOVs of the CT and PET systems may differ significantly. Commonly, the PET system has a much larger radial FOV than the CT, although at least one manufacturer offers a system in which the PET and CT systems have equal FOVs. If part of a patient, for example a patient of large girth or a patient imaged with the arms by his or her side, extends outside the FOV of the CT, there will be error in the attenuation correction of the PET images because attenuation by the portion of the patient outside the CT's FOV is not considered.

SPECT/X-ray CT Systems

Several manufacturers provide imaging systems incorporating two scintillation camera heads capable of planar imaging and SPECT and an x-ray CT system with a single patient bed. Some of these systems have very simple x-ray CT systems that provide x-ray CT information for attenuation correction of the SPECT information and image co-registration only, whereas others can produce diagnostic quality CT images.

The advantages and disadvantages of using the x-ray CT system for attenuation correction and image coregistration are the same as in the case of the PET/CT systems described above. The x-ray CT system acquires the attenuation information much more quickly than does a system using radioactive sealed sources and the attenuation information has less statistical noise, but the linear attenuation coefficients for the energies of the gamma rays must be estimated from the CT attenuation information. The methods for doing this are similar to those used in PET/CT, which were discussed earlier in this chapter. Artifacts can occur when the calculation produces the wrong attenuation coefficient. This can be caused by high atomic number material in the patient, such as metal objects and concentrated contrast material. Furthermore, as in PET/CT, the SPECT and x-ray CT information are not acquired simultaneously and patient organ motion can result in the misregistrations of SPECT and PET image information.

A common use of SPECT/CT is myocardial perfusion imaging. In myocardial perfusion imaging, nonuniform attenuation, particularly by the diaphragm and, in women, the breasts, can cause apparent perfusion defects in the SPECT images. Attenuation correction using the CT information has been reported to improve diagnostic accuracy by compensating for these artifacts. However, spatial misregistration between the heart in the CT and SPECT images can cause artifacts (Goetze et al., 2007). An important quality assurance step in myocardial perfusion SPECT/CT is to verify alignment of the SPECT and CT image information.

PET/MRI Systems

Dual modality PET/MRI systems have very recently been developed. These include small systems for imaging of animals and larger systems for imaging humans for research. As in PET/CT, the MRI system provides tomographic images with excellent depiction of anatomic detail and the PET information is spatially coregistered with the MRI information. The MRI information is also used to estimate attenuation coefficients in each voxel of the patient for correction of the PET information for attenuation of the annihilation photons.

A problem that must be addressed in the design of PET/MRI imaging systems is that photomultiplier tubes (PMTs) are adversely affected by magnetic fields, particularly very strong ones such as those produced by MRI magnets. Furthermore, PMTs are very bulky. Two methods have been used to address this problem. In one approach, the rings of PET detectors are inside the bore of the MRI system's main magnet. These detectors consist of scintillation crystals optically coupled to avalanche photodiodes, which are not affected by the strong magnetic field. (Avalanche photodiodes were briefly discussed in Chapter 17.) In the other approach, the PET system is at one end of the patient couch and the MRI system is at the other end of the patient couch, with the two systems being separated by a distance of about 2 m. In this latter approach, the PET detectors consist of scintillation crystals coupled to PMTs. A system with the PET detectors inside the MRI permits simultaneous image acquisition, whereas the other design requires sequential imaging.

Quality Control of Dual Modality Imaging Systems

There are three aspects to the quality control of dual modality imaging systems. There is quality control testing of the SPECT or PET imaging system; these were discussed in the relevant sections earlier in this chapter. Then, there should be the quality control testing of the CT or MRI system. Lastly, there should be testing of the operation of the combined systems. The two major items to be tested are the accuracy of the spatial coregistration of the two modalities and the accuracy of the attenuation correction.

19.5 Clinical Aspects, Comparison of PET and SPECT, and Dose

As mentioned in the first chapter of this textbook, nuclear medicine imaging produces images depicting function. The function depicted may be a mechanical function, such as the ability of the heart to contract, but very often is a physiological or biochemical function. However, a disadvantage is that the images may lack sufficient anatomic information to permit determination of the organ or tissue containing a feature of interest. Fusion of the nuclear medicine images with those from another modality, such as CT, providing good depiction of anatomy can resolve this problem. Another disadvantage of imaging radiopharmaceuticals is that attenuation by the patient of the emitted photons can cause artifacts. CT attenuation information can be used to largely correct these artifacts.

F-18 Fluorodeoxyglucose and Other PET Radiopharmaceuticals

As discussed in the previous chapter, the utility of nuclear medicine is as much determined by the radiopharmaceutical as it is by the imaging device. For example, the success of the Anger scintillation camera was in part due to the development of many radiopharmaceuticals incorporating Tc-99m.

An advantage of PET is that there are positron-emitting radioisotopes of the common biochemical elements carbon, nitrogen, and oxygen, but these have short half-lives (20, 10, and 2 min, respectively). The use of radiopharmaceuticals incorporating them requires a nearby or on-site cyclotron and so their use has largely been restricted to research.

The widespread clinical adoption of PET and now PET/CT has been driven by the remarkable radiochemical (F-18)2-fluoro-2-deoxy-D-glucose (F-18 FDG). F-18 FDG is a glucose analog; it is transported by facilitated diffusion into cells that utilize glucose and phosphorylated, as is glucose. However, the phosphorylated F-18 FDG cannot proceed further along the metabolic path of glucose and therefore remains in the cells. Thus, F-18 accumulates in cells at a rate proportional to local extracellular concentration and glucose uptake. (Some cells have an enzyme that dephosphorylates glucose-6-phosphate and some F-18 FDG escapes these cells.) F-18 has a half-life of 110 min, permitting a cyclotron-equipped radiopharmacy to provide F-18 FDG throughout a metropolitan area or even over larger distances. FDG has shown clinical utility for differentiating Alzheimer's disease from other forms of dementia, identifying foci responsible for epileptic seizures, and for differentiating hypoperfused myocardium from scar tissue. However, its most common application today is in oncology, in which it is used to evaluate and assess the efficacy of treatment for the many forms of cancer that accumulate glucose. However, F-18 FDG is only of limited use in some forms of cancer, notably prostate cancer.

The FDA has approved a few other PET radiopharmaceuticals, which are described in Chapter 16. Other PET radiopharmaceuticals are under study.

Radiation Doses

As mentioned in Chapter 16, the radiation doses from the administration of a radiopharmaceutical depends on the physiological behavior of the radiopharmaceutical, the physical half-life of the radionuclide, the activity administered, and the types and energies of the radiations emitted. Positrons deposit nearly all of their kinetic energies within millimeters of the sites of their emission. Much, but not all, of the energy of the annihilation photons escapes the patient. To keep the doses to patients sufficiently low, the radionuclides commonly used in PET have been restricted to ones with relatively short half-lives. The intravenous administration of 370 MBq (10 mCi) of F-18 FDG to an adult imparts an effective dose of about 7 mSv (Appendix F-2).

The radiation dose from a PET/CT or SPECT/CT examination includes that of the CT scan. In oncologic PET/CT, the CT scan is typically performed on a length of the body from just below the eyes to the symphysis pubis. The effective dose from this CT scan is relatively large because of the length of the body that is scanned. The CT scan can be a high x-ray tube current scan that produces images of diagnostic quality, or it can be a low dose scan that produces images only for attenuation correction and anatomic correlation. The effective dose from the former may be about 16 mSv, whereas that from the latter may be about 4 mSv (Brix et al., 2005). Innovations in CT such as automatic tube current modulation and iterative image reconstruction may reduce these doses.

Comparison of SPECT and PET

In single photon emission imaging, the spatial resolution and the detection efficiency are primarily determined by the collimator. Both are ultimately limited by the compromise between collimator efficiency and collimator spatial resolution that is a consequence of collimated image formation. It is the use of ACD instead of collimation that makes the PET scanner much more efficient than the scintillation camera and also yields its superior spatial resolution.

In systems that use collimation to form images, the spatial resolution rapidly deteriorates with distance from the face of the imaging device. This causes the spatial resolution to deteriorate from the edge to the center in transverse SPECT images. In contrast, PET is not subject to this limitation and the spatial resolution in a transverse PET image is best in the center.

TABLE 19-5   COMPARISON OF SPECT AND PET

	SPECT	PET
Principle of projection data collection	Collimation.	Annihilation coincidence detection (ACD).
Transverse image reconstruction	Iterative methods or filtered backprojection.	Iterative methods or filtered backprojection.
Radionuclides	Any emitting x rays, gamma rays, or annihilation photons. Optimal performance for photon energies of 100–200 keV.	Positron emitters only.
Spatial resolution	Depends upon collimator and camera orbit.	Relatively constant across transaxial image, best at center.
	Within a transaxial image, the resolution in the radial direction is relatively uniform, but the tangential resolution is degraded toward the center.	Typically 4.5–5 mm FWHM at center.
	Typically about 10 mm FWHM at center for a 30 cm diameter orbit and ^{99m}Tc.	
	Larger camera orbits produce worse resolution.	
Attenuation	Attenuation less severe.	Attenuation more severe.
	Radioactive attenuation correction sources or x-ray CT can correct for attenuation.	Radioactive attenuation correction sources or x-ray CT can correct for attenuation.

The cost of a dual-head SPECT system is typically a few hundred thousand dollars. The cost of a SPECT-CT system depends greatly on the capabilities of the CT system. As mentioned previously, some have slow low-dose CT systems that are not capable of producing diagnostic quality CT images, whereas others have multirow detector, subsecond rotation CT systems that can produce diagnostic quality images. The cost of the latter system may be more than twice that of a SPECT system without CT. The cost of a PET/CT system is about twice that of a SPECT/CT system capable of diagnostic quality CT imaging. Table 19-5 compares SPECT and PET systems.

Quantitative Imaging

It is desirable, for research studies and many clinical studies, that each pixel value in a SPECT or PET image be proportional to the number of nuclear transformations occurring during imaging in the corresponding voxel of the patient. For example, in myocardial perfusion imaging, it is desirable that the count in each pixel depicting left ventricular myocardium be proportional to the concentration of radioactive tracer in the corresponding voxel in the patient's heart.

The primary factors limiting the quantitative accuracy of SPECT and PET are imperfect spatial resolution and photon attenuation and scattering in the patient. At high interaction rates in the imaging system, other effects such as dead-time count losses and, in PET, random coincidences may also contribute to divergence from proportionality. Yet another reason is patient motion. Because SPECT and PET imaging occur for lengthy time intervals, spatial resolution is degraded by motion, particularly respiratory motion. PET with radioactive sources for attenuation correction and PET/CT are considered quantitative imaging modalities and the reconstructed voxel values can be calibrated in units of activity.

The *partial volume effect* is a reduction in the apparent activity concentration in smaller objects caused by averaging of the actual activity concentration with that of surrounding tissues. Causes of the partial volume effect are blurring caused by the imaging device; blurring by the tomographic reconstruction process (e.g., the spatial filtering used in filtered backprojection or after iterative reconstruction); and the sizes of the pixels in the resultant images. PET's higher spatial resolution causes it to suffer less from the partial volume effect than SPECT.

A physiological model was developed by Sokoloff and colleagues that enables the rate of local tissue glucose utilization to be calculated from the amount of radiolabeled FDG that accumulates in the tissue (Sokoloff et al., 1977). The model has been extended to permit non-invasive measurements of this rate using F-18 FDG and PET imaging (Phelps et al., 1979). This latter method has been used extensively in research studies of the brain, heart, and other organs. However, the method requires blood sampling, which has hindered its clinical use.

The standardized uptake value (SUV) is a calculated quantity used in F-18 FDG imaging in an attempt to normalize the uptake of F-18 FDG for administered activity, radioactive decay from the time of dosage administration, and patient body mass (Keyes, 1995; Thie, 2004). Some physicians use the SUV to assist in characterizing tissues that accumulate the radiopharmaceutical, particularly in distinguishing benign from malignant lesions or in monitoring tumor therapy. It is defined as

$$SUV = \frac{\text{activity concentration in a voxel or group of voxels}}{\text{activity administered/body mass}}$$

where either the administered activity or the activity concentration is corrected for radioactive decay from the time of dosage assay until imaging.

The SUV has units of density, for example, g/cm^3. Some institutions use lean body mass or body surface area instead of body mass in the denominator of this equation. Because the SUV is not based upon a physiological model, such as the Sokoloff model, it is regarded as an approximate or semiquantitative index of FDG uptake.

The SUV measurement is affected by many factors:

1. Accuracy of the assay of activity to be administered. This includes correction for activity remaining in the syringe after administration
2. Extravasation of activity during administration, which occurs in a small fraction of administrations
3. Calibration of the PET/CT and accuracy of attenuation correction
4. Elapsed time from activity administration until imaging, including correct recording of time of administration
5. Accuracy of patient body mass
6. Physiological state of patient at time of administration. This includes preparation of the patient, including fasting before administration and possibly insulin administration
7. Patient body composition (e.g., ratio of fatty to lean tissue)
8. Size of lesion. The partial volume affect can reduce the measured SUV for very small lesions
9. Motion, such as respiratory motion, during image acquisition, particularly for smaller lesions
10. User region-of-interest (ROI) selection

Clinicians using the SUV for making decisions regarding patient workup, staging, treatment, and treatment planning should discuss with their nuclear medicine physicians the potential uncertainties in the SUV as it is determined in their nuclear medicine service or PET/CT provider and apply caution in using SUVs from different institutions.

SUGGESTED READINGS

Bax JJ, Wijns W. Editorial—fluorodeoxyglucose imaging to assess myocardial viability: PET, SPECT, or gamma camera coincidence imaging. *J Nucl Med* 1999;40:1893–1895.

Carney JPJ, Townsend DW, Rappoport V, Bendriem B. Method for transforming CT images for attenuation correction in PET/CT imaging. *Med Phys* 2006;33(4):976–983.

Cherry SR, Phelps ME. Positron emission tomography: methods and instrumentation. In: Sandler MP, et al., eds. *Diagnostic nuclear medicine.* 4th ed. Baltimore, MD: Lippincott Williams & Wilkins, 2003:61–83.

EANM Physics Committee: Sokole EB, Płachcínska A, Britten A with contribution from the EANM Working Group on Nuclear Medicine Instrumentation Quality Control: Georgosopoulou ML, Tindale W, Klett R. Routine quality control recommendations for nuclear medicine instrumentation *Eur J Nucl Med Mol Imaging* 2010;37:662–671.

Gelfand MJ, Thomas SR. *Effective use of computers in nuclear medicine.* New York, NY: McGraw-Hill, 1988.

Groch MW, Erwin WD. SPECT in the Year 2000: Basic principles. *J Nucl Med Technol* 2000;28:233–244.

Groch MW, Erwin WD, Bieszk JA. Single photon emission computed tomography. In: Treves ST, ed. *Pediatric nuclear medicine.* 2nd ed. New York, NY: Springer-Verlag, 1995:33–87.

Hines H, Kayayan R, Colsher J, Hashimoto D, Schubert R, Fernando J, Simcic V, Vernon P, Sinclair RL. NEMA recommendations for implementing SPECT instrumentation quality control. *J Nucl Med* 2000;41:383–389.

Patton JA, Turkington TG. SPECT/CT physical principles and attenuation correction. *J Nucl Med Technol* 2008;36:1–10.

Sureshbabu W, Mawlawi O. PET/CT imaging artifacts. *J Nucl Med Technol* 2005;33:156–161.

Thie JA. Understanding the standardized uptake value, its methods, and implications for usage. *J Nucl Med* 2004;45(9):1431–1434.

Yester MV, Graham LS, eds. Advances in nuclear medicine: the medical physicist's perspective. Proceedings of the 1998 Nuclear Medicine Mini Summer School, American Association of Physicists in Medicine, June 21–23, 1998, Madison, WI.

Zaidi H, ed. *Quantitative analysis in nuclear medicine imaging.* New York, NY: Springer, 2006.

Zanzonico P. Routine quality control of clinical nuclear medicine instrumentation: a brief review. *J Nucl Med* 2008;49:1114–1131.

SELECTED REFERENCES

Boren EL Jr., Delbeke D, Patton JA, Sandler MP. Comparison of FDG PET and positron coincidence detection imaging using a dual-head gamma camera with 5/8-inch NaI(Tl) crystals in patients with suspected body malignancies. *Eur J Nucl Med Mol I* 1999;26(4):379–387.

Brix G, Lechel U, Glatting G, Ziegler SI, Münzing W, Müller SP, Beyer T. Radiation exposure of patients undergoing whole-body dual-modality ^{18}F-FDG PET/CT examinations. *J Nucl Med* 2005;46:608–613.

Chang LT. A method for attenuation correction in radionuclide computed tomography. *IEEE Trans Nucl Sci* 1978;NS-25:638.

Delbeke D, Patton JA, Martin WH, Sandler MP. FDG PET and dual-head gamma camera positron coincidence detection imaging of suspected malignancies and brain disorders. *J Nucl Med* 1999;40(1):110–117.

Goetze S, Brown TL, Lavely WC, Zhang Z, Bengel FM. Attenuation correction in myocardial perfusion SPECT/CT: effects of misregistration and value of reregistration. *J Nucl Med* 2007;48(7):1090–1095.

Hendel RC, et al. The value and practice of attenuation correction for myocardial perfusion SPECT imaging: a joint position statement from the American Society of Nuclear Cardiology and the Society of Nuclear Medicine. *J Nuclear Med* 2002;43(2):273–280.

Hudson HM, Larkin RS. Accelerated image reconstruction using ordered subsets of projection data. *IEEE Trans Med Imaging* 1994;13:601–609.

Keyes JW Jr. SUV: Standard Uptake or Silly Useless Value? *J Nucl Med* 1995; 36:1836–1839.

Kuhl DE, Edwards RQ. Image separation radioisotope scanning. *Radiology* 1963;80:653–662.

Liu Y-H, Lam PT, Sinusas AJ, Wackers FJTh. Differential effect of 180° and 360° acquisition orbits on the accuracy of SPECT imaging: quantitative evaluation in phantoms. *J Nuclear Med* 2002;43(8):1115–1124.

Macfarlane DJ, Cotton L, Ackermann RJ, Minn H, Ficaro EP, Shreve PD, Wahl RL. Triple-head SPECT with 2-[fluorine-18]fluoro-2-deoxy-D-glucose (FDG): initial evaluation in oncology and comparison with FDG PET. *Radiology* 1995;194:425–429.

Masood Y, et al. Clinical validation of SPECT attenuation correction using x-ray computed tomography– derived attenuation maps: multicenter clinical trial with angiographic correlation. *J Nuclear Cardiol* 2005;12(6);676–686.

Mawlawi O, Erasmus JJ, et al. Quantifying the effect of iv contrast media on integrated PET/CT: clinical evaluation. *AJR* 2006;186:308–319.

National Electrical Manufacturers Association, NEMA NU 1-2007, Performance Measurements of Gamma Cameras.

National Electrical Manufacturers Association, NEMA NU 2-2007, Performance Measurements of Positron Emission Tomographs.

Nichols KJ. Editorial: How serious a problem for myocardial perfusion assessment is moderate misregistration between SPECT and CT? *J Nuclear Cardiol* 2007;14(2):150–152.

Otero HJ, Yap JT, et al. Evaluation of low-density neutral oral contrast material in PET/CT for tumor imaging: results of a randomized clinical trial. *AJR* 2009;193:326–332.

Oturai PS, Mortensen J, Enevoldsen H, Eigtved A, Backer V, Olesen KP, Nielsen HW, Hansen H, Stentoft P, Friberg L. γ-camera ^{18}F-FDG PET in diagnosis and staging of patients presenting with suspected lung cancer and comparison with dedicated PET. *J Nucl Med* 2004;45(8):1351–1357.

Phelps ME, Huang SC, Hoffman EJ, Selin C, Sokoloff L, Kuhl DE. Tomographic measurement of local cerebral glucose metabolic rate in humans with (F-18)2-fluoro-2-deoxy-D-glucose: validation of method. *Ann Neurol* 1979;6:371–388.

Sokoloff L, Reivich M, Kennedy C, Des Rosiers MH, Patlak CS, Pettigrew KD, Sakurada O, Shinohara M. The [14C]deoxyglucose method for the measurement of local cerebral glucose utilization: theory, procedure, and normal values in the conscious and anesthetized albino rat. *J Neurochem* 1977;28:897–916.

Tiepolt C, Beuthien-Baumann B, Hlises R, Bredow J, Kühne A, Kropp J, Burchert W, Franke WG. 18F-FDG for the staging of patients with differentiated thyroid cancer: comparison of a dual-head coincidence gamma camera with dedicated PET. *Ann Nucl Med* 2000;14(5):339–345.

Yutani K, Tatsumi M, Shiba E, Kusuoka H, Nishimura T. Comparison of dual-head coincidence gamma camera FDG imaging with FDG PET in detection of breast cancer and axillary lymph node metastasis. *J Nucl Med* 1999;40(6):1003–1008.

Zhang H, Tian M, Oriuchi N, Higuchi T, Tanada S, Endo K. Oncological diagnosis using positron coincidence gamma camera with fluorodeoxyglucose in comparison with dedicated PET. *Brit J Radiol* 2002;75:409–416.

Zimny M, Kaiser HJ, Cremerius U, Sabri O, Schreckenberger M, Reinartz P, Büll U. F-18-FDG positron imaging in oncological patients: gamma camera coincidence detection versus dedicated PET. *Nuklearmed* 1999;38(4):108–114.

Radiation Biology and Protection

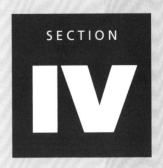

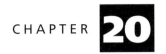
Radiation Biology

20.1 Overview

Rarely have beneficial applications and hazards to human health followed a major scientific discovery more rapidly than with the discovery of ionizing radiation. Shortly after Roentgen's discovery of x-rays in 1895 and Becquerel's discovery of natural radioactivity in 1896, adverse biological effects from ionizing radiation were observed. Within months after their discovery, x-rays were being used in medical diagnosis and treatment. Unfortunately, the development and implementation of radiation protection techniques lagged behind the rapidly increasing use of radiation sources. Within the first 6 months of their use, several cases of erythema, dermatitis, and alopecia were reported among x-ray operators and their patients. Becquerel himself observed radiation induced erythema on his abdomen from a vial of radium he carried in his vest pocket during a trip to London to present his discovery. Many years later, this effect was referred to as a "Becquerel burn". The first report of a skin cancer ascribed to x-rays was in 1902, to be followed 8 years later by experimental confirmation. However, it was not until 1915 that the first radiation protection recommendations were made by the British Roentgen Society, followed by similar recommendations from the American Roentgen Ray Society in 1922.

The study of the action of ionizing radiation on healthy and diseased tissue is the scientific discipline known as radiation biology. Radiation biologists seek to understand the nature and sequence of events that occur following the absorption of energy from ionizing radiation, the biological consequences of any damage that results, and the mechanisms that enhance, compensate for, or repair the damage. A century of radiobiologic research has amassed more information about the effects of ionizing radiation on living systems than is known about almost any other physical or chemical agent.

This chapter reviews the consequences of ionizing radiation exposure, beginning with the chemical basis by which radiation damage is initiated and its subsequent effects on cells, organ systems, and the whole body. This is followed by a review of the concepts and risks associated with radiation-induced carcinogenesis, hereditary effects, and the special concerns regarding radiation exposure of the fetus.

Determinants of the Biologic Effects of Radiation

There are many factors that determine the biologic response to radiation exposure. In general, these factors include variables associated with the radiation source and the biologic system being irradiated. The identification of these biologic effects depends on the method of observation and the time following irradiation. Radiation-related factors include the absorbed dose (quantity) and dose rate as well as the type and energy (quality) of the radiation. The radiosensitivity of a complex biologic system is determined by a number of variables some of which are inherent to the cells themselves while others relate to the conditions in the cells at the time of irradiation. Damage observed at the molecular or cellular level may or may not result in clinically detectable adverse effects.

Furthermore, although some responses to radiation exposure appear instantaneously or within minutes to hours, others take weeks, years, or even decades to appear.

Classification of Biologic Effects

Biologic effects of radiation exposure can be classified as either *stochastic* or *deterministic*. A stochastic effect is one in which the probability of the effect occurring, (rather than its severity), increases with dose. Radiation-induced cancer and hereditary effects are stochastic in nature. For example, the probability of radiation-induced leukemia is substantially greater after an exposure to 1 Gy than to 10 mGy, but there will be no difference in the severity of the disease if it occurs. Stochastic effects are believed not to have a dose threshold, because damage to a few cells or even a single cell could theoretically result in production of the disease. Therefore even minor exposures may carry some, albeit small, increased risk (i.e., increased probability of radiation induced cancer or genetic effect). It is this basic, but unproven, assumption that *risk increases with dose and there is no threshold dose below which the magnitude of the risk goes to zero,* that is the basis of modern radiation protection programs, the goal of which is to keep exposures *as low as reasonably achievable* (see Chapter 21). Stochastic effects are regarded as the principal health risk from low-dose radiation, including exposures of patients and staff to radiation from diagnostic imaging procedures.

If a radiation exposure is very high, the predominant biologic effect is cell killing, which presents clinically as degenerative changes in the exposed tissue. In this case, the effects are classified as deterministic for which the severity of the injury, (rather than its probability of occurrence), increases with dose. Deterministic effects (also referred to as tissue reactions) differ from stochastic effects in that they require much higher doses to produce a clinically observable effect and there is a *threshold* dose below which the effect does not occur or is subclinical. Skin erythema, fibrosis, and hematopoietic damage are some of the deterministic effects that can result from large radiation exposures. As there is substantial individual variability in response to radiation, the "threshold dose" is really just an approximation of the dose that would likely result in the specified effect. Many of these effects are discussed in the sections entitled "Response of Organ Systems to Radiation" and "The Acute Radiation Syndrome." Deterministic effects can be caused by severe radiation accidents and can be observed in healthy tissue that is unavoidably irradiated during radiation therapy. However, with the exception of some lengthy, fluoroscopically guided interventional procedures (see Chapter 9), they are unlikely to occur as a result of routine diagnostic imaging procedures or occupational exposure.

20.2 Interaction of Radiation with Tissue

As discussed in Chapter 3, x-ray and gamma-ray photon interactions in tissue, as well as radiations emitted during radionuclide decay, result in the production of energetic electrons. These electrons transfer their kinetic energy to their environment via excitation, ionization, and thermal heating. Energy is deposited randomly and rapidly (in less than 10^{-8} seconds) and the secondary ionizations set many more low-energy electrons in motion causing additional excitation and ionization along the path of the initial energetic electron. For example, a single 30 keV electron, set in motion following the photoelectric absorption of a single x-ray or gamma-ray photon, can result in the production of over 1,000 low-energy secondary electrons (referred to as *delta rays*), each of which may cause additional excitation or ionization events in the tissue. This chain of ionizations ultimately gives rise to subexcitation electrons (i.e., electrons with kinetic energies less than the first excitation potential of liquid water,

7.4 eV) that become thermalized as they transfer their remaining kinetic energy by vibrational, rotational, and collisional energy exchanges with the water molecules. Observable effects such as chromosome breakage, cell death, oncogenic transformation, and acute radiation sickness, all have their origin in radiation-induced chemical changes in important biomolecules.

Low Energy Electrons and Complex Damage

The delta rays and other lower energy electrons, set in motion following an initial ionizing event, result in a unique ionization pattern in which closely spaced ionizations occur over a very short range (~4 to 12 nm) along the path of the primary ionization track. The energy deposition (~100 ev) along the shorter tracks referred to as *spurs,* whose diameters are approximately 4 to 5 nm, result in an average of three ionizing events. It is estimated that 95% of the energy deposition events from x-rays and gamma rays occurs in spurs (Hall, 2006). Longer and less frequent pear shaped tracks called *blobs* deposit more energy (~300 to 500 ev) and thus on average result in more ionization events (~12 ion pairs) over their path (~12 nm). The high concentrations of reactive chemical species (such as free radicals—discussed below) produced by these spurs and blobs increase the probability of molecular damage at these locations (Fig. 20-1A,B). If ionizing events occur near the DNA, whose diameter (~2 nm)

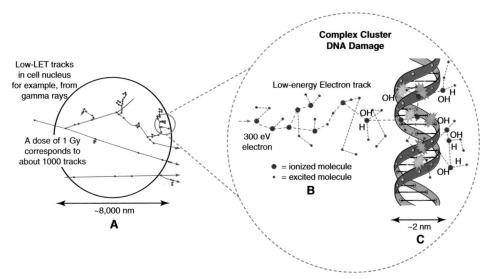

■ **FIGURE 20-1 A.** Low-LET radiation like x-rays and gamma rays is considered sparsely ionizing on average; however, a majority of the radiation energy is deposited in small regions (on the scale of nanometers) via denser clusters of ionizations from low-energy secondary electrons. This illustration depicts primary and secondary electron tracks producing clusters of ionization events. The calculated number of tracks is based on a cell nucleus with a diameter of 8 μm. The track size is enlarged relative to the nucleus to illustrate the theoretical track structure. **B.** A segment of the electron track is illustrated utilizing a Monte Carlo simulation of clustered damage produced by ionizations and excitations along the path of a low-energy (300 eV) electron. Excitation and ionization along with secondary electrons are shown until the electron energy drops below the ionization potential of water (~ 10 eV). **C.** DNA double helix drawn on the same scale as the ionization track. Complex clustered damage can result from closely spaced damage to the DNA sugar-phosphate backbone and bases from both direct ionizations and diffusion of OH radicals produced by the radiolysis of water molecules in close proximity (few mm) with the DNA (i.e., indirect effect). Multiple damaged sites are shown as green, or orange, explosion symbols that denote DNA strand breaks, or damaged bases, respectively. In this example, the result is a complex double strand break, consisting of three strand breaks and three damaged bases, all within ten base pairs along the DNA. This type of complex DNA lesion is more difficult for the cell to repair and can lead to cell death, impaired cell function, or transformations with oncogenic potential, (Adapted from Goodhead 2006, 2009).

is on the same order as that of these short ionization tracks, they can produce damage in multiple locations in the DNA in close proximity to one another. These lesions, initially referred to as *locally multiply damaged sites* are more difficult for the cell to repair or may be repaired incorrectly, Figure 20-1C (Goodhead, 1994; Ward, 1988).

Synonyms for this type of damage in more common use today include *clustered damage, complex damage,* and *multiply damaged sites (MDS)*. While endogenous processes mainly produce isolated DNA lesions, the complex clustered damage, in which groups of several damaged nucleotides occur within one or two helical turns of the DNA, is a hallmark of ionizing radiation—induced DNA damage. While the ionization pattern and radiation chemistry of the microenvironment produced by radiation is different from other oxidative events in the cell of endogenous (e.g., oxidative metabolism) and exogenous (e.g., chemotherapy) origin, the functional changes produced in molecules, cells, tissues, and organs cannot be distinguished from damage produced by other sources.

Repair of radiation damage occurs at molecular, cellular, and tissue levels. A complex series of enzymes and cofactors repair most radiation-induced DNA lesions within hours and, to the extent possible, damaged cells are often replaced within days following irradiation. However, clinical manifestation of radiation-induced damage may appear over a period of time that varies from minutes to weeks and even years depending on the radiation dose, cell type, and the nature and scope of the damage. Only a fraction of the radiation energy deposited brings about chemical changes; the vast majority of the energy is deposited as heat. The heat produced is of little biologic significance compared with the heat generated by normal metabolic processes. For example, it would take more than 4,000 Gy, a supralethal dose, to raise the temperature of tissue by 1°C.

Free Radical Formation and Interactions

Radiation interactions that produce biologic changes are classified as either *direct* or *indirect*. The change is said to be due to direct action if a biologic macromolecule such as DNA, RNA, or protein becomes ionized or excited by an ionizing particle or photon passing through or near it. Indirect action refers to effects that are the result of radiation interactions within the medium (e.g., cytoplasm) that create mobile, chemically reactive species that in turn interact with nearby macromolecules. Because approximately 70% of most cells in the body are composed of water, the majority (~60%) of radiation-induced damage from medical irradiation is caused by radiation interactions with water molecules. The physical and chemical events that occur when radiation interacts with a water molecule lead to the formation of a number of different highly reactive chemical species. Initially, water molecules are ionized to form, H_2O^+ and e^-. The e^- rapidly thermalizes and becomes hydrated, with a sphere of water molecules orienting around the e^- to form the hydrated or aqueous electron (e^-_{aq}). The e^-_{aq} then reacts with another water molecule to form a negative water ion ($H_2O + e^-_{aq} \rightarrow H_2O^-$). These waters ions very unstable; each rapidly forms another ion and a *free radical*:

$$H_2O^+ + H_2O \rightarrow H_3O^+ + \cdot OH \text{ (Hydroxyl Radical)}$$
$$H_2O^- \rightarrow OH^- + H\cdot \text{(Hydrogen Radical)}$$

Free radicals, denoted by a dot next to the chemical symbol, are atomic or molecular species that have unpaired orbital electrons. Thus, free radicals can be radical ions (e.g., H_2O^+ and H_2O^-), or electrically neutral ($\cdot OH$). The hydrogen and hydroxyl radicals can be created by other reaction pathways, the most important of which is the radiation-induced excitation and disassociation of a water molecule (H_2O^* excitation $\rightarrow H\cdot$ and $\cdot OH$). The H^+ and OH^- ions do not typically produce significant biologic damage because of their extremely short lifetimes ($\sim10^{-10}$ seconds) and their tendency to recombine to form water. Free radicals are extremely reactive chemical species that can undergo a variety of chemical reactions. Free radicals can combine with other free radicals to form nonreactive chemical species such as water (e.g., $H\cdot + \cdot OH \rightarrow H_2O$), in which case no biologic damage occurs, or with each other to form other molecules such as hydrogen peroxide (e.g., $\cdot OH + \cdot OH \rightarrow H_2O_2$), which is highly toxic to the cell. However, for low linear energy transfer (LET) radiation like x-rays and gamma rays, the molecular yield of H_2O_2 is low and the majority of indirect effects are due to the interactions of the hydroxyl radicals with biologically important molecules.

The damaging effect of free radicals is enhanced by the presence of oxygen. Oxygen stabilizes free radicals and reduces the probability of free radical recombination into nontoxic chemicals such as water or molecular hydrogen. Oxygen can combine with the hydrogen radical to form a highly reactive oxygen species (ROS) such as the hydroperoxyl radical (e.g., $H\cdot + O_2 \rightarrow HO_2\cdot$). Free radicals can act as strong oxidizing or reducing agents by combining directly with macromolecules. Free radicals can attack biomolecules (R) in a number of ways including hydrogen abstraction (RH + $\cdot OH \rightarrow R\cdot + H_2O$) and $\cdot OH$ addition (R + $\cdot OH \rightarrow ROH\cdot$). Chemical repair of the damaged biomolecules can occur via radical recombination (e.g., $R\cdot + H\cdot \rightarrow RH$) or more commonly, by hydrogen donation from thiol compounds (RSH + $R\cdot \rightarrow RH + RS\cdot$), producing the much less reactive or damaging thiyl radical. In the presence of oxygen, repair is inhibited by the chemical transformation into peroxyradicals ($R\cdot + O_2 \rightarrow RO_2\cdot$). Although their lifetimes are limited (less than 10^{-5} seconds), free radicals can diffuse sufficiently far in the cell (on the order of ~4 nm), to produce damage at locations other than their origin. Free radical-induced damage to DNA is the primary cause of biologic damage from low-LET radiation. While radiation exposure from medical imaging does result in some direct ionization of critical cellular targets, approximately two thirds of the total radiation damage is due to the free radical-mediated indirect effects of ionizing radiation.

Many enzymatic repair mechanisms exist within cells that are capable, in most cases, of returning the cell to its preirradiated state. For example, if a break occurs in a single strand of DNA, the site of the damage is identified and the break may be repaired by rejoining the broken ends. If the damage is too severe or these repair mechanisms are compromised or overwhelmed by excessive radiation exposure, the DNA could suffer mutations. The clinical consequence of such DNA damage depends on a number of variables. For example, if the damage were to the DNA at a location that prevented the cell from producing albumin, the clinical consequences would be insignificant considering the number of cells remaining with the ability to produce this serum protein. If, however, the damage were to the DNA at a location that was responsible for controlling the rate of cell division (e.g., in an oncogene or tumor suppressor gene), the clinical consequences could be the formation of a tumor or cancer. Heavily irradiated cells, however, often die during mitosis, thus preventing the propagation of seriously defective cells. Figure 20-2 summarizes the physical and biologic responses to ionizing radiation.

Experiments with cells and animals have shown that the biologic effect of radiation depends not only on factors such as the dose, dose rate, environmental conditions at the time of irradiation, and radiosensitivity of the biologic system, but also on the spatial distribution of the energy deposition at the molecular level (microdosimetry). The LET is a parameter that describes the average energy deposition per unit path length of the incident radiation (see Chapter 3). Although all ionizing radiations are capable of producing the same types of biologic effects, the magnitude of the effect per unit dose differs. To evaluate the effectiveness of different types and energies of radiation and their associated LETs, experiments are performed that compare the dose required for the test radiation to produce the same specific biologic

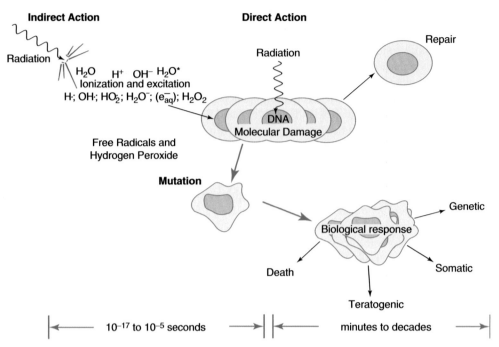

■ **FIGURE 20-2** Physical and biologic responses to ionizing radiation. Ionizing radiation causes damage either directly by damaging the molecular target or indirectly by ionizing water, which in turn generates free radicals that attack molecular targets. The physical steps that lead to energy deposition and free radical formation occur within 10^{-5} to 10^{-6} seconds, whereas the biologic expression of the physical damage may occur from seconds to decades later.

response produced by a particular dose of a reference radiation (typically, x-rays produced by a potential of 250 kV). The term relating the effectiveness of the test radiation to the reference radiation is called the *relative biological effectiveness* (RBE). The RBE is defined, for identical exposure conditions, as follows:

$$RBE = \frac{\text{Dose of 250-kV x-rays required to produce effect X}}{\text{Dose of test radiation required to produce effect X}}$$

The RBE is initially proportional to LET: As the LET of the radiation increases, so does the RBE (Fig. 20-3). The increase is attributed to the higher specific ionization (i.e., ionization density) associated with high-LET radiation (e.g., alpha particles) and its relative advantage in producing cellular damage (increased number and complexity of clustered DNA lesions) compared with low-LET radiation (e.g., x-rays and gamma rays). However, beyond approximately 100 keV/μm in tissue, the RBE decreases with increasing LET, because of the overkill effect. Overkill (or *wasted dose*) refers to the deposition of radiation energy in excess of that necessary to produce the maximum biologic effect. The RBE ranges from less than 1 to more than 20. For a particular type of radiation, the RBE depends on the biologic end point being studied. For example, chromosome aberrations, cataract formation, or acute lethality of test animals may be used as end points. Compared to high-energy gamma rays, the increased effectiveness of diagnostic x-rays in producing DNA damage is suggested not only by the differences in their microdosimetric energy deposition patterns but has also been demonstrated experimentally with an RBE of about 1.5 to 3. However, these differences do not necessarily imply (nor have epidemiological studies been able to confirm) any associated increase in cancer risk. The RBE also depends on the total dose and the dose rate. Despite these limitations, the

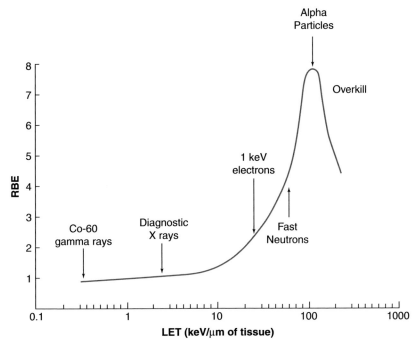

■ **FIGURE 20-3** The RBE of a given radiation is an empirically derived value that, in general (with all other factors being held constant), increases with the LET of the radiation. However, beyond approximately 100 keV/μm, the radiation becomes less efficient due to overkill (i.e., the maximal potential damage has already been reached), and the increase in LET beyond this point results in wasted dose.

RBE is a useful radiobiologic tool that helps to characterize the potential damage from various types of and energies of ionizing radiation. The RBE is an essential element in establishing the radiation weighting factors (w_R) discussed in Chapter 3.

20.3 Molecular and Cellular Response to Radiation

Although all critical lesions responsible for cell killing have not been identified, it has been established that the radiation-sensitive targets are located in the nucleus and not in the cytoplasm of the cell. Cells contain numerous macromolecules, only some of which are essential for cell survival. For example, there are many copies of various enzymes within a cell; the loss of one particular copy would not significantly affect the cell's function or survival. However, if a key molecule, for which the cell has no replacement (e.g., DNA), is damaged or destroyed, the result may be cell death. In the context of diagnostic x-ray exposure, cell death does not mean the acute physical destruction of the cell by radiation but rather a radiation-induced loss of mitotic capacity (i.e., reproductive death) or premature activation of apoptotic pathways (i.e., programmed cell death). There is considerable evidence that damage to DNA is the primary cause of radiation-induced cell death.

Radiation-Induced DNA Damage and Response

Spectrum of DNA Damage

The deposition of energy (directly or indirectly) by ionizing radiation induces chemical changes in large molecules that may then undergo a variety of structural changes. These structural changes include (1) hydrogen bond breakage, (2) molecular degradation or breakage, and (3) intermolecular and intramolecular cross-linking. The rupture of the hydrogen bonds that link base pairs in DNA may lead to irreversible changes in the secondary and tertiary structure of the molecule that compromise genetic transcription and translation. Molecular breakages also may involve the sugar-phosphate polymers that comprise the backbones of the two helical DNA strands. They may occur as single-strand breaks (SSBs), double-strand breaks (DSBs) (in which both strands of the double helix break simultaneously at approximately the same nucleotide pair), base loss, base changes, or cross-links between DNA strands or between DNA and proteins. A SSB between the sugar and the phosphate can rejoin, provided there is no opportunity for the broken portion of the strands to separate. While the rejoining is not typically immediate, because the broken ends require the action of a series of enzymes (endonuclease, polymerase, ligase) to rejoin, the rejoining is fast and the repair typically occurs with high fidelity. The presence of oxygen potentiates the damage by causing peroxidation of a base, which then undergoes radical transfer to the sugar, causing damage that prevents rejoining.

A DSB can occur if two SSBs are juxtaposed or when a single, densely ionizing particle (e.g., an alpha particle) produces a break in both strands. DNA DSBs are very genotoxic lesions that can result in chromosome aberrations. The genomic instability resulting from persistent or incorrectly repaired DSBs can lead to carcinogenesis through activation of oncogenes, inactivation of tumor suppressor genes, or loss of heterozygosity. SSBs (caused in large part by the OH radical) are more easily repaired than DSBs and are more likely to result from the sparse ionization pattern that is characteristic of low-LET radiation. For mammalian cells, an absorbed dose of one Gy from x-rays will cripple the mitotic capability of approximately half of the cells exposed. Each cell would experience approximately 40 DSBs, 1,000 SSBs, and 3,000 damaged bases. While DSBs and complex DNA damage are often associated with high-LET radiation, in reality, all ionizing radiation is capable of producing a substantial number of complex DSBs. In the case of low-LET radiations, used in diagnostic imaging, about a quarter to a third of the absorbed dose in tissue is deposited via low-energy secondary electrons with energies on the order of 0.1 to 5 keV. These low-energy electrons produce high ionization densities over very short tracks that are of the same scale as the DNA double helix. The result is an increased probability of complex DNA damage that may contain not only SSBs and DSBs but localized base damage as well. These complex DNA lesions are less likely to be repaired correctly than an isolated SSB, DSB, or base damage which may lead to permanent DNA modifications or losses (Goodhead, 1988, 1994). The increased effectiveness of alpha particles in producing biological damage is not due to an increased yield of DNA damage but rather the ability of the higher ionization density to produce more complex DNA lesions (Brenner and Ward, 1992). This ability to produce several MDS in proximity in the chromatin structure is referred to as regional multiply damaged sites (RMDS). These lesions are repaired more slowly, if at all, and may serve as a signal for gene induction for a longer time than following low-LET irradiation (Löbrich et al., 1996). In addition, the production of RMDS increases the probability that short double-stranded oligonucleotides will be released, making high fidelity repair without the loss of sequence information problematic. Figure 20-4 illustrates some of the common forms of damage to DNA.

Regardless of its severity or consequences, the loss or change of a base is considered a type of *mutation*. Although mutations can have serious implications, changes in the DNA are discrete and do not necessarily result in structural changes in the chromosomes. However, chromosome breaks produced by radiation do occur and can be observed microscopically during anaphase and metaphase, when the chromosomes

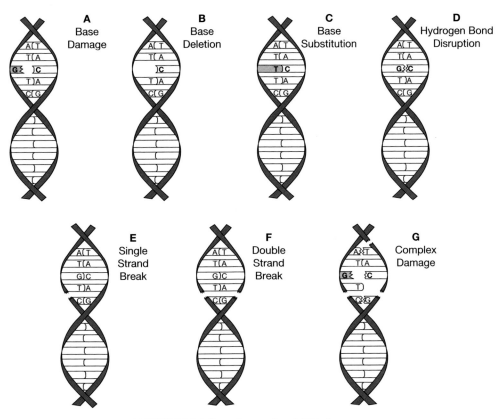

■ **FIGURE 20-4** Several examples of DNA damage.

are condensed. Radiation-induced chromosomal lesions can occur in both somatic and germ cells and, if not repaired before DNA synthesis, may be transmitted during mitosis and meiosis. Chromosomal damage that occurs before DNA replication is referred to as *chromosome aberrations*, whereas that occurring after DNA synthesis is called *chromatid aberrations*. Unlike chromosomal aberrations, in chromatid aberrations only one of the daughter cells will be affected if only one of the chromatids of a pair is damaged.

DNA Repair

Even in the absence of radiation, DNA damage is a relatively common event in the life of a cell. Mammalian cells experience many thousands of DNA lesions per cell per day as a result of a number of common cellular functions such as respiration (e.g., oxidative damage induced by ROS during metabolism) and mitosis (e.g., errors during base replication). Yet the mutation rate is surprisingly low due to the effectiveness of the cell's response and the varied and robust DNA repair mechanisms operating within the cell. DNA damage induces several cellular responses that enable the cell either to repair or to cope with the damage. For example, the cell may activate the G1/S *checkpoint* (which arrests cell cycle progression), to allow for repair of damaged or incompletely replicated chromosomes. In the case of potentially catastrophic mutations, the cell may initiate *apoptosis* (programmed cell death), effectively eliminating the damaged genetic material. Apoptosis is a form of cell death that is characteristically different from cell necrosis in morphology and biochemistry, leading to the elimination of cells without releasing inflammatory substances into the surrounding area. Apoptosis results in cell shrinkage via nuclear condensation and extensive membrane blebbing ultimately resulting in the fragmentation of the cell into membrane bound apoptotic bodies composed of cytoplasm and tightly packed organelles that are eliminated by phagocytosis. The checkpoint and apoptosis responses utilize many of the same sensor molecules or complexes involved in DNA damage recognition and signal transduction. Many types of DNA repair mechanisms exist, including direct repair of a damaged nucleotide, short and long patch base excision repair (SP BER, LP BER), nucleotide excision repair (NER), SSB and DSB repair, and cross-link repair. The repair of DNA damage depends on several factors, including the stage of the cell cycle and the type and location of the lesion. For example, if there is base damage on a single strand, enzymatic

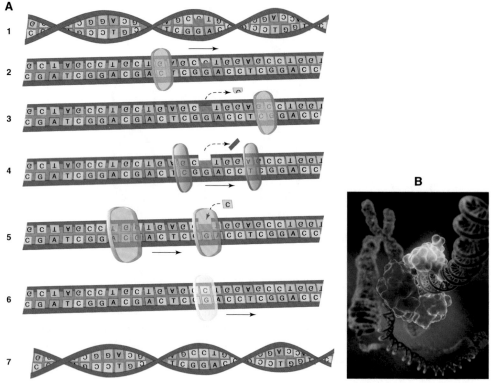

■ **FIGURE 20-5** **A.** A schematic of short patch base excision repair (SP BER), which is one of several DNA repair pathways. *(1)* A cytosine base is damaged by one of several possible agents such as ROS or directly ionizing radiation. *(2,3)* A DNA glycosylase detects the damaged base and removes it, creating an abasic site. *(4)* A specific endonuclease is brought to the damage site where it cleaves the segment of the sugar-phosphate backbone resulting in a SSB that can then be processed by short-patch repair. *(5)* DNA polymerase accompanied by the scaffolding protein resynthesizes the DNA segment using the complementary base as a template *(6)* DNA ligase joins the DNA segments. *(7)* At this point the BER is complete and the DNA resumes its normal helical shape. **B.** Scientists have recently been able to visualize the complicated and dynamic structures of DNA ligase using a combination of x-ray crystallography and small angle x-ray scattering techniques. These experiments revealed the crystal structure of the human DNA ligase I protein bound to a short DNA oligonucleotide. The ring-shaped structure in the center of the figure is the solvent-accessible surface of the protein. The extended, chromosomal DNA (long coils) are an artist's representation of the high-level organization of DNA structure. The figure illustrates the ring-shaped ligase protein sliding along the DNA searching for a break in the phosphodiester backbone of the DNA that is the substrate for the enzyme's DNA end joining activity. The enzyme, DNA ligase, repairs millions of DNA breaks generated during the normal course of a cell's life, for example, linking together the abundant DNA fragments formed during replication of the genetic material in dividing cells. DNA ligase switches from an open, extended shape to a closed, circular shape as it joins DNA strands together. (Courtesy of Dr. Tom Ellenberger, Department of Biochemistry and Molecular Biophysics at Washington University School of Medicine, St. Louis. MO.)

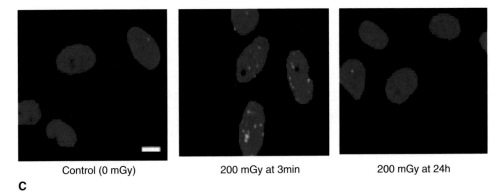

| Control (0 mGy) | 200 mGy at 3min | 200 mGy at 24h |

C

■ **FIGURE 20-5** (*Continued*) **C.** DSB induction and repair in primary human fibroblasts. Using immunofluorescence techniques, a fluorescent antibody specific for γ-H2AX (a phosphorylated histone) forms discrete nuclear foci that can be visualized at sites of DSBs. DSB repair was evaluated at 3 minutes and 24 hours after exposure to 200 mGy; repair was almost complete at 24 hours. The length of the white scale bar shown in the unirradiated control panel equals 10 μm. (From Rothkamm K, Löbrich M. Evidence for a lack of DNA double-strand break repair in human cells exposed to very low x-ray doses. *Proc Natl Acad Sci U S A* 2003;100:5057–5062.)

excision occurs, and the intact complementary strand of the DNA molecule provides the template on which to reconstruct the correct base sequence (Fig. 20-5A,B).

There are specific endonucleases and exonucleases that, along with other proteins or complexes of proteins, are capable of repairing damage to the DNA. Most DNA base damage and SSBs are repaired by the base excision repair pathway. NER is the major pathway for the repair of bulky, helix-distorting lesions such as thymine dimers produced by exposure to ultraviolet radiation. While the repair of simple DNA lesions caused by metabolism and the actions of ROS are considered the primary substrates for the BER pathway, these lesions can also be recognized and repaired via the NER pathway. LP BER and NER may play a more significant role in the repair of clustered damage where significant distortions in the DNA structure may occur. DNA repair occurs rapidly, and approximately 90% of SSB and base damage is repaired within an hour after the initial damage. Even with DSBs, DNA rejoining is virtually complete with 24 hours (Fig. 20-5C).

While most DSBs are repaired correctly, a few undergo binary misrepair. DSBs can be repaired with high fidelity via homologous recombination repair (HRR) involving exchanges with homologous DNA strands (from sister chromatids after replication or from homologous chromosomes). More often DSBs are repaired by the error prone nonhomologous end-joining (NHEJ) that involves end-to-end joining of broken strands (Fig. 20-6).

HRR can preserve the genetic integrity of the chromosome while NHEJ repair results in loss of DNA fidelity. There is a strong force of cohesion between broken ends of chromatin material. Interchromosomal and intrachromosomal recombination may occur in a variety of ways, yielding many types of aberrations such as rings and dicentrics. Figure 20-7 illustrates some of the more common chromosomal aberrations and the consequences of replication and anaphasic separation. In about half the binary misrepair events, the two DSB lead to a translocation (Fig. 20-7C). Translocations involve large scale rearrangements and can cause potentially precarcinogenic alterations in cellular phenotype, but most do not impair cellular survival. Binary misrepair can also result in a dicentric chromosome aberration (Fig. 20-7D), which generally destroys the clonogenic viability of the cell.

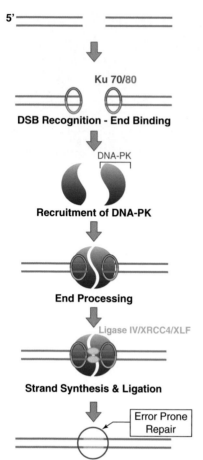

5′

Ku 70/80

DSB Recognition - End Binding

DNA-PK

Recruitment of DNA-PK

End Processing

Ligase IV/XRCC4/XLF

Strand Synthesis & Ligation

Error Prone Repair

NHEJ does not require a homologous template for DSB repair and usually results in the correction of the break in an error-prone manner.

Essential to the NHEJ pathway is the activity of the Ku70/Ku80 heterodimeric protein which initiates NHEJ by binding to the free ends of the DNA.

The Ku heterodimer recruits other NHEJ factors such as DNA-dependent protein kinase (DNA-PK), XRCC4, and DNA Ligase IV to the site of injury

DNA-PK becomes activated upon DNA binding, and phosphorylates a number of substrates including p53, Ku, and the DNA Ligase IV cofactor XRCC4/XLF. Phosphorylation of these factors is believed to further facilitate the repair process.

Most DSBs generated by genotoxic agents are damaged and unable to be directly ligated, they often have to undergo limited processing by nucleases and/or polymerases before NHEJ can proceed.

NHEJ is the simplest, fastest and most predominant mechanism for DSB repair in humans. However, it is not as accurate as other forms of DSB DNA repair and often results in small deletions and insertions at the repair site.

■ **FIGURE 20-6** Model of the key steps required for NHEJ of two ends of double strand DNA break. This repair greatly improves the cells' chance of successful replication, and any loss of DNA fidelity is limited and thus has a low probability of compromising regulatory control or gene expression. (Adapted from Helleday T, Lo J, van Gent DC, et al. DNA double-strand break repair: From mechanistic understanding to cancer treatment. DNA Repair. (March 14, 2007) See animation at http://web.mit.edu/engelward-lab/animations/NHEJ.html)

Chromosomal Aberrations

The extent of the total genetic damage transmitted with chromosomal aberrations depends on a variety of factors, such as the cell type, the number and kind of genes deleted, and whether the lesion occurred in a somatic or in a gametic cell.

Chromosomal aberrations are known to occur spontaneously. In certain circumstances the scoring of chromosomal aberrations in human lymphocytes can be used as a biologic dosimeter to estimate the dose of radiation received after an accidental exposure. Lymphocytes are cultured from a sample of the patient's blood and then stimulated to divide, allowing a karyotype to be performed. The cells are arrested at metaphase, and the frequency of rings and dicentrics are scored. Whole-body doses from penetrating radiation in excess of 250 mGy for acute exposure and 400 mGy for chronic exposure can be detected with confidence limits that do not include zero. Although many chromosomal aberrations are unstable and gradually lost from circulation, this assay is generally considered the most sensitive method for estimating recent exposure (i.e., less than 6 months). More persistent, stable reciprocal translocations can be measured using fluorescence in situ hybridization (FISH).

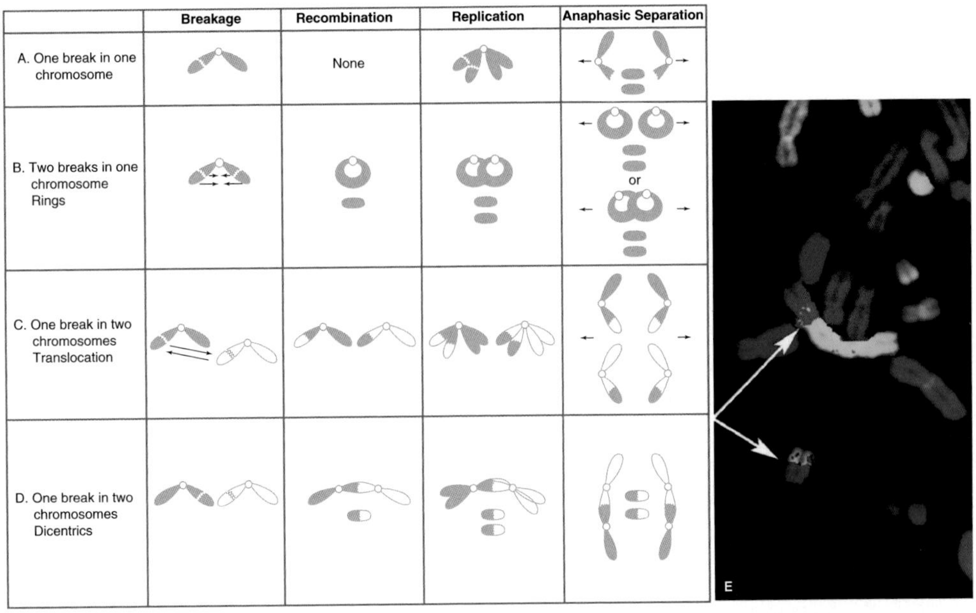

FIGURE 20-7 Several examples of chromosomal aberrations and the effect of recombinations, replication, and anaphasic separation. **A.** Single break in one chromosome, which results in centric and acentric fragments. The acentric fragments are unable to migrate and are transmitted to only one of the daughter cells. These fragments are eventually lost in subsequent divisions. **B.** Ring formation may result from two breaks in the same chromosome in which the two broken ends of the centric fragment recombine. The ring-shaped chromosome undergoes normal replication, and the two (ring-shaped) sister chromatids separate normally at anaphase—unless the centric fragment twists before recombination, in which case the sister chromatids will be interlocked and unable to separate. **C.** Translocation may occur when two chromosomes break and the acentric fragment of one chromosome combines with the centric fragment of the other and vice versa, or **D.** the two centric fragments recombine with each other at their broken ends, resulting in the production of a dicentric. **E.** Metaphase spread, containing a simple dicentric interchange between chromosomes 2 and 8 visualized with multiplex fluorescence in situ hybridization (mFISH). This technique utilizes fluorescently labeled DNA probes with markers specific to regions of particular chromosomes which allows for the identification of each homologous chromosome pair by its own color. The color is computer generated based on differences in fluorescence wavelength among probes. (From Cornforth MN, et al. *J Cell Biol* 2002;159:237–244).

In this method, chromosomes are labeled with chromosome-specific fluorescent DNA probes, allowing translocations to be identified using fluorescent microscopy (Fig. 20-7E). Reciprocal translocations are believed to persist for a considerable period after the exposure, and this approach has been used as one of the methods to estimate the doses to survivors of the atomic bombs detonated in Hiroshima and Nagasaki decades ago.

Response to Radiation at the Cellular Level

There are a number of potential responses at the cellular level following radiation exposure. Depending on a variety of inherent and conditional biologic variables related to the cell and its environment (e.g., cell type, oxygen tension, cell cycle at time of exposure) as well as a number of physical factors related to the radiation exposure (e.g., dose, dose rate, LET) a number of responses are possible such as delayed cell division, apoptosis, reproductive failure, genomic instability (delay expression of radiation damage), DNA mutations, phenotypic (including potentially oncogenic) transformations, bystander effects (damage to neighboring unirradiated cells), and adaptive responses (irradiated cells become more radioresistant). Many of these effects are discussed in more detail below. While a wide variety of the biologic responses to radiation have been identified, the study of radiation-induced reproductive failure (also referred to as clonogenic cell death or loss of reproductive integrity) is particularly useful in assessing the relative biologic impact of various types of radiation and exposure conditions. The use of reproductive integrity as a biologic effects marker is somewhat limited, however, in that it is applicable only to proliferating cell systems (e.g., stem cells). For differentiated cells that no longer have the capacity for cell division (e.g., muscle and nerve cells), cell death is often defined as loss of specific metabolic functions or functional capacity.

Cell Survival Curves

Cells grown in tissue culture that are lethally irradiated may fail to show evidence of morphologic changes for long periods; however, reproductive failure eventually occurs. The most direct method of evaluating the ability of a single cell to proliferate is to wait until enough cell divisions have occurred to form a visible colony. Counting the number of *colonies* that arise from a known number of individual cells irradiated *in vitro* and cultured provides a way to easily determine the relative radiosensitivity of particular cell lines, the effectiveness of different types of radiation, or the effect of various environmental conditions. The loss of the ability to form colonies as a function of radiation exposure can be described by cell survival curves.

Several mathematical methods have been developed to model biologic response to radiation. The shape of a cell survival curve reflects the relative radiosensitivity of the cell line and the random nature of energy deposition by radiation. Survival curves are usually presented with the radiation dose plotted on a linear scale on the x-axis and the surviving fraction (SF) of cells plotted on a logarithmic scale on the y-axis. In the *multitarget model*, the response to radiation is defined by three parameters: the extrapolation number (n), the quasithreshold dose (D_q), and the D_0 dose (Fig. 20-8).

The D_0 describes the radiosensitivity of the cell population under study. The D_0 dose is the reciprocal of the slope of the linear portion of the survival curve, and it is the dose of radiation that produces, along the linear portion of the curve, a 37%

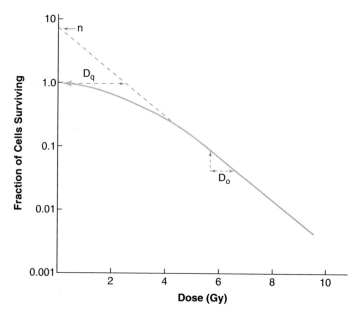

■ FIGURE 20-8 Typical cell survival curve illustrating the portions of the curve used to derive the extrapolation number (n), the quasithreshold dose (D_q), and the D_0 dose.

reduction in the number of viable cells. Radioresistant cells have a higher D_0 than radiosensitive cells. A lower D_0 implies less survival per dose. The D_0 for mammalian cells ranges from approximately 1 to 2 Gy for low LET radiation.

In the case of low-LET radiation, the survival curve is characterized by an initial "shoulder" before the linear portion of the semilogarithmic plot. The extrapolation number, which gives a measure of the "shoulder" is found by extrapolating the linear portion of the curve back to its intersection with the y-axis. The extrapolation number for mammalian cells ranges between 2 and 10; the larger the n, the larger the shoulder. D_q also defines the width of the shoulder region of the cell survival curve and is a measure of sublethal damage. Sublethal damage is a concept based on experiments that show that when radiation dose is split into two or more fractions, with sufficient time between fractions, the cell survival increases after low-LET radiation. The presence of the shoulder in a cell survival curve is taken to indicate that more than one ionizing event "hit", on average, is required to kill a cell and the reappearance of the shoulder when a large dose is delivered in fractions indicates that the cells are capable of repairing sublethal damage between fractions.

The linear quadratic (LQ) model is now the most often used to describe cell survival studies where the SF is generally expressed as

$$SF(D) = e^{-\alpha D + \beta D^2}$$

where D is the dose in Gy, α is the coefficient of cell killing that is proportional to dose (i.e., the initial linear component on a log-linear plot) and β is the coefficient of cell killing that is proportional to the square of the dose (i.e., the quadratic component of the survival curve). The two constants (α and β) can be determined for specific tissues and cancers to predict dose response. As described previously, cell killing (i.e., loss of clonogenic viability) occurs via misrepaired or unrepaired chromosome damage such as dicentric aberrations that are formed when pairs of nearby DSBs wrongly rejoin to one another. The double helix can undergo a DSB as the result of two different mechanisms: (1) both DNA strands are broken by the same radiation track (or "event") and (2) each strand is broken independently, but the breaks are close enough in time and space to lead to a DSB. The linear (alpha) component of the survival curve represents the damage done by individual radiation particle tracks and is thus independent of dose rate. While the damage is partially repairable over time, α still represents the probability of cell death due to individual, noninteracting, particle tracks. This linear (single-hit kinetics) dose-response relationship dominates with high-LET radiation. The quadratic (beta) component of the survival curve represents the probability of cell death due to interactions between two or more individual particle tracks (i.e., dominates with low-LET radiation and follows multiple-hit kinetics) causing the curve to bend at higher doses and is sensitive to dose rate. The LQ (or alpha-beta model, as many call it) is more commonly used than the previously described n-D_0 model, for several reasons: the LQ model is mechanistically based, it is more useful in radiotherapy for explaining fractionation effect differences between late responding normal tissues and early responding tissues or tumors and the LQ model seems to fit most experimental data on human cell lines. The dose at which cell killing is equal from the linear (αD) and quadratic (βD^2) contribution is referred to as the α/β ratio. The α/β ratio is a measure of the curvature of the cell survival curve and, thus, a measure of the sensitivity of different cell types to fractionation of radiation dose, Figure 20-9. For example, late responding normal tissues such as spinal cord or lung that have smaller α/β ratios of 3 or 4 are preferentially "spared" by fractionation compared to tumors and early responding normal tissues (gut, skin, bone marrow) where the α/β ratio is larger (8 to 12), indicating less ability to repair (i.e., more alpha component and less effect of fractionating the dose).

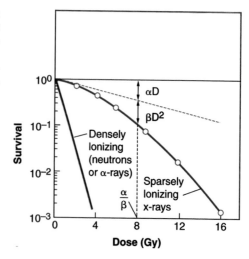

■ **FIGURE 20-9** The LQ model. The experimental data are fitted to a LQ function. There are two components to cell killing: One is proportional to dose (αD); the other is proportional to the square of the dose βD^2. The dose at which the linear and quadratic components are equal is the ratio α/β. The LQ curve bends continuously but is a good fit to the experimental data for the first few decades of survival. (From Hall EJ, Giaccia AJ. *Radiobiology for the radiologist.* 7th ed. Philadelphia, PA: Lippincott Williams and Wilkins, 2012, with permission.)

Factors Affecting Cellular Radiosensitivity

Cellular radiosensitivity can be influenced by a variety of factors that can enhance or diminish the response to radiation or alter the temporal relationship between the exposure and a given response. These factors can be classified as either *conditional* or *inherent*. Conditional radiosensitivities are those physical or chemical factors that exist before and/or at the time of irradiation. Some of the more important conditional factors affecting dose-response relationships are discussed in the following paragraphs, including dose rate, LET, and the presence of oxygen. Inherent radiosensitivity includes those biologic factors that are characteristics of the cells themselves, such as the mitotic rate, the degree of differentiation, and the stage of the cell cycle.

Conditional Factors

The rate at which a dose of low-LET radiation is delivered has been shown to affect the degree of biologic damage for a number of biologic end points including chromosomal aberrations, reproductive delay, and cell death. In general, high dose rates are more effective at producing biologic damage than low dose rates. The primary explanation for this effect is the diminished potential for repair of radiation damage. Cells have a greater opportunity to repair sublethal damage at low dose rates than at higher dose rates, reducing the amount of damage and increasing the survival fraction. Figure 20-10 shows an example of the dose rate effect on cell survival.

Note that the broader shoulder associated with low-dose-rate exposure indicates its diminished effectiveness compared with the same dose delivered at a higher dose rate. This dose-rate effect is diminished or not seen with high-LET radiation primarily because the dense ionization tracks typically produce more complex, clustered DNA damage that cannot be repaired correctly. However, for a given dose rate, high-LET radiation is considerably more effective in producing cell damage than low-LET radiation (Fig. 20-11).

For a given radiation dose, a reduction in radiation damage is also observed when the dose is *fractionated* over a period of time. This technique is fundamental to the practice of radiation therapy. The intervals between doses (hours to a few days) allow the repair mechanisms in healthy tissue to gain an advantage over the tumor by repairing some of the sublethal damage. Figure 20-12 shows an idealized experiment

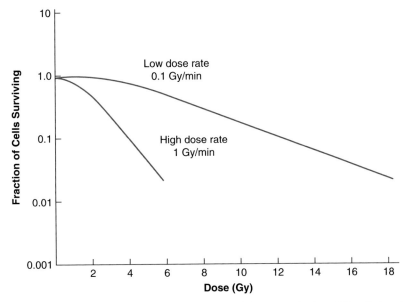

■ **FIGURE 20-10** Cell survival curves illustrating the effect of dose rate for low LET radiation. Lethality is reduced because repair of sublethal damage is enhanced when a given dose of radiation is delivered at a low versus a high dose rate.

in which a dose of 10 Gy is delivered either all at once or in five fractions of 2 Gy with sufficient time between fractions for repair of sublethal damage.

For low-LET radiation, the decreasing slope of the survival curve with decreasing dose rate (see Fig. 20-10) and the reoccurrence of the shoulder with fractionation (see Fig. 20-12) are clear evidence of repair.

The presence of oxygen increases the damage caused by low-LET radiation by inhibiting the recombination of free radicals to form harmless chemical species and

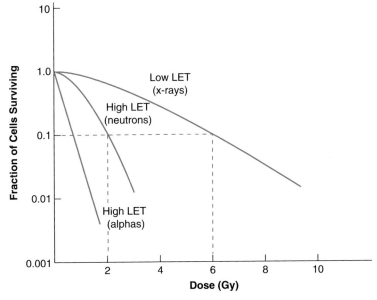

■ **FIGURE 20-11** Cell survival curves illustrating the greater damage produced by radiation with high-LET. At 10% survival, high-LET radiation is three times as effective as the same dose of low-LET radiation in this example.

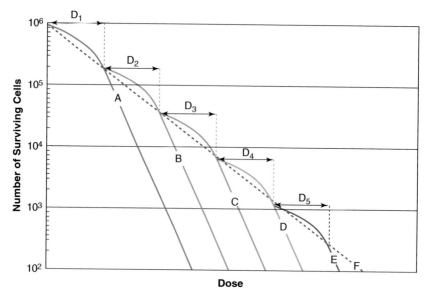

FIGURE 20-12 Idealized fractionation experiment depicting the survival of a population of 10^6 cells as a function of dose. Curve A represents one fraction of 10 Gy. Curve F represents the same total dose as in curve A delivered in equal fractionated doses (D_1 through D_5) of 2 Gy each, with intervals between fractions sufficient to allow for repair of sublethal damage. (Modified from Hall EJ. *Radiobiology for the radiologist.* 5th ed. Philadelphia, PA: Lippincott Williams & Wilkins, 2000.)

by inhibiting the chemical repair of damage caused by free radicals. This effect is demonstrated in Figure 20-13, which shows a cell line irradiated under aerated and hypoxic conditions.

The relative effectiveness of radiation to produce damage at various oxygen tensions is described by the oxygen enhancement ratio (OER). The OER is defined

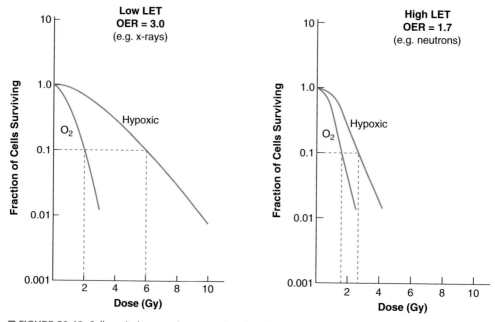

FIGURE 20-13 Cell survival curves demonstrating the effect of oxygen during high (*blue*) and low (*green*) oxygen tension on the OER for high and low-LET irradiation.

as the dose of radiation that produces a given biologic response in the absence of oxygen divided by the dose of radiation that produces the same biologic response in the presence of oxygen. Increasing the oxygen concentration at the time of irradiation has been shown to enhance the killing of otherwise hypoxic (i.e., radioresistant) cells that can be found in some tumors. The OER for mammalian cells in cultures is typically between 2 and 3 for *low*-LET radiation. High-LET damage is not primarily mediated through free radical production, and therefore the OER for high-LET radiation can be as low as 1.0.

Inherent Factors

In 1906, two French scientists, J. Bergonie and L. Tribondeau, performed a series of experiments that evaluated the relative radiosensitivity of rodent germ cells at different stages of spermatogenesis. From these experiments, some of the fundamental characteristics of cells that affect their relative radiosensitivities were established. The Law of Bergonie and Tribondeau states that radiosensitivity is greatest for those cells that (1) have a high mitotic rate, (2) have a long mitotic future, and (3) are undifferentiated. With only a few exceptions (e.g., lymphocytes), this law provides a reasonable characterization of the relative radiosensitivity of cells *in vitro* and *in vivo*. For example, the pluripotential stem cells in the bone marrow have a high mitotic rate, a long mitotic future, are poorly differentiated, and are extremely radiosensitive compared with other cells in the body. On the other end of the spectrum, the fixed postmitotic cells that comprise the central nervous system (CNS) are relatively radioresistant (Fig.20-14).

This classification scheme was refined in 1968 by Rubin and Casarett, who defined five cell types according to characteristics that affect their radiosensitivity (Table 20-1).

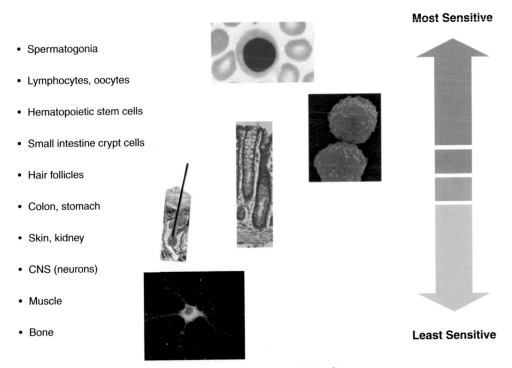

Most Sensitive

- Spermatogonia

- Lymphocytes, oocytes

- Hematopoietic stem cells

- Small intestine crypt cells

- Hair follicles

- Colon, stomach

- Skin, kidney

- CNS (neurons)

- Muscle

- Bone

Least Sensitive

■ **FIGURE 20-14** Relative radiosensitivity of tissues.

TABLE 20-1   CLASSIFICATION OF CELLULAR RADIOSENSITIVITY

CELL TYPE	CHARACTERISTICS	EXAMPLES	RADIOSENSITIVITY
VIM	Rapidly dividing; undifferentiated; do not differentiate between divisions	Type A spermatogonia Erythroblasts Crypt cells of intestines Basal cells of epidermis	Most radiosensitive
DIM	Actively dividing; more differentiated than VIMs; differentiate between divisions	Intermediate spermatogonia Myelocytes	Relatively radiosensitive
MCT	Irregularly dividing; more differentiated than VIMs or DIMs	Endothelial cells Fibroblasts	Intermediate in radiosensitivity
RPM	Do not normally divide but retain capability of division; differentiated	Parenchymal cells of the liver and adrenal glands Lymphocytes[a] Bone Muscle cells	Relatively radioresistant
FPM	Do not divide; differentiated	Some nerve cells Erythrocytes Spermatozoa	Most radioresistant

[a]Lymphocytes, although classified as relatively radioresistant by their characteristics, are in fact very radiosensitive.
VIM, vegetative intermitotic cells; DIM, differentiating intermitotic cells; MCT, multipotential connective tissue cells; RPM, reverting postmitotic cells; FPM: fixed postmitotic cells.
Source: Rubin P, Casarett GW. Clinical radiation pathology as applied to curative radiotherapy. *Clin Pathol Radiat* 1968;22:767–768.

The stage of the cells in the reproductive cycle at the time of irradiation greatly affects their radiosensitivity. Figure 20-15 shows the phases of the cell reproductive cycle and several checkpoints that can arrest the cell cycle or interrupt the progression to allow for the integrity of key cellular process to be evaluated and if necessary, repaired. Experiments indicate that, in general, cells are most sensitive to radiation during mitosis (M phase) and the "gap" between S phase and mitosis (G_2), less sensitive during the preparatory period for DNA synthesis (G_1), and least sensitive during late DNA synthesis (S phase).

Adaptive Response, Bystander Effect, and Genomic Instability

A number of other responses to radiation have been observed *in vitro* that raise interesting questions about the applicability of the LQ dose-response model for low-dose low-LET radiation used in medical imaging. An adaptive response to radiation has been demonstrated in which an initial exposure or "priming dose" reduced the effectiveness of a subsequent exposure. For example, it has been demonstrated in vitro with human lymphocytes, which compared to controls did not receive a small initial exposure, a priming dose of 10 mGy significantly reduced the frequency of chromosomal aberrations in the same cells exposed to several Gy a few hours later (Shadley, 1987). However, the magnitude of this adaptive response varies considerably with dose and dose rate as well as among lymphocytes from different individuals and with other variables. Many other end points for adaptive response have been studied such as cell lethality, mutations, and defects in embryonic development for which the evidence for an adaptive response was highly variable. While many

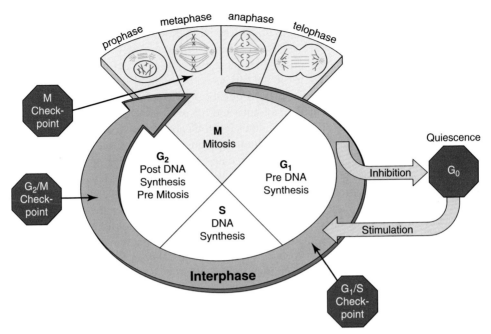

■ **FIGURE 20-15** Phases of the cell's reproductive cycle. The time between cell divisions is called interphase. Interphase includes the period after mitosis but before DNA synthesis (G_1), which is the most variable in length of the phases; followed by S phase, during which DNA synthesis occurs; followed by G_2, all leading up to mitosis (M phase), the events of which are differentiated into prophase, metaphase, anaphase, and telophase. Much of the control of the progression through the phases of a cell cycle is exerted by specific cell cycle control genes at checkpoints. Checkpoints are critical control points in the cell cycle that have built-in stop signals that halt the cell cycle until overridden by external chemical signals to proceed. There are three major checkpoints in the cell cycle, G_1 checkpoint between G_1 and S phase (G_1/S), the G_2 checkpoint between G_2 and mitosis (G_2/M) and the M (metaphase) checkpoint. The G_1/S checkpoint is where the cell monitors its size, available nutrients, and the integrity of DNA (e.g., prevents copying of damaged bases, which would fix mutations in the genome) to assure all are adequate for cell division. In the absence of a proceed signal, the cell will enter a quiescent state G_0 (the state of most cells in the body) until it receives a stimulation signal to continue. Following DNA synthesis, the G_2/M checkpoint occurs at the end of the G_2 phase, during which DNA damage induced during replication, such as mismatched bases and double-stranded breaks, is repaired. The cell ensures that DNA synthesis (S-Phase) has been successfully completed before triggering the start of the mitosis, and at the metaphase (spindle) checkpoint the cell monitors spindle formation and ensures all chromosomes are attached to the mitotic spindle by kinetochores prior to advancing to anaphase. The tumor-suppressor gene p53 (so named because it encodes a phosphorylated protein with a molecular weight of 53 kDa), operates at the G_1/S and G_2/M checkpoints. The p53 protein (discussed again in relation to radiation-induced carcinogenesis later in the chapter) induces cell-cycle arrest through the inhibition of cyclin dependent protein kinases (required for cell cycle advancement) and thus allows for repair of DNA damage. This protein also activates DNA repair mechanisms, or (in the case of severe DNA damage) induces cell death via apoptosis.

theories have been advanced to explain this phenomenon, there is still insufficient evidence to use these results to modify the dose-response relationship for human exposure to radiation.

The bystander effect is another fascinating phenomenon in which irradiated cells or tissues can produce deleterious effects on nonirradiated cells or tissues. This so-called *abscopal* ("out-of-field") effect of radiation has been demonstrated in a variety of experiments. One of the earliest examples was the ability of plasma from patients who had received radiation therapy to induce chromosomal aberrations in lymphocytes from nonirradiated patients (Hollowell, 1968). Among the most compelling evidence for the bystander effect are *in vitro* experiments in which an α-particle microbeam, with the ability to irradiate a single cell, can produce a host of deleterious effects in neighboring unirradiated cells. Examples of induced changes in the unirradiated cells include evidence of DNA damage such as micronuclei formation, sister-chromatid exchanges, cell killing, as well as up and down regulation of a number of important genes (e.g., p53 and rad51), genomic instability (discussed below) and even malignant transformation. Like adaptive response, the sequence of events following exposure is varied and complex and while many molecular mechanisms have been proposed to explain the bystander effects, relationship of this phenomenon to low-dose, low-LET radiation effects characteristic of medical radiation exposure in humans is still an open question.

While the vast majority of unrepaired and misrepaired radiation-induced lesions are expressed as chromosomal damage at the first division, a certain fraction of cells can express chromosomal damage such as chromosomal rearrangements, chromatid breaks and gaps, and micronuclei over many cell cycles after they are irradiated. The biological significance and molecular mechanism surrounding this persistent *genomic instability* has been an area of active research for many years. Genomic instability has been demonstrated *in vitro* as delayed lethality in which cell cloning efficiency is reduced several generations after irradiation. Another interesting aspect is the differences in the types of mutations associated with radiation-induced genomic instability. Experiments have shown that the unirradiated progeny of the irradiated cells primarily demonstrate a *de novo* increase in lethal point mutations several generations after the initial irradiation. These mutations are more typical of spontaneous mutations than deletions and other mutations induced directly by ionizing radiation. There is evidence that suggests that errors induced during DNA repair may contribute to genomic instability. For example, experiments with cells deficient in the repair enzymes needed for NHEJ repair of radiation-induced DSBs demonstrate greater genomic instability than normal cells of the same type (Little, 2003). However, there are data to suggest that many other factors such as ROS, alterations in signal transduction pathways, centrosome defects and other factors also play a role in radiation-induced genomic instability. Despite the many experimental models that have revealed different aspects of this phenomenon, the search for the relevance of radiation-induced genomic instability to radiation-induced cancer continues.

While radiation-induced responses such as genomic instability, adaptation, bystander effects, (as well as others which have not been discussed such as low-dose hypersensitivity) are fascinating in their own right, the results obtained are often restricted to specific experimental conditions and clear mechanistic understanding about these phenomena is still lacking. It has been suggested that these effects may alter the responses of cells and tissues to low doses of radiation, especially for carcinogenesis induction; however, at this time, they cannot be reliably used as a modifying factor to predict the biological consequences of radiation exposure in humans. On the other hand, the nonlinear nature of these and other multicellular and tissue-level responses raise serious questions regarding the current paradigm of linear extrapolation of risk based on the individual cell and the target. Addressing these complex responses to radiation interactions requires a multidimensional, systems-level approach and is an active area of current radiobiological research.

20.4 Organ System Response to Radiation

The response of an organ system to radiation depends not only on the dose, dose rate, and LET of the radiation but also on the relative radiosensitivities of the cells that comprise both the functional parenchyma and the supportive stroma. In this case, the response is measured in terms of morphologic and functional changes of the organ system as a whole rather than simply changes in cell survival and kinetics.

The response of an organ system after irradiation occurs over a period of time. The higher the dose, the shorter the interval before the physiologic manifestations of the damage become apparent (latent period) and the shorter the period of expression during which the full extent of the radiation-induced damage is evidenced. There are practical threshold doses below which no significant changes are apparent. In most cases, the pathology induced by radiation is undistinguishable from naturally occurring pathology.

Regeneration and Repair

Healing of tissue damage produced by radiation occurs by means of cellular *regeneration* (repopulation) and *repair* (Fig. 20-16). Regeneration refers to replacement of the damaged cells in the organ by cells of the same type, thus replacing the lost functional capacity. Repair refers to the replacement of the damaged cells by fibrotic scar tissue, in which case the functionality of the organ system is compromised. The types of response and the degree to which they occur are functions of the dose, the volume of tissue irradiated, and the relative radiosensitivity and regenerative capacity of the cells that comprise the organ system. In so far as repopulation at the cellular level occurs within days after irradiation (Trott, 1991) fractionation of the dose (e.g., multiple fluoroscopically guided interventional procedures separated by days or weeks) allows for cellular repair and typically results in less extensive tissue damage than if the same total dose were to be delivered all at once. In radiation therapy, fractionation increases the effectiveness of the radiation by allowing for reoxygenation of the tumor cells and reassortment (redistribution) of the irradiated cells into more radiosensitive phases of the cell cycle. If the exposures are excessive, the ability of the cells to affect any type of healing may be lost, resulting in tissue fibrosis and necrosis.

Radiation dose

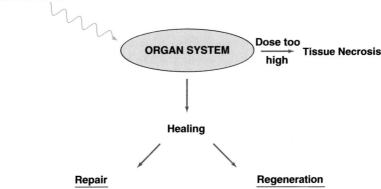

■ **FIGURE 20-16** Schematic diagram of organ system response to radiation.

Characterization of Radiosensitivity

The characterization of an organ system as radioresistant or radiosensitive depends in large part on the radiosensitivity of cells that comprise the functional parenchyma. The cells of the supportive stromal tissue consist mainly of cells of intermediate radiosensitivity. Therefore, when the parenchyma contains radiosensitive cell types (e.g., stem cells), the initial hypoplasia and concomitant decrease in functional integrity will be the result of damage to these radiosensitive cell populations. Functional changes are typically apparent within days or weeks after the exposure. However, if the parenchyma is populated by radioresistant cell types (e.g., nerve or muscle cells), damage to the functional layer occurs indirectly by compromise of the cells in the vascular stroma. In this case, the hypoplasia of the parenchymal cells is typically delayed several months and is secondary to changes in the supportive vasculature. Late radiation effects on the vasculature include fibrosis, proliferation of myointimal cells, and hyaline sclerosis of arterioles, the effect of which is a gradual narrowing of the vessels and reduction in the blood supply to the point that the flow of oxygen and nutrients is insufficient to sustain the cells comprising the functional parenchyma (Fig. 20-17). The relative radiosensitivity of various tissue and organs and the primary mechanism for radiation-induced parenchymal hypoplasia is shown in Table 20-2.

Specific Organ System Responses

This section focuses on radiation-induced changes to the skin, reproductive organs, and eyes. Effects on the hematopoietic, gastrointestinal, and cardiovascular systems, and the CNS are addressed in the context of the acute radiation syndrome (ARS). Additional information on radiation effects on these and other tissues and organ systems can be found in several textbooks and review publications listed at the end of the chapter under sections for suggested reading and references (e.g., Hall, 2012; ICRP, 2011; Mettler, 2008).

Skin

While radiation-induced skin damage is a relatively rare event, it is still the most commonly encountered tissue reaction (deterministic effect) following high-dose image guided interventional procedures. Acute radiation-induced skin changes were recognized soon after the discovery of x-rays and were reported in the literature as early as 1896 (Codman, 1896; Daniel, 1896). The first evidence of biologic effects

■ FIGURE 20-17 Histopathology showing radiation-induced arteriole fibrosis (**left**). (From Zaharia M, Goans RE, Berger ME, et al. Industrial radiography accident at the Yanango hydroelectric power plant. In: Ricks RC, et al., eds. *The medical basis for radiation-accident preparedness, the clinical care of victims.* New York: The Parthenon Publishing Group, 2001:267–281.)

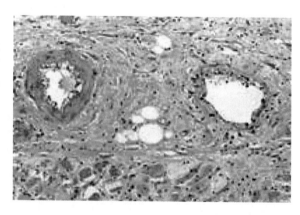

TABLE 20-2   RELATIVE ORGAN AND TISSUE RADIOSENSITIVITY AND PRIMARY MECHANISM FOR RADIATION-INDUCED PARENCHYMAL HYPOPLASIA

ORGANS	RELATIVE RADIOSENSITIVITY	CHIEF MECHANISM OF PARENCHYMAL HYPOPLASIA
Lymphoid organs; bone marrow; testes and ovaries; small intestines	High	Destruction of parenchymal cells, especially the vegetative and differentiating cells
Skin and other organs with epithelial cell lining (cornea, lens, oral cavity, esophagus, GI organs, bladder, vagina, uterine cervix, uterus, rectum)	Fairly high	Destruction of radiosensitive vegetative and differentiating parenchymal cells of the epithelial lining
Growing cartilage; the vasculature; growing bones	Medium	Destruction of proliferating chondroblasts or osteoblasts; damage to the endothelium; destruction of connective tissue cells and chondroblasts or osteoblasts
Mature cartilage or bone; lungs; kidneys; liver; pancreas; adrenal gland; pituitary gland; thyroid; salivary glands	Fairly low	Hypoplasia secondary to damage to the fine vasculature and connective tissue elements
Muscle; brain; spinal cord	Low	Hypoplasia secondary to damage to the fine vasculature and connective tissue elements, with little contribution by the direct effect on parenchymal tissues

Note: Cells of the testes are more sensitive than ovaries. Skin radiosensitivity is particularly high around the hair follicles.
Source: Adapted from Rubin P, Casarett GW. *Clinical radiation pathology.* Philadelphia, PA: W.B. Sanders, 1968.

of ionizing radiation appeared on exposed skin in the form of erythema and acute radiation dermatitis. In fact, before the introduction of the roentgen as the unit of radiation exposure, radiation therapists evaluated the intensity of x-rays by using a quantity called the "skin erythema dose," which was defined as the dose of x-rays necessary to cause a certain degree of erythema within a specified time. This quantity was unsatisfactory for a variety of reasons, not least of which was that the response to skin from radiation exposure is quite variable. Malignant skin lesions from chronic radiation exposure were reported as early as 1902 (Frieben, 1902).

The reaction of skin to ionizing radiation (often referred to as the *cutaneous radiation syndrome*) has been studied extensively, and the degree of damage has been found to depend not only on the radiation quantity, quality, and dose rate but also on the location and extent of the exposure. Radiation-induced skin injuries can be severe, debilitating, and in some cases, the dose has been high enough to cause chronic ulceration and necrosis requiring surgical intervention and a prolonged course of intense care lasting years.

While radiation oncologists are well versed in the potential for skin injury from radiotherapy, most physicians (including radiologists) are unfamiliar with the appearance, time course, and doses necessary to produce clinically significant skin damage. There are often no immediate clinical symptoms from a high skin dose and when initial symptoms do develop (e.g., erythema, xerosis, pruritus) they are often delayed by weeks or even months. Primary care physicians evaluating their patients often fail to consider the patient's past radiologic procedure as a potential cause of their symptoms. Fortunately, serious skin injuries are rare and with the exception of prolonged, fluoroscopically guided interventional procedures and rare cases where excessive doses have been received from CT it is highly unlikely that the radiation dose from carefully performed (i.e., optimized) diagnostic examinations will be high enough to produce any of the effects discussed below.

Skin damage is a consequence of acute radiation-induced oxidative stress resulting in a cascade of inflammatory responses, reduction and impairment of functional stem cells, endothelial cell changes, and epidermal cell death via apoptosis and necrosis. The most sensitive structures in the skin include the germinal epithelium, sebaceous glands, and hair follicles. The cells that make up the germinal epithelium, located between the dermis and the epidermis, have a high mitotic rate and continuously replace sloughed epidermal cells. Complete turnover of the epidermis normally occurs within approximately 4 to 6 weeks. Skin reactions to radiation exposure are deterministic and have a threshold of approximately 1 Gy below which no effects are seen. At higher doses, radiation can interfere with normal maturation, reproduction, and repopulation of germinative epidermal cell populations. At very high doses, the mitotic activity in the germinal cells of the sebaceous glands, hair follicles, basal cell layer, and intimal cells of the microvasculature can be compromised.

A generalized erythema can occur within hours following an acute dose of 2 Gy or more of low-LET radiation and will typically fade within a few hours or days. This inflammatory response, often referred to as *early transient erythema,* is largely caused by increased capillary dilatation and permeability secondary to the release of vasoactive amines (e.g., histamine). Higher doses produce earlier and more intense erythema. A later wave of erythema can reappear as early as 2 weeks after a high initial exposure or after repeated lower exposures (e.g., 2 Gy/day as in radiation therapy), reaching a maximal response about the third week, at which time the skin may be edematous, tender, and often exhibit a burning sensation. This secondary or *main erythema* is believed to be an inflammatory reaction secondary to release of proteolytic enzymes from damaged epithelial basal cells as well as reflecting loss of those epithelial cells. The oxidative stress resulting from a burst of radiation-induced free radicals is known to upregulate numerous pathways pertinent to vascular damage, including adhesion molecules, proinflammatory cytokines, smooth muscle cell proliferation, and apoptosis. A third or *late erythema* wave may also be seen between between 8 and 52 weeks after exposure. The dermal ischemia present at this stage produces an erythema with a bluish or mauve tinge.

Temporary hair loss (epilation) can occur in approximately 3 weeks after exposure to 3 to 6 Gy, with regrowth beginning approximately 2 months later and complete within 6 to 12 months. After moderately large doses—40 Gy over a period of 4 weeks or 20 Gy in a single dose—intense erythema followed by an acute radiation dermatitis and moist desquamation occurs and is characterized by edema, dermal hypoplasia, inflammatory cell infiltration, damage to vascular structures, and permanent hair loss. Moist desquamation, which implies a total destruction of the epidermis, is a clear predictor of late delayed injuries, particularly telangiectasia. Provided the vasculature and germinal epithelium of the skin have not been too severely damaged, reepithelialization occurs within 6 to 8 weeks, returning the skin to normal within 2 to 3 months. If these structures have been damaged but not destroyed, healing may occur although the skin may be atrophic, hypo- or hyper-pigmented, and easily damaged by minor physical trauma. Recurring lesions and infections at the site of irradiation are common in these cases, and necrotic ulceration can develop. Chronic radiation dermatitis can also be produced by repeated low-level exposures (10 to 20 mGy/d) where the total dose approaches 20 Gy or more. In these cases the skin may become hypertrophic or atrophic and is at increased risk for development of skin neoplasms (especially squamous cell carcinoma). Erythema will not result from chronic exposures in which the total dose is less than 6 Gy.

The National Cancer Institute (NCI) has defined four grades of radiation-induced skin toxicity where grade 1 is the least severe and grade 4 is the most severe. The range or "band" of doses associated with each grade and the anticipated skin damage as well as the temporal character of the response is shown in Table 20-3. Figure 20-18 illustrates several grades of radiation-induced skin reactions from exposure to diagnostic and interventional imaging procedures.

Skin contamination with radioactive material can also produce skin reactions. The extent of the reaction will depend on the quantity of radioactive material, characteristics of the radionuclide including the types and energy of the radiations emitted, the half-life and specific activity, region of the skin that was contaminated and how long the contamination remained on the skin. Radionuclides with high specific activity and high-energy beta particle emissions such as F-18 are more likely to illicit skin reactions (see Figure 20-18B).

For all end points, the higher the dose and dose rate (beyond the threshold for effects) the shorter the latency and more severe the effect. However, it is important to recognize that the dose ranges shown in Table 20-3 are not to be interpreted as clear demarcations between various skin reactions and their associated dose. There are a number of factors that may cause the individual patient to be more or less sensitive to radiation exposure. Biologic factors, such as diabetes mellitus, systemic lupus erythematous, scleroderma, or mixed connective tissue disease, and homozygosity for ataxia-telangiectasia (A-T), have increased sensitivity and potential for severe skin reactions. Other physical and biological variables that can substantially modify the severity of radiation-induced skin damage include size of the exposure area, anatomical location, fractionation, patient health, and medications (Table 20-4).

Reproductive Organs

In general, the gonads are very radiosensitive. The testes contain cell populations that range from the most radiosensitive germ cells (i.e., spermatogonia) to the most radioresistant mature spermatozoa. The other cell populations with progressively greater differentiation during the 10-week maturation period (i.e., primary and secondary spermatocytes and spermatids) are of intermediate radiosensitivity compared to the germ cells and mature sperm. The primary effects of radiation on the male reproductive system are reduced fertility, temporary, and permanent sterility (azoospermia) (Clifton and Bremner, 1983). Temporary and permanent sterility can occur after acute doses of approximately 500 mGy and 6 Gy, respectively. The duration of temporary sterility is dose dependent with recovery beginning at 1 and as long as 3.5 years after doses of 1 and 2 Gy, respectively. However, following exposure (and provided the dose is not excessive), there will be a window of fertility before the onset of sterility, as long as mature sperms are available. Chronic exposures of 20 to 50 mGy/wk can result in permanent sterility when the total dose exceeds 2.5 to 3 Gy. The reduced threshold for affect following chronic versus acute exposure is unusual (i.e., an inverse fractionation effect) and is believed to be due to stem cells progressing into radiosensitive stages (Lushbaugh and Ricks, 1972). Reduced fertility due to decreased sperm count (oligospermia) and motility (asthenozoospermia) can occur

TABLE 20-3 TISSUE REACTIONS FROM A SINGLE-DELIVERY RADIATION DOSE TO THE SKIN OF THE NECK, TORSO, PELVIS, BUTTOCKS, OR ARMS[a,b]

SINGLE-SITE ACUTE SKIN-DOSE RANGE (Gy)[c-e]	NCI (2006) SKIN REACTION GRADE	APPROXIMATE TIME OF ONSET OF EFFECTS[e,f]			
		PROMPT <2 wk	EARLY 2-8 wk	MID TERM 6-52 wk	LONG >40 wk
0–2	Not applicable	No observable effects expected at any time			
2–5	1	Transient erythema	Epilation	Recovery from hair loss	None expected
5–10	1–2	Transient erythema	Erythema, epilation	• Recovery • At higher doses: prolonged erythema, permanent partial epilation	• Recovery • At higher doses: dermal atrophy induration
10–15	2–3	Transient erythema	• Erythema, epilation • Possible dry or moist desquamation • Recovery from desquamation	• Prolonged erythema • Permanent epilation	• Telangiectasia[g] • Dermal atrophy induration • Skin likely to be weak; atrophic
>15	3–4	• Transient erythema • After very high doses: edema and acute ulceration, long-term surgical intervention likely to be required	• Erythema, epilation • Moist desquamation	• Dermal atrophy • Secondary ulceration due to failure of moist desquamation to heal, surgical intervention likely to be required • At higher doses: dermal necrosis, surgical intervention likely to be required	• Telangiectasia[g] • Dermal atrophy induration • Possible late skin breakdown • Wound might be persistent and progress into a deeper lesion • Surgical intervention likely to be required

[a]This table is applicable to the normal range of patient radiosensitivities in the absence of mitigating or aggravating physical or clinical factors.
[b]This table does not apply to the skin of the scalp.
[c]Skin dose refers to actual skin dose (including backscatter). This quantity is *not* air kerma at the reference point ($K_{a,r}$).
[d]Skin dosimetry based on $K_{a,r}$ or P_{KA} is unlikely to be more accurate than ±50%.
[e]The dose range and approximate time period are not rigid boundaries. Also, signs and symptoms can be expected to appear earlier as the skin dose increases.
[f]Abrasion or infection of the irradiated area is likely to exacerbate radiation effects.
[g]Refers to radiation-induced telangiectasia. Telangiectasia associated with an area of initial moist desquamation or the healing of ulceration may be present earlier.
Source: Radiation dose management for fluoroscopically-guided interventional procedures. NCRP Report No. 168. Bethesda, MD: National Council on Radiation Protection, 2010.

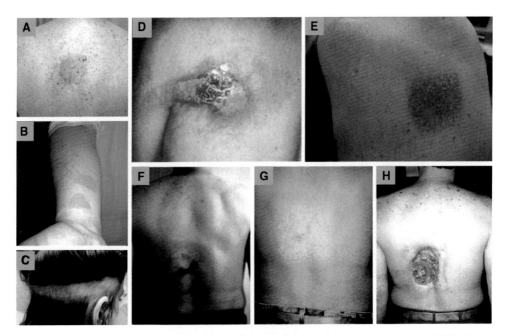

■ **FIGURE 20-18** Examples of radiation-induced effects on skin. **A.** National Cancer Institute (NCI) skin toxicity grade 1: Two fluoroscopically guided procedures were performed through overlapping skin ports in a 65-year-old man. Note enhanced reaction in the overlap zone. The first procedure was performed 6 weeks before and the second procedure, 2 weeks before this photograph was obtained (Balter S, Hopewell JW, Miller DL, et al. Fluoroscopically guided interventional procedures: a review of radiation effects on patients' skin and hair. *Radiology* 2010;254(2):326–341). **B.** Radionuclide skin contamination. Slight erythema after accidental contamination by F-18 fluorodeoxyglucose (https://rpop.iaea.org/rpop/rpop/content/information-for/healthprofessionals/5_interventionalcardiology/phaseserythema.htm, Accessed July 11, 2011). **C.** Epilation following unnecessarily high-dose CT perfusion scan. (Photo courtesy of New York Times: The Radiation Boom After Stroke Scans, Patients Face Serious Health Risks by Walt Bogdanich Published: July 31, 2010.) **D.** NCI skin toxicity grade 3. Chronic radiodermatitis after interventional cardiac catheterization. Grade 3 is classified as moist desquamation in areas other than skinfolds and creases. Note the increased severity of reaction in an area of radiation field overlap (Henry FA, et al. Fluoroscopy-induced chronic radiation dermatitis: A report of three cases. *Dermatol Online* J 2009). **E.** Dry desquamation (poikiloderma) at one month in a patient receiving approximately 11 Gy calculated peak skin dose (Chambers C, Fetterly K, Holzer R, et al. Radiation safety program for the cardiac catheterization laboratory. *Catheter Cardiovasc Interv.* 2011;77). **F–H.** NCI skin toxicity grade 4. A 40-year-old male who underwent multiple coronary angiography and angioplasty procedures. The photographs show the time sequence of a major radiation injury (Shope TB. Radiation-induced skin injuries from fluoroscopy. *RadioGraphics* 1996;16:1195–1199). **(F)** Six to eight weeks postexposure (prolonged erythema with mauve central area, suggestive of ischemia). The injury was described as "turning red about 1 month after the procedure and peeling a week later." By 6 weeks, it had the appearance of a second-degree burn; **(G)** sixteen to twenty-one weeks postexposure (depigmented skin with central area of necrosis); and **(H)** eighteen to twenty-one months postexposure (deep necrosis with atrophic borders). Skin breakdown continued over the following months with progressive necrosis. The injury eventually required a skin graft. While the magnitude of the skin dose received by this patient is not known, from the nature of the injury it is probable that the dose exceeded 20 Gy. This sequence is available on the FDA Web site (NCRP 168, 2010).

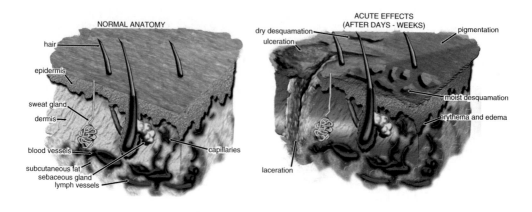

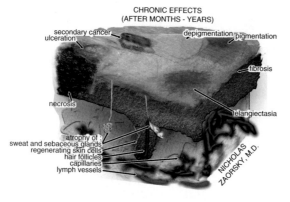

I

■ **FIGURE 20-18** *(Continued)* **I.** A three dimensional view depicting the spectrum of radiation-induced effects on skin as shown in the previous photos (Figures 20-18A–H) and discussed in the text. (Source: Courtesy of Nicholas Zaorsky, MD.)

6 weeks after a dose of 150 mGy. These effects are not related to diagnostic examinations, because acute gonadal doses exceeding 100 mGy are unlikely.

The ova within ovarian follicles (classified according to their size as small, intermediate, or large) are sensitive to radiation. The intermediate follicles are the most radiosensitive, followed by the large (mature) follicles and the small follicles, which are the most radioresistant. Therefore, after a radiation dose as low as 1.5 Gy, fertility may be temporarily preserved owing to the relative radioresistance of the mature follicles, and this may be followed by a period of reduced fertility. Fertility will recur provided the exposure is not so high as to destroy the relatively radioresistant small primordial follicles. The dose that will produce permanent sterility is age dependent, with higher doses (~10 Gy) required to produce sterility prior to puberty than in premenopausal women over 40 years old (~2 to 3 Gy).

Another concern regarding gonadal irradiation is the induction of genetic mutations and their effect on future generations. This subject is addressed later in the chapter.

Ocular Effects

The lens of the eye contains a population of radiosensitive cells that can be damaged or destroyed by radiation. Insofar as there is no removal system for these damaged cells, they can accumulate to the point at which they cause vision impairing cataracts. A unique aspect of cataract formation is that, unlike senile cataracts, which typically develop in the anterior pole of the lens, radiation-induced cataracts are

TABLE 20-4   PHYSICAL AND BIOLOGICAL MODIFIERS OF RADIATION-INDUCED SKIN DAMAGE

FACTOR	EXAMPLES	COMMENT
Location of irradiated skin	Relative radiosensitivity: anterior aspect of the neck > flexor surfaces of the extremities > trunk > back > extensor surfaces of extremities > nape of the neck > scalp > palms of the hands > soles of feet	See Figure 20-18C demonstrating focal scalp epilation
Size of exposed area	Smaller lesions heal faster due to cell migration from skin margin surrounding the exposure area thus accelerating wound closure	Benefit only significant for relatively small lesions. Not typically a factor for medical exposures where field sizes are larger.
Dose Fractionation	Dry Desquamation Threshold: Single expsoure ~14 Gy 3 Fractionations in 3 d ~27 Gy	Repair of sublethal damage to DNA is completed within ~24 h, however repopulation can take days, weeks or even months to complete.
Patient-related	Increased radiosensitivity examples: smoking, poor nutritional status, compromised skin integrity, light colored skin, obesity, DNA repair defects, prior irradiation on the same area, UV exposure	DNA repair defect examples: ataxia telangiectasia, Fanconi anemia, Bloom syndrome and xeroderma pigmentosum. Other diseases, e.g., scleroderma, hyperthyroidism, diabetes mellitus. Patients are more prone to sun burns and should minimize sun exposure following radiation-induced skin injury.
Drugs	Some drugs are known to increase radiosensitivity, e.g., actinomycin D, doxorubicin, bleomycin, 5-fluorouracil and methotrexate	Some chemotherapeutic agents, (e.g., doxorubicin, etoposide, paclitaxel, epirubicin), antibiotics (e.g., cefotetan), statins (e.g., simvastatin), and herbal preparations can produce an inflammatory skin reaction at the site of prior irradiation (*radiation recall*) weeks to years after exposure at the same location.

Source: Adapted from information provided in Balter S, Hopewell JW, Miller DL, et al. fluoroscopically guided interventional procedures: a review of radiation effects on patients' skin and hair. *Radiology* 2010;254(2):326–341.

caused by abnormal differentiation of damaged epithelial cells that begin as a small opacities (abnormal lens fibers) in the anterior subcapsular region and migrate posteriorly. Even at relatively minor levels of visual acuity loss, these posterior subcapsular cataracts can impair vision by causing glare or halos around lights at night. While the degree of the opacity and the probability of its occurrence increases with the dose, the latent period is inversely related to dose. High-LET radiation is more efficient for cataractogenesis by a factor of 2 or more. There have been a number of recent studies of mechanistic models of radiation-induced cataractogenesis. In addition, more recent epidemiological studies have included several additional occupational exposure populations and longer periods of observation for previously studied populations. These studies have raised concern regarding the previous scientific consensus that regarded radiation-induced cataracts as a deterministic effect with dose thresholds for detectable opacities of 2 for acute and 5 Gy for chronic exposures respectively. The view that cataractogenesis is a deterministic event, exhibiting a dose threshold below which lens opacities would not develop, served as the basis for ICRP and NCRP recommended occupational dose limit to the lens of the eye of 150 mSv/y (ICRP, 1991, 2007; NCRP, 2000). Studies of A-bomb survivors who were young at the time of exposure and followed for longer periods than previous studies and other exposed populations such as the workers involved in the cleanup around the Chernobyl nuclear reactor accident site and radiologic technologists in the United States (Gabriel, 2008), suggest that if there is a threshold for cataract development, it is likely to be substantially lower than previously believed (Ainsbury, 2009; ICRP, 2011). These data, and the presumption that subclinical, but detectable opacities will, if given enough time, eventually progress to impair vision led the ICRP to conclude in a recent statement that the threshold for acute and chronic exposure may be more on the order of 0.5 Gy (ICRP, 2011a). Furthermore, some suggest that the dose response may be more accurately described by a linear no-threshold stochastic (rather than a deterministic) model. ICRP's recent review of the scientific evidence regarding the risk of radiation-induced cataract has led the commission to propose a much more conservative occupational equivalent dose limit for the lens of the eye (20 mSv/y averaged over 5 years, with no single year exceeding 50 mSv).

Cataracts among early radiation workers were common because of the extremely high doses resulting from long and frequent exposures from poorly shielded x-ray equipment and the absence of any substantial shielding of the eyes. Today, radiation-induced cataracts are much less common; however, there is concern that for radiation workers receiving higher lens exposures in a medical setting (typically from interventional fluoroscopic procedures) there may be a risk for clinically significant lens opacities over an occupational lifetime. Considering the mounting evidence of a substantially lower threshold for radiation-induced cataracts, the current US regulatory limit of 150 mSv/y to the lens of the eye may need to be reevaluated. However, the proposed ICRP limit is almost a factor of 10 lower than current limits and lower than the whole body dose limit in the United States of 50 mSv/y. Adoption of ICRP recommendations by regulatory bodies would present new challenges for radiation protection in health care settings, especially for those involved in performing fluoroscopically guided interventional procedures. In any case, the use of eye protection in the form of leaded glasses or ceiling mounted lead acrylic shielding is imperative for workers whose careers will involve long-term exposure to scattered radiation.

Summary

There is general agreement that acute doses below 100 mGy will not result in any functional impairment of tissues or organ systems. This can also be considered generally applicable to the risk of clinically significant lenticular opacities with the caveat that the existence of a true deterministic threshold for radiation-induced cataracts remains uncertain. The previous discussion has been limited to tissues and organ systems that are often the focus of concerns for patients and for staff performing diagnostic and interventional fluoroscopic procedures. A more complete discussion of these and other organ and tissue reactions to radiation exposure can be found in the current draft of the ICRP report devoted to this subject (ICRP, 2011). A summary from this report of threshold doses (defined as ~1% incidence in morbidity) in tissues and organs in adults exposed to acute, fractionated or protracted, and chronic irradiation is reproduced in Table 20-5.

TABLE 20-5   THRESHOLD DOSES IN TISSUES AND ORGANS IN ADULTS EXPOSED TO ACUTE, FRACTIONATED OR PROTRACTED, AND CHRONIC RADIATION EXPOSURE[a]

EFFECT	ORGAN/TISSUE	TIME TO DEVELOP EFFECT	ACUTE EXPOSURE (Gy)	HIGHLY FRACTIONATED (2 Gy PER FRACTION) OR EQUIVALENT PROTRACTED EXPOSURES (Gy)[b]	ANNUAL (CHRONIC) DOSE RATE FOR MANY YEARS (Gy y⁻¹)
Temporary sterility	Testes	3–9 wk	~0.1	NA	0.4
Permanent sterility	Testes	3 wk	~6	<6	2.0
Permanent sterility	Ovaries	<1 wk	~3	6.0	>0.2
Depression of hematopoiesis	Bone marrow	3–7 d	~0.5	~10–14 Gy	>0.4
Xerostomia	Salivary glands	1 wk	NA	<20	NA
Dysphasia, stricture	Esophagus	3–8 mo	NA	55	NA
Dyspepsia, ulceration	Stomach	2 y	NA	50	NA
Stricture	Small intestine	1.5 y	NA	45	NA
Stricture	Colon	2 y	NA	45	NA
Anorectal dysfunction	Rectum	1 y	NA	60	NA
Hepatomegaly, ascites	Liver	2 wk to 3 mo	NA	<30–32	NA
Main phase of skin reddening	Skin (large areas)	1–4 wk	<3–6	30	NA
Skin burns	Skin (large areas)	2–3 wk	5–10	35	NA
Temporary hair loss	Skin	2–3 wk	~4	NA	NA
Late atrophy	Skin (large areas)	>1 y	10	40	NA
Telangiectasia @ 5 y	Skin (large areas)	>1 y	10	40	NA
Cataract (visual impairment)	Eye	>20 y	~0.5	~0.5	~0.5 divided by years of duration[c]
Acute pneumonitis	Lung	1–3 mo	6–7	18	NA
Edema	Larynx	4–5 mo	NA	70	NA
Renal failure	Kidney	>1 y	7–8	18	NA
Fibrosis/necrosis	Bladder	>6 mo	15	55	NA
Stricture	Ureters	>6 mo	NA	55–60	NA
Fracture	Adult bone	>1 y	NA	50	NA
Fracture	Growing bone	<1 y	NA	25	NA
Necrosis	Skeletal Muscle	Several years	NA	55	NA
Endocrine dysfunction	Thyroid	>10 y	NA	>18	NA

(Continued)

TABLE 20-5 **THRESHOLD DOSES IN TISSUES AND ORGANS IN ADULTS EXPOSED TO ACUTE, FRACTIONATED OR PROTRACTED, AND CHRONIC RADIATION EXPOSURE**[a] *(continued)*

EFFECT	ORGAN/TISSUE	TIME TO DEVELOP EFFECT	ACUTE EXPOSURE (Gy)	HIGHLY FRACTIONATED (2 Gy PER FRACTION) OR EQUIVALENT PROTRACTED EXPOSURES (Gy)[b]	ANNUAL (CHRONIC) DOSE RATE FOR MANY YEARS (Gy y^{-1})
Endocrine dysfunction	Pituitary	>10 y	NA	≤10	NA
Paralysis	Spinal cord	>6 mo	NA	55	NA
Necrosis	Brain	>1 y	NA	55–60	NA
Cognitive defects	Brain	Several years	1–2	<20	NA
Cognitive defects infants <18 mo	Brain	Several years	0.1–0.2	NA	NA

[a]Defined as 1% incidence in morbidity. Most values rounded to nearest Gy; ranges indicate area dependence for skin and differing medical support for bone marrow.
[b]Derived from fractionated radiotherapeutic exposures, generally using 2 Gy per fraction. For other fraction sizes, the following formula can be used, where D is total dose (number of fractions multiplied by d), d is dose per fraction (2 Gy in the case of D_1, and new value of d in the case of D_2), and the ratio α/β can be found in the appropriate section of the ICRP (2011) report: $D_1[1+2/(\alpha/\beta)] = D_2[1+d_2/(\alpha/\beta)]$.
Note: Protracted doses at a low dose rate of around 10 mGy per minute are approximately isoeffective to doses delivered in 2 Gy fractions at high dose rate for some tissues, but this equivalence is dependent on the repair half-time of the particular tissue. Further details can be found in ICRP (2011) report references Joiner and Bentzen, 2009; Bentzen and Joiner, 2009; van der Kogel, 2009.
[c]The values quoted for the lens assume the same incidence of injury irrespective of the acute or chronic nature of the exposure, with more than 20 years follow up. It is emphasized that great uncertain is attached to these values.
NA, Not Available.

20.5 Whole Body Response to Radiation: The Acute Radiation Syndrome

As previously discussed, the body consists of cells of differing radiosensitivities and a large radiation dose delivered acutely yields greater cellular damage than the same dose delivered over a protracted period. When the whole body (or large portion of the body) is subjected to a high acute radiation dose, there are a series of characteristic clinical responses known collectively as the *acute radiation syndrome* (ARS). The ARS is an organismal response quite distinct from isolated local radiation injuries such as epilation or skin ulcerations.

The ARS refers to a group of subsyndromes occurring in stages over a period of hours to weeks after the exposure as the injury to various tissues and organ systems is expressed. These subsyndromes result from the differing radiosensitivities of these organ systems. In order of their occurrence with increasing radiation dose, the ARS is divided into the hematopoietic, gastrointestinal, and neurovascular syndromes. These syndromes identify the organ system, the damage to which is, primarily responsible for the clinical manifestation of disease. The ARS can occur when a high radiation dose is (1) delivered acutely; (2) involves exposure to the whole body (or at least a large portion of it), and (3) is from external penetrating radiation, such as x-rays, gamma rays, or neutrons. Accidental internal or external contamination with radioactive material is unlikely to result in a sufficiently acute dose to produce the ARS in the organ systems. However, as the widely publicized death of Alexander Litvinenko in 2006 from Po-210 (an alpha emitter) poisoning demonstrated, ARS can be observed when internal contamination with large quantities of highly radiotoxic material (~2 GBq in this case) are widely distributed in the body. Mr. Litvinenko died approximately 3 weeks after the poisoning from the complications of profound panocytopenia that is characteristic of severe hematopoietic damage.

Sequence of Events

The clinical manifestation of each of the subsyndromes occurs in a predictable sequence of events that includes the *prodromal, latent, manifest illness,* and, if the dose is not fatal, *recovery* stages (Fig. 20-19).

The onset of prodromal symptoms is dose dependent and can begin within minutes to hours after the exposure. As the whole-body exposure increases above a threshold of approximately 0.5 to 1 Gy, the prodromal symptoms, which (depending on dose) can include anorexia, nausea, lethargy, fever, vomiting, headache, diarrhea and altered mental status, begin earlier and are more severe. Table 20-6 summarizes

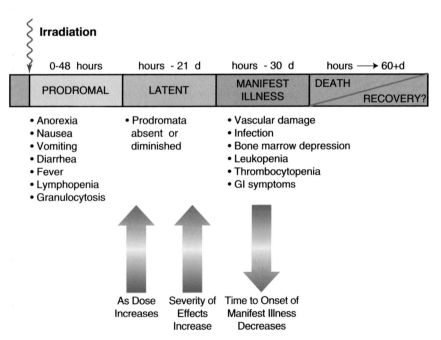

■ FIGURE 20-19 ARS follows a clinical pattern that can be divided into three phases: (1) an initial or prodromal phase that presents as nonspecific clinical symptoms, such as nausea, vomiting, and lethargy (hematological changes may also occur during this period); (2) the latent phase, during which the prodromal symptoms typically subside; and (3) the manifest illness phase, during which the underlying organ system damage is expressed. The type, time of onset, and severity of prodromal symptoms are dose dependent. The duration of the latent period, as well as the time of onset and severity of the manifest illness phase, and ultimate outcome are all, to a variable extent, dependent upon total dose, uniformity of the exposure, and individual radiation sensitivity. As a rule, higher doses shorten the time of onset and duration of all three phases and increase the severity of the prodrome and the manifest illness phases.

TABLE 20-6   CLINICAL FINDINGS DURING PRODROMAL PHASE OF ARS

SYMPTOMS AND MEDICAL RESPONSE	ARS DEGREE AND THE APPROXIMATE DOSE OF ACUTE WHOLE BODY EXPOSURE				
	MILD (1–2 Gy)	MODERATE (2–4 Gy)	SEVERE (4–6 Gy)	VERY SEVERE (6–8 Gy)	LETHAL (>8 Gy)[a]
Vomiting Onset	2 h after exposure or later	1–2 h after exposure	Earlier than 1 h after exposure	Earlier than 30 min after exposure	Earlier than 10 min after exposure
Incidence, %	10–50	70–90	100	100	100
Diarrhea	None	None	Mild	Heavy	Heavy
Onset			3–8 h	1–3 h	Within minutes or 1 h
Incidence, %			<10	>10	Almost 100
Headache	Slight	Mild	Moderate	Severe	Severe
Onset			4–24 h	3–4 h	1–2 h
Incidence, %			50	80	80–90
Consciousness	Unaffected	Unaffected	Unaffected	May be altered	Unconsciousness (may last seconds to minutes)
Onset					Seconds/minutes
Incidence, %					100 (at <50 Gy)
Body temperature	Normal	Increased	Fever	High fever	High fever
Onset		1–3 h	1–2 h	<1 h	<1 h
Incidence, %		10–80	80–100	100	100
Medical response	Outpatient observation	Observation in general hospital, treatment in specialized hospital if needed	Treatment in specialized hospital	Treatment in specialized hospital	Palliative treatment (symptomatic only)

ARS, Acute radiation syndrome;
[a]With intensive medical support and marrow resuscitative therapy, individuals may survive for 6 to 12 months with whole-body doses as high as 12 Gy.
Source: Adapted from *Diagnosis and Treatment of Radiation Injuries*, Safety Report Series No. 2. Vienna, Austria: International Atomic Energy Agency, 1998 and Koenig KL, Goans RE, Hatchett RJ, et al. Medical treatment of radiological casualties: current concepts. *Ann Emerg Med* 2005;45:643–652.

some of the clinical findings, probability of occurrence, and time of onset that may be anticipated during the prodromal phase of ARS as a function of whole body dose.

The time of onset and the severity of these symptoms were used during the initial phases of the medical response to the Chernobyl (Ukraine) nuclear reactor accident in 1986 to triage patients with respect to their radiation exposures. The prodromal symptoms subside during the latent period, whose duration is shorter for higher doses and may last for up to 4 weeks for modest exposures less than 1 Gy. The latent period can be thought of as an "incubation period" during which the organ system damage is progressing. The latent period ends with the onset of the clinical expression of organ system damage, called the *manifest illness stage*, which can last for approximately 2 to 4 weeks or in some cases even longer. This stage is the most difficult to manage from a therapeutic standpoint, because of the overlying immunoincompetence that results from damage to the hematopoietic system. Therefore, treatment during the first 6 to 8 weeks after the exposure is essential to optimize the chances for recovery. If the patient survives the manifest illness stage, recovery is likely; however, the patient will be at higher risk for cancer and, to a lesser extent, his or her future progeny may have an increased risk of genetic abnormalities.

Hematopoietic Syndrome

Hematopoietic stem cells are very radiosensitive. However, with the exception of lymphocytes, their mature counterparts in circulation are relatively radioresistant. Hematopoietic tissues are located at various anatomic sites throughout the body; however, posterior radiation exposure maximizes damage because the majority of the active bone marrow is located in the spine and posterior region of the ribs and pelvis. The hematopoietic syndrome is the primary acute clinical consequence of an acute radiation dose between 0.5 and 10 Gy. Healthy adults with proper medical care almost always recover from doses lower than 2 Gy, whereas doses greater than 8 Gy are almost always fatal unless advanced therapies such as the use of colony-stimulating factors or bone marrow transplantation are successful. Growth factors such as granulocyte-macrophage colony-stimulating factor and other glycoproteins that induce bone marrow hematopoietic progenitor cells to proliferate and differentiate into specific mature blood cells have shown promise in the treatment of severe stem cell depletion. Even with effective stem cells therapy, however, it is unlikely that patients will survive doses in excess of 12 Gy because of irreversible damage to the gastrointestinal tract and the vasculature. In the absence of medical care, the human $LD_{50/60}$ (the dose that would be expected to kill 50% of an exposed population within 60 days) is approximately 3.5 to 4.5 Gy to the bone marrow. The $LD_{50/60}$ may extend to 5 to 6 Gy with supportive care such as the use of transfusions and antibiotics and may be as high as 6 to 8 Gy with effective use of hematopoietic growth factors in an intensive care setting. In contrast to whole body high-dose penetrating radiation exposures, radiation exposure during some accident scenarios may result in nonuniform or inhomogeneous exposures for which the potential for spontaneous hematopoietic regeneration from unirradiated or only mildly irradiated stem cells is much greater. The probability of recovering from a large radiation dose is reduced in patients who are compromised by trauma or other serious comorbidities. The severe burns and trauma received by some of the workers exposed during the Chernobyl nuclear accident resulted in a lower $LD_{50/60}$ than would have been predicted from their radiation exposures alone. In addition, patients with certain inherited diseases that compromise DNA repair, such as A-T, Fanconi's anemia, and Bloom's syndrome, are known to have an increased sensitivity to radiation exposure.

The prodromal symptoms associated with the hematopoietic syndrome can occur within a few hours after exposure and may consist of nausea, vomiting, headache, and diarrhea. If these symptoms appear early and severe diarrhea occurs within the first 2 days, the radiation exposure may prove to be fatal. The prodromal and latent periods may each last for weeks. Although the nausea and vomiting may subside during the latent period, patients may still feel fatigued and weak. During this period, damage to the stem cells reduces their number and thus their ability to maintain normal hematologic profiles by replacing the circulating blood cells that eventually

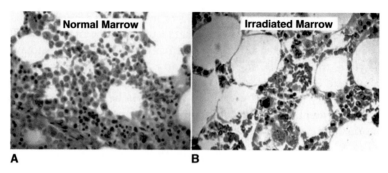

■ **FIGURE 20-20 A.** Normal bone marrow stem cells. **B.** Pyknotic stem cell damage following a bone marrow dose of approximately 2 Gy. (Adapted from *Medical management of radiological casualties*, Online Third Edition June 2010 Armed Forces Radiobiology Research Institute, Bethesda, MD http://www.usuhs.mil/afrri/outreach/pdf/3edmmrchandbook.pdf)

die by senescence. The kinetics of this generalized pancytopenia are accelerated with higher (acute) exposures. An example of radiation-induced stem cell damage following a bone marrow dose of 2 Gy is shown in Figure 20-20. Figure 20-21 illustrates the time course of the hematological consequences of bone marrow doses of 1 and 3 Gy.

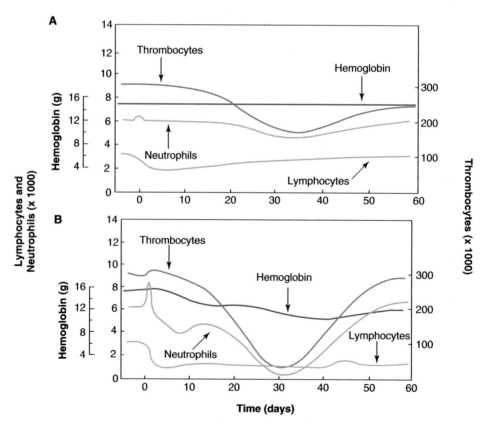

■ **FIGURE 20-21** Hematological changes following an acute bone marrow dose of 1 Gy (**A**) and 3 Gy (**B**). One Gy causes a transient and 3 Gy an extended period of neutropenia, and thrombocytopenia. The lymphopenia is a consequence of radiation-induced apoptosis in some types of lymphocytes. (Adapted from *Medical management of radiological casualties*. Online Third Edition June 2010 Armed Forces Radiobiology Research Institute, Bethesda, MD http://www.usuhs.mil/afrri/outreach/pdf/3edmmrchandbook.pdf)

The initial rise in the neutrophil count is presumably a stress response in which neutrophils are released from extravascular stores. The decline in the lymphocyte count occurs within hours after exposure and is a crude early biologic marker of the magnitude of exposure. The threshold for a measurable depression in the blood lymphocyte count is approximately 0.25 Gy; an absolute lymphocyte count lower than 1,000/mm^3 in the first 48 hours indicates a severe exposure.

The clinical manifestation of bone marrow depletion peak 3 to 4 weeks after the exposure as the number of cells in circulation reaches its nadir. Hemorrhage from platelet loss and opportunistic infections secondary to severe neutropenia are the potentially lethal consequences of severe hematopoietic compromise. Overall, the systemic effects that can occur from the hematopoietic syndrome include mild to profound immunologic compromise, sepsis, hemorrhage, anemia, and impaired wound healing.

Gastrointestinal Syndrome

At higher doses the clinical expression of the gastrointestinal syndrome becomes the dominant component of the radiation response, the consequences of which are more immediate, severe, and overlap with those of the hematopoietic syndrome. At doses greater than 12 Gy, this syndrome is primarily responsible for lethality. Its prodromal stage includes severe nausea, vomiting, watery diarrhea, and cramps occurring within hours after the exposure, followed by a much shorter latent period (5 to 7 days). The manifest illness stage begins with the return of the prodromal symptoms that are often more intense than during their initial presentation. The intestinal dysfunction is the result of the severe damage to the intestinal mucosa. Severely damaged crypt stem cells lose their reproductive capacity. As the mucosal lining ages and eventually sloughs, the differentiated cells in the villi are not adequately replaced by cells from the progenitor compartment in the crypt. The denuding of bowel villi, in turn, causes a host of pathophysiological sequelae. The breakdown of the mucosal barrier allows for the entry of luminal contents such as antigens, bacterial products, and digestive enzymes into the intestinal wall ultimately resulting in a radiation-induced intestinal mucositis. The net result is a greatly diminished capacity to regulate the absorption of electrolytes and nutrients and, at the same time, a portal is created for intestinal flora to enter the systemic circulation. These changes in the gastrointestinal tract are compounded by equally drastic changes in the bone marrow. The most potentially serious effect is the severe decrease in circulating white cells at a time when bacteria are invading the bloodstream from the gastrointestinal tract.

Overall, intestinal pathology includes mucosal ulceration and hemorrhage, disruption of normal absorption and secretion, alteration of enteric flora, depletion of gut lymphoid tissue, and disturbance of gut motility. The systemic effects of acute radiation enteropathy include malnutrition resulting from malabsorption; vomiting and abdominal distention from paralytic ileus; anemia from gastrointestinal bleeding; sepsis resulting from invasion of intestinal bacteria into the systemic circulation; and dehydration and acute renal failure from fluid and electrolyte imbalance. The patient may not become profoundly panocytopenic, because death will likely occur before radiation-induced damage to the bone marrow causes a significant decrease in cell types with longer life spans (e.g., platelets and red cells). Lethality from the gastrointestinal syndrome is essentially 100%. Death occurs within 3 to 10 days after the exposure if no medical care is given or as long as 2 weeks afterward with intensive medical support.

It is important to appreciate that even at doses within the hematopoietic syndrome dose range (2 to 10 Gy), damage to the gastrointestinal tract is occurring. It is responsible for many of the prodromal symptoms and contributes to the toxicity of the radiation-induced myelosuppression that is the signature of the hematopoietic component of the ARS. While a whole body dose of 6 Gy does not result in the full gastrointestinal sequelae described above, damage to the mucosal barrier causes cytokines and other inflammatory mediators to be released into the circulation. In addition, sepsis resulting from the entry of bacteria from the bowel into the systemic circulation during a period of progressive neutropenia is an important cause of death from doses in the hematopoietic syndrome dose range.

Neurovascular Syndrome

Death occurs within 2 to 3 days after supralethal doses in excess of 50 Gy. Doses in this range result in cardiovascular shock with a massive loss of serum and electrolytes into extravascular tissues. The ensuing circulatory problems of edema, increased intracranial pressure, and cerebral anoxia cause death before damage to other organ systems and tissues can become clinically significant.

The stages of the neurovascular syndrome are extremely compressed. Patients may experience transitory incapacitation or unconsciousness. The prodromal

TABLE 20-7   CLINICAL FEATURES DURING THE MANIFEST ILLNESS PHASE OF ARS

	DEGREE OF ARS AND APPROXIMATE DOSE OF ACUTE WHOLE-BODY EXPOSURE				
	MILD (1–2 Gy)	MODERATE (2–4 Gy)	SEVERE (4–6 Gy)	VERY SEVERE (6–8 Gy)	LETHAL (>8 Gy)
Onset of signs	>30 d	18–28 d	8–18 d	<7 d	<3 d
Lymphocytes, G/L[a]	0.8–1.5	0.5–0.8	0.3–0.5	0.1–0.3	0.0–0.1
Platelets, G/L[a]	60–100	30–60	25–35	15–25	<20
Percent of patients with cytopenia	10%–25%	25%–40%	40%–80%	60%–80%	80%–100%[b]
Clinical manifestations	Fatigue, weakness	Fever, infections, bleeding, weakness, epilation	High fever, infections, bleeding, epilation	High fever, diarrhea, vomiting, dizziness and disorientation, hypotension	High fever, diarrhea, unconsciousness
Lethality, %	0	0–50	20–70	50–100	100
Onset		6–8 wk	4–8 wk	1–2 wk	1–2 wk
Medical response	Prophylactic	Special prophylactic treatment from d 14–20; isolation from d 10–20	Special prophylactic treatment from d 7–10; isolation from the beginning	Special treatment from the first day; isolation from the beginning	1–2 wk Symptomatic only

[a]G/L, SI units for concentration and refers to 10^9 per liter.
[b]In very severe cases, with a dose greater than 50 Gy, death precedes cytopenia.
Source: Adapted from *Diagnosis and Treatment of Radiation Injuries. Safety Report Series No. 2.* Vienna, Austria: International Atomic Energy Agency, 1998 and Koenig KL, Goans RE, Hatchett RJ, et al. Medical treatment of radiological casualties: current concepts. *Ann Emerg Med* 2005;45:643–652.

period may include a burning sensation of the skin that occurs within minutes, followed by nausea, vomiting, confusion, ataxia, and disorientation within 1 hour. There is an abbreviated latent period (4 to 6 hours), during which some improvement is noted, followed by a severe manifest illness stage. The prodromal symptoms return with even greater severity, coupled with respiratory distress and gross neurologic changes (including tremors and convulsions) that inevitably lead to coma and death. Many other aspects of this syndrome are not understood because human exposures to supralethal radiation are rare. Experimental evidence suggests that the initial hypotension may be caused by a massive release of histamine from mast cells, and the principal pathology may result from massive damage to the microcirculation.

Summary of Clinical Features During the Manifest Illness Phase of the Acute Radiation Syndrome

Table 20-7 summarizes the clinical features of the ARS within several dose ranges with respect to hematological changes, manifestations of clinical symptoms, latency as well as the medical response, and probability of survival. The previously discussed relationships among various elements of the ARS are summarized in Figure 20-22.

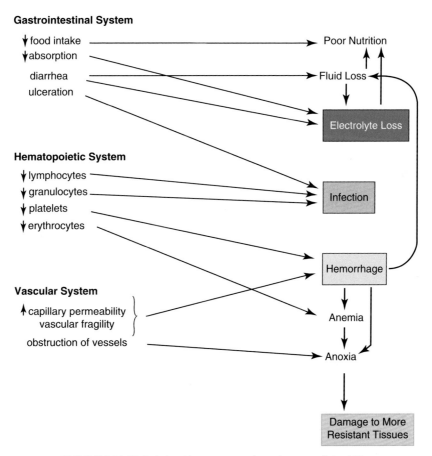

■ FIGURE 20-22 Relationships among various elements of the ARS.

Radiation-Induced Carcinogenesis

Introduction

Most of the radiation-induced biologic effects discussed thus far are detectable within a relatively short time after the exposure. Ionizing radiation can, however, cause damage whose expression is delayed for years or decades. The ability of ionizing radiation to increase the risk of cancer years after exposure has been well established. Cancer, unfortunately, is not a rare disease; indeed, it is the second most likely cause of death, after cardiovascular disease, in the United States. According to a recent report on cancer in the U.S. from the American Cancer Society (ACS, 2011) the lifetime probability of developing an invasive cancer is 41% (44.3% male and 37.8% female) and the probability of dying from cancer is about half that, 22% (23.2% males and 19.7% female). Incidence rates are defined as the number of people per 100,000 who are diagnosed with cancer during a given time period (typically provided as an annual age-adjusted rate per 100,000). The National Center for Health Statistics recommends that the U.S. 2000 standard population be used when calculating and comparing age-adjusted rates for specific population groups. If one compares age-adjusted rates from different populations, it is important that the same standard population is used for the comparison. The annual cancer incidence and mortality age-adjusted rates, for the U.S. population, are approximately 465 and 178 per 100,000, respectively, with males having a higher incidence rate (543 per 100,000) than females (409 per 100,000), (CDC, 2011). Subsequent sections of this chapter address estimates of radiation-induced cancer (incidence and mortality). To help place these numbers in perspective, the baseline lifetime risk of cancer incidence, mortality and average years of life lost are shown in Table 20-8. As previously discussed, ICRP tissue weighting factors (w_T) were developed to account for inherent differences in tissue sensitivity to "detriment" caused by radiation exposure. Part of the detriment values are based on average years of life lost, which, even in the absence of additional radiation exposure, can vary between sex and by type of cancer by almost a factor of two (e.g., prostate and breast cancer).

Although the etiologies of most cancers are not well defined, diet, lifestyle, genetic, and environmental conditions appear to be among the most important factors affecting specific cancer risks. For example, the total cancer incidence among populations around the world varies by only a factor of 2 or so, but the incidences of specific cancers can vary by a factor of 200 or more!

Cancer is the most important delayed somatic effect of radiation exposure. However, radiation is a relatively weak carcinogen at low doses (e.g., occupational and diagnostic exposures). While moderate doses of radiation cause well-documented effects, one cannot detect significantly increased effects at the doses typically encountered in diagnostic imaging. In fact, the body's robust capacity to repair radiation damage means that the possibility of no increased risk at low doses cannot be ruled out. The effectiveness of different DNA repair systems was discussed above. The determinants of radiation-induced cancer risk are discussed in greater detail later in the chapter.

Molecular Biology and Cancer

Cancer arises from abnormal cell division. Cells in a tumor are believed to descend from a common ancestral cell that at some point (typically decades before a tumor results in clinically noticeable symptoms) loses its control over normal reproduction. The malignant transformation of such a cell can occur through the accumulation of

TABLE 20-8   BASELINE LIFETIME RISK ESTIMATES OF CANCER INCIDENCE AND MORTALITY

CANCER SITE	INCIDENCE		MORTALITY	
	MALES	FEMALES	MALES	FEMALES
Solid cancer[a]	45,500	36,900	22,100 (11)	17,500 (11)
Stomach	1,200	720	670 (11)	430 (12)
Colon	4,200	4,200	2,200 (11)	2,100 (11)
Liver	640	280	490 (13)	260 (12)
Lung	7,700	5,400	7,700 (12)	4,600 (14)
Breast	—	12,000	—	3,000 (15)
Prostate	15,900	—	3,500 (8)	—
Uterus	—	3,000	—	750 (15)
Ovary	—	1,500	—	980 (14)
Bladder	3,400	1,100	770 (9)	330 (10)
Other solid cancer	12,500	8,800	6,800 (13)	5,100 (13)
Thyroid	230	550	40 (12)	60 (12)
Leukemia	830	590	710 (12)	530 (13)

Note: Number of estimated cancer cases or deaths in population of 100,000 (No. of years of life lost per death).
[a]Solid cancer incidence estimates exclude thyroid and nonmelanoma skin cancers.
Source: BEIR. *Health risks from exposure to low levels of ionizing radiation: BEIR VII, Phase 2. Committee to Assess Health Risks from Exposure to Low Levels of Ionizing Radiation*, Board of Radiation Effects, Research Division on Earth and Life Studies, National Research Council of the National Academies. National Academy of Sciences, Washington, DC: National Academies Press, 2006.

mutations in specific classes of genes. Mutations in these genes are a critical step in the development of cancer.

Any protein involved in the control of cell division may also be involved in cancer. However, two classes of genes, *tumor suppressor genes* and *protooncogenes*, which respectively inhibit and encourage cell growth, play major roles in triggering cancer. Tumor suppressor genes such as the p53 gene, in its nonmutated or "wild-type state", promotes the expression of certain proteins. One of these halts the cell cycle and gives the cell time to repair its DNA before dividing. Alternatively, if the damage cannot be repaired, the protein pushes the cell into apoptosis. The loss of normal function of the p53 gene product may compromise DNA repair mechanisms and lead to tumor development. Defective p53 genes can cause abnormal cells to proliferate and as many as 50% of all human tumors have been found to contain p53 mutations.

Protooncogenes code for proteins that stimulate cell division. Mutated forms of these genes, called *oncogenes*, can cause the stimulatory proteins to be overactive, resulting in excessive cell proliferation. For example, mutations of the Ras protooncogenes (H-Ras, N-Ras, and K-Ras) are found in about 25% of all human tumors. The Ras family of proteins plays a central role in the regulation of cell growth and the integration of regulatory signals. These signals govern processes within the cell cycle and regulate cellular proliferation. Most mutations result in abrogation of the normal enzymatic activity of Ras, which causes a prolonged activation state and unregulated stimulation of Ras signaling pathways that either stimulate cell growth or inhibit apoptosis.

Stages of Cancer Development

Cancer is thought to occur as a multistep process in which the initiation of damage in a single cell leads to a preneoplastic stage followed by a sequence of events that permit the cell to successfully proliferate. All neoplasms and their metastases are thought to be derivatives or clones of a single cell and are characterized by unrestrained growth, irregular migration, and genetic diversity. For the purpose of setting radiation protection standards, it is assumed that there is no threshold dose for the induction of cancer, because even a single ionization event could theoretically lead to molecular changes in the DNA that result in malignant transformation and ultimately cancer. However, the probability of cancer development is far lower than would be expected from the number of initiating events. For example, a whole body dose of 3 mGy of low-LET radiation (equivalent to the average annual background in the United States) generates multiple DNA lesions (including on average, three SSBs and five to eight damaged bases) in every cell (BEIR, 2006). However, cancer may never arise because a host of defense mechanisms are initiated following radiation-induced damage to prevent cancer development (e.g., activation of DNA repair systems; free radial scavenging; cell cycle checkpoint controls; induced apoptosis, mitotic failure, etc.). Additionally, all of the subsequent steps required for expression of the malignant potential of the cell may not occur.

Cancer formation can be thought of (albeit in a greatly oversimplified way) as occurring in three stages: (1) *initiation*, (2) *promotion*, and (3) *progression*. During initiation, a somatic mutational event occurs that is misrepaired. This initial damage can be produced by radiation or any of a variety of other environmental or chemical carcinogens. During the promotion stage, the preneoplastic cell is stimulated to divide. A promoter is an agent that by itself does not cause cancer but, once an initiating carcinogenic event has occurred, promotes or stimulates the cell containing the original damage. Unlike many carcinogens, radiation may act as an initiator or a promoter. Some hormones act as promoters by stimulating the growth of target tissues. For example, estrogen and thyroid-stimulating hormone may act as promoters of breast cancer and thyroid cancer, respectively. The final stage is progression, during which the transformed cell produces a number of phenotypic clones, not all of which are neoplastic. Eventually, one phenotype acquires the selective advantage of evading the host's defense mechanisms, thus allowing the development of a tumor and possibly a metastatic cancer. Radiation may also enhance progression by immunosuppression resulting from damage to lymphocytes and macrophages that are essential to the humoral antibody response.

Environmental Risk Factors

Environmental factors implicated in the promotion of cancer include tobacco, alcohol, diet, sexual behavior, air pollution, and bacterial and viral infections. Support for the role of environmental factors comes from observations such as the increased incidence of colon and breast cancer among Japanese immigrants to the United States compared with those living in Japan. Among the best known and striking modifiers of cancer risk is smoking. For men, relative risk (RR) of developing lung cancer is 20 to 40 times greater in smokers than nonsmokers. In addition, agents that compromise the immune system, such as the human immunodeficiency virus, increase the probability of successful progression of a preneoplastic cell into cancer. A number of chemical agents, when given alone, are neither initiators nor promoters but when given in the presence of an initiator will enhance cancer development. Many of these agents are present in cigarette smoke, which may in part account for its potent carcinogenicity. Environmental exposure to nonionizing radiation, such as radiofrequency radiation from cellular telephones and their base stations or magnetic field exposures from power lines, has been an area of intense research in the last few decades. While reports of possible associations between sources of nonionizing radiation and cancer have received considerable media attention, the evidence of any causal connection is weak and inconsistent and no biologically plausible mechanism of action has been identified.

A number of national and international agencies and organizations such as the World Health Organization's International Agency for Research on Cancer (IARC) and the National Toxicology Program (NTP) (an inter-agency program within the U.S. Department of Health and Human Services) report on the carcinogenic potential of various physical and chemical agents. Each organization has its own rules and classification schemes, which often lead to confusion in the public and the media regarding the potential health impact of a substance that appears in one of these reports. Periodically, the NTP publishes an update of its *Report on Carcinogens* (RoC). This report, now in its 12th edition (NTP, 2011), identifies substances that are considered to have carcinogenic potential in humans. The NTP lists more than 240 substances, which are classified into one of two categories: "known to be carcinogenic in humans", of which there are 54 in the current report including benzene, smoking tobacco, vinyl chloride, asbestos and of course, ionizing radiation; and another 186 agents that are classified as "reasonably anticipated to be human carcinogens" including exogenous progesterone used for contraception, chemotherapeutic agents adriamycin and cisplatin as well as a naturally occurring contaminants such as aflatoxin, formed by certain fungi on agricultural crops.

Risk Expressions

One way of expressing the risk from radiation (or any other agent) in an exposed population is in terms of its *relative risk* (RR). RR is the ratio of the disease (e.g., cancer) incidence in the exposed population to that in the general (unexposed) population; thus, a RR of 1.2 would indicate a 20% increase over the spontaneous rate that would otherwise have been expected. The *excess relative risk* (ERR) is simply RR − 1; in this case, 1.2 − 1 = 0.2. While the RR of a specific cancer following some exposure is informative about the magnitude of the increased risk relative to its natural occurrence, it does not provide a sense of perspective of the risk in terms of the overall health impact the risk represents. For example, a study showing that a particular exposure resulted in a 300% increase (i.e., RR of 4) in the incidence of a very rare cancer with a natural incidence of 2 per 100,000 means that the cancer risk is now 8 per 100,000. When compared to total incidence of cancer in the population of approximately 43,000 per 100,000, a 300% increase of a rare disease does not seem so impressive as a potential health threat. *Absolute risk* (AR) is another way of expressing risk, as the number of excess cancer cases per 100,000 in a population. In radiation epidemiology, it may be expressed as a rate such as the number of excess cases per 10^4 or 10^5 people per Sv per year (e.g., #/10^4/Sv/y). For a cancer with a radiation-induced risk of 4/10^4/Sv/y (or 4×10^{-4} Sv^{-1} y^{-1}) and a minimum latency period of about 10 years, the risk of developing cancer within the next 40 years from a dose of 0.1 Sv would be 30 years $\times$ 0.1 Sv $\times$ 4 $\times$ 10^{-4} Sv^{-1} y^{-1} = 12 per 10,000 or 0.12%. In other words, if 10,000 people (with the same age and gender distribution as in the general population) each received a dose of 0.1 Sv, 12 additional cases of cancer would be expected to develop in that population over the subsequent 40 years. *Excess Absolute Risk* (EAR), also referred to as *excess attributable risk*, is the difference between two absolute risks and is commonly used in radiation epidemiology expressed as the EAR per unit dose. Thus if the absolute risk in a population exposed to 1 Sv was 95 $\times 10^{-5}$ y^{-1} and 20 $\times$ 10^{-5} y^{-1} in the unexposed population, the EAR would be (95 per 100,000 per year) − (20 per 100,000 per year) = 75 $\times 10^{-5}$ y^{-1} Sv^{-1}.

Modifiers of Radiation-Induced Cancer Risk

Radiation-induced cancers can occur in most tissues of the body and are indistinguishable from those that arise from other causes. The probability of development of a radiation-induced cancer depends on a number of physical and biological factors. Physical factors include the radiation quality (e.g., LET), total dose and, in some instances, the rate at which the dose was received (e.g., acute versus chronic). Research on the biological factors that may influence the carcinogenic effectiveness of radiation has been undertaken in numerous biomolecular, cellular, animal, and epidemiological studies. The influence of radiation quality, dose fractionation, age, tumor type, and gender on radiation-induced cancer risks following exposure and the influence of genetic susceptibility to cancer will be discussed briefly below. Many of these topics will be revisited in the context of specific results from major epidemiological investigations of radiation-induced cancer discussed in this chapter.

Radiation Quality

The RBE of radiation as a function of LET for a variety of biological end points (e.g., double strand DNA breaks, clonogenic potential of cells in culture) was discussed earlier in this chapter. The high ionizations density of high-LET radiation is more effective in producing DNA damage and is less likely to be faithfully repaired than damage produced by low-LET radiation. Consequently, for a given absorbed dose, the probability of inducing a cancer-causing mutation is higher for high-LET radiation, but so is the probability of cell killing. Although the RBE values and their modifying factors for radiocarcinogenesis are not known with great certainty, high-LET radiation has been shown to produce more cancers of the lung, liver, thyroid, and bone than an equal dose of low-LET radiation in human populations. The uncertainty in α-particle risk is large, with a median value of 14.1 and a 90% CI from 5 to 40, (EPA, 2011). The EPA, ICRP, and the NCRP recommend risk coefficients for α-particles that are based on an RBE of 20. RBE values obtained from epidemiological studies vary greatly. For example, studies of the patients injected with thorium-232 dioxide (a primordial alpha emitting radionuclide with a half-life of billions of years) as a diagnostic contrast agent (Thorotrast) for cerebral angiography from about 1930 to the mid 1950s, found an RBE of approximately 20 for liver cancer, but an RBE of only about 1 for leukemia.

It has been demonstrated that for certain biological end points, such as efficiency of producing dicentrics in human lymphocytes, that low-energy photons are more effective than high-energy photons (Fig. 20-23). Presumably this is a result of the higher LET of lower energy secondary electrons (e.g., 30 keV electron LET ~ 1 keV/μm) compared to that of higher energy electrons (e.g., 500 keV electron LET ~ 0.2 keV/μm) and the resultant increase in complex DNA damage generated by ionization and excitation events of these low-energy electrons near the ends of their tracks.

While there is experimental and theoretical evidence supporting higher RBEs of low-photon and low-electron energies, epidemiological support for such an effect is lacking. In fact, risk coefficients for x-rays derived from studies of medically irradiated cohorts are in some cases lower than what has been observed for the A-bomb survivors. However, there are a number of potential confounders that may have prevented detection of an elevated risk if it were present. Thus any difference in carcinogenic risk, per unit dose, from low-energy x-rays compared to that of higher energy photons remains to be determined (BEIR, 2006; ICRP, 2003a,b).

Dose Rate and Fractionation

It has long been recognized that the biological effectiveness of the radiation-induced damage to cells and tissues generally decreases at lower dose rates. This effect is due

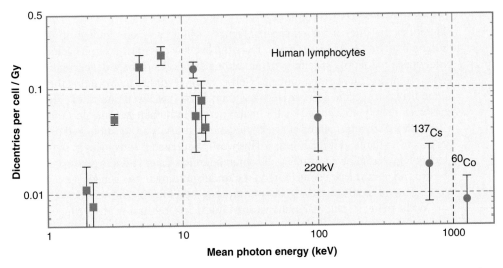

■ **FIGURE 20-23** The photon energy dependence for efficacy of producing dicentric chromosomes per unit dose in human peripheral blood lymphocytes. Data points and standard errors of number of dicentrics per cell per Gy for monoenergetic photons at low and high energies (x-axis) Squares are for monoenergetic photons; circles are x-ray spectra or γ-rays. (Source Sasaki MS, Kobayashi K, Hieda K, et al. Induction of chromosome aberrations in human lymphocytes by monochromatic x-rays of quantum energy between 4.8 and 14.6 keV. *Int J Radiat Biol* 1989;56:975–988; Sasaki MS. Primary damage and fixation of chromosomal DNA as probed by monochromatic soft x-rays and low-energy neutrons. In: Fielden EM, O'Neil P, eds. *The Early Effects of Radiation on DNA*. Vol. H54. NATO ASI Series, Berlin: Springer-Verlag, 1991:369–384; and BEIR VII.)

at least in part to the ability of cells to repair damage during exposure or between exposures in the case of fractionated exposures. The effect of fractionating large doses to increase the probability of cellular repair has been well characterized *in vitro* and has been shown to reduce the incidence of carcinogenesis in some cases such as leukemia. Currently, a dose and dose-rate effectiveness factor (DDREF) are used to convert high-dose-rate risk estimates to estimates for exposure at low dose rates for the purposes of radiation protection. However, at the low doses associated with diagnostic examinations and occupational exposures, dose rate may not affect cancer risk.

Age at Exposure, Gender, Tumor Type, and Latency

Latency (the period between exposure and clinical expression of disease) and the risk of radiation-induced cancers vary with the type of cancer and age at the time of exposure. For example, the risk of ovarian cancer from an acute exposure at age 10 is approximately three times greater than if the exposure occurred at age 50. For whole body exposure, females on average have a 40% higher risk of radiogenic cancer than males. This is due in large part to the high risks for radiation-induced breast, ovarian, and lung cancer in women and the substantially lower risks for radiation-induced testes and prostate cancer in men. Breast cancer occurs almost exclusively in women, and absolute risk estimates for lung cancer induction by radiation are (unlike the normal incidence) approximately twice as high for women than for men. However, for some specific cancers, the radiation-induced cancer risk is lower for women than for men (e.g., liver cancer ~50% lower risk in females than males). The organs at greatest risk for radiogenic cancer induction and mortality are breast and lung for women and lung and colon for men. The minimal latent period is 2 to 3 years for leukemia, with a period of expression (i.e., the time interval required for full expression of the radiogenic cancer increase) proportional to the age at the time of exposure, ranging from approximately 12 to 25 years. Latent periods for solid tumors range from 5 to 40 years, with a period of expression for some cancers longer than 50 years.

Genetic Susceptibility

Mutations in one or more specific genes, while rare, are known to increase susceptibility to developing cancer. Over the last few decades, extensive efforts have been made to identify specific gene mutations that act as sources of genetic susceptibility to cancer. Increasing numbers of observational studies investigating the association between specific gene variants and cancer risk have been published. This effort has been greatly accelerated by the mapping of the human genome and the results from related advances aimed at identifying the quantity, type, location, and frequency of genetic variants in human genes. This work, facilitated by advances in sequencing technology, has allowed results to be obtained much faster and less expensively than before and continues to contribute to the understanding of the genetic susceptibility to cancer and to advance the goal of improved, individualized gene therapy.

While there are still many unanswered questions, the ability of specific inherited gene mutations to substantially increase risk of developing specific cancers (i.e., high penetrance genes) has been well documented. For example, women with inherited mutations in the breast cancer susceptibility genes 1 or 2 (BRCA1 or BRCA2) and a family history of multiple cases of breast cancer carry a lifetime risk of breast cancer that is approximately 5 times higher than for women in the general population, (i.e., 60% and 12%, respectively) (NCI 2011).

Ataxia-telangiectasia (A-T), a rare, recessive genetic disorder of childhood, occurs in 1–2 of every 100,000 people. Patients with the ataxia-telangiectasia mutation (ATM) have trouble walking as children (ataxia) and have small red spider-like veins (telangiectasia). These patients are at substantially higher risk of infection and of developing cancer (especially leukemias and lymphomas) than the general population. These patients are also hypersensitive to ionizing radiation exposure because of defective DNA repair mechanisms. The products of the ATM gene plays a central role in the recognition and repair of double-strand DNA breaks and in the activation of cell cycle checkpoints. A-T patients exhibit unusual susceptibility to injury by radiation and often suffer more severe reactions to radiotherapy than other radiotherapy patients. While physicians who treat A-T patients limit their x-ray exposures to the extent possible, they do recommend diagnostic x-ray imaging procedures when needed, if there are not appropriate alternative procedures that do not use ionizing radiation.

There are still many open questions regarding these single gene human genetic disorders and their influence on cancer risks. One such question is to what extent radiation exposure modifies the cancer risk in patients with these inherited mutations. The BEIR VII committee concluded that, while there is evidence to suggest that many of the known, strongly expressing, cancer-prone human genetic disorders are likely to show an elevated risk of radiation-induced cancer, the rarity of these disorders in the population will not significantly distort current population-based cancer risk estimates. Their view was that the more practical issue associated with these high penetrance genes was their impact on the risk of second cancers in such patients following radiotherapy.

Epidemiologic Investigations of Radiation-Induced Cancer

Although the dose-response relationship for cancer induction at high dose (and dose rate) has been fairly well established for several cancers the same cannot be said for low doses like those resulting from typical diagnostic and occupational exposures. Insufficient data exist to determine accurately the risks of low-dose radiation exposure to humans. Animal and epidemiologic investigations indicate that the risks of low-level exposure are small, but how small is still (despite decades of research) a matter of great debate in the scientific community. Nevertheless, there is general agreement that above cumulative doses of 100 to 150 mSv (acute or protracted exposure), direct epidemiological evidence from human populations demonstrates that exposure to ionizing radiation increases the risk of some cancers.

The populations that form the bases of the epidemiologic investigation of radiation bioeffects come from four principal sources: (1) Life Span Study (LSS) cohort of survivors of the atomic bomb explosions in Hiroshima and Nagasaki; (2) patients with medical exposure during treatment of a variety of neoplastic and nonneoplastic diseases; (3) persons with occupational exposures; and (4) populations with high natural background exposures (Fig. 20-24).

It is very difficult to detect a small increase in the cancer rate due to radiation exposure at low doses (less than ~100 mSv) because radiation is a relatively weak carcinogen; the natural incidence of many types of cancer is high and the latent period for most cancers is long. To rule out simple statistical fluctuations, a very large irradiated population is required. To be able to detect a relative cancer risk of 1.2 with a statistical confidence of 95% (i.e., $p < 0.05$) when the spontaneous incidence is 2% in the population (typical of many cancers), a study population in excess of 10,000 is required. More than 1 million people would be required to identify a RR of 1.01 (i.e., a 1% cancer rate increase) in this same population! A simplified hypothetical example that demonstrates the limited statistical power faced by many epidemiological studies of radiation exposure at low doses was provided in an ICRP report on low-dose extrapolation of radiation-related cancer risk (ICRP, 2006). Statistical power calculations were performed to assess the population size needed for 80% power to detect an excess risk at the 5% significance level in which baseline cancer risk, for an unspecified and hypothetical subset of cancers, is known to be 10%, and the "unknown" radiation-related excess risk is actually 10% at 1 Gy and proportional to dose between 0 and 1 Gy. As shown in Table 20-9, the population size necessary to be able to detect an increased risk at doses typical of many diagnostic imaging exams (organ dose less than 10 mGy) would require a very large population and enormous resources to accomplish. As pointed out by ICRP, the calculation is actually unrealistically optimistic since, as one can never be that sure of the baseline rate in any exposed population, it may be necessary to estimate the baseline rate by including an equal number of nonexposed subjects (i.e., twice the population size would be required to have equal power for detecting the difference). Confounding factors take on much greater importance when excess risks are low, and spurious results can occur by chance alone that result in exaggerated estimates of risk. Commenting on this problem, the ICRP stated, "At low and very low radiation doses, statistical and other variations in baseline risk tend to be the dominant sources of error in both epidemiological and experimental carcinogenesis studies, and estimates of radiation-related risk tend to be highly uncertain because of a weak signal-to-noise ratio and because it is difficult to recognize or to control for subtle confounding factors. At such dose levels, and with the absence of bias from uncontrolled variation in baseline rates, positive and negative estimates of radiation-related risk tend to be almost equally likely on statistical grounds, even under the LNT theory. Also, by definition, statistically significant positive or negative findings can be expected in about one in 20 independent studies when the underlying true excess risk is close to zero. Thus, even under the LNT theory, the smaller the dose, the more likely it is that any statistically significant finding will be a purely chance occurrence, and that it will be consistent with either beneficial effects of radiation (hormesis) or a grossly exaggerated risk (Land, 1980)…….. A result predictable under both of two opposing hypotheses supports neither of them against the other. Thus, for example, failure of epidemiological studies to demonstrate a statistically significant excess cancer risk associated with exposures of the order of 1 mGy does not imply that there is no risk, although it does suggest that any such risk is small relative to baseline cancer rates.", ICRP 2006.

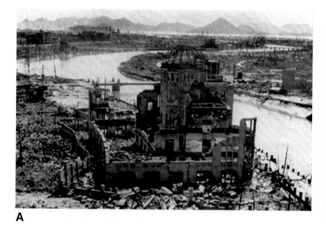
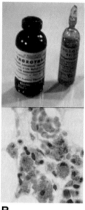

A

B

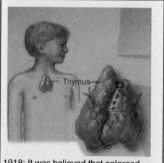

1918: It was believed that enlarged Thymus gland in children was abnormal and radiation was suggested to shrink it.

C

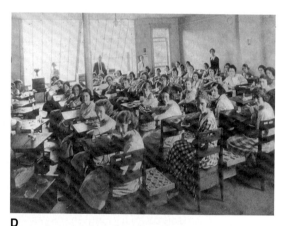

D

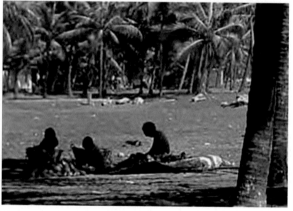

E

■ **FIGURE 20-24** Sources of data on exposure of humans to radiation. The most important source of epidemiological data is the LSS of the Japanese atomic bomb survivors, who received acute doses of radiation, over a range of doses up to 2 Gy, beyond which errors in dose reconstruction and mortality from complications of the ARS provided limited radioepidemiological information. The studies of cancer mortality in the LSS began in 1950, and have formed the basis of radiation protection guidelines ever since. More recently, cancer incidence data have been included by the ICRP in the formulation of radiation detriment, which is used to establish tissue weighting factors for calculating effective dose in their radiation protection system. **A.** There was widespread destruction following the detonation of the atomic bomb in Hiroshima, Japan at 8:15 AM on August 6, 1945. The building shown was the former Hiroshima Prefecture Industrial Promotion Hall, where special products of Hiroshima were exhibited and various gatherings were held.

(Continued)

■ **FIGURE 20-24.** (*Continued*) Located just under the hypocenter, blast pressure was vertically exerted on the building and only the dome-shaped framework and part of the outer wall remained. **B.** From 1931 to the mid 1950s, Thorotrast, a colloidal suspention of radioactive thorium dioxide (**top panel**), was commonly used as a diagnostic contrast agent for cerebral angiography. Thorotrast (containing thorium, a long lived alpha emitter) remains in the body, accumulates in the liver and results in liver cancer and leukemia. Thorotrast-laden macrophages in the bone marrow shown at 1000× (**bottom panel**). (Graham et al., Whole-body pathologic analysis of a patient with thorotrast-in-induced myelodysplasia. *Health Phys* 1992;63(1):20–26.) **C.** Radiation has also been used in the past to treat benign medical conditions with unfortunate consequences such as the increase in thyroid cancer in children who were unnecessarily irradiated to reduce the size of the thymus gland. During a review of children with thyroid cancer, Dr. Fitzgerald noticed that nine out of the first ten patients he reviewed had had a history of thymic radiation. Drs. Duffy and Fitzgerald's report, *Cancer of the thyroid in children,* in the *Journal of Endocrinology* in 1950 was the first demonstration of an association between radiation treatment and thyroid cancer. **D.** In the 1920s, bone cancer was linked with ingestion of large quantities of radium by young women who painted dials on watches and clocks with radium-laden paints. The type of bone cancer (osteogenic sarcoma) is rare, but it occurred with alarming incidence in radium-dial painters and its location (often in the mandible) is an extremely unusual location for this type of cancer. **E.** Several areas of the world have high natural background due to being at high elevation or having high concentrations of naturally occurring radioactive material in the ground. High concentrations of radioactive thorium-containing monazite sands are found in the coastal belt of Karunagappally, Kerala, India. The median outdoor radiation levels are more than 4 mGy/y and, in some locations, as high as 70 mGy/y. A cohort of all 385,103 residents in Karunagappally was established in the 1990s to evaluate the health effects of living in a high background radiation area. Studies to date however have not shown any excess cancer risk from this chronic exposure to gamma radiation (Nair RR, Rajan B, Akiba S, et al. Background radiation and cancer incidence in Kerala, India-Karanagappally cohort study. *Health Phys.* 2009;96:55–66; and Boice JD Jr, Hendry JH, Nakamura N, et al. Low-dose-rate epidemiology of high background radiation areas. *Radiat Res* 2010;173:849–854.)

Considering the limitations (both practical and inherent) to epidemiological investigation (which are by nature, observational not experimental), there is no such thing as a perfect epidemiology study. Some epidemiologic investigations have been complicated by such factors as failure to adequately control exposure to other known carcinogens or an inadequate period of observation to allow for full expression of cancers with long latent periods. Other studies suffer from inadequate design, resulting in problems such as small study size or biased selection of case and control populations or poor assessment of estimated exposure. Exposure assessment that relies on data that are incomplete, inaccurate, or a surrogate for the actual exposure of interest can lead to flawed conclusions. In retrospective studies in particular, the use of questionnaires that relied on people's recollections to estimate exposure can be a particularly problematic, especially if there is a high likelihood of recall bias among cases compared to controls. For example, the case subjects may have more reliable memories than the control subjects because they have been searching for a plausible explanation of the cause of their disease. These methodological issues notwithstanding, epidemiology has made invaluable contributions to public health, espe-

TABLE 20-9   STATISTICAL POWER CALCULATIONS FOR A HYPOTHETICAL STUDY IN WHICH THE BASELINE CANCER RISK, FOR AN UNSPECIFIED SUBSET OF CANCER SITES, IS KNOWN TO BE 10%, AND THE UNKNOWN RADIATION-RELATED EXCESS RISK IS 10% AT 1 Gy AND PROPORTIONAL TO DOSE BETWEEN 0 AND 1 Gy

RADIATION DOSE	EXCESS RISK	TOTAL RISK	POPULATION SIZE N
1 Gy	10%	20%	80
100 mGy	1%	11%	6,390
10 mGy	0.1%	10.1%	620,000
1 mGy	0.01%	10.01%	61.8 million

N, the population size needed for 80% power to detect the excess risk at the 5% significance level.
Source: Adapted from International Commission on Radiological Protection. Low-dose extrapolation of radiation-related cancer risk. ICRP Publication 99. *Ann ICRP* 2006;35:1–140.

cially in cases where the exposures, such as in smoking, resulted in widespread adverse public health consequences. The situations where epidemiological investigations have the most difficulty are where the risks are small compared to the normal incidence of the disease and where exposures in cases and controls are difficult to quantify. Table 20-10 summarizes details of some of the principal epidemiologic investigations on which current dose-response estimates are based. Several excellent overviews on radiation epidemiology

TABLE 20-10   SUMMARY OF MAJOR EPIDEMIOLOGIC INVESTIGATIONS THAT FORM THE BASIS OF CURRENT CANCER DOSE-RESPONSE ESTIMATES IN HUMAN POPULATIONS

POPULATION AND EXPOSURE	EFFECTS OBSERVED	STRENGTHS AND LIMITATIONS
A-bomb survivors: The LSS of the Japanese A-bomb survivors has provided detailed epidemiological data from a study of this population for about 50 y. Three cohorts currently being studied are: (1) A cancer (and noncancer) incidence and mortality study of ~105,000 residents of Hiroshima and Nagasaki (1950) with doses ranging from 0 (e.g., not in the city at time of the bombing) to 4 Gy (42% received a dose between 5 and 100 mGy); (2) those exposed *in utero* (~3,600) and (3) F1 generation children of those exposed (~77,000). The cancer incidence and mortality assessment through 1998 has been completed. Mean organ doses have been calculated for 12 organs. Risk estimates were revised in 2006 by the National Academy of Sciences / National Research Council Committee on the Biological Effects of Ionizing Radiation. Their reanalysis of the scientific data on low-dose radiation health effects was undertaken in light of a reassessment of the doses received by the Japanese atomic-bomb survivors, referred to as the DS02 dose estimate, (Young, 2005), additional information on nontargeted effects of radiation (e.g., bystander effect, low-dose hypersensitivity) as well as an additional decade of follow-up of the A-bomb survivors.	A-bomb survivor data demonstrates an undeniable increase in cancer for doses >100 mSv (some say 50 while others say 200 mSv). Excess risks of most cancer types have been observed, the major exceptions being chronic lymphocytic leukemia, multiple myeloma, non-Hodgkin's lymphoma, pancreatic, prostate and gall bladder cancer. A total of 853 excess solid cancers from a total of 17,488 cases are thought to have been induced by radiation exposure. Table 20-11 lists, for each dose category, the observed and expected numbers of cancers, the excess number of cancers, and the percent of cancers that can be attributed to radiation exposure (attributable fraction). The small but statistically significant increase in the 5–100 mGy exposure group is of particular interest in medical imaging as it is similar to organ dose experienced in many diagnostic imaging studies. In more than 50 y of follow-up of the 105,427 atomic-bomb survivors, the percent of cancers attributed to their radiation exposure is 10.7%. Estimates of the site-specific solid cancer risks are shown in Figure 20-25. The influence of sex and age at the time of exposure, and the risk as a function of attained age following exposure can be very significant and examples of their influence are shown in Figure 20-26.	The analysis of the data from the atom-bomb survivors cohort is the single most important factor that has influenced current radiation-induced cancer risk estimates. The population is large and there is a wide range of doses from which it is possible to determine the dose-response and the effects of modifying factors such as age on the induction of cancer. Data at high doses are limited; thus the analysis only included individuals in whom the doses were 2 Gy or less. The survivors were not representative of a normal Japanese population insofar as many of the adult males were away on military service while those remaining presumably had some physical condition preventing them from active service. In addition, the children and the elderly perished shortly after the detonation in greater numbers than did young adults, suggesting the possibility that the survivors may represent a hardier subset of the population. Another important uncertainty is the transfer of site-specific cancer risk estimates to the U.S. population, based on results obtained on the LSS population, for cancers with substantially different baseline incidence rates.

TABLE 20-10 SUMMARY OF MAJOR EPIDEMIOLOGIC INVESTIGATIONS THAT FORM THE BASIS OF CURRENT CANCER DOSE-RESPONSE ESTIMATE IN HUMAN POPULATIONS (continued)

POPULATION AND EXPOSURE	EFFECTS OBSERVED	STRENGTHS AND LIMITATIONS
Ankylosing spondylitis: This cohort consists of ~14,000 patients treated with radiotherapy to the spine for ankylosing spondylitis throughout the United Kingdom between 1935 and 1954. Although individual dose records were not available for all patients, estimates were made ranging from 1 to 25 Gy to the bone marrow and other various organs.	Mortality has been reported through 1982, at which point 727 cancer deaths had been reported. Excess leukemia rates were reported from which an absolute risk of 80 excess cases/Gy/y per million was estimated.	This group represents one of the largest bodies that has provided data on radiation-induced leukemia in humans for which fairly good dose estimates exist. Control groups were suboptimal, however, and doses were largely unfractionated. In addition, only cancer mortality (not incidence) was available for this cohort.
Postpartum mastitis study: This group consists of ~600 women, mostly between the ages of 20 and 40 y, treated with radiotherapy for postpartum acute mastitis in New York in the 1940s and 1950s for which ~1,200 nonexposed women with mastitis and siblings of both groups of women served as controls. Breast tissue doses ranged from 0.6 to 14 Gy.	Forty-five year follow-up identified excess breast cancer in this population as compared with the general female population of New York.	A legitimate objection to using the data from this study to establish radiation-induced breast cancer risk factors is the uncertainty as to what effect the inflammatory changes associated with postpartum mastitis and the hormonal changes due to pregnancy have on the risk of breast cancer.
Radium dial painters: Young women who ingested radium (Ra-226 and Ra-228 with half-lives of ~1,600 and 7 y, respectively) while licking their brushes (containing luminous radium sulfate) to a sharp point during the application of luminous paint on dials and clocks in the 1920s and 1930s. Over 800 were followed.	Large increase in osteogenic sarcoma. Osteogenic sarcoma is a rare cancer (incidence, ~5 per 10^6 population). RR in the population was >100×s. No increase was seen below doses of 5 Gy but a sharp increase was noticed thereafter.	One of only a few studies that analyzed the radiocarcinogenic effectiveness of internal contamination with high-LET radiation in humans.
Thorotrast: Several populations were studied in which individuals were injected intravascularly with an x-ray contrast medium, Thorotrast, used between 1931 and 1950. Thorotrast contains 25% by weight radioactive colloidal Th-232 dioxide. Th-232 is an alpha emitter with a half-life of ~14 billion y.	Particles were deposited in the reticuloendothelial systems. Noted increase in number of cancers, particularly liver cancer (angiosarcoma, bile duct carcinomas, and hepatic cell carcinomas) and leukemia. Evaluation of the data resulted in estimates of alpha radiation-induced liver cancer risk of ~8 × 10^{-2} per Gy which appears to be linear with dose. Alpha RBE ~20. An increase in leukemia was also seen, however, the RBE was much lower (~1).	Dose estimates are fairly good. However, the extent to which the chemical toxicity of the Thorotrast may have influenced the risk is not known. Thorotrast administration resulted in chronic alpha particle irradiation from radionuclides in the thorium decay series. Organs of deposition of Th-232 and from the daughter products of radon-220 in the lungs and of radium-224 and its decay products in the skeletal system.

Source: Adapted and updated and from National Academy of Sciences/National Research Council Committee on the Biological Effects of Ionizing Radiation. The health effects of exposure to low levels of ionizing radiation (BEIR V). Washington, DC: NAS/NRC, 1990.

TABLE 20-11 SOLID CANCERS CASES BY DOSE CATEGORY

DOSE CATEGORY[a]	SUBJECTS	OBSERVED	BACKGROUND[B]	FITTED EXCESS[B]	ATTRIBUTABLE FRACTION (%)
<0.005	60,792	9,597	9,537	3	0
0.005–0.1	27,789	4,406	4,374	81	1.8
0.1–0.2	5,527	968	910	75	7.6
0.2–0.5	5,935	1,144	963	179	15.7
0.5–1	3,173	688	493	206	29.5
1–2	1,647	460	248	196	44.2
2–4[b]	564	185	71	111	61
Total	**105,427**	**17,448**	**16,595**	**853**	**10.7**

[a]Weighted colon dose in Gy.
[b]Note Estimates of background and fitted excess cases are based on an ERR model with a linear dose response with effect modification by gender, age at exposure and attained age.
[c]Note that the most reliable source of epidemiological data in the LSS include doses range up to 2Gy, beyond which, errors in dose reconstruction and mortality from complications of the ARS provided limited radioepidemiological information.
Source: Modified from (Preston, 2007).

and perspective on the relative strength of the evidence supporting current risk estimates for radiation-induced cancers and future challenges are available in the literature and are highly recommended (Boice, 2006, 2011; UNSCEAR, 2008).

Estimates of Radiation-Induced Cancer Risks from Low-Dose, Low-LET Radiation

Numerous national and international scientific organizations periodically report on the state of scientific knowledge regarding the carcinogenic risk and other biological

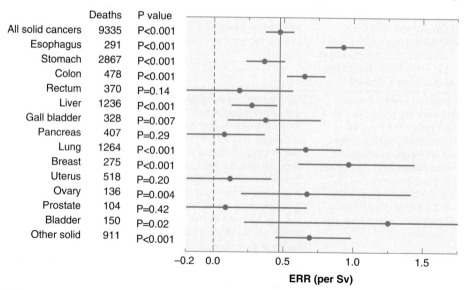

■ **FIGURE 20-25** Estimates of the site-specific solid cancer mortality ERR with 90% confidence intervals. Except for gender-specific cancers (breast, ovary, uterus, and prostate), the estimates are averaged over gender. The *dotted vertical line* at 0 corresponds to no excess risk, while the *solid vertical line* indicates the gender-averaged risk for all solid cancers. Some cancer sites such as brain, testes, cervix, oral cavity, and kidney are not included. (Source Preston DL, Shimizu Y, Pierce DA, et al. Studies of mortality of atomic bomb survivors. Report 13: Solid cancer and noncancer disease mortality: 1950–1997. *Radiat Res* 2003;160:381–407).

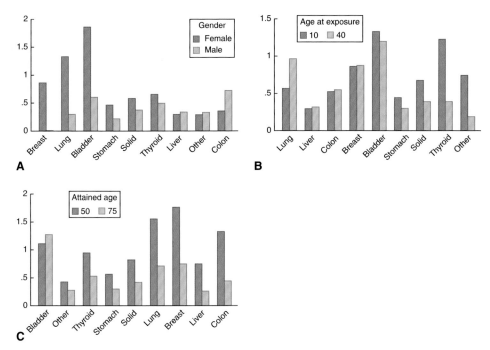

■ **FIGURE 20-26** Comparison of gender (**A**), age-at-exposure (**B**), and attained-age (**C**) effects on standardized $ERR_{1\,Gy}$ for selected sites and all solid cancers in the LSS. The ERR estimates for the "Other" category are based on the results of analyses of the 5,396 cancer cases not included in the sites explicitly considered here. The gender-specific estimates correspond to the fitted ERR per Gy at age 70 for a person exposed at age 30. The age-at-exposure specific estimates are gender-averaged ERR estimates at age 70 after exposure at age 10 (*red* bar) or age 40 (*green* bar). Attained-age-specific estimates are gender averaged ERR estimates at ages 50 (*red* bar) and 75 (*green* bar) after exposure at age 30. Within each panel, the sites are ordered based on the magnitude of the ratio of the effect pairs (Preston, 2007).

effects of ionizing radiation. Most recently, these include the United Nations Scientific Committee on the Effects of Atomic Radiation (UNSCEAR, 2006, 2008, 2009, 2011) report; the National Research Council, Committee on the Biological Effects of Ionizing Radiations (BEIR VII) report entitled *Health Effects of Exposure to Low Levels of Ionizing Radiation* in 2006 (BEIR, 2006); the U.S. Environmental Protection Agency's report on *Radiogenic Cancer Risk Models and Projections for the U.S. Population* (EPA, 2011); as well as reports focused on specific radiation health and radiation protection related topics by the NCRP, ICRP, and others. While there are some differences in the interpretation of specific aspects in the scientific literature among these various expert bodies, it is fair to say that there is general agreement on the most important aspects of radiation-induced risks, including the magnitude of the risk for the general population and its uncertainty at low doses. General points of agreement that are consistent with the results from the A-bomb survivor LSS include (1) risk varies according to cancer site; (2) risk is greater when exposures occur at younger ages; (3) risk is greater for females than males; (4) solid cancer risk is consistent with a linear function of dose when all cancers are combined; (5) leukemia risk is consistent with a nonlinear function of dose; (6) with the exception of leukemia for which there is a fairly well-defined risk interval following exposure, risk remains elevated for 50+ years after exposure; and (7) there is no convincing epidemiological evidence of radiation causing genetic (inherited) effects. In as much as there is not a major divergence of opinions expressed in the reports cited above, information on radiation-induced cancer risks and genetic effects will be presented based on the analysis and perspectives contained in the BEIR VII committee report.

BEIR VII Report

The *BEIR VII* report was an update of their previous 1990 report (BEIR V) on the same topic and a report focused on risk from radon exposure (BEIR VI), which was published in 1999. The primary objective of the report was to provide a comprehensive reassessment of the health risks resulting from exposures to low-dose, low-LET radiation in humans. The report provided updated risk estimates based on a review of the relevant scientific evidence from epidemiology and the vast array of data from laboratory experiments that included everything from long term animal studies to molecular mechanisms of radiation-induced damage and response. For the purpose of the report, "low dose" was defined as less than 100 mGy. The report also considered chronic exposure, defined as dose rates less than 0.1 mGy/min, irrespective to total dose. The report provided risk estimates of cancer incidence and mortality from radiation in the U.S. population as well as population and organ-specific risk estimates adjusted for gender, age at exposure, and time interval following exposure including lifetime risks. Heritable effects and risk from *in utero* radiation exposure were also considered. For most cancer risk estimates, the BEIR VII committee relied on the most recent cancer incidence and mortality data from the A-bomb survivor LSS. For breast and thyroid cancer, the committee used a pooled analysis of data from the LSS and studies of medically exposed persons.

Modeling of Epidemiological Data

Within the context of the limitations of epidemiology described earlier, scientists have developed dose-response models to predict the risk of cancer in human populations from exposure to low levels of ionizing radiation. While the data from the LSS are without doubt the most robust data set from which cancer risk estimates can be made, their use requires answers to several important questions such as (1) how can the effects demonstrated at high dose and high dose rate be compared to low dose and low dose rate exposures typical of most medical, occupational, and environmental exposures; (2) what is the effect of age at time of exposure on risk estimates; (3) how well do the risk estimates based on exposure in the Japanese population translate to what might be expected in the US population; (4) how representative is a population exposed in 1945 in a war-torn country with nutritional and other deficiencies to a modern healthy population of today?

Dose-Response Models

Several models have been proposed to characterize dose-response relationships of radiation exposure in humans. The shapes of the dose-response curves have been characterized as *linear nonthreshold* (LNT), *linear-quadratic* (LQ), and *threshold* (Fig. 20-27). The two LNT extrapolations represent the high dose and dose rate (black) and low dose (orange) components of the dose-response data. The LQ dose-response curve (red) demonstrates a reduced effectiveness for radiogenic cancer induction at lower dose and higher effectiveness at higher dose that eventually flattens out, reflecting doses associated with substantial cell killing.

In addition to the experimental evidence previously mentioned, there is also epidemiological evidence for a threshold for some cancers (e.g., blue dashed line in Fig. 20-27). For example, a threshold model provides the best fit for the osteogenic sarcoma risk among dial painters who had substantial internal radium contamination (discussed previously in this chapter). Other cancers, for which the evidence for radiation-induced risk is consistent with a threshold, include bone, soft tissue sarcoma, rectum, and nonmelanoma skin cancer. In addition, there are sites for

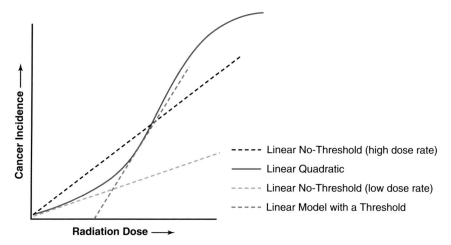

■ **FIGURE 20-27** Possible dose response relationship for radiation-induced cancer. (Adapted from BEIR. *Health risks from exposure to low levels of ionizing radiation: BEIR VII, Phase 2. Committee to Assess Health Risks from Exposure to Low Levels of Ionizing Radiation*, Board of Radiation Effects, Research Division on Earth and Life Studies, National Research Council of the National Academies. National Academy of Sciences, Washington, DC: National Academies Press, 2006.)

which there is no convincing evidence for a radiation-induced increase in cancer risk (e.g., prostate, pancreas, testes, cervix).

However, even though there is evidence for a threshold dose for some types of radiation exposure in specific tissues below which no radiogenic cancer risk is evident, the evidence supporting this model is not sufficient to be accepted for general use in assessing cancer risk from radiation exposure. Both the ICRP and BEIR VII committee concluded that, although there are alternatives to linearity, there is no strong evidence supporting the choice of another form of the dose response relationship. The statement in ICRP publication 99 captured the essence of the consensus view in this regard: ".... while existence of a low-dose threshold does not seem to be unlikely for radiation-related cancers of certain tissues, the evidence does not favor the existence of a universal threshold. The LNT hypothesis, combined with an uncertain DDREF for extrapolation from high doses, remains a prudent basis for radiation protection at low doses and low dose rates" (ICRP, 2006).

Figure 20-28, adapted from BEIR VII, shows the point estimates (orange dots) of ERRs of solid cancer incidence, (averaged over gender and standardized to represent individuals exposed at age 30 who have attained age 60) for specific dose intervals from the A-bomb survivor LSS. Vertical lines represent the 95% confidence intervals around each point estimate. The orange solid line and the green dashed line are linear and LQ dose-response models (respectively) for ERR of solid tumors, estimated from all subjects with doses in the range 0 to 1.5 Sv. The LQ dose-response function was discussed previously in the context of cell survival curves. Here the probability of an effect (cancer induction in this case) is proportional to the sum of two coefficients, one that is proportional to dose (αD) and one that is proportional to square of the dose (βD^2). Just as with the cell survival curves, the linear and quadratic components represent the response to low dose and high dose and dose rate effects, respectively. The degree of curvature is the ratio of the quadratic and linear coefficients. These coefficients can be estimated for different cancers reflecting their unique dose-response relationships.

As discussed previously, the biological effectiveness of the radiation-induced damage to cells and tissues generally decreases at lower dose and lower dose rates. This effect is due, at least in part, to the ability to repair damage during low dose

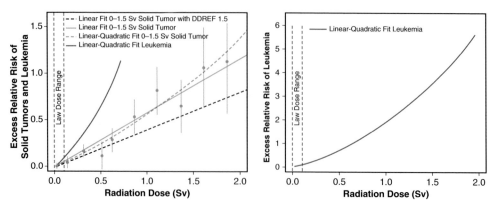

■ **FIGURE 20-28** Dose-response models of ERR for solid cancer and leukemia from cancer incidence data of Japanese A-bomb survivors. (Adapted from BEIR VII, 2006).

exposure or between exposures in the case of a higher total dose delivered in smaller dose fractions. A DDREF has been used to convert risk from exposures at high dose and high dose rate to estimates of risk at low doses for the purposes of radiation protection. The BEIR VII committee applied a DDREF of 1.5 to adjust the response observed in the high dose range making it roughly equivalent to the line representing the LNT low-dose response (black dashed line in Fig. 20-28). This line represents an extension of the linear portion (i.e., zero-dose tangent) of the LQ model (seen more clearly as the low-dose LNT line in Fig. 20-27). The value of the DDREF was derived based on a 95% confidence interval of a Bayesian statistical analysis of the solid cancer incidence data from the A-bomb survivor LSS, as well as the results from selected laboratory animal data. The BEIR VII committee, however, noted the uncertainty in their estimate of a DDREF because of the substantial inconsistency and imprecision in the animal data and because the DDREF estimate was particularly sensitive to the selection of the dose range used for estimation, the particular studies chosen for analysis, and the approach used for estimating curvature that is presumed to be the same across all studies. While it would be equally correct to use the LQ fit to the solid cancer risk data, the BEIR VII committee chose to use the DDREF-adjusted linear dose-response model for cancer risk estimates with the exception of leukemia, for which the LQ model was a better fit. In the absence of a superior dose-response model, the decision was made because it was simple to apply and is widely used by other organizations for this purpose, albeit with a somewhat different DDREF value (e.g., DDREF of 2 was used by UNSCEAR and ICRP). Note that in the low-dose range of interest in medical imaging and occupational exposure to radiation (less than 100 mSv), the difference between the linear fit to the solid tumor data (incorporating a DDREF 1.5–black dashed line) and the LQ fit to the same data (green dashed line) is relatively small compared to the 95% confidence intervals. The red lines in the left and right panels of Figure 20-28 show the ERR for leukemia which best fit a LQ dose-response model. The left panel shows the ERR for leukemia plotted on the same ERR scale as the solid cancer risk data up to approximately 0.7 Sv while the panel on the right shows the same dose-response up to 2 Sv on a broader ERR scale. One can appreciate the greater ERR per unit dose (i.e., the degree of curvature) observed for this cancer.

Multiplicative and Additive Risk Models: (Transport of Risk Between Populations)

Previous estimates of radiation-induced cancer have employed both the *multiplicative* and the *additive* risk models. The multiplicative risk-projection model (also referred to as the *relative risk* model) is based on the assumption that the excess cancer risk increases in proportion to the baseline cancer rate. Thus, the multiplicative risk model predicts that, after the latent period (e.g., 10 years), the excess risk is a multiple of the natural age-specific risk for the specific cancer and population in question (Fig. 20-29A). The alternative *additive* (or *absolute*) risk model (expressed in in terms of EAR) is based on the assumption that, following the latent period, the excess cancer rate is constant and independent of the spontaneous population and age-specific natural cancer risk (see Fig. 20-29B). While neither of these two simple models appears adequate to completely describe the risk of radiation-induced cancer, the multiplicative risk model is consistent with the scientific evidence that radiation acts predominantly as an initiator, rather than a promoter, of carcinogenesis. In addition, the copious epidemiological evidence, which indicates that exposure of children to radiation carries a greater risk than exposures later in life, further supports its role as an initiator rather than promoter. The multiplicative risk model was used by the BEIR VII committee for deriving tissue-specific solid cancer risk estimates as a function of gender, age at time of exposure, and time elapsed since exposure.

The multiplicative and additive risk-projection models can be used to transport risk calculated from one population to another dissimilar population. This is a critical issue, insofar as the LSS of the Japanese A-bomb survivors serves as the foundation of many radiation risk estimates and radiation protection regulations. The problem is especially important for U.S. population based radiation risk estimates because the natural incidence of several types of cancer in the U.S. and in Japan are very dissimilar. For example, the incidence of breast cancer in the U.S. is 3 times that of Japan while the incidences of liver and stomach cancer are 7.5 and 10 times higher respectively in

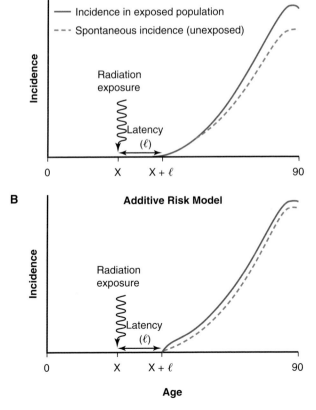

■ **FIGURE 20-29** Comparison of multiplicative and additive risk models. Radiation-induced risk increments are seen after a minimal latent period (ℓ); X is age at exposure. **A.** In the multiplicative risk model, the excess risk is a multiple of the natural age-specific cancer risk for a given population which increases with age. **B.** The additive risk model is shown in which a fixed incremental increased risk is added to the spontaneous disease incidence which is assumed to be constant over the remaining lifetime. The multiplicative risk model predicts the greatest increment in incidence at older ages.

TABLE 20-12   BASELINE CANCER INCIDENCE RATES IN UNITED STATES AND JAPAN (FEMALES)[a]

	U.S.	JAPAN
All	280	185
Stomach	3.5	34
Colon	22	17
Liver	1.3	9.8
Lung	34	12
Breast	89	30
Bladder	5.9	2.6

Source: Correa CN, Wu X-C, Andrews P, et al., eds. *Cancer incidence in five continents*, vol VIII. Lyon, France: IARC Scientific Publications No. 155, 2002.
[a]Incidence rates per 100,000 women.

Japan than in the U.S. (Table 20-12). The previous BEIR committee (BEIR V) based its estimates on multiplicative risk transport, where it is assumed that the excess risk due to radiation is proportional to baseline cancer risks. BEIR VII took a hybrid approach using the multiplicative risk model for some cancers (e.g., thyroid); the absolute risk model for others (e.g., breast); and, for most, a weighted average between the values calculated using the absolute and multiplicative risk models.

Age and Gender Specific Radiation Risk Estimates

A summary of the BEIR VII preferred estimates of lifetime attributable risk of solid cancer (incidence and mortality) along with their 95% confidence intervals for different exposure scenarios is shown in Table 20-13. Tables of lifetime attributable

TABLE 20-13   BEIR VII PREFERRED ESTIMATES OF LIFETIME ATTRIBUTABLE RISK OF SOLID CANCER INCIDENCE AND MORTALITY WITH 95% CONFIDENCE INTERVALS[a]

EXPOSURE SCENARIO	INCIDENCE		MORTALITY	
	MEN	WOMEN	MEN	WOMEN
0.1 Gy to population of mixed ages	800 (400–1,590)	1,310 (690–2,490)	410 (200–830)	610 (300–1,230)
0.1 Gy at age 10	1,330 (660–2,660)	2,530 (1,290–4,930)	640 (300–1,390)	1,050 (470–2,330)
0.1 Gy at age 30	600 (290–1,290)	1,000 (500–2,020)	320 (150–650)	490 (250–950)
0.1 Gy at age 50	510 (240–1,100)	680 (350–1,320)	290 (140–600)	420 (210–810)
1 mGy/y throughout life	550 (280–1,100)	970 (510–1,840)	290 (140–580)	460 (230–920)
10 mGy/y from ages 18 to 65	2,600 (1,250–5,410)	4,030 (2,070–7,840)	1,410 (700–2,860)	2,170 (1,130–4,200)

[a]Cancer incidence and mortality per 100,000 exposed persons. 95% Confidence intervals shown in parentheses.
Source: BEIR. *Health risks from exposure to low levels of ionizing radiation: BEIR VII, Phase 2.* Committee to Assess Health Risks from Exposure to low levels of Ionizing Radiation, Board of Radiation Effects, Research Division on Earth and Life Studies, National Resarch Council of the National Academies. National Academy of Sciences, Washington, DC: National Academies Press, 2006.

cancer incidence and mortality risk by age at exposure and cancer site are provided in the BEIR VII report. The cancer incidence data from that document are shown below in Table 20-14 and the mortality data table can be found in Chapter 11, Table 11.6.

The risks in these tables are expressed as the number of additional cases per 100,000 per 100 mGy to the specified tissue. From this information, organ-specific risk estimates can be derived. For example, if a 10-year-old girl received a 20 mGy

TABLE 20-14   LIFETIME ATTRIBUTABLE RISK OF SITE-SPECIFIC CANCER INCIDENCE

	NUMBER OF CASES PER 100,000 PERSONS EXPOSED TO A SINGLE DOSE OF 0.1 Gy										
	AGE AT EXPOSURE (y)										
Cancer Site	0	5	10	15	20	30	40	50	60	70	80
Men											
Stomach	76	65	55	46	40	28	27	25	20	14	7
Colon	336	285	241	204	173	125	122	113	94	65	30
Liver	61	50	43	36	30	22	21	19	14	8	3
Lung	314	261	216	180	149	105	104	101	89	65	34
Prostate	93	80	67	57	48	35	35	33	26	14	5
Bladder	209	177	150	127	108	79	79	76	66	47	23
Other	1,123	672	503	394	312	198	172	140	98	57	23
Thyroid	115	76	50	33	21	9	3	1	0.3	0.1	0.0
All solid	2,326	1,667	1,325	1,076	881	602	564	507	407	270	126
Leukemia	237	149	120	105	96	84	84	84	82	73	48
All cancers	2,563	1,816	1,445	1,182	977	686	648	591	489	343	174
Women											
Stomach	101	85	72	61	52	36	35	32	27	19	11
Colon	220	187	158	134	114	82	79	73	62	45	23
Liver	28	23	20	16	14	10	10	9	7	5	2
Lung	733	608	504	417	346	242	240	230	201	147	77
Breast	1,171	914	712	553	429	253	141	70	31	12	4
Uterus	50	42	36	30	26	18	16	13	9	5	2
Ovary	104	87	73	60	50	34	31	25	18	11	5
Bladder	212	180	152	129	109	79	78	74	64	47	24
Other	1,339	719	523	409	323	207	181	148	109	68	30
Thyroid	634	419	275	178	113	41	14	4	1	0.3	0.0
All solid	4,592	3,265	2,525	1,988	1,575	1,002	824	678	529	358	177
Leukemia	185	112	86	76	71	63	62	62	57	51	37
All cancers	4,777	3,377	2,611	2,064	1,646	1,065	886	740	586	409	214

Source: Adapted from BEIR VII Table 12 D-1, BEIR. *Health risks from exposure to low levels of ionizing radiation: BEIR VII, Phase 2. Committee to Assess Health Risks from Exposure to Low Levels of Ionizing Radiation*, Board of Radiation Effects, Research Division on Earth and Life Studies, National Research Council of the National Academies. National Academy of Sciences, Washington, DC: National Academies Press, 2006.

breast dose from a chest CT exam, the lifetime risk of being diagnosed with breast cancer as a result of the exam would be:

> From Table 20-14, the radiation-induced breast cancer risk at age 10 is 712 cases per 100,000 per 100 mGy. Thus the risk would be calculated as (712) (20 mGy/100 mGy) = 142 per 100,000 or approximately 1 in 700.

If the same dose were received by a 50-year-old woman the risk would drop by approximately a factor of 10 (~1 in 7,000). It is important to understand that the risk coefficients presented in these tables have large uncertainties associated with them and there are many other risk factors for breast cancer (discussed below). Furthermore, the evidence that radiation causes breast cancer at 100 mSv is equivocal and this uncertainty is even greater for doses less than 20 mSv, implying that the statistical uncertainty of risk estimates at these low doses is large and the possibility of no increase in risk cannot be excluded. Nevertheless they can be used to provide a perspective of the magnitude of the risk engendered from the dose received for a particular exam in a given patient population. A number of such risks estimates have been made in recent years for a variety of imaging studies. The result from one such study evaluating the change in dose and risk with age of exposure for CT exams of the head and abdomen is shown in Figure 20-30. As discussed in Chapter 21, the use of medical imaging using ionizing radiation has increased dramatically in the last 20 years. There has been a growing awareness of the potential for overutilization of this technology and the attendant radiation risk to patients (Brenner, 2007; Frazel, 2009). This issue is particularly troubling for the pediatric patient population who have inherently higher cancer risks from a given dose and (depending on the imaging study) may receive higher organ doses than adults for the same procedure (Brenner, 2001; Brody, 2007). Efforts to educate physicians and patients about these issues continue and will no doubt be necessary for many years to come. Optimization of imaging procedures in this context includes not only the technical factors related to image acquisition but also (and often most importantly) the appropriateness of the requested examination to resolve the particular clinical question. The pressure in some cases from parents who may insist on a CT exam for the child being evaluated for relatively minor head injury adds to this problem. The use of clear evidence based guidelines and appropriateness criteria for medical imaging procedures is an important quality care goal and their implementation in an emergency department setting when evaluating pediatric patients is especially important (Kuppermann, 2009).

Estimates of the total cancer incidence and mortality risk as a function of sex and age at exposure are presented graphically in Figure 20-31. The increased cancer risk associated with exposure to radiation of children and infants is easily appreciated. Compared to the risk to adults, the cancer risk for a 12-month-old infant is three to four times higher. The increased risk of radiation exposure in females compared to males at all ages is also shown; however, the magnitude of the difference decreases with age.

Population Radiation Risk Estimates

The population averaged radiation-induced cancer incidence and mortality risk estimates, calculated from data provided in the BEIR VII report, are shown in Table 20-15. The risk estimates of the International Commission on Radiological Protection (ICRP), (derived from evaluation of the radiation-induced cancer incidence and mortality data), are in general agreement with those in the BEIR VII report. As mentioned earlier the ICRP risk estimates were made for the purpose of radiation protection (see Chapter 3) and are not directly comparable to the BEIR VII cancer risk estimates. The current

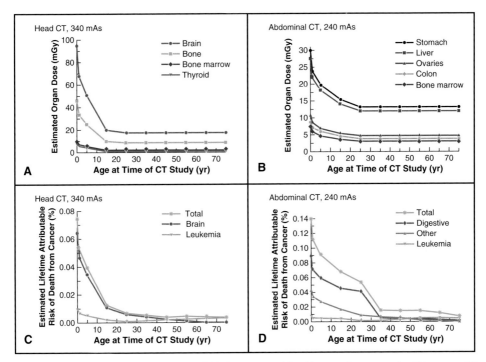

■ **FIGURE 20-30** Estimated organ doses and lifetime cancer risk with age of exposure for CT exams of the head and abdomen. **A, B** show estimated radiation doses for selected organs from a single CT scan of the head or the abdomen. As discussed in Chapter 10, for a given mAs, pediatric doses are typically larger than adult doses, because there is less self shielding of organs during the tube rotation. Exposure parameters and other aspects of imaging studies should be optimized for each patient. However, it is especially important for children due to their increased risk of radiogenic cancer and often higher organ doses. Optimization of imaging procedures in this context includes not only the technical factors related to the image acquisition but also (and often most importantly) the appropriateness of the requested examination to resolve the particular clinical question. Panels **C, D** show the corresponding estimated lifetime percent cancer mortality risk attributable to the radiation from a single CT scan; the risks (both for selected individual organs and overall) have been averaged for male and female patients. One can appreciate that even though doses are higher for the head CT scans, the risks are higher for abdominal scans because organs exposed are more sensitive than the brain to radiation-induced cancer. It should be noted that the mAs (and resultant doses) used in these examples are from the source cited below and are higher than typical doses for similar exams performed with image acquisition parameters optimized for smaller patients. Contrary to current practice, these data assume that no tube current adjustment for patient size has been applied, which of course would substantially reduce the dose (and thus risk) in the pediatric population. (From Brenner DJ, Hall EJ. Computed tomography—an increasing source of radiation exposure. *N Engl J Med* 2007;357:2277–2284.)

ICRP risk estimates of radiation-induced "detriment"[1] (e.g., cancer and genetic effects) at low dose are 4.2% per Sv for a population of adult workers and 5.7% per Sv for the whole population (which includes more radiosensitive subpopulations, such as children). The majority of this detriment is assigned to a cancer risk of 4.1% and 5.5% per Sv for adult workers and the general population, respectively. Even though the definitions and methodology of calculating radiation-induced cancer risk are different for the ICRP and the BEIR VII committee, the ICRP population estimate of cancer detriment from radiation exposure (5.5%/Sv) corresponds fairly well to BEIR VII lifetime attributable cancer mortality projections averaged for the U.S. population (5.7%/Sv).

---

[1]The total harm to health experienced by an exposed group and its decendants as a result of the group's exposure to a radiation source. Detriment is a multimentional concept. Its principal components are the stochastic quantities: probability of attributable fatal cancer, weighted probability of attributable non-fatal cancer, weighted probability of severe heritable effects, and length of life lost if the harm occurs.

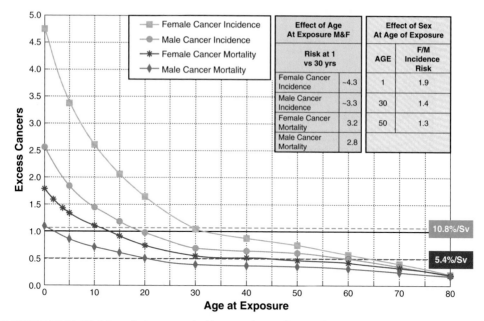

FIGURE 20-31 Lifetime radiation cancer incidence and mortality as a function of sex and age at exposure. Excess cancer cases per 1,000 following a whole body dose 10 mSv (multiply by 10 to convert to percent per Sv). The table inserts shows the relative effect on cancer incidence and mortality for exposures at ages 1 and 30 years old (**left**) and the relative increased radiogenic cancer risk for females compared to males as a function of exposure at 1,30, and 50 years old (**right**). The population averaged cancer incidence of 11.4%/Sv (*green line*) and mortality 5.7%/Sv (*red line*) as calculated from the BEIR VII data is superimposed over the age and sex-specific risk estimates. (Adapted from BEIR. *Health risks from exposure to low levels of ionizing radiation: BEIR VII, Phase 2. Committee to Assess Health Risks from Exposure to Low Levels of Ionizing Radiation*, Board of Radiation Effects, Research Division on Earth and Life Studies, National Research Council of the National Academies. National Academy of Sciences, Washington, DC: National Academies Press, 2006.)

To estimate risk to the general population from radiation exposure at low exposure levels the approximate values of 11% and 6% per Sv, respectively for cancer incidence and mortality can be used. As mentioned earlier, the lifetime probability of developing or dying from cancer in the United States (averaged for both sexes) is approximately 41% and 22%, respectively. According to the linear risk-projection model, an acute exposure of 100 people to 100 mSv would add approximately 1 additional

TABLE 20-15   THE US POPULATION AVERAGED RADIATION-INDUCED CANCER INCIDENCE AND MORTALITY RISK ESTIMATES IN PERCENT PER Sv

	INCIDENCE	MORTALITY
Female	13.7	6.6
Male	9.0	4.8
U.S. population average	11.4	5.7

Source: Calculated from: Health risks from exposure to low levels of ionizing radiation: BEIR VII, Phase 2. Committee to Assess Health Risks from Exposure to Low Levels of Ionizing Radiation, Board of Radiation Effects, Research Division on Earth and Life Studies, National Research Council of the National Academies. National Academy of Sciences, Washington, DC: National Academies Press, 2006.

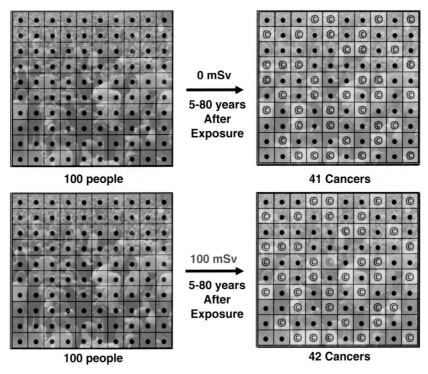

0 mSv

→

5-80 years
After
Exposure

100 people

41 Cancers

100 mSv

→

5-80 years
After
Exposure

100 people

42 Cancers

■ **FIGURE 20-32** Cancer incidence for two identical groups of 100 people with age and sex distributions similar to the general population. An acute exposure to 100 mSv for each person in one group would be expected to add approximately 1 additional cancer case (occurring anytime after a latent period of approximately 5 years) to the 41 normally expected to occur in the identical unexposed group over the group's lifetime.

cancer case to the 41 normally expected to occur over the lifetime of a group with an age and sex distribution similar to the general population (Fig. 20-32).

Of course there would be no way of identifying which person had the additional cancer (if it occurred at all) that was caused by the radiation exposure and given the small number of individuals exposed, the natural variation associated with the average incidence of cancer would be larger than one. The number of exposed individuals and the dose in the example above were chosen to provide a simple example of the LNT dose-response relationship. However, it would be very unusual for such a group to receive such a large whole body dose at one time. Using a more realistic dose from an (albeit unlikely) exposure scenario, one could imagine an accidental release of radioactive material into the environment exposing a population of 10,000 to 10 mSv in 1 year (i.e., ten times the annual public exposure limit in the U.S.). The LNT model would project 11 additional cancer cases (approximately one half of which would be fatal) over the life time of the population. This represents an increase of less than 0.3% above the spontaneous cancer incidence rate. UNSCEAR and ICRP, however, argue against using collective dose to predict future cancer deaths when the average dose to the population is small and below the doses where excess risks have been convincingly demonstrated. An additional perspective on cancer risks is presented in Table 20-16, which compares adult cancers with respect to their spontaneous and radiation-induced incidence.

Cancer Risk for Selected Organs and Tissues

Leukemia

Leukemia is a relatively rare disease, with an incidence in the general U.S. population of approximately 1 in 10,000 per year. However, genetic predisposition to

TABLE 20-16   SPONTANEOUS INCIDENCE AND SENSITIVITY OF VARIOUS TISSUES TO RADIATION-INDUCED CANCER

SITE OR TYPE OF CANCER	SPONTANEOUS INCIDENCE	RADIATION SENSITIVITY
Most frequent radiation-induced cancers		
Female breast	Very high	High in children and young women
Thyroid	Low	Very high in children, especially in females, but very low in adults
Lung (bronchus)	Very high	Moderate
Leukemia	Moderate	Very high
Alimentary tract	High	Moderate
Less frequent radiation-induced cancers		
Pharynx	Low	Moderate
Liver and biliary tract	Low	Moderate
Lymphomas	Moderate	Moderate
Kidney and bladder	Moderate	Low
Brain and nervous system	Low	Low
Salivary glands	Very low	Low
Bone	Very low	Low
Skin	High	Low
Magnitude of radiation risk uncertain		
Larynx	Moderate	Low
Nasal sinuses	Very low	Low
Parathyroid	Very low	Low
Ovary	Moderate	Low
Connective tissue	Very low	Low
Radiation risk not demonstrated		
Prostate	Very high	Absent?
Uterus and cervix	Very high	Absent?
Testis	Low	Absent?
Mesothelium	Very low	Absent?
Chronic lymphocytic leukemia	Low	Absent?

Source: Modified from Committee on Radiological Units, Standards and Protection: *Medical Radiation: A Guide to Good Practice*. Chicago, IL: American College of Radiology, 1985.

leukemia can dramatically increase the risk. For example, an identical twin of a leukemic child has a one in three chance of developing leukemia. Although it is rare in the general population, leukemia is one of the most frequently observed radiation-induced cancers. Leukemia may be acute or chronic, and it may take a lymphocytic or myeloid form. With the exception of chronic lymphocytic leukemia and viral-induced leukemia, increases in all forms of leukemia have been detected in human populations exposed to radiation and in animals experimentally irradiated.

Within a few years after the detonation of the A-bombs, an increase in the incidence of leukemia was apparent in the survivor population. This evidence, together with subsequent studies of medically and occupationally exposed cohorts, indicate

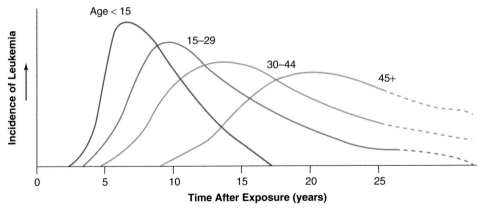

■ **FIGURE 20-33** Effect of age at the time of exposure on the incidence of leukemia (all forms except chronic lymphocytic leukemia) among the A-bomb survivors. (From Ichuimaru et al. Incidence of leukemia in atomic-bomb survivors, Hiroshima and Nagasaki 1950 to 1971, by radiation dose, years after exposure, age, and type of leukemia. Technical Report RERF 10-76. Hiroshima, Japan: Radiation Effects Research Foundation, 1976.)

that excess leukemia cases can be detected as early as 1 to 2 years after exposure and reach a peak approximately 12 years after the exposure. The incidence of leukemia is influenced by age at the time of exposure. The younger the person is at the time of exposure, the shorter are the latency period and the period of expression (Fig. 20-33).

Although the incidence of radiation-induced leukemia decreases with age at the time of exposure, the interval of increased risk is protracted. The BEIR VII committee's preferred model for leukemia risk was a LQ function of dose and, like models for solid cancers, leukemia risk is expressed as a function of age at exposure. However, the unique temporal wave-like character of the elevated risk for leukemia makes it more useful to express risk as a function of time since exposure rather than attained age (Fig. 20-34).

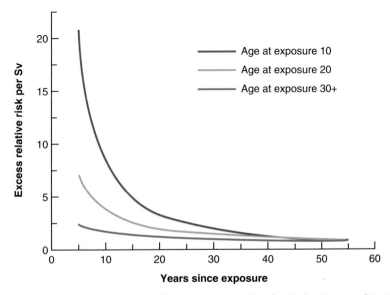

■ **FIGURE 20-34** Age-time patterns in radiation-associated risks for leukemia mortality. Curves are sex-averaged estimates of the risk at 1 Sv for people exposed at age 10 (*red line*), age 20 (*orange line*), and age 30 or more (*blue line*). (Adapted from BEIR VII.)

Another unique feature of the risk model is that there was no need to apply a DDREF as the estimates are already based on a LQ function of dose. The BEIR VII preferred model for leukemia estimates an excess lifetime risk from an exposure to 0.1 Gy for 100,000 persons with an age distribution similar to that of the U.S. population to be approximately 70 and 100, for females and males, respectively (i.e., ~1% per Sv).

Thyroid Cancer

Distinct from the previously discussed cancer risk estimates, the preferred BEIR VII models for thyroid and breast cancers are based on pooled analyses of the LSS data and medically irradiated cohorts. Spontaneous and radiation-induced thyroid cancer shows a greater difference by gender than most cancers, with women having a risk approximately two to three times as great as that for men (presumably because of hormonal influences on thyroid function). Persons of Jewish and North African ancestry also appear to be at greater risk than the general population. Thyroid cancer accounts for only approximately 2% of the yearly total cancer incidence. In addition, the mortality is low, resulting in only approximately 0.2% of all cancer deaths each year. Even though there is a large relative risk for thyroid cancer from radiation exposure in childhood, the absolute risks (even in children and young adults) are lower than for breast, colon and lung cancer. There is also a rapid decrease in radiogenic cancer risk with age, with the lifetime absolute risk per Gy for thyroid cancer at age 40 and beyond lower than the risk to all but a few other organs and tissues. Most studies do not indicate any elevation in risk when exposure occurs in adulthood.

The majority of radiation-induced thyroid neoplasms are well-differentiated papillary adenocarcinomas, with a lower percentage being of the follicular form. Because of improved diagnostic procedures and the fact that radiation-induced thyroid cancers do not usually include the anaplastic and medullary types, the associated mortality rate is very low ($\sim5/10^6$ per year for all races and both genders). The dose-response data for thyroid cancer fit a linear pattern. The latency period for benign nodules is approximately 5 to 35 years, and for thyroid malignancies it is approximately 10 to 35 years. While recent studies of the risk of radiation-induced thyroid cancer have taken different modeling approaches to estimate the risk (BEIR VII, 2006; NCRP, 2008; EPA, 2011), the results differ by less than a factor of 2 and all estimates had a range representing the 95% confidence interval that were a factor of 4 or more from their point of estimate.

The relative effectiveness of producing radiogenic thyroid cancer from internally deposited radionuclides has been shown to be approximately 60% to 100% as effective as external irradiation from x-rays. A comprehensive update of a previous NCRP report on radiation effects on the thyroid (NCRP, 2008), found that for the same absorbed dose, I-131 and I-125 were no more than 30% to 60% as effective as external radiation in causing thyroid cancer with the higher effectiveness applicable to radioiodine exposure in children. However, the report concluded that other radionuclides including I-123 and Tc-99m were equally effective (per unit thyroid dose) as external radiation in causing thyroid cancer.

Irradiation of the thyroid may produce other responses, such as hypothyroidism and thyroiditis. Threshold estimates for adult populations range from 2 Gy for external irradiation to 50 Gy for internal (low-dose-rate) irradiation. Lower threshold estimates exist for children. Approximately 10% of persons with thyroid doses of 200 to 300 Gy from radioactive iodine will develop symptoms of thyroiditis and/or a sore throat, and higher doses may result in thyroid ablation.

Due to the considerable ability of the thyroid gland to concentrate iodine, the thyroid dose from radioiodine is typically 1,000 times greater than in other organs in the body. The relatively large thyroid dose per unit activity administered explains why thyroid cancer is a major concern following exposure to radioiodine, especially in children. The Chernobyl nuclear plant accident released large quantities of radio-iodine that resulted in a substantial increase in the incidence of thyroid cancer among children living in heavily contaminated regions. The cows concentrated the radioio-dine in their milk by eating contaminated foliage, which was further concentrated in the thyroid glands of people who consumed the milk. The thyroid dose to children was higher because they consume more milk and their thyroid glands had higher concentrations of radioiodine than in adult thyroid glands. Decreased dietary levels of stable iodine dramatically increase radioiodine uptake by the thyroid. It appears that dietary iodine deficiency was an important factor in the elevated occurrence of thyroid cancer observed in children exposed to radioiodine from the Chernobyl disaster. The increase so far has been almost entirely papillary carcinoma, which is the most common malignant tumor of the thyroid in adults, adolescents, and chil-dren. There has been no increase in thyroid cancer in cohorts made up of adults at the time of the accident, consistent with the absence of a thyroid cancer excess among patients treated with I-131 for Graves and other thyroid disorders. In addi-tion, no other cancers have shown an increased incidence thus far, and no increase has been detected in the incidence of birth defects.

Breast Cancer

For women exposed to ionizing radiation during mammography, the potential for an increase in the risk of breast cancer is of particular concern. The high prevalence and morbidity of breast cancer in the female population, and the often differing profes-sional opinions about the risk and benefits of screening mammography only serve to exacerbate these concerns. Breast cancer is the most commonly diagnosed cancer among women regardless of race or ethnicity. According to National Cancer Institute, one out of every eight women (12%) in the U.S, develops breast cancer with approxi-mately 230,000 new cases of invasive breast cancer and 54,000 cases of noninvasive (*in situ*) breast cancer expected to be diagnosed in women each year (SEER, 2011). The lifetime breast cancer mortality risk for women is approximately 2.8% with significant variation by race and ethnicity (e.g., annual mortality rates for Black and Hispanic populations are 32.4 and 15.3 per 100,000 respectively). Other etiologic factors in the risk of breast cancer include age at first full-term pregnancy, family history of breast cancer, and estrogen levels in the blood. Women who have had no children or only one child are at greater risk for breast cancer than women who have had two or more children. In addition, reduced risks are associated with women who conceive earlier in life and who breast-fed for a longer period of time. Familial history of breast cancer can increase the risk twofold to fourfold, with the magnitude of the risk increasing as the age at diagnosis in the family member decreases. As shown previously for Japan and the United States, there is also considerable racial and geographic variation in breast cancer risk. Several investigations have suggested that the presence of estrogen, acting as a promoter, is an important factor in the incidence and latency associated with spontaneous and radiation-induced breast cancer.

The BEIR VII committee utilized a pooled analysis of data on A-bomb survivors and medically exposed persons to evaluate the breast cancer risk for low-LET radia-tion. The data fit a linear dose-response model, with a dose of approximately 800 mGy required to double the natural incidence of breast cancer. The data from acute and fractionated (but high dose rate) exposure studies indicate that fractionation of the dose reduces the risk of breast cancer induced by low-LET radiation. There is some evidence that protracted exposure to radiation in children reduces the risk of radiation-induced breast cancer compared with acute or highly fractionated exposures (Preston, 2002). The latent period ranges from 10 to 40 years, with younger women having longer latencies. In contrast to leukemia, there is no identifiable window of expression; therefore the risk seems to continue throughout the life of the exposed individual. The lifetime attributable risk of developing breast cancer in a population of women with an age distribution similar to that of the U.S. general population is 310/10⁵/0.1 Gy The risk is very age dependent, being approximately 13 times higher for exposure at age 5 (914/10⁵/0.1 Gy) than at age 50 (70/10⁵/0.1 Gy), (BEIR VII, 2006). Using the age-specific values in the BEIR VII report, the lifetime attributable risks of developing breast cancer for females receiving a breast dose of 20 mGy from a chest CT at age 10, 30, or 50 are approximately 0.14%, 0.06%, and 0.014%, respectively. Use of the tube current modulation (TCM) capability of modern scanners has substantially lowered the dose and subsequent cancer risk, especially for younger patients. The following example illustrates the benefit of TCM compared to fixed mA for chest CT in 50-, 30-, and 10-year-old patients. In this example, we will assume a nominal breast dose of 15 mGy for a chest CT scan of a 50-year-old woman using fixed mA. In the absence of any other changes except decreasing body habitus with age, the breast dose might increase to 20 and 25 mGy for similar exams in the 30- and 10-year-old patients, receptively. As seen in Table 20-17, the increase in future cancer risk in the 10-year-old is 17 times that of the 50-year-old due to the combined effects of both increased dose and greater risk per unit dose associated with her scan. With TCM activated, the dose to 50-year-old women might increase somewhat but the dose (and associated risk) reductions in the other two age groups relative to that for the 50-year-old patient is substantial. It can also be appreciated that while the relative reduction in risk can be dramatic as shown in the example above, the change to the baseline breast cancer risk at the age of exposure is much less so. Thus, while the difference in dose reduction techniques illustrated above has only a minor influence on the cancer risk for an individual patient, considering the high utilization of CT in the United States and elsewhere, the overall public health impact could be quite important. Further discussion of the effect of TCM on dose reduction can be found in Chapter 10 and in the literature (Angel, 2009a,b).

Improvements in quality assurance and the introduction of digital mammography have resulted in a substantial reduction in dose to the breast (see Chapter 8). Women participating in large, controlled mammographic screening studies have been shown to have a decreased risk of mortality from breast cancer. The American Cancer Society, the American College of Obstetricians and Gynecologists, and the American College of Radiology currently recommend annual mammography examination for women beginning at age 40. We started this section mentioning that there has been concern

TABLE 20-17   EFFECT OF AGE AND USE OF AUTO MA ON BREAST DOSE AND LIFETIME ATTRIBUTABLE CANCER RISK FROM CHEST CT

AGE	CT mA (FIXED/ AUTO)	BREAST DOSE (mGy)	LAR BEIR VII PER 10⁵ PER 0.1 Gy	LIFETIME RISK AT AGE	% LAR RISK	LIFETIME RISK AT AGE + % LAR	RISK RATIO AGE/50	RISK RATIO FIX/AUTO mA AT AGE
10	Fixed	25	712	12.3	0.178	12.478	17.0	2.50
	Auto	10	712	12.3	0.071	12.371	5.1	
30	Fixed	20	253	12.3	0.051	12.351	4.8	1.33
	Auto	15	253	12.3	0.038	12.338	2.7	
50	Fixed	15	70	10.9	0.011	10.911	1.0	0.75
	Auto	20	70	10.9	0.014	10.914	1.0	

over radiation risks associated with mammographic screening examinations. It is reassuring that the risk of radiation-induced breast cancer decreases substantially with age at exposure and, despite the models used for risk estimation, there is no consistent epidemiologic evidence for significant risks for exposures once a woman has passed the menopausal ages. Further, the exposures for mammographic images are substantially below the levels for which significantly increased risks have been detected.

Noncancer Radiation Effects

Studies of some radiotherapy patient populations have demonstrated increased risks for diseases other than cancer, particularly cardiovascular disease. There is also evidence of an increase in cardiovascular disease at much lower doses among A-bomb survivors; however, there is no statistically significant increase at doses below 0.5 Sv. This evidence notwithstanding, there is no direct evidence for an increased risk of cardiovascular disease or other noncancer effects at the low doses associated with typical occupational exposures and diagnostic imaging procedures and thus far, the data are inadequate to quantify this risk, if it exists.

20.7 Hereditary Effects of Radiation Exposure

Conclusive evidence of the ability of ionizing radiation to produce genetic effects was first obtained in 1927 with the experimental observations of radiation-induced genetic effects in fruit flies (Muller, 1927). Extensive laboratory investigations since that time (primarily large-scale studies in mice (Russell W, et al, 1958)) have led scientists to conclude that (1) radiation is a mutagenic agent; (2) most mutations are harmful to the organism; (3) radiation does not produce unique mutations; (4) chronic radiation exposure produces fewer heritable effects in offspring than the same dose delivered acutely; and (5) radiation-induced genetic damage can theoretically occur (like cancer) from a single mutation and appears to be linearly related to dose (i.e., LNT dose-response model). However, it is reassuring that no human study has demonstrated transgenerational effects following parental exposure. Specifically, the studies of over 70,000 children, of A-bomb survivors and the children of cancer survivors treated with radiotherapy find no evidence for increased risks of malformations, neonatal deaths, stillbirths, chromosomal abnormality, or gene changes that could be related to the exposure to radiation of fathers and mothers (Signorello, 2010; Winther, 2009). Although genetic effects were initially thought to be the most significant biologic effect of ionizing radiation, it is clear that, for doses associated with occupational and medical exposure, the risks are small compared with the spontaneous incidence of genetic anomalies and are secondary to their carcinogenic potential.

Epidemiologic Investigations of Radiation-Induced Hereditary Effects

Epidemiologic investigations have failed to demonstrate radiation-induced hereditary effects, although mutations of human cells in culture have been shown. For a given exposure, the mutation rates found in the progeny of irradiated humans are significantly lower than those previously identified in insect populations. The largest population studied is the A-bomb survivors and their progeny. Based on current risk estimates, failure to detect an increase in radiation-induced mutations in this population is not surprising considering how few are predicted in comparison to the spontaneous incidence. Screening of 28 specific protein loci in the blood of 27,000 children of A-bomb survivors resulted in only two mutations that might have been caused by radiation exposure of the parents.

Earlier studies of survivors' children to determine whether radiation exposure caused an increase in sex-linked lethal gene mutations that would have resulted in increased prenatal death of males or alteration of the gender birth ratio were negative. Irradiation of human testes has been shown to produce an increase in the incidence of translocations in spermatogonial stem cells, although no additional chromosomal aberrations have been detected in children of A-bomb survivors. A large cohort study of more than 90,000 U.S. radiologic technologists (RTs) examined the risk of childhood cancer (less than 20 years) among more than 100,000 offspring born between 1921 and 1984 to the technologists (Johnson, 2008). Parental occupational radiation exposure of the testis or ovary prior to conception was estimated from work history data, dosimetry records, and by estimate from the literature for exposure prior to 1960. Despite the size of the study population, no convincing evidence of an increase in radiation exposure-related risk of childhood cancer in the offspring of RTs was found. The result from a number of recent studies evaluating the potential for trans-generational effects in the children of cancer survivors treated with radiotherapy have also been consistently negative (Signorello, 2010; Tawn, 2011; Winther, 2009).

Estimating Genetic Risk

The *genetically significant dose* is an index of the presumed genetic impact of radiation-induced mutation in germ cells in an exposed population. The sensitivity of a population to radiation-induced genetic damage can be measured by the *doubling dose*, defined as the dose required per generation to double the spontaneous mutation rate. The spontaneous mutation rate is approximately 5×10^{-6} per locus and 7 to 15×10^{-4} per gamete for chromosomal abnormalities. The doubling dose for humans is estimated to be approximately 1 Gy per generation; however, this represents an extrapolation from animal data. The BEIR VII committee estimated that an exposure of 10 mGy to the parental generation would cause 30 to 47 additional genetic disorders per 1 million births in the succeeding generation, as a result of increases in the number of autosomal dominant and (to a much lesser degree) sex-linked dominant mutations.

Variations in exposure to natural background do not contribute significantly to a population's genetic risk. Even a dose of 100 mGy would only be estimated to produce about 400 additional genetic disorders per 1 million live births in the first generation (0.4%/Gy), compared with the normal incidence of approximately 1 in 20 or 5% (some estimates are 1 in 10). Therefore, the 100-mGy dose would cause an increase in the spontaneous rate of genetic disorders of less than 0.8%.

While the estimates of cancer risk attributable to radiation exposure published in authoritative reports from the BEIR committees, UNSCEAR, NCRP, and ICRP have not changed greatly in the past two decades, new data and risk modeling have resulted in a substantial reduction in the estimated radiation-induced risk of heritable disease. According to a review by the ICRP, previous estimates of radiation-induced genetic effects from experiments in mice, and the study of genetic data from A-bomb survivors likely overestimated the risk of heritable disease from radiation exposure (ICRP, 2006). Taking into consideration substantial advances in the understanding of human genetic diseases and the process of germ line mutagenesis after radiation exposure, the ICRP substantially reduced the proportion of detriment ascribed to the potential heritable effects of radiation exposure. The ICRP currently estimates the genetic risks, up to the second generation, to be about 0.2% per Gy. The change in the ICRP estimates of the relative contribution to the total detriment from cancer and

TABLE 20-18   DETRIMENT-ADJUSTED NOMINAL RISK COEFFICIENTS FOR STOCHASTIC EFFECTS AT LOW DOSE RATE (UNIT, % Sv⁻¹)

	CANCER		HERITABLE		TOTAL	
EXPOSED	1990	2007	1990	2007	1990	2007
All	6.0	5.5	1.3	0.2	7.3	5.7
Adult	4.8	4.1	0.8	0.1	5.6	4.2

heritable effects is shown in Table 20-18. For the population at large, the contribution of heritable effects to the total detriment from radiation exposure has been reduced from 23% in 1990 to 3.5% in 2006. This has of course also been reflected in a similar reduction to the tissues weighting factor for the gonads from 0.2 to 0.08.

Typical diagnostic and occupational radiation exposures, although increasing the dose to the gonads of those exposed, would not be expected to result in any significant genetic risk to their progeny. Although delaying conception after therapeutic doses of radiation to reduce the probability of transmission of genetic damage to offspring is effective, it is not a commonly recommended practice for the relatively low gonadal doses from most diagnostic imaging procedures.

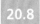 ## Radiation Effects *In Utero*

Developing organisms are highly dynamic systems that are characterized by rapid cell proliferation, migration, and differentiation. Thus, the developing embryo is extremely sensitive to ionizing radiation, as would be expected based on Bergonie and Tribondeau's early characterization of cellular radiosensitivity. The response after exposure to ionizing radiation depends on a number of factors including (1) total dose, (2) dose rate, (3) radiation quality, and (4) the stage of development at the time of exposure. Together, these factors determine the likelihood of potential consequences (if any) of *in utero* radiation exposure, including such effects as prenatal or neonatal death, congenital abnormalities, growth impairment, reduced intelligence, genetic aberrations, and an increase in future risk of cancer.

Radiation Effects and Gestation

The gestational period can be divided into three stages: a relatively short *preimplantation* stage, followed by an extended period of *major organogenesis,* and finally the *fetal growth* stage, during which differentiation is complete and growth occurs. Each of these stages is characterized by different responses to radiation exposure, owing principally to the relative radiosensitivities of the tissues at the time of exposure.

Preimplantation

The preimplantation stage begins with the union of the sperm and egg and continues through day 9 in humans, when the zygote becomes embedded in the uterine wall. During this period, the two pronuclei fuse, cleave, and form the morula and blastula.

The conceptus is very sensitive during the preimplantation stage and susceptibility to the lethal effects of irradiation is a concern. However, for doses less than 100 mGy, the risks are very low. Embryos exhibit the so-called *all-or-nothing response*, to radiation exposure at this stage of development, in which, if the exposure is not lethal, the damaged cells are repaired or replaced to the extent that there is unlikely to be any additional radiation-induced risk of congenital abnormalities beyond that which would occur for other reasons. Several factors, including repair capability, lack of cellular differentiation, and the relatively hypoxic state of the embryo, are thought to contribute to its resistance to radiation-induced abnormalities. During the first few divisions, the cells are undifferentiated and lack predetermination for a particular organ system. If radiation exposure were to kill some cells at this stage, the remaining cells could continue the embryonic development without gross malformations because they are indeterminate. However, any misrepaired chromosomal damage at this point may be expressed at some later time. When cells become specialized and are no longer indeterminate, loss of even a few cells may lead to anomalies, growth retardation, or prenatal death. The most sensitive times of exposure in humans are at 12 hours after conception, when the two pronuclei fuse to the one-cell stage, and again at 30 and 60 hours when the first two divisions occur. Chromosomal aberrations from radiation exposure at the one-cell stage could result in loss of a chromosome in subsequent cell divisions that would then be uniform throughout the embryo. Most chromosomal loss at this early stage is lethal. Loss of a sex chromosome in female embryos may result in Turner syndrome, although there is no evidence that this has occurred following radiation exposure.

A woman may not know she is pregnant during the preimplantation period, the time at which the conceptus is at greatest risk of lethal effects. Animal experiments have demonstrated an increase in the spontaneous abortion (prenatal death) rate after doses as low as 50 to 100 mGy delivered during the preimplantation period. After implantation, doses in excess of 250 mGy are required to induce prenatal death. The risk of spontaneous abortion following a dose of 10 mGy to the conceptus is approximately 1%, compared to the naturally occurring rate, which is reported to be between 30% and 50%. The LD_{50} for stages from the zygote to expanded blastocysts is in the range of 1 Gy (ICRP, 2003a).

Organogenesis

Embryonic malformations occur more frequently during the period of major organogenesis (second to eighth week after conception). The initial differentiation of cells to form certain organ systems typically occurs on a specific gestational day. For example, neuroblasts (stem cells of the CNS) appear on the 18th gestational day, the forebrain and eyes begin to form on day 20, and primitive germ cells are evident on day 21. Each organ system is not at equal risk during the entire period of major organogenesis. In general, the greatest probability of a malformation in a specific organ system (the so-called *critical period*) exists when the radiation exposure is received during the period of peak differentiation of that system. This may not always be the case however, because damage can occur to adjacent tissue, which has a negative effect on a developing organ system. Some anomalies may have more than one critical period. For example, cataract formation has been shown to have three critical periods in mice.

The only organ system (in humans or laboratory rodents) that has shown an association between malformations and low-LET radiation doses less than 250 mGy is the CNS. Embryos exposed early in organogenesis exhibit the greatest intrauterine growth retardation, presumably because of cell depletion. *In utero* exposure to doses greater than 100–200 mGy of mixed neutron and gamma radiation from the Hiroshima atomic bomb resulted in a significant increase in the occurrence of microcephaly.

In general, radiation-induced teratogenic effects are less common in humans than in animals. This is primarily because, in humans, a smaller fraction of the gestational

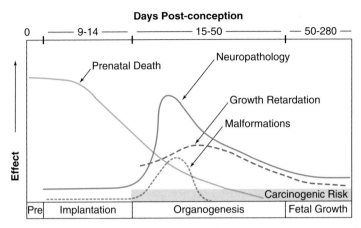

Days Post-conception

■ **FIGURE 20-35** Relative sensitivity for radiation-induced effects during different stages of fetal development. (Adapted from Mettler FA, Upton AC. *Medical effects of ionizing radiation.* 3rd ed. Philadelphia, PA: Saunders, Co., 2008.)

period is taken up by organogenesis (about $\frac{1}{15}$ of the total, compared with $\frac{1}{3}$ for mice). Nevertheless, development of the CNS in humans takes place over a much longer gestational interval than in experimental animals, and therefore the CNS is more likely to be a target for radiation-induced damage. An important distinguishing characteristic of teratogenic effects in humans are the concomitant effects on the CNS and/or fetal growth. All cases of human *in utero* irradiation that have resulted in gross malformations have been accompanied by CNS abnormalities or growth retardation or both. The response of each organ to the induction of radiation-induced malformations is unique. Such factors as gestational age; radiation quantity, quality, and dose rate; oxygen tension; the cell type undergoing differentiation and its relationship to surrounding tissues; and other factors influence the outcome.

Fetal Growth Stage

The fetal growth stage in humans begins after the end of major organogenesis (day 50) and continues until term. During this period the occurrence of radiation-induced prenatal death and congenital anomalies is, for the most part, negligible, unless the exposures are exceptional high and in the therapeutic range. Anomalies of the nervous system and sense organs are the primary radiation-induced abnormalities observed during this period, which coincides with their relative growth and development. Much of the damage induced at the fetal growth stage may not be manifested until later in life as behavioral alterations or reduced intelligence (e.g., IQ). Figure 20-35 summarizes the relative sensitivity for radiation-induced *in utero* effects during different gestational periods.

Epidemiologic Investigations of Radiation Effects *In Utero*

Teratogenic Effects

Two groups that have been studied for teratogenic effects of *in utero* irradiation are the children of the A-bomb survivors and children whose mothers received medical irradiation (diagnostic and/or therapeutic) during pregnancy. The predominant effects that were observed included microcephaly and mental and growth retardation. Eye, genital, and skeletal abnormalities occurred less frequently. Excluding the mentally retarded, individuals exposed *in utero* at Hiroshima and Nagasaki between the 8th and 25th week after conception demonstrated poorer IQ scores and school performance than did unexposed children. No such effect was seen in those exposed before the 8th week or after the 25th week. The decrease in IQ was dose dependent (~25 points/Gy), with an apparent threshold at approximately 100 mGy below which, if there was any effect, it was considered negligible. The greatest sensitivity for radiation-induced mental retardation is seen between the 8th and 15th weeks, during which the risk for severe mental retardation (SMR) to the fetus is approximately 44% per Gy with a threshold for SMR of approximately 200 to 300 mGy (ICRP, 2003a).

Microcephaly was observed in children exposed *in utero* at the time of the atomic bomb detonations. For those exposed before the 16th week, the incidence of microcephaly was proportional to the dose, from about 100–200 mGy up to 1.5 Gy, above which the decreased occurrence was presumably due to the increase in fetal mortality. The occurrence of microcephaly increased when exposures occurred during the first or second trimester and decreased dramatically for exposure in the third trimester. For exposure prior to 16 weeks, the occurrence of microcephaly for a fetal dose in the range of 100 to 190 mGy was approximately 11% and increased to approximately 40% for doses of approximately 1 Gy. Due to differences in the periods of rapid proliferation and radiosensitivity of the glial and neuronal cells, microcephaly can appear without SMR between 0 and 7 weeks whereas they appear together at 8 to 15 weeks and SMR can occur without microcephaly at 16 to 25 weeks.

Similar effects have been reported after *in utero* exposure during medical irradiation of the mother. Twenty of twenty-eight children irradiated *in utero* as a result of pelvic radium or x-ray therapy were mentally retarded, among which sixteen were also microcephalic (Goldstein, 1929). Other deformities, including abnormal appendages, hydrocephaly, spina bifida, blindness, cataracts, and microphthalmia have been observed in humans exposed *in utero* to high (radiotherapy) doses.

Although each exposure should evaluated individually, the prevailing scientific opinion is that there are thresholds for most congenital abnormalities. Doses lower than 100 mGy to perhaps 200 mGy are generally thought to carry negligible risk compared with the reported occurrence of congenital anomalies (4% to 6%) in liveborn children. **Recommendation of therapeutic abortion for fetal doses less than 100 mGy, regardless of the gestational age, would not usually be justified.** At one time, radiation was widely used to induce therapeutic abortion in cases where surgery was deemed inadvisable. The standard treatment was 3.5 to 5 Gy given over 2 days, which typically resulted in fetal death within 1 month. However, in diagnostic imaging, even several abdominal/pelvic CT scans or dozens of chest CT scans would not expose the fetus to doses in excess of 100 mGy. In fact, in most instances, fetal irradiation from diagnostic procedures rarely exceeds 50 mGy (see Appendix E-8), which has not been shown to place the fetus at any significant increased risk for congenital malformation or growth retardation.

Carcinogenic Effects

According to the U.S. National Cancer Institute, a newborn male and female have 0.25% and 0.22% probability of developing cancer by age 15, respectively (i.e., 1 in 400 males and 1 in 450 in females, respectively) (NIH, 2009). The majority of these cancers are leukemia and CNS neoplasms. A correlation between childhood leukemia and solid tumors and *in utero* diagnostic radiation was reported by Stewart in 1956 in a retrospective study of childhood cancer in Great Britain (often referred to as the "Oxford Survey of Childhood Cancers" [OSCC]; Stewart, 1956).

This observation was supported by similar case-control studies reporting a RR of approximately 1.4 for childhood cancer based on interviewing mothers of children with and without cancer (UNSCEAR, 1996; Doll and Wakeford, 1997; Wakeford and Little, 2003). However, no childhood leukemias and only one childhood cancer were observed among survivors of the atomic bombs who were irradiated *in utero*. Absence of a positive finding in the A-bomb survivors could have been predicted on a statistical basis, owing to the relatively small sample size, but the much higher fetal dose compared with diagnostic radiography points to an inconsistency in the studies (1 childhood cancer observed versus 8.8 predicted based on fetal dose). These positive studies have been criticized based on a variety of factors, including the influence of the preexisting medical conditions for which the examinations were required; the lack of individual dosimetry and the possibility of recall bias in that mothers with children who died of cancer may have had more reliable memories of their prenatal exposures than mothers who did not have such a traumatic experience.

A small increase of approximately 40% in the risk of childhood cancer is associated with acute exposure to diagnostic radiation *in utero* at doses in the range of 10 mGy, based on results from case-control studies of subjects born between late 1940s and early 1980s (Doll and Wakeford, 1997). If these estimates are correct, they represent a notable exception to the previously mentioned limit on the general sensitivity of radioepidemiological studies to detect cancer from acute exposures less than approximately 100-mGy. This may reflect the combined effect of a low background incidence of, and an increased fetal radiosensitivity to, childhood cancer.

Doll and Wakeford reviewed the scientific evidence and concluded that irradiation of the fetus *in utero* (particularly in the last trimester) does increase the risk of childhood cancer; that the increase in risk is produced by doses on the order of 10 mGy, and that the excess risk is approximately 6% per Gy. However, the reported association with prenatal x-ray and childhood cancer is not uniformly accepted as causal (ICRP, 2003a). The argument against causality is that the Oxford survey reported the same risk (odds ratio) for each childhood malignancy, including leukemia, lymphoma, CNS, Wilms tumor, or neuroblastoma. Such a commonality of risks has never been reported in any radiation study, even among atomic bomb survivors exposed in childhood. The biological implausibility of the case-control studies is indicated by the high risks seen for Wilms tumor and neuroblastoma, which are embryonic malignancies and not likely to be induced following pelvimetry examinations occurring shortly before birth. High dose exposures among children and newborns have not been correlated with increases in Wilms tumor or neuroblastoma. In addition, no cohort study has reported an increase in childhood leukemia following prenatal x-rays, even a large series of over 30,000 exposed mothers followed in the United Kingdom. This finding is further supported by animal studies that also failed to demonstrate an increased risk of leukemia following *in utero* exposures. Summarizing their view of the increased RR reported in the OSCC, the ICRP stated, "Although the arguments fall short of being definitive because of the combination of biological and statistical uncertainties involved, they raise a serious question of whether the great consistency in elevated RRs, including embryonal tumors and lymphomas, may be due to biases in the OSCC study rather than a causal association." (ICRP, 2003a) Thus the cancer risk associated with *in utero* exposure and the often cited risk estimate of 6% per Gy for childhood cancer remain controversial.

This controversy notwithstanding, it is instructive to place the possibly increased risk of childhood cancer from medical x-rays into perspective by evaluating the magnitude of the potential risk from common diagnostic imaging procedures. Recall that the baseline risk of a male developing a malignancy through age 15 years is 1/400. If a two view chest x-ray delivered 2 μGy to the conceptus, (and employing the conservative assumption of a causal association between exposure and increased cancer risk at low dose of 6% per Gy) the probability of developing cancer during childhood from the exposure would be less than 1 in 8.3 million! Even a chest CT, which might deliver a dose to the conceptus that is on the order of 100 times greater than a chest x-ray (i.e., 200 μGy) still results in a small additional statistical risk of approximately 1/83,000 (0.0012%) of developing a childhood cancer. Using the 6%/Gy risk coefficient suggested by Doll, the doubling dose for childhood malignancies induced by radiation *in utero* would be on the order of 35 to 40 mGy. However, current estimates of the risk coefficient, based on further study of atomic bomb survivors, are on the order of 0.6%/Gy and may be lower than the risk following exposures in early childhood (Preston 2008).

The lifetime risk of cancer is also believed to be elevated following radiation exposure *in utero*. ICRP considers the risk to be of the same order of magnitude as the estimated increased risk from radiation exposure during childhood compared to exposures as adults. The Commission's 2006 report states that it *"considers that it is prudent to assume that life-time cancer risk following* in utero *exposure will be similar to that following irradiation in early childhood, i.e., at most, about three times that of the population as a whole,* ICRP, 2006. However, the most recent data from the *in utero* exposed atomic bomb survivors indicates an increased risk of cancer later in life, it is much lower than the incidence seen for survivors exposed under the age of 6 years, (Preston 2008). While there is little doubt about the relative increase in cancer risk (compared with adult populations) from childhood exposures of some organs and tissues early in life (e.g., breast, thyroid) the magnitude of the increase and the applicability of these data for all radiogenic cancers (and for *in utero* exposures) remains open to debate. A summary of fetal effects from low-level radiation exposure is shown in Table 20-19.

U.S. regulatory agencies limit occupational radiation exposure of the fetus to no more that 5 mSv during the gestational period, provided that the dose rate does not substantially exceed 0.5 mSv in any 1 month. If twice the maximally allowed dose were received, the statistical probability of developing cancer during childhood from the exposure would be approximately 1 in 1,600. Table 20-20 presents a comparison of the risks of radiation exposure with other risks encountered during pregnancy. It is clear from these data that, although unnecessary radiation exposure should be minimized, its risk at levels associated with occupational and diagnostic exposures is nominal when compared with other potential risk factors.

Risks from *In Utero* Exposure to Radionuclides

Radiopharmaceuticals may be administered to pregnant women if the diagnostic information to be obtained outweighs the risks associated with the radiation dose. The principal risk in this regard is the dose to the fetus. Radiopharmaceuticals can be divided into two broad categories: those that cross the placenta and those that remain on the maternal side of the circulation. Radiopharmaceuticals that do not cross the placenta irradiate the fetus by the emission of penetrating radiation (mainly gamma rays and x-rays). Early in the pregnancy, when the embryo is small and the radiopharmaceutical distribution is fairly uniform, the dose to the fetus can be approximated by the dose to the ovaries. Estimates of early-pregnancy fetal doses from commonly used radiopharmaceuticals are listed in Appendix F-4A. Radiopharmaceuticals that cross the placenta may be distributed in the body of the fetus or be concentrated locally if the fetal target organ is mature enough. A classic (and important) example of such a radiopharmaceutical is radioiodine.

Radioiodine rapidly crosses the placenta, and the fetal thyroid begins to concentrate radioiodine around the 11th to 12th week post conception. The ability of

TABLE 20-19   FETAL EFFECTS FROM LOW-LEVEL RADIATION EXPOSURE

EFFECT	MOST SENSITIVE PERIOD AFTER CONCEPTION WEEKS (DAYS)	THRESHOLD DOSE AT WHICH AN EFFECT WAS OBSERVED (mGy) ANIMAL STUDIES	HUMAN STUDIES	ABSOLUTE INCIDENCE[a]	COMMENTS
Prenatal death	0–1 (0–8)		ND	ND	If the conceptus survives, it is thought to develop fully, with no radiation damage.
Preimplantation		50–100			
Postimplantation		250			
Growth retardation	1–8 (8–56)	10	200	ND	A-bomb survivors who received >200 mGy were 2–3 cm shorter and 3 kg lighter than controls and had, on average, head circumferences 1 cm smaller.
Organ malformation[b]	2–8 (14–56)	250	250	ND	Coincides with period of peak organ system development
Microcephaly (MC)	2–15 (14–105)	100	ND	5%–10%	MC can appear without severe SMR between 0–7 wks (see text)
Severe Mental Retardation (SMR)	8–15 (56–105)	ND	200–300	4%	At 8–15 wk 95% CI (2.2%–5.7%) No increase in absolute incidence was observed for exposure in the first 7 weeks or after the 25th wk.
	16–25 (112–175)	ND	600–900	0.9%	At 16–25 wk 95% CI (0%–1.8%)
Reduction of IQ	8–15 (56–105)	ND	100	2.5 IQ pts	Effects from a dose of 100 mGy or less were statistically unrecognizable. At 8–15 wk 2.5 pts 95% CI (1.8–3.3) At 16–25 wk 2.1 pts 95% CI (1.2–3.1)
Childhood cancer	2–term (14–term)	No threshold observed	No threshold observed	0.06–0.6[c]	Leukemia is the most common type of childhood cancer. Magnitude of the risk is controversial.

Note: IQ, intelligence quotient; ND, no data or inadequate data; CI, confidence interval; wk, weeks; d, days.

[a]Absolute incidence is defined as the percentage of exposed fetuses in which an effect is expected to be observed with an equivalent dose of 100 mGy.

[b]Organ malformation is defined as malformation of an organ outside the CNS. Data regarding the most sensitive period after conception are from animal studies.

[c]The baseline risk of childhood cancer up to age 15 for unexposed fetuses is approximately 0.25% (1 in 400).

Source: Adapted and modified from McCollough, 2007; ICRP, 2003a.

TABLE 20-20   EFFECT OF RISK FACTORS ON PREGNANCY-OUTCOME

EFFECT	APPROXIMATE NUMBER OCCURRING FROM NATURAL CAUSES	RISK FACTOR	ESTIMATED EXCESS OCCURRENCES FROM RISK FACTORS
Radiation Risks			
Childhood Cancer			
Cancer incidence in children (0–15)	~3/1,000	Radiation dose of 10 mGy received before birth	0.06/1,000 to 0.6/1,000
Abnormalities		Radiation dose of 10 mGy received during specific periods after conception:	
Small head size	40/1,000	4–7 wk	5/1,000
Small head size	40/1,000	8–11 wk	9/1,000
Mental retardation	4/1,000	8–15 wk	BT
Nonradiation Risks			
Occupation			
Stillbirth or spontaneous abortion	200/1,000	Work in high-risk occupations	90/1,000
Alcohol Consumption			
Fetal alcohol syndrome	1–2/1,000[a]	2–4 drinks/d	100/1,000
Fetal alcohol syndrome	1–2/1,000[a]	More than 4 drinks/d	200/1,000
Fetal alcohol syndrome	1–2/1,000[a]	Chronic alcoholic (>10 drinks/d)	350/1,000
Perinatal infant death	23/1,000	Chronic alcoholic (>10 drinks/d)	170/1,000
Smoking			
Perinatal infant death	23/1,000	<1 pack/d	5/1,000
Perinatal infant death	23/1,000	≥ 1 pack/d	10/1,000

[a]There is a naturally occurring syndrome that has the same symptoms as a fetal alcohol syndrome that occurs in children born to mothers who have not consumed alcohol.
BT, Below threshold for established effects.
Source: Apdapted from U.S. Nuclear Regulatory Commission. *Instruction concerning prenatal radiation exposure.* Regulatory Guide 8.13, Rev. 2.

the fetal thyroid to concentrate iodine remains relatively low until the 22nd week, after which it increases progressively and eventually exceeds that of the mother. The biologic effect on the fetal thyroid is activity dependent and can result in hypothyroidism or ablation if the dose administered to the mother is high enough. For I-131, estimates of dose to the fetal thyroid range from 230 to a maximum of 580 mGy/MBq (851 to 2,146 rad/mCi) for gestational ages between 3 and 5 months. Total body fetal dose ranges from 0.072 mGy/MBq (0.266 rad/mCi) early in pregnancy to a maximum of 0.27 mGy/MBq (1 rad/mCi) near term. Table 20-21 presents the fetal thyroid dose from various radioiodines and Tc-99m.

TABLE 20-21   ABSORBED DOSE mGy/MBq (rad/mCi) IN FETAL THYROID FROM RADIONUCLIDES GIVEN ORALLY TO MOTHER

FETAL AGE (mo)	IODINE-123	IODINE-125	IODINE-131	TECHNETIUM-99ᵐ
3	2.7 (10)	290 (1,073)	230 (851)	0.032 (0.12)
4	2.6 (10)	240 (888)	260 (962)	
5	6.4 (24)	280 (1,036)	580 (2,146)	
6	6.4 (24)	210 (777)	550 (2,035)	0.15 (0.54)
7	4.1 (15)	160 (592)	390 (1,443)	
8	4.0 (15)	150 (555)	350 (1,295)	
9	2.9 (11)	120 (444)	270 (1,000)	0.38 (1.40)

Source: Watson EE. Radiation absorbed dose to the human fetal thyroid. In: Watson EE, Schlaske-Stelson A, eds. *5th International Radiopharmaceutical Dosimetry Symposium.* Oak Ridge, TN. May 7–10, 1991. Oak Ridge, TN: Oak Ridge Associated Universities, 1992.

Summary

Radiation exposure of the embryo at the preimplantation stage usually leads to an all-or-nothing phenomenon (i.e., either fetal death and resorption or normal fetal risk). During the period of organogenesis, the risk of fetal death decreases substantially, whereas the risk of congenital malformation coincides with the peak developmental periods of various organ systems. Exposures in excess of 1 Gy are associated with a high incidence of CNS abnormalities. During the fetal growth stage *in utero*, exposure poses little risk of congenital malformations; however, growth retardation, abnormalities of the nervous system, and the risk of childhood cancer can be increased depending on fetal dose. Growth retardation after *in utero* fetal doses in excess of 200 mGy has been demonstrated. Fetal doses from most diagnostic x-ray and nuclear medicine examinations are typically much lower than 50 mGy (see Appendices E-8 and F-4A) and have not been demonstrated to produce any significant impact on fetal growth and development. A number of epidemiologic studies have evaluated the association between *in utero* radiation exposure and childhood neoplasms. Although these studies show conflicting results and remain open to varying interpretations, a reasonable estimate of the excess risk of childhood cancer from *in utero* irradiation is approximately 0.6% to 6% per Gy. Figure 20-35 and Table 20-19 summarize the relative incidence of radiation-induced health effects at various stages in fetal development.

While there has been a justifiable concern, both in public opinion and among health care providers regarding the potential for overutilization of x-rays in medical imaging, the concern regarding radiation exposure during pregnancy is often disproportionate to the actual risks involved. In one study evaluating perceptions of teratogenic risk with the use of medical x-rays, approximately 6% of primary care physicians and gynecologists suggested that therapeutic abortion would be appropriate for women having undergone an abdominal CT scan (Ratnapalan, 2004). Pregnant patients have also been shown to greatly overestimate the radiation-related risk to the fetus (Cohen-Kerem, 2006). The risk of *in utero* radiation exposure can be placed in perspective by considering the probability of birthing a healthy child after a given dose the conceptus (Table 20-22).

Clearly, even a conceptus dose of 100 mGy does not significantly affect the risks associated with pregnancy. Fetal doses from diagnostic examinations rarely, if ever, justify therapeutic abortion; however, some patients may receive one or more high-dose interventional exams or radiation therapy where the fetal doses

TABLE 20-22   PROBABILITY OF BIRTHING HEALTHY CHILDREN

DOSE TO CONCEPTUS mGy[a]	CHILD WITH NO MENTAL RETARDATION (%)	CHILD WITH NO BIRTH DEFECT (%)	CHILD WILL NOT DEVELOP CANCER (%)[b,c]	CHILD WILL NOT DEVELOP CANCER OR HAVE MENTAL RETARDATION OR BIRTH DEFECT (%)[c]
0	99.6	96	99.77	95.40
1.0	99.6	96	99.76	95.39
2.5	99.6	96	99.75	95.38
5	99.6	96	99.74	95.37
10	99.6	96	99.71	95.34
100	99.6	96	99.17	94.82

[a]Refers to equivalent dose above natural background. Dose assumed to be delivered during the most sensitive period of gestation (mental retardation: 8–15 weeks post conception; malformation: 2–7 weeks post conception).
[b]Assumes conservative risk estimates, and it is possible that there is no added radiation-induced cancer risk. Childhood (0–15 years) cancer risk from fetal irradiation of 6%/Gy Source: Doll R, Wakeford R. Risk of childhood cancer from fetal irradiation Br J Radiol 1997;70:130–139; Wakeford R, Little MP. Risk coefficients for childhood cancer after intrauterine irradiation: a review. Int J Radiat Biol 2003;79:293–309; and ICRP 84 (2000) Pregnancy and Medical Radiation Vol 30, No 1.
[c]Precision displayed is only for the purpose of showing the magnitude of the potential change in risk as a function of dose and should not be interpreted as a measure of precision with which these outcomes can be predicted.
Source: Adapted and modified from Wagner LK, Hayman LA. Pregnancy in women radiologists. Radiology 1982;145:559–562 and ICRP Publication 84 (ICRP, 2000).

are significant. Each case should be evaluated individually and the risks should be explained to the patient. Many professional organizations including the NCRP, ICRP, the American College of Radiology (ACR) and the American College of Obstetricians and Gynecologists (ACOG) have issued policy statements regarding the use of therapeutic abortion and the relatively low risk of diagnostic imaging procedures resulting in radiation exposure of the fetus. The ACR policy states "The interruption of pregnancy is rarely justified because of radiation risk to the embryo or fetus from a radiologic examination." (ACR, 2005). The ACOG policy, which was revised in 2004, states "Women should be counseled that x-ray exposure from a single diagnostic procedure does not result in harmful fetal effects. Specifically, exposure to less than 5 rad [50 mGy] has not been associated with an increase in fetal anomalies or pregnancy loss." (ACOG, 2004).

Every effort should be made to optimize radiation exposure of the patient and to reduce or avoid fetal exposure whenever possible. However, considering the relatively small risk associated with diagnostic examinations, postponing clinically necessary examinations or scheduling examinations around the patient's menstrual cycle to avoid irradiating a potential conceptus are unwarranted measures. Nevertheless, every fertile female patient should be asked whether she might be pregnant before diagnostic examinations or therapeutic procedures using ionizing radiation are performed. If the patient is pregnant and alternative diagnostic or therapeutic procedures are inappropriate, the risks and benefits of the procedure should be discussed with the patient.

SUGGESTED READINGS

Alliance for Radiation Safety in Pediatric Imaging. Image Gently. http://www.pedrad.org/associations/5364/ig/. Accessed August 1, 2011.

Amundson S, et al. Low-dose radiation risk assessment. Report of an International Workshop on Low Dose Radiation Effects held at Columbia University Medical Center, New York, April 3–4, 2006. Radiat Res 2006;166:561–565.

Boice JD Jr., Miller RW. Childhood and adult cancer after intrauterine exposure to ionizing radiation. *Teratology* 1999;59(4):227–233.

Boice JD Jr. Ionizing radiation. In: Schottenfeld D, Fraumeni JF Jr, eds. *Cancer epidemiology and prevention.* 3rd ed. New York: Oxford University Press, 2006.

Boice JD Jr. Lauriston S. Taylor lecture: Radiation epidemiology: the golden age and future challenges. *Health Phys* 2011;100:59–76.

Brenner DJ, Doll R, Goodhead DT, et al. Cancer risks attributable to low doses of ionizing radiation: assessing what we really know. *Proc Natl Acad Sci USA* 2003;100:13761–13766.

Brent RL. Saving lives and changing family histories: appropriate counseling of pregnant women and men and women of reproductive age, concerning the risk of diagnostic radiation exposures during and before pregnancy. *Am J Obstetr Gynecol* 2009;200(1):4–24.

Dauer LT, Brooks AL, Hoel DG, et al. Review and evaluation of updated research on the health effects associated with low-dose ionising radiation. *Radiat Prot Dosimetry* 2010;140(2):103–136.

Douple EB, Mabuchi K, Cullings HM, Preston DL, Kodama K, Shimizu Y, Fujiwara S, Shore RE. Long-term radiation-related health effects in a unique human population: lessons learned from the atomic bomb survivors of Hiroshima and Nagasaki. *Disaster Med Public Health Prep* 2011;5(Suppl 1):S122–S133.

Fry RJM, Boice JD Jr. Radiation carcinogenesis. In: Souhami RL, Tannock I, Hohenberger P, Horiot JC, eds. *Oxford textbook of oncology.* 2nd ed. New York: Oxford Press, 2002:167–184.

Hall EJ, Giaccia AJ. *Radiobiology for the radiologist.* 7th ed. Philadelphia, PA: Lippincott Williams and Wilkins, 2012.

Hall EJ, Metting N, Puskin J, et al. Low dose radiation epidemiology: what can it tell us? *Radiat Res* 2009;172:134–138.

International Agency for Research on Cancer. *IARC monographs on the evaluation of carcinogenic risks to humans. Vol 75. Ionizing Radiation, Part 1: X- and Gamma (γ) – Radiation, and Neutrons.* Lyon, France: IARC, 2000.

ICRP Report 90. Biological Effects after Prenatal Irradiation (Embryo and Fetus). *Ann ICRP* 2003;33(1–2).

IAEA: Radiation Protection of Patients https://rpop.iaea.org/RPOP/RPoP/Content/index.htm

Joiner M, van der Kogel A. *Basic clinical radiobiology.* 4th ed. London: Hodder Arnold, 2009.

Mettler FA, Upton AC. *Medical effects of ionizing radiation.* 3rd ed. Philadelphia, PA: W.B. Saunders Co., 2008.

National Research Council, Committee on the Biological Effects of Ionizing Radiations, Health Effects of Exposure to Low Levels of Ionizing Radiation (BEIR VII). Washington, DC: National Academy Press, 2006.

Wagner LK, et al. *Radiation bioeffects and management test and syllabus.* American College of Radiology Professional Self-Evaluation and Continuing Education Program, Number 32. Reston, VA: American College of Radiology, 1991.

Wagner LK, Lester RG, Saldana LR. *Exposure of the pregnant patient to diagnostic radiations: a guide to medical management.* 2nd ed. Madison, WI: Medical Physics Publishing, 1997.

West CM, Martin CJ, Sutton DG, et al. 21st L H Gray Conference: the radiobiology/radiation protection interface. *Br J Radiol* 2009;82(977):353–362.

REFERENCES

ACOG (2004) ACOG Committee on Obstetric Practice. Guidelines for diagnostic imaging during pregnancy. ACOG Committee opinion no. 299, September 2004 (replaces no. 158, September 1995). *Obstet Gynecol* 2004;104:647–651.

Ainsbury EA, et al. Radiation cataractogenesis: A review of recent studies. *Radiat Res.* 2009; 172:1–9.

American College of Radiology. *ACoR 04–05 bylaws.* Reston, VA: American College of Radiology, 2005.

American Cancer Society. *Cancer facts and figures 2011.* Atlanta, GA: American Cancer Society, 2011.

Angel E, Yaghmai N, Jude CM, et al. Monte Carlo simulations to assess the effects of tube current modulation on breast dose for multidetector CT. *Phys Med Biol* 2009a;54:497–512.

Angel E, Yaghmai N, Jude CM, et al. Monte Carlo simulations to assess the effects of tube current modulation on breast dose for multidetector CT. *Phys Med Biol* 2009b54(3):497–512; doi: 10.1088/0031-9155/54/3/003.

Balter S, Hopewell JW, Miller DL, et al. Fluoroscopically guided interventional procedures: a review of radiation effects on patients' skin and hair. *Radiology* 2010;254(2):326–341.

BEIR. *Health risks from exposure to low levels of ionizing radiation: BEIR VII, Phase Committee to Assess Health Risks from Exposure to Low Levels of Ionizing Radiation,* Board of Radiation Effects, Research Division on Earth and Life Studies, National Research Council of the National Academies. National Academy of Sciences, Washington, DC: National Academies Press, 2006.

Boice JD Jr, Hendry JH, Nakamura N, et al. Low-dose-rate epidemiology of high background radiation areas. *Radiat Res* 2010;173:849−854.

Bernstein JL, Thomas DC, Shore RE, et al. Radiation-induced second primary breast cancer and BRCA1 and BRCA2 mutation carrier status: A report from the WECARE Study. [JNCI In press?]

Brenner D, Elliston C, Hall E, et al. Estimated risks of radiation-induced fatal cancer from pediatric CT. *AJR Am J Roentgenol* 2001;176(2):289−296.

Brenner DJ, Hall EJ. Computed tomography—an increasing source of radiation exposure. *N Engl J Med* 2007;357:2277−2284.

Brenner DJ, Ward JF. Constraints on energy deposition and target size of multiply-damaged sites associated with DNA double-strand breaks. *Int J Radiat Biol* 1992;61:737.

Brody AS, Frush DP, Huda W, et al.; American Academy of Pediatrics Section on Radiology. Radiation risk to children from computed tomography. *Pediatrics* 2007;120(3):677−682.

Chambers C, Fetterly K, Holzer R, et al. Radiation safety program for the cardiac catheterization laboratory. *Catheter Cardiovasc Interv.* 2011;77:546–556

Clifton DK, Bremner WJ. The effect of testicular x-irradiation on 6872 spermatogenesis in man. A comparison with the mouse. *J Androl* 1983;4:387–392.

Cohen-Kerem R, Nulman I, Abramow- Newerly M, et al. Diagnostic radiation in pregnancy: Perception versus true risks. *J Obstet Gynaecol Can* 2006;28:43−48.

Correa CN, Wu X-C, Andrews P, et al., eds. *Cancer incidence in five continents*, vol VIII Lyon, France: IARC Scientific Publications No. 155, 2002.

Court Brown WM, Doll R, Hill RB. Incidence of leukaemia after exposure to diagnostic radiation in utero. *Br Med J* 1960;2(5212):1539–1545.

Dekaban AS. Abnormalities in children exposed to x-irradiation during various stages of gestation: tentative time table of radiation injury to human fetus. *J Nucl Med.* 1968;9:471−477.

De Santis M, Di Gianantonio E, Straface G, et al. Ionizing radiations in pregnancy and teratogenesis. A review of literature. *Reprod Toxicol* 2005;20:323−329.

Doll R, Wakeford E. Risk of childhood cancer from fetal irradiation. *Br J Radiol* 1997;70:130−139.

EPA. U.S. Environmental Protection Agency. EPA Radiogenic Cancer Risk Models and Projections for the U.S. Population, EPA 402-R-11-001, April 2011. *Fed Reg* 2011;76(104).

Fazel R, Krumholz HM, Wang Y, et al. Exposure to low-dose ionizing radiation from medical imaging procedures. *N Engl J Med* 2009;361(9):849−857.

FDA (1995). U.S. Food and Drug Administration. Radiation-Induced Skin Injuries from Fluoroscopy, http://www.fda.gov/Radiation-EmittingProducts/ RadiationEmittingProductsandProcedures/MedicalImaging/MedicalX-Rays/ucm116682.htm (accessed July 11, 2011) (U.S. Food and Drug Administration, Rockville, Maryland).

Frieben H. Demonstration eines Cancroid des rechten Handruckens, das sich nach langdauernder Einwirkung von Rontgenstrahlen entwickelt hatte. *Fortschr Rontgenstr* 1902;6:106−111.

Gabriel C. Risk of cataract after exposure to low doses of ionizing radiation: A 20-year prospective cohort study among US radiologic technologists. *Am J Epidemiol.* 2008;168(6): 620−631.

Goldstein L, Murphy DP. Etiology of ill-health in children born after postconceptional maternal irradiation. *Am J Roentgenol* 1929;22:322–331.

Goodhead DT. Initial events in the cellular effects of ionizing radiations: Clustered damage in DNA. *Int J Radiat Biol* 1994;65:7−17.

Goodhead DT. Spatial and temporal distribution of energy. *Health Phys* 1988;55:231−240.

Graham SJ, et al. Whole-body pathologic analysis of a patient with thorotrast-in-induced myelodysplasia. *Health Phys* 1992;63(1):20−26.

Granel F, Barbaud A, Gillet-Terver MN,et al. Chronic radiodermatitis after interventional cardiac catheterization: Four cases [in French]. *Ann Dermatol Venereol.* 1998;125:405−407.

Hall EJ, Giaccia AJ. *Radiobiology for the radiologist.* 7th ed. Philadelphia, PA: Lippincott Williams and Wilkins, 2012.

Henry FA, et al. Fluoroscopy-induced chronic radiation dermatitis: A report of three cases. *Dermatol Online J.* 2009;15(1):1–6.

Hollowell JG Jr, Littlefield LG. Chromosome damage induced by plasma of x-rayed patients: an indirect effect of x ray. *Proc Soc Exp Biol Med* 1968;129:240−244

Howlader N, Noone AM, Krapcho M, et al., eds. SEER Cancer Statistics Review, 1975–2008, Bethesda, MD:National Cancer Institute. http://seer.cancer.gov/csr/1975_2008/, based on November 2010 SEER data submission, posted to the SEER web site, 2011.

International Commission on Radiological Protection. *1990 recommendations of the international commission on radiological protection.* ICRP Publication 60. Elsevier, New York: Ann ICRP 21(1−3), 1991.

International Commission on Radiological Protection. *Genetic susceptibility to cancer.* ICRP publications 79. Tarrytown, NY:Ann. ICRP Permagon Press, 1999.

International Commission on Radiological Protection. *Pregnancy and medical radiation*. ICRP Publication 84. Elsevier, New York: Ann. ICRP 30(1), 2000.

International Commission on Radiological Protection. *Biological effects after prenatal irradiation (embryo and fetus)*. ICRP Publication 90. *Ann ICRP* 2003a;33(1/2).

International Commission on Radiological Protection. Relative Biological Effectiveness (RBE), Quality Factor (Q), and Radiation Weighting Factor (w_R). ICRP Publication 92. *Ann ICRP* 2003b;33(4).

International Commission on Radiological Protection. Low-dose extrapolation of radiation-related cancer risk. ICRP Publication 99. *Ann ICRP* 2006;35:1−140.

International Commission on Radiological Protection. *The 2007 Recommendations of the International Commission on Radiological Protection*. ICRP Publication 103. *Ann ICRP* 2007a;37:1−332.

International Commission on Radiological Protection. *Radiological Protection in Medicine*, ICRP Publication 105. *Ann ICRP* 2007b;37(6).

International Commission on Radiological Protection. ICRP reference 4825-3093-1464. Statement on Tissue Reactions Approved by the Commission on April 21, 2011. 2011a.

International Commission on Radiological Protection. *Early and late effects of radiation in normal 16 tissues and organs: threshold doses for tissue reactions and other non-cancer effects of radiation in a radiation protection context* ICRP Draft Report For Consultation: reference 4844-6029-7736, January 20, 2011. 2011b.

Johnson KJ, Alexander BH, Doody MM, et al. Childhood cancer in the offspring born in 1921−1984 to US radiologic technologists. *Br J Cancer* 2008;99:545–550.

Kuppermann N, Holmes JF, Dayan PS; et al, Pediatric Emergency Care Applied Research Network (PECARN). Identification of children at very low risk of clinically-important brain injuries after head trauma: a prospective cohort study. *Lancet* 2009;374(9696):1160−1170.

Little JB. Genomic instability and bystander effects: a historical perspective. *Oncogene* 2003;22: 6978−6987.

Löbrich M, Cooper PK, Rydberg B. Non-random distribution of DNA double-strand breaks induced by particle irradiation. *Int J Radiat Biol* 1996;70:493.

Lushbaugh CC, Ricks RC. Some cytokinetic and histopathologic considerations of irradiated male and female gonadal tissues. *Front Radiat Ther Oncol* 1972;6:228–248.

McCollough CH, Schueler BA, Atwell TD, et al. Radiation exposure and pregnancy: When should we be concerned? *Radiographics* 2007;27:909−917.

Mettler FA, Upton AC. *Medical effects of ionizing radiation*. 3rd ed. Philadelphia, PA: W.B. Saunders Co., 2008.

Muller HJ, Artificial transmutation of the gene. *Science* 1927;66:84–87

Nair RR, Rajan B, Akiba S, et al. Background radiation and cancer incidence in Kerala, India-Karanagappally cohort study. *Health Phys*. 2009;96:55−66.

National Cancer Institute;. PDQ® Cancer Information Summary. Genetics of Breast and Ovarian Cancer (PDQ®)—Health Professional. Bethesda, MD Date last modified 06/23/2011. Available at: http://www.cancer.gov/cancertopics/pdq/genetics/breast-and-ovarian/healthprofessional, 2011. Accessed 07/15/2011.

National Council on Radiation Protection and Measurements. *Limitation of exposure to ionizing radiation*. NCRP Report No. 116. National Council on Radiation Protection and Measurements, Bethesda, MD, 1993.

National Council on Radiation Protection and Measurements. *Radiation protection guidance for activities in low-earth orbit*. NCRP Report No. 132. Bethesda, MD: National Council on Radiation Protection and Measurements, 2000.

National Council on Radiation Protection and Measurements. *Extrapolation of radiation-induced cancer risks from nonhuman experimental systems to humans*. NCRP Report No. 150. Bethesda, MD: National Council on Radiation Protection and Measurements, 2005.

National Council on Radiation Protection and Measurements. *Risk to thyroid from ionizing radiation*. NCRP Report No. 159. Bethesda, MD: National Council on Radiation Protection and Measurements, 2008.

National Council on Radiation Protection and Measurements. *Radiation dose management for fluoroscopically-guided interventional procedures*. NCRP Report No. 168. Bethesda, MD: National Council on Radiation Protection, 2010.

NIH. Probability of Developing or Dying of Cancer Software, Version 6.4.1. Statistical Research and Applications Branch, National Cancer Institute, 2009. http://srab.cancer.gov/devcan.

NTP. Report on Carcinogens, Twelfth Edition. Research Triangle Park, NC: U.S. Department of Health and Human Services, Public Health Service, National Toxicology Program, 2011.

Preston DL, Cullings H, Suyama A, Funamoto S, Nishi N, Soda M, Mabuchi K, Kodama K, Kasagi F, Shore RE. Solid cancer incidence in atomic bomb survivors exposed in utero or as young children. *J Natl Cancer Inst* 2008;100(6):428–436.

Preston DL, Mattsson A, Holmberg E, Shore R, Hildreth NG, Boice JD Jr. Radiation effects on breast cancer risk: a pooled analysis of eight cohorts. *Radiat Res* 2002;158:220–235.

Preston DL, Pierce DA, Shimizu Y, et al. Effect of recent changes in atomic bomb survivor dosimetry on cancer mortality., risk estimates. *Radiat Res* 2004;162:377–389.

Preston DL, Shimizu Y, Pierce DA, et al. Studies of mortality of atomic bomb survivors. Report 13: Solid cancer and noncancer disease mortality: 1950–1997. *Radiat Res* 2003;160:381–407.

Preston DL, et al. Solid cancer incidence in atomic bomb survivors: 1958–1998. *Radiat Res* 2007;168:1.

Russell WL, Russell LB, Kelly EM. Radiation dose rate and mutation frequency. *Science* 1958;128:1546–1550.

Sasaki MS. Primary damage and fixation of chromosomal DNA as probed by monochromatic soft x-rays and low-energy neutrons. In: Fielden EM, O'Neil P, eds. *The Early Effects of Radiation on DNA*. Vol. H54. NATO ASI Series, Berlin: Springer-Verlag, 1991:369–384.

Sasaki MS, Kobayashi K, Hieda K, et al. Induction of chromosome aberrations in human lymphocytes by monochromatic x-rays of quantum energy between 4.8 and 14.6 keV. *Int J Radiat Biol* 1989;56:975–988.

Schull WJ, Neel JV. Atomic bomb exposure and the pregnancies of biologically related parents. A prospective study of the genetic effects of ionizing radiation in man. *Am J Public Health Nations Health* 1959;49(12):1621–1629.

Shadley JD, Afzal V, Wolff S. Characterization of the adaptive response to ionizing radiation induced by low doses of x rays to human lymphocytes. *Radiat Res* 1987;111:511–517.

Shope TB. Radiation-induced skin injuries from fluoroscopy. *RadioGraphics* 1996;16:1195–1199.

Shrieve, Loeffler. *Human radiation injury*. Philadelphia, PA: Wolters Kluwer Health/Lippincott Williams & Wilkins, 2011.

Signorello LB, Mulvihill JJ, Green DM, Munro HM, Stovall M, Weathers, RE, Mertens AC, Whitton JA, Robison LL, Boice JD Jr. Stillbirth and neonatal death in relation to radiation exposure before conception: a retrospective cohort study. *Lancet* 2010;376:624–630.

Stewart A, Webb J, Hewitt D. A survey of childhood malignancies. *Brit Med J* 1958;30:1495–1508.

Tawn EJ, Rees GS, Leith C, Winther JF, Curwen GB, Stovall M, Olsen JH, Rechnitzer C, Schroeder H, Guldberg P, Boice JD Jr. Germline minisatellite mutations in survivors of childhood and young adult cancer treated with radiation. *Int J Radiat Biol* 2011;87:330–340.

United Nations Scientific Committee on the Effects of Atomic Radiation (UNSCEAR). UNSCEAR 1996. Sources and Effects of Ionizing Radiation. 1996 Report to the General Assembly with Scientific Annex. New York: United Nations.

United Nations Scientific Committee on the Effects of Atomic Radiation (UNSCEAR). UNSCEAR 2006 Report to the General Assembly with Scientific Annexes, Effects of Ionizing Radiation. Vol 1: Report and Annexes A and B, 2008. Vol 2: Annexes C, D and E, 2009, 2011, New York: United Nations.

Upton AC, Odell TT Jr., Sniffen EP. Influence of age at time of irradiation on induction of leukemia and ovarian tumors in RF mice. *Proc Soc Exp Biol Med* 1960;104:769–772.

Wakeford R, Little MP. Risk coefficients for childhood cancer after intrauterine irradiation: a review. *Int J Radiat Biol* 2003;79:293–309.

Ward JF. DNA damage produced by ionizing radiation in mammalian cells: Identities, mechanisms of formation, and repairability. *Prog Nucleic Acid Res Mol Biol* 1988;35:95–125.

Ward JF. The complexity of DNA damage: Relevance to biological consequences. *Int J Radiat Biol* 1994;66:427–432.

Winther JF, Boice JD Jr, Fredericksen K, Bautz A, Mulvihill JJ, Stovall M, Olsen JH. Radiotherapy for childhood cancer and risk for congenital malformations in offspring: a population-based cohort study. *Clin Genet* 2009;75:50–56.

Young R, Kerr G. Report of the joint US-Japan working group. Reassessment of the atomic bomb radiation dosimetry for Hiroshima and Nagasaki: dosimetry system DS02. Radiation Effects Research Foundation, 2005.

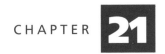

CHAPTER **21**

Radiation Protection

It is incumbent upon all individuals who use radiation in medicine to strive for an optimal compromise between its clinical utility and the radiation doses to patients, staff, and the public. Federal and state governments and even some large municipalities have agencies that promulgate regulations regarding the safe use of radiation and radioactive material. Another goal of radiation protection programs is to ensure compliance with these regulations. To a large degree, the success of radiation protection programs depends on the development of procedures for the safe use of radiation and radioactive material and on the education of staff about radiation safety principles, the risks associated with radiation exposure and contamination, and the procedures for safe use. This chapter discusses the application of radiation protection principles (also known as health physics) in diagnostic x-ray and nuclear imaging, image-guided interventional procedures, and therapy with unsealed radioactive material.

21.1 Sources of Exposure to Ionizing Radiation

According to the National Council on Radiation Protection and Measurements (NCRP) Report No. 160, the average annual per capita effective dose, exclusive of doses to patients from external beam radiation therapy, from exposure to ionizing radiation in the United States in 2006 was approximately 6.2 millisievert (mSv). Approximately half of this, about 3.1 mSv, was from naturally occurring sources, whereas about 48%, 3.0 mSv, was from medical exposure of patients. Only about 2%, 0.14 mSv, was from other sources, such as consumer products and activities and occupational exposure. These averages apply to the entire population of the United States. Doses to individuals from these sources vary considerably with a variety of factors discussed below.

Ubiquitous Background Exposure

Naturally occurring sources of radiation include (1) cosmic rays, (2) cosmogenic radionuclides, and (3) primordial radionuclides and their radioactive decay products. Cosmic radiation includes both the primary extraterrestrial radiation that strikes the Earth's atmosphere and the secondary radiations produced by the interaction of primary cosmic rays with the atmosphere. Primary cosmic rays predominantly consist of extremely penetrating high-energy (mean energy ~10 GeV) particulate radiation, approximately 80% of which is high-energy protons. Almost all primary cosmic radiation collides with our atmosphere before reaching the ground, producing showers of secondary particulate radiations (e.g., electrons and muons) and electromagnetic radiation. The average per capita effective dose from cosmic radiation is approximately 0.33 mSv per year or approximately 11% of natural background radiation. However, the range of individual exposures is considerable. The majority of the population of the United States is exposed to cosmic radiation near sea level where the outdoor effective dose rate is approximately 0.3 mSv per year. However, smaller populations receive much more than this amount (e.g., Colorado Springs, Colorado, at 1,840 m, ~0.82 mSv per year). Exposures increase with altitude, approximately doubling every 1,500 m, as there is less atmosphere to attenuate the cosmic radiation. Cosmic radiation is also greater at the Earth's magnetic poles than at the equator, as charged particles encountered by the Earth's magnetic field are forced to travel along the field lines to either the North or South Pole. Structures provide some protection from cosmic radiation; the indoor effective dose rate is approximately 20% lower than outdoors.

Some of the secondary cosmic ray particles collide with stable atmospheric nuclei producing "cosmogenic" radionuclides (e.g., $^{14}_{7}N[n,p]^{14}_{6}C$). Although many cosmogenic radionuclides are produced, they contribute very little (~0.01 mSv per year or less than 1%) to natural background radiation. The majority of the effective dose caused by cosmogenic radionuclides is from carbon 14.

The radioactive materials that have been present on the Earth since its formation are called *primordial radionuclides*. Primordial radionuclides with physical half-lives comparable to the age of the Earth (~4.5 billion years) and their radioactive decay products are the largest sources of terrestrial radiation exposure. The population radiation dose from primordial radionuclides is the result of external radiation exposure, inhalation, and incorporation of radionuclides in the body. Primordial radionuclides with half-lives less than 10^8 years have decayed to undetectable levels since their formation, whereas those with half-lives greater than 10^{10} years do not significantly contribute to background radiation levels because of their long physical half-lives (i.e., slow rates of decay). Most radionuclides with atomic numbers greater than lead decay to stable isotopes of lead through a series of radionuclide decays called *decay chains*. The radionuclides in these decay chains have half-lives ranging from seconds to many thousands of years. Other primordial radionuclides, such as potassium 40 (K-40, T½ = 1.28 × 10^9 years), decay directly to stable nuclides. The decay chains of uranium 238 (U-238), T½ = 4.51 × 10^9 years (uranium series), and thorium 232 (Th-232), T½ = 1.41 × 10^{10} years (thorium series), produce several dozen radionuclides that together with K-40 are responsible for most of the external terrestrial average effective dose of 0.21 mSv per year or approximately 7% of natural background. Individuals may receive much higher or lower exposures than the average, depending on the local concentrations of terrestrial radionuclides. The range in the United States is approximately 0.1 to 0.4 mSv per year. There are a few regions of the world where terrestrial radionuclides are highly concentrated. For example, as discussed in Chapter 20, monazite sand deposits, containing high concentrations of radionuclides from the Th-232 decay series, are found along certain beaches in India. The external radiation levels on these black sands range up to 70 mGy per year (Nair et al., 2009), which is more than 300 times the average level from terrestrial sources in the United States.

The short-lived alpha particle-emitting decay products of radon 222 (Rn-222) are believed to be the most significant source of exposure from the inhalation of naturally occurring radionuclides. Radon-222, a noble gas, is produced in the U-238 decay chain by the decay of radium 226 (Ra-226). Rn-222 decays by alpha emission, with a half-life of 3.8 days, to polonium 218 (Po-218), followed by several other alpha and beta decays, eventually leading to stable lead-206 (Pb-206). When the short-lived daughters of radon are inhaled, most of the dose is deposited in the tracheobronchial region of the lung. Radon concentrations in the environment vary widely. There are both seasonal and diurnal variations in radon concentrations. Radon gas emanates primarily from the soil in proportion to the quantity of natural uranium deposits; its dispersion can be restricted by structures, producing much higher indoor air concentrations than found outdoors in the same area. Radon gas dissolved in domestic water supplies can be released into the air within a home during water usage, particularly when the water is from a well or another ground water source. Weatherproofing of homes and offices and other energy conservation measures typically decrease outside air ventilation, resulting in higher indoor radon concentrations.

The radiation from exposure to Rn-222 and its daughters in the United States results in an average effective dose of approximately 2.1 mSv per year or approximately 68% of natural background. The dose from inhalation of radon decay products is primarily to the bronchial epithelium. In order to convert the absorbed dose from the alpha particles to effective dose, a tissue weighting factor (w_T) of 0.08 is applied along with a radiation weighting factor (w_R) of 20 to account for increased risk from exposure to high LET radiation.

The average indoor air concentration of Rn-222 in homes in the United States is approximately 46 Bq/m^3 (1.24 pCi/L); however, levels can exceed 2.75 kBq/m^3 (75 pCi/L) in poorly ventilated structures with high concentrations of U-238 in the soil. Outdoor air concentrations are approximately three times lower, 15 Bq/m^3 (0.41 pCi/L). The U.S. Environmental Protection Agency recommends taking action to reduce radon levels in homes exceeding 147 Bq/m^3 (4 pCi/L), whereas other countries have somewhat different limits (e.g., the United Kingdom and Canada have higher action levels, 200 Bq/m^3 [5.4 pCi/L]). Although Rn-222 accounts for about two thirds of the natural radiation effective dose, it can be easily measured and exposures can be reduced when necessary.

The third largest source of natural background radiation is from ingestion of food and water containing primordial radionuclides (and their decay products), of which K-40 is the most significant. K-40 is a naturally occurring isotope of potassium (~0.01%). Skeletal muscle has the highest concentration of potassium in the body. K-40 produces an average effective dose of approximately 0.15 mSv per year, or approximately 5% of natural background. Th-232 and U-238 and their decay products are found in food and water and result in an average annual effective dose of approximately 0.13 mSv.

Long-lived radionuclides released to or created in the environment from the atmospheric testing of nuclear weapons (450 detonations between 1945 and 1980) consist mainly of carbon 14, tritium (H-3), cesium 134 and 137 (Cs-134, Cs-137), strontium 90, plutonium, and transplutonium elements. A large fraction of these radionuclides have since decayed and/or have become progressively less available for biologic uptake. Today, the dose from this radioactive material is minimal and results in an average annual effective dose less than 10 µSv (NCRP, 1987).

Medical Exposure of Patients

The single greatest controllable source of radiation exposure in the US population is from medical imaging. The majority of the exposure is from x-ray imaging (primarily from diagnostic radiology), with a smaller contribution from nuclear medicine. Doses from individual medical imaging procedures are summarized in Appendices E and F. In 2006, the medical use of radiation, not including radiation therapy, produced an average annual effective dose to the population of the United States of approximately 3 mSv, which is about 97% of the total from artificial radiation sources and nearly half of the average annual effective dose from all sources (NCRP, 2009). There have been significant changes in medical imaging technology and its uses since 1980, when the estimated average annual effective dose equivalent from the medical exposure of patients was about 0.53 mSv (NCRP, 1987). The two largest factors that increased the average effective dose from 1980 until 2006 are the increased utilization of computed tomography (CT) and nuclear medicine imaging procedures

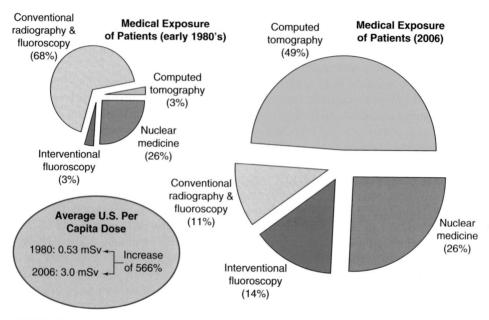

■ **FIGURE 21-1** Average annual per capita effective doses in the United States from medical imaging procedures, showing the large increase from 1980 to 2006. (NCRP, 1987; NCRP, 2009.)

(Fig. 21-1). While CT and nuclear medicine procedures collectively account for only approximately 22% of all medical imaging procedures using ionizing radiation, they deliver approximately 75% of the collective effective dose. The CT and nuclear medicine procedures that contribute the most to this dose are CT of the abdomen and of the pelvis and Tc-99m and Tl-201 myocardial perfusion imaging, which together account for more than half of the effective dose to the population from medical imaging. Conversely, conventional radiographic and noninterventional fluoroscopic imaging procedures, which account for approximately 74% of the imaging procedures, result in only 11% of the collective effective dose (Table 21-1). Data from the State of Michigan from 2002 to 2006 indicate that there has been an increase in the entrance skin exposure of 67% for a PA chest projection and 28% for an AP lumbar spine projection for digital imaging when compared with screen-film imaging

TABLE 21-1   RADIATION EXPOSURE TO US POPULATION IN 2006—MEDICAL EXPOSURES (EXCLUDING RADIATION THERAPY)

	NUMBER OF PROCEDURES (MILLIONS)	%	COLLECTIVE EFFECTIVE DOSE (person Sv)	%	EFFECTIVE DOSE (mSv)
Computed Tomography	67	(17)	440,000	(49)	1.5
	22%		75%		
Nuclear Medicine	18	(5)	231,000	(26)	0.8
Interventional Fluoroscopy	17	4	128,000		0.4
Conventional Radiography and Fluoroscopy	293	(74)	99,000	(11)	0.3
TOTALS	**395**	**100**	**898,000**	**100**	**~3**

Data from NCRP (2009).

(NCRP, 2009). Studies have shown that the per-image doses to patients when photo-stimulable phosphor (computed radiography [CR]) image receptors are used are on the order of twice the doses when modern 400-speed rare-earth screen-film image receptors are used (Compagnone et al., 2006; Seibert et al., 1996) and it is likely that this is the cause of the increase. However, digital radiography equipment with much more detection efficient thin-film-transistor flat-panel arrays is now replacing many CR systems, and this equipment can produce images with lower patient doses than CR or even state of the art film-screen systems (Compagnone et al., 2006; Williams et al., 2007). If this technology is used effectively, the per procedure and population doses from radiography may decline significantly.

Consumer Products and Activities

This category includes a variety of sources, most of which are consumer products. The largest contribution in this category is from tobacco products. Two alpha-emitting radionuclides Pb-210 and Po-210 (which occur naturally from the decay of Ra-226) have been measured in both tobacco leaves and cigarette smoke. It has been estimated that a one-pack-a-day smoker increases his or her annual effective dose by approximately 0.36 mSv. The NCRP estimates the average annual effective dose to an exposed individual is 0.3 mSv and, based on a smoking population of 45 million in the United States, this results in an average annual effective dose to the entire population of 0.045 mSv, which is about 35% of the effective dose from all consumer products and activities.

Many building materials contain radioisotopes of uranium, thorium, radium, and potassium. These primordial radionuclides and their decay products are found in higher concentration in such materials as brick, concrete, and granite, and thus structures built from these materials will cause higher exposures than structures constructed primarily from wood. The average annual per capita effective dose is estimated to be approximately 0.035 mSv from this source.

Air travel can substantially add to an individual's cosmic ray exposure. For example, a 5-h transcontinental flight in a commercial jet aircraft will result in an equivalent dose of approximately 0.025 mSv. The average annual per capita effective dose to passengers from commercial air travel is estimated to be approximately 0.034 mSv.

There are many other less important sources of enhanced natural radiation exposure, such as mining and agricultural activities (primarily from fertilizers containing members of the uranium and thorium decay series and K-40); combustible fuels, including coal and natural gas (radon); and consumer products, including smoke alarms (americium-241), gas lantern mantles (thorium), and dental prostheses, certain ceramics, and optical lenses (uranium). These sources contribute less than 12% of the average annual effective dose from consumer products and activities.

Occupational and Other Sources of Exposure

Occupational exposures are received by some people employed in medicine, including veterinary medicine; by aircraft crew in commercial aviation; by workers in some industrial and commercial activities; by workers in the commercial nuclear power industry; by workers in some educational and research institutions; and by some individuals in the military, some in governmental agencies, and some in U.S. Department of Energy facilities. Since most individuals are not occupationally exposed to radiation and the majority of those who are exposed typically receive fairly low annual doses, the contribution to the average annual per capita effective dose to the population from occupational exposure is very low, 0.005 mSv (less than 0.1%). However, among those occupationally exposed to radiation, the average annual effective dose was 1.1 mSv.

In 2006, medical personnel, whose occupational exposures were monitored, received an average annual effective dose of approximately 0.75 mSv (NCRP, 2009). This average is somewhat lower than might be expected because the doses to many staff members are quite low (e.g., radiology supervisors and radiologists who perform few if any fluoroscopic procedures). For example, occupational doses to radiologists not routinely performing interventional procedures have been declining in recent years and an average annual effective dose of approximately 0.1 to 0.2 mSv is common (Linet et al., 2010). Similarly, full-time technologists working in large hospitals performing mostly CT and radiography examinations will typically have annual effective doses of approximately 0.5 to 1 mSv. However, medical staff involved in fluoroscopically guided interventional procedures will typically have much higher occupational exposures. The actual doses received by the staff will depend on a number of factors including their roles in the procedures (i.e., performing or assisting), the number of procedures performed, the type and difficulty (which determines the lengths) of the cases, as well as the availability and use of radiation protection devices and techniques. Annual doses recorded by the dosimeters worn at the collar (outside the lead apron) in the range of 5 to 15 mSv are typical for personnel routinely performing these procedures. In reality, these are only partial body exposures (i.e., to the head and extremities) because the use of radiation-attenuating aprons greatly reduces the exposure to most of the body. Adjusting their measured exposures to account for the shielding provided is discussed in the following section on dosimetry. After making adjustments to account for shielding, the effective dose is typically reduced by a factor of 3 or more compared to that recorded on the collar dosimeter.

For most routine nuclear medicine procedures, the effective doses to the technologists are typically less than 1 µSv per procedure, putting typical annual exposures in the range 2 to 3 mSv. However for positron emission tomography (PET) procedures, an effective dose of 1 to 5 µSv per procedure has been reported (Guillet, 2005). Nuclear medicine technologists whose routine workload also includes dose preparation and imaging of patients for PET may have annual effective doses in the range of 10 to 15 mSv.

Airline crew members are estimated to receive an additional average annual effective dose of approximately 3.1 mSv; some receive effective doses of more than twice this value. It is interesting to note that the average annual effective dose of airline crew exceeds the annual effective doses of many diagnostic radiology personnel.

The contribution to the annual effective dose of members of the public (those not working in the industry) from activities related to commercial nuclear power production is minimal, approximately 0.5 µSv. Population radiation exposure from nuclear power production occurs during all phases of the fuel cycle, including uranium mining and processing, uranium enrichment, manufacturing of uranium fuel, reactor operations, and radioactive waste disposal.

Summary

The average annual effective dose to the US population from all radiation sources is obtained by dividing the annual collective effective dose by the size of the US population. The result in 2006 was approximately 6.2 mSv per year or approximately 17 µSv per day for all people in the United States from all sources, exclusive of radiation therapy. It is interesting to note that, although nuclear power, fallout from atomic weapons, and a variety of consumer products receive considerable attention in the popular media, they in fact cause only a small fraction of the average population exposure to radiation.

The average annual effective dose is somewhat misleading for categories such as the medical use of radiation, in that many people in the population are neither occupationally nor medically exposed, yet are included in the average. Figure 21-2

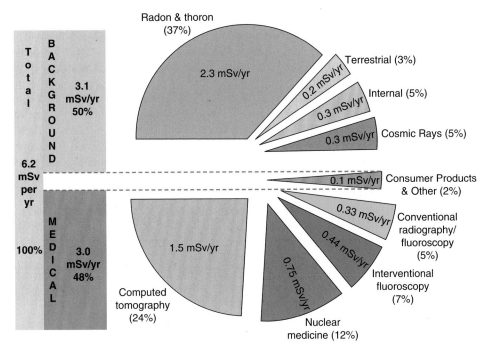

■ **FIGURE 21-2** Percent contributions of various sources of exposure to the annual collective effective dose (1,870,000 person-Sv) and the average annual effective dose per person in the US population (6.2 mSv) in 2006. Percentages have been rounded to the nearest 1%. (Adapted from NCRP 2006.)

presents a summary of the average annual effective dose for the US population from the radiation sources previously discussed.

21.2 Personnel Dosimetry

The radiation exposures of some people must be monitored for both safety and regulatory purposes. Such assessments may need to be made over periods of several minutes to several months. There are three main types of individual radiation recording devices called *personnel dosimeters* used in diagnostic radiology and nuclear medicine: (1) *film badges*, (2) *dosimeters using storage phosphors* (e.g., thermoluminescent dosimeters [TLDs]), and (3) *pocket dosimeters*, each with its own advantages and disadvantages.

Ideally, one would like to have a single personnel dosimeter capable of meeting all of the dosimetry needs in medical imaging. The ideal dosimeter would instantaneously respond, distinguish among different types of radiation, and accurately measure the dose equivalent from all forms of ionizing radiation with energies from several keV to MeV, independent of the angle of incidence. In addition, the dosimeter would be small, lightweight, rugged, easy to use, inexpensive, and unaffected by environmental conditions (e.g., temperature, humidity, pressure) and nonionizing radiation sources. Unfortunately, no such dosimeter exists; however, most of these characteristics can be satisfied to some degree by selecting the dosimeter best suited for a particular application.

Film Badges

A film badge consists of a small sealed packet of radiation sensitive film, similar to dental x-ray film, placed inside a special plastic holder that can be clipped to clothing. Radiation striking the emulsion causes a darkening of the developed film (see Chapter 7). The amount of darkening increases with the absorbed dose to the film emulsion and is measured with a densitometer. The film emulsion contains grains of silver bromide, resulting in a higher effective atomic number than tissue; therefore, the dose to the film is not equal to the dose to tissue. However, with the selective use of several metal filters over the film (typically lead, copper, and aluminum), the relative optical densities of the film underneath the metal filters can be used to identify the approximate energy range of the radiation and to calculate the dose to soft tissue. Film badges typically have an area where the film is not covered by a metal filter or plastic and thus is directly exposed to the radiation. This "open window" is used to detect medium and high-energy beta radiation that would otherwise be attenuated (Fig. 21-3).

Most film badges can record doses from about 100 µSv to 15 Sv (10 mrem to 1,500 rem) for photons and from 500 µSv to 10 Sv (50 mrem to 1,000 rem) for beta radiation. The film in the badge is usually replaced monthly and sent to the commercial supplier for processing. The developed film is usually kept by the vendor, providing a permanent record of radiation exposure.

Film badges are small, lightweight, inexpensive, and easy to use. However, exposure to excessive moisture or temperature can damage the film emulsion, making dose estimates difficult or impossible.

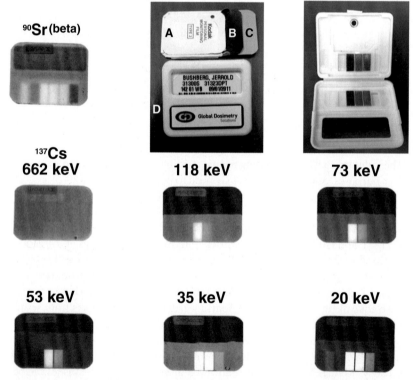

■ **FIGURE 21-3** A film pack (**A**) consists of a light opaque envelope (**B**) containing the film (**C**). The film pack is placed in the plastic film badge (**D**) sandwiched between two sets of Teflon (**E**), lead (**F**), copper (**G**), and aluminum (**H**) filters. Film badges typically have an area where the film pack is not covered by a filter or the plastic of the badge and thus is directly exposed to the radiation. This "open window" area (**I**) is used to detect medium and high-energy beta radiation that would otherwise be attenuated. The relative darkening of the developed film (filter pattern) provides a crude but useful assessment of the energy of the radiation. The diagram shows typical filter patterns from exposure to a high-energy beta emitter (Sr-90), a high-energy gamma emitter (Cs-137), and x-rays with effective energies from 20 to 118 keV. (Film badge and filter patterns courtesy of Global Dosimetry Solutions, Irvine, CA.)

Thermoluminescent and Optically Stimulated Luminescent Dosimeters

Some dosimeters contain storage phosphors in which a fraction of the electrons, raised to excited states by ionizing radiation, become trapped in excited states. When these trapped electrons are released, either by heating or by exposure to light, they fall to lower energy states with the emission of light. The amount of light emitted can be measured and indicates the radiation dose received by the phosphor material.

TLDs, discussed in Chapter 17, are excellent personnel and environmental dosimeters; however, they are somewhat more expensive than film badges. The most commonly used TLD material for personnel dosimetry is lithium fluoride (LiF). LiF TLDs have a wide dose response range of 100 μSv to 10 Sv and are reusable (Fig. 21-4). These dosimeters can be used over a long time interval (up to 6 months if necessary) before being returned to the vendor for analysis. The energy response is 0.766 to 5 MeV (E_{max}) for beta radiation and 20 keV to 6 MeV for x-ray and gamma-ray radiation.

Another advantage of LiF TLDs is that their effective atomic number is close to that of the tissue; therefore, the dose to the LiF chip is close to the tissue dose over a wide energy range. TLDs do not provide a permanent record, because heating the chip to read the exposure removes the deposited energy. TLDs are routinely used in nuclear medicine as extremity dosimeters; a finger ring containing a chip of LiF worn on the hand is expected to receive the highest exposure during radiopharmaceutical preparation and administration. Figure 21-5 shows a finger ring dosimeter and a LiF chip.

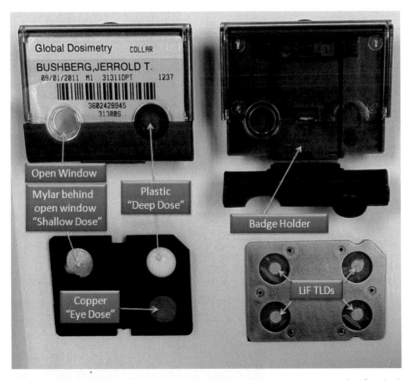

■ **FIGURE 21-4** TLD dosimeter with four LiF TLDs. The filters in this dosimeter are made of mylar (7 mg/cm²), copper (300 mg/cm²), and polypropylene plastic (1,000 mg/cm²), representing the specified depths for determination of dose to the skin ("shallow dose") at a depth of 0.007 cm, lens of the eye at a depth of 0.3 cm, and deep dose at a depth of 1.0 cm, respectively. (Technical specifications from Global Dosimetry Solutions Irvine, CA.)

Dosimeters using optically stimulated luminance (OSL) have recently become commercially available as an alternative to TLDs. The principle of OSL is similar to that of TLDs, except that the release of trapped electrons and light emission are stimulated by laser light instead of by heat. Crystalline aluminum oxide activated with carbon (Al_2O_3:C) is commonly used. Like LiF TLDs, these OSL dosimeters have a broad dose response range, and are capable of detecting doses as low as 10 µSv. As in film dosimeters, the Al_2O_3 has a higher effective atomic number than soft tissue and so an OSL dosimeter has filters over the sheet of OSL material that are used to estimate dose to soft tissue, as in film badges. However, OSL dosimeters have certain advantages over TLDs in that they can be reread several times and an image of the filter pattern can be produced to differentiate between static (i.e., instantaneous) and dynamic (i.e., normal) exposure. TLDs or OSL dosimeters are the dosimeters of choice when longer dose assessment intervals (e.g., quarterly) are required.

Direct Ion Storage Dosimeters

Direct ion storage dosimeters are a relatively new technology in which a nonvolatile analog memory cell, surrounded by a gas-filled ion chamber, is used to record radiation exposure (Fig. 21-6). The initial interactions of the x-ray and gamma-ray photons occur in the wall material, and secondary electrons ionize the gas of the chamber. The positive ions are collected on a central negative electrode resulting in a reduction in voltage that is proportional to the dose received by the dosimeter. The dose recorded by the dosimeter can be read at any time by connecting it to the USB port of any computer with Internet access. Analysis of the deep, shallow, and lens of the eye dose is accomplished by a computer algorithm that takes into consideration the typical photon energy spectrum experience of the user. The advantages of this technology include a broad dose and photon energy response range (0.01 mSv to 5 Sv and 5 keV to 6 MeV), unlimited real-time dose readings by the user without the need for a special reader, online management of dosimeter assignment and dosimetry reports, and elimination of the periodic distribution and collection of dosimeters as well as the delay and cost associated with returning the dosimeters for processing by the dosimetry vendor. Disadvantages include initial cost of the dosimeters, more costly replacement of lost dosimeters, and the need for users to upload dosimetry information periodically. In addition, the current version of this dosimeter cannot be used to measure exposure to beta radiation.

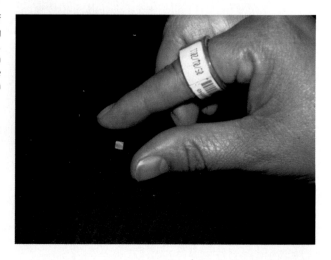

■ **FIGURE 21-5** A small chip of LiF (**right**) is sealed in a finger ring (underneath the identification label). In nuclear medicine, the ring is worn with the LiF chip on the palmar surface such that the chip would be facing a radiation source held in the hand.

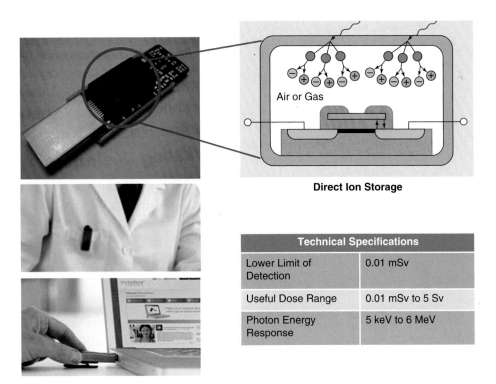

Direct Ion Storage

Technical Specifications	
Lower Limit of Detection	0.01 mSv
Useful Dose Range	0.01 mSv to 5 Sv
Photon Energy Response	5 keV to 6 MeV

■ **FIGURE 21-6** Direct ion storage dosimeter. (Photos courtesy of Mirion Technologies San Ramon, CA, www. mirion.com.)

Practical Aspects of Dosimeter Use

Nearly every medical facility obtains non–self-reading dosimeters, whether film badges, TLD dosimeters, and/or OSL dosimeters, from a commercial vendor monthly or quarterly. One or more control dosimeters are shipped with each batch. At the beginning of a wear period, typically at the beginning of a month, the new dosimeters are issued to staff and the used dosimeters from the previous wear period are collected. The used dosimeters are returned to the dosimeter vendor for reading. At least one control dosimeter from the same batch is included in the shipment. Control dosimeters are stored in an area away from radiation sources. The vendor subtracts the reading from the control dosimeter from the readings of the dosimeters that were used. An exposure report is received from the vendor in about 2 weeks. However, reporting of unusual exposures or exposures over regulatory limits is expedited. The dosimetry report lists the "shallow" dose, corresponding to the skin dose, the "eye" dose corresponding to the dose to the lens of the eye and the "deep" dose, corresponding to penetrating radiations. Most vendors post dosimetry results on password-secured Web sites.

Placement of Dosimeters on the Body

A dosimeter is typically worn on the part of the torso that is expected to receive the largest radiation exposure or is most sensitive to radiation damage. Most radiologists, x-ray technologists, and nuclear medicine technologists wear a dosimeter at waist or shirt-pocket level. During fluoroscopy, a dosimeter is typically placed at collar level in front of the lead apron to measure the dose to the thyroid and lens of the eye because most of the body is shielded from exposure. Alternatively, a dosimeter can be placed at the collar level in front of the radiation-protective apron, and a second dosimeter can be worn on the torso underneath the apron. A pregnant radiation worker typically wears an additional dosimeter at waist level (behind the lead apron, if worn) to assess the fetal dose.

Estimating Effective Dose and Effective Dose Equivalent for Staff Wearing Protective Aprons

When protective aprons, which shield the torso and upper legs, are worn during diagnostic and interventional x-ray imaging procedures, the effective dose and effective dose equivalent can be estimated by using methods that take the protection from the shielding into account. When a single dosimeter is worn at collar level outside the apron, the NCRP (NCRP, 1995) recommends that effective dose equivalent (H_E) be calculated from the dose recorded by the collar dosimeter (H_N) using Equation 21-1:

$$H_E = 0.18 \, H_N \qquad [21\text{-}1]$$

When a dosimeter is worn at collar level outside the protective apron and another dosimeter is worn underneath the apron at the waist or chest, the recommended method for calculating H_E is to use H_N and the dose (H_W) recorded by the dosimeter worn under the lead apron in Equation 21-2:

$$H_E = 1.5 \, H_W + 0.04 \, H_N \qquad [21\text{-}2]$$

Similar equations for estimating the effective dose can be found in NCRP Report No. 122 (NCRP, 1995).

Pocket Dosimeters

The major disadvantage to film, thermoluminescent, and OSL dosimeters is that the accumulated dose is not immediately displayed. Pocket dosimeters measure radiation exposure and can be read immediately. The analog version of the pocket dosimeter is the pocket ion chamber. It utilizes a quartz fiber suspended within an air-filled chamber on a wire frame, on which an electrical charge is placed. The fiber is bent away from the frame because of coulombic repulsion and is visible through an optical lens system upon which an exposure scale is superimposed. When radiation strikes the detector, ion pairs produced in the air partially neutralize the charge, thereby reducing coulombic repulsion and allowing the fiber to move closer to the wire frame. This movement is seen as an up-range excursion of the hairline fiber on the exposure scale (Fig. 21-7).

Pocket ion chambers can typically detect photons of energies greater than 20 keV. Pocket ion chambers commonly display the quantity exposure (defined in Chapter 3). Pocket ion chambers are available in a variety of ranges; the most commonly used models measure exposures from 0 to 200 mR or 0 to 5 R. These devices are small (the size of a pen) and easy to use; however, they may produce erroneous readings if bumped or dropped and, although reusable, do not provide a permanent record of exposure.

Digital pocket dosimeters can be used in place of pocket ion chambers. These dosimeters use solid-state electronics and either Geiger-Mueller (GM) tubes or radiation-sensitive semiconductor diodes to measure and display radiation dose in a range from approximately 10 μSv to 100 mSv. Figure 21-8 shows analog and digital pocket dosimeters.

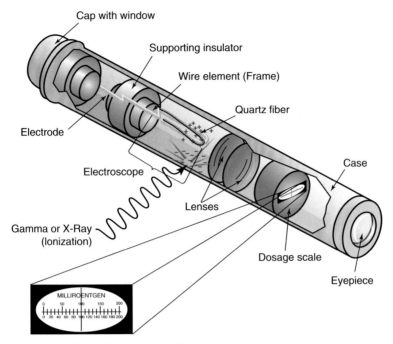

Cap with window

Supporting insulator

Wire element (Frame)

Quartz fiber

Electrode

Case

Electroscope

Lenses

Gamma or X-Ray
(Ionization)

Dosage scale

Eyepiece

MILLIROENTGEN

0   50   100   150   200

0 20 40 60 80 100 120 140 160 180 200

■ **FIGURE 21-7** Cross-sectional diagram of an analog pocket ion chamber.

Pocket dosimeters can be utilized when high doses are expected, such as during cardiac catheterization or manipulation of large quantities of radioactivity. Table 21-2 summarizes the characteristics of the various personnel monitoring devices discussed above.

Problems with Dosimetry

Common problems associated with dosimetry include dosimeters being left in radiation fields when not worn, contamination of a dosimeter itself with radioactive material, lost and damaged dosimeters, and people not wearing dosimeters when working with radiation sources. If a dosimeter is positioned so that the body is between it and the radiation source, attenuation will cause a significant underestimation of the true

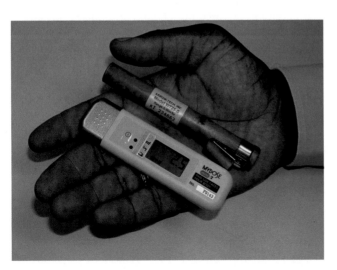

■ **FIGURE 21-8** Examples of analog and digital pocket dosimeters. Pocket ion chamber courtesy of Arrow-Tech, Inc. Rolla, ND, and electronic personnel dosimeter courtesy of Cone Instruments, Solon, OH.

TABLE 21-2 SUMMARY OF PERSONNEL MONITORING METHODS

METHOD	MEASURES	USEFUL RANGE (X-AND GAMMA RAY)		PERMANENT RECORD	USES AND COMMENTS
Film badge	Beta; gamma and x-ray	0.1–15,000 mSv[a] (beta) 0.5–10,000 mSv[a]		Yes	Routine personnel monitoring; most common in diagnostic radiology and nuclear medicine
TLD	Beta; gamma and x-ray	0.01–10^6 mSv[a]		No	Becoming more common but still more expensive than film; used for phantom and patient dosimetry
OSL	Beta; gamma and x-ray	0.01–10^6 mSv[a]		No[b]	Advantage over TLD includes the ability to reread the dosimeters and distinguish between dynamic and static exposures
Pocket dosimeter	Gamma and x-ray	Analog 0–0.2 R 0–0.5 R 0–5 R	Digital 0–100 mSv[a]	No	Special monitoring (e.g., cardiac cath); permits direct (i.e., real-time) reading of exposure

[a]Multiply mSv by 100 to obtain mrem.
[b]OSL dosimeters are typically retained and can be reread by the manufacturer for approximately 1 year.
OSL, optically stimulated luminance; TLD, thermoluminescent dosimeter.

exposure. Most personnel do not remain in constant geometry with respect to the radiation sources they use. Consequently, the dosimeter measurements are usually representative of the individual's average exposure. For example, if a dosimeter is worn properly and the radiation field is multidirectional or the wearer's orientation toward it is random, then the mean exposure over a period of time will tend to be a good approximation (±10% to 20%) of the individual's true exposure.

21.3 Radiation Detection Equipment in Radiation Safety

A variety of portable radiation detection instruments, the characteristics of which are optimized for specific applications, are used in radiology and nuclear medicine. The portable GM survey meter and portable ionization chamber survey meter satisfy most of the requirements for radiation protection measurements in nuclear medicine. X-ray machine evaluations require specialized ion chamber instruments capable of recording exposure, exposure rates, and exposure durations. All portable radiation detection instruments should be calibrated at least annually. A small radioactive check source can be used to verify an instrument's response to radiation.

Geiger-Mueller Survey Instruments

GM survey instruments are used to detect the presence and provide semiquantitative estimates of the intensities of radiation fields. Measurements from GM survey meters typically are in units of counts per minute (cpm) rather than mR/h, because the GM detector does not duplicate the conditions under which exposure is defined. In addition, the relationship between count rate and exposure rate with most GM probes is a complicated function of photon energy. If a GM survey meter is calibrated to indicate exposure rate (most commonly performed using a sealed source containing Cs-137 [662 keV gamma rays]), one should refer to the detector's energy response curve before making quantitative measurements of photons whose energies significantly differ from the energy for which it was calibrated. However, with specialized energy–compensated probes, GM survey instruments can provide approximate measurements of exposure rate (typically in mR/h) over a wide range of photon energies, although with reduced sensitivity. The theory of operation of GM survey instruments was presented in Chapter 17.

A common application of GM survey meters is to perform surveys for radioactive contamination in nuclear medicine. A survey meter coupled to a thin window (~1.5 to 2 mg/cm^2), large surface area GM probe (called a "pancake" probe) is ideally suited for contamination surveys (see Fig. 17-7). Thin window probes can detect alpha (greater than 3 MeV), beta (greater than 45 keV), and x- and gamma (greater than 6 keV) radiations.

These detectors are extremely sensitive to charged particulate radiations with sufficient energy to penetrate the window, but are less sensitive to x- and gamma radiations. These detectors will easily detect natural background radiation (on the order of ~50 to 100 cpm at sea level). These instruments have long dead times resulting in significant count losses at high count rates. For example, a typical dead time of 100 μs will result in, approximately, a 20% loss at 100,000 cpm. Some GM survey instruments will saturate in high-radiation fields and read zero, which, if unrecognized, could result in significant overexposures. Portable GM survey instruments are best suited for low-level contamination surveys and should not be used in high-radiation fields or when accurate measurements of exposure rate are required unless specialized energy–compensated probes or other techniques are used to account for these inherent limitations.

Portable Ionization Chamber Survey Meters

Portable ionization chamber survey meters are used when accurate measurements of radiation exposure rates are required (see Figure 17-6). These ionization chambers approximate the conditions under which the roentgen is defined (see Chapter 3). They have a wide variety of applications including assessment of radiation fields near brachytherapy or radionuclide therapy patients, and surveys of radioactive material packages. The principles of operation of ion chambers are discussed in Chapter 17.

The ion chambers of some survey meters are filled with ambient air, whereas others have sealed ion chambers. Some of those with sealed chambers are pressurized to increase the sensitivity. Ionization chamber measurements are influenced by photon energy and exposure rate and ambient air chambers are also affected by temperature and atmospheric pressure. However, these limitations are not very significant for conditions typically encountered in medical imaging. For example, a typical portable ion chamber survey meter will experience only approximately 5% loss for exposure rates approaching 10 R/h; specialized detectors can measure much higher exposure rates. Most portable ionization chamber survey meters respond slowly to rapidly changing radiation exposure rates. These instruments must be allowed to warm up and stabilize before accurate measurements can be obtained. Some are also affected by orientation and strong magnetic fields (e.g., from magnetic resonance imaging [MRI] scanners). Ionization chamber survey meters are typically capable of measuring exposure rates between 1 mR/h and 50 R/h for photons of energies greater than approximately 20 keV. Some ionization chambers have a cover over one end of the detector, which serves as a buildup cap to establish electronic equilibrium for accurate measurement of higher-energy x- and gamma rays; it can be removed to improve the accuracy when measuring low-energy x- and gamma rays. Removing the cap also permits assessment of the contribution of beta particles to the radiation field. The slow response time and limited sensitivity of these detectors preclude their use as low-level contamination survey instruments or to locate a lost low-activity radiation source.

21.4 Fundamental Principles and Methods of Exposure Control

Principles of Justification, Optimization, and Limitation

The International Commission on Radiological Protection (ICRP) has formulated a set of principles that apply to the practice of radiation protection (ICRP, 2007):

- The principle of justification: Any decision that alters the radiation exposure situation, for example, by introducing a new radiation source or by reducing existing exposure, should do more good than harm, that is, yield an individual or societal benefit that is higher than the detriment it causes.
- The principle of optimization of protection: Optimization of protection should ensure the selection of the best protection option under the prevailing circumstances, that is, maximizing the margin of good over harm. Thus, optimization involves keeping exposures as low as reasonably achievable (ALARA), taking into account economic and societal factors.
- The principle of limitation of maximum doses: In planned situations, the total dose to any individual from all the regulated sources should not exceed the appropriate regulatory limits.

The ICRP recommends that the last principle, limitation of maximal doses, not apply to medical exposure of patients or emergency situations. However, the other two principles do apply to medical exposure of patients and emergency situations.

Methods of Exposure Control

There are four principal methods by which radiation exposures to persons can be minimized: (1) reducing time of exposure, (2) increasing distance, (3) using shielding, and (4) controlling contamination by radioactive material. Although these methods are widely used in radiation protection programs, their application to medical imaging is addressed below.

Time

Although it is obvious that reducing the time spent near a radiation source will reduce one's radiation exposure, techniques to minimize time in a radiation field are not always recognized or practiced. First, not all sources of radiation produce constant exposure rates. Diagnostic x-ray machines typically produce high exposure rates during brief time intervals. For example, a typical chest x-ray produces an entrance skin exposure of approximately 20 mR in less than $^1/_{20}$ of a second, an exposure rate of 1,440 R/h. In this case, exposure is minimized by not activating the x-ray tube when staff are near the radiation source. Nuclear medicine procedures, however, typically produce lower exposure rates for extended periods of time. The time spent near a radiation source can be minimized by having a thorough understanding of the tasks to be performed and the appropriate equipment to complete them in a safe and timely manner. Similarly, radiation exposure to staff and patients can be reduced during fluoroscopy if the operator is proficient in the procedure to be performed.

Distance

The exposure rate from a source of radiation decreases with increasing distance from the source, even in the absence of an attenuating material. In the case of a point source of radiation (i.e., a source whose physical dimensions are much less than the distance from which it is being measured), the exposure rate decreases as the distance from the source is squared. This principle is called *the inverse square law* and is the result of the geometric relationship between the surface area (A) and the radius (r) of a sphere: $A = 4\pi r^2$. Thus, if one considers an isotropic point radiation source at the center of the sphere, the surface area over which the radiation is distributed increases as the square of the distance from the source (i.e., the radius). If the exposure rate from a point source is X_1 at distance d_1, at another distance d_2 the exposure rate X_2 will be

$$X_2 = X_1 \left(d_1 / d_2 \right)^2$$ [21-3]

For example, if the exposure rate at 20 cm from a source is 90 mR/h, doubling the distance will reduce the exposure by $(\tfrac{1}{2})^2 = \tfrac{1}{4}$ to 22.5 mR/h; increasing the distance to 60 cm decreases the exposure by $(\tfrac{1}{3})^2 = \tfrac{1}{9}$ to 10 mR/h (Fig. 21-9).

This relationship is only valid for point sources (i.e., sources whose dimensions are small with respect to the distances d_1 and d_2). Thus, this relationship would not be valid near (e.g., less than 1 m from) a patient injected with radioactive material. In this case, the exposure rate decreases less rapidly than $1/(\text{distance})^2$.

This rapid change in radiation intensity with distance is familiar to all who have held their hand over a heat source, such as a stove top or candle flame. There is only a fairly narrow range over which the infrared (thermal, nonionizing) radiation felt is comfortable. A little closer and the heat is intolerable; a little further away and the heat is barely perceptible. Infrared radiation, like all electromagnetic radiation, follows the inverse square law.

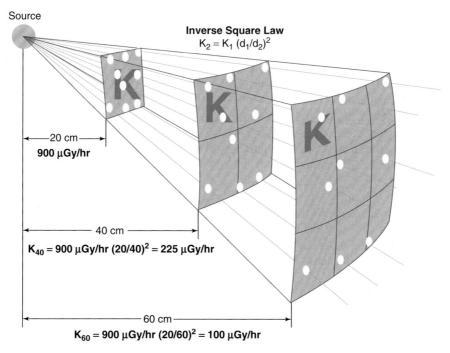

■ **FIGURE 21-9** The inverse square law, showing the decreasing air kerma rate with distance from a point source.

Scattered radiation from a patient, x-ray tabletop, or shield is also a source of personnel radiation exposure. For diagnostic energy x-rays, a good rule of thumb is that at 1 m from a patient at 90 degrees to the incident beam, the radiation intensity is approximately 0.1% to 0.15% (0.001 to 0.0015) of the intensity of the beam incident upon the patient for a 400 cm^2 x-ray field area on the patient (typical field area for fluoroscopy). All personnel should stand as far away from the patient as practicable during x-ray imaging procedures and behind a shielded barrier or out of the room, whenever possible. The NCRP recommends that personnel should stand at least 2 m from the x-ray tube and the patient during radiography with mobile equipment (NCRP, 1989).

Because it is often not practical to shield the technologist from the radiation emitted from the patient during a nuclear medicine exam (see "Shielding"), distance is the primary dose reduction technique. The majority of the nuclear medicine technologist's annual whole-body radiation dose is received during patient imaging. Imaging rooms should be designed to allow a large distance between the imaging table and the computer terminal where the technologist spends most of the time during image acquisition and processing.

Shielding

Shielding is used in diagnostic radiology and nuclear medicine to reduce exposures of patients, staff, and the public. The decision to utilize shielding, and its type, thickness, and location for a particular application, are functions of the photon energy, intensity and geometry of the radiation sources, exposure rate goals at various locations, and other factors. The principles of attenuation of x- and gamma rays are reviewed in Chapter 3.

Shielding may be installed in a wall, floor, or ceiling of a room; this is commonly done for rooms containing x-ray imaging machines, PET/CT machines, and sometimes rooms housing patients administered large activities. It may be in the walls of a cabinet used to store radioactive sources. It may be installed around a work area, such as the dose preparation area in a nuclear medicine radiopharmacy. It may be around individual sources, such as an x-ray tube or a vial or syringe of radioactive material in nuclear medicine. It is incorporated behind the image receptors of fluoroscopes and radiographic machines and in the gantries of CT devices. It may be worn as protective aprons by people performing fluoroscopy. It may also be in movable barriers, such as the freestanding and ceiling-mounted shields in fluoroscopic procedure rooms.

The x-rays from nearly all medical x-ray machines used for diagnostic and interventional imaging have photon energies that do not exceed 140 keV and the average energies are much less. The gamma rays emitted by the radionuclides used in nuclear medicine mostly have energies less than 365 keV, although some of these radionuclides emit higher-energy gamma rays of low abundance. The annihilation photons used in PET have energies of 511 keV. For photons of these energies, use of a high atomic number material for shielding, due to photoelectric absorption, requires less mass of shielding than a material of lower atomic number. The use of a material of high density permits a thinner shield. Thus, lead is commonly used for shielding, because of its very high atomic number, density, and reasonable cost. In general, placing shielding closer to a source of radiation does not reduce the thickness needed, but does reduce the mass of shielding necessary by reducing the area of the shielding.

21.5 Structural Shielding of Imaging Facilities

The purpose of radiation shielding of rooms containing x-ray machines is to limit radiation exposures of employees and members of the public to acceptable levels. Several factors must be considered when determining the amount and type of radiation shielding. Personnel exposures may not exceed limits established by regulatory agencies. Furthermore, personnel radiation exposures must be kept *ALARA*.

Methods and technical information for the design of shielding for diagnostic and interventional x-ray rooms are found in NCRP Report No. 147, *Structural Shielding Design for Medical X-ray Imaging Facilities* (NCRP, 2004). The recommended quantity for shielding design calculations is *air kerma* (K), with the unit of Gy; typical annual amounts of air kerma in occupied areas are commonly expressed in mGy. The recommended radiation protection quantity for the limitation of exposure of people to sources of ionizing radiation is *effective dose* (E), defined as the sum of the weighted equivalent doses to specific organs or tissues (the equivalent dose to each organ or tissue being multiplied by a corresponding tissue weighting factor, w_T), expressed in Sv (see Chapter 3 for definition); for protection purposes, typical levels of E are expressed in mSv.

Areas to be protected by shielding are designated as *controlled* and *uncontrolled areas*; a controlled area is an area to which access is controlled for the purpose of radiation protection and in which the occupational exposure of personnel to radiation is under the supervision of a person responsible for radiation protection. Controlled areas, such as procedure rooms and control booths, are usually in the immediate vicinity of the x-ray and nuclear medicine imaging devices. The workers in controlled areas are usually radiologic technologists, nurses, radiologists, and other physicians trained in the use of ionizing radiation and whose radiation exposures are typically individually monitored. Uncontrolled areas for radiation protection purposes are most other areas in the hospital or clinic, such as offices adjacent to x-ray rooms.

Shielding design goals, P, are amounts of air kerma delivered over a specified time at a stated reference point that are used in the design and evaluation of barriers constructed for the protection of employees and members of the general public from a medical x-ray or radionuclide imaging source or sources. Shielding design goals are stated in terms of K (mGy) at a reference point beyond a protective barrier (e.g., 0.3 m for a wall, a conservative assumption of the distance of closest approach). Because of conservative assumptions, achieving the design goals will ensure that the respective annual recommended values for E are not exceeded. The relationship between E and K is complex, and depends on several factors, including x-ray energy spectrum and the posture (e.g., standing or sitting) of the exposed individual. Because E cannot be directly measured, it is impractical to use it for a shielding design goal, and therefore, shielding design goals P are stated in terms of K.

There are different shielding design goals for controlled and uncontrolled areas. Radiation workers, typically employees, have significant potential for exposure to radiation in the course of their jobs, and as a result are subject to routine monitoring by personal dosimeters. On the other hand, many people in uncontrolled areas have not voluntarily chosen to be irradiated and may not be aware that they are being irradiated. NCRP Report No. 147 recommends that the shielding design goal P for controlled areas be 5 mGy per year, and that for uncontrolled areas be 1 mGy per year. These are equivalent to shielding design goals, P, of 0.1 mGy per week for controlled areas and 0.02 mGy per week for uncontrolled areas.

There are also air-kerma design goals for stored radiographic film and loaded film-screen cassettes to avoid film fogging. A shielding design goal, P, less than 0.1 mGy is recommended for the period in which radiographic film is stored. Since loaded screen-film cassettes and CR cassettes awaiting use are more sensitive to radiation, a P not to exceed 0.5 µGy for the period of storage (on the order of a few days) is recommended.

These shielding design methods are based upon conservative assumptions that will result in the actual air kerma transmitted through each barrier being much less than the applicable shielding design goal. These assumptions include (1) neglecting the attenuation of the primary x-ray beam by the patient (the patient typically attenuates the x-ray beam by a factor of 10 to 100); (2) assuming perpendicular incidence of the radiation on the barrier, which has the greatest transmission through the barrier; (3) ignoring the presence of other attenuating materials in the path of the radiation; (4) assuming a large x-ray beam field size for scattered radiation levels; and (5) assuming high occupancy factors for uncontrolled areas.

Shielding designed by these methods will keep the effective doses or effective dose equivalents received by workers in these areas much less than a tenth of the current occupational dose limits in the United States, will keep the dose to an embryo or fetus of a pregnant worker much less than 5 mGy over the duration of gestation, and will keep the effective doses to members of the public and employees, who are not considered radiation workers, less than 1 mSv per year.

Sources of Exposure

The sources of exposure that must be shielded in a diagnostic or interventional x-ray room are *primary radiation, scattered radiation,* and *leakage radiation* (Fig. 21-10).

Scatter and leakage radiation are together called *secondary* or *stray radiation.* Primary radiation, also called the *useful beam,* is the radiation passing through the open area defined by the collimator of the x-ray source. The amount of primary radiation depends on the output of the x-ray tube (determined by the kV, mGy/mAs, and mAs) per examination, the average number of examinations performed during a week, the fraction of time the x-ray beam is directed toward any particular barrier, the distance to the point to be protected, and the presence (or absence) of a primary barrier built into the imaging equipment. Scattered radiation arises from the interaction of the useful beam with the patient, causing a portion of the primary x-rays to be redirected. For radiation protection purposes scatter is considered as a separate radiation source with essentially the same photon energy spectrum (and penetrability) as the primary beam. In general, the exposure from scattered radiation at 1 m from the patient is approximately 0.1% to 0.15% of the incident exposure to the patient for typical diagnostic x-ray energies with a 20 cm × 20 cm (400 cm²) field area. The scattered radiation is proportional to the field size, and can be calculated as a fraction of the reference field area. For CT applications,

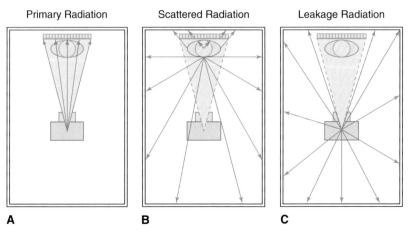

■ **FIGURE 21-10** The sources of exposure in a diagnostic x-ray room. **A.** Primary radiation emanating from the focal spot. **B.** Scattered radiation emanating from the patient. **C.** Leakage radiation emanating from the x-ray tube housing (other than the collimated primary radiation).

the rectangular collimation over a smaller volume will have a distinct scattered radiation distribution, and is considered separately, as discussed below. Leakage is the radiation that emanates from the x-ray tube housing other than the useful beam. Because leakage radiation passes through the shielding of the housing, its effective energy is very high (only the highest energy photons are transmitted). The exposure due to leakage radiation is limited by FDA regulations to 0.87 mGy/h (100 mR/h) at 1 m from the tube housing when the x-ray tube is operated at the maximum allowable continuous tube current (usually 3 to 5 mA) at the maximum rated kV, typically 150 kV.

The primary and secondary radiation exposure of an individual in an adjacent area to be protected depends primarily on (1) the amount of radiation produced by the source; (2) the distance between the patient and the radiation source; (3) the amount of time a given individual spends in an adjacent area; (4) the amount of protective shielding between the source of radiation and the individual; and (5) the distance between the source of radiation and the individual.

Types of Medical X-ray Imaging Facilities

General purpose radiographic installations produce intermittent radiographic exposures using tube potentials of 50 to 150 kV, with the x-ray beam directed toward the patient and the image receptor. Depending on the type of procedures, a large fraction of the exposures will be directed towards the floor or to an upright image receptor, and sometimes to other barriers (as in cross-table lateral image acquisitions). Barriers that can intercept the unattenuated primary beam are considered primary barriers. A protected control area for the technologist is required, with the ability to observe and communicate with the patient. The viewing window of the control booth should be of similar attenuation as the wall and large enough to allow unobstructed viewing. The configuration of the room should not depend on the control area shielding as a primary barrier, and in no situation should there be an unprotected direct line of sight from the patient or x-ray tube to the x-ray machine operator or to loaded screen-film or CR cassettes, regardless of the distance from the radiation sources. Also, the switch that energizes the x-ray tube should be installed so that the operator cannot stand outside of the shielded area and activate the switch.

Fluoroscopic imaging systems are typically operated over a range of 60 to 120 kV. Since the image receptor is designed to also be a primary barrier, only secondary radiation barriers need to be considered in the shielding design. In some cases, a radiographic and fluoroscopic combined unit is installed, and the shielding requirements are based on the combination of the workloads of both units. In this case, the radiographic room issues discussed above must also be taken into account.

Interventional facilities include angiography and vascular interventional, neuroangiography, and cardiovascular and electrophysiology imaging suites. Like other fluoroscopic rooms, the walls, floors, and ceilings of interventional suites are considered to be secondary radiation barriers. However, they may have multiple x-ray tubes and the procedures often require long fluoroscopy times, and include cine and digital fluorography image sequences that have large workload factors and so the rooms may require more shielding than general fluoroscopy rooms.

A dedicated chest radiography installation has the x-ray tube directed at the image receptor assembly on a particular barrier all of the time. Since the receptor can be used at various heights above the floor, the area behind the image receptor from the finished floor to a height of 2.1 m must be considered to be a primary barrier. All other areas in this room are secondary barriers, and any portion of the wall that the primary beam cannot be directed toward can also be considered a secondary barrier.

Mammography employs a very low kV in the range of 25 to 35 kV, and the breast support provides the primary barrier for the incident radiation. Thus, radiation barriers protect from secondary radiation only, and given the low x-ray energies and the small volume of tissue irradiated, often all that is needed in a permanent mammography room is the installation of a second layer of a gypsum wallboard. Doors for mammography rooms might need special consideration, because wood attenuates much less than typical gypsum wallboard; a metal door may be advisable. Regarding operator safety, mammography machines have lead acrylic barriers to protect the control area.

CT uses a collimated x-ray fan beam intercepted by the patient and by the detector array; thus, only secondary radiation reaches protective barriers. The x-ray tube voltage used for most scans is 120 kV, over a range of 80 to 140 kV. As mentioned in Chapter 10, modern wide-beam multirow detector CT scanners (MDCTs) make more efficient use of the radiation produced by the x-ray tubes than did the now-obsolete single detector row scanners. MDCTs can perform extensive scanning without exceeding their heat limits, allowing more procedures per day, more contrast phases per procedure, and scans that cover more patient anatomy. Although the amount of scattered radiation per equivalent scan is not significantly more than that produced by a single-row scanner, a large number of scans per day can require a greater thickness of shielding for walls, and perhaps even additional shielding of floors and ceilings. Secondary scatter emanating from the scanner is not isotropic, as there are much higher radiation levels along the axis of the patient table than in the direction of the gantry (see Fig. 21-14). Assuming an isotropic scatter distribution is conservative in terms of the amount of shielding for the various barriers in a room, it provides flexibility for future CT scanner installations when different orientations are considered.

Mobile radiography and fluoroscopy systems (used in situations in which patients cannot be transported to fixed imaging systems or used in operating rooms or intensive care units) present a challenge for protecting nearby individuals. For bedside radiography, protection is chiefly accomplished by maintaining a distance from the source of radiation and keeping the primary beam directed away from anyone

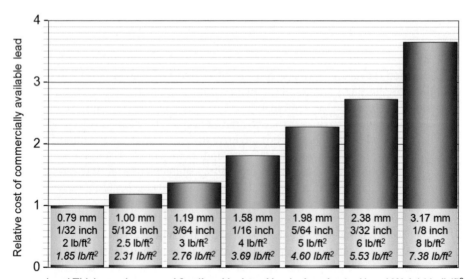

■ FIGURE 21-11 Cost of lead (adapted from Fig. 2-3, NCRP Report No.147). Lead is commercially sold by nominal weight in pounds per square foot (lb/ft²). Equivalent thickness in inches and millimeters are also stated. The height of each bar is the relative cost of lead sheet compared to 2 lb/ft², normalized to a value of 1.

nearby. For mobile fluoroscopy, all individuals within 2 m of the patient should wear protective aprons, and if available, protective mobile shielding should be positioned between the patient and attending personnel.

A *bone mineral densitometry x-ray system* typically uses a well-collimated scanning beam and, due to the low beam intensity and correspondingly low x-ray scatter, such a scanner will not produce scattered radiation levels above 1 mGy per year at 1 m for a busy facility, which is the shielding design goal for a fully occupied, uncontrolled area (NCRP, 2004). Thus, structural shielding is not required in most situations. The control console, however, should be placed as far away as practicable to minimize exposure to the operator.

Dental and veterinary x-ray facilities require special consideration depending on the scope and unique attributes of the procedures. The NCRP has published reports that describe shielding and radiation protection requirements for these facilities. For these and all other applications and future developments, sources of ionizing radiation should be evaluated by a qualified expert in order to determine the type and nature of the shielding required in the facility.

Shielding Materials

X-ray shielding is accomplished by interposing an attenuating barrier between the source(s) of radiation and the area to be protected in order to reduce the exposures to below acceptable limits. The thickness of shielding needed to achieve the desired attenuation depends on the shielding material selected. Lead is the most commonly used material because of its high-attenuation properties and relatively low cost. Commercially available thicknesses of lead sheet are commonly specified in nominal weight per area (in pounds per square foot), with corresponding thicknesses specified in inches and millimeters, as shown in Figure 21-11. The actual masses per area are considerably less than the nominal values. The least thickness commonly installed is 2 lb/ft² equal to 1/32 inch or 0.79 mm; there is little cost savings from using a lesser thickness. Other thicknesses and relative costs are compared in the figure. For typical shielding installations, the lead sheet is glued to a sheet of gypsum wallboard and installed with nails or screws on wood or metal studs. Where the edges of two lead sheets meet, continuity of shielding must be ensured by overlapping lead, as well as for gaps and inclusions in the wall (e.g., electrical junction boxes and switches.).

Other shielding materials are also used, such as gypsum wallboard, concrete, glass, leaded glass, and leaded acrylic. Gypsum wallboard (sheetrock) is used for wall construction in medical facilities, and a nominal 5/8 inch thickness (14 mm minimum) is most often used. While there is little protection provided at higher energies, significant attenuation occurs at the low x-ray energies used for mammography. Because of possible non-uniformity of the gypsum sheets, it is prudent to specify an extra layer (e.g., two sheets of wallboard) when using this material for shielding. Concrete is a common construction material used in floors, wall panels, and roofs, and is usually specified as standard-weight (147 lb/ft³, 2.4 g/cm³) or light-weight (115 lb/ft³, 1.8 g/cm³). The concrete density must be known to determine the thickness needed to provide the necessary attenuation. When concrete is poured on a ribbed-profile steel deck, the thickness is not constant and the minimum concrete thickness should be used for attenuation specifications. Glass, leaded glass, and leaded acrylic are transparent shielding materials. Ordinary plate glass may be used when protection requirements are low; its attenuation may be increased by laminating two or more 6 mm glass sections. More common and useful are leaded glass (glass with a high lead content) and leaded acrylic (impregnated with lead during manufacturing) that are specified in various thicknesses of lead equivalent, such as 0.5, 0.8, 1.0, and 1.5 mm.

Computation of X-ray Imaging Shielding Requirements

Terminology

As stated above, the shielding design goals, P, are 0.1 mGy/wk for controlled areas and 0.02 mGy/wk for uncontrolled areas. The distance from the radiation source to the nearest approach to the barrier of the sensitive organs of a person in the occupied area must be chosen; the point of closest approach to the barrier is assumed to be 0.3 m for a wall, 1.7 m above the floor below, and, for transmission through the ceiling, at least 0.5 m above the floor of the room above, as shown in Figure 21-12.

The occupancy factor, T, for an area is defined as the average fraction of time that the maximally exposed individual is present while the x-ray beam is on. The maximally exposed individuals will usually be employees of the facility, or residents or employees of an adjacent facility. Recommended values for T are listed in Table 21-3, for use when information about actual occupancy for a specific situation is not known. The occupancy factor modifies the shielding design goal allowable at a given point by 1/T; in other words, the attenuation of a barrier must lower the radiation to a level given by the ratio P/T.

The *workload* (W) is the time integral of the x-ray tube current in milliampere-minutes over a period of 1 week (mA-min/wk). In NCRP Report No. 147, a normalized average workload per patient, W_{norm}, is also described; it includes multiple exposures depending on the type of radiographic exam and clinical goal. The total workload per week, W_{tot}, is the product of W_{norm} and the average number of patients per week (N).

Unlike earlier shielding methods that assumed a single, fixed high kV value for the workload, the *workload distribution* described in NCRP Report No. 147 is a function of the kV, which is spread over a wide range of operating potentials for extremity examinations (e.g., about 1/3 of the total exams in a general radiographic room) at 50 to 60 kV, abdominal exams at 70 to 80 kV, and chest exams at greater than

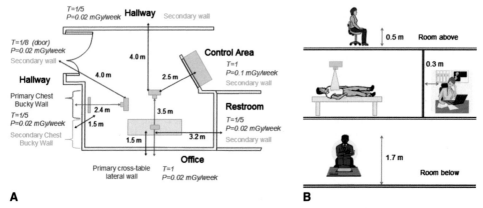

A **B**

■ **FIGURE 21-12 A.** Floor plan of a general purpose radiographic room shows the location of the x-ray source, orientation and location of the x-ray beam for various acquisitions, and the adjacent areas with typical occupancy factors, T; shielding design goals, P; and indication of primary and secondary barriers. Distances to each barrier are determined for the primary beam, leakage radiation from the x-ray tube, and scattered radiation from the patient. For secondary radiation, the closest distance is used. **B.** The elevation diagram provides information to determine the distances to adjacent areas above and below the x-ray room to be shielded. The floor-to-floor heights in multi-story buildings must be known.

TABLE 21-3 SUGGESTED OCCUPANCY FACTORS FOR ADJACENT AREAS

OCCUPANCY LEVEL	LOCATION	OCCUPANCY FACTOR (T)
Full	Administrative or clerical offices; laboratories, pharmacies, and other work areas fully occupied by an individual; receptionist areas, attended waiting rooms, children's indoor play areas, adjacent x-ray rooms, film-reading areas, nurse's stations, x-ray control rooms	1
Partial	Rooms used for patient examinations and treatments	1/2
	Corridors, patient rooms, employee lounges, staff rest rooms	1/5
	Corridor doors	1/8
Occasional	Public toilets, unattended vending areas, storage rooms, outdoor areas with seating, unattended waiting rooms, patient holding areas	1/20
	Outdoor areas with only transient pedestrian or vehicular traffic, unattended parking lots, vehicular drop-off areas (unattended), attics, stairways, unattended elevators, janitor's closets	1/40

National Council on Radiation Protection and Measurements. *Structural shielding design for medical x-ray imaging facilities*. NCRP Report No. 147. National Council on Radiation Protection and Measurements, Bethesda, MD, 2004.

100 kV (with reduced tube current-time product). Workload distributions are specific for a given type of radiological installation, including radiographic room (all barriers, chest bucky, floor, or other barriers), fluoroscopy tube (R&F room), radiographic tube (R&F room), chest room, mammography room, cardiac angiography, and peripheral angiography. For shielding design, the magnitude of the workload is less important than the distribution of the workload as a function of kV, since attenuation properties of the barriers have a strong kV dependence.

The *use factor* (U) is the fraction of the primary beam workload that is directed toward a given primary barrier, and will depend on the type of radiographic room and the orientation of the equipment. In a dedicated chest room, the primary barrier has U = 1, since the x-ray beam is always directed toward the wall-mounted chest receptor, and all other walls are secondary radiation barriers. In a general radiographic room, U must be estimated for the types of procedures and the amount of time the x-ray beam will be used for a specific orientation. Most often, the x-ray beam is pointed at the floor for acquiring images with patients on the table, occasionally pointed at a wall for a cross-table acquisition, and at a chest receptor stand for a combined room. For a general radiographic room, a survey of clinical sites (NCRP Report No. 147) yielded, for radiography not using a vertical chest receptor, U = 0.89 for the floor, U = 0.09; for the cross-table lateral wall, and U = 0.02 for an unspecified wall; for procedures using a vertical chest receptor stand, U = 1 for the chest receptor stand; and U = 0 for the ceiling and the control area barrier in that same room. For fluoroscopy and mammography, the primary beam stop is the image receptor assembly, so U = 0 and only secondary radiation must be considered.

The *primary barrier*, found in radiographic, dedicated chest, and radiographic-fluoroscopic rooms, is designed to attenuate the primary beam to the shielding design goal. Unshielded primary air kerma at the point to be protected per week is dependent on the average number of patients per week (N), the use factor (U) for that barrier, the primary air kerma per patient at 1 m, and the distance to the point (inverse square law correction is applied).

The *secondary barrier* is designed to attenuate the unshielded secondary air kerma from leakage and scatter radiation to the shielding design goal (or less). All walls not considered primary barriers are secondary barriers. Scattered radiation from the patient increases with the intensity and area of the useful beam, and is a function of the scattering angle. The total contribution from unshielded secondary air kerma, proportional to W_{tot}, is calculated from the clinical workload distributions, determined at 1 m, and modified by the inverse square law to the distance of the point to be protected, similar to that described for primary radiation. In certain orientations such as lateral acquisitions, the distance from the scattering source (the patient) will be different than the distance from the leakage radiation source (the x-ray tube) to the point to be protected.

Example Shielding Calculation

Room diagrams of a radiographic room are shown in Figure 21-12, with distances in meters from each of the radiation sources (primary, x-ray tube leakage, and scatter from the patient), as well as adjacent areas that are defined in terms of T, P, and primary or secondary barriers.

There are many complexities involved in calculating the necessary attenuation of the primary and secondary barriers to achieve the shielding design goals that are beyond the scope of this book. Many of the details regarding workloads, workload distributions, normalized workloads per patient (W_{norm}), field size area, attenuation of primary radiation by the image receptor, and other nuances are incorporated into shielding thickness charts found in NCRP Report No. 147, which display the required shielding thicknesses for the various barriers as a function of $N \times T/(P \times d^2)$, where as stated previously, N is the number of patients per week, T is the occupancy factor (see Table 21-3), P is the shielding design goal in mGy/wk, and d is the distance in meters from the radiation source to the point to be protected. In abbreviated notation, this is NT/Pd^2. These charts, which assume specific normalized workloads per patient (W_{norm}) as described in NCRP Report No. 147, are provided for radiographic and radiographic/fluoroscopic rooms for both lead and concrete shielding materials. If the site-normalized workload per patient (W_{site}) is different, then the values of NT/Pd^2 are scaled by W_{site}/W_{norm}. Primary beam use factors U are identified by specific curves in each chart for primary barriers.

Three of these charts are shown in Figure 21-13 for a radiographic room, considering (A) no primary beam preshielding, (B) primary beam preshielding, and (C) secondary radiation. The required lead thickness in millimeters is a function of NT/Pd^2. The term "preshielding" refers to attenuation of the primary beam by the image receptor. The graphs for primary beam preshielding consider the attenuation of the image receptor in the radiographic table or wall-mounted cassette holder due to the grid, cassette, and support structures, equivalent to 0.85 mm lead, and for cross-table laterals attenuation due to the grid and cassette, equivalent to 0.3 mm lead. Note the decreased requirement for lead thickness with primary beam preshielding (e.g., for the chest bucky wall barrier and $NT/Pd^2 = 1,000$, without preshielding the thickness is 1.95 mm lead and with preshielding is 1.13 mm lead, as shown in Fig. 21-13A,B, respectively).

For determination of barrier thicknesses using NT/Pd^2 methods, scale drawings of the room, including elevation drawings, location of the equipment, designations of adjacent areas as controlled or uncontrolled, occupancy factors of adjacent areas, and distances to adjacent areas are necessary, in addition to the average number of patients, N, per week. Charts are selected according to room type and shielding materials. For example, using the diagrams in Figure 21-12, if N = 120 patients per week for a general radiographic room, then NT/Pd^2 can be calculated for each barrier and

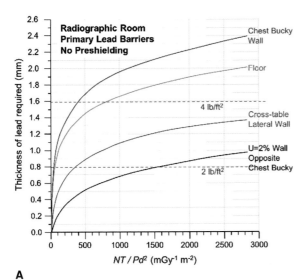

A

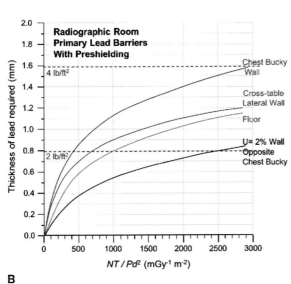

B

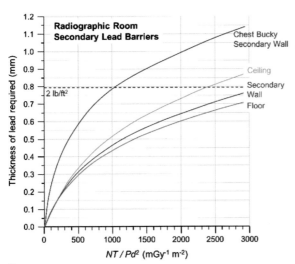

C

■ **FIGURE 21-13** Required lead barrier thickness for a radiographic room as a function of NT/Pd^2, using W_{norm} = 0.6 mA min patient^{-1} for the chest bucky and 1.9 mA min patient^{-1} for the floor and other barriers. **A.** No preshielding for primary barriers. **B.** Preshielding for primary barriers. **C.** Secondary lead barriers. In each of the graphs, the horizontal dotted lines indicate the common lead thicknesses of 0.79 and 1.58 mm, corresponding to 2 lb/ft^2 and 4 lb/ft^2 lead sheet. (Adapted from Fig 4.5A–C, NCRP Report No. 147.)

the required lead thickness is determined from the graph. For the chest bucky wall primary radiation barrier with T = 0.2, P = 0.02 mGy/wk, and d = 2.4 m, NT/Pd^2 = 120 × 0.2/(0.02 × 2.4²) = 208 and, using the blue curve labeled *chest bucky wall*, the lead thickness required is about 1.3 mm to achieve the shielding design goal. Therefore, the primary barrier to be installed is specified as 4 lb/ft² (1.6 mm) over the indicated area, which is from the finished floor to a height of 2.1 m (7 ft), with lateral margins around the image receptor of at least 0.5 m (e.g., a leaded drywall sheet 4 ft wide).

Shielding for secondary barriers is determined in a similar manner; however, because the total amount of secondary radiation emanates from a variety of locations and distances, the calculations can be very complex. A conservative approach is to assume that all of the secondary radiation in the room emanates from the closest distance to the barrier, which would increase the shielding thickness. Thus, for the wall adjacent to the chest wall bucky designated as a secondary barrier, the closest distance is 1.5 m, and NT/Pd^2 = 120 × 0.2/(0.02 × 1.5²) = 533. From Figure 21-11C, the thickness of lead (using the chest bucky secondary wall curve) is about 0.6 mm, and therefore the secondary barrier is specified as 2 lb/ft², installed continuously and seamlessly with the adjacent primary radiation barrier. For the control area barrier with T = 1, P = 0.1 mGy/wk, d = 2.5 m, NT/Pd^2 = 120 × 1/(0.1 × 2.5²) = 192, and using the curve labeled "secondary wall," the lead thickness is 0.15 mm, so 2 lb/ft² of lead is specified. For the control area window, leaded acrylic is often used, and would be specified as having an equivalent attenuation as the surrounding wall of 2 lb/ft² or 0.8 mm lead. Note that in these situations, the conservative approach ensures more than adequate protection for individuals in adjacent areas, and allows for increased room workload in the future. The shielding for each other radiation barrier, including doors, the floor, and ceiling, is similarly calculated and specified.

In walls, the shielding (e.g., leaded drywall, leaded doors, leaded acrylic, and sheet lead) is installed from the finished floor to a height of 2.1 m (7 ft) with overlapping lead at the seams of at least 1 cm, and lead backing at electrical outlets and other access points (electrical junction boxes, plumbing, etc.) into the wall to ensure continuous protection. Attachment screws used for mounting leaded drywall do not need lead backing (the steel that displaces the lead combined with the length of the screw provides adequate attenuation), but care must be taken to ensure that the screws that penetrate the lead sheet remain in place to maintain shielding integrity.

Surveys after Shielding Installation

After installation of shielding, a radiation protection survey should be performed by a qualified expert to ensure the adequacy of the installed shielding. The survey should verify that the barriers are contiguous and free of voids and defects and provide sufficient attenuation to meet the relevant shielding design goal divided by the occupancy factor (P/T). Visual inspection during installation should be part of the evaluation, followed by transmission measurements using a gamma-ray source of suitable energy (e.g., Tc-99m) and a detector with high sensitivity and fast response (e.g., GM survey meter). Alternatively, the x-ray source in the room can be used to generate a primary beam and secondary radiation, and measurements performed with a suitable high-sensitivity integrating survey meter.

Computed Tomography Scanner Shielding

For a CT scanner, all walls in the room are secondary barriers, because the detector array within the gantry is the primary radiation barrier. The scatter distribution emanating from the scanner is highly directional, being highest along the scanner axis

(Fig. 21-14). Because most CT scans are acquired at 120 and 140 kV with a highly filtered beam, the scattered radiation is highly penetrating. There are three methods that can be used to determine the shielding requirements, one based upon $CTDI_{vol}$, another based upon typical dose length product (DLP) values per acquisition, and the third based on the measured scatter distribution isodose maps provided by the manufacturer. For instance, using typical values for DLP, the scatter intensity (air kerma in mGy/acquisition) at 1 m is estimated for head and body scans, and then multiplied by the number of acquisitions (much greater than the number of patients due to multiple acquisitions being performed of many patients) expected over a typical work week for an 8-h shift (the busiest shift if the scanner is operated over extended hours). This is the total unshielded peak air kerma at 1 m from the gantry. For each barrier, the distance from the gantry to the calculation point beyond the barrier is determined, and the inverse square law is applied. A thickness of shielding is then determined to reduce the radiation level to the design goal modified by the inverse of the occupancy factor (P/T) by the use of specific transmission charts (Fig. 21-15).

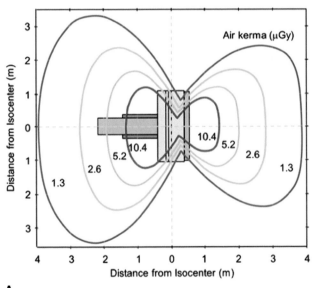

A

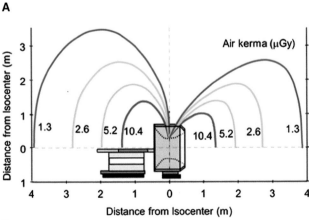

B

■ **FIGURE 21-14** Secondary (scatter and leakage) radiation distributions for a 32-cm-diameter PMMA phantom, 40-mm collimation, 64-channel MDCT, 140 kV, 100 mA, 1 s scan. Actual secondary radiation levels must be scaled to the techniques used for the acquisition. **A.** Horizontal isodose scatter distribution at the height of the isocenter. **B.** Elevational isodose scatter distribution; the distribution is vertically symmetric above and below the level of the table.

Example Barrier Calculation for a CT Scanner

A CT scanner performs 125 head procedures/week and 150 body procedures/week using a tube voltage of 120 kV, and produces a scatter air kerma of 63.8 mGy/wk at 1 m from the gantry isocenter. A barrier that is 3.3 m (11 ft) from the gantry isocenter to an uncontrolled corridor with P = 0.02 mGy/wk and an occupancy factor T = 0.2 requires a transmission factor to reduce the radiation to a level less than P/T = 0.02/0.2 = 0.1 mGy/wk. At 3.3 m, the unshielded air kerma is $63.8/3.3^2$ = 5.86 mGy/wk, and the transmission factor through the lead must therefore be less than 0.1/5.86 = 0.017 Consulting Figure 21-15, this transmission factor requires a minimum of 1.0 mm lead. This is greater than 2 lb/ft², so 4 lb/ft² is specified for this barrier. The shielding for other barriers of the CT scanner room is calculated similarly. For the floors and ceilings, a transmission chart with varying thicknesses of concrete should be used; if the thickness of concrete is insufficient, a sheet of lead should be installed above or below the concrete.

For multirow detector array scanners with collimator widths of 40 mm (and in some cases greater, up to 160 mm), the amount of scatter per gantry rotation for a specific kV and mAs will typically be much higher than that of a single-slice scanner. However, because of the increased axial coverage per rotation, the total mAs per scan will be a fraction of the single-slice scanner's, on the order of two to four times lower, and thus, the amount of scatter per scan will be comparable. On the other hand, the acquisition speed allows a larger number of patients to be scanned, which can significantly increase the total amount of scatter that must be considered for shielding calculations. It is therefore prudent to determine the shielding for the peak patient workloads expected over a given work shift (8 h is typical, but in some cases this can be up to 12 h on the job) to ensure adequate protection from secondary radiation in adjacent areas. Dose-reducing features on CT scanners, such as automatic tube current modulation, may reduce shielding requirements in the future.

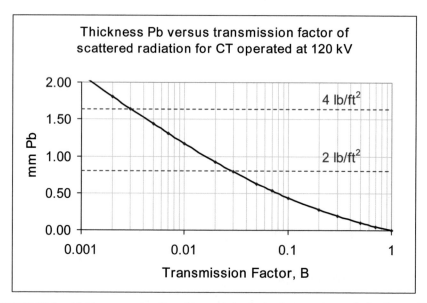

■ **FIGURE 21-15** Lead thickness as a function of transmission factor for secondary radiation from a CT scanner operated at 120 kV. (National Council on Radiation Protection and Measurements. *Structural shielding design for medical x-ray imaging facilities.* NCRP Report No. 147. National Council on Radiation Protection and Measurements, Bethesda, MD, 2004.)

PET/CT and SPECT/CT Shielding

Most PET today is performed using the radiopharmaceutical F-18 fluorodeoxy-glucose (FDG). In PET imaging with F-18 FDG, the radiopharmaceutical is administered to a patient, the patient rests for a period of about 45 to 90 min to allow uptake by cells and washout from other physiologic compartments, the patient urinates to remove activity from the bladder, and then is imaged. The installation of shielding must be considered for the room containing the PET/CT system and for the uptake rooms where patients rest after radiopharmaceutical administration and before imaging. It is common for a PET/CT facility to have three uptake rooms per PET/CT system because a modern PET/CT system can scan about three patients an hour. Required shielding depends upon the patient workload, the activity administered per patient, the uses of areas near the PET/CT room and uptake rooms, and the distances to these nearby occupied areas. Because of the high energies (511 keV) of annihilation photons, the shielding thicknesses can be very large and consideration must be given to whether the building can support the weight of the shielding. The amount of shielding needed can be minimized by placing the PET/CT and uptake rooms on the lowest floor (no shielding needed below) or on the top floor (no shielding needed above) and against an exterior wall or walls, thereby reducing or eliminating the need for shielding of one or two walls. Placing the uptake rooms adjacent to each other also reduces the weight of shielding needed. The amount of needed shielding can be further reduced by designing the area so that areas of low occupancy (e.g., storage rooms, mechanical and electrical equipment rooms, and bathrooms) are immediately adjacent to the uptake and PET/CT rooms. The shielding design methods for PET/CT facilities are described in AAPM Report No. 108, *PET and PET/CT Shielding Requirements* (AAPM, 2005).

The shielding design for a PET/CT or a SPECT/CT facility must also consider the radiation from the x-ray CT system. In most PET/CT installations, the thick shielding for the annihilation photons is more than sufficient for the lower-energy secondary radiation from the x-ray CT system. SPECT imaging rooms are often not shielded; for a SPECT/CT, a shielding calculation should be performed for the x-ray CT system and shielding should be installed if needed. In some SPECT/CT scanners, a cone-beam detector is utilized to acquire the CT projection data, and will have scatter distributions that might require specific considerations when determining the barrier thickness. If a nuclear medicine imaging room is near a PET/CT room or a PET uptake room, shielding of greater thickness than needed for the protection of people may be required so that the high-energy photons emanating from patients do not interfere with imaging procedures in the nearby room.

21.6 Radiation Protection in Diagnostic and Interventional X-ray Imaging

Personnel Protection in Medical X-ray Imaging

During CT, radiographic, and remote fluoroscopic procedures, medical staff are seldom in the room with the patient while x-rays are being produced, although there may be exceptions for pediatric and critically ill patients and those who are incapable of following instructions. During most procedures, staff are protected from radiation by the structural shielding installed in the walls of the room. However, physicians and assisting staff are in the room for most procedures utilizing fluoroscopy, particularly angiographic and interventional procedures, and during some CT-guided diagnostic and interventional procedures. Figure 21-16 shows the varying intensity of stray radiation, primarily scattered x-rays from the patient, during fluoroscopy. Understanding the spatial pattern of stray radiation can help staff to reduce the doses by where they stand during the procedure and how they position movable shielding. In particular, when the x-ray beam is in a lateral angulation, the stray radiation intensity is much higher on the side of the patient toward the x-ray source than on the side toward the image receptor. The x-ray doses to the heads and arms of staff tend to be least when the x-ray tube is beneath the patient.

Several items provide protection for staff during a fluoroscopic or radiographic imaging procedure. The first and foremost is the *protective apron* worn by all individuals who must work in the room when the x-ray tube is operated. Lead equivalent thicknesses from 0.25 to 0.50 mm are typical. Usually, the lead is in the form of a rubber material to provide flexibility and handling ease. Aprons protect the torso of the body and the upper legs and are available in designs with only frontal shielding or with wrap-around shielding, the latter being important when the back is exposed to the scattered radiation for a considerable portion of the time. Greater than 90% of the scattered radiation incident on the apron is attenuated by the 0.25-mm thickness at standard x-ray energies (e.g., tube voltage less than 100 kV). Aprons of 0.35 and 0.50 mm lead equivalents give greater protection (up to 95% to 99% attenuation), but weigh 50% to 100% more than the 0.25-mm lead equivalent aprons. Since the k-absorption edge of lead is at 88 keV and the average energy of typical diagnostic x-rays is about 35 to 40 keV, materials in the middle range of atomic numbers (Z) such as tin and barium are more efficient per unit weight in absorbing those x-rays than is lead. Several types of non-lead and lead composite aprons for shielding personnel from diagnostic x-rays are available (Murphy et al., 1993; Zuguchi et al., 2008). The shielding capabilities of the lighter aprons are commonly specified in mm lead equivalent, but such a specification is valid only for a specific x-ray energy spectrum. These lighter aprons are typically adequate for x-rays generated at tube potentials up to 120 kV, but their effectiveness compared to conventional lead aprons declines at tube potentials above about 100 kV. For long fluoroscopic procedures, the weight of the apron may become a limiting factor in the ability of the physician and the attending staff to complete the case without substitutions. Some

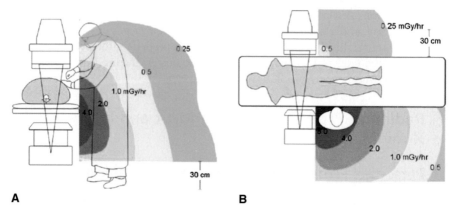

A   **B**

■ **FIGURE 21-16** Dose rates from scattered radiation during fluoroscopy, with the x-ray beam in PA (**A**) and lateral (**B**) orientations. These diagrams show the decrease in dose rate with distance from the location where the x-ray beam enters the patient. When the x-ray tube is beneath the patient (**A**), the highest scatter intensity is to the lower part of the operator's body. When the x-ray beam has a lateral angulation (**B**), the scatter intensity is much less on the side of the patient toward the image receptor. (From: National Council on Radiation Protection and Measurements. *Radiation dose management for fluoroscopically guided interventional medical procedures.* NCRP Report No. 168. National Council on Radiation Protection and Measurements, Bethesda, MD, 2010a.)

apron designs, such as skirt-vest combinations, place much of the weight on the hips instead of the shoulders. The areas not covered by the apron include the arms, lower legs, the head and neck, and the back (except for wrap-around aprons).

Aprons also do not protect the thyroid gland or the eyes. Accordingly, there are *thyroid shields* and *leaded glasses* that can be worn by the personnel in the room. The leaded thyroid shield wraps around the neck to provide attenuation similar to that of a lead apron. Leaded glasses attenuate the incident x-rays to a lesser extent, typically 30% to 70%, depending on the content (weight) of the lead. Unfortunately, their weight is a major drawback. Normal, everyday glasses provide only limited protection, typically much less than 20% attenuation. During fluoroscopy, the operator commonly looks at the display monitor while x-rays are produced and the x-rays typically strike his or her head from the side and below. Therefore, the protective glasses or goggles should provide shielding on the sides, or the glasses should be of wrap-around designs. Whenever the hands must be near the primary beam, *protective gloves* of 0.5-mm thick lead (or greater) should be considered when use does not interfere with the dexterity required to carry out the procedure.

In high workload angiographic and interventional laboratories, *ceiling-mounted, table-mounted, and mobile radiation barriers* are often used (Fig. 21-17). These devices are placed between the location where the x-ray beam intercepts the patient and the personnel in the room. The ceiling-mounted system is counterbalanced and easily positioned. Leaded glass or leaded acrylic shields are transparent and usually provide greater attenuation than the lead apron.

Only people whose presence is necessary should be in the imaging room during imaging. All such people must be protected with lead aprons or portable shields. In addition, no persons, especially individuals who are pregnant or under the age of 18 years, should routinely hold patients during examinations. Mechanical supporting or restraining devices must be available and used whenever possible. In no instance should the holder's body be in the useful beam, and it should be as far away from the primary beam as possible.

Protection of the Patient in Medical X-ray Imaging

The two main methods for limiting the radiation doses to patients in medical imaging are to avoid unnecessary examinations and to ensure the doses from examinations are no larger than necessary. The goal of a radiological examination should be to produce images of adequate quality for the clinical task, not images of unnecessarily high quality if that increases the radiation dose to the patient. On the other hand, using too low a dose can also be harmful, if it results in images that cause a clinical error or must be repeated.

Tube Voltage and Beam Filtration

An important goal in diagnostic imaging is to achieve an optimal balance between image quality and dose to the patient. *Increasing the kV* will result in a greater transmission (and therefore less absorption) of x-rays through the patient. Even though the air kerma (or exposure) per mAs increases as the kV is increased, an accompanying reduction in the mAs to produce a similar signal to the image receptor will decrease the incident exposure to the patient. Unfortunately, there is a concomitant reduction in image contrast due to the higher effective energy of the x-ray beam. Within limits, this compromise is acceptable. Therefore, the patient exposure can be reduced by using a higher kV and lower mAs. However, in procedures such as angiography and CT angiography in which contrast material is to be visualized and not soft tissue,

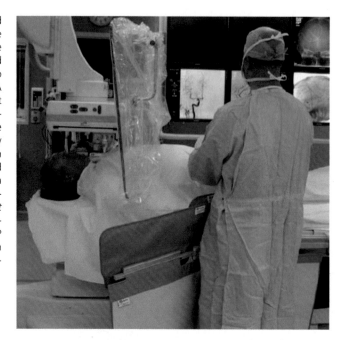

■ **FIGURE** 21-17 Shielding used with a C-arm fluoroscope. The optimal position of the movable ceiling-mounted transparent shield is approximately perpendicular to and in contact with the patient. A table-mounted shield (seen in front and to the left of the operator) protects the lower part of his body. The operator is looking at the display monitors and scattered radiation striking his face is from the side and below. (Source: National Council on Radiation Protection and Measurements. *Radiation dose management for fluoroscopically-guided interventional medical procedures.* NCRP Report No. 168. National Council on Radiation Protection and Measurements, Bethesda, MD, 2010a.)

greater beam filtration and lower kV can dramatically improve the contrast to noise ratio, which can result in a lower dose to the patient for these applications.

Filtration of the polychromatic x-ray energy spectrum can significantly reduce exposure by selectively attenuating the low-energy x-rays in the beam that would otherwise be absorbed in the patient with little or no contribution to image formation. These low-energy x-rays mainly impart dose to the skin and shallow tissues where the beam enters the patient. As the beam filtration is increased, the beam becomes "hardened" (the average photon energy increases) and the dose to the patient *decreases* because fewer low-energy photons are in the incident beam. The amount of filtration that can be added is limited by the increased x-ray tube loading necessary to offset the reduction in tube output, and the decreased contrast that occurs with excessive beam hardening. Except for mammography, a moderate amount of beam filtration does not significantly decrease subject contrast. The *quality* (effective energy) of the x-ray beam is assessed by measuring the HVL. State and federal regulations require the HVL of the beam to exceed a minimum value (see Chapter 6, Table 6-3, and for mammography systems, Chapter 8, Table 8-2). Adequate filtration helps to avoid or minimize skin injuries from prolonged fluoroscopically guided interventional procedures.

Field Area, Organ Shielding, and Geometry

Restriction of the field size by collimation to just the necessary volume of interest is an important dose reduction technique. While it does not significantly reduce the entrance dose to the area in the primary beam, it reduces the volume of tissue in the primary beam and thus the energy imparted to the patient. It also reduces the amount of scatter and thus the radiation doses to adjacent organs. From an image quality perspective, the scattered radiation incident on the detector is also reduced, thereby improving image contrast and the signal-to-noise ratio.

When possible, particularly radiosensitive organs of patients undergoing radiographic examinations should be shielded. For instance, when imaging a limb (such as a hand), a lap apron should be provided to the patient. When the gonads are in the primary beam, *gonadal shielding* should be used to protect the gonads when the shadow of the shield does not interfere with the anatomy under investigation. Because the gonadal shield must attenuate primary radiation, its thickness must be equivalent to at least 0.5 mm of lead. In any situation, the use of patient protection must not interfere with the examination. Other organs that may benefit from shielding if they must be in the primary beam include the lenses of the eyes and breast tissue in female children and young women. Care must be taken regarding proper placement of organ-specific shielding; distracted technologists have been known to place it on the x-ray receptor side of the patient instead of the x-ray tube side. Care also must be taken to ensure that gonadal and other organ-specific shielding does not block an active sensor for the automatic exposure control system. When critical organs must be in the beam, their doses can be reduced by orienting the beam so that the critical organ is on the side of the patient away from the x-ray tube.

Increasing the distance from the x-ray source to the patient (source-to-object distance [SOD]) helps reduce dose. As this distance is increased, a reduced beam divergence limits the volume of the patient being irradiated, thereby reducing the integral dose. Increasing this distance also reduces entrance dose due to the inverse square law. The exposure due to tube leakage is also reduced since the distance from the tube to the patient is increased, although this is only a minor consideration. With C-arm fluoroscopic systems that have fixed source-to-image receptor distances, patient dose is reduced by increasing the SOD as much as possible and moving the patient as close to the image receptor as possible. Federal regulations (21 CFR 1020.32[g]) specify a minimum patient (or tabletop) to focal spot distance of 20 cm. Furthermore, maintaining at least 30 cm is strongly recommended to prevent excessive radiation exposure.

X-ray Image Receptors

For film-screen image receptors, the speed of the image receptor determines the number of x-ray photons and thus the patient dose necessary to achieve an appropriate film darkening. Relative speed values are based on a par speed screen-film system, assigned a speed of 100; a higher speed system requires less exposure to produce the same optical density (e.g., a 400-speed screen-film-receptor requires four times less exposure than a 100-speed system). Specialized film processing can also affect the speed of the system. Either a faster screen or a faster film will reduce the incident exposure to the patient. In the case of a faster film, the disadvantage is increased quantum mottle and, in the case of a thicker intensifying screen, the disadvantage is reduced spatial resolution. Thus, increasing the speed of the screen-film image receptor reduces patient exposure, but the exposure reduction possible is limited by image-quality requirements. In modern film-screen imaging, a 400-speed system is typically used for head and body imaging and a 100-speed system may be used for imaging the extremities.

Digital radiography devices using photostimulable storage phosphor (PSP) plates, phosphor plates optically coupled to CCD cameras, or flat-panel thin-film transistor array image receptors have wide exposure latitudes. Postacquisition image scaling (adjustments to brightness and contrast) and processing modify the image for optimal viewing. Thus, these detectors can compensate (to a large degree) for under- and overexposure and can reduce retakes caused by inappropriate radiographic techniques. However, underexposed images may contain excessive quantum mottle, hindering the ability to discern contrast differences, and overexposed images result in needless exposure to the patient. In comparison to screen-film receptors, PSP receptors are roughly equivalent to a 200-speed screen-film receptor in terms of quantum mottle and noise (e.g., for adult examinations of the abdomen and chest [Compagnone et al., 2006; Seibert et al., 1994]), whereas digital flat-panel detectors have higher detection efficiencies, equivalent to 400- to 600-speed screen-film receptors. Techniques for extremity imaging with digital radiographic receptors should deliver higher exposure levels (similar to extremity screen-film cassettes with speeds of 75 to 100). In pediatric imaging, there are many examinations and corresponding technique protocols that allow low-dose, high-speed imaging; however, there are also situations requiring high spatial resolution and high signal-to-noise ratio which, in turn, require higher dose. The flexibility of the digital detector response can be used to advantage in these situations to achieve optimal image quality at appropriate patient doses.

Conventional screen-film radiographic image receptors have an inherent safety feature. If the film processor is operating properly and the kV is adequate, using an excessive quantity of radiation to produce an image results in an overly dark film. On the other hand, when digital image receptors are used for radiography, fluoroscopy, and CT, excessive incident radiation may not have an adverse effect on image quality, and unnecessarily high exposures to patients may go unnoticed. Routine monitoring of the exposures to the digital image receptors in radiography, particularly in mobile radiography in which automatic exposure control is commonly not possible, is therefore necessary as a quality assurance measure. Similarly, careful calibration of the automatic exposure control system in radiography, calibration of the automatic exposure rate control system in fluoroscopy, and attention to several factors, discussed below, in CT are necessary to avoid unnecessarily high doses to patients.

The image intensifier is a detector system with a wide dynamic range, whereby the necessary entrance exposure is determined by a light-limiting aperture or the electronic gain of a subsequent detector (e.g., TV camera). Entrance exposures to the image intensifier as low as one μR per image for fluoroscopy or as high as 4 mR per image for digital subtraction angiography are possible. The amount of exposure reduction is limited by the quantum statistics (i.e., too little exposure will produce an image with excessive quantum mottle which hinders the ability to discern subtle, low-contrast anatomical features).

Fluoroscopy

Fluoroscopy imparts a moderate fraction of the cumulative effective dose delivered in medical imaging (~18% of the total in 2006), but imparts some of the largest tissue doses to individual patients. Even though the fluoroscopic techniques are quite modest (e.g., 1 to 3 mA continuous tube current at 75 to 85 kV or higher mA, short exposure pulsed fluoroscopy at 7.5 to 15 frames per second), a fluoroscopic examination can require several minutes and, in some difficult cases, can exceed hours of "on" time. For example, a procedure using 2 mA at 80 kV for 10 min of fluoro time (1,200 mAs) delivers an air kerma of 60 mGy at 1 m (assuming 50 μGy/mAs for 80 kV at 1 m). If the focal spot is 30 cm from the skin, the patient entrance air kerma is $(100/30)^2 \times 60$ mGy ≈ 670 mGy! In the United States, fluoroscopic patient entrance air kerma (exposure) rates at 30 cm from the x-ray source for C-arm systems and at 1 cm above the table for systems with the x-ray tube fixed under the table are limited to a maximum of 87.3 mGy/min (10 R/min) for systems with automatic brightness control (ABC) and to 44 mGy/min (5 R/min) for systems without ABC. Some systems have a high air-kerma-rate fluoroscopic ("turbo") mode delivering up to 175 mGy/min (20 R/min) output at this reference point, a factor of five to ten times greater than the typical fluoro levels. This capability, which requires continuous manual activation of a switch by the operator (and produces a continuous audible signal), must be used very judiciously. Cineangiography studies deliver high dose rates of 175 to 600 mGy/min (20 to 70 R/min) at high frame rates (15 to 30 frames per s) but typically with short acquisition times. The patient entrance air-kerma rate depends on the angulation of the beam through the patient, with the air-kerma rate increasing with the thickness of the body traversed by the beam (e.g., the air kerma rate is greater for lateral projections than for anteroposterior [AP] or posteroanterior [PA] projections).

Severe x-ray–induced skin injuries to patients have been reported following prolonged fluoroscopically guided interventional procedures, such as percutaneous transluminal coronary angioplasty, radiofrequency cardiac catheter ablation, vascular embolization, transjugular interhepatic portosystemic shunt placement, and other percutaneous endovascular reconstruction (Koenig et al., 2001). The cumulative skin doses in difficult cases or from a series of procedures of a single area of the body can exceed 10 Gy, which can lead to severe radiation-induced skin injuries (see Specific Organ System Responses—Skin in Chapter 20). Figure 20-18 shows severe skin injuries following several fluoroscopically-guided interventional procedures. Such injuries may not become fully apparent until many weeks or even months after the procedure. It is recommended that each medical facility determine the procedures that may impart doses that exceed the threshold for skin injury. Prior to each such procedure, it is recommended that each patient be screened for factors that may decrease the dose threshold for skin injury; these include large radiation exposures to the same part of the body from fluoroscopically guided interventional procedures or radiation therapy; some drugs; some hereditary diseases affecting DNA repair; and possibly other diseases such as connective tissue disorders, diabetes mellitus, and hyperthyroidism (Balter et al., 2010; Koenig et al., 2001). While large radiation doses may be unavoidable in difficult cases, care should be taken during all examinations to employ techniques that will minimize the radiation exposure. Methods for minimizing the radiation exposure to the patient were described in Chapter 9 (see the section entitled "Dose Reduction"). Chapter 9 discusses the metrics of patient dose that are displayed by fluoroscopes. Fluoroscopes manufactured since June 10, 2006, display the cumulative air kerma at a reference point (for C-arm fluoroscopes, this reference point is 15 cm from the isocenter of rotation, toward the x-ray source), typically the kerma-area product or dose-area product, and the cumulative fluoro time. Older systems may display only the cumulative fluoro time. Studies have shown that cumulative air kerma and kerma area product correlate better with peak skin dose than does the total fluoro time (Fletcher et al., 2002; Miller et al., 2003). Ideally, a map of skin doses would be generated after each procedure, but this is not available at this time. Implementation of this feature in future systems will greatly assist in dose management. "Gafchromic" films that self-develop can be placed between the patient and support table to provide a postexamination map of surface peak skin dose. Dosimeters may be placed on the patients' skin to measure skin dose. In any dose-monitoring system, the real-time display of accumulated patient dose provides the physician with the ability to modify the procedure, if necessary, to minimize the potential for radiation-induced skin injuries. The dose metrics (e.g., cumulative air kerma, kerma-area product, or total fluoro time) recorded at the completion of the procedures allow physicians to identify patients who may be at risk for radiation-induced skin damage. After all procedures, areas of the patients' skin that received large doses should be documented in the patients' medical records. The patients should be notified and arrangements made for clinical follow-up if there is the potential for significant skin injury.

Physicians using or directing the use of fluoroscopic systems should be trained and credentialed to ensure they understand the technology of fluoroscopy machines, particularly the dose implications of the different modes of operation; the biological effects of x-rays; and the techniques used to minimize patient and personnel exposure. In addition, the physicians should be familiar with radiation control regulations. NCRP Report No. 168 is an excellent resource for all radiation protection aspects of fluoroscopically guided interventional procedures, including the management of radiation exposure to patient and staff (NCRP, 2010a).

Computed Tomography

As mentioned earlier in this chapter, the average annual effective dose to the population of the United States from medical imaging increased by a factor more than five from about 1980 until 2006 and about half of this effective dose in 2006 was from CT imaging. In 2001, it was reported in the medical literature that at least some medical facilities in the United States were using adult technique factors for the CT examinations of children and even infants (Patterson et al., 2001); it has been estimated that this practice causes a risk of cancer to the patients on the order of ten times the risk to adult patients (Brenner et al., 2001). In recent years, professional societies, advisory bodies such as the ICRP and NCRP, and governmental agencies have urged that efforts be made to reduce the doses to patients from medical imaging. Because of the large fraction from CT imaging and the relatively large dose per examination, much of this effort should be focused on CT imaging.

In CT, many operator-selectable parameters determine the patient dose. These include the kV and mA applied to the x-ray tube, time per x-ray tube rotation, detector-table motion pitch, and beam filter. As mentioned in Chapter 10, these are not usually individually selected by a technologist for each patient procedure, but are instead specified in organ- and procedure-specific protocols, such as "chest (routine)," "three-phase liver," and "brain (CTA)." A technologist selects the appropriate protocol for a patient and indication, although the technologist may have to modify the technique in the protocol for patient-specific circumstances. Modern CT scanners provide the capability to protect protocols with passwords, which should be restricted to only a few individuals. The use of passwords can protect protocols from inadvertent or deliberate modification.

Most radiographic images, other than those acquired with mobile machines, are acquired utilizing automatic exposure control (phototiming). However, older CT scanners use a fixed kV and mAs selected by the technologist, regardless of the size of the patient, unless the CT technologist changes them. The fixed techniques in CT for a given protocol often lead to unnecessarily high mAs values for thinner patients, particularly neonatal and young children. A way to avoid this unnecessary radiation dose to the patient is to train the CT technologists to reduce the mAs (and perhaps the kV) for thinner patients. A technique chart can be devised for each such CT scanner showing kV and mAs values for different diameter patients as a guide to achieving good image quality at proper dose levels. Table 21-4 shows the dose reductions that can be achieved if the CT protocols (mAs values) are adjusted to the patient's size.

New scanners have the ability to modulate the tube current as a function of tube rotation angle and axial position on the patient, to compensate for the attenuation variations along the beam path through the patient. Some CTs use the localizer images (scout scan or topogram) to determine the mA, whereas others also measure the amount of transmitted radiation during the scan itself. Automatic tube current modulation can markedly reduce exposure without decreasing image quality. However, each implementation of automatic tube current modulation requires information to be provided to the CT regarding the amount of random noise in the resultant images tolerated by the interpreting physicians. The various CT manufacturers specify this differently (e.g., for one manufacturer, a parameter called "noise index" and the reconstructed slice thickness must be selected, whereas for another manufacturer, a parameter called the "reference mAs" and a setting of "weak," "average," or "strong"

TABLE 21-4 DOSE REDUCTION POTENTIAL IN CT

PATIENT DIAMETER (cm)	PERCENT mAs	mAs
14	0.3	1
16	0.6	2
18	1.2	4
20	2.2	7
22	4.2	13
24	7.9	24
26	15	45
28	28	85
30	53	160
32	100	300
34	188	564
36	352	1,058
38	661	1,983
40	1,237	3,712

Note: If a CT technique of 120 kV and 300 mAs delivers good image quality (low noise images) for a 32-cm-diameter patient, the same image quality (signal to noise ratio [SNR]) can be achieved by reducing the mAs to the levels indicated for patients smaller than 32, and increasing the mAs for patients larger than 32 cm. The large mA values for very large diameters are not possible; alternatively a higher kV could be used. Large patients have greater amounts of abdominal fat that results in improved conspicuity of organ boundaries, and a lesser SNR might be tolerable.

must be selected). This information is commonly stored in the organ and procedure specific CT protocols and can vary among protocols.

Another innovation in CT that has the potential to significantly reduce doses to patients is iterative image reconstruction, discussed in Chapter 10. It addresses random noise more effectively than filtered backprojection and can produce images of equal quality with significantly lower radiation doses.

Two indices of dose to a patient displayed by modern CT scanners are the $CTDI_{VOL}$ and the DLP, the DLP being the $CTDI_{VOL}$ multiplied by the scanned length of the patient (see Chapter 11). For scans of a significant length, the $CTDI_{VOL}$ is approximately the average dose that would be imparted to a cylindrical acrylic phantom from the scan being given to the patient. Therefore, the $CTDI_{VOL}$ and DLP provide information about the amount of radiation being given to a specific patient, but do not reflect the actual doses to the patient.

Modern CT scanners display the $CTDI_{VOL}$ and DLP before and after each scan and have the ability to send this dose information to a PACS or other digital information system after a scan, either as a secondary capture image with the study or as a DICOM Radiation Dose Structured Report (RDSR). If automatic tube current modulation is used, the $CTDI_{VOL}$ and DLP displayed before a scan may not be identical to those displayed after the scan. The display of these dose metrics before a scan provides the technologist the ability to assess the approximate magnitude of the radiation exposure before performing a scan. The RDSR has a full description of the procedure with radiation dose metrics and includes many details not found in the DICOM metadata associated with the images; however, because the RDSR is a separate DICOM object, reading or storing the information as a RDSR is a separate DICOM transaction. To ensure compatibility in dose reporting, the Integrating the Healthcare Enterprise (IHE) Radiation Exposure Monitoring integration profile should be specified when purchasing new imaging systems (IHE integration profiles are discussed in Chapter 5).

CT scanners that comply with the National Electrical Manufacturers Association (NEMA) XR 25 Computed Tomography Dose Check standard have the capability of displaying alerts when the $CTDI_{VOL}$ or DLP of a CT study about to be performed is expected to exceed preset values. A "notification value" is the dose metric of an individual scan or series of a study that causes a notification warning to be displayed. An "alert value" is the cumulative dose metric of the entire study already acquired plus that for the scan or series about to be performed that causes a warning to be displayed. By setting notification and alert values, the technologist is warned if the scan he or she is planning to acquire exceeds the user-configured level of dose. The alert value is intended to be set to avoid a patient injury and is different from a diagnostic reference level. The FDA has recommended that the alert value be set at $CTDI_{VOL} = 1$ Gy. This is an unusually high dose for a CT scan—about one-half the level that could result in skin erythema. If an alert is displayed, the technologist should review the acquisition parameters for an error. If the alert cannot be resolved, radiologist approval should be obtained before proceeding, except in a dire emergency. The notification level could be set to the DRL level. However that would result in numerous notifications, particularly for obese patients. The American Association of Physicists in Medicine (AAPM) has recommended that the notification level be set higher than the DRL so that notifications are issued only for doses that are "higher than usual," thereby warning the technologist that an acquisition parameter may be set incorrectly. The following AAPM recommended notification values are shown below, (AAPM 2011). This document also contains recommendations for notification levels for pediatric CT examinations.

EXAMINATION	$CTDI_{VOL}$ (mGy)
Adult head	80
Adult torso	50
Brain perfusion	600
Cardiac—retrospective gating	150
Cardiac—prospective gating	50

Dose Optimization in CT

The key to optimizing dose in CT imaging is to review and optimize the CT protocols. This is a substantial and complicated task and an overview will be provided herein. Each protocol should be reviewed from several perspectives. Many scans consist of a noncontrast scan and one or more scans after the administration of contrast material. Eliminating one or more phases from a protocol will greatly reduce patient dose.

■ Thin slices are usually noisier and in some cases may require a higher mA. One should consider whether high spatial resolution is diagnostically necessary. One might overcome the noise of thin slices by calculating thicker slices but at intervals smaller than the slice thickness (i.e., overlapping). Thin slices exhibit less partial volume effect and so benefit from higher tissue contrast which could allow dose to be reduced through lower mAs (ICRP, 2007).

■ Tissues with inherently high tissue contrast may be acquired at low dose without loss of diagnostic value. These include lung and bone. A renal stone protocol, for example, could be acquired at lower dose than a liver protocol.

- Patients who are obese generally require greater dose. However, a factor that balances this effect is that adipose tissue better delineates soft tissues, which causes acceptable contrast to be more easily achieved in obese than in thin patients. A kV of 140 could be selected for the most obese patients.
- Create separate abdominal protocols for obese patients.
- Lower kV can increase the visibility of contrast material in angiography or brain perfusion imaging. The k-absorption edge of iodine—where its attenuation coefficient reaches a maximum—is at about 30 keV. Improved images and lower patient dose may be achieved with a tube voltage of 100 kV instead of 120 kV in angiography. A tube voltage of 80 kV is commonly used in brain perfusion imaging.
- Scan only the z-axis length you need.
- When possible, avoid radiation directly to the eyes.
- Review the clinical necessity of multiple contrast phases.
- Only scan the contrast phases necessary for the diagnostic task. For example, follow-up exams may not require precontrast images.
- Vary tube current according to contrast phase. You may be able to use a lower mA for noncontrast phases.
- Compare your protocols with optimized protocols for the same model of CT. Sample CT protocols are available from the CT manufacturer, AAPM, and other sources. (See the Image Wisely Web site.)
- Look to see that protocols of similar body parts have similar dose indices, taking into consideration that some indications can tolerate less relative noise.
- Use iterative reconstruction, if available.
- Use automatic tube current modulation (see below) for procedures for which it will reduce dose. Most procedures should use it. (Not all procedures, e.g., brain perfusion imaging, benefit from it.)
- Ensure body imaging protocols that do not use automatic mA modulation require technique adjustment for patient body habitus.
- Create low-dose protocols (e.g., low-dose chest protocol, low-dose kidney stone protocol, low-dose AAA protocol) for use when indicated, particularly for follow-up examinations.
- Most automatic mA modulation systems have a maximum allowable mA setting. Ensure this is set to a reasonable value, beyond which you increase the kV.
- Ensure the $CTDI_{VOL}$ for brain perfusion CT does not exceed 0.5 Gy.
- Record the $CTDI_{VOL}$ and DLP for a patient of average size in each protocol document. You may need to average the values from several patients.
- Compare these dose indices with DRLs.

For cardiac CT protocols, significant reduction in dose can be achieved by the following strategies:

- Minimize the scan range.
- Use heart rate reduction.
- Prospective triggering results in lower dose than does retrospective gating.
- If one is using retrospective gating, employ ECG-gated mA modulation.
- Reduce tube voltage whenever possible to 100 kV or even 80 kV.

Miscellaneous Considerations

Careful identification of the patient and, for female patients of reproductive age, determination of pregnancy status are necessary before an examination is performed. For higher-dose studies (e.g., fluoroscopy and multiphase CT examinations) of the abdomen or pelvis, a pregnancy test within 72 h before the examination should be performed in addition to the usual screening for pregnancy, unless the possibility of pregnancy is eliminated by certain premenarche in a child, certain postmenopausal state, or documented hysterectomy or tubal ligation.

A significant reduction in population dose can be achieved by eliminating screening exams that only rarely detect pathology. Standing-order x-rays, such as presurgical chest exams for hospital admissions or surgeries not involving the chest, are inappropriate. Frequent screening examinations are often not indicated without a specific reason or a reasonable amount of time elapsed (e.g., years) from the previous exam. A good example is the "yearly" dental x-ray. While yearly exams are appropriate for some patients, a 2-year interval between x-ray examinations in noncavity-prone adult patients with a healthy mouth is appropriate. Another opportunity for significant patient dose reduction in dentistry is the use of high-speed film (e.g., E-speed film) or digital image receptors. Many dental offices still use slower D-speed films that require approximately twice the exposure (and thus patient dose). Periodic screening mammography examinations are not appropriate for women younger than 35 to 40 years old, unless there is a familial history of breast cancer or other indication. However, as the probability of cancer increases with age, and the fact that survival is drastically enhanced by early detection makes yearly screening mammograms sensible for the general population of women 40 to 50 years old.

Each radiology department should have a program to monitor examinations that must be repeated. The frequency of repeat exams due to faulty technique or improper position is primarily determined by the skill and diligence of the x-ray technologists. Training institutions often have higher repeat rates, mainly attributed to lack of experience. The largest numbers of studies that must be repeated are from mobile exams, in which positioning difficulty causes the anatomy of interest to be improperly represented on the image, and lack of automatic exposure control increases the likelihood of improper optical densities or dose to the image receptor.

Programmed techniques for examinations are commonly available on radiographic equipment, and can eliminate the guesswork in many radiographic situations (of course, provided that the techniques are properly set up). Technique charts for various examinations should be posted conspicuously at the control panel to aid the technologist in the correct selection of radiographic technique. The use of photostimulable phosphor imaging plates or direct digital image receptors (Chapter 7) can significantly reduce the number of exams that must be repeated because of improper radiographic technique. The examinations with the highest retake rates are portable chests; lumbar spines; thoracic spines; kidneys, ureters, and bladders; and abdomens. Continuous monitoring of retakes and inadequate images and identification of their causes are important components of a quality assurance program, so that appropriate action may be taken to improve quality.

Equipment problems, such as improperly loaded cassettes, excessive fog due to light leaks or poor film storage conditions, processor artifacts caused by dirty components or contaminated chemicals, uncalibrated x-ray equipment, or improper imaging techniques can also lead to retakes. Many of these errors are eliminated by a quality control program that periodically tests the performance of the x-ray equipment, image receptors, and processing systems.

Reference Levels

A reference level, also known as a diagnostic reference level, is a particular value of a metric of dose to a patient or a phantom, such as entrance air kerma in radiography or $CTDI_{VOL}$ in CT, to be used in a quality assurance program to identify possibly excessive doses to patients or protocols or equipment that may be imparting excessive doses. A dose value from an imaging procedure that exceeds a reference level should be investigated, but would not be presumed as excessive until so determined by an investigation. Reference levels were mentioned in Chapter 11. In the case of fluoroscopically guided interventional procedures, comparing dose metrics from actual clinical procedures to reference levels may help to identify clinicians who are not making full use of the dose-optimizing features of the imaging devices or who are less adept at the clinical procedures.

Reference levels may be based upon measurements made with a phantom, such as CTDI measurements made using the FDA CT body or head phantom, or they may be based upon dose metrics, such as $CTDI_{VOL}$ and DLP, from clinical imaging of patients. There are advantages and disadvantages, discussed below, to each approach.

A reference level is typically determined from a study of a dose metric from many institutions and imaging systems. A reference level is typically set at the seventy-fifth percentile of the set of data from the study, meaning that three fourths of the measurements in the data set were less than the reference level.

In the United States, the Nationwide Evaluation of X-ray Trends (NEXT) Program, conducted jointly by the US Food and Drug Administration, the Conference of Radiation Control Program Directors, and most state radiation regulatory agencies, periodically performs measurements of doses from x-ray imaging devices. NEXT studies have been of phantom-based dose measurements. The American College of Radiology (ACR) publishes reference levels determined from dose data from its imaging modality accreditation program. The ACR's reference levels are also based upon measurements using phantoms. A possible limitation of the ACR's reference levels is that they are determined only from dose measurements from imaging facilities seeking accreditation. European governmental agencies are also a source of reference levels. Reference levels may also be provided by studies reported in the professional literature (e.g., Hausleiter et al., 2009).

There are shortcomings to the use of reference levels as a quality assurance tool. Reference levels for dose measurements made using phantoms may not fully test an imaging device and imaging protocol. For example, the cylindrical FDA CT dose phantoms have shapes very different from patients and do not assess the effect of automatic tube current modulation. For another example, a measurement of a fluoroscope with a phantom does not assess the clinician's knowledge in the proper use of the imaging system or his or her skill in the clinical procedure. On the other hand, using dose measurements and reference levels determined from actual patient studies involves uncertainty due to factors such as patient body size and, in the case of fluoroscopically guided interventional procedures, the difficulty of individual patient procedures. The studies used to determine reference levels may lag current technology and uses; furthermore, because the studies used to determine reference levels are costly of resources, there are many clinical imaging protocols for which there are no appropriate reference levels. Lastly, comparisons of dose metrics to reference levels identify high outliers; a dose metric that is less than a reference level does not imply that the protocol or procedure is fully optimized.

Nonetheless, reference levels are a useful tool in identifying imaging protocols, equipment, and practices imparting unnecessarily high doses to patients. As mentioned in Chapter 11, the automated collection of dose information, using standard DICOM and IHE protocols, from clinical procedures and its collection by dose registries may facilitate the timely creation and updating of reference levels and the comparison of dose metrics from clinical procedures with reference levels.

21.7 Radiation Protection in Nuclear Medicine

Minimizing Time of Exposure to Radiation Sources

Nuclear medicine procedures typically produce low exposure rates for extended periods of time. For example, the typical exposure rate at 1 m from a patient after the injection of approximately 740 MBq (20 mCi) of technetium 99m methylenediphosphonate (Tc-99m MDP) for a bone scan is approximately 1 mR/h, which, through radioactive decay and urinary excretion, will be reduced to approximately 0.5 mR/h at 2 h after injection, when imaging typically begins. Therefore, knowledge of both the exposure rate and how it changes with time are important in minimizing personnel exposure. Table 21-5 shows the typical exposure rates at 1 m from adult nuclear medicine patients after the administration of commonly used radiopharmaceuticals.

The time spent near a radiation source can be minimized by having a thorough understanding of the tasks to be performed and the appropriate equipment to complete them in a safe and timely manner. For example, elution of a Mo-99/Tc-99m generator and subsequent radiopharmaceutical preparation requires several steps with a high-activity source. It is important to have practiced these steps with a nonradioactive source to learn how to manipulate the source proficiently and use the dose measurement and preparation apparatus.

Minimizing Exposure with Distance from Radiation Sources

Other than low-activity sealed sources (e.g., a 370-kBq [10 μCi] Co 57 marker), unshielded radiation sources should never be manipulated by hand. The use of tongs or other handling devices to increase the distance between the source and the hand substantially reduces the exposure rate. Table 21-6 lists the exposure rates from radionuclides commonly used in nuclear medicine and the 100-fold exposure rate reduction achieved simply by increasing the distance from the source from 1 to 10 cm.

Radiation exposure rates in the nuclear medicine laboratory can range from over 100 R/h (e.g., contact exposure from an unshielded vial containing approximately 37 GBq [1 Ci] of Tc-99m generator eluate or a therapeutic dosage of approximately

TABLE 21-5 TYPICAL EXPOSURE RATE AT 1 METER FROM AN ADULT NUCLEAR MEDICINE PATIENT AFTER RADIOPHARMACEUTICAL ADMINISTRATION

STUDY	RADIOPHARMACEUTICAL	ACTIVITY MBq (mCi)	EXPOSURE RATE AT 1 m μGy/h (mR/h)
Thyroid cancer therapy	I-131 (NaI)	7,400 (200)	~306 (35)
Tumor imaging	F-18 (FDG)	370 (10)	~43.7 (5.0)
Cardiac-gated imaging	Tc-99m RBC	740 (20)	~7.9 (0.9)
Bone scan	Tc-99m MDP	925 (25)	~10.5 (1.2)
Tumor imaging	Go-67 citrate	111 (3)	~3.5 (0.4)
Liver-spleen scan	Tc-99m sulfur colloid	148 (4)	~1.8 (0.2)
Myocardial perfusion imaging	Tl-201 chloride	111 (3)	~0.87 (0.1)

Exposure rate measurements courtesy of M. Hartman, University of California, Davis.

TABLE 21-6   EFFECT OF DISTANCE ON EXPOSURE WITH COMMON RADIONUCLIDES USED IN NUCLEAR MEDICINE

RADIONUCLIDE 370 MBq (10 mCi)	EXPOSURE RATE[a] mGy/h[b] (R/h) AT 1 cm	EXPOSURE RATE[a] mGy/h[b] (R/h) AT 10 cm (~4 inches)
Ga-67	65.5 (7.5)	0.65 (0.075)
Tc-99m	54.1 (6.2)	0.54 (0.062)
I-123	143 (16.3)	1.43 (0.163)
I-131	190 (21.8)	1.90 (0.218)
Xe-133	46.3 (5.3)	0.46 (0.053)
Tl-201	39.3 (4.5)	0.39 (0.045)
F-18	494 (56.6)	4.9 (0.57)

[a]Calculated from the Γ_{20}.
[b]Air kerma rate.

11 GBq [300 mCi] of I-131) to natural background. The air kerma rate at any distance from a small container of a particular radionuclide can be calculated using the air-kerma-rate constant (Γ_δ), of the radionuclide. The air-kerma-rate constant for a photon-emitting radionuclide is defined by the ICRU as the quotient of $l^2 \dot{K}_\delta$ by A, where $\dot{K}_\delta$ is the air kerma rate due to photons of energy greater than δ, at a distance l from a point source of the nuclide having an activity A,

$$\Gamma_\delta = \frac{l^2 \dot{K}_\delta}{A} \qquad [21\text{-}4]$$

The air-kerma-rate constant has units of m^2 Gy Bq^{-1} s^{-1}. For convenience, the air-kerma-rate constant is sometimes expressed in m^2 μGy GBq^{-1} h^{-1}.

Because very low energy photons are significantly attenuated in air and other intervening materials, air kerma rate constants usually ignore photons below a particular energy. For example, Γ_{20} represents the air-kerma-rate constant for photons $\geq$ 20 keV.

EXAMPLE: An unshielded vial containing 3.7 GBq of Tc-99m pertechnetate is left on a lab bench. For Tc-99m, Γ_{20} = 14.6 $m^2 \cdot \mu$Gy$\cdot$GBq$^{-1} \cdot$h^{-1} What would be the air kerma (K_{air}) if a technologist were standing 0.5 m away for 30 min?

SOLUTION:

$$\dot{K}_{air} = (14.6 \; m^2 \cdot \mu Gy \cdot GBq^{-1} \cdot h^{-1}) \; (3.7 \; GBq) \; (0.5 \; h)/(0.5 \; m)^2 = 108 \; \mu Gy$$

Multiplying the air kerma in μGy by 0.1145 mR/μGy will convert it to exposure in units of mR; thus 108 μGy is equivalent to (108 μGy $\times$ 0.1145 mR/μGy) = 12.4 mR.

The air-kerma-rate constant has largely replaced the older *exposure rate constant* (expressed in units of R$\cdot$cm$^2 \cdot$mCi$^{-1} \cdot$h^{-1}) where the exposure rate in R/h at 1 cm from 1 mCi of the specified radionuclide was expressed as

$$\text{Exposure rate (R/h)} = \Gamma_x A / d^2 \qquad [21\text{-}5]$$

where Γ_x is the exposure rate constant R$\cdot$cm$^2 \cdot$mCi$^{-1} \cdot$h^{-1} for photons of energy greater than x, A is the activity in mCi, and d is the distance in centimeters from a point source of radioactivity.

One can multiply the exposure rate constant in $R \cdot cm^2 \cdot mCi^{-1} \cdot h^{-1}$ by 21.69 to convert to air-kerma-rate constant in $\mu Gy \cdot GBq^{-1} \cdot h^{-1}$. This conversion assumes that the photon energy cutoff (i.e., δ and x) is the same.

Shielding in Nuclear Medicine

Tungsten, lead, leaded glass, and leaded acrylic shields are used in nuclear medicine to reduce the radiation exposure from vials and syringes containing radioactive material. Table 21-7 shows exposure rate constants and lead HVLs for radionuclides commonly used in nuclear medicine.

Syringe shields (Fig. 21-18) are used to reduce personnel exposure from syringes containing radioactivity during dose preparation and administration to patients. Syringe shields can reduce hand exposure from Tc-99m by as much as 100-fold.

Leaded glass or acrylic shields are used in conjunction with solid lead shields in radiopharmaceutical preparation areas. Radiopharmaceuticals are withdrawn from vials surrounded by thick lead containers (called "lead pigs") into shielded syringes behind the leaded glass shield in the dose preparation area (Fig. 21-19).

Persons handling radionuclides should wear laboratory coats, disposable gloves, finger ring TLD dosimeters, and body dosimeters. The lead aprons utilized in diagnostic radiology are of limited value in nuclear medicine because, in contrast to their effectiveness in reducing exposure from low-energy scattered x-rays, they do not attenuate enough of the medium-energy photons emitted by Tc-99m (140 keV) to be practical (Table 21-8).

Radioactive material storage areas are shielded to minimize exposure rates. Mirrors mounted on the back walls of high-level radioactive material storage areas are often used to allow retrieval and manipulation of sources without direct exposure to the head and neck. Beta radiation is best shielded by low atomic number (Z) material (e.g., plastic or glass), which provides significant attenuation while minimizing bremsstrahlung x-ray production. For high-energy beta emitters (e.g., P-32), the low Z shield can be further shielded by lead to attenuate bremsstrahlung. With the exception of PET facilities, which often shield surrounding areas from the 511-keV annihilation radiation, most nuclear medicine laboratories do not find it necessary to shield the walls within or surrounding the department.

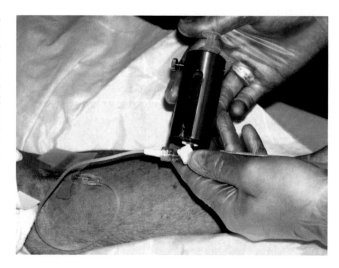

■ **FIGURE 21-18** A butterfly needle and three-way stopcock connected to a syringe with normal saline and a syringe shield containing the syringe with the radiopharmaceutical for injection. The barrel of the syringe shield is made of a high-Z material (e.g., lead or tungsten) in which a leaded glass window is inserted so that the syringe scale and the contents of the syringe can be seen.

TABLE 21-7   EXPOSURE RATE CONSTANTS (Γ_{20} AND Γ_{30})[a] AND HALF VALUE LAYERS (HVL) OF LEAD FOR RADIONUCLIDES OF INTEREST TO NUCLEAR MEDICINE

RADIONUCLIDE	Γ_{20}[b,c]	D_{20}[d]	Γ_{30}[c]	HVL IN Pb (cm)[e,f]
C-11, N-13, O-15	139 (5.85)	153.10	5.85	0.39
Co-57	13.2 (0.56)	14.51	0.56	0.02
Co-60	303 (12.87)	333.41	12.87	1.2
Cr-51	4.24 (0.18)	4.66	0.18	0.17
Cs-137/Ba-137m	76.5 (3.25)	84.19	3.25	0.55
F-18	135 (5.66)	148.44	5.66	0.39
Ga-67	17.7 (0.75)	19.43	0.75	0.1
I-123	38.4 (1.63)	42.23	0.86	0.04
1-125	34.6 (1.47)	38.08	0.26	0.002
I-131	51.3 (2.18)	56.47	2.15	0.3
In-111	75.4 (3.20)	82.90	2.0	0.1
Ir-192	108.6 (4.61)	119.43	4.61	0.60
Mo-99/Tc-99m[g]	34.6 (1.47)	38.08	1.43	0.7
Rb-82	134 (5.65)	159	5.65	0.7
Tc-99m	14.6 (0.62)	16.06	0.60	0.03
Tl-201	10.6 (0.45)	11.66	0.45	0.02
Xe-133	12.5 (0.53)	13.73	0.53	0.02

[a](Γ_{20} and Γ_{30}) calculated from the absorption coefficients of Hubbell and Seltzer (1995) and the decay data table of Kocher (1981): Hubbell JH, Seltzer SM. Tables of x-ray mass attenuation coefficients and mass energy-absorption coefficients 1 keV to 20 MeV for elements Z = 1 to 92 and 48 additional substances of dosimetric interest. NISTIR 5632, National Institute of Standards and Technology, May 1995 and Kocher DC. Radioactive decay data tables. DOE/TIC-11026, Technical Information Center, U.S. Department of Energy, 1981.
[b]Air kerma rate constant, 20 keV photon energy cutoff, in μGy m^2 GBq^{-1} h^{-1}.
[c](R·cm^2/mCi·h): Multiply by 23.69 to obtain air kerma rate constant in μGy·m^2/GBq·h.
[d]Equivalent dose rate μSv m^2 GBq^{-1} h^{-1}.
[e]The first HVL will be significantly smaller than subsequent HVLs for those radionuclides with multiple photon emissions at significantly different energies (e.g., Ga-67) because the lower-energy photons will be preferentially attenuated in the first HVL.
[f]Some values were adapted from Goodwin PN. Radiation safety for patients and personnel. In: Freeman and Johnson's clinical radionuclide imaging. 3rd ed. Philadelphia, PA: WB Saunders, 1984:370. Other values were calculated by the authors.
[g]In equilibrium with Tc-99m.

Contamination Control and Surveys

Contamination is simply uncontained radioactive material located where it is not wanted. Contamination control methods are designed to prevent radioactive material from coming into contact with people and to prevent its spread to other work surfaces. Protective clothing and handling precautions to control contamination are similar to the "universal precautions" that are taken to protect hospital personnel from pathogens. In most cases, disposable plastic gloves, laboratory coats, and closed-toe shoes offer adequate protection. One advantage of working with radioactive material, in comparison to other hazardous substances, is that small quantities can be easily detected. Personnel and work surfaces must be routinely surveyed for contamination. Nonradioactive work areas near radioactive material use areas (e.g., reading rooms and patient exam areas) should be posted as "clean areas" where radioactive materials

■ **FIGURE 21-19 A.** Dose preparation workstation. The technologist is placing a syringe containing a radiopharmaceutical into a syringe shield. Protection from radiation exposure is afforded by working behind the lead "L-shield" with a 1.8-mm lead equivalent glass window that reduces the radiation exposure from Tc-99m by approximately 100. The technologist is wearing a lab coat and disposable gloves to protect his skin and clothing from contamination. A film badge is worn on the lab coat to record body exposure and a TLD finger ring dosimeter is worn inside the glove with the TLD chip facing the source to record the extremity exposure. **B.** A much thicker syringe shield is required for PET radiopharmaceuticals to attenuate the 511 keV annihilation photons (**left**) compared to the typical syringe shields used for shielding the 140 keV photons from Tc-99m (**right**).

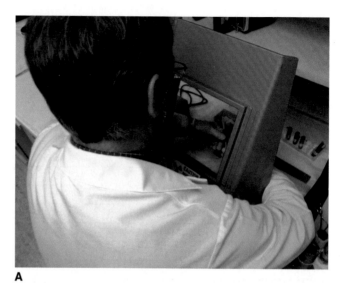

A

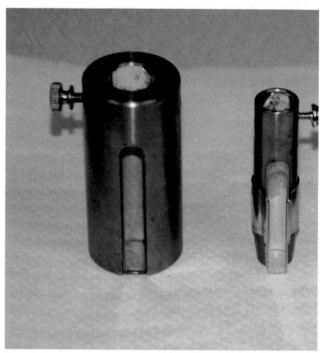

B

TABLE 21-8 EXPOSURE REDUCTION ACHIEVED BY A 0.5-mm LEAD EQUIVALENT APRON FOR VARIOUS RADIATION SOURCES

SOURCE	ENERGY (keV)	EXPOSURE REDUCTION WITH 1 APRON	NO. OF APRONS TO REDUCE EXPOSURE BY 90% (I.E., 1 TVL)	WEIGHT (lb)
Scattered x-rays	10–30	>90%	~1	~15
Tc-99m	140	~70%	~2	~30
Cs-137	662	~6%	~36	~540

are prohibited. Work surfaces where unsealed radioactive materials are used should be covered by plastic-backed absorbent paper that is changed when contaminated or worn. Volatile radionuclides (e.g., I-131 and Xe-133 gas) should be stored in a fume hood with 100% exhaust to the exterior of the building to prevent airborne contamination and subsequent inhalation. Personnel should discard gloves into designated radioactive waste receptacles after working with radioactive material and monitor their hands, shoes, and clothing for contamination periodically. All personnel should wash their hands after handling radioactive materials and especially before eating or drinking to minimize the potential for internal contamination. If the skin becomes contaminated, the best method of decontamination is washing with soap and warm water. The skin should not be decontaminated too aggressively to avoid creating abrasions that can enhance internal absorption. External contamination is rarely a serious health hazard; however, internal contamination can lead to significant radiation exposures. Good contamination control techniques help prevent inadvertent internal contamination.

The effectiveness of contamination control is monitored by periodic GM meter surveys (after handling unsealed radioactive material, whenever contamination is suspected, and at the end of each workday) and wipe tests (typically weekly) of radionuclide use areas. Wipe tests are performed by wiping surfaces using small pieces of filter paper or cotton-tipped swabs to check for removable contamination at various locations throughout the nuclear medicine laboratory. These wipe test samples (called "swipes") are counted in a NaI (Tl) gamma well counter. Areas that are demonstrated to be in excess of twice background radiation levels are typically considered to be contaminated. The contaminated areas are immediately decontaminated followed by additional wipe tests to confirm the effectiveness of decontamination efforts. GM meter surveys are also performed throughout the department at the end of the day to detect areas of contamination. In addition, exposure rate measurements (with a portable ion chamber survey meter) are made near areas that could produce high exposure rates (e.g., radioactive waste and material storage areas).

Laboratory Safety Practices

The following are other laboratory safety practices that minimize the potential for personnel or facility contamination. Examples of these radiation safety practices are shown in Figure 21-20.

- Label each container of radioactive material with a "Caution – Radioactive Material" label and the radionuclide, measurement or calibration date, activity, and chemical form.
- Wear laboratory coats or other protective clothing at all times in areas where radioactive materials are used.
- Wear disposable gloves at all times while handling radioactive material.
- Either after each procedure or before leaving the area, monitor hands and clothing for contamination in a low-background area using an appropriate survey instrument.
- Use syringe shields for reconstitution of radiopharmaceutical kits and administration of radiopharmaceuticals to patients, except when their use is contraindicated (e.g., recessed veins, infants). In these and other exceptional cases, use other protective methods, such as remote delivery of the dose (e.g., use a butterfly needle).
- Wear personnel monitoring devices, if required, at all times while in areas where radioactive materials are used or stored. When not being worn to monitor occupational exposures, personnel monitoring devices shall be stored in the work place in a designated low-background area.
- Wear extremity dosimeters, if required, when handling radioactive material.

■ **FIGURE 21-20** Routine radiation safety practices in nuclear medicine. **A.** Disposal of radioactive waste into a shielded container and proper posting of caution radioactive material signs. **B.** Unit dosages of radiopharmaceuticals come from a commercial radiopharmacy in lead shielded tubes that are cushioned for transport. **C.** Package survey with ion chamber survey meter to verify the shielding of the radioactive material is intact. **D.** Package labels state the radionuclides, the activity, and the maximum exposure rates expected at one meter from the package surface.

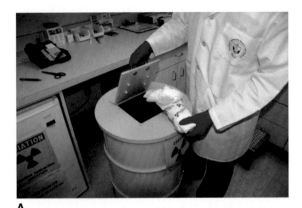

A

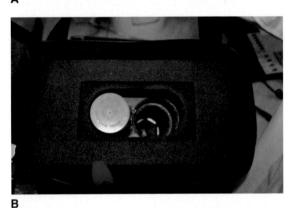

B

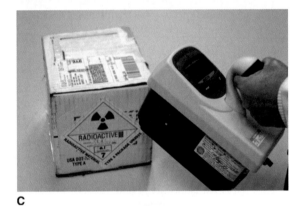

C

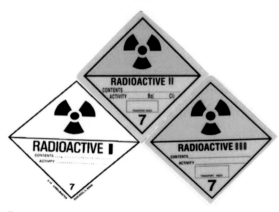

D

- Dispose of radioactive waste only in designated, labeled, and properly shielded receptacles.
- Shield sources of radioactive material to reduce potential exposure to people.
- Perform package receipt survey to assure the source shielding has not been damaged in transport and that the package is not leaking or contaminated.
- Do not eat, store food, drink, smoke, or apply cosmetics in any area where radioactive material is stored or used.
- Perform Xe-133 ventilation studies in a room with negative pressure with respect to the hallway. (Negative pressure will occur if the room air exhaust rate substantially exceeds the supply rate. The difference is made up by air flowing from the hallway into the room, preventing the escape of the xenon gas.) Xe-133 exhaled by patients undergoing ventilation studies must be exhausted into a Xe trap. Xe traps have large shielded activated charcoal cartridges, which adsorb xenon on the large surface areas presented by the charcoal, thus slowing its migration through the cartridge and allowing significant decay to occur before it is exhausted to the environment.
- Report serious spills or accidents to the radiation safety officer (RSO) or health physics staff.

Radioactive Material Spills

Urgent first aid takes priority over decontamination after an accident, and personnel decontamination takes priority over facility decontamination efforts. Individuals in the immediate area should be alerted to a spill and remain until they can be monitored with a GM survey instrument to ensure that they have not been contaminated. Radioactive material spills should be contained with absorbent material and the area isolated and posted with warning signs indicating the presence of radioactive contamination. Disposable shoe covers and plastic gloves should be donned before beginning decontamination. Decontamination should be performed from the perimeter of the spill toward the center to limit the spread of contamination. Decontamination is usually accomplished by simply absorbing the spill and cleaning the affected areas with detergent and water. A meter survey and wipe test should be used to verify successful decontamination. Personnel participating in decontamination should remove their protective clothing and be surveyed with a GM survey instrument to assure that they are not contaminated. If the spill involves volatile radionuclides or if other conditions exist that suggest the potential for internal contamination, bioassays should be performed by the radiation safety staff. Common bioassays for internal contamination include external counting with a NaI (Tl) detector (e.g., thyroid bioassay for radioiodine) and measurement of radioactivity in urine (e.g., tritium bioassay).

Protection of the Patient in Nuclear Medicine

Sometimes nuclear medicine patients are administered the wrong radiopharmaceutical or the wrong activity. Depending upon the activity, dose, and other specifics, these accidents may meet the regulatory criteria for what are referred to as *medical events* (see Chapter 16) which have prescriptive reporting and quality improvement requirements. The following event has occurred at several institutions: a patient referred for a whole-body bone scan (typically 740 MBq [20 mCi] of Tc-99m MDP) has been mistakenly administered up to 370 MBq (10 mCi) of I-131 sodium iodide for a whole-body thyroid cancer survey [thyroidal dose for 370 MBq and 20% uptake is ~100 Gy (10,000 rad)]. The cause has often been a verbal miscommunication. In another case, a mother who was nursing an infant was administered a therapeutic dose of I-131 sodium iodide without being instructed to discontinue breast-feeding, resulting in an estimated dose of 300 Gy (30,000 rad) to the infant's thyroid. The following precautions, most of which are mandated by the U.S. Nuclear Regulatory Commission (NRC), are intended to reduce the frequency of such incidents.

Each syringe or vial that contains a radiopharmaceutical must be conspicuously labeled with the name of the radiopharmaceutical or its abbreviation. Each syringe or vial shield must also be conspicuously labeled, unless the label on the syringe or vial is visible. It is prudent to also label each syringe or vial containing a dosage of a radiopharmaceutical with the patient's name. The patient's identity must be verified, whenever possible by two means (e.g., by having the patient recite his or her name and birth date). The possibility that a female adolescent or a woman is pregnant or nursing an infant by breast must be ascertained before administering the radiopharmaceutical. In the case of activities of I-131 sodium iodide exceeding 30 µCi and therapeutic radiopharmaceuticals, pregnancy should be ruled out by a pregnancy test within 72 h before the procedure, certain premenarche in a child, certain postmenopausal state, or documented hysterectomy or tubal ligation.

Before the administration of activities exceeding 1.1 MBq (30 µCi) of I-131 in the form of sodium iodide and any radionuclide therapy, a written directive must be prepared by the nuclear medicine physician identifying the patient, the radionuclide, the radiopharmaceutical, the activity to be administered, and the route of administration. The written directive must be consulted at the time of administration and the patient's identity should be verified by two methods. Although not required by the NRC, similar precautions should be taken when reinjecting autologous radiolabeled blood products to prevent transfusion reactions and the transmission of pathogens.

In some cases, women who are nursing infants by breast at the time of the examination may need to be counseled to discontinue breast-feeding until the radioactivity in the breast milk has been reduced to a safe level. Table 21-9 contains recommendations for cessation of breast-feeding after the administration of radiopharmaceuticals to mothers.

Radiation doses from the activity ingested by a nursing infant have been estimated for the most common radiopharmaceuticals used in diagnostic nuclear medicine (Stabin and Breitz, 2000). In many cases, no interruption in breast-feeding is needed to maintain a radiation dose to the infant well below 1 mSv. Only brief interruption (hours to days) of breast-feeding was advised for other Tc-99m radiopharmaceuticals: macroaggregated albumin, pertechnetate, red blood cells, white blood cells, as well as I-123 metaiodobenzylguanidine, and Tl-201. Complete cessation is suggested for Ga-67 citrate and I-131, however prior recommendation for cessation following I-123 NaI administration were based on a 2.5% contamination with I-125, which is no longer applicable (Siegel, 2002).

The NRC requires written instructions be given to nursing mothers if the total effective dose equivalent (TEDE) to a nursing infant could exceed 1 mSv (Code of Federal Regulations Title 10 Part 35.75). The instructions include guidance on the interruption or discontinuation of breast-feeding, and information on the potential consequences, if any, of failure to follow the guidance.

Radionuclide Therapy

Treatment of thyroid cancer and hyperthyroidism with I-131 sodium iodide is a proven and widely utilized form of radionuclide therapy. NaI-131 is manufactured in liquid and capsule form. I-131 in capsules is incorporated into a waxy or crystalline matrix or bound to a gelatin substance, all of which reduce the volatility of the I-131. In recent years, advances in monoclonal antibody and chelation chemistry

TABLE 21-9 RECOMMENDED DURATION OF INTERRUPTION OF BREAST-FEEDING FOLLOWING RADIOPHARMACEUTICAL ADMINISTRATION TO A PATIENT WHO IS NURSING AN INFANT OR CHILD

RADIOPHARMACEUTICAL	ADMINISTERED ACTIVITY MBq (mCi)	DURATION OF INTERRUPTION OF BREAST-FEEDING[a]
Tc-99m DTPA, MDP, PYP, RBC, or GH	740 (20)	None
Tc-99m sestamibi or tetrofosmin	1,110 (30)	None
Tc-99m disofenin	300 (8)	None
Tc-99m MAG3	370 (10)	None
Tc-99m sulfur colloid	444 (12)	None
I-123OIH	74 (2)	None
Tc-99m sodium pertechnetate	185 (5)	4 h
Tc-99m MAA	148 (4)	12 h
F-18 FDG[b]	740 (20)	12 h[b]
I-123 NaI	14.8 (0.4)	24 h
I-123 MIBG	370 (10)	48 h
Tc-99m WBC	185 (5)	48 h
In-111 WBC	18.5 (0.5)	1 wk
Tl-201 chloride	111 (3)	96 h
Ga-67 citrate	185 (5)	Discontinue[c]
I-131 NaI	1 (0.027)	Discontinue[c]

"None" means that interruption of breast-feeding need not be recommended, given criterion of a limit of 1 mSv effective dose to infant and these administered activities. However, even this low dose may be reduced by a 12 to 24-h interruption of breast-feeding.
[a]Adapted from NUREG 1556, Vol. 9, Rev. 2, Program-Specific Guidance About Medical Use Licenses, Appendix U, U.S. Nuclear Regulatory Commission, January 2008. (See Romney BM, Nickloff EL, Esser PD, et al. Radionuclide administration to nursing mothers: mathematically derived guidelines. *Radiology* 1986;160: 549–554; for derivation of milk concentration values for radiopharmaceuticals.)
[b]Minimal F-18 FDG in breast milk (*J Nucl Med* 2001;42(8):1238–1242). Waiting 6 half-lives (12 h) lowers the exposure to the infant from the mother.
[c]Discontinuance is based not only on the long duration recommended for cessation of breast-feeding but also on the high dose the breasts themselves would receive during the radiopharmaceutical breast transit. Stabin MG, Breitz HB. Breast milk excretion of radiopharmaceuticals: mechanisms, findings, and radiation dosimetry. *J Nucl Med* 2000;41(5):863–873.
DTPA, diethylenetriaminepentaaceticacid; MAA, macroaggregated albumin; disofenin is an iminodiacetic acid derivative; FDG, fluorodeoxyglucose; MIBI, methoxyisobutylisonitrile; MDP, methylene diphosphonate; PYP, pyrophosphate; RBC, red blood cells; WBC, white blood cells; OIH, orthoiodohippurate; MIBG, metaiodobenzylguanidine; GH, glucoheptonate; MAG3, mercaptoacetyltriglycine.

technology have produced a variety of radioimmunotherapeutic agents, many labeled with I-131. I-131 decays with an 8-day half-life and emits high-energy beta particles and gamma rays. These decay properties, together with the facts that I-131 can be released as a gas under certain conditions, can be absorbed through the skin, and concentrates and is retained in the thyroid, necessitate a number of radiation protection precautions with the administration of therapeutic quantities of I-131.

Following administration, I-131 is secreted or excreted in all body fluids including urine, saliva, and perspiration. In some cases the patient may need to be hospitalized as a radiation safety precaution or because of comorbidities (criteria for hospitalization are discussed below). If a patient is to be hospitalized, before I-131 is administered, surfaces of the patient's room likely to become contaminated, such as the floor, bed controls, mattress, light switches, toilet, and telephone, are covered with plastic or absorbent plastic-backed paper to prevent contamination. In addition, the patient's meals are served on disposable trays. Containers are placed in the patient's room to dispose of used meal trays and to hold contaminated linens for decay. Radiation safety staff will measure exposure rates at the bedside, at the doorway, and in neighboring rooms. In some cases, immediately adjacent rooms must be posted off limits to control radiation exposure to other patients and nursing staff. These measurements are posted, together with instructions to the nurses and visitors including maximal permissible visiting times. Nursing staff are required to wear dosimeters and are trained in the radiation safety precautions necessary to care for these patients safely. Visitors are required to wear disposable shoe covers, and staff members wear both shoe covers and disposable gloves to prevent contamination. Visiting times are limited and patients are instructed to stay in their beds during visits and avoid direct physical contact with visitors to keep radiation exposure and contamination to a minimum. Visitors and staff are usually restricted to nonpregnant adults. After the patient is discharged, the health physics or nuclear medicine staff decontaminates the room and verifies through wipe tests and GM surveys that the room is sufficiently decontaminated. Federal or state regulations may require thyroid bioassays of staff technologists and physicians directly involved with dose preparation or administration of large activities of I-131.

The NRC regulations (Title 10 Part 35.75) require that patients receiving therapeutic radionuclides be hospitalized until or unless it can be demonstrated that the TEDE to any other individual from exposure to the released patient is not likely to exceed 5 mSv. Guidance on making this determination can be found in two documents from the NRC: NUREG-1556, Vol. 9, entitled "A Consolidated Guidance about Materials Licenses: Program-Specific Guidance about Medical Licenses" and Regulatory Guide 8.39, entitled "Release of Patients Administered Radioactive Materials." These documents describe methods for calculating doses to other individuals and contain tables of activities not likely to cause doses exceeding 5 mSv. For example, patients may be released from the hospital following I-131 therapy when the activity in the patient is at or below 1.2 GBq (33 mCi) or when the dose rate at 1 m from the patient is at or below 70 μSv/h.

To monitor the activity of I-131 in a patient, an initial exposure measurement is obtained at 1 m from the patient soon after the administration of the radiopharmaceutical. This exposure rate is proportional to the administered activity. Exposure rate measurements are repeated daily until the exposure rate associated with 1.2 GBq (33 mCi) is obtained. The exposure rate from 33 mCi in a patient will vary with the mass of the patient. The activity remaining in the patient can be estimated by comparing initial and subsequent exposure rate measurements made at a fixed, reproducible geometry. The exposure rate equivalent to 1.2 GBq (33 mCi) remaining the patient ($X_{1.2}$) is

$$X_{1.2} = \frac{(1.2 \text{ GBq})X_0}{A_0}$$

where X_0 is the initial exposure rate (~15 min after radiopharmaceutical administration) and A_0 is the administered activity (GBq).

For example, a thin patient is administered 5.55 GBq (150 mCi) I-131, after which an exposure rate measurement at 1 m reads 37 mR/h. The patient can be discharged when the exposure rate at 1 m falls below:

$$X_{1.2} = \frac{(1.2 \text{ GBq}) (37 \text{ mR/h})}{5.5 \text{ GBq}} = 8.0 \text{ mR/h}$$

Once below 1.2 GBq (33 mCi), assuming a stable medical condition, the patient may be released. If the TEDE to any other individual is likely to exceed 1 mSv (0.1 rem), the NRC requires the licensee to provide the released individual, or the individual's parent or guardian, with radiation safety instructions. These instructions must be provided in writing and include recommended actions that would minimize radiation exposure to, and contamination of, other individuals. Typical radiation safety precautions for home care following radioiodine therapy are shown in Appendix H. These precautions also apply to patient therapy with less than 1.2 GBq (33 mCi) of I-131 for hyperthyroidism. On the rare occasions when these patients are hospitalized for medical or radiation safety reasons (e.g., small children at home), contamination control procedures similar to thyroid cancer therapy with I-131 should be observed.

Phosphorus-32 as sodium phosphate is used for the treatment of polycythemia vera and some leukemias, and palliation of pain from cancerous metastases in bone; P-32 in colloidal form is used to treat malignant effusions and other diseases. Strontium-89 chloride and samarium-153 lexidronam are used to treat intractable pain from metastatic bone disease. The primary radiation safety precaution for these radionuclide therapies is contamination control. For example, the wound and bandages at the site of an intra-abdominal instillation of P-32 should be checked regularly for leakage. The blood and urine will be contaminated and universal precautions should be observed. Exposure rates from patients treated with pure beta emitters like P-32 are not significant. Likewise the exposure rates from patients treated with Sr-89 and Y-90, both of which emit gamma rays with very low abundances, are insignificant compared to the risk of contamination.

Iodine-131 and yttrium-90, bound to monoclonal antibodies, are used to treat non-Hodgkin's lymphomas that exhibit a particular antigen. The precautions for therapy with I-131 antibodies are similar to those for therapies using I-131 sodium iodide. The precautions for therapies with Y-90 antibodies are similar to those in the previous paragraph.

Radioactive Waste Disposal

Minimizing radioactive waste is an important element of radioactive material use. Most radionuclides used in nuclear medicine have short half-lives that allow them to be held until they have decayed. As a rule, radioactive material is held for at least 10 half-lives and then surveyed in an area of low radiation background with an appropriate radiation detector (typically a GM survey instrument with a pancake probe) to confirm the absence of any detectable radioactivity before being discarded as nonradioactive waste. Disposal of decayed radioactive waste in the nuclear medicine department is made easier by segregating the waste into short half-life (e.g., F-18 and Tc-99m), intermediate half-life (e.g., Ga-67, In-111, I-123, Xe-133, Tl-201), and long half-life (e.g., P-32, Cr-51, Sr-89, I-131) radionuclides.

Small amounts of radioactive material may be disposed of into the sanitary sewer system if the material is water soluble and the total amount does not exceed regulatory limits. Records of all radioactive material disposals must be maintained for inspection by regulatory agencies. Radioactive excreta from patients receiving diagnostic or therapeutic radiopharmaceuticals are exempt from these disposal regulations and thus may be disposed into the sanitary sewer. The short half-lives and large dilution in the sewer system provide a large margin of safety with regard to environmental contamination and public exposure.

Many solid waste and medical waste disposal facilities have radiation detection systems to monitor incoming waste shipments. It is prudent for hospitals to take measures to ensure that radioactive patient waste such as diapers are not inadvertently placed into non-radioactive waste containers. Many hospitals have radiation waste monitoring systems and housekeepers take solid waste containers past them before discarding the waste into dumpsters.

 ## 21.8 Regulatory Agencies and Radiation Exposure Limits

Regulatory Agencies

A number of regulatory agencies have jurisdiction over various aspects of the use of radiation in medicine. The regulations promulgated under their authority carry the force of law. These agencies can inspect facilities and records, levy fines, suspend activities, and issue and revoke radiation use authorizations.

The U.S. NRC regulates *special nuclear* material (plutonium and uranium enriched in the isotopes U-233 and U-235), *source* material (thorium, uranium, and their ores), and *by-product* material used in the commercial nuclear power industry, research, medicine, and a variety of other commercial activities. Under the terms of the Atomic Energy Act of 1954, which established the Atomic Energy Commission whose regulatory arm now exists as the NRC, the agency was given regulatory authority only for special nuclear, source, and by-product material. The term by-product material originally referred primarily to radioactive by-products of nuclear fission in nuclear reactors, that is, fission products and radioactive materials produced by neutron activation. However, the federal Energy Policy Act of 2005 modified the definition of by-product material to include material made radioactive by use of a particle accelerator. Thus, accelerator-produced radioactive materials (e.g., cyclotron-produced radionuclides such as F-18, Tl-201, I-123, and In-111) are now subject to NRC regulation.

Most states administer their own radiation control programs for radioactive materials and other radiation sources. These states have entered into agreements with the NRC, under the Atomic Energy Act of 1954, to promulgate and enforce regulations similar to those of the NRC and are known as "agreement states." These agreement states conduct the same regulatory oversight, inspection, and enforcement actions that would otherwise be performed by the NRC. In addition, the agencies of the agreement states typically regulate all sources of ionizing radiation, including diagnostic and interventional x-ray machines and linear accelerators used in radiation oncology.

While NRC and agreement state regulations are not identical, there are many essential aspects that are common to all of these regulatory programs. Workers must be informed of their rights and responsibilities, including the risks inherent in utilizing radiation sources and their responsibility to follow established safety procedures. The NRC's regulations are contained in Title 10 (Energy) of the Code of Federal Regulations (CFR). The most important sections for medical use of radionuclides are the "Standards for Protection against Radiation" (Part 20) and "Medical Use of By-Product Material" (Part 35). Part 20 contains the definitions utilized in the radiation control regulations and requirements for radiation surveys; personnel monitoring (dosimetry and bioassay); radiation warning signs and symbols; and shipment, receipt, control, storage, and disposal of radioactive material. Part 20 also specifies the maximal permissible doses to radiation workers and the public; environmental release limits; and documentation and notification requirements after a significant radiation accident or event, such as the loss of a brachytherapy source or the release of a large quantity of radioactive material to the environment.

Part 35 lists the requirements for the medical use of by-product material. Some of the issues covered in this section include the medical use categories, training requirements, precautions to be followed in the medical use of radiopharmaceuticals, testing and use of dose calibrators, and requirements for the reporting of medical events involving specified errors in the administrations of radiopharmaceuticals to patients. The NRC also issues regulatory guidance documents, which provide the licensee with methods acceptable to NRC for satisfying the regulations. The procedures listed in these documents may be adopted completely or in part with the licensee's own procedures, which will be subject to NRC review and approval.

The FDA regulates the development and manufacturing of radiopharmaceuticals as well as the manufacturing of medical x-ray equipment. Its regulations regarding the manufacture of medical x-ray imaging equipment contain extensive design and performance requirements for the equipment. Although this agency does not directly regulate the end user (except for mammography), it does maintain a strong involvement in both the technical and regulatory aspects of human research with radioactive materials and other radiation sources and publishes guidance documents in areas of interest including radiologic health, design and use of x-ray machines, and radiopharmaceutical development. FDA regulations, specifically 21 CFR 803, require the reporting of serious injuries and deaths that a medical device has or may have caused or contributed to.

The U.S. Department of Transportation (DOT) regulates the transportation of radioactive materials. Other regulations and recommendations related to medical radiation use programs are promulgated by other federal, state, and local agencies.

Advisory Bodies

Several advisory organizations exist that periodically review the scientific literature and issue recommendations regarding various aspects of radiation protection. While their recommendations do not constitute regulations and thus do not carry the force of law, they are usually the origin of most of regulations adopted by regulatory agencies and are widely recognized as "standards of good practice." Many of these recommendations are voluntarily adopted by the medical community even in the absence of a specific legal requirement. The two most widely recognized advisory bodies are the National Council on Radiation Protection and Measurements (NCRP) and the International Commission on Radiological Protection (ICRP). The NCRP is a nonprofit corporation chartered by Congress to collect, analyze, develop, and disseminate, in the public interest, information and recommendations about radiation protection, radiation measurements, quantities, and units. In addition, it is charged with working to stimulate cooperation and effective utilization of resources regarding radiation protection with other organizations including the ICRP.

The ICRP is similar in scope to the NCRP; however, its international membership brings to bear a variety of perspectives on radiation health issues. The dose limits of the countries in the European Union are based upon its recommendations. The NCRP and ICRP have published over 300 monographs containing recommendations on a wide variety of radiation health issues that serve as the reference documents from which many regulations are crafted.

NRC "Standards for Protection against Radiation"

As mentioned above, the NRC has established "Standards for Protection against Radiation" (10 CFR 20) to protect radiation workers and the public. The regulations incorporate a twofold system of dose limitation: (1) the doses to individuals shall not exceed limits established by the NRC, and (2) all exposures shall be kept ALARA, social and economic factors being taken into account. The regulations adopt a system recommended by the ICRP, which permits internal doses (from ingested or inhaled radionuclides) and doses from radiation sources outside the body to be summed, with a set of limits for the sum.

Summing Internal and External Doses

There are significant differences between external and internal exposures. The dose from an internal exposure continues after the period of ingestion or inhalation, until the radioactivity is eliminated by radioactive decay or biologic removal. The exposure may last only a few minutes, for example, in the case of the radionuclide O-15 ($T\frac{1}{2}$ = 122 s), or may last the lifetime of the individual, as is the case for the ingestion of long-lived Ra-226. The *committed dose equivalent* ($H_{50,T}$) is the dose equivalent to a tissue or organ over the 50 years following the ingestion or inhalation of radioactivity. The committed effective dose equivalent (CEDE) is a weighted average of the committed dose equivalents to the various tissues and organs of the body:

$$CEDE = \Sigma \ w_T H_{50,T} \qquad \text{[21-6]}$$

The NRC adopted the quantity *effective dose equivalent* and the tissue weighting factors (w_T) from ICRP Publication 26 (1977) and the annual limits on intake (ALI) of radionuclides by workers (discussed below) from ICRP Publication 30 (1978 to 1988), which predate those in the most current ICRP recommendations (ICRP Publication 103, see Chapter 3: Effective Dose).

To sum the internal and external doses to any individual tissue or organ, the deep dose equivalent (indicated by a dosimeter worn by the exposed individual) and the committed dose equivalent to the organ are added. The sum of the external and internal doses to the entire body, called the total effective dose equivalent (TEDE), is the sum of the deep dose equivalent and the CEDE.

Occupational Dose Limits

The NRC's radiation dose limits are intended to limit the risks of stochastic effects, such as cancer and genetic effects, and to prevent deterministic effects, such as cataracts, skin damage, sterility, and hematologic consequences of bone marrow depletion (deterministic and stochastic effects are discussed in Chapter 20). To limit the risk of stochastic effects, the sum of the external and internal doses to the entire body, the TEDE, may not exceed 0.05 Sv (5 rem) in a year. To prevent deterministic effects, the sum of the external dose and committed dose equivalent to any individual organ except the lens of the eye may not exceed 0.5 Sv (50 rem) in a year. The dose limit to the lens of the eye is 0.15 Sv (15 rem) in a year (Fig. 21-21). As discussed in Chapter 20, the ICRP recently reviewed the scientific evidence regarding the risk of radiation-induced cataract and proposed a much more conservative occupational equivalent dose limit for the lens of the eye (20 mSv per year averaged over 5 years, with no single year dose >50 mSv).

The dose to the fetus of a declared pregnant radiation worker may not exceed 5 mSv (0.5 rem) over the 9-month gestational period and should not substantially exceed 500 µSv (50 mrem) in any 1 month. Table 21-10 lists the most important ICRP and NRC radiation dose limits.

Annual Limits on Intake and Derived Air Concentrations

In practice, the committed dose equivalent and CEDE are seldom used in protecting workers from ingesting or inhaling radioactivity. Instead, the NRC has established annual limits on intake (ALIs), which limit the inhalation or ingestion of radioactive

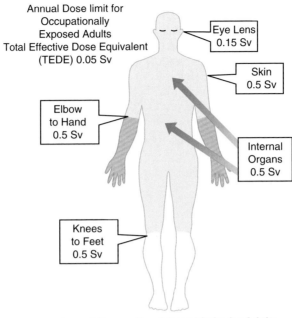

Annual Dose limit for
Occupationally
Exposed Adults
Total Effective Dose Equivalent
(TEDE) 0.05 Sv

Eye Lens
0.15 Sv

Skin
0.5 Sv

Elbow
to Hand
0.5 Sv

Internal
Organs
0.5 Sv

Knees
to Feet
0.5 Sv

**Annual Occupational Dose Limits for Adults
NRC 10CFR20**

■ **FIGURE 21-21** NRC's occupational radiation dose limits.

material to activities that will not cause radiation workers to exceed any of the limits in Table 21-10. The ALIs are calculated for the "standard person" and expressed in units of microcuries. ALIs are provided for the inhalation and oral ingestion pathways for a wide variety of radionuclides, some examples of which, relevant to nuclear medicine, are shown in Table 21-11.

Exposure to airborne activity is also regulated via the derived air concentration (DAC), which is that concentration of a radionuclide that, if breathed under conditions of light activity for 2,000 h (the average number of hours worked in a year), will result in the ALI; DACs are expressed in units of μCi/mL. Table 21-11 lists DACs and ALIs for volatile radionuclides of interest in medical imaging. In circumstances in which either the external exposure or the internal deposition does not exceed 10% of its respective limits, summation of the internal and external doses is not required to demonstrate compliance with the dose limits; most nuclear medicine departments will be able to take advantage of this exemption.

As Low as Reasonably Achievable Principle

Dose limits to workers and the public are regarded as upper limits rather than as acceptable doses or thresholds of safety. In fact, the majority of occupational exposures in medicine and industry result in doses far below these limits. In addition to the dose limits specified in the regulations, all licensees are required to employ good health physics practices and implement radiation safety programs to ensure that radiation exposures to workers and members of the public are kept *ALARA*, taking societal and economic factors into consideration. The ALARA doctrine is the driving force for many of the policies, procedures, and practices in radiation laboratories and represents a commitment by both employee and employer to minimize radiation exposure to staff and the public. For example, the *L*-shield in the nuclear pharmacy

TABLE 21-10 NUCLEAR REGULATORY COMMISSION REGULATORY REQUIREMENTS (NRC 2011) AND INTERNATIONAL COMMISSION ON RADIOLOGICAL PROTECTION RECOMMENDATIONS (ICRP 2007) FOR MAXIMUM PERMISSIBLE DOSE

LIMITS[a]	MAXIMUM PERMISSIBLE ANNUAL DOSE LIMITS	
	ICRP 2007 mSv	NRC mSv (rem)
Occupational Limits		
Effective dose (total effective dose equivalent)	20/y, averaged over 5 y; 50 in any 1 y	50 (5)
Equivalent dose (Dose equivalent) to any individual organ (except lens of eye) including skin; hands, feet	500	500 (50)
Equivalent dose (Dose equivalent) to the lens of the eye	20/y, averaged over 5 y; 50 in any 1 y	150 (15)
Minor (<18 years old)	Public limits	10% of adult limits
Equivalent dose (Dose equivalent) to an embryo or fetus[b]	1 in 9 mo	5 (0.5) in 9 mo
Non-occupational (public) Limits	1	1.0 (0.1)
Effective dose (total effective dose equivalent)	1	1 (0.1)
Effective dose (total effective dose equivalent) to medical caregivers (e.g., at home with I-131 therapy patient)	5 per episode; 20/y maximum	5 (0.5)
Dose equivalent in an unrestricted area	NA	0.02 (0.002) in any 1 h[c]

[a]These limits are exclusive of natural background and any dose the individual receives for medical purposes; inclusive of internal committed dose equivalent and external effective dose equivalent (i.e., total effective dose equivalent). As explained in the text, ICRP and NRC use different (although similar) dose quantities. In this column the first quantity is the ICRP quantity and the NRC quantity is in parentheses.
[b]Applies only to a conceptus of a worker who declares her pregnancy. If the limit exceeds 4.5 mSv (450 mrem) at declaration, conceptus dose for remainder of gestation is not to exceed 0.5 mSv (50 mrem).
[c]This means the dose to an unrestricted area (irrespective of occupancy) shall not exceed 0.02 mSv (2 mrem) in any 1 h. This is not a restriction of instantaneous dose rate to 0.02 mSv/h (2 mrem/h).
ICRP. The 2007 Recommendations of the International Commission on Radiological Protection. ICRP Publication 103. *Ann ICRP* 2007;37:1–332.

TABLE 21-11 EXAMPLES OF DACs AND ALI FOR OCCUPATIONALLY EXPOSED WORKERS (NRC REGULATIONS: 10 CFR 20)

RADIONUCLIDE	DAC (μCi/mL)[a]	ALI (μCi)[a] INGESTION
I-125	3×10^{-8}	40
I-131	2×10^{-8}	30
Tc-99m	6×10^{-5}	8×10^4
Xe-133 (gas)	1×10^{-4}	N/A

[a]Multiply μCi/mL (or μCi) by 37 to obtain kBq/mL (or kBq).
N/A, not applicable.

may not be specifically required by a regulatory agency; however, its use has become common practice in nuclear medicine departments and represents a "community standard" against which the department's practices will be evaluated.

The ALARA principle is equivalent to the ICRP's principle of optimization of protection, stated in Section 21.4. While the NRC's regulations only apply the ALARA principle to the radiation doses of workers and members of the public, the ICRP and many other advisory bodies, professional societies, and governmental agencies recommend the application of the ALARA principle to the radiation doses received by patients in diagnostic and interventional imaging.

21.9 Prevention of Errors

A goal of radiation protection programs is to reduce the likelihood and severity of accidents involving radiation and radioactive materials. Although this pertains to the protection of staff, patients, and members of the public, this section focuses on protection of the patient. However, the principles discussed apply to all of these categories of people.

Error prevention is certainly not a field exclusive to medical radiation protection or even medicine in general. Most of the principles have been developed in other industries such as aviation and nuclear power. The report, To Err Is Human, by the Institute of Medicine in 2000 (Kohn et al., 2004) focused attention on errors in the delivery of care to patients. There has been national media attention regarding the delivery of excessive doses to patients by CT (Bogdanich, 2009) and the professional literature has reported the delivery of unnecessarily high doses to children and infants from CT due to the use of adult technique factors (Patterson et al., 2001). Methods for the prevention of errors in the delivery of care to patients are only briefly discussed in this section.

Efforts in error prevention can be prospective, to avoid errors in the future, or retrospective, in response to an error or "near miss" that has occurred, with the goal of preventing a recurrence. The efforts directed toward prevention of a particular error should be in proportion to the severity of the consequences of the error and of the likelihood of the error. Methods for the prevention of errors include the development of written procedures and training of staff initially, periodically thereafter, and in response to incidents or changes in procedures. Policies and procedures may incorporate the use of a "time out" in which the staff about to perform a clinical procedure jointly verify that the intended procedure is to be properly performed on the intended patient; the use of written or computerized checklists to ensure that essential actions are not omitted; checks of critical tasks by a second person; requiring that certain critical communications be in writing; employing readback in verbal communications, whereby the person hearing information repeats it aloud; and measures to avoid distractions and interruptions during critical tasks, such as prohibiting unnecessary conversations unrelated to a task. In developing procedures, it is advisable to consider what errors might occur, procedures developed at other institutions, and errors that have occurred in the past. The incorporation of engineered safety features, such as interlocks that prevent unsafe actions, and automated checks, such as the dose notifications and alerts provided by newer CT scanners, help avoid accidents due to human errors. The Joint Commission (TJC) has included similar recommendations in a universal protocol to prevent error prior to surgery, which is one of a number of its national patient safety goals (TJC, 2010).

When an error or a "near miss" occurs, an analysis should be performed to determine the causes and to devise actions to reduce the likelihood of a recurrence and possibly, the severity of a recurrence. These analyses attempt to identify the most basic correctable causes, called "root causes." Methods for such root cause analyses may be found in several texts. The actions implemented to avoid a recurrence should be designed with the root causes in mind.

Safety culture is a set of attributes of an organization, such as a radiology or nuclear medicine department, that are believed to reduce the likelihood of errors. There are varying, but similar definitions or descriptions by various organizations focusing on safety. Safety culture may be defined as the behavior and practices resulting from a commitment by leaders and individuals to emphasize safety over competing goals to protect patients, staff, and the public. The following list of traits of a safety culture was adapted from an NRC policy statement (NRC, 2011):

- Leaders demonstrate a commitment to safety in their decisions and behaviors.
- All individuals take personal responsibility for safety.
- Issues potentially impacting safety are promptly identified, evaluated, and corrected commensurate with their significance.
- Work activities are planned and conducted so that safety is maintained.
- Opportunities to learn about ways to ensure safety are sought out and implemented.
- A work environment is maintained in which people feel free to raise safety concerns.
- Communications maintain a focus on safety.
- Trust and respect permeate the organization.
- Workers avoid complacency and continuously challenge, in a spirit of cooperation, conditions and activities in order to identify discrepancies that might result in error.

The Joint Commission

The Joint Commission (TJC), formerly the Joint Commission on Accreditation of Healthcare Organizations, is a not-for-profit organization that accredits thousands of hospitals and other health care facilities in the United States. Most state governments have conditioned receipt of Medicaid reimbursement on accreditation by TJC or a similar organization.

TJC defines a *sentinel event* as "an unexpected occurrence involving death or serious physical or psychological injury, or the risk thereof." A sentinel event does not necessarily indicate that a medical error has occurred. However, each sentinel event should be promptly investigated and action taken if warranted.

TJC defines as a sentinel event prolonged fluoroscopy with a cumulative dose exceeding 15 Gy to a single field, "a single field" being a location on the skin onto which the x-ray beam is directed. The issue here is the magnitude of the dose to that portion of the skin that receives the maximal dose. The maximal dose may result from using several different x-ray beam projections whose beam areas on the patient's skin overlap in a specific location to produce a region of highest radiation dose. It may also result from two or more procedures days or even months apart.

TJC issues sentinel event alerts (SEAs) which identify serious unanticipated incidents in a health care setting that could or did harm patients. TJC expects accredited facilities to consider information in an SEA when evaluating similar processes and consider implementing relevant suggestions contained in the SEA or reasonable alternatives. TJC has issued a SEA, *Radiation Risks of Diagnostic Imaging* (TJC, 2011). It warns that health care organizations must seek new ways to reduce exposure to repeated doses of harmful radiation from these diagnostic procedures. The SEA urges greater attention to the risk of long-term damage and cumulative harm that can occur if a patient is given repeated doses of diagnostic radiation. TJC suggests that health care organizations can reduce risks due to avoidable diagnostic radiation by raising awareness among staff and patients of the increased risks associated with cumulative doses and by providing the right test and the right dose through effective processes, safe technology and a culture of safety. The actions suggested include

- Use of imaging techniques other than CT, such as ultrasound or MRI, and collaboration between radiologists and referring physicians about the appropriate use of diagnostic imaging.
- Adherence to the ALARA principle, as well as guidelines from the Society for Pediatric Radiology, American College of Radiology and the Radiological Society of North America, for imaging for children and adults.
- Assurance by radiologists that the proper dosing protocol is in place for the patient being treated and review of all dosing protocols either annually or every 2 years.
- Expansion of the RSO's role to explicitly include patient safety as it relates to radiation and dosing, as well as education on proper dosing and equipment usage for all physicians and technologists who prescribe diagnostic radiation or use diagnostic radiation equipment.
- Use of a diagnostic medical physicist in designing and altering CT scan protocols; centralized quality and safety performance monitoring of all diagnostic imaging equipment that may emit high amounts of cumulative radiation; testing imaging equipment initially and annually or every 2 years thereafter; and designing a program for quality control, testing (including daily functional tests) and preventive maintenance activities.
- Investing in technologies that optimize or reduce dose.

21.10 Management of Radiation Safety Programs

The goals of a radiation safety program were discussed in the introductory paragraph of this chapter. They include maintaining the safety of staff, patients, and members of the public; compliance with regulations of governmental agencies; and preparedness for emergencies involving radiation and/or radioactive material. In particular, the radiation doses of staff and members of the public must not exceed regulatory limits and should conform to the ALARA principle (equivalent to the ICRP's principle of optimization), as described earlier in this chapter. Although there are no regulatory limits to the radiation doses that patients may receive as part of their care, the doses to patients should be optimized. The methods for achieving these goals are described in the other sections of this chapter.

A license from a state regulatory agency, or the US NRC, is required to possess and use radioactive materials in medicine. The license lists the radioactive materials that may be used, the amounts that may be possessed, and the uses that are allowed. The licenses for most institutions list the physicians permitted to use and supervise the use of radioactive material. Licenses also contain requirements, in addition to the regulations of the state regulatory agency or NRC, regarding procedures and record-keeping requirements for radioactive material receipt, transportation, use, and disposal. Radioactive material use regulations require "cradle-to-grave" control of all radiation sources.

Each institution must designate a person, called the RSO, who is responsible for the day-to-day oversight of the radiation safety program and is named on the institution's radioactive material license. At a smaller institution, the RSO may be a physician or a consultant. A larger institution may have a person whose main duty is to be the RSO. At very large institutions, the RSO is assisted by a health physics department.

An institution with complex uses of radiation and radioactive material will have a radiation safety committee that oversees the radiation safety program. A radiation safety committee typically meets quarterly and approves policies and procedures, periodically reviews the program, and reviews corrective actions after adverse incidents involving radiation or radioactive material. The radiation safety committee is comprised of the RSO, representatives from departments with substantial radiation and radioactive material use (e.g., nuclear medicine, radiology, cardiology, radiation oncology, and nursing), and a member representing hospital management.

A radiation safety program should include an audit program to ensure compliance with regulatory requirements, accepted radiation safety practices, and institutional procedures. The audit program should evaluate people's knowledge and performance of radiation safety–related activities in addition to reviewing records. This is best accomplished by observing people while they perform tasks related to radiation safety. Personnel dosimetry reports should be reviewed when they arrive from the dosimetry vendor and larger or unusual doses should be investigated. The radiation safety program should ensure the training of staff in regulatory requirements, good radiation safety practices, and institutional procedures; training should be provided initially, periodically thereafter, and as needed, for example, following incidents, changes in regulations, or changes in uses of radiation or radioactive material. A review should be performed of the radiation safety program at least annually, with the findings presented to the radiation safety committee and executive management. The radiation safety program should be "risk informed," that is, the efforts devoted to radiation safety regarding a particular use should be in proportion to the risks associated with that use.

A diagnostic medical physicist is essential to the radiation safety program of a medical facility performing radiological imaging. A diagnostic medical physicist has expertise in the diagnostic and interventional applications of x-rays, gamma rays, ultrasonic radiation, radiofrequency radiation, and magnetic fields; the equipment associated with their production, use, measurement, and evaluation; the doses of radiation to patients from these sources; the quality of images resulting from their production and use; and medical health physics associated with their production and use. A duty of the diagnostic medical physicist is testing imaging equipment initially, annually thereafter, and after repairs or modifications that may affect the radiation doses to patients or the quality of the images. The diagnostic medical physicist should also participate in the creation and evaluation of the organization's technical quality assurance programs, safety programs (e.g., radiation safety and MRI safety) regarding diagnostic and interventional imaging, and optimization of clinical imaging protocols. Diagnostic medical physicists commonly design the structural shielding for rooms containing radiation-producing equipment and perform shielding evaluations, based upon measurements of transmitted radiation, after the installation of the shielding. Another task occasionally performed is the estimation of the radiation dose to the embryo or fetus after a pregnant patient received an examination before her pregnancy was known or when a procedure on a pregnant patient is being considered. The RSO may be a diagnostic medical physicist.

Another task of a radiation safety program is to respond to adverse incidents or regulatory violations. When such an incident or violation is identified, an analysis of the causes should be performed and actions to prevent a recurrence should be implemented. In some cases, such as a medical event involving a patient, serious injury or death of a patient involving medical equipment, or a person receiving a radiation dose exceeding a regulatory limit, notification of the pertinent state or federal regulatory agency may be required. When such an incident occurs, action to protect the patient, staff, or other people should take priority over meeting regulatory requirements.

IMAGING OF PREGNANT AND POTENTIALLY PREGNANT PATIENTS

The risks of ionizing radiation to the embryo and fetus must be considered when imaging female patients of childbearing age using ionizing radiation and performing therapies using radiopharmaceuticals. These risks vary with the radiation dose and the stage of gestation and have been discussed in Chapter 20. Each department performing imaging or treatments with ionizing radiation should have policies and procedures regarding this issue.

In general, the pregnancy status of a patient of childbearing age should be determined prior to an imaging examination or treatment involving ionizing radiation. Pregnancy status should be determined for female patients from about 12 to 50 years of age. The measures to determine whether a patient is pregnant depend upon the radiation dose that an embryo or fetus would receive. For most examinations, a technologist asks the patient whether she could possibly be pregnant, inquiring about the last menstruation, and documents this information on a form. For a patient who is a minor, it is best to obtain this information in a private setting without the parents or a guardian present. For some procedures that would or might impart doses to an embryo or fetus exceeding 100 mSv, such as possibly prolonged fluoroscopically guided procedures and multi-phase diagnostic CT examinations of the abdomen or pelvis, a pregnancy test should also be obtained within 72 hours before the examination or procedure, unless the examination is medically urgent or the possibility of pregnancy can be eliminated by factors such as a documented hysterectomy. Pregnancy tests should always be obtained before radiopharmaceutical therapies. Pregnancy tests can produce false-negative results and should not preclude questioning the patient regarding the possibility of pregnancy. There are some examinations that can be performed without regard to pregnancy due to the very low dose that an embryo or fetus would receive if the patient were pregnant. These include mammograms and diagnostic x-ray imaging of the head, arms and hands, and lower legs and feet.

Occasionally imaging is considered for a patient who is known to be pregnant or suspected of being pregnant. In this case, the radiation dose and potential risks to the embryo or fetus should be estimated and presented to the imaging physician. Consideration should be given to whether the examination or procedure can be delayed until after the pregnancy, alternative examinations or procedures that would not involve ionizing radiation, or that would deliver less radiation to the embryo or fetus, and ways to modify the examination to reduce the radiation dose to the embryo or fetus. However, care should be taken to ensure that modifications to reduce the radiation dose do not cause an inadequate examination that must be repeated. The imaging physician must obtain informed consent from the patient.

Occasionally it is discovered, after an examination or treatment with ionizing radiation was performed, that the patient was pregnant at the time of the examination or treatment. In this case, fetal age, the radiation dose to the embryo or fetus, and the potential effects on the embryo or fetus should be estimated. The dose estimation is commonly performed by a diagnostic medical physicist. The patient is then counseled by a physician. In most cases, the risks to the embryo or fetus are small in comparison with the other risks of gestation. Professional consensus is that in no cases should medical intervention with a pregnancy be considered for estimated doses to the embryo or fetus that do not exceed 100 mSv; if the dose exceeds 100 mSv, decisions would be guided by the fetal age and individual circumstances. All x-ray imaging examinations, in which the embryo or fetus is not close to the area being imaged, impart doses much less that 100 mSv to the embryo or fetus and most x-ray examinations of the abdomen and pelvis, including single phase diagnostic CT examinations, impart doses less than 100 mSv. More detailed guidance regarding the pregnant or possibly pregnant patient is available in ACR, 2008; Wagner et al., 1997.

21.12 Medical Emergencies Involving Ionizing Radiation

Medical institutions should be prepared to respond to emergencies involving radiation and radioactive materials. These may include incidents within the institution, such as spills of radioactive material, contamination of personnel with radioactive material, and medical events involving errors in the administration of radioactive material to patients; these also include external incidents, such as transportation accidents involving shipments of radioactive material, accidents at nuclear facilities, and radiological or nuclear terrorism, which could result in contaminated and injured people arriving at medical facilities. Serious accidents involving substantial radiation exposure or contamination are rare. Hence, most health care providers are unfamiliar with (and may have unjustified fear of) treating patients who have been exposed to radiation or contaminated with radioactive material. Radiologists and other health care professionals familiar with the properties of radiation, its detection, and biological effects (e.g., radiation oncologists, radiation therapists, health and medical physicists, and nuclear medicine and radiology technologists) may be called upon to assist in such emergencies and should be prepared to provide guidance and technical assistance to medical staff managing such patients; they should also assist the medical institution's emergency planner in preparing for such emergencies. The overarching goal in these incidents is to ensure that critically ill or injured patients are not denied effective medical care due to unfounded concerns of medical personnel about risk from providing care to the patients.

Potential Sources of Radiation Exposure and Contamination

Radiation Accidents

Incidents have occurred in which people have been injured by inadvertently coming into contact with objects or material that they did not realize contained large quantities of radioactive material. Small metal capsules containing high-intensity gamma-emitting radioactive sources are commonly used for industrial radiography. Failure to realize or report the loss of such sources has resulted in a number of severe radiation injuries to individuals who found the sources but did not recognize the danger. In two cases, stolen radioactive sources once used for cancer therapy were opened, causing widespread contamination and injury to people (Juarez Mexico in 1983 and 1984, Goiânia Brazil in 1987).

A nuclear reactor accident, in which an accidental prompt-critical power excursion caused a steam explosion (Chernobyl in the Ukraine in 1986), killed workers and emergency responders and released massive amounts of fission products to the environment. In 2011, a tsunami following a massive earthquake off the coast of Japan caused the loss of core cooling of multiple reactors at the Fukushima Daiichi nuclear power facility. Even though the reactors shut down during the earthquake (stopping further fissioning of the fuel in the reactors), there was still a tremendous amount of heat being produced by the decay of the fission products already created. The inability to adequately remove this heat ultimately led to partial core meltdowns.

The release of large quantities of fission products from the damaged reactors resulted in widespread environmental contamination requiring the evacuation of large populations living within 30 to 50 km from the site.

Radiological and Nuclear Terrorism

There has been increasing concern that radioactive material or an improvised nuclear device (an improvised nuclear weapon, less likely but potentially much more devastating) could be used as a weapon of terrorism. A hidden radioactive source, referred to as a radiation exposure device, could be used to expose people to large doses of radiation. Victims of such a device might exhibit the signs and symptoms of the acute radiation syndrome and possibly also localized radiation skin injuries. Alternatively, a large activity of radioactive material could be dispersed in a populated area. A device to do this is referred to as a radiological dispersal device (RDD). An RDD that uses a chemical explosion to accomplish the dispersion is called a "dirty bomb." An RDD, to be effective, would require a large activity of a radioactive material with a relatively long half-life and that emits abundant penetrating radiation and/or has a high radiotoxicity if ingested or inhaled. Radionuclides having these qualities and which are commonly used in very large activities are Co-60 ($T_{1/2}$ = 5.27 years, 1.17 and 1.33 MeV gamma rays), Sr-90 ($T_{1/2}$ = 28.8 years, no gamma rays, very high–energy beta rays), Cs-137 ($T_{1/2}$ = 30.1 years, 662 keV gamma rays), Ir-192 ($T_{1/2}$ = 73.8 days, 296 to 612 keV gamma rays), and Am-241 ($T_{1/2}$ = 433 years, 59.5 keV gamma rays, alpha particles). A dirty bomb detonation could result in a few or dozens of casualties with trauma and radioactive contamination and a much larger number of uninjured people with radioactive contamination. Attack on or sabotage of a nuclear power facility or shipments of large quantities of radioactive material could also cause widespread contamination; attacks of this nature have the potential to release a much larger quantity of radioactive material. In recent years, many countries have greatly increased the security of nuclear facilities and of sources containing large activities of radioactive material (including those in hospitals and research facilities) to prevent or discourage radiological terrorism.

The detonation of an improvised or stolen nuclear weapon in a city is much less likely than other forms of terrorism because construction of such a device requires several kilograms of plutonium or highly enriched uranium and considerable technical expertise, and access to nuclear weapons is tightly controlled. However, with the proliferation of nuclear weapons and nuclear weapons technology, such an attack may become more likely in the future. The successful use of such a device in a major metropolitan area would be devastating, with an area around the weapon demolished by blast and prompt thermal radiation. If the weapon were detonated at ground level or a low altitude, there would be extensive radioactive fallout in a pattern determined by surface and higher-altitude winds. A large number of casualties would be created rapidly by the blast wave, collapses of structures, injuries from shrapnel and falling objects, prompt thermal radiation, fires caused by the explosion and prompt radiation consisting of x- and gamma rays, and neutrons from the detonation. Delayed radiation injuries, particularly the acute radiation syndrome from exposure to gamma rays from radioactive fallout and cutaneous injuries from beta radiation from fallout on the skin, would also occur to some people in the fallout zone. The mass casualties, widespread infrastructure failure, and initial inability to operate in the fallout zone would greatly impede the response to the incident.

Each medical facility has or should have a plan for responding to radiation emergencies of varying types and scopes. In particular, the emergency department (ED) should be expected to receive and treat injured patients with radioactive contamination. Radioactive contamination has only very rarely been an immediate health

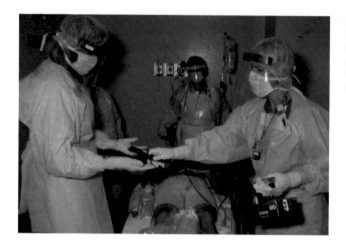

■ **FIGURE 21-22** Standard protective clothing commonly worn by ED staff and periodic surveys with a GM survey meter protect staff from contamination with radioactive material.

threat to patients and almost never to medical staff. Treatment of severe injuries or life-threatening medical conditions should take priority over decontamination, although very simple and quick measures, such as removal of the patients' clothing and wiping exposed skin with mild soap, tepid water, and a damp cloth, will likely remove most of the contamination. Standard protective clothing commonly worn by ED staff is sufficient to protect them from radioactive contamination. Periodic surveys with a GM detector and methods similar to common infection prevention techniques will prevent significant contamination with radioactive material (Fig. 21-22).

Concern for radiation exposure or radioactive material contamination should not prevent the use of any of a hospital's diagnostic and treatment capabilities including the use of medical imaging facilities and operating rooms. Most contamination can be prevented and any contamination that does occur can be managed and would not render any of these facilities inoperable or unsuitable for other critically ill patients.

Following a large-scale emergency involving radiation and/or radioactive material, it is possible that many people, perhaps some with radioactive contamination, but without serious injuries or medical conditions requiring emergency treatment, will arrive at medical centers seeking care. The medical centers' plans should include measures to prevent the emergency departments from becoming overwhelmed by these people. Each community should prepare to establish decontamination centers away from hospitals. However, each medical center should prepare to promptly establish a triage, monitoring, and decontamination center away from the emergency department and to divert to this center people not requiring emergency care. More detailed information on developing a radiological emergency response plan, staff training, and sources of expert consultation are widely available (ACR, 2006; Bushberg et al., 2007; HPS, 2011; NCRP, 2001, 2005, 2009, 2010b; REAC/TS, 2011; REMM, 2011).

Decontamination of People

External radioactive contamination is contamination of a person's clothing, skin, and perhaps other parts of the body surface with radioactive material. An incident involving external radioactive contamination may be as simple as a single nuclear medicine or research laboratory worker who has spilled radioactive material on a small part of his or her body or it could involve dozens or hundreds of people, some injured and many contaminated, arriving at a medical center after a radiological terrorist incident.

Decontamination is commonly performed by removing contaminated clothing and washing the contaminated area with soap and water, taking care not to spread contamination to other parts of the body or onto other people and to ensure that people do not inhale or ingest the radioactive material. If the radioactive material is not water soluble, another solvent may be needed. Uncontaminated wounds should be protected by waterproof dressings during decontamination. Thermal burns of the skin should be decontaminated by gentle rinsing with sterile saline solution, but should not be scrubbed to avoid further injury. The progress of decontamination is assessed by surveys using a portable radiation survey meter. Decontamination is performed until the amount of remaining radioactive contamination approaches background levels or until decontamination efforts cease to reduce the amount of remaining contamination. If large numbers of people are contaminated, a greater amount of residual contamination may have to be accepted. Decontamination efforts should not abrade the skin to avoid the absorption of radioactive material through the injured skin.

Contaminated wounds are decontaminated by flushing with sterile saline and mild scrubbing. Excision of viable tissue to remove radioactive contamination should be performed only after consulting with an expert.

Personnel with external radioactive contamination, particularly on the upper parts of their bodies, may also have internal contamination. Radioactive contamination of a person should never delay critical medical care.

Treatment for Internal Radioactive Contamination

The term *internal contamination* refers to radioactive material in the body. It may enter the body by inhalation, ingestion, through a wound, by injection, or, for some radioactive material, by absorption through the skin. It may result from an accident, poor contamination control in the workplace, a terrorist act or an act of war, or an administration error in nuclear medicine.

Effective treatment of internal contamination varies with the radionuclide, its chemical and physical form, and, in some cases, its route into the body. In general, treatment is more effective the sooner it is begun after the radioactive material is introduced into the body. Hence, it may be best to begin treatment before definitive information is available. NCRP Report No. 161, *Management of Persons Contaminated with Radionuclides*, provides detailed guidance on the treatment of internal contamination (NCRP, 2008).

An accident in nuclear medicine or a research laboratory or a nuclear reactor accident with a release of fission products can cause internal contamination with radioactive iodine. Radioactive iodine is sequestered by the thyroid gland and retained with a long biological half-life. The most effective treatment is to administer nonradioactive iodine to block thyroidal uptake of the radioactive iodine. This treatment is most effective the sooner it is begun, becoming much less effective with time after an intake. Table 21-12 provides guidance for the treatment of internal contamination with radioactive iodine.

The amount of internal contamination and the effectiveness of treatment may be assessed by bioassays. Bioassays are usually either measurements of radiation from the body (e.g., thyroid counts using a thyroid probe or whole-body counts using a whole-body counter) or assays of excreta, usually urine.

TABLE 21-12   GUIDANCE FOR KI ADMINISTRATION: THRESHOLD THYROID RADIOACTIVE EXPOSURES AND RECOMMENDED DOSAGES OF KI FOR DIFFERENT RISK GROUPS

	PREDICTED THYROID GLAND EXPOSURE (cGy)[d]	KI DOSE (mg)	NUMBER OR FRACTION OF 130 mg TABLETS	NUMBER OR FRACTION OF 65 mg TABLETS	MILLILITERS (mL) OF ORAL SOLUTION, 65 mg/mL[a]
Adults over 40 y	≥500	130	1	2	2 mL
Adults over 18 through 40 y	≥10	130	1	2	2 mL
Pregnant or Lactating Women	≥5	130	1	2	2 mL
Adolescents, 12 through 18 y[b]	≥5	65	½	1	1 mL
Children over 3 y through 12 y	≥5	65	½	1	1 mL
Children 1 mo through 3 y	≥5	32	Use KI oral solution[c]	½	0.5 mL
Infants birth through 1 mo	≥5	16	Use KI oral solution[c]	Use KI oral solution[c]	0.25 mL

[a]See the Home Preparation Procedure for Emergency Administration of Potassium Iodide Tablets to Infants and Small Children at the URL below.
[b]Adolescents approaching adult size (≥150 lbs) should receive the full adult dose (130 mg)
[c]Potassium iodide oral solution is supplied in 1 oz (30 mL) bottles with a dropper marked for 1, 0.5, and 0.25 mL dosing. Each mL contains 65 mg potassium iodide.
[d]A centigray (cGy) is a hundredth of a gray (Gy) and is equal to one rad.
NAS: National Research Council. *Distribution and administration potassium iodide in the event of a nuclear incident.* Washington, DC: National Academies Press, 2004.
http://www.fda.gov/Drugs/EmergencyPreparedness/BioterrorismandDrugPreparedness/ucm072248.htm

Treatment of the Acute Radiation Syndrome

The acute radiation syndrome, discussed in Chapter 20, is typically caused by the irradiation of the entire body or a large portion of the body to a very large dose of penetrating radiation, such as x-rays, gamma rays, or neutrons. An acute dose of x- or gamma rays to the bone marrow exceeding 0.5 Gy is usually necessary to cause the syndrome; an acute dose of about 3.5 gray will kill about half of exposed individuals without medical care; and an acute dose exceeding 10 gray will kill nearly all individuals even with medical care. The lethality is increased by skin burns or trauma. The most significant adverse effects, for individuals receiving doses that they may survive, are injury to the lining of the gastrointestinal tract and the red bone marrow, causing a loss of electrolytes, the entry of intestinal flora into the body, and a depression or even elimination of white blood cells, increasing the risk of infection.

The dose received by an individual can be crudely estimated by the severity of the prodromal phase, particularly the time to emesis. It can be more accurately estimated by the kinetics of circulating white blood cells, particularly lymphocytes, and by a cytogenetic assay of circulating lymphocytes, which requires a blood sample to be sent to a specialized laboratory. Treatment involves reverse isolation, support of electrolytes, support of bone marrow recovery by the administration of cytokines, perhaps the administration of irradiated red blood cells and platelets, prophylactic treatment with antibiotics, and treatment of infections (Waselenko et al., 2004). If surgery is needed for injuries, it should either be performed in the first 2 days after the exposure or should be delayed until the hematopoietic system recovers.

SUGGESTED READINGS

American College of Radiology, ACR Practice Guideline for Imaging Pregnant or Potentially Pregnant Adolescents and Women with Ionizing Radiation, 2008.

Brateman L. The AAPM/RSNA physics tutorial for residents: radiation safety considerations for diagnostic radiology personnel. *RadioGraphics* 1999;19:1037–1055.

Bushberg JT, Leidholdt EM Jr. Radiation protection. In: Sandler MP et al., eds. *Diagnostic nuclear medicine.* 4th ed. Philadelphia, PA: Lippincott Williams & Wilkins, 2001.

International Commission on Radiological Protection. ICRP Publication 102: Managing patient dose in multi-detector computed tomography (MDCT) Annals of the ICRP Volume 37/1 2007

International Commission on Radiological Protection. *ICRP Publication 105: Radiological Protection in Medicine Annals of the ICRP Volume 37 Issue 6.*

Miller DL, Vano E, Bartel G, et al. Occupational radiation protection in interventional radiology: A joint guideline of the cardiolvascular and interventional society of Europe and the society of interventional radiology. *Cardiovasc Intervent Radiol* 2010;33:230–239.

National Council on Radiation Protection and Measurements. *Medical x-ray, electron beam, and gamma-ray protection for energies up to 50 MeV (equipment design, performance, and use).* NCRP Report No. 102. Bethesda, MD: National Council on Radiation Protection and Measurements, 1989.

National Council on Radiation Protection and Measurements. *Radiation protection for medical and allied health personnel.* NCRP Report No. 105. Bethesda, MD: National Council on Radiation Protection and Measurements, 1989.

National Council on Radiation Protection and Measurements. *Limitation of exposure to ionizing radiation.* NCRP Report No. 116. Bethesda, MD: National Council on Radiation Protection and Measurements, 1993.

National Council on Radiation Protection and Measurements. *Sources and magnitude of occupational and public exposures from nuclear medicine procedures.* NCRP Report No. 124. Bethesda, MD: National Council on Radiation Protection and Measurements, 1996.

National Council on Radiation Protection and Measurements. *Radionuclide exposure of the embryo/fetus.* NCRP Report No. 128. Bethesda, MD: National Council on Radiation Protection and Measurements, 2000.

National Council on Radiation Protection and Measurements. *Radiation protection for procedures performed outside the radiology department.* NCRP Report No. 133. Bethesda, MD: National Council on Radiation Protection and Measurements, 2000.

National Council on Radiation Protection and Measurements. *Ionizing Radiation Exposure of the Population of the United States.* NCRP Report No. 160. Bethesda, MD: National Council on Radiation Protection and Measurements, 2009.

National Council on Radiation Protection and Measurements. *Radiation Dose Management for Fluoroscopically-Guided Interventional Medical Procedures.* NCRP Report No. 168. Bethesda, MD: National Council on Radiation Protection and Measurements, 2010.

National Council on Radiation Protection and Measurements. Proceedings of the 43rd Annual NCRP Meeting (2007). *Adv Radiat Protect Med Health Phys* 2008;95(5).

Schueler BA, Vrieze TJ, Bjarnason H, et al. An investigation of operator exposure in interventional radiology. *Radiographics* 2006;26:1533–1541.

Siegel JA. *Guide for diagnostic nuclear medicine.* Reston, VA: Society of Nuclear Medicine, 2002.

Title 10 (Energy) of the Code of Federal Regulations (CFR), Part 20: Standards for Protection Against Radiation.

Title 10 (Energy) of the Code of Federal Regulations (CFR), Part 35: Medical Use of By-product Material.

Wagner LK, Archer BR. *Minimizing risks from fluoroscopic x-rays; bioeffects, instrumentation and examination, a credentialing program for physicians.* 4th ed. Houston, TX: Partners in Radiation Management, 2004.

Wagner LK, Lester RG, Saldana LR. *Exposure of the pregnant patient to diagnostic radiations.* 2nd ed. Madison, WI: Medical Physics Publishing, 1997.

REFERENCES

American Association of Physicists in Medicine. AAPM Task Group 108: PET and PET/CT shielding requirements. *Med Phys* 2006;33(1).

American Association of Physicists in Medicine. AAPM Dose Check Guidelines version 1.0 04/27/2011, http://www.aapm.org/pubs/CTProtocols/documents/NotificationLevelsStatement_2011-04-27.pdf, accessed October 1, 2011

American College of Radiology, *Disaster Preparedness for Radiology Professionals, Response to Radiological Terrorism: A Primer for Radiologists, Radiation Oncologists and Medical Physicists*, version 3, 2006. www.acr.org

Bogdanich W. *Radiation Overdoses Point Up Dangers of CT Scans*, New York Times, October 15, 2009.

Brenner DJ, Hall EJ. Computed tomography: an increasing source of radiation exposure. *N Engl J Med* 2007;357(22):2277–2284.

Brenner DJ, Elliston CD, Hall EJ, Berdon WE. Estimated Risks of Radiation-Induced Fatal Cancer from Pediatric CT. AJR 2001; 176:289–296.

Bushberg JT, Kroger LA, Hartman MB, et al. Nuclear/radiological terrorism: Emergency department management of radiation casualties. *J Emerg Med* 2007;32(1):71–85.

Compagnone G, Baleni MC, Pagan L, et al. Comparison of radiation doses to patients undergoing standard radiographic examinations with conventional screen–film radiography, computed radiography and direct digital radiography. *Br J Radiol*. 2006;79:899–904.

Fletcher DW, Miller DL, Balter S, Taylor MA. Comparison of four techniques to estimate radiation dose to skin during angiographic and interventional radiology procedures. *J Vasc Interv Radiol* 2002;13:391–397.

Guillet B, et al. Technologist radiation exposure in routine clinical practice with ^{18}F-FDG PET. *J Nucl Med Technol* 2005;33:175–179.

Hausleiter J, Meyer T, Hermann F, et al. Estimated radiation dose associated with cardiac CT angiography. *JAMA* 2009;301(5):500–507.

HPS. "*Emergency Department Management of Radiation* Casualties," Health Physics 2011. Society http://hps.org/hsc/responsemed.html

International Commission on Radiological Protection. The 2007 Recommendations of the International Commission on Radiological Protection. ICRP Publication 103. *Ann ICRP* 2007;37:1–332.

The Joint Commission *2010 Universal Protocol*: http://www.jointcommission.org/standards_information/up.aspx

The Joint Commission. *Sentinel event alert, radiation risks of diagnostic imaging*, Issue 47, August 24, 2011

Kohn LT, Corrigan JM, Donaldson MS, eds.; Committee on Quality of Health Care in America, Institute of Medicine. *To err is human: Building a safer health system*. Washington DC: National Academies Press, 2000. Accessed January 30, 2004.

Miller DL, Balter S, Cole PE, Lu HT, Berenstein A, Albert R, Schueler BA, Georgia JD, Noonan PT, Russell EJ, Malisch TW, Vogelzang RL, Geisinger M, Cardella JF, St. George J, Miller GL III, Anderson J. Radiation doses in interventional radiology procedures: the RAD-IR study Part II: Skin dose. *J Vasc Interv Radiol* 2003;14:977–990.

Murphy PH, Wu Y, Glaze SA. Attenuation properties of lead composite aprons. *Radiology* 1993;186:269–272.

Nair RR, Rajan B, Akiba S, et al. Background radiation and cancer incidence in Kerala, India-Karanagappally cohort study. *Health Phys* 2009;96:55–66.

NAS: National Research Council. *Distribution and administration potassium iodide in the event of a nuclear incident*. Washington, DC: National Academies Press, 2004.

National Council on Radiation Protection and Measurements. *Ionizing Radiation Exposure of the Population of the United States*, NCRP Report No. 93 National Council on Radiation Protection and Measurements, Bethesda, MD, 1987.

National Council on Radiation Protection and Measurements. *Use of Personal Monitors to Estimate Effective Dose Equivalent and Effective Dose to Workers for External Exposure to Low-LET Radiation*, NCRP Report No. 122. National Council on Radiation Protection and Measurements, Bethesda, MD, 1995.

National Council on Radiation Protection and Measurements. *Management of terrorist events involving radioactive material*. NCRP Report No. 138 National Council on Radiation Protection and Measurements, Bethesda, MD, 2001.

National Council on Radiation Protection and Measurements. *Structural shielding design for medical x-ray imaging facilities*. NCRP Report No. 147 National Council on Radiation Protection and Measurements, Bethesda, MD, 2004.

National Council on Radiation Protection and Measurements. *Key elements of preparing emergency responders for nuclear and radiological terrorism*. NCRP Commentary No. 19 National Council on Radiation Protection and Measurements, Bethesda, MD, 2005.

National Council on Radiation Protection and Measurements. *Management of persons contaminated with radionuclides*. NCRP Report No. 161 National Council on Radiation Protection and Measurements, Bethesda, MD, 2008.

National Council on Radiation Protection and Measurements. *Ionizing radiation exposure of the population of the United States*. NCRP Report No. 160 National Council on Radiation Protection and Measurements, Bethesda, MD, 2009.

National Council on Radiation Protection and Measurements. *Radiation dose management for fluoroscopically-guided interventional medical procedures*. NCRP Report No. 168. National Council on Radiation Protection and Measurements, Bethesda, MD, 2010a.

National Council on Radiation Protection and Measurements. *Responding to a radiological or nuclear terrorism incident: a guide for decision makers*. NCRP Report No. 165. National Council on Radiation Protection and Measurements, Bethesda, Maryland, 2010b.

Paterson A, Donald P. Frush DP, Donnelly LF. Helical CT of the body: Are settings adjusted for pediatric patients? *Am J Roentgenol* 2001;176:297–301.

Proceedings of the Thirty-third Annual Meeting of the National Council on Radiation Protection and Measurements. The effects of pre- and postconception exposure to radiation. *Teratology* 1999;59(4).

Radiation Emergency Assistance Center/Training Site (REAC/TS), Oak Ridge Institute for Science and Education (ORISE) positions the U.S. Department of Energy (DOE), 2011; http://orise.orau.gov/reacts/

Radiation Emergency Medical Management (REMM), Department of Health and Human Services, 2011; http://www.remm.nlm.gov/

Seibert JA, Shelton DK, Elizabeth H, et al. Computed radiography x-ray exposure trends. *Acad Radiol* 1996;3:313–318.

Stabin MG, Breitz HB. Breast milk excretion of radiopharmaceuticals: Mechanisms, findings, and radiation dosimetry. *J Nucl Med* 2000;41(5):863–873.

US Nuclear Regulatory Commission, NUREG-1556. Consolidated Guidance about Materials Licenses. Volume 9, Program-Specific Guidance about Medical Use Licenses. Revision 2, U.S. Nuclear Regulatory Commission, Washington, DC, January 2008.

US Nuclear Regulatory Commission, Safety Culture Policy Statement, NUREG/BR-0500, June 2011.

Waselenko JK, MacVittie TJ, BlakelyWF, et al. Medical Management of the Acute Radiation Syndrome: Recommendations of the Strategic National Stockpile Radiation Working Group K. *Ann Intern Med* 2004;140(12):1037–1051.

Williams MB, Krupinski EA, Strauss KJ, et al. Digital radiography image quality: image acquisition. *J Am Coll Radiol* 2007;4:371–388.

Zuguchi M, Chida K, Taura M, Inaba Y, Ebata A, Yamada S. Usefulness of non-lead aprons in radiation protection for physicians performing interventional procedures. *Radiat Prot Dosimetry* 2008;131(4):531–534.

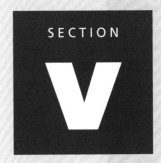

SECTION

V

Appendices

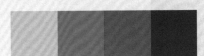

APPENDIX **A**

Fundamental Principles of Physics

A.1   Physics Laws, Quantities, and Units

Laws of Physics

Physics is the study of the physical environment around us—from the smallest quarks to the galactic dimensions of black holes and quasars. Much of what is known about physics can be summarized in a set of laws that describe physical reality. These laws are based on reproducible results from physical observations that are consistent with theoretical predictions. A well-conceived law of physics is applicable in a wide range of circumstances. A physical law that states that the force exerted by gravity on an individual on the surface of the Earth is 680 N is a poor example, because it is a description of a single situation only. Newton's law of gravity, however, describes the gravitational forces between any two bodies at any distance from each other and is an example of a well-conceived, generally usable law.

Vector Versus Scalar Quantities

For some quantities, such as force, velocity, acceleration, and momentum, direction is important, in addition to the magnitude. These quantities are called *vector* quantities. Quantities that do not incorporate direction, such as mass, time, energy, electrical charge, and temperature, are called *scalar* quantities.

A vector quantity is represented graphically by an arrow whose length is proportional to the magnitude of the vector. A vector quantity is represented by boldface type, as in the equation $\mathbf{F} = m\mathbf{a}$, where $\mathbf{F}$ and $\mathbf{a}$ are vector quantities and m is a scalar quantity.

In many equations of physics, such as $\mathbf{F} = m\mathbf{a}$, a vector is multiplied by a scalar. In vector-scalar multiplication, the magnitude of the resultant vector is the product of the magnitude of the original vector and the scalar; however, the direction of the vector is not changed by the multiplication. If the scalar has units, the multiplication may also change the units of the vector. Force, for example, has different units than acceleration. Vector-scalar multiplication is shown in Figure A-1.

Two or more vectors may be added. This addition is performed graphically by placing the tail of one vector against the head of the other, as shown in Figure A-2. The resultant vector is that reaching from the tail of the first to the head of the

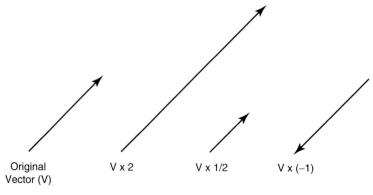

Original Vector (V)   V x 2   V x 1/2   V x (−1)

■ **FIGURE A-1** Vector-scalar multiplication.

second. The order in which vectors are added does not affect the result. A special case occurs when one vector has the same magnitude but opposite direction of the other; in this case, the two vectors cancel, resulting in no vector.

International System of Units

As science has developed, many disciplines have devised their own specialized units for measurements. An attempt has been made to establish a single set of units to be used across all disciplines of science. This set of units, called the *Systeme International* (SI), is gradually replacing the traditional units. The SI establishes a set of seven base units—the kilogram, meter, second, ampere, kelvin, candela, and mole—whose magnitudes are carefully described by standards laboratories. Two supplemental units, the radian and steradian, are used to describe angles in two and three dimensions, respectively. All other units, called *derived units,* are defined in terms of these fundamental units. For representing quantities much greater than or much smaller than an SI unit, the SI unit may be modified by a prefix. Commonly used prefixes are shown in Table A-1. A more complete list of prefixes is provided in Appendix C along with physical constants, geometric formulae, conversion factors, and radiologic data for elements 1 through 100.

■ **FIGURE A-2** Vector addition.

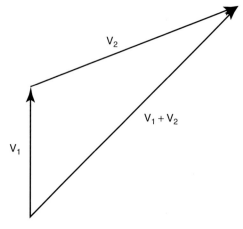

V_2

$V_1 + V_2$

V_1

TABLE A-1   COMMONLY USED PREFIXES FOR UNITS

PREFIX	MEANING	PREFIX	MEANING
centi (c)	10^{-2}		
milli (m)	10^{-3}	kilo (k)	10^{+3}
micro (μ)	10^{-6}	mega (M)	10^{+6}
nano (n)	10^{-9}	giga (G)	10^{+9}
pico (p)	10^{-12}	tera (T)	10^{+12}
femto (f)	10^{-15}	peta (P)	10^{+15}

 ## A.2 Classical Physics

Mass, Length, and Time

Mass is a measure of the resistance a body has to acceleration. It should not be confused with weight, which is the gravitational force exerted on a mass. The SI unit for mass is the kilogram (kg). The SI unit for length is the meter (m) and for time is the second (s).

Velocity and Acceleration

Velocity, a vector quantity, is the rate of change of position with respect to time:

$$v = \Delta x/\Delta t \qquad \text{[A-1]}$$

The magnitude of the velocity, called the *speed,* is a scalar quantity. The SI unit for velocity and speed is the meter per second (m/s). *Acceleration,* also a vector quantity, is defined as the rate of change of velocity with respect to time:

$$a = \Delta v/\Delta t \qquad \text{[A-2]}$$

The SI unit for acceleration is the meter per second per second (m/s^2).

Forces and Newton's Laws

Force, a vector quantity, is a push or pull. The physicist and mathematician Isaac Newton proposed three laws regarding force and velocity:

1. Unless acted upon by external force, an object at rest remains at rest and an object in motion remains in uniform motion. That is, an object's velocity remains unchanged unless an external force acts upon the object.
2. For every action, there is an equal and opposite reaction. That is, if one object exerts a force on a second object, the second object also exerts a force on the first that is equal in magnitude but opposite in direction.
3. A force acting upon an object produces an acceleration in the direction of the applied force:

$$F = ma \qquad \text{[A-3]}$$

The SI unit for force is the newton (N): 1 N is defined as 1 kg-m/s². There are four types of forces: *gravitational, electrical, magnetic,* and *nuclear.* These forces are discussed later.

Energy

Kinetic Energy

Kinetic energy, a scalar quantity, is a property of moving matter that is defined by the following equation:

$$E_k = \tfrac{1}{2}mv^2 \qquad \text{[A-4]}$$

where E_k is the kinetic energy, m is the mass of the object, and v is the speed of the object. (Einstein discovered a more complicated expression that must be used for objects with speeds approaching the speed of light.) The SI unit for all forms of energy is the joule (J): 1 J is defined as 1 kg-m²/s².

Potential Energy

Potential energy is a property of an object in a force field. The force field may be a gravitational force field. If an object is electrically charged, it may be an electrical force field caused by nearby charged objects. If an object is very close to an atomic nucleus, it may be influenced by nuclear forces. The potential energy (E_p) is a function of the position of the object; if the object changes position with respect to the force field, its potential energy changes.

Conservation of Energy

The total energy of an object is the sum of its kinetic and potential energies:

$$E_{total} = E_k + E_p \qquad \text{[A-5]}$$

Aside from friction, the total energy of the object does not change. For example, consider a brick held several feet above the ground. It has a certain amount of gravitational potential energy by virtue of its height, but it has no kinetic energy because it is at rest. When released, it falls downward with a continuous increase in kinetic energy. As the brick falls, its position changes and its potential energy decreases. The sum of its kinetic and potential energies does not change during the fall. One may think of the situation as one in which potential energy is converted into kinetic energy.

Momentum

Momentum, like kinetic energy, is a property of moving objects. However, unlike kinetic energy, momentum is a vector quantity. The momentum of an object is defined as follows:

$$\mathbf{p} = m\mathbf{v} \qquad \text{[A-6]}$$

where $\mathbf{p}$ is the momentum of an object, m is its mass, and $\mathbf{v}$ is its velocity. The momentum of an object has the same direction as its velocity. The SI unit of momentum is the kilogram-meter per second (kg-m/s). It can be shown from Newton's laws that, if no external forces act on a collection of objects, the total momentum of the set of objects does not change. This principle is called the law of conservation of momentum.

Electricity and Magnetism

Electricity

Electrical Charge

Electrical charge is a property of matter. Matter may have a positive charge, a negative charge, or no charge. The charge on an object may be determined by observing how it behaves in relation to other charged objects. The *coulomb* (C) is the SI derived unit of electric charge. It is defined in terms of two SI base units as the charge transported by a steady current of one ampere in one second. The smallest magnitude of charge is that of the electron. There are approximately 10^{19} electron charges per coulomb.

A fundamental law of physics states that electrical charge is conserved. This means that, if charge is neither added to nor removed from a system, the total amount of charge in the system does not change. The signs of the charges must be considered in calculating the total amount of charge in a system. If a system contains two charges of the same magnitude but of opposite sign—for example, in a hydrogen atom, in which a single electron (negative charge) orbits a single proton (positive charge)—the total charge of the system is zero.

Electrical Forces and Fields

The force (**F**) exerted on a charged particle by a second charged particle is described by the equation:

$$\mathbf{F} = kq_1q_2/r^2 \tag{A-7}$$

where q_1 and q_2 are the charges on the two particles, r is the distance between the two particles, and k is a constant. The direction of the force on each particle is either toward or away from the other particle; the force is attractive if one charge is negative and the other positive, and it is repulsive if both charges are of the same sign.

An electrical field exists in the vicinity of electrical charges. To measure the electrical field strength at a point, a small test charge is placed at that point and the force on the test charge is measured. The electrical field strength (**E**) is then calculated as follows:

$$\mathbf{E} = \mathbf{F}/q \tag{A-8}$$

where **F** is the force exerted on the test charge and q is the magnitude of the test charge. Electrical field strength is a vector quantity. If the test charge q is positive, **E** and **F** have the same direction; if the test charge is negative, **E** and **F** have opposite directions.

An electrical field may be visualized as lines of electrical field strength existing between electrically charged entities. The strength of the electrical field is depicted as the density of these lines. Figure A-3 shows the electrical fields surrounding a point charge and between two parallel plate electrodes.

An *electrical dipole* has no net charge but does possess regional distribution of positive and negative charge. When placed in an electrical field, the dipole tends to align with the field because of the torque exerted on it by that field (attraction by unlike charges, repulsion by like charges). The electrical dipole structure of certain natural and man-made crystals is used in ultrasound imaging devices to produce and detect sound waves, as described in Chapter 16.

Electrical Forces on Charged Particles

When a charged particle is placed in an electrical field, it experiences a force that is equal to the product of its charge q and the electrical field strength E at that location:

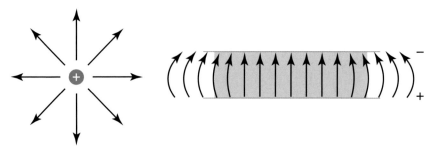

■ **FIGURE A-3** Electrical fields around a point charge (**left**) and between two parallel charged electrodes (**right**).

$$F = qE$$

If the charge on the particle is positive, the force is in the direction of the electrical field at that position; if the charge is negative, the force is opposite to the electrical field. If the particle is not restrained, it experiences an acceleration:

$$a = qE/m$$

where m is the mass of the particle.

Electrical Current

Electrical current is the flow of electrical charge. Charge may flow through a solid, such as a wire; through a liquid, such as the acid in an automobile battery; through a gas, as in a fluorescent light; or through a vacuum, as in an x-ray tube. Current may be the flow of positive charges, such as positive ions or protons in a cyclotron, or it may be the flow of negative charges, such as electrons or negative ions. In some cases, such as an ionization chamber radiation detector, there is a flow of positive charges in one direction and a flow of negative charges in the opposite direction. Although current is often the flow of electrons, the direction of the current is defined as the flow of positive charge (Fig. A-4). The SI unit of current is the *ampere* (A): 1 A is 1 C of charge passing a point in an electric circuit per second.

Electrical Potential Difference

Electrical potential, more commonly called *voltage,* is a scalar quantity. Voltage is the difference in the electrical potential energy of an electrical charge at two positions, divided by the charge:

$$V_{ab} = (E_{pa} - E_{pb})/q \qquad [A-9]$$

where E_{pa} is the electrical potential energy of the charge at location a, E_{pb} is the electrical potential energy of the same charge at location b, and q is the amount of charge. It is meaningless to specify the voltage at a single point in an electrical circuit; it must be specified in relation to another point in the circuit. The SI unit of electrical potential is the volt (V): 1 V is defined as 1 J/C, or 1 kg m²/s²−C.

Potential is especially useful in determining the final kinetic energy of a charged particle moving between two electrodes through a vacuum, as in an x-ray tube. According to the principle of conservation of energy (Equation A-5), the gain in kinetic energy of the charged particle is equal to its loss of potential energy:

$$E_{k-final} - E_{k-initial} = E_{p-initial} - E_{p-final} \qquad [A-10]$$

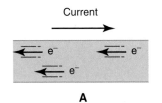

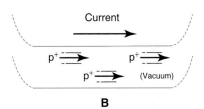

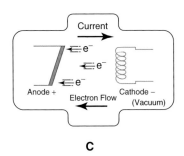

■ **FIGURE A-4** Direction of electrical current. **A.** A situation is shown in which electrons are flowing to the left. **B.** Positive charges are shown moving to the right. In both cases, the direction of current is to the right. **C.** Although the electrons in an x-ray tube pass from cathode to anode, current technically flows in the opposite direction.

Assuming that the charged particle starts with no kinetic energy ($E_{k-initial} = 0$) and using Equations A-9, and A-10 becomes

$$E_{k-final} = qV \qquad [A-11]$$

where q is the charge of the particle and V is the potential difference between the two electrodes.

For example, the final kinetic energy of an electron (charge = 1.602×10^{-19} C) accelerated through an electrical potential difference of 100 kV is

$$E_{k-final} = qV\ (1.602 \times 10^{-19}\ \text{C})\ (100\ \text{kV}) = 1.602 \times 10^{-14}\ \text{J}$$

The joule is a rather large unit of energy for subatomic particles. In atomic and nuclear physics, energies are often expressed in terms of the *electron volt* (eV). One electron volt is the kinetic energy developed by an electron accelerated across a potential difference of 1 V. One electron volt is equal to 1.602×10^{-19} J.

For example, the kinetic energy of an electron, initially at rest, that is accelerated through a potential difference of 100 kV is

$$E_k = qV = (1\ \text{electron charge})\ (100\ \text{kV}) = 100\ \text{keV}$$

One must be careful not to confuse the units of potential difference (V, kV, and MV) with units of energy (eV, keV, and MeV).

Electrical Power

Power is defined as the rate of the conversion of energy from one form to another with respect to time:

$$P = \Delta E / \Delta t \qquad \text{[A-12]}$$

For an example, an automobile engine converts chemical energy in gasoline into kinetic energy of the automobile. The amount of energy converted into kinetic energy per unit time is the power of the engine. The SI unit of power is the watt (W): 1 W is defined as 1 J/s.

When electrical current flows between two points of different potential, the potential energy of each charge changes. The change in potential energy per unit charge is the potential difference (V), and the amount of charge flowing per unit time is the current (i). Therefore, the electrical power (P) is equal to

$$P = iV \qquad \text{[A-13]}$$

where i is the current and V is the potential difference. Because 1 V = 1 J/C and 1 A. = 1 C/s, 1 W = 1 A−V:

$$(1 \text{ A})(1 \text{ V}) = (1 \text{ C/s})(1 \text{ J/C}) = 1 \text{ J/s} = 1 \text{ W}$$

For example, if a potential difference of 12 V applied to a heating coil produces a current of 1 A, the rate of heat production is

$$`P = iV = (1 \text{ A}) (12 \text{ V}) = 12 \text{ W}$$

Direct and Alternating Current

Electrical power is normally supplied to equipment as either *direct current* (DC) or *alternating current* (AC). DC power is provided by two wires connecting the equipment to a power source. The power source maintains a constant potential difference between the two wires (Fig. A-5A). Many electronic circuits require DC, and chemical batteries produce DC.

AC power is usually provided as *single-phase* or *three-phase* AC. Single-phase AC is supplied using two wires from the power source. The power source produces a potential difference between the two wires that varies sinusoidally with time (see Fig. A-5B). Single-phase AC is specified by its amplitude (the maximal voltage) and its frequency (the number of cycles per unit time). Normal household and building power is single-phase 117-V AC. Its actual peak amplitude is 1.4 × 117 V, or 165 V.

AC power is usually supplied to buildings and to heavy-duty electrical equipment as *three-phase* AC. It uses three or four wires between the power source and the

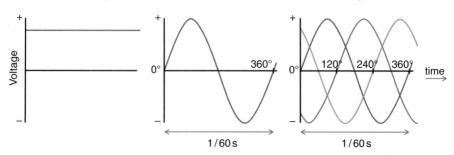

■ FIGURE A-5 **A.** Direct current. **B.** Single-phase AC. **C.** Three-phase AC, comprised of three single-phase AC sources, each separated by 120 degrees over the repeating 360 degrees cycle.

equipment. When present, the fourth wire, called the *neutral wire,* is maintained at ground potential (the potential of the earth). The power source provides a sinusoidally varying potential on each of the three wires with respect to the neutral wire. Voltages on these three wires have the same amplitudes and frequencies; however, each is a third of a cycle *out of phase* with respect to the other two, as shown in Figure A-5C. Each cycle is assigned a total of 360 degrees, and therefore each cycle in a three-phase circuit is 120 degrees out of phase with the others.

AC is produced by electric generators and used by electric motors. The major advantage of AC over DC is that its amplitude may be easily increased or decreased using devices called *transformers,* as described later. AC is converted to DC for many electronic circuits.

Ground potential is the electrical potential of the earth. One of the two wires supplying single-phase AC is maintained at ground potential, as is the neutral wire used in supplying three-phase AC. These wires are maintained at ground potential by connecting them to a metal spike driven deep into the earth.

Conductors, Insulators, and Semiconductors

When a potential difference is applied across a conductor, it causes an electrical current to flow. In general, increasing the potential difference increases the current. The quantity *resistance* is defined as the ratio of the applied voltage to the resultant current:

$$R = V/i \qquad \text{[A-14]}$$

The SI unit of resistance is the ohm (Ω): 1 Ω is defined as 1 volt per ampere.

Current is defined as the flow of positive charge. In solid matter, however, current is caused by the movement of negative charges (electrons) only. Based on the amount of current generated by an applied potential difference, solids may be roughly classified as conductors, semiconductors, or insulators. Metals, especially silver, copper, and aluminum, have very little resistance and are called conductors. Some materials, such as glass, plastics, and fused quartz, have very large resistances and are called insulators. Other materials, such as selenium, silicon, and germanium, have intermediate resistances and are called *semiconductors.*

The band theory of solids explains the conduction properties of solids. The outer-shell electrons in solids exist in discrete energy bands. These bands are separated by gaps; electrons cannot possess energies within the gaps. For an electron to be mobile, there must be a nearby vacant position in the same energy band into which it can move. In conductors, the highest energy band occupied by electrons is only partially filled, so the electrons in it are mobile. In insulators and semiconductors, the highest occupied band is completely filled and electrons are not readily mobile.

The difference between insulators and semiconductors is the width of the forbidden gap between the highest occupied band and the next higher band; in semiconductors, the gap is about 1 eV, whereas in insulators, it is typically greater than 5 eV. At room temperature, thermal energy temporarily promotes a small fraction of the electrons from the valence band into the next higher band. The promoted electrons are mobile. Their promotion also leaves behind vacancies in the valence band, called *holes,* into which other valence band electrons can move. Because the band gap of semiconductors is much smaller than that of insulators, a much larger number of electrons exist in the higher band of semiconductors, and the resistance of semiconductors is therefore less than that of insulators. Reducing the temperature of insulators and semiconductors increases their resistance by reducing the thermal energy available for promoting electrons from the valence band.

For certain materials, including most metallic conductors, the resistance is not greatly affected by the applied voltage. In these materials, the applied voltage and resultant current are nearly proportional:

$$V = iR \qquad\qquad [A\text{-}15]$$

This equation is called Ohm's law.

Magnetism

Magnetic Forces and Fields

Magnetic fields can be caused by moving electrical charges. This charge motion may be over long distances, such as the movement of electrons through a wire, or it may be restricted to the vicinity of a molecule or atom, such as the motion of an unpaired electron in a valence shell. The basic features of magnetic fields can be illustrated by the bar magnet. First, the bar magnet, made of an iron ferromagnetic material, has a unique atomic electron orbital packing scheme that gives rise to an intense magnetic field due to the constructive addition of magnetic fields arising from *unpaired* spinning electrons in different atomic orbital shells. The resultant "magnet" has two poles and experiences a force when placed in the vicinity of another bar magnet or external magnetic field. By convention, the pole that points north under the influence of the earth's magnetic field is termed the *north pole,* and the other is called the *south pole.* Experiments demonstrate that like poles of two magnets repel each other and unlike poles attract. When a magnet is broken in two, each piece becomes a new magnet, with a north and a south pole. This phenomenon continues on to the atomic level. Therefore, the simplest magnetic structure is the magnetic *dipole.* In contrast, the simplest electrical structure, the isolated point charge, is unipolar.

Magnetic fields may be visualized as lines of magnetic force. Because magnetic poles exist in pairs, the magnetic field lines have no beginning or end and, in fact, circle upon themselves. Figure A-6A shows the magnetic field surrounding a bar magnet. A current-carrying wire also produces a magnetic field that circles the wire, as shown in Figure A-6B. Increasing the current flowing through the wire increases the magnetic field strength. The *right-hand rule* allows the determination of the magnetic field direction by grasping the wire with the thumb pointed in the direction of the current (opposite the electron flow). The fingers will then circle the wire in the direction of the magnetic field. When a current carrying wire is curved in a loop, the resultant concentric lines of magnetic force overlap and augment the total local magnetic field strength inside the loop, as shown in Figure A-6C. A coiled wire, called a *solenoid,* results in even more augmentation of the magnetic lines of force within the coil, as shown in Figure A-6D. The field strength depends on the number of turns in the coil over a fixed distance. An extreme example of a solenoid is found in most magnetic resonance scanners; in fact, the patient resides inside the solenoid during the scan. A further enhancement of magnetic field strength can be obtained by applying a greater current through the wire or by placing a ferromagnetic material such as iron inside the solenoid. The iron core in this instance confines and augments the magnetic field. The solenoid is similar to the bar magnet discussed previously; however, the magnetic field strength may be changed by varying the current. If the current remains fixed (e.g., DC), the magnetic field also remains fixed; if the current varies (e.g., AC), the magnetic field varies. Solenoids are also called *electromagnets.*

Current loops behave as magnetic dipoles. Like the simple bar magnet, they tend to align with an external magnetic field, as shown in Figure A-7. An electron in an atomic

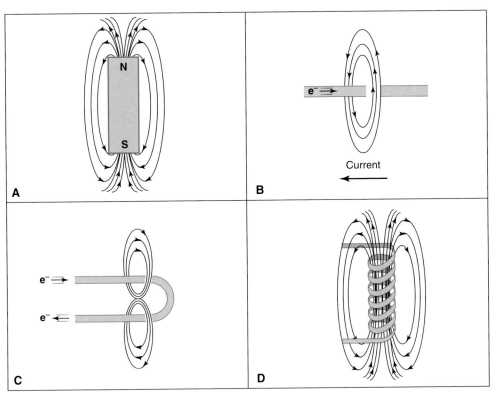

■ **FIGURE A-6** Magnetic field descriptions: surrounding a bar magnet (**A**), around a wire (**B**), about a wire loop (**C**), and about a coiled wire (**D**).

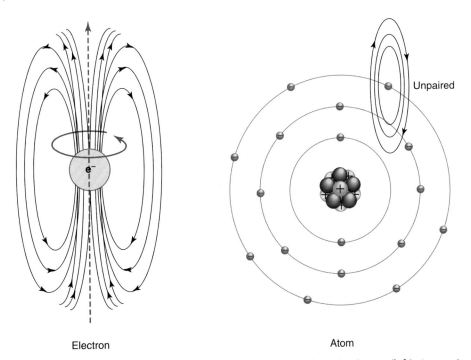

Electron   Atom

■ **FIGURE A-7** A spinning charge has an associated magnetic field, such as the electron (**left**). An unpaired electron in an atomic orbital produces a magnetic field (**right**). Each produces magnetic dipoles that will interact with an external magnetic field.

orbital is a current loop about the nucleus. A spinning charge such as the proton also may be thought of as a small current loop. These current loops act as magnetic dipoles and tend to align with external magnetic fields, a tendency that gives rise to the macroscopic magnetic properties of materials (discussed further in Chapter 12.).

The SI unit of magnetic field strength is the *tesla* (T). An older unit of magnetic field strength is the *gauss* (G): 1 T is equal to 10^4 G. By way of comparison, the earth's magnetic field is approximately 0.05 to 0.1 mT whereas magnetic fields used for magnetic resonance imaging typically range from 1 T.

Magnetic Forces on Moving Charged Particles

A magnetic field exerts a force on a moving charge, provided that the charge crosses the lines of magnetic field strength. The magnitude of this force is proportional to (a) the charge; (b) the speed of the charge; (c) the magnetic field strength, designated B; and (d) the direction of charge travel with respect to the direction of the magnetic field. The direction of the force on the moving charge can be determined through the use of the right-hand rule. It is perpendicular to both the direction of the charge's velocity and the lines of magnetic field strength. Because an electrical current consists of moving charges, a current-carrying wire in a magnetic field will experience a force (a torque). This principle is used in devices such as electric motors.

Electromagnetic Induction

In 1831, Michael Faraday discovered that a *moving* magnet induces an electrical current in a nearby conductor. His observations with magnets and conducting wires led to the findings listed here. The major ideas are illustrated in Figure A-8.

1. A *changing* magnetic field induces a voltage (electrical potential difference) in a nearby conducting wire and causes a current to flow. An identical voltage is induced whether the wire moves with respect to the magnetic field position or the magnetic field moves with respect to the wire position. A *stationary* magnetic field *does not* induce a voltage in a stationary wire.
2. A stronger magnetic field results in a stronger induced voltage. The voltage is proportional to the number of magnetic field lines cutting across the wire conductor per unit time. If the relative speed of the wire or the magnet is increased with respect to the other, the induced voltage will be larger because an increased number of magnetic field lines will be cutting across the wire conductor per unit time.
3. A 90-degree angle of the wire conductor relative to the magnetic field will provide the greatest number of lines to cross per unit distance, resulting in a higher induced voltage than for other angles.
4. When a solenoid (wire coil) is placed in a magnetic field, the magnetic field lines cut by each turn of the coil are additive, causing the resultant induced voltage to be directly proportional to the number of turns of the coil.

The direction of current flow caused by an induced voltage is described by Lenz's law (Fig. A-9: *An induced current flows in a direction such that its associated magnetic field opposes the magnetic field that induced it.* Lenz's law is an important concept that describes self-induction and mutual induction.

Self-Induction

A time-varying current in a coil wire produces a magnetic field that varies in the same manner. By Lenz's law, the varying magnetic field induces a potential difference across the coil that opposes the source voltage. Therefore, a rising and falling source voltage (AC) creates an *opposing* falling and rising induced voltage in the coil. This

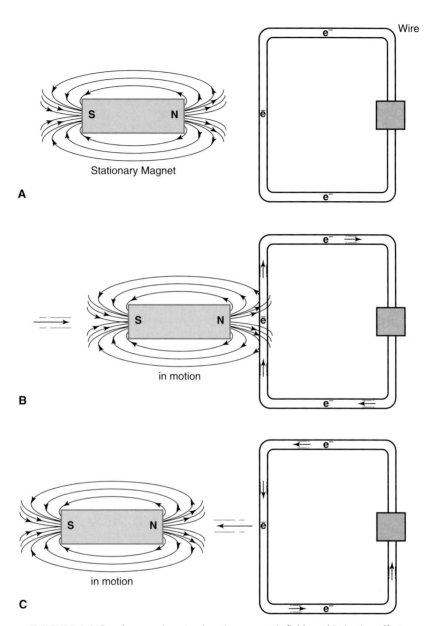

FIGURE A-8 Faraday experiments: changing magnetic fields and induction effects. **A.** A stationary magnetic field is depicted, with no electron flow occurring. **B.** The magnetic field is moving towards the wire loop, resulting in the induction of an electromotive force that results in electron flow in a clockwise direction. **C.** The magnetic field is moving away from the position indicated in (**B**), resulting in the reverse, counterclockwise flow of electrons in the wire loop.

phenomenon, called *self-induction*, is used in autotransformers that provide a variable incremental voltage.

Mutual Induction

A *primary* wire coil carrying AC produces a time-varying magnetic field. When a *secondary* wire coil is located under the influence of this magnetic field, a time-varying potential difference across the secondary coil is similarly induced, as shown in

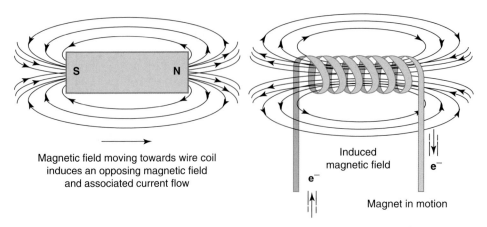

■ FIGURE A-9 Lenz's law, demonstrating mutual induction between a moving magnetic field and a coiled wire conductor.

Figure A-9. The amplitude of the induced voltage, V_s, can be determined from the following equation, known as the law of transformers:

$$\left(\frac{V_p}{N_p}\right) = \left(\frac{V_s}{N_s}\right) \qquad [A-16]$$

where V_p is the voltage amplitude applied to the primary coil, V_s is the voltage amplitude induced in the secondary coil, N_p is the number of turns in the primary coil, and N_s is the number of turns in the secondary coil. With a predetermined number of "turns" on the primary and secondary coils, this *mutual inductance* property can increase or decrease the voltage in electrical circuits. The devices that provide this change of voltage (current changes in the opposite direction) are called *transformers*. Further explanation of their use in x-ray generators is covered in Chapter 6.

Electric Generators and Motors

The electric generator utilizes the principles of electromagnetic induction to convert mechanical energy into electrical energy. It consists of a coiled wire mounted on a rotor between the poles of a strong magnet, as shown in Figure A-10A. As an external mechanical energy source rotates the coil (e.g., hydroelectric turbine generator), the wires in the coil cut across the magnetic force lines, resulting in a sinusoidally varying potential difference, the polarity of which is determined by the wire approaching or receding from one pole of the magnet. The generator serves as a source of AC power.

The electric motor converts electrical energy into mechanical energy. It consists of a coil of wires mounted on a freely rotating axis (rotor) between the poles of a fixed magnet, as shown in Figure A-10B. When AC flows through the coil, an increasing and decreasing magnetic field is generated, the coil acting as a magnetic dipole. This dipole tends to align with the external magnetic field, causing the rotor to turn. As the dipole approaches alignment, however, the AC and thus, the magnetic field of the rotor reverse polarity, causing another half-turn rotation to achieve alignment. The alternating polarity of the rotor's magnetic field causes a continuous rotation of the coil wire mounted on the rotor as long as AC is applied.

Magnetic Properties of Matter

The magnetic characteristics of materials are determined by atomic and molecular structures related to the behavior of the associated electrons. Three categories of

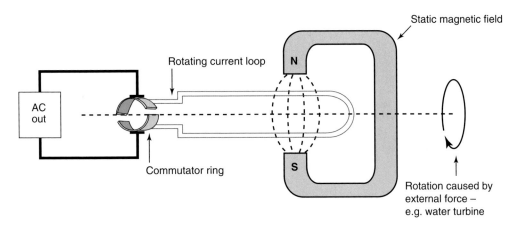

The rotating current wire loop in the static magnetic field creates an induced current occuring with an alternating potential difference.

A

Induced rotation of the current loop is caused by the variable magnetic field within current loop associated with the applied alternating current interacting with the static magnetic field.

B

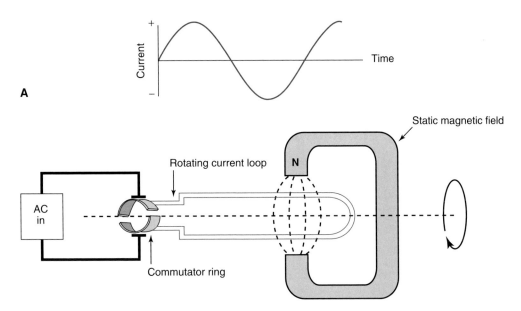

■ **FIGURE A-10** Electrical and mechanical energy conversion: electric generators (**A**) and electric motors (**B**).

magnetic properties are defined: diamagnetic, paramagnetic, and ferromagnetic. Their properties arise from the association of moving charges (electrons) and magnetic fields.

Diamagnetic Materials

Individual electrons orbiting in atomic or molecular shells represent a current loop and give rise to a magnetic field. The various electron orbits do not fall in any preferred plane, so the superposition of the associated magnetic fields results in a net magnetic field that is too small to be measured. When these atoms or molecules are placed in a changing magnetic field, however, the electron motions are altered by the induced electrical motive force to form a reverse magnetic field *opposing* the applied magnetic field. *Diamagnetic materials,* therefore, cause a depletion of the applied magnetic field in the local micromagnetic environment. An example of a diamagnetic material is calcium, and its magnetic properties are described in Chapter 12.

Paramagnetic Materials

Based on the previous discussion, it would seem likely that all elements and molecules would behave as diamagnetic agents. In fact, all have diamagnetic properties, but some have additional properties that overwhelm the diamagnetic response. Electrons in atomic or molecular orbitals orient their magnetic fields in such a way as to cancel in pairs; however, in those materials that have an *odd* number of electrons, one electron is unpaired, exact cancellation cannot occur, and a magnetic field equivalent to one electron orbital results. Depending on orbital structures and electron filling characteristics, *fractional* unpaired electron spins can also occur, resulting in variations in the magnetic field strength. When placed in an external magnetic field, the magnetic field of the material caused by the unpaired electron aligns with the applied field. *Paramagnetic materials,* having unpaired electrons, locally *augment* the micromagnetic environment. The magnetic overall properties o the atom result from these paramagnetic effects as well as the diamagnetic effects discussed earlier, with the paramagnetic characteristics predominating. An example of a paramagnetic material is gadolinium, an element used in magnetic resonance imaging contrast agents, as described in Chapters 12 and 13.

Ferromagnetic Materials

Iron, nickel, and cobalt can possess intrinsic magnetic fields and will react strongly in an applied magnetic field. These *ferromagnetic materials* are transition elements that have an unorthodox atomic orbital structure: electrons will fill the outer orbital shells before the inner orbitals are completely filled. The usual spin cancellation of the electrons does not occur, resulting in an unusually high atomic magnetic moment. While they are in a random atomic (elemental) or molecular (compound) arrangement, cancellation of the dipoles occurs and no intrinsic magnetic field is manifested; however, when the individual magnetic dipoles are nonrandomly aligned by an external force (e.g., a strong electrical field), a constructive enhancement of the individual atomic magnetic moments gives rise to an intrinsic magnetic field that reacts strongly in an applied magnetic field. Permanent magnets are examples of a permanent *nonrandom* arrangement of local "magnetic domains" of the transition elements. Ferromagnetic characteristics dominate over paramagnetic and diamagnetic interactions. These materials become dangerous in the vicinity of a strong magnetic field, and must be carefully identified and avoided in an around magnetic resonance imaging scanners, as explained in the MR safety section of Chapter 13.

Digital Computers

Digital computers were originally designed in the 1940s and early 1950s to perform mathematical computations and other information processing tasks very quickly. Since then, they have come to be used for many other purposes, including information display, information storage, and, in conjunction with computer networks, information transfer and communications.

Computers, mechanical, electrical, or part mechanical and part electrical, were constructed that represented numerical data in analog form. They have been almost entirely supplanted by digital electronic computers. The explosive growth of such computers was made possible by the development of the integrated electronic circuit ("chip"), which today can have billions of microscopic electronic components such as transistors and capacitors. In this appendix, the term "computer" will refer exclusively to programmable digital electronic computers. Analog and digital representation of information was discussed in Chapter 5.

Computers were introduced in medical imaging in the early 1970s and have become increasingly important since that time. Their first uses in medical imaging were mostly in nuclear medicine, where they were used to acquire series of images depicting the organ-specific kinetics of radiopharmaceuticals and to extract physiological information from the images. Today, computers are essential to many imaging modalities, including x-ray computed tomography (CT), magnetic resonance imaging (MRI), single photon emission computed tomography (SPECT), and positron emission tomography (PET).

Any function that can be performed by a computer can also be performed by a hardwired electronic circuit. The advantage of the computer over a hardwired circuit is its flexibility. The function of the computer can be modified merely by changing the program that controls the computer, whereas modifying the function of a hardwired circuit usually requires replacing the circuit. Although the computer is a very complicated and powerful data processing device, the actual operations performed by a computer are very simple. The power of the computer is mainly due to its speed in performing these operations and its ability to store large volumes of data.

A *workstation* is a computer designed for use by a single person at a time. A workstation is usually equipped with one or more display monitors for the visual display of information, a keyboard for the entry of alphanumeric information, and a pointing device, such as a mouse.

B.1 Components and Operation of Computers

A computer consists of a central processing unit (CPU), main memory, and input/output (I/O) devices, connected by data pathways called data buses (Fig. B-1). The main memory of the computer stores the program (sequence of instructions) being executed and the data being processed. The CPU executes the instructions in the program to process the data.

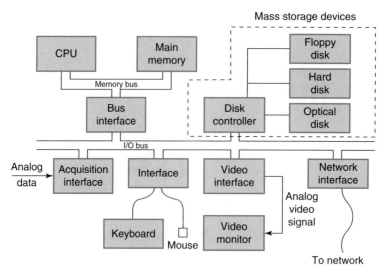

■ **FIGURE B-1** Components of a computer.

Digital signals and binary digital signals in particular are discussed in Chapter 5. Although digital signals need not be binary and some very fast computer networks use nonbinary digital signals, essentially all computers today store and transfer information in binary form.

A group of wires used to transfer data between several devices is called a *data bus*. Each device connected to the bus is identified by an address or a range of addresses. Only one device at a time can transmit information on a bus, and in most cases, only one device receives the information. The sending device transmits both the information and the address of the device that is intended to receive the information. Some buses use separate wires for the data and addresses, whereas others transmit both over the same wires. The width of a bus refers to the number of wires used to transmit data. For example, a 32-bit bus transmits 32 bits of data simultaneously. Buses usually have additional wires, such as a ground wire to establish a reference potential for the voltage signals on the other wires, wires to carry control signals, and wires at one or more constant voltages to provide electrical power to circuit boards attached to the bus.

I/O devices enable information to be entered into and retrieved from the computer and to be stored. The I/O devices of a computer usually include a keyboard, a mouse or other pointing device, a display interface and display monitor, several mass storage devices, and often a printer. The keyboard, pointing device, display interface, and display monitor enable an operator to communicate with the computer. Mass storage devices permit the storage of large volumes of programs and data. They include magnetic disk drives, optical disk drives, and magnetic tape drives.

When the CPU or another device sends data to memory or a mass storage device, it is said to be *writing* data, and when it requests data stored in memory or on a storage device, it is said to be *reading* data. Computer memory and data storage devices permit either random access or sequential access to the data. The term *random access* describes a storage medium in which the locations of the data may be read or written in any order, and *sequential access* describes a medium in which data storage locations can only be accessed in a serial manner. Most solid-state memories, magnetic disks, and optical disks are random access, whereas magnetic tape typically permits only sequential access.

Main Memory

Main memory provides temporary storage for the instructions of the computer program being executed and the information being processed by the computer. Main memory is used for these functions instead of mass storage devices because the access time is much shorter and the data transfer rate between the CPU and the main memory is much faster than those between the CPU and the mass storage devices.

Main memory consists of a large number of data storage locations, each of which contains the same number of bits (usually 1 byte, which is composed of 8 bits). Each bit can store only one of two values, represented by the binary digits 0 and 1. Bits and bytes are discussed in Chapter 5. A unique number, called a *memory address*, identifies each storage location. When a CPU performs a memory write, it sends both a memory address, designating the desired storage location, and the data to be stored to the memory. When it performs a memory read, it sends the address of the desired data to the memory and, in return, is sent the data at that location.

One type of memory is commonly called *random access memory* (RAM). In common usage, RAM refers to memory onto which the CPU can both read and write data. A better name for such memory is read-write memory. A disadvantage of most read-write memory is that it is *volatile*, meaning that data stored in it are lost when electrical power is turned off.

Another type of memory is called *read-only memory* (ROM). The CPU can only read data from ROM; it cannot write or erase data on ROM. The main advantage to ROM is that data stored in it are not lost when power is lost to the computer. ROM is usually employed to store frequently used programs provided by the manufacturer that perform important functions such as setting up the computer for operation when power is turned on. Although the term *RAM* is commonly used to distinguish read-write memory from ROM, ROM does permit random access.

The size of the main memory can affect the speed at which a program is executed. A very large program or one that processes large volumes of information will usually be executed more quickly on a computer with a large memory. A computer with a small memory can fit only small portions of the program and information into its memory at one time and must frequently interrupt the processing of information to load other portions of the program and information into the memory from the magnetic disk or another storage device.

It would be very expensive to have a large main memory that could provide program instructions and data to the CPU as fast as the CPU can process them. The main memories of most computers today use a relatively slow but inexpensive type of memory called dynamic RAM (DRAM). DRAM uses one capacitor (an electrical charge storage device) and one transistor for each bit. It is called dynamic because each bit must be read and refreshed several times a second to maintain the data. To compensate for the low speed of DRAM with respect to the CPU clock speed, many computers contain one or more smaller but faster memories, called *cache memories*, between the main memory and the CPU. They maintain exact copies of small portions of the program and data in the main memory. A cache memory usually consists of static RAM (SRAM), which uses several transistors to represent each bit. SRAM stores data while power is on without requiring refreshing and can be read or written several times faster than DRAM but requires more space and is more expensive. Cache memories are effective because program segments and data that were recently read from the memory by the CPU are very likely to be read again soon.

Computer Program and Central Processing Unit

A computer program is a sequence of instructions and the CPU is a set of electronic circuits that executes them. A CPU fetches and executes the instructions in a program sequentially; it fetches an instruction from the main memory, executes that instruction, and then fetches the next instruction in the program sequence. A CPU contained in a single computer chip is called a *microprocessor.*

The CPU contains a small number of data storage locations, called *storage registers,* for storing data and memory addresses. For example, one computer system has 16 registers, each containing 32 bits. Operations can be performed on data in the registers much more quickly than on data in memory. The CPU also contains an *arithmetic logic unit* (ALU) that performs mathematical operations and comparisons between data stored in the registers or memory. In addition, the CPU contains a clock. This clock is not a time-of-day clock (although the computer may have one of these as well), but a circuit that produces a periodic stream of logic pulses that serve as timing marks to synchronize the operation of the various components of the computer. CPU clock speeds today are usually several gigahertz (GHz); a GHz is 10^9 hertz (Hz) and a Hz is defined as one cycle per second.

An instruction can cause the CPU to perform one or a combination of four actions:

Transfer a unit of data (e.g., a 16- or 32-bit word) from a memory address, CPU storage register, or I/O device to another memory address, register, or I/O device.

Perform a mathematical operation, such as addition or multiplication, between two numbers in storage registers in the CPU or in memory.

Compare two numbers or other pieces of data in registers or in memory.

Change the address of the next instruction to be executed in the program to another location in the program. This type of instruction is called a branching instruction.

A CPU fetches and executes the instructions in a program sequentially until it fetches a branching instruction. The CPU then jumps to a new location in the program that is specified by the branching instruction and, starting at the new location, again executes instructions sequentially. There are two types of branching instructions, unconditional and conditional. *Conditional branching instructions* cause a branch to occur only if a specified condition is met. For example, a conditional branching instruction may specify that a branch is to occur only if the number stored in a particular CPU storage register is zero. Conditional branching instructions are especially important because they permit the computer to make "decisions" by allowing the data to alter the order of instruction execution.

Each instruction in a program has two parts. The first part specifies the operation, such as a data transfer, an addition of two numbers, or a conditional branch, to be performed. The second part describes the location of the data to be operated on or compared and the location where the result is to be stored. In the case of an addition, it contains the locations of the numbers to be added and the locations where the sum is to be stored. In the case of a branching instruction, the second part is the memory address of the next instruction to be fetched and executed.

A computer or microprocessor manufacturer creates an *architecture* for its computers; this term refers to the set of instructions that a CPU can execute and the formats for data of different types (unsigned integers, signed integers, floating point numbers, alphanumeric characters, etc.) that the instructions cause the CPU to process. If the computers or microprocessors incorporating an architecture are commercially successful, software companies and individuals write programs for that architecture. When the computer or microprocessor manufacturer creates a faster CPU or microprocessor (e.g., with a higher clock speed or a design that requires fewer clock cycles to execute an instruction), if the instruction architecture is not changed, the new computer or microprocessor will be capable of executing existing programs. A person or an organization may have a large financial investment in software and store information in that format and will likely prefer to purchase new computers that can execute this software and access existing data. On the other hand, such a computer architecture may restrict the ability to take advantage of new developments in computer technology. A partial solution to this dilemma is to design new microprocessors that add additional instructions and data formats but continue to execute all existing instructions and accept existing data formats. Such processors are said to be "backward compatible."

A CPU or microprocessor may be described as being an 8-, 16-, 32-, or 64-bit design. Modern systems commonly are 32- or 64-bit designs. This terminology is somewhat ambiguous; the number of bits may refer to the number of bits in each storage or address register in the CPU, the number of address lines in the data bus, or the number of data lines in the data bus. For example, if 32 bits are allotted for address registers and there are 32 address lines in the bus, 4 gigabytes of memory can be directly accessed. If 32 bits are allotted for storage registers and there are 32 data lines in the bus, 32 bits of information can be read from or written to memory simultaneously. In general, the number of bits refers to the amount of information that can be read, written, or processed in a single operation and the number of memory addresses that can be accessed without schemes like memory segmentation. Thus, a CPU or microprocessor described as being of a design with more bits will, in general, process information more quickly, all other factors such as clock speed being equal. However, this improvement in efficiency requires software that effectively utilizes these capabilities.

The CPU is a bottleneck in a conventional computer. A computer may have many megabytes of data to be processed and a program requiring the execution of instructions many billions of times. However, the CPU executes the instructions only one or a few at a time. One way to increase speed is to build the circuits of the CPU and memory with faster components so the computer can run at a higher clock speed. This makes the computer more expensive and there are practical and technical limits to how fast a circuit can operate.

The other method of relieving the bottleneck is to design the CPU to perform *parallel processing*. This means that the CPU performs some tasks simultaneously rather than sequentially. Most modern general-purpose CPUs incorporate limited forms of parallel processing. One form of parallel processing is pipelining. Several steps, each requiring one clock cycle, are required for a CPU to execute a single instruction. Older CPUs, such as the Intel 8088, 80286, and 80386 microprocessors, completed only one instruction every few cycles. The instruction execution circuits of newer microprocessors are organized into pipelines, a pipeline having several stages that operate simultaneously. Instructions enter the pipeline one at a time and are passed from one stage to the next. Several instructions are in different stages of execution at the same time. It takes several clock cycles to fill the pipeline, but, once full, it completes the execution of one instruction per cycle. Pipelining permits a CPU to attain an average instruction execution rate of almost one instruction per cycle. (Pipelining does not yield exactly one instruction per cycle because some instructions interfere with its operation, in particular ones that modify the data to be operated on by immediately subsequent instructions, and branching instructions, because they change the order of instruction execution.)

Superscalar CPU architectures incorporate several pipelines in parallel and can attain average instruction execution rates of two to five instructions per CPU clock cycle.

Modern microprocessors may contain more than one CPU. These are called multicore microprocessors. To effectively use their processing capability, the software must provide threads of instructions that can be processed simultaneously.

However, many common tasks performed by general-purpose computers are not well suited to large-scale parallel processing. On the other hand, many tasks in image processing are very well suited for parallel processing and so some specialized processors for image processing, described later in this chapter, are designed to perform extensive parallel processing.

Input/Output Bus and Expansion Slots

Data buses have been described earlier in this chapter. The input/output buses of most computers are provided with several expansion slots into which printed circuit boards can be installed. The boards installed in these slots can include cards to connect the computer to a computer network, controllers for mass storage devices, display interface cards to provide a signal to a display monitor, sound cards to provide audio signals to speakers, and acquisition interfaces to other devices such as scintillation cameras. The provision of expansion slots on this bus makes it possible to customize a general-purpose computer for a specific application and to add additional functions and capabilities.

Mass Storage Devices

Mass storage devices permit the nonvolatile (i.e., data are not lost when power is turned off) storage of information. Mass storage devices include hard magnetic disk drives (nonremovable hard disks are called fixed disks), flash memory, magnetic tape drives, and optical (laser) disk units. Each of these devices, except flash memory, consists of a mechanical drive; the storage medium, which may be removable; and an electronic controller. Despite the wide variety of storage media, there is not one best medium for all purposes, because they differ in storage capacity, data access time, data transfer rate, cost, and other factors. Mass storage devices were discussed in detail in Chapter 5.

Display Interface

An important use of many computers, particularly workstations, is to display information in visual form. The information is usually displayed on one or more display monitors, although it may also be presented in hard-copy form, most commonly using photographic film or paper. Such a computer has a display interface; the display interface is a collection of electronic circuits that receives information in digital form from the memory of a computer via the computer's bus and provides it, in analog or digital form, to one or more display monitors. Display interfaces and display devices are described in detail in Chapter 5.

Acquisition Interface

A computer's acquisition interface accepts data from an attached device and transfers it to memory via the computer's bus. An acquisition interface that accepts analog data first converts it into digital form using one or more analog-to-digital converters

(ADCs) (ADCs were described in Chapter 5.). Until perhaps a decade ago, many medical imaging devices, such as scintillation cameras, sent analog data directly to attached computers. In most cases today, the analog data are converted into digital form by the imaging device, which sends data in digital form to the computer. Some acquisition interfaces store the received information in their own dedicated memories to permit the computer to perform other tasks during data acquisition. An imaging computer that is not directly connected to an imaging device may instead receive images over a computer network, as described below.

Communications Interfaces

Computers serve not only as information processing and display devices but also as communications devices. A computer may be connected to a network by a network interface. The interface converts digital signals from the computer into the digital form required by the network and vice versa. Various forms of the local area network standard Ethernet have become so common that most computers today are equipped with Ethernet interfaces. There are also wireless interfaces, such as WiFi, which use radio signals to connect portable computers to a network. For example, in bedside radiography, such wireless network technology may be used to transfer information between a portable image receptor and a mobile radiographic system. A computer may have a modem (contraction of "modulator-demodulator") to permit it to transfer information to another computer or to a network using analog telephone lines. These interfaces and computer networks are discussed in detail in Chapter 5.

Specialized Processors

The speed of a general-purpose computer in performing mathematical operations can be greatly enhanced by adding a specialized processor. A specialized processor is a specialized computer designed to perform the mathematical manipulation of data very quickly. It typically consists of a CPU, a small high-speed memory, a high-speed bus, and an interface to connect it to the bus of the main computer. The main computer is called the *host computer*. Most specialized processors rely heavily on parallel processing for their speed. Parallel processing is particularly efficient for many image processing tasks. The host computer sends the data from its memory to the specialized processor's memory along with the instructions for processing the information. The specialized processor processes the data and returns the processed information to the memory of the host computer. Alternatively, digital information from an imaging device, such as the digital projection data from a CT scanner, may be sent directly to a specialized processor, with the processed information, such as transverse images, sent to the host computer. Figure B-2 shows a computer with a specialized processor. Uses of specialized processors in medical imaging include the production of tomographic image sets from projection images in CT, SPECT, and PET and the production of surface- and volume-rendered images from tomographic image data sets. Specialized processors for image processing are commonly used on display cards; these are known as graphics processing units (GPUs).

B.2   Performance of Computers

There are many factors that affect the time required for a computer to complete a task. These include the speed of the CPU (as reflected by its clock speed); how extensively the CPU uses parallel processing; the number of independent CPUs, called

■ **FIGURE B-2** Specialized high-capacity parallel processor (*arrows*) for reconstructing tomographic images from projection image data for a modern multirow detector CT system. The parallel processor is mounted above the motherboard of a very powerful, but conventional personal computer that receives the image data from the specialized processor. (Image courtesy of Philips Healthcare.)

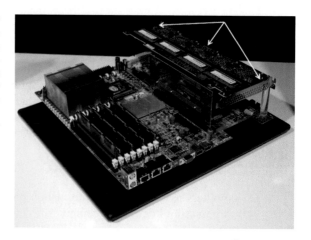

"cores," that a microprocessor contains (four or more cores are now typical); the width and the clock speed of the data bus between the CPU and the main memory; the size of the memory; and the access times and data transfer rates of mass storage devices. A larger memory permits more of the program being executed and the data being processed to reside in memory, thereby reducing the time that the CPU is idle while awaiting the transfer of program segments and data from mass storage devices into memory. The widths (number of data wires) of the data buses affect the speed of the computer; a 32-bit bus can transfer twice as much data per clock cycle as a 16-bit bus. A program that is "multithreaded" divides a processing task into separate "threads" of instructions that are sent to individual cores in a multicore microprocessor, thereby distributing individual tasks for simultaneous processing. Multitasking (running more than one process at one time) can also take advantage of multiple core microprocessor designs, thus enhancing the data and processing throughput.

There are several ways to compare the performance of computer systems. One indicator of CPU speed is the speed of its clock. If two computers are otherwise identical, the computer with the faster clock speed is faster. For example, if the CPUs of two computers are otherwise identical, a CPU running at 2 gigahertz (GHz) is faster than a CPU running at 1 GHz.

The clock speed of a CPU is not as useful in comparing computers with different microprocessors, because one microprocessor architecture may execute more instructions per clock cycle than another. To avoid this problem, the speed of a CPU may be measured in *millions of instructions per second* (MIPS). If a computer is used to performing extensive mathematical operations, it may be better to measure its performance in millions or billions of floating-point operations per second (megaflops or gigaflops). Another way to compare the performance of computers is to compare the times it takes them to execute standard programs. Programs used for this purpose are called *benchmarks*.

The ability of a computer to execute a particular program in less time than another computer or to perform a greater number of MIPS or megaflops does not prove that it is faster for all applications. For example, the execution speed of one application may rely primarily on CPU speed and CPU-memory transfer rates, whereas another application's speed of execution may largely depend on the rate of transfer of data between the hard disk and main memory. When evaluating computers for a particular purpose, such as reconstructing tomographic images, it is better to compare their speed in performing the actual tasks expected of them than to compare them solely on the basis of clock speed, MIPS, megaflops, or benchmark performance.

B.3   Computer Software

Computer Languages

Machine Language

The actual binary instructions that are executed by the CPU are written in *machine language*. There are disadvantages to writing a program in machine language. The programmer must have a very detailed knowledge of the computer's construction to write such a program. Also, machine-language programs are very difficult to read and understand. For these reasons, programs are seldom written in machine language today

High-Level Languages

To make programming easier and to make programs more readable, *high-level languages,* such as Fortran, Basic, Pascal, C, and Java, have been developed. These languages enable computer programs to be written using statements similar to simple English, resulting in programs that are much easier to read than those in machine language. Also, much less knowledge of the particular computer is required to write a program in a high-level language. Using a program written in a high-level language requires a program called a *compiler* or an *interpreter* to convert the statements written in the high-level language into machine-language instructions that the CPU can execute.

Applications Programs

An *applications program*, commonly referred to as an *application*, is a program that performs a specific function for a user. Examples of applications are e-mail programs, word processing programs, web browsers, and image display programs.

Operating System

Even when a computer is not executing an assigned program and seems to be idle, there is a fundamental program, called the *operating system*, being executed. When the user instructs a computer to run a particular program, the operating system copies the program into memory from a disk, transfers control to it, and regains control of the computer when the program has finished. The operating system also handles most of the complex aspects of input/output operations and controls the sharing of resources on multiuser computers. Common operating systems include Windows and Linux for IBM-compatible PCs; the Mac OS X on Apple computers; and Unix, used on a wide variety of computers.

Most operating systems store information on mass storage devices as *files.* A single file may contain a program, one or more images, patient data, or a manuscript. Each storage device or unit of storage media has a *directory* that lists all files on the device and describes the location of each.

The operating system can be used to perform many utility functions. These utility functions include listing the files on a mass storage device, determining how much unused space remains on a mass storage device, deleting files, and making a copy of a file on another device.

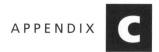
Physical Constants, Prefixes, Geometry, Conversion Factors, and Radiologic Data

TABLE C-1 PHYSICAL CONSTANTS, PREFIXES, AND GEOMETRY

A: PHYSICAL CONSTANTS

Acceleration due to gravity	9.80665 m/s^2
Gyromagnetic ratio of proton	42.5764 MHz/T
Avogadro's number	6.0221415×10^{23} particles/mole
Planck's constant	6.62607×10^{-34} J-s
Planck's constant	4.13567×10^{-15} eV-s
Charge of electron	1.602177×10^{-19} C
Mass of electron	9.109382×10^{-31} kg
Mass of proton	1.672623×10^{-27} kg
Mass of neutron	1.674929×10^{-27} kg
Atomic mass unit	1.660539×10^{-27} kg
Molar volume	22.465 L/mol (at 25°C)
Speed of light (c)	2.99792458×10^{8} m/s

B: PREFIXES

yotta (Y)	10^{24}
zetta (Z)	10^{21}
exa (E)	10^{18}
peta (P)	10^{15}
tera (T)	10^{12}
giga (G)	10^{9}
mega (M)	10^{6}
kilo (k)	10^{3}
hecto (h)	10^{2}
deca (da)	10^{1}
deci (d)	10^{-1}
centi (c)	10^{-2}

(Continued)

TABLE C-1 PHYSICAL CONSTANTS, PREFIXES, AND GEOMETRY (Continued)

milli (m)	10^{-3}
micro (μ)	10^{-6}
nano (n)	10^{-9}
pico (p)	10^{-12}
femto (f)	10^{-15}
atto (a)	10^{-18}
zepto (z)	10^{-21}
yocto (y)	10^{-24}

C: GEOMETRY

Area of circle	πr^2
Circumference of circle	$2\pi r$
Surface area of sphere	$4\pi r^2$
Volume of sphere	$(4/3)\pi r^3$
Area of triangle	$(1/2)$ base $\times$ height

TABLE C-2 DEFINITIONS AND CONVERSION FACTORS

ENERGY

1 electron volt (eV)	1.6022×10^{-19} J
1 calorie	4.187 J

POWER

1 watt (W)	J/s

CURRENT

1 ampere	1 C/s
1 ampere	6.241×10^{18} electrons/s

VOLUME

1 US gallon	3.7854 L
1 liter (L)	1,000 cm³

TEMPERATURE

°C (Celsius)	$5/9 \times (°F - 32)$
°F (Fahrenheit)	$9/5 \times °C + 32$
°K (Kelvin)	$°C + 273.16$

MASS

1 pound	0.45359 kg
1 kg	2.2 pound

LENGTH

1 inch	25.4 mm
1 inch	2.54 cm

(Continued)

TABLE C-2   DEFINITIONS AND CONVERSION FACTORS (Continued)

ANGLE

1 radian	$360°/2\pi \approx 57.2958$ degrees

RADIOLOGIC UNITS

1 roentgen (R)	2.5×10^{-4} C/kg
1 roentgen (R)	8.73 mGy air kerma
1 mGy air kerma	114.5 mR
1 gray (Gy)	100 rad
1 sievert (Sv)	100 rem
1 curie (Ci)	3.7×10^{10} becquerel (Bq)
1 becquerel (Bq)	1 disintegration s^{-1} (dps)

TABLE C-3   RADIOLOGIC DATA FOR ELEMENTS 1 THROUGH 100

Z	SYM	ELEMENT	DENSITY (g/cm³)	AT MASS (g/mol)	K-EDGE (KeV)	L-EDGES: L_I (KeV)	L-EDGES: L_{II} (KeV)	L-EDGES: L_{III} (KeV)	$K\alpha_1$ (KeV)	$K\alpha_2$ (KeV)	$K\beta_1$ (KeV)	$K\beta_2$ (KeV)
1	H	Hydrogen	8.988E-05	1.008	0.0136	–	–	–	–	–	–	–
2	He	Helium	0.0001785	4.003	0.0246	–	–	–	–	–	–	–
3	Li	Lithium	0.534	6.939	0.0550	–	–	–	0.052	0.052	–	–
4	Be	Beryllium	1.85	9.012	0.115	–	–	0.006	0.109	0.109	–	–
5	B	Boron	2.34	10.811	0.188	–	–	0.005	0.183	0.183	–	–
6	C	Carbon	2.267	12.011	0.282	–	–	0.005	0.277	0.277	–	–
7	N	Nitrogen	0.0012506	14.007	0.397	–	–	0.004	0.393	0.393	–	–
8	O	Oxygen	0.001429	15.999	0.533	–	–	0.008	0.525	0.525	–	–
9	F	Fluorine	0.001696	18.998	0.692	–	–	0.015	0.677	0.677	–	–
10	Ne	Neon	0.0008999	20.179	0.874	–	–	0.026	0.848	0.848	0.858	0.858
11	Na	Sodium	0.971	22.99	1.080	0.06	–	0.039	1.041	1.041	1.071	1.071
12	Mg	Magnesium	1.738	24.312	1.309	0.062	0.08	0.056	1.253	1.253	1.302	1.302
13	Al	Aluminum	2.698	26.982	1.840	0.118	0.076	0.075	1.487	1.486	1.557	1.557
14	Si	Silicon	2.3296	28.086	2.143	0.153	0.101	0.100	1.740	1.739	1.836	1.836
15	P	Phosphorus	1.82	30.974	2.471	0.193	0.130	0.129	2.014	2.013	2.139	2.139
16	S	Sulfur	2.067	32.064	2.824	0.237	0.164	0.163	2.308	2.307	2.464	2.464
17	Cl	Chlorine	0.003214	35.453	3.203	0.286	0.204	0.202	2.622	2.620	2.816	2.816
18	Ar	Argon	0.0017837	39.948	3.607	0.340	0.247	0.245	2.958	2.956	3.19	3.19
19	K	Potassium	0.862	39.102	4.034	0.403	0.296	0.293	3.314	3.311	3.59	3.59
20	Ca	Calcium	1.54	40.08	4.486	0.462	0.346	0.342	3.692	3.688	4.013	4.013
21	Sc	Scandium	2.989	44.958	4.965	0.529	0.400	0.396	4.090	4.086	4.461	4.461

(Continued)

TABLE C-3 RADIOLOGIC DATA FOR ELEMENTS 1 THROUGH 100 (Continued)

Z	SYM	ELEMENT	DENSITY (g/cm³)	AT MASS (g/mol)	K-EDGE (KeV)	L-EDGES: L_I (KeV)	L-EDGES: L_{II} (KeV)	L-EDGES: L_{III} (KeV)	$K\alpha_1$ (KeV)	$K\alpha_2$ (KeV)	$K\beta_1$ (KeV)	$K\beta_2$ (KeV)
22	Ti	Titanium	4.54	47.9	5.463	0.626	0.460	0.454	4.511	4.505	4.932	4.932
23	V	Vanadium	6.11	50.942	5.987	0.694	0.519	0.511	4.952	4.944	5.427	5.427
24	Cr	Chromium	7.15	51.996	6.537	0.768	0.582	0.572	5.415	5.405	5.947	5.947
25	Mn	Manganese	7.44	54.938	7.112	0.846	0.649	0.638	5.899	5.888	6.49	6.49
26	Fe	Iron	7.874	55.847	7.712	0.929	0.721	0.708	6.404	6.391	7.058	7.058
27	Co	Cobalt	8.86	58.933	8.339	1.016	0.797	0.782	6.930	6.915	7.649	7.649
28	Ni	Nickel	8.912	58.71	8.993	1.109	0.878	0.861	7.478	7.461	8.265	8.265
29	Cu	Copper	8.96	63.54	9.673	1.208	0.965	0.945	8.048	8.028	8.905	8.93
30	Zn	Zinc	7.134	65.37	10.386	1.316	1.057	1.034	8.639	8.616	9.572	9.6581
31	Ga	Gallium	5.907	69.72	11.115	1.426	1.155	1.134	9.252	9.231	10.271	10.3661
32	Ge	Germanium	5.323	72.59	11.877	1.536	1.259	1.228	9.887	9.856	10.983	11.1011
33	As	Arsenic	5.776	74.922	12.666	1.662	1.368	1.333	10.544	10.509	11.727	11.8641
34	Se	Selenium	4.809	78.96	13.483	1.791	1.485	1.444	11.222	11.181	12.496	12.6521
35	Br	Bromine	3.122	79.909	14.330	1.923	1.605	1.559	11.924	11.878	13.292	13.4701
36	Kr	Krypton	0.003733	83.8	15.202	2.067	1.732	1.680	12.650	12.598	14.113	14.3151
37	Rb	Rubidium	1.532	85.47	16.106	2.217	1.866	1.806	13.396	13.336	14.962	15.1851
38	Sr	Strontium	2.64	87.62	17.037	2.372	2.008	1.940	14.166	14.098	15.836	16.0851
39	Y	Yttrium	4.469	88.905	17.997	2.535	2.155	2.079	14.958	14.882	16.737	17.0151
40	Zr	Zirconium	6.506	91.22	18.985	2.698	2.305	2.227	15.770	15.692	17.662	17.9631
41	Nb	Niobium	8.57	92.906	20.002	2.867	2.464	2.370	16.615	16.521	18.623	18.9471
42	Mo	Molybdenum	10.22	95.94	21.048	3.047	2.628	2.523	17.479	17.374	19.608	19.960
43	Tc	Technetium	11.5	99	22.123	3.230	2.797	2.681	18.367	18.251	20.619	21.002
44	Ru	Ruthenium	12.37	101.7	23.229	3.421	2.973	2.844	19.279	19.150	21.656	22.072

45	Rh	Rhodium	12.41	102.905	24.365	3.619	3.156	3.013	20.216	20.073	22.723	23.173
46	Pd	Palladium	12.02	106.4	25.531	3.822	3.344	3.187	21.178	21.021	23.819	24.303
47	Ag	Silver	10.501	107.87	26.727	4.034	3.540	3.368	22.163	21.991	24.943	25.463
48	Cd	Cadmium	8.69	112.4	27.953	4.250	3.742	3.554	23.173	22.985	26.095	26.653
49	In	Indium	7.31	114.82	29.211	4.475	3.951	3.744	24.209	24.002	27.275	27.872
50	Sn	Tin	7.287	118.69	30.499	4.706	4.167	3.939	25.272	25.044	28.491	29.122
51	Sb	Antimony	6.685	121.75	31.817	4.942	4.389	4.140	26.359	26.110	29.725	30.402
52	Te	Tellurium	6.232	127.6	33.168	5.186	4.616	4.345	27.472	27.201	30.995	31.712
53	I	Iodine	4.93	126.904	34.551	5.442	4.851	4.556	28.612	28.317	32.295	33.054
54	Xe	Xenon	0.005887	131.3	35.966	5.700	5.092	4.772	29.779	29.459	33.625	34.428
55	Cs	Cesium	1.873	132.905	38.894	6.235	5.341	4.993	30.973	30.625	34.985	35.833
56	Ba	Barium	3.594	137.34	40.410	6.516	5.597	5.220	32.194	31.817	36.378	37.270
57	La	Lanthanum	6.145	138.91	41.958	6.802	5.860	5.452	33.442	33.034	37.802	38.739
58	Ce	Cerium	6.77	140.12	43.538	7.095	6.131	5.690	34.720	34.279	39.258	40.243
59	Pr	Praseodymium	6.773	140.907	45.152	7.398	6.408	5.932	36.026	35.550	40.748	41.778
60	Nd	Neodymium	7.007	144.24	46.801	7.707	6.691	6.177	37.361	36.847	42.272	43.345
61	Pm	Promethium	7.26	145	48.486	8.024	6.981	6.427	38.725	38.171	43.825	44.947
62	Sm	Samarium	7.52	150.35	50.207	8.343	7.278	6.683	40.118	39.523	45.413	46.584
63	Eu	Europium	5.243	151.96	51.965	8.679	7.584	6.944	41.542	40.902	47.036	48.256
64	Gd	Gadolinium	7.895	157.25	53.761	9.013	7.898	7.211	42.996	42.309	48.696	49.964
65	Tb	Terbium	8.229	158.924	55.593	9.365	8.221	7.484	44.481	43.744	50.382	51.709
66	Dy	Dysprosium	8.55	162.5	57.464	9.725	8.553	7.762	45.999	45.208	52.119	53.491
67	Ho	Holmium	8.795	164.93	59.374	10.097	8.894	8.046	47.547	46.699	53.878	55.308
68	Er	Erbium	9.066	167.26	61.322	10.479	9.243	8.336	49.128	48.221	55.681	57.164

(Continued)

TABLE C-3   RADIOLOGIC DATA FOR ELEMENTS 1 THROUGH 100 (Continued)

Z	SYM	ELEMENT	DENSITY (g/cm³)	AT MASS (g/mol)	K-EDGE (KeV)	L-EDGES: L_I (KeV)	L-EDGES L_{II} (KeV)	L-EDGES: L_{III} (KeV)	$K\alpha_1$ (KeV)	$K\alpha_2$ (KeV)	$K\beta_1$ (KeV)	$K\beta_2$ (KeV)
69	Tm	Thulium	9.321	168.934	63.311	10.869	9.601	8.632	50.742	49.773	57.513	59.059
70	Yb	Ytterbium	6.965	173.04	65.345	11.262	9.968	8.933	52.389	51.354	59.374	60.991
71	Lu	Lutetium	9.84	174.97	67.405	11.672	10.346	9.241	54.070	52.965	61.286	62.960
72	Hf	Hafnium	13.31	178.49	69.517	12.092	10.734	9.555	55.790	54.611	63.236	64.973
73	Ta	Tantalum	16.654	180.948	71.670	12.522	11.128	9.872	57.533	56.277	65.221	67.011
74	W	Tungsten	19.25	183.85	73.869	12.968	11.535	10.199	59.318	57.982	67.244	69.100
75	Re	Rhenium	21.02	186.2	76.111	13.416	11.952	10.530	61.140	59.718	69.309	71.230
76	Os	Osmium	22.61	190.2	78.400	13.880	12.382	10.868	63.001	61.487	71.416	73.404
77	Ir	Iridium	22.56	192.2	80.729	14.353	12.824	11.215	64.896	63.287	73.560	75.620
78	Pt	Platinum	21.46	195.09	83.109	14.835	13.277	11.568	66.832	65.123	75.751	77.883
79	Au	Gold	19.282	196.967	83.532	15.344	13.739	11.925	68.804	66.990	77.985	80.182
80	Hg	Mercury	13.5336	200.5	88.008	15.863	14.215	12.290	70.819	68.894	80.261	82.532
81	Tl	Thallium	11.85	204.37	90.540	16.391	14.700	12.660	72.872	70.832	82.575	84.924
82	Pb	Lead	11.342	207.19	93.113	16.940	15.204	13.039	74.969	72.804	84.936	87.367
83	Bi	Bismuth	9.807	208.98	95.730	17.495	15.725	13.422	77.118	74.815	87.354	89.866
84	Po	Polonium-209	9.32	208.98	98.402	18.047	16.250	13.812	79.301	76.863	89.801	92.403
85	At	Astatine-210	7	209.983	101.131	18.630	16.787	14.207	81.523	78.943	92.302	94.983

86	Rn	Radon-222	0.00973	222.018	103.909	19.222	17.337	14.609	83.793	81.065	94.866	97.617
87	Fr	Francium-223	1.87	223.02	106.738	19.823	17.900	15.017	86.114	83.231	97.477	100.306
88	Ra	Radium-226	5.5	226.025	109.641	20.449	18.475	15.433	88.476	85.434	100.130	103.039
89	Ac	Actinium-227	10.07	227.028	112.599	21.088	19.063	15.854	90.884	87.675	102.846	105.837
90	Th	Thorium-232	11.72	232.038	115.606	21.757	16.689	16.283	93.358	89.952	105.611	108.690
91	Pa	Protactinium-231	15.37	231.036	118.678	22.427	20.312	16.716	95.883	92.287	108.435	111.606
92	U	Uranium-238	18.95	238.051	121.818	23.097	20.947	17.166	98.440	94.659	111.303	114.561
93	Np	Neptunium-237	20.45	237.048	125.027	23.773	21.601	17.610	101.068	97.077	114.243	117.591
94	Pu	Plutonium-239	19.84	239.052	128.220	24.460	22.266	18.057	103.761	99.552	117.261	120.703
95	Am	Americium-241	13.69	241.05	131.590	25.275	22.944	18.504	106.523	102.083	120.360	123.891
96	Cm	Curium-247	13.51	247.07	135.960	26.110	23.779	18.930	109.290	104.441	123.423	127.066
97	Bk	Berkelium-247	14.79	247.07	139.490	26.900	24.385	19.452	112.138	107.205	126.663	130.355
98	Cf	Californium-251	15.1	251.08	143.090	27.700	25.250	19.930	116.030	110.710	130.851	134.681
99	Es	Einsteinium-252	13.5	252.083	146.780	28.530	26.020	20.410	119.080	113.470	134.238	138.169
100	Fm	Fermium-257	—	257.095	150.540	29.380	26.810	20.900	122.190	116.280	137.693	141.724

APPENDIX D

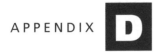

Mass Attenuation Coefficients

D.1 Mass Attenuation Coefficients for Selected Elements

TABLE D-1 MASS ATTENUATION COEFFICIENTS IN cm²/g (DENSITY (ρ) IN g/cm³)

ENERGY (keV)	ALUMINUM Z = 13 ρ = 2.699	CALCIUM Z = 20 ρ = 1.55	COPPER Z = 29 ρ = 8.96	MOLYBDENUM Z = 42 ρ = 10.22	RHODIUM Z = 45 ρ = 12.41	IODINE Z = 53 ρ = 4.93	TUNGSTEN Z = 74 ρ = 19.3	LEAD Z = 82 ρ = 11.35
3	7.83E+02	2.71E+02	7.47E+02	2.01E+03	4.42E+02	7.49E+02	1.92E+03	1.96E+03
4	3.58E+02	1.20E+02	3.46E+02	9.65E+02	1.17E+03	3.56E+02	9.54E+02	1.25E+03
5	1.92E+02	5.97E+02	1.89E+02	5.42E+02	6.55E+02	8.30E+02	5.51E+02	7.28E+02
6	1.15E+02	3.74E+02	1.15E+02	3.38E+02	4.11E+02	6.10E+02	3.55E+02	4.73E+02
7	7.37E+01	2.46E+02	7.48E+01	2.23E+02	2.72E+02	4.13E+02	2.36E+02	3.16E+02
8	5.04E+01	1.72E+02	5.18E+01	1.56E+02	1.90E+02	2.89E+02	1.69E+02	2.27E+02
9	3.56E+01	1.25E+02	2.76E+02	1.13E+02	1.39E+02	2.13E+02	1.24E+02	1.68E+02
10	2.60E+01	9.30E+01	2.14E+02	8.55E+01	1.05E+02	1.62E+02	9.33E+01	1.29E+02
12	1.53E+01	5.60E+01	1.35E+02	5.22E+01	6.44E+01	1.00E+02	2.10E+02	8.15E+01
14	9.73E+00	3.62E+01	8.91E+01	3.40E+01	4.21E+01	6.61E+01	1.65E+02	1.33E+02
16	6.58E+00	2.48E+01	6.20E+01	2.37E+01	2.92E+01	4.61E+01	1.17E+02	1.51E+02
18	4.65E+00	1.76E+01	4.49E+01	1.72E+01	2.10E+01	3.35E+01	8.63E+01	1.10E+02
20	3.42E+00	1.30E+01	3.36E+01	7.89E+01	1.57E+01	2.52E+01	6.56E+01	8.61E+01
25	1.83E+00	6.88E+00	1.82E+01	4.78E+01	5.29E+01	1.37E+01	3.66E+01	4.93E+01
30	1.13E+00	4.07E+00	1.09E+01	2.82E+01	3.32E+01	8.38E+00	2.28E+01	3.06E+01
35	7.69E-01	2.63E+00	7.05E+00	1.85E+01	2.21E+01	3.10E+01	1.51E+01	2.02E+01
40	5.67E-01	1.83E+00	4.85E+00	1.29E+01	1.54E+01	2.20E+01	1.06E+01	1.43E+01

45	4.46E−01	1.34E+00	3.51E+00	9.38E+00	1.12E+01	1.62E+01	7.72E+00	1.05E+01
50	3.68E−01	1.02E+00	2.62E+00	7.07E+00	8.42E+00	1.23E+01	5.84E+00	7.98E+00
55	3.15E−01	8.07E−01	2.01E+00	5.42E+00	6.52E+00	9.56E+00	4.54E+00	6.20E+00
60	2.78E−01	6.61E−01	1.60E+00	4.29E+00	5.18E+00	7.61E+00	3.62E+00	4.98E+00
65	2.52E−01	5.56E−01	1.30E+00	3.46E+00	4.20E+00	6.18E+00	2.92E+00	4.04E+00
70	2.30E−01	4.72E−01	1.06E+00	2.80E+00	3.39E+00	5.02E+00	1.09E+01	3.30E+00
75	2.14E−01	4.12E−01	9.00E−01	2.33E+00	2.84E+00	4.19E+00	9.21E+00	2.77E+00
80	2.02E−01	3.66E−01	7.63E−01	1.96E+00	2.37E+00	3.53E+00	7.80E+00	2.32E+00
85	1.92E−01	3.33E−01	6.71E−01	1.70E+00	2.05E+00	3.05E+00	6.78E+00	1.98E+00
90	1.83E−01	3.00E−01	5.80E−01	1.44E+00	1.74E+00	2.57E+00	5.78E+00	7.20E+00
95	1.77E−01	2.79E−01	5.20E−01	1.27E+00	1.53E+00	2.26E+00	5.10E+00	6.38E+00
100	1.71E−01	2.58E−01	4.60E−01	1.10E+00	1.32E+00	1.95E+00	4.42E+00	5.54E+00
110	1.61E−01	2.28E−01	3.78E−01	8.66E−01	1.04E+00	1.52E+00	3.47E+00	4.36E+00
120	1.53E−01	2.06E−01	3.23E−01	7.10E−01	8.43E−01	1.22E+00	2.83E+00	3.55E+00
130	1.47E−01	1.90E−01	2.81E−01	5.88E−01	6.95E−01	1.00E+00	2.29E+00	2.90E+00
140	1.42E−01	1.77E−01	2.47E−01	4.91E−01	5.77E−01	8.26E−01	1.89E+00	2.38E+00
150	1.38E−01	1.67E−01	2.23E−01	4.23E−01	4.94E−01	7.00E−01	1.59E+00	2.02E+00
160	1.34E−01	1.59E−01	2.03E−01	3.69E−01	4.29E−01	6.01E−01	1.36E+00	1.72E+00
170	1.31E−01	1.53E−01	1.89E−01	3.31E−01	3.82E−01	5.31E−01	1.18E+00	1.50E+00

(Continued)

TABLE D-1 MASS ATTENUATION COEFFICIENTS IN cm²/g (DENSITY (ρ) IN g/cm³) (Continued)

ENERGY (keV)	ALUMINUM Z = 13 ρ = 2.699	CALCIUM Z = 20 ρ = 1.55	COPPER Z = 29 ρ = 8.96	MOLYBDENUM Z = 42 ρ = 10.22	RHODIUM Z = 45 ρ = 12.41	IODINE Z = 53 ρ = 4.93	TUNGSTEN Z = 74 ρ = 19.3	LEAD Z = 82 ρ = 11.35
180	1.27E−01	1.47E−01	1.75E−01	2.93E−01	3.36E−01	4.61E−01	1.02E+00	1.29E+00
190	1.25E−01	1.42E−01	1.65E−01	2.68E−01	3.06E−01	4.14E−01	9.03E−01	1.15E+00
200	1.22E−01	1.37E−01	1.56E−01	2.43E−01	2.75E−01	3.68E−01	7.90E−01	1.00E+00
250	1.12E−01	1.22E−01	1.28E−01	1.73E−01	1.91E−01	2.40E−01	4.75E−01	6.02E−01
300	1.04E−01	1.11E−01	1.12E−01	1.38E−01	1.49E−01	1.80E−01	3.26E−01	4.07E−01
350	9.76E−02	1.04E−01	1.01E−01	1.18E−01	1.25E−01	1.43E−01	2.43E−01	2.97E−01
400	9.26E−02	9.75E−02	9.39E−02	1.04E−01	1.10E−01	1.22E−01	1.92E−01	2.33E−01
450	8.82E−02	9.26E−02	8.82E−02	9.52E−02	9.90E−02	1.07E−01	1.60E−01	1.90E−01
500	8.43E−02	8.83E−02	8.35E−02	8.83E−02	9.11E−02	9.67E−02	1.37E−01	1.61E−01
550	8.10E−02	8.45E−02	7.94E−02	8.27E−02	8.49E−02	8.89E−02	1.21E−01	1.40E−01
600	7.80E−02	8.13E−02	7.61E−02	7.82E−02	8.02E−02	8.31E−02	1.10E−01	1.26E−01
650	7.52E−02	7.83E−02	7.30E−02	7.45E−02	7.60E−02	7.79E−02	9.98E−02	1.13E−01
700	7.27E−02	7.56E−02	7.04E−02	7.13E−02	7.25E−02	7.37E−02	9.16E−02	1.02E−01
750	7.05E−02	7.34E−02	6.81E−02	6.86E−02	6.97E−02	7.05E−02	8.59E−02	9.53E−02
800	6.83E−02	7.11E−02	6.59E−02	6.61E−02	6.70E−02	6.73E−02	8.02E−02	8.82E−02

D-2 Mass Attenuation Coefficients for Selected Compounds

TABLE D-2 MASS ATTENUATION COEFFICIENTS IN cm²/g (DENSITY (ρ) IN g/cm³)

ENERGY (keV)	AIR $\rho = 0.001293$	WATER $\rho = 1.00$	PLEXIGLAS[a] $\rho = 1.19$	MUSCLE $\rho = 1.06$	BONE $\rho = 1.5$ TO 3.0	ADIPOSE[b] $\rho = 0.930$	50/50[b] $\rho = 0.982$	GLANDULAR[b] $\rho = 1.040$
2	5.20E+02	6.17E+02	4.04E+02	5.67E+02	5.24E+02	3.70E+02	4.60E+02	5.41E+02
3	1.63E+02	1.95E+02	1.26E+02	1.87E+02	2.42E+02	1.15E+02	1.44E+02	1.71E+02
4	7.43E+01	8.24E+01	5.23E+01	8.16E+01	1.06E+02	4.77E+01	6.04E+01	7.17E+01
5	3.84E+01	4.24E+01	2.66E+01	4.22E+01	1.34E+02	2.43E+01	3.09E+01	3.68E+01
6	2.24E+01	2.47E+01	1.54E+01	2.47E+01	8.26E+01	1.41E+01	1.79E+01	2.14E+01
7	1.40E+01	1.54E+01	9.66E+00	1.55E+01	5.36E+01	8.81E+00	1.12E+01	1.34E+01
8	9.42E+00	1.03E+01	6.46E+00	1.04E+01	3.71E+01	5.90E+00	7.50E+00	8.94E+00
9	6.62E+00	7.23E+00	4.54E+00	7.32E+00	2.68E+01	4.15E+00	5.28E+00	6.28E+00
10	4.84E+00	5.30E+00	3.34E+00	5.37E+00	1.99E+01	3.06E+00	3.87E+00	4.60E+00
12	2.87E+00	3.16E+00	2.01E+00	3.21E+00	1.19E+01	1.85E+00	2.33E+00	2.75E+00
14	1.85E+00	2.02E+00	1.31E+00	2.05E+00	7.67E+00	1.22E+00	1.51E+00	1.77E+00
16	1.29E+00	1.40E+00	9.36E-01	1.43E+00	5.26E+00	8.74E-01	1.07E+00	1.24E+00
18	9.55E-01	1.04E+00	7.12E-01	1.06E+00	3.78E+00	6.71E-01	8.03E-01	9.22E-01
20	7.43E-01	8.08E-01	5.70E-01	8.23E-01	2.82E+00	5.42E-01	6.37E-01	7.23E-01
25	4.66E-01	5.09E-01	3.86E-01	5.16E-01	1.56E+00	3.74E-01	4.22E-01	4.64E-01
30	3.46E-01	3.75E-01	3.04E-01	3.79E-01	9.80E-01	3.00E-01	3.26E-01	3.49E-01
35	2.80E-01	3.07E-01	2.60E-01	3.09E-01	6.86E-01	2.59E-01	2.75E-01	2.90E-01
40	2.44E-01	2.68E-01	2.34E-01	2.69E-01	5.20E-01	2.35E-01	2.46E-01	2.55E-01
45	2.21E-01	2.44E-01	2.19E-01	2.44E-01	4.18E-01	2.21E-01	2.28E-01	2.34E-01

(Continued)

TABLE D-2 MASS ATTENUATION COEFFICIENTS IN cm²/g (DENSITY (ρ) IN g/cm³) (Continued)

ENERGY (keV)	AIR ρ = 0.001293	WATER ρ = 1.00	PLEXIGLAS[a] ρ = 1.19	MUSCLE ρ = 1.06	BONE ρ = 1.5 TO 3.0)	ADIPOSE[b] ρ = 0.930	50/50[b] ρ = 0.982	GLANDULAR[b] ρ = 1.040
50	2.05E-01	2.27E-01	2.07E-01	2.26E-01	3.53E-01	2.10E-01	2.15E-01	2.19E-01
55	1.94E-01	2.14E-01	1.98E-01	2.14E-01	3.07E-01	2.02E-01	2.05E-01	2.08E-01
60	1.86E-01	2.06E-01	1.92E-01	2.05E-01	2.75E-01	1.96E-01	1.98E-01	2.00E-01
65	1.80E-01	1.99E-01	1.87E-01	1.98E-01	2.52E-01	1.91E-01	1.92E-01	1.94E-01
70	1.74E-01	1.93E-01	1.82E-01	1.92E-01	2.34E-01	1.86E-01	1.87E-01	1.88E-01
75	1.69E-01	1.88E-01	1.78E-01	1.86E-01	2.20E-01	1.82E-01	1.83E-01	1.84E-01
80	1.65E-01	1.83E-01	1.75E-01	1.82E-01	2.08E-01	1.79E-01	1.79E-01	1.80E-01
85	1.62E-01	1.79E-01	1.72E-01	1.78E-01	2.00E-01	1.76E-01	1.76E-01	1.76E-01
90	1.59E-01	1.76E-01	1.69E-01	1.75E-01	1.92E-01	1.73E-01	1.73E-01	1.73E-01
95	1.56E-01	1.73E-01	1.66E-01	1.72E-01	1.86E-01	1.70E-01	1.70E-01	1.70E-01
100	1.54E-01	1.71E-01	1.64E-01	1.69E-01	1.80E-01	1.68E-01	1.68E-01	1.68E-01
110	1.49E-01	1.65E-01	1.59E-01	1.64E-01	1.71E-01	1.63E-01	1.63E-01	1.63E-01
120	1.45E-01	1.61E-01	1.55E-01	1.60E-01	1.64E-01	1.60E-01	1.59E-01	1.59E-01
130	1.42E-01	1.57E-01	1.52E-01	1.56E-01	1.58E-01	1.56E-01	1.55E-01	1.55E-01
140	1.38E-01	1.54E-01	1.49E-01	1.52E-01	1.53E-01	1.52E-01	1.52E-01	1.51E-01
150	1.35E-01	1.50E-01	1.46E-01	1.49E-01	1.49E-01	1.49E-01	1.49E-01	1.48E-01
160	1.33E-01	1.47E-01	1.43E-01	1.46E-01	1.45E-01	1.46E-01	1.46E-01	1.45E-01
170	1.30E-01	1.44E-01	1.40E-01	1.43E-01	1.42E-01	1.44E-01	1.43E-01	1.42E-01
180	1.27E-01	1.42E-01	1.37E-01	1.40E-01	1.38E-01	1.41E-01	1.40E-01	1.40E-01
190	1.25E-01	1.39E-01	1.35E-01	1.38E-01	1.36E-01	1.39E-01	1.38E-01	1.37E-01
200	1.23E-01	1.37E-01	1.32E-01	1.35E-01	1.33E-01	1.36E-01	1.35E-01	1.35E-01

250	1.14E−01	1.27E−01	1.23E−01	1.25E−01	1.22E−01	1.26E−01	1.25E−01	1.25E−01
300	1.07E−01	1.18E−01	1.15E−01	1.17E−01	1.14E−01	1.18E−01	1.17E−01	1.17E−01
350	1.00E−01	1.11E−01	1.08E−01	1.10E−01	1.07E−01	1.11E−01	1.11E−01	1.10E−01
400	9.53E−02	1.06E−01	1.03E−01	1.05E−01	1.02E−01	1.06E−01	1.05E−01	1.04E−01
450	9.09E−02	1.01E−01	9.82E−02	1.00E−01	9.68E−02	1.01E−01	1.00E−01	9.97E−02
500	8.70E−02	9.67E−02	9.39E−02	9.58E−02	9.26E−02	9.65E−02	9.60E−02	9.54E−02
550	8.36E−02	9.29E−02	9.03E−02	9.21E−02	8.89E−02	9.27E−02	9.22E−02	9.17E−02
600	8.05E−02	8.96E−02	8.70E−02	8.87E−02	8.56E−02	8.94E−02	8.89E−02	8.83E−02
650	7.77E−02	8.64E−02	8.39E−02	8.56E−02	8.26E−02	8.62E−02	8.57E−02	8.52E−02
700	7.51E−02	8.35E−02	8.11E−02	8.27E−02	7.98E−02	8.34E−02	8.29E−02	8.24E−02
750	7.29E−02	8.10E−02	7.87E−02	8.03E−02	7.75E−02	8.09E−02	8.04E−02	7.99E−02
800	7.06E−02	7.85E−02	7.63E−02	7.78E−02	7.51E−02	7.84E−02	7.79E−02	7.75E−02

^{a}Polymethyl methacrylate, $C_5H_8O_2$.

^{b}Composition data from Hammerstein GR, Miller DW, White DR, et al. Absorbed radiation dose in mammography. *Radiology* 1979;130:485–491. The 50% adipose data is presented here for reference. More recent information suggests that the typical breast is not 50%–50%, but much lower in terms of volume glandular fraction. See: MJ Yaffe, JM Boone, N Packard, O Alonzo-Proulx, Peressotti K, Al-Mayah A, Brock K. The Myth of the 50%–50% breast. *Med Phys* 2009;36:5437–5443.

D.3

Mass Energy Attenuation Coefficients for Selected Detector Compounds

TABLE D-3 MASS ENERGY ATTENUATION COEFFICIENTS IN cm²/G (DENSITY (ρ) IN G/CM³)

ENERGY (keV)	SI (ELEMENTAL) $\rho = 2.33$	Se (ELEMENTAL) $\rho = 4.79$	BaFBr $\rho = 4.56$	CsI $\rho = 4.51$	Gd_2O_2S $\rho = 7.34$	$YTaO_4$ $\rho = 7.57$	$CaWO_4$ $\rho = 6.12$	AgBr $\rho = 6.47$
2	2.75E+03	3.09E+03	2.48E+03	2.11E+03	2.88E+03	2.37E+03	2.76E+03	2.24E+03
3	9.81E+02	1.11E+03	9.20E+02	7.96E+02	1.22E+03	1.49E+03	1.31E+03	8.14E+02
4	4.51E+02	5.22E+02	4.37E+02	3.80E+02	5.90E+02	7.28E+02	6.47E+02	9.89E+02
5	2.44E+02	2.88E+02	2.93E+02	5.20E+02	3.35E+02	4.14E+02	4.46E+02	5.62E+02
6	1.47E+02	1.78E+02	4.96E+02	6.44E+02	2.12E+02	2.64E+02	2.85E+02	3.52E+02
7	9.49E+01	1.16E+02	3.39E+02	4.33E+02	1.39E+02	1.74E+02	1.88E+02	2.33E+02
8	6.44E+01	8.08E+01	2.37E+02	3.04E+02	3.44E+02	1.23E+02	1.34E+02	1.63E+02
9	4.57E+01	5.81E+01	1.73E+02	2.25E+02	2.96E+02	9.01E+01	9.81E+01	1.19E+02
10	3.37E+01	4.34E+01	1.32E+02	1.71E+02	2.27E+02	1.46E+02	7.39E+01	8.99E+01
12	2.02E+01	2.64E+01	8.16E+01	1.06E+02	1.43E+02	1.38E+02	1.43E+02	5.51E+01
14	1.26E+01	1.22E+02	8.54E+01	6.97E+01	9.47E+01	9.29E+01	1.11E+02	8.36E+01
16	8.49E+00	8.66E+01	6.01E+01	4.87E+01	6.64E+01	6.70E+01	7.87E+01	5.88E+01
18	6.02E+00	6.39E+01	4.39E+01	3.54E+01	4.86E+01	6.93E+01	5.78E+01	4.31E+01
20	4.44E+00	4.80E+01	3.32E+01	2.66E+01	3.68E+01	5.26E+01	4.39E+01	3.27E+01
25	2.37E+00	2.62E+01	1.82E+01	1.45E+01	2.02E+01	2.93E+01	2.44E+01	1.77E+01
30	1.43E+00	1.60E+01	1.11E+01	8.87E+00	1.25E+01	1.82E+01	1.52E+01	2.83E+01
35	9.63E-01	1.04E+01	9.20E+00	1.82E+01	8.22E+00	1.20E+01	1.01E+01	1.91E+01
40	7.00E-01	7.17E+00	1.77E+01	2.29E+01	5.72E+00	8.40E+00	7.06E+00	1.33E+01

45	5.41E−01	5.18E+00	1.30E+01	1.69E+01	4.15E+00	6.11E+00	5.17E+00	9.68E+00
50	4.39E−01	3.88E+00	9.91E+00	1.29E+01	3.07E+00	4.61E+00	3.92E+00	7.29E+00
55	3.70E−01	2.98E+00	7.72E+00	1.00E+01	1.23E+01	3.57E+00	3.05E+00	5.64E+00
60	3.22E−01	2.35E+00	6.17E+00	7.96E+00	9.83E+00	2.84E+00	2.44E+00	4.50E+00
65	2.87E−01	1.90E+00	5.01E+00	6.46E+00	8.05E+00	2.30E+00	1.98E+00	3.62E+00
70	2.59E−01	1.54E+00	4.07E+00	5.25E+00	6.59E+00	6.42E+00	7.06E+00	2.93E+00
75	2.40E−01	1.29E+00	3.39E+00	4.37E+00	5.55E+00	5.40E+00	5.98E+00	2.44E+00
80	2.23E−01	1.09E+00	2.86E+00	3.68E+00	4.69E+00	4.57E+00	5.07E+00	2.05E+00
85	2.11E−01	9.37E−01	2.47E+00	3.18E+00	4.06E+00	3.97E+00	4.41E+00	1.77E+00
90	2.00E−01	8.12E−01	2.10E+00	2.69E+00	3.44E+00	3.40E+00	3.77E+00	1.51E+00
95	1.92E−01	7.22E−01	1.85E+00	2.37E+00	3.02E+00	3.00E+00	3.33E+00	1.33E+00
100	1.84E−01	6.31E−01	1.60E+00	2.04E+00	2.61E+00	2.61E+00	2.90E+00	1.15E+00
110	1.72E−01	5.07E−01	1.25E+00	1.59E+00	2.04E+00	2.06E+00	2.28E+00	9.05E−01
120	1.63E−01	4.23E−01	1.01E+00	1.28E+00	1.65E+00	1.68E+00	1.87E+00	7.36E−01
130	1.56E−01	3.59E−01	8.38E−01	1.05E+00	1.36E+00	1.37E+00	1.52E+00	6.13E−01
140	1.50E−01	3.08E−01	6.93E−01	8.65E−01	1.12E+00	1.13E+00	1.26E+00	5.12E−01
150	1.45E−01	2.72E−01	5.91E−01	7.33E−01	9.44E−01	9.57E−01	1.07E+00	4.40E−01
160	1.40E−01	2.43E−01	5.10E−01	6.28E−01	8.09E−01	8.21E−01	9.18E−01	3.84E−01
170	1.37E−01	2.21E−01	4.51E−01	5.54E−01	7.11E−01	7.22E−01	8.07E−01	3.43E−01
180	1.33E−01	2.02E−01	3.95E−01	4.80E−01	6.15E−01	6.26E−01	6.98E−01	3.04E−01

(Continued)

TABLE D-3   MASS ENERGY ATTENUATION COEFFICIENTS IN cm²/G (DENSITY (ρ) IN G/CM³) (Continued)

ENERGY (keV)	SI (ELEMENTAL) ρ = 2.33	Se (ELEMENTAL) ρ = 4.79	BaFBr ρ = 4.56	CsI ρ = 4.51	Gd₂O₂S ρ = 7.34	YTaO₄ ρ = 7.57	CaWO₄ ρ = 6.12	AgBr ρ = 6.47
250	1.16E−01	1.35E−01	2.14E−01	2.48E−01	3.06E−01	3.14E−01	3.46E−01	1.77E−01
300	1.08E−01	1.14E−01	1.63E−01	1.84E−01	2.21E−01	2.27E−01	2.48E−01	1.41E−01
350	1.01E−01	1.02E−01	1.33E−01	1.46E−01	1.72E−01	1.78E−01	1.92E−01	1.19E−01
400	9.59E−02	9.27E−02	1.15E−01	1.24E−01	1.42E−01	1.47E−01	1.58E−01	1.06E−01
450	9.14E−02	8.63E−02	1.02E−01	1.09E−01	1.23E−01	1.27E−01	1.35E−01	9.61E−02
500	8.73E−02	8.11E−02	9.30E−02	9.78E−02	1.09E−01	1.13E−01	1.19E−01	8.88E−02
550	8.38E−02	7.68E−02	8.61E−02	8.97E−02	9.91E−02	1.02E−01	1.08E−01	8.31E−02
600	8.07E−02	7.33E−02	8.09E−02	8.37E−02	9.16E−02	9.45E−02	9.93E−02	7.87E−02
650	7.78E−02	7.02E−02	7.62E−02	7.84E−02	8.51E−02	8.78E−02	9.19E−02	7.48E−02
700	7.52E−02	6.75E−02	7.23E−02	7.40E−02	7.99E−02	8.22E−02	8.58E−02	7.14E−02
750	7.29E−02	6.52E−02	6.94E−02	7.08E−02	7.60E−02	7.81E−02	8.13E−02	6.88E−02
800	7.07E−02	6.30E−02	6.64E−02	6.75E−02	7.21E−02	7.40E−02	7.69E−02	6.62E−02

aSource of these coefficients is described in: Boone JM, Chavez AE. Comparison of x-ray cross sections for diagnostic and therapeutic medical physics. *Med Phys* 1996;23:1997–2005.

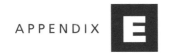

Effective Doses, Organ Doses, and Fetal Doses from Medical Imaging Procedures

Estimates of effective dose and organ doses for a specific diagnostic procedure extend over a range of values, and are dependent on many parameters such as image quality (signal to noise and contrast to noise ratios), patient size, x-ray acquisition techniques, and the application of dose reduction technologies. Methods to reduce radiation dose include utilization of higher quantum detection efficiency digital radiographic detectors and application of image processing algorithms to reduce noise. In CT, they include implementation of automatic tube current modulation as a function of tube angle and patient attenuation, and deployment of statistical iterative reconstruction techniques. As technology advances and improves, a trend towards lower radiation dose should occur, which for many procedures will result in lower effective doses than the values listed in these tables. The numbers of days of typical background radiation equal to the average effective dose of the examination are provided to help to place the magnitude of the exposure into perspective.

Table E-1 lists typical adult effective doses for various diagnostic radiology procedures. Table E-2 provides specific information for interventional examinations, Table E-3 lists dose information for common CT procedures, and Table E-4 presents information on dose from dental imaging procedures.

Table E-5 provides information on *organ doses* based on typical techniques for radiography and CT procedures. Table E-6 lists *organ doses* determined from direct measurements of a 6-year-old pediatric anthropomorphic phantom for "routine" abdominal and chest CT examination techniques at seven different sites in Japan, along with effective dose. Table E-7 lists *effective dose* estimates of various pediatric examinations including the common chest radiograph as well as CT of the head and abdomen as a function of age, from neonate to 15 years old. Table E-8 lists the conceptus dose for various CT, radiography and fluoroscopy imaging procedures.

TABLE E-1 ADULT EFFECTIVE DOSES FOR VARIOUS DIAGNOSTIC RADIOLOGY PROCEDURES (2008)

EXAMINATION	AVERAGE EFFECTIVE DOSE (mSv)	VALUES REPORTED IN LITERATURE (mSv)	DAYS OF EQUIVALENT BACKGROUND RADIATION
Skull	0.1	0.03–0.22	12
Cervical spine	0.2	0.07–0.3	24
Thoracic spine	1	0.6–1.4	118
Lumbar spine	1.5	0.5–1.8	177
Posteroanterior and lateral study of chest	0.1	0.05–0.24	12

(Continued)

TABLE E-1 ADULT EFFECTIVE DOSES FOR VARIOUS DIAGNOSTIC RADIOLOGY PROCEDURES (2008) (Continued)

EXAMINATION	AVERAGE EFFECTIVE DOSE (mSv)	VALUES REPORTED IN LITERATURE (mSv)	DAYS OF EQUIVALENT BACKGROUND RADIATION
Posteroanterior study of chest	0.02	0.007–0.050	2
Two view digital mammography	0.4	0.10–0.60	47
Abdomen	0.7	0.04–1.1	82
Pelvis	0.6	0.2–1.2	73
Hip	0.7	0.18–2.71	82
Shoulder	0.01	—	1
Knee	0.005	—	1
Other extremities	0.001	0.0002–0.1	<1
Dual x-ray absorptiometry (without CT)	0.001	0.001–0.035	<1
Dual x-ray absorptiometry (with CT)	0.04	0.003–0.06	5
Intravenous urography	3	0.7–3.7	350
Upper gastrointestinal series	6	1.5–12	710
Small-bowel series	5	3.0–7.8	590
Barium enema	8	2.0–18.0	940

Source: Mettler FA, et al.: Effective doses in radiology and diagnostic nuclear medicine: a catalog. *Radiology* 2008;248:254–263.

TABLE E-2 ADULT EFFECTIVE DOSES FOR VARIOUS INTERVENTIONAL RADIOLOGY PROCEDURES (2008)

EXAMINATION	AVERAGE EFFECTIVE DOSE (mSv)[a]	VALUES REPORTED IN LITERATURE (mSv)	DAYS OF EQUIVALENT BACKGROUND RADIATION
Head and/or neck angiography	5	0.8–19.6	590
Coronary angiography (diagnostic)	7	2.0–15.8	820
Coronary percutaneous transluminal angioplasty, stent placement, or radiofrequency ablation	15	6.9–57	1,770
Thoracic angiography of pulmonary artery or aorta	5	4.1–9.0	590
Endoscopic retrograde cholangiopancreatography	4	2.0–8.0	470
Abdominal angiography or aortography	12	4.0–48.0	1,410
Transjugular intrahepatic portosystemic shunt placement	70	20–180	8,240
Pelvic vein embolization	60	44–78	7,060

[a]*Source*: Mettler FA, et al.: Effective doses in radiology and diagnostic nuclear medicine: a catalog. *Radiology* 2008;248:254–263.

TABLE E-3   ADULT EFFECTIVE DOSES FOR VARIOUS CT PROCEDURES (2008)

EXAMINATION	AVERAGE EFFECTIVE DOSE (mSv)	RANGE REPORTED IN LITERATURE (mSv)	DAYS OF EQUIVALENT BACKGROUND RADIATION
Head	2	0.9–4.0	240
Neck	3	—	350
Chest	7	4.0–18.0	820
Chest for pulmonary embolism	15	13–40	1,770
Abdomen	8	3.5–25	940
Pelvis	6	3.3–10	710
Three-phase liver study	15	—	1,880
Spine	6	1.5–10	710
Coronary angiography	16	5.0–32	1,880
Calcium scoring	3	1.0–12	350
Virtual colonoscopy	10	4.0–13.2	1,180
Extremities	<0.025	—	<3

Source: Mettler FA, et al.: Effective doses in radiology and diagnostic nuclear medicine: a catalog. *Radiology* 2008;248:254–263.

TABLE E-4   ADULT EFFECTIVE DOSE FOR VARIOUS DENTAL RADIOLOGY PROCEDURES (2008)

EXAMINATION	AVERAGE EFFECTIVE DOSE (mSv)	VALUES REPORTED IN LITERATURE (mSv)	DAYS OF EQUIVALENT BACKGROUND RADIATION
Intraoral radiography	0.005	0.0002–0.010	1
Panoramic radiography	0.01	0.007–0.090	1
Dental CT	0.2	—	20

Source: Mettler FA, et al.: Effective doses in radiology and diagnostic nuclear medicine: a catalog. *Radiology* 2008;248:254–263.

TABLE E-5   TYPICAL ORGAN-SPECIFIC RADIATION DOSES RESULTING FROM VARIOUS RADIOLOGY PROCEDURES

EXAMINATION	ORGAN	ORGAN SPECIFIC RADIATION DOSE (mGy)
PA chest radiography	Lung	0.01
Mammography	Breast	3.5
CT chest	Breast	21.4
CT coronary angiography	Breast	51.0
Abdominal radiography	Stomach	0.25
CT abdomen	Stomach	10.0
	Colon	4.0
Barium enema	Colon	15.0

Source: Davies HE, Wathen CG, Gleeson FV. *BMJ* 2011;342:d947.

TABLE E-6 ORGAN DOSE AVERAGES FOR A 6-YEAR-OLD PEDIATRIC ANTHROPOMORPHIC PHANTOM USING ROUTINE TECHNIQUES AT SEVEN CT SCANNER SITES

	ORGAN DOSE (mGy) ± σ	
TISSUE OR ORGAN	PEDIATRIC ABDOMEN	PEDIATRIC CHEST
Thyroid gland	0.3 ± 0.2	10.5 ± 6.6
Lung	4.2 ± 2.1	9.1 ± 4.2
Breast	2.3 ± 1.8	8.4 ± 4.7
Esophagus	4.2 ± 2.0	9.0 ± 4.4
Liver	8.8 ± 3.5	8.0 ± 3.7
Stomach	9.5 ± 3.9	4.7 ± 2.8
Kidneys	9.0 ± 3.5	4.3 ± 2.2
Colon	9.4 ± 3.5	0.6 ± 0.3
Ovary	9.0 ± 3.1	0.1 ± 0.1
Bladder	9.1 ± 3.3	0.1 ± 0.0
Testis	7.8 ± 3.7	0.1 ± 0.0
Bone surface	8.1 ± 2.8	8.5 ± 3.8

Source: Fujii K, Aoyama T, Koyama S, et al. Comparative evaluation of organ and effective doses for paediatric patients with those for adults in chest and abdominal CT examinations. *Br J Radiol* 2007;80:657–667.
σ, standard deivation

TABLE E-7 EFFECTIVE DOSE ESTIMATES FROM PEDIATRIC DIAGNOSTIC EXAMS AS A FUNCTION OF AGE

EXAMINATION	EFFECTIVE DOSE (mSv)	DAYS OF EQUIVALENT BACKGROUND RADIATION
Chest (PA and Lat)	0.06	7
CT Head[a]		
neonate	4.2	490
1 y	3.6	420
5 y	2.4	280
10 y	2.0	240
15 y	1.4	160
CT Abdomen[a]		
neonate	13.1	1,540
1 y	11.1	1,310
5 y	8.4	990
10 y	8.9	1,050
15 y	5.9	690

[a]Data from Thomas KE, Wang B. Age specific effective doses for pediatric MSCT examinations at a large children's hospital using DLP conversion coefficients: a simple estimation method. *Pediatr Radiol* 2008;38(6):645–656.

TABLE E-8 ESTIMATED CONCEPTUS DOSES FROM COMMON RADIOGRAPHIC, FLUOROSCOPIC, AND CT EXAMINATIONS

ESTIMATED CONCEPTUS DOSES FROM SINGLE CT ACQUISITION

EXAMINATION	DOSE LEVEL	TYPICAL CONCEPTUS DOSE (mGy)
EXTRA-ABDOMINAL		
Head CT	Standard	0
Chest CT		
Routine	Standard	0.2
Pulmonary embolus	Standard	0.2
CT angiography of coronary arteries	Standard	0.1
ABDOMINAL		
Abdomen, routine	Standard	4
Abdomen/pelvis, routine	Standard	25
CT angiography of aorta (chest through pelvis)	Standard	34
Abdomen/pelvis, stone protocol[a]	Reduced	10

[a]Anatomic coverage is the same as for routine abdominopelvic CT, but the tube current is decreased and the pitch is increased because standard image quality is not necessary for detection of high-contrast stones.

ESTIMATED CONCEPTUS DOSES FROM RADIOGRAPHIC AND FLUOROSCOPIC EXAMINATIONS

EXAMINATION	TYPICAL CONCEPTUS DOSE (mGy)
Cervical spine (AP, lat)	<0.001
Extremities	<0.001
Chest (PA, lat)	0.002
Thoracic spine (AP, lat)	0.003
Abdomen (AP)	
21-cm patient thickness	1
33-cm patient thickness	3
Lumbar spine (AP, lat)	1
Limited IVP[a]	6
Small-bowel study[b]	7
Double-contrast barium enema study[c]	7

AP, anteroposterior projection, lat, lateral projection, PA, posteroanterior projection.

[a]Limited IVP is assumed to include four abdominopelvic images. A patient thickness of 21 cm is assumed.

[b]A small-bowel study is assumed to include a 6-min fluoroscopic examination with the acquisition of 20 digital spot images.

[c]A double-contrast barium enema study is assumed to include a 4-min fluoroscopic examination with the acquisition of 12 digital spot images.

Source: McCollough CH, Schueler BA, Atwell TD, et al. Radiation exposure and pregnancy: when should we be concerned? *Radiographics* 2007;27:909–917.

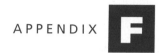

APPENDIX **F**

Radiopharmaceutical Characteristics and Dosimetry

APPENDIX F-1 METHOD OF ADMINISTRATION, LOCALIZATION, CLINICAL UTILITY, AND OTHER CHARACTERISTICS OF COMMONLY UTILIZED RADIOPHARMACEUTICALS

(1)RADIOPHARMACEUTICAL (DI/DNI/T)[a]	METHOD OF ADM[b]	DELAY BEFORE IMAGING	METHOD OF LOCALIZATION	CLINICAL UTILITY	COMMENTS
Co-57 Vitamin B$_{12}$ (DNI)	ORL	NA In vitro measurement of radioactivity in urine	Complexed to intrinsic factor and absorbed by distal ileum.	Diagnosis of pernicious anemia and intestinal absorption deficiencies.	Wait ≥24 h following more than 1 mg IV/IM vitamin B$_{12}$. Have patient fast ≥8 h before test.
Cr-51 Sodium Chromate RBCs (DNI)	IV	NA 20 mL blood sample @ 24 h and every 2–3 d for ≥30 d	Cr^{6+} attaches to hemoglobin and reduced to Cr^{3+}. Cr-RBC is a blood pool marker.	Most commonly used for red cell mass and survival. Also used for splenic sequestration studies. Non-imaging in vitro assay via counting serial blood samples.	RBC labeling efficiency 80%–90%. Free Cr^{3+} will not tag RBCs and is rapidly eliminated in the urine. Splenic sequestration study. ~111 MBq (~3 mCi) of heat denatured RBC.
F-18 Fluorodeoxyglucose (DI)	IV	45–60 min	Glucose analogue, increased uptake correlates with increased glucose metabolism. Crosses blood-brain barrier, taken up by cells where it is trapped due to phosphorylation of FDG 6-phosphate.	Major clinical application in oncology imaging. Used to assess recurrence and to differentiate between recurring tumor and necrotic tissue. Also used for the localization of epileptogenic focus and evaluation of dementias. Cardiac applications in determining metabolic activity and viability of myocardium.	PET Radiopharmaceutical. 511-keV annihilation photons require substantial shielding of source vials and care to prevent cross-talk between other imaging devices.

(Continued)

APPENDIX F-1   METHOD OF ADMINISTRATION, LOCALIZATION, CLINICAL UTILITY, AND OTHER CHARACTERISTICS OF COMMONLY UTILIZED RADIOPHARMACEUTICALS (Continued)

(i)RADIOPHARMACEUTICAL (DI/DNI/T)[a]	METHOD OF ADM[b]	DELAY BEFORE IMAGING	METHOD OF LOCALIZATION	CLINICAL UTILITY	COMMENTS
F-18 Sodium fluoride (DI)	IV	1–2 h	Fluorine ions accumulate in the skeleton with deposition being greater around active areas (e.g., arthritis, trauma, malignancies).	Bone scan. Uptake of F-18 reflects blood flow and bone remodeling. The CT component of PET/CT systems have significantly improved the specificity, allowing for morphologic characterization of the functional lesions and more accurate differentiation between benign lesions and metastases.	Cleared rapidly in urine. Patient should be well hydrated prior to dosing. Patient should void 30 min after injection and again immediately prior to imaging to reduce background.
Ga-67 Citrate (DI)	IV	Typically 24–72 h range 6–120 h	Exact mechanism unknown. Accumulates in lysosomes and is bound to transferrin blood.	Tumor, abscess imaging; Hodgkin's disease; lymphoma, and acute inflammatory lesions. Interstitial lung diseases and fever of unknown origin.	Ga-67 uptake influenced by vascularity, increased permeability of tumor cells, rapid proliferation, and low pH. Used in lieu of WBC in patients with leukemias or white cell deficiencies. Ga-67 secreted in large intestine; bowel activity interferes with abdominal imaging.
I-123 ioflupane also known as DaTscan (DI)	IV	3–6 h	Ioflupane binds to dopamine transporter in the brain.	Brain SPECT for dopamine transporter allows visualization of brain striata to evaluate patients with suspected parkinsonian syndromes. Helps differentiate essential tremor from tremor due to Parkinson's.	Supersaturated potassium iodide (SSKI) is administered to block the thyroid. Inject slowly over not less than 15–20 s

Radiopharmaceutical	Route	Time	Localization	Clinical Utility	Comments
I-123 Metaiodobenzylguanidine MIBG (DI)	IV	18–24 h	Uptake and accumulation by the norepinephrine transporter in adrenergically innervated tissues.	Detection of primary or metastatic pheochromocytoma or neuroblastoma.	SSKI is administered to block the thyroid. Weight adjust for pediatric use, see Appendix F-3B. SPECT may be performed after planar imaging. False negatives seen in patients with impaired renal function. MIBG is not cleared by dialysis. I-131 MIBG for therapy is in clinical trials.
I-123 Sodium Iodide (DI & DNI)	ORL	4–6 h	Rapidly absorbed from GI tract. Trapped and organically bound by thyroid.	Evaluation of thyroid function and/or morphology. Uptake determined by NaI (Tl) thyroid probe.	Dose range 3.7 MBq (100 μCi) (uptake study only) to 14.8 MBq (400 μCi) (uptake and imaging). Up to 2 mCi for metastatic disease imaging. Administered as a capsule.
I-125 Albumin (DNI)	IV	N/A ~20 mL blood withdrawn ~10 min after dose administration	Blood pool marker.	Blood and plasma volume determinations.	Dilution principle and hematocrit used to determine blood and plasma volume.
I-131 Sodium Iodide (DI, DNI, T)	ORL	24 h	Rapidly absorbed from GI tract, trapped and organically bound by thyroid.	~370 kBq (~10 μCi) used for uptake studies (DNI). ~74–185 MBq (~2–5 mCi) for diagnostic thyroid carcinoma metastatic survey. ~185–555 MBq (~5–15 mCi) or hyperthyroidism therapy. ~1.1–7.4 GBq (~30–200 mCi) for thyroid carcinoma therapy.	Liquid doses should be manipulated in 100% exhaust fume hood. Iodine is volatile at low pH. 90% of local radiation dose is from beta; 10% gamma.

(Continued)

APPENDIX F-1 METHOD OF ADMINISTRATION, LOCALIZATION, CLINICAL UTILITY, AND OTHER CHARACTERISTICS OF COMMONLY UTILIZED RADIOPHARMACEUTICALS (Continued)

(a)RADIOPHARMACEUTICAL (DI/DNI/T)a	METHOD OF ADMb	DELAY BEFORE IMAGING	METHOD OF LOCALIZATION	CLINICAL UTILITY	COMMENTS
I-131 Tositumomab also known as Bexxar (T)	IV	Whole-body counts are obtained on day 1 and 3 following imaging dose ~74–185 MBq (~2–5 mCi) to determine residence time and calculate therapeutic dose	This agent is a radiolabeled murine IgG2a monoclonal antibody directed against the CD20 antigen on B cells.	Radioimmunotherapic monoclonal antibody for the treatment of chemotherapy-refractory low-grade or transformed low-grade Non-Hodgkin's Lymphoma	Cytotoxic effect is the result of both direct antitumor effects of the antibody and the radiation dose delivered by the I-131. 90% of local radiation dose is from beta; 10% gamma. SSKI is administered to block the thyroid. Can typically be administered on an outpatient basis.
In-111 Capromab Pendetide also known as ProstaScint (DI)	IV	72–120 h	This agent is a monoclonal antibody to a membrane specific antigen expressed in many primary and metastatic prostate cancer lesions.	Indicated for patients with biopsy proven prostate cancer that is thought to be clinically localized following standard diagnostic imaging tests. Also indicated in postprostatectomy patients with high clinical suspicion of occult metastatic disease.	High false positive rate. Best results when imaged on a SPECT/CT. Patient management should not be based on ProstaScint results without confirmatory studies. May induce human anti-mouse antibodies which may interfere with some immunoassays (e.g., PSA and dioxin).
In -111 Pentetreotide also known as Octreoscan (DI)	IV	24–48 h	Pentetreotide is a DTPA conjugate of octreotide, a long acting analog of the human hormone somatostatin. Pentetreotide binds to somatostatin receptors on the cell surfaces throughout the body.	Localization of primary and metastatic neuroendocrine tumors bearing the somatostatin receptor.	Incubate In-111 Pentetreotide at 25°C for at lease 30 min. Do not administer in TPN admixtures or lines as complex glycosyl octreotide conjugates may form. Patients should be well hydrated prior to dose administration. Clinical trials underway for use of this as a therapeutic agent with Y-90.

In-111 White Blood Cells (DI)	IV	4–24 h	In-111 oxyquinoline is a neutral lipid-soluble complex that can penetrate cell membranes where the In-111 translocates to cytoplasmic components.	Detection of occult inflammatory lesions not visualized by other modalities. Confirmation of active infection in a known area. Careful isolation and labeling of WBCs is essential to maintain cell viability labeling efficiency ~80%. Better for deep abscesses or vertebral osteomyelitis than Tc-99m WBC.	In-111 WBC prepared in vitro with In-111 Oxyquinoline (Indium Oxine) and isolated plasma free suspension of autologous WBCs. ~30% dose in spleen, ~30% liver, ~5% lung (clears ~4 h). ~20% in circulation after injection. In-111 WBC has a longer $T_{1/2}$ and holds the label longer than Tc-99m WBC.
Kr-81m Krypton Gas (DI)	INH	None	No equilibrium or washout phase, thus Kr-81m distribution reflects only regional ventilation.	Lung ventilation studies; however, availability of Rb-81/Kr-81m generator is limited due to short parent $T_{1/2}$ (4.6 h). Used infrequently due to expense for the generator.	Due to ultrashort half life (13 s) only wash-in images can be obtained, however, repeat studies and multiple views can be obtained; radiation dose and hazard is minimal.
P-32 Chromic Phosphate Colloid (T)	IC	NA	Instilled directly into the body cavity containing a malignant effusion. Dose range (IP) 370–740 MBq (10–20 mCi) (IPL) 222–444 MBq (6–12 mCi).	Intraperitoneal (IP) or intrapleural (IPL) instillation.	Bluish green colloidal suspension. Never given IV. Do not use in the presence of ulcerative tumors.
P-32 Sodium Phosphate (T)	IV	NA	Concentration in blood cell precursors.	Treatment of polycythemia vera (PCV) most common; also myelocytic leukemia, chronic lymphocytic leukemia.	Clear colorless solution, typical dose range (PCV) 37–296 MBq (1–8 mCi) Do not use sequentially with chemotherapy. WBC should be ≥5,000/mm³; platelets should be ≥150,000 mm³.

(Continued)

APPENDIX F-1   METHOD OF ADMINISTRATION, LOCALIZATION, CLINICAL UTILITY, AND OTHER CHARACTERISTICS OF COMMONLY UTILIZED RADIOPHARMACEUTICALS (Continued)

⁽¹⁾RADIOPHARMACEUTICAL (DI/DNI/T)ᵃ	METHOD OF ADMᵇ	DELAY BEFORE IMAGING	METHOD OF LOCALIZATION	CLINICAL UTILITY	COMMENTS
Rb-82 also known as CardioGen-82 (DI)	IV	Infused into patient while on camera. Begin imaging 10–60 s after infusion when count rate reaches ~ 550 kcpm.	Accumulates in viable myocardium analogous to potassium. Myocardial extraction fraction is 60% at rest and 30% at peak stress.	Myocardial perfusion agent that is useful in distinguishing normal from abnormal myocardium in patients with suspected myocardial infarction. Short half life allows rest and stress to be performed in less than 1 h.	Better imaging agent for large patients (i.e., less attenuation). No ability to perform exercise stress tests. Must have a generator on site so high patient volume is essential to be cost effective. Sr-82/Sr-85 breakthrough was recently the subject of an FDA safety advisory.
Sm-153 EDTMP also known as Quadramet (T)	IV Over 1 to 2 min period	103-keV photon can be imaged however this is not essential	This therapeutic agent is formulated as a tetraphosphate chelate (EDTMP: ethylenediaminetetra methylenephosphonic acid) with an affinity for areas of high bone turnover associated with the hydroxyapatite (i.e., primary and metastatic bone tumors).	Therapy only. Indicated for the palliative relief of bone pain in patients with painful skeletal metastases. Beta and gamma. Gamma allows imaging if desired.	The patient should be well hydrated. Bone marrow toxicity is expected. Requires assessment of WBC/platelet count prior to use. Peripheral blood cell counts should be monitored at least once every other week. Pain relief expected 7–21 days following dose.
Sr-89 Chloride also known as Metastron (T)	IV Over a 1–2 min period	N/A	Calcium analog selectively localizing in bone mineral. Preferential absorption occurs in sites of active osteogenesis (i.e., primary and metastatic bone tumors).	Therapy only. Indicated for the palliative relief of bone pain in patients with painful skeletal metastasis. Pure beta so radiation safety concerns for caregivers are less than for Sm-153.	Bone marrow toxicity is expected. Requires minimum WBC/platelet count. Peripheral blood cell counts should be monitored at least once every other week. Pain relief expected 7–21 days following dose. Due to longer half-life, Metastron is not recommended in patients with very short life expectancy.

Tc-99m Disofenin also known as HIDA (iminodiacetic acid™) (DI)	IV	~5 min serial images every 5 min for ~30 min; and @ 40 & 60 min.	Excreted through the hepatobiliary tract into the intestine. Clearance mechanism: hepatocyte uptake, binding and storage. Excretion into canaliculi via active transport.	Hepatobiliary imaging agent, hepatic duct and gallbladder visualization occurs ~20 min after administration as liver activity decreases. The patient should be fasting >4 h. Delayed images are obtained @ ~4 h for acute/chronic cholecystitis.	Biliary system not well visualized when serum bilirubin values are over ~8 mg/dL; do not use if over 10 mg/dL. Normal study: visualized common duct and intestinal tract by ~30 min. CCK routinely used for gall bladder ejection fraction.
Tc-99m DMSA (dimercaptosuccinic acid) also known as Succimer (DI)	IV	1–2 h	After IV administration Tc-99m succimer is bound to plasma proteins. Cleared from plasma with a $T_{1/2}$ of about 60 min. and concentrates in the renal cortex.	Evaluation of renal parenchymal disorders.	Should be administered within 10 min to 4 h following preparation. Best cortical imaging agent. Only renal tracer for use with SPECT/CT.
Tc-99m Exametazime also known as Ceretec™ and HMPAO (DI)	IV	~30–300 min. When used for inflammatory bowel or appendicitis, imaging must start immediately.	Rapidly cleared from blood. Lipophilic complex, brain uptake ~4% of injected dose occurs ~1 min after injection.	Ceretec is used to radiolabel leukocytes as an adjunct in the localization of intra-abdominal infection and inflammatory bowel disease. Good for superficial lesions such as diabetic ulcers. Also used in detection of altered regional cerebral perfusion in stroke, Alzheimer's disease, seizures, etc.	Administer ASAP after preparation. SPECT images only. High photon flux and fast uptake in sites of infection permits early imaging. Short half-life limits delayed imaging.

(Continued)

APPENDIX F-1   METHOD OF ADMINISTRATION, LOCALIZATION, CLINICAL UTILITY, AND OTHER CHARACTERISTICS OF COMMONLY UTILIZED RADIOPHARMACEUTICALS (Continued)

(¹)RADIOPHARMACEUTICAL (DI/DNI/T)[a]	METHOD OF ADM[b]	DELAY BEFORE IMAGING	METHOD OF LOCALIZATION	CLINICAL UTILITY	COMMENTS
Tc-99m Macro aggregated albumin (MAA) (DI)	IV	None	~85% Tc-99m MAA mechanically trapped in arterioles and capillaries. Particle size (~15–80 μm). Distribution in lungs is a function of regional pulmonary blood flow.	Scintigraphic evaluation of pulmonary perfusion. ~0.6 million (range 0.2–1.2) particles are injected with an adult dose. Not be used in patients with severe pulmonary hypertension or history of hypersensitivity to human serum albumin. Also used to assess liver perfusion before chemoembolization or sphere therapy.	Mix reagent thoroughly before withdrawing dose; avoid drawing blood into syringe or injecting through IV tubing to prevent nonuniform distribution of particles. Inject patients supine.
Tc-99m phosphonates also known as Tc-99m Methyenediphosphonate (MDP) (DI)	IV	2–4 h	Specific affinity for areas of altered osteogenesis uptake related to osteogenic activity and skeletal perfusion. ~50% bone ~50% bladder in 24 h.	Skeletal imaging agent. Three-phase (flow, blood pool, bone uptake) used to distinguish between cellulitis and osteomyelitis. Theory of bone uptake: (1) hydroxyapatite crystal binding; (2) collagen dependent uptake in organic bone matrix.	Normal increase in activity in distal aspect of long bones compared to diaphyses. Higher target to background than pyrophosphate; 85% urinary excretion w/MDP versus 65% w/pyrophosphate in 24 h.
Tc-99m Mertiatide also known as MAG3 (DI)	IV	None	Reversible plasma protein binding. Excreted by kidneys via active tubular secretion and glomerular filtration.	Renal imaging agent. Diagnostic aid for assessment of renal function; split function; renal angiograms; renogram curves, whole kidney and renal cortex. Best tubular agent with high extraction faction. MAG3 clearance provides estimate of effective renal plasma flow.	~90% of dose excreted in 3 h. Preparation involves injection of ~2 mL of air in reaction vial and 10-min incubation in boiling water bath within 5 min after Tc-99m is added. Kits are light sensitive therefore must be stored in dark.

Name	Route	Time	Mechanism/Localization	Use	Comments
Tc-99m Bicisate also known as Neurolite (DI)	IV	30–60 min	This is a lipophilic complex that crosses the blood-brain barrier and intact cells by passive diffusion. Cells metabolize this agent to a polar (i.e., less diffusible) compound.	SPECT imaging with Neurolite used as an adjunct to CT and MRI in the localization of stroke in patients in whom stroke has been diagnosed.	Localization depends upon both perfusion and regional uptake by brain cells. Use caution in patients with hepatic or renal impairment.
Tc-99m Pentetate also known as Tc-99m DTPA (DI)	IV	None	Cleared by glomerular filtration, little to no binding to renal parenchyma.	Kidney imaging; assess renal perfusion; estimate glomerular filtration rate (GFR; f ~20% filtered per pass). Historically used as a brain imaging agent to identity excessive vascularity or altered blood-brain barrier.	~5% bound to serum proteins, which leads to GFR lower than that determined by inulin clearance. Can be used in aerosol form for ventilation side of VQ scan.
Tc-99m Pyrophosphate (DI)	IV	1–6 h bone imaging; 1–2 h myocardial imaging.	Specific affinity for areas of altered osteogenesis and injured/infarcted myocardium. 50% (bone) and ~50% (bladder) in 24 h.	Skeletal imaging agent used to demonstrate areas of hyper or hypo osteogenesis and/or osseous blood flow; cardiac agent as an adjunct in diagnosis of acute myocardial infarction.	Pyrophosphate also has an affinity for red blood cells. Administered IV ~30 min before Tc-99m for in vivo RBC cell labeling. ~75% of activity remains in blood pool.
Tc-99m Red Blood Cells (DI)	IV	None	Blood pool marker ~25% excreted in 24 h. 95% of blood pool activity bound to RBC @ 24 h.	Blood pool imaging including cardiac first pass and gated equilibrium imaging and detection of sites of G.I. bleeding. Heat damaged RBC are used for diagnosis of splenosis and accessory spleen. Also used for diagnosis of hemangiomas.	In vitro cell labeling with kit containing lyophilized tin chloride dihydrate, Na citrate and dextrose. Blood collection with 19–21 gauge needle to prevent hemolysis. Use heparin or ACD for anticoagulants, not EDTA or oxalate. Two syringe method and gentle mixing complete the radiolabeling; administered within 30 min. labeling efficiency ~95%.

(Continued)

APPENDIX F-1 METHOD OF ADMINISTRATION, LOCALIZATION, CLINICAL UTILITY, AND OTHER CHARACTERISTICS OF COMMONLY UTILIZED RADIOPHARMACEUTICALS (Continued)

(1)RADIOPHARMACEUTICAL (DI/DNI/T)a	METHOD OF ADMb	DELAY BEFORE IMAGING	METHOD OF LOCALIZATION	CLINICAL UTILITY	COMMENTS
Tc-99m Sestamibi also known as Cardiolite (DI)	IV	30–60 min	Accumulates in viable myocardium in a manner analogous to Tl-201 chloride. Major clearance pathway is the hepatobiliary system.	Diagnosis of myocardial ischemia and infarct. Also used for tumor imaging and parathyroid imaging.	The patient should not have fatty foods (e.g., milk) following injection. Low-dose/high-dose regime (typical 3:1 activity ratio) allows obtaining same day rest/stress images.
Tc-99m Sodium Pertechnetate (DI)	IV	None (Angio/Venography). Other applications ~0.5–1 h.	Pertechnetate ion distributes similarly to the iodide ion; it is trapped but not organified by the thyroid gland.	Primary agent for radiopharmaceutical preparations, thyroid imaging, salivary gland imaging, placental localization, detection of vesicourethral reflux, radionuclide angiography/venography.	Eluate should not be used greater than 12 h after elution. Tc-99m produced as daughter of Mo/Tc generator.
Tc-99m Sulfur Colloid (DI)	IV	~20 min	Rapidly cleared by reticuloendothelial (RE) system. ~85% colloidal particles are phagocytized by Kupffer's cells of liver. ~10% in RE system of spleen; ~5% in bone marrow.	Relative functional assessment of liver, spleen, bone marrow RE system; also used for gastroesophageal reflux imaging; esophageal transit time following oral administration. When used as a marrow agent, correlates with WBC imaging. Patency evaluation of peritoneovenous (LeVeen) shunt, administered in shunt.	Preparation requires addition of acidic solution; 5 min in boiling water bath followed by addition of a buffer to bring pH to 6–7. Plasma clearance T ½ ~2–5 min. Larger particles (~100 nm) accumulate in liver and spleen; small particles less than 20 nm in bone marrow.

APPENDIX F-2 SUMMARY OF TYPICALLY ADMINISTERED ADULT DOSE; ORGAN RECEIVING THE HIGHEST RADIATION DOSE AND ITS DOSE; GONADAL DOSE; EFFECTIVE DOSE AND EFFECTIVE DOSE PER ADMINISTERED ACTIVITY FOR SOME COMMONLY USED DIAGNOSTIC AND THERAPEUTIC RADIOPHARMACEUTICALS

RADIOPHARMACEUTICAL	TYPICAL ADULT DOSE MBq	TYPICAL ADULT DOSE mCi	ORGAN RECEIVING HIGHEST DOSE	ORGAN DOSE mGy	ORGAN DOSE rad	GONADAL DOSE mGy	GONADAL DOSE ov/ts	GONADAL DOSE rad	EFFECTIVE DOSE mSv	EFFECTIVE DOSE rem	EFFECTIVE DOSE PER ADMINISTERED ACTIVITY mSv/MBq	EFFECTIVE DOSE PER ADMINISTERED ACTIVITY rem/mCi	SOURCE
Co-57 Vitamin B$_{12}$ also known as Schilling's test	0.037	0.001	Liver	0.89	0.09	0.03 / 0.02	ov / ts	0.003 / 0.002	0.1	0.01	2.7	9.99	3
Cr-51 Sodium chromate denatured RBC's	7.4	0.2	Spleen	41.44	4.14	0.13 / 0.04	ov / ts	0.013 / 0.004	2.96	0.296	0.4	1.48	3
F-18 Sodium fluoride	185	5	Bladder	40.7	4.07	2.41 / 2.04	ov / ts	0.24 / 0.20	5	0.5	0.027	0.1	3
F-18 Fluoro-deoxyglucose	740	20	Bladder	96.2	9.62	10.36 / 8.14	ov / ts	1.04 / 0.81	14.06	1.406	0.019	0.07	1
Ga-67 Citrate	185	5	Bone surfaces	116.55	11.66	15.17 / 10.36	ov / ts	1.52 / 1.04	18.5	1.85	0.1	0.37	2
I-123 Loflupane also known as DaTscan	185	5	Bladder	9.81	0.98	2.96 / 1.57	ov / ts	0.3 / 0.16	3.94	0.394	0.021	0.079	5
I-123 Metaiodobenzylguanidine (MIBG)	185	5	Liver	12.4	1.24	1.52 / 1.05	ov / ts	0.15 / 0.11	2.41	0.241	0.013	0.048	2
I-123 Sodium iodide (35% uptake)	14.8	0.4	Thyroid	66.6	6.66	0.16 / 0.07	ov / ts	0.02 / 0.007	2.22	0.222	0.15	0.555	3
I-125 Albumin	0.74	0.02	Heart	0.51	0.05	0.15 / 0.12	ov / ts	0.02 / 0.01	0.25	0.03	0.34	1.258	3
I-131 Bexxar	3,145	85	Thyroid	8,523	852.3	786.3 / 2,610	ov / ts	78.63 / 261			NA[4]		5

(Continued)

APPENDIX F-2 SUMMARY OF TYPICALLY ADMINISTERED ADULT DOSE; ORGAN RECEIVING THE HIGHEST RADIATION DOSE AND ITS DOSE; GONADAL DOSE; EFFECTIVE DOSE AND EFFECTIVE DOSE PER ADMINISTERED ACTIVITY FOR SOME COMMONLY USED DIAGNOSTIC AND THERAPEUTIC RADIOPHARMACEUTICALS (Continued)

RADIOPHARMACEUTICAL	TYPICAL ADULT DOSE		ORGAN RECEIVING HIGHEST DOSE	ORGAN DOSE		GONADAL DOSE				EFFECTIVE DOSE		EFFECTIVE DOSE PER ADMINISTERED ACTIVITY		SOURCE
	MBq	mCi		mGy	rad	mGy		rad		mSv	rem	mSv/MBq	rem/mCi	
I-131 Sodium iodide (35% uptake)	3,700	100	Thyroid	2.66E+05	2.66E+04	162.8 ov 107.3 ts		16.28 ov 10.73 ts				NA⁴		3
In-111 Octreotide also known as Octreoscan	222	6	Spleen	126.54	12.65	5.99 ov 3.77 ts		0.60 ov 0.38 ts		11.99	1.20	0.054	0.200	2
In-111 White blood cells	19	0.5	Spleen	101.75	10.18	2.22 ov 0.83 ts		0.22 ov 0.08 ts		10.92	1.09	0.59	2.183	3
Kr-81m Krypton gas	370	10	Lung	0.08	0.008	6.3E-05 ov 6.3E-06 ts		6.3E-06 ov 6.3E-07 ts		0.01	0.001	2.70E-05	9.99E-05	3
P-32 Sodium phosphate	148	4	Red marrow	1,628	162.8	109.52 ov 109.52 ts		10.95 ov 10.95 ts				NA⁴		3
Rb-82	1,480	40	Kidney	13.79	1.38	0.48 ov 0.29 ts		0.05 ov 0.03 ts		2.55	0.26	1.72E-03	6.36E-03	6
Sm-153 EDTMP also known as Quadramet	2,590	70	Bone surfaces	1.75E+04	1.75E+03	22.27 ov 13.99 ts		2.23 ov 1.40 ts				NA⁴		5
Sr-89 Chloride also known as Metastron	148	4	Bone surfaces	2.52E+03	2.52E+02	115.44 ov 115.44 ts		11.54 ov 11.54 ts				NA⁴		3
Tc-99m Disofenin also known as HIDA (iminodiacetic acid)	185	5	Gall bladder	20.35	2.04	3.52 ov 0.28 ts		0.35 ov 0.03 ts		3.15	0.32	0.017	0.063	2
Tc-99m DMSA (dimercaptosuccinic acid) also known as Succimer	185	5	Kidneys	33.3	3.33	0.65 ov 0.33 ts		0.07 ov 0.03 ts		1.63	0.16	0.009	0.033	2

Tc-99m Exametazime also known as Ceretec and HMPAO	740	20	Kidneys	25.16	2.52	4.88 1.78	ov ts	0.49 0.18	6.88	0.69	0.009	0.034	2
Tc-99m Macroaggregated albumin (MAA)	148	4	Lungs	9.77	0.98	0.27 0.16	ov ts	0.03 0.02	1.63	0.16	0.011	0.041	2
Tc-99m phosphonates also known as Tc-99m MDP	740	20	Bone surfaces	46.62	4.66	2.66 1.78	ov ts	0.27 0.18	4.22	0.42	0.006	0.021	2
Tc-99m Mertiatide also known as MAG3	370	10	Bladder	40.7	4.07	2.0 1.37	ov ts	0.20 0.14	2.59	0.26	0.007	0.026	2
Tc-99m Bicisate also known as ECD and Neurolite	740	20	Bladder	37.0	3.70	5.85 2.0	ov ts	0.59 0.20	5.70	0.57	0.008	0.029	1
Tc-99m Pentetate also known as Tc-99m DTPA	370	10	Bladder	22.94	2.30	1.55 1.07	ov ts	0.16 0.11	1.81	0.18	0.005	0.018	2
Tc-99m Pyrophosphate	555	15	Bone surfaces	34.97	3.50	2.0 1.33	ov ts	0.2 0.13	3.16	0.32	0.006	0.021	2
Tc-99m Red blood cells	740	20	Heart	17.02	1.70	2.74 1.70	ov ts	0.27 0.17	5.18	0.52	0.007	0.026	2
Tc-99 Sestamibi also known as Cardiolite (rest)	296	8	Gall bladder	11.54	1.54	2.69 1.12	ov ts	0.27 0.11	2.66	0.27	0.009	0.033	2
Tc-99 Sestamibi also known as Cardiolite (stress)	1,110	30	Gall bladder	36.63	3.66	8.99 4.11	ov ts	0.90 0.41	8.77	0.88	0.008	0.029	2
Tc-99m Sodium pertechnetate	370	10	Upper large intestine	21.09	2.11	3.7 1.04	ov ts	0.37 0.10	4.81	0.48	0.013	0.048	2

(Continued)

APPENDIX F-2   SUMMARY OF TYPICALLY ADMINISTERED ADULT DOSE; ORGAN RECEIVING THE HIGHEST RADIATION DOSE AND ITS DOSE; GONADAL DOSE; EFFECTIVE DOSE AND EFFECTIVE DOSE PER ADMINISTERED ACTIVITY FOR SOME COMMONLY USED DIAGNOSTIC AND THERAPEUTIC RADIOPHARMACEUTICALS (Continued)

RADIOPHARMACEUTICAL	TYPICAL ADULT DOSE		ORGAN RECEIVING HIGHEST DOSE	ORGAN DOSE		GONADAL DOSE				EFFECTIVE DOSE		EFFECTIVE DOSE PER ADMINISTERED ACTIVITY		SOURCE
	MBq	mCi		mGy	rad		mGy		rad	mSv	rem	mSv/MBq	rem/mCi	
Tc-99m Sulfur colloid	185	5	Spleen	13.88	1.39	ov ts	0.41 0.1		0.04 0.01	1.74	0.17	0.010	0.035	2
Tc-99m Tetrofosmin also known as Myoview (rest)	296	8	Gall bladder	7.99	0.80	ov ts	2.28 1.01		0.23 0.101	2.04	0.20	0.007	0.026	1
Tc-99m Tetrofosmin also known as Myoview (stress)	1,110	30	Gall bladder	29.97	3.00	ov ts	8.44 3.22		0.84 0.32	7.66	0.77	0.007	0.026	1
Tl-201 Thallous chloride	74	2	Kidneys	35.52	3.55	ov ts	8.88 13.32		0.89 1.33	10.36	1.04	0.140	0.518	1
Xe-133 Xenon gas (rebreathing for 5 min)	555	15	Lungs	0.61	0.06	ov ts	0.41 0.38		0.04 0.04	0.44	0.04	0.0008	0.003	3
Y-90 Zevalin	38,332	1,036	Spleen	360,320	36,032	ov ts	15,332 34,822		1,533 34,882			NA[4]		5

1. Annals of the International Commission on Radiological Protection Publication 106: Radiation Dose to Patients from Radiopharmaceuticals, Elsevier Science Inc., Tarrytown, NY, 2009. Note: Effective dose calculated utilizing weighting factors from ICRP Report 60.

2. Annals of the International Commission on Radiological Protection Publication 80: Radiation Dose to Patients from Radiopharmaceuticals, Elsevier Science Inc., Tarrytown, NY, 1999. Note: Effective dose calculated utilizing weighting factors from ICRP Report 60.

3. Annals of the International Commission on Radiological Protection Publication 53: Radiation Dose to Patients from Radiopharmaceuticals, Pergamon Press, Elmsford, NY, 1988. Note: The value provided in the Effective Dose column is the effective dose equivalent as defined on pages 10–11 of the report and utilizing weighting factors from ICRP Report 26.

4. The effective dose is not a relevant quantity for therapeutic doses of radionuclides because it provides an estimate of effective stochastic risk (e.g., cancer and genetic detriment) and is not relevant to effects at high tissue/organ doses such as deterministic (i.e., nonstochastic) risks.

5. Information supplied by the manufacturer.

6. Stabin Michael G. Proposed Revision To the Radiation Dosimetry of ^{82}Rb. Health Physics. 99(6):811–813, December 2010.

NA Not applicable

E, exponential (e.g., 2.66 E+055 = 2.66×10^5.)

APPENDIX F-3A   EFFECTIVE DOSE PER UNIT ACTIVITY ADMINISTERED TO 15;10;5 AND 1-YEAR-OLD PATIENTS FOR SOME COMMONLY USED DIAGNOSTIC RADIOPHARMACEUTICALS

RADIOPHARMACEUTICAL	EFFECTIVE DOSE								SOURCE
	15 YEARS OLD		10 YEARS OLD		5 YEARS OLD		1 YEAR OLD		
	mSv/MBq	rem/mCi	mSv/MBq	rem/mCi	mSv/MBq	rem/mCi	mSv/MBq	rem/mCi	
F-18 Sodium fluoride	0.034	0.126	0.052	0.192	0.086	0.318	0.170	0.629	3
F-18 Fluorodeoxyglucose	0.024	0.089	0.037	0.137	0.056	0.207	0.095	0.352	1
Ga-67 Citrate	0.130	0.481	0.200	0.740	0.330	1.221	0.640	2.368	2
I-123 Metaiodobenzylguanidine (MIBG)	0.017	0.063	0.026	0.096	0.037	0.137	0.068	0.252	2
I-123 Sodium iodide (35% uptake)	0.230	0.851	0.350	1.295	0.740	2.738	1.400	5.180	3
In-111 Octreotide also known as Octreoscan	0.071	0.263	0.100	0.370	0.160	0.592	0.280	1.036	2
In-111 White blood cells	0.459	1.700	0.703	2.600	1.054	3.900	1.919	7.100	2
Tc-99m Disofenin also known as HIDA (iminodiacetic acid)	0.021	0.078	0.029	0.107	0.045	0.167	0.100	0.370	2
Tc-99m DMSA (dimercaptosuccinic acid) also known as Succimer	0.011	0.041	0.015	0.056	0.021	0.078	0.037	0.137	2
Tc-99m Exametazime also known as Ceretec and HMPAO	0.011	0.041	0.017	0.063	0.027	0.100	0.049	0.181	2
Tc-99m Macroaggregated albumin (MAA)	0.016	0.059	0.023	0.085	0.034	0.126	0.063	0.233	2
Tc-99m phosphonates also known as Tc-99m MDP	0.007	0.026	0.011	0.041	0.014	0.052	0.027	0.100	2

(Continued)

APPENDIX F-3A EFFECTIVE DOSE PER UNIT ACTIVITY ADMINISTERED TO 15;10;5 AND 1-YEAR-OLD PATIENTS FOR SOME COMMONLY USED DIAGNOSTIC RADIOPHARMACEUTICALS (Continued)

RADIOPHARMACEUTICAL	EFFECTIVE DOSE								SOURCE
	15 YEARS OLD		10 YEARS OLD		5 YEARS OLD		1 YEAR OLD		
	mSv/MBq	rem/mCi	mSv/MBq	rem/mCi	mSv/MBq	rem/mCi	mSv/MBq	rem/mCi	
Tc-99m Mertiatide also known as MAG3	0.009	0.033	0.012	0.044	0.012	0.044	0.022	0.081	2
Tc-99m Bicisate also known as ECD and Neurolite	0.010	0.037	0.015	0.056	0.022	0.081	0.040	0.148	1
Tc-99m Pentetate also known as Tc-99m DTPA	0.006	0.022	0.008	0.030	0.009	0.033	0.016	0.059	2
Tc-99m Pyrophosphate	0.007	0.026	0.011	0.041	0.014	0.052	0.027	0.100	2
Tc-99m Red blood cells	0.009	0.033	0.014	0.052	0.021	0.078	0.039	0.144	2
Tc-99 Sestamibi also known as Cardiolite (rest)	0.012	0.044	0.018	0.067	0.028	0.104	0.053	0.196	2
Tc-99 Sestamibi also known as Cardiolite (stress)	0.010	0.037	0.016	0.059	0.023	0.085	0.045	0.167	2
Tc-99m Sodium pertechnetate	0.017	0.063	0.026	0.096	0.042	0.155	0.079	0.292	2
Tc-99m Sulfur colloid	0.012	0.044	0.018	0.067	0.028	0.104	0.050	0.185	2
Tc-99m Tetrofosmin also known as Myoview (rest)	0.009	0.033	0.013	0.048	0.021	0.078	0.039	0.144	1
Tc-99m Tetrofosmin also known as Myoview (stress)	0.009	0.033	0.013	0.048	0.021	0.078	0.039	0.144	1
Tl-201 Thallous chloride	0.200	0.740	0.560	2.072	0.790	2.923	1.300	4.810	1
Xe-133 Xenon gas (5 min)	0.001	0.004	0.002	0.006	0.003	0.010	0.005	0.020	3

1. Annals of the International Commission on Radiological Protection Publication 106: Radiation Dose to Patients from Radiopharmaceuticals, Elsevier Science Inc., Tarrytown, NY, 2009. Note: Effective dose calculated utilizing weighting factors from ICRP Report 60.

2. Annals of the International Commission on Radiological Protection Publication 80: Radiation Dose to Patients from Radiopharmaceuticals, Elsevier Science Inc., Tarrytown, NY, 1999. Note: Effective dose calculated utilizing weighting factors from ICRP Report 60.

3. Annals of the International Commission on Radiological Protection Publication 53: Radiation Dose to Patients from Radiopharmaceuticals, Pergamon Press, Elmsford, NY, 1988. Note: The value provided in the Effective Dose column is the effective dose equivalent as defined on pages 10–11 of the report and utilizing weighting factors from ICRP Report 26.

APPENDIX F-3B   NORTH AMERICAN CONSENSUS GUIDELINES FOR ADMINISTERED RADIOPHARMACEUTICAL ACTIVITIES IN CHILDREN AND ADOLESCENTS[a,b]

RADIOPHARMACEUTICAL	RECOMMENDED ADMINISTERED ACTIVITY (BASED ON WEIGHT ONLY)	MINIMUM ADMINISTERED ACTIVITY	MAXIMUM ADMINISTERED ACTIVITY	COMMENTS
^{123}I-MIBG	5.2 MBq/kg (0.14 mCi/kg)	37 MBq (1.0 mCi)	370 MBq (10.0 mCi)	[c]EANM Paediatric Does Card (2007 version) may also be used in patients weighing more than 10 kg
^{99m}Tc-MDP	9.3 MBq/kg (0.25 mCi/kg)	37 MBq (1.0 mCi)		[c]EANM Paediatric Does Card (2007 version) may also be used.
^{18}F-FDG	Body, 3.7–5.2 MBq/kg (0.10–0.14 mCi/kg) Brain, 3.7 MBq/kg (0.10 mCi/kg)	37 MBq (1.0 mCi)		Low end of dose range should be considered for smaller patients. Administered activity may take into account patient mass and time available on PET scanner. [c]EANM Paediatric Does Card (2007 version) may also be used.
[99m]Tc-dimercaptosuccinic acid	1.85 MBq/kg (0.05 mCi/kg)	18.5 MBq (0.5 mCi)		
^{99m}Tc-MAG3	Without flow study, 3.7 MBq/kg (0.10 mCi/kg) With flow study, 5.55 MBq/kg (0.15 mCi/kg)	37 MBq (1.0 mCi)	148 MBq (4 mCi)	Administered activities at left assume that image data are reframed at 1 min/image. Administered activity may be reduced if image data are reframed at longer time per image. [c]EANM Paediatric Dose Card (2007 version) may also be used.
[99m]Tc-iminodiacetic acid	1.85 MBq/kg (0.05 mCi/kg)	18.5 MBq (0.5 mCi)		Higher administered activity of 37 MBq (1 mCi) may be considered for neonatal jaundice. [c]EANM Paediatric Does Card (2007 version) may be used.
[99m]Tc-macroaggregated albumin	If ^{99m}Tc used for ventilation, 2.59 MBq/kg (0.07 mCi/kg) No ^{99m}Tc ventilation study, 1.11 MBq/kg (0.03 mCi/kg)	14.8 MBq (0.4 mCi)		[c]EANM Paediatric Does Card (2007 version) may be also be used.

(Continued)

APPENDIX F-3B   NORTH AMERICAN CONSENSUS GUIDELINES FOR ADMINISTERED RADIOPHARMACEUTICAL ACTIVITIES IN CHILDREN AND ADOLESCENTS[a,b] (Continued)

RADIOPHARMACEUTICAL	RECOMMENDED ADMINISTERED ACTIVITY (BASED ON WEIGHT ONLY)	MINIMUM ADMINISTERED ACTIVITY	MAXIMUM ADMINISTERED ACTIVITY	COMMENTS
^{99m}Tc-pertechnetate (Meckel diverticulum imaging)	1.85 MBq/kg (0.05 mCi/kg)	9.25 MBq (0.25 mCi)		[c]EANM Paediatric Dose Card (2007 version) may also be used.
^{18}F-sodium fluoride	2.22 MBq/kg (0.06 mCi/kg)	18.5 MBq (0.5 mCi)		
^{99m}Tc (for cystography)	No weight-based dose		No more than 37 MBq (1.0 mCi) for each bladder-filling cycle	^{99m}Tc-sulfur colloid, ^{99m}Tc-pertechnetate, ^{99m}Tc-diethylene triamine pentaacetic acid, or possibly other ^{99m}Tc radiopharmaceuticals may be used. There are a wide variety of acceptable administration techniques for ^{99m}Tc, many of which will work well with lower administered activities.
^{99m}Tc-sulfur colloid For oral liquid gastric emptying	No weight-based dose	9.25 MBq (0.25 mCi)	37 MBq (1.0 mCi)	Administered activity will depend on age of child, volume to be fed to child, and time per frame used for imaging.
For solid gastric emptying	No weight-based dose	9.25 MBq (0.25 mCi)	18.5 MBq (0.5 mCi)	^{99m}Tc-sulfur colloid is usually used to label egg.

[a]This information is intended as a guideline only. Local practice may vary depending on patient population, choice of collimator, and specific requirements of clinical protocols. Administered activity may be adjusted when appropriate by order of the nuclear medicine practitioner. For patients who weigh more than 70 kg, it is recommended that maximum administered activity not exceed product of patient's weight (kg) and recommended weight-based administered activity. Some practitioners may choose to set fixed maximum administered activity equal to 70 times the recommended weight-based administered activity, for example, approximately 370 MBq (10 mCi), for ^{18}F body imaging. The administered activities assume the use of a low energy high resolution collimator for Tc-99m radiopharmaceuticals and a medium energy collimator for I-123-MIBG. Individual practitioners may use lower administered activities if their equipment or software permits them to do so. Higher administered activities may be required in certain patients. No recommended dose is given for ^{67}Ga-citrate. Intravenous ^{67}Ga-citrate should be used infrequently and only in low doses.

[b]Reproduced with permission from: M. Gelfand, M. Parisi, T. Treves: Pediatric Radiopharmaceutical Administered Doses: 2010 North American Consensus Guidelines *J Nucl Med* Vol. 52, No. 2 February 2011

[c]The European Association of Nuclear Medicine (ENAM) Paediatric Dose Card (2007 Version) Reference: Lassmann M, Biassoni L, Monsieurs M, Franzius C, Jacobs F. The new EANM paediatric dosage card. 2007; 34:796–798. Additional notes and erratum related to the Lassmann reference can found in Eur J Nucl Med Mol Imaging. 2008;35:1666–1668 and Eur J Nucl Med Mol Imaging. 2008;35:2141.

APPENDIX F-4A SUMMARY OF ABSORBED DOSE ESTIMATES TO THE EMBRYO/FETUS PER UNIT ACTIVITY ADMINISTERED TO THE MOTHER FOR SOME COMMONLY USED RADIOPHARMACEUTICALS[a]

| RADIOPHARMACEUTICAL | DOSE AT DIFFERENT STAGES OF GESTATION | | | | | | | |
| | EARLY | | 3 MONTHS | | 6 MONTHS | | 9 MONTHS | |
	mGy/MBq	rad/mCi	mGy/MBq	rad/mCi	mGy/MBq	rad/mCi	mGy/MBq	rad/mCi
Co-57 Vitamin B_{12} also known as Schilling's test	1.0	3.7	0.68	2.516	0.84	3.108	0.88	3.256
F-18 Sodium fluoride	0.022	0.081	0.017	0.063	0.008	0.028	0.007	0.025
F-18 Fluoro-deoxyglucose	0.022	0.081	0.022	0.081	0.017	0.063	0.017	0.063
Ga-67 Citrate	0.093	0.344	0.2	0.74	0.18	0.666	0.13	0.481
I-123 Sodium iodide	0.02	0.074	0.014	0.052	0.011	0.041	0.01	0.036
I-125 Albumin	0.25	0.925	0.078	0.289	0.038	0.141	0.026	0.096
I-131 Sodium iodide	0.072	0.266	0.068	0.252	0.23	0.851	0.27	0.999
In-111 Pentetreotide also known as Octreoscan	0.082	0.303	0.06	0.222	0.035	0.13	0.031	0.115
In-111 White blood cells	0.13	0.481	0.096	0.355	0.096	0.355	0.094	0.348
Tc-99m Disofenin also known as HIDA (iminodiacetic acid)	0.017	0.0629	0.0150	0.056	0.012	0.044	0.007	0.025
Tc-99m DMSA (dimercapto-succinic acid) also known as Succimer	0.005	0.019	0.005	0.017	0.004	0.015	0.003	0.013
Tc-99m Exametazime also known as Ceretec and HMPAO	0.009	0.032	0.007	0.025	0.005	0.018	0.004	0.013
Tc-99m Macroaggregated albumin (MAA)	0.003	0.01	0.004	0.015	0.005	0.019	0.004	0.015

(Continued)

APPENDIX F-4A   SUMMARY OF ABSORBED DOSE ESTIMATES TO THE EMBRYO/FETUS PER UNIT ACTIVITY ADMINISTERED TO THE MOTHER FOR SOME COMMONLY USED RADIOPHARMACEUTICALS[a] (Continued)

RADIOPHARMACEUTICAL	DOSE AT DIFFERENT STAGES OF GESTATION							
	EARLY		3 MONTHS		6 MONTHS		9 MONTHS	
	mGy/MBq	rad/mCi	mGy/MBq	rad/mCi	mGy/MBq	rad/mCi	mGy/MBq	rad/mCi
Tc-99m Medronate also known as Tc-99m Methylene diphosphonate (MDP)	0.006	0.023	0.005	0.02	0.003	0.01	0.002	0.009
Tc-99m Mertiatide also known as MAG3	0.018	0.067	0.014	0.052	0.006	0.02	0.005	0.019
Tc-99m Bicisate also known as ECD and Neurolite	0.011	0.041	0.008	0.03	0.004	0.014	0.004	0.013
Tc-99m Pentetate also known as Tc-99m DTPA	0.012	0.044	0.009	0.032	0.004	0.015	0.005	0.017
Tc-99m Pyrophosphate	0.006	0.022	0.007	0.024	0.004	0.013	0.003	0.011
Tc-99m Red blood cells	0.006	0.024	0.004	0.016	0.003	0.012	0.003	0.01
Tc-99 Sestamibi also known as Cardiolite (rest)	0.015	0.056	0.012	0.044	0.008	0.031	0.005	0.02
Tc-99 Sestamibi also know as Cardiolite (stress)	0.012	0.044	0.01	0.035	0.007	0.026	0.004	0.016
Tc-99m Sodium pertechnetate	0.011	0.041	0.022	0.081	0.014	0.052	0.009	0.034
Tc-99m Sulfur colloid	0.002	0.007	0.002	0.008	0.003	0.012	0.004	0.014
Tc-99 Tetrofosmin also known as Myoview	0.01	0.036	0.007	0.026	0.005	0.02	0.004	0.013
Tc-99m WBC	0.004	0.014	0.003	0.01	0.003	0.011	0.003	0.01
Tl-201 Thallous chloride (rest)	0.097	0.359	0.058	0.215	0.047	0.174	0.027	0.1
Xe-133 Xenon gas (rebreathing for 5 min)	0.00041	0.00152	0.00005	0.00018	0.00004	0.00013	0.00003	0.0001

[a]Source: Stabin M.G., Blackwell R., Brant R.L., Donnelly E., Kinf V.A., Lovins K., Stovall M. Fetal Radiation Dose Calculations. ANSI N13.54 2008, Washington, DC: American National Standards Institute, 2008.

APPENDIX F-4B EFFECTIVE DOSE TO THE NEWBORN AND INFANT PER UNIT ACTIVITY ADMINISTERED FROM THE MOTHER'S BREAST MILK[a]

Radiopharmaceutical	Newborn mSv/MBq (rem/mCi)	1-y-old mSv/MBq (rem/mCi)
^{67}Ga-citrate	1.2 (4.4)	0.490 (1.81)
^{99m}Tc-DTPA	0.030 (0.111)	0.014 (0.052)
^{99m}Tc-MAA	0.17 (0.63)	0.068 (0.252)
^{99m}Tc-pertechnetate	0.14 (0.52)	0.062 (0.229)
^{131}I-NaI[†]	5,400 (20,000)	3,900 (14,400)
^{51}Cr-EDTA	0.028 (0.104)	0.012 (0.044)
^{99m}Tc-DISIDA	0.22 (0.81)	0.095 (0.35)
^{99m}Tc-glucoheptonate	0.080 (0.30)	0.036 (0.13)
^{99m}Tc-HAM	0.20 (0.74)	0.083 (0.31)
^{99m}Tc-MIBI	0.14 (0.52)	0.065 (0.24)
^{99m}Tc-MDP	0.063 (0.23)	0.026 (0.096)
^{99m}Tc-PYP	0.066 (0.24)	0.028 (0.10)
^{99m}Tc-RBC in vivo labeling	0.070 (0.26)	0.031 (0.12)
^{99m}Tc-RBC in vitro labeling	0.071 (0.26)	0.031 (0.12)
^{99m}Tc-sulfur colloid	0.092 (0.34)	0.042 (0.16)
^{111}In-white blood cells	5.5 (20)	2.2 (8.1)
^{123}I-NaI	2.7 (10)	1.9 (7.0)
^{123}I-OIH	0.051 (0.19)	0.022 (0.081)
^{123}I-MIBG	2.7 (10)	1.9 (7.0)
^{125}I-OIH	0.20 (0.74)	0.082 (0.30)
^{131}I-OIH	0.23 (0.85)	0.093 (0.34)
^{99m}Tc-DTPA aerosol	0.052 (0.19)	0.022 (0.081)
^{99m}Tc-MAG3	0.027 (0.10)	0.012 (0.044)
^{99m}Tc-white blood cells	0.20 (0.74)	0.074 (0.27)
^{201}Tl-chloride	3.6 (13)	2.1 (7.8)

[a]Effective Dose to infant per unit activity administered intravenously to infant. (i.e., assumes 100% of the activity ingested by the infant is instantaneously absorbed. Calculation based on ICRP 60 methodology. See below for narrative and sample calculation of effective dose to the infant based on serial measurements of activity in the breast milk.

[†]Dose to infant's thyroid per unit activity administered intravenously (or orally) to infant.

DTPA, diethylenetriamine pentaacetic acid; MAA, macroaggregated albumin; EDTA, ethylenediaminetetraacetic acid; DISIDA, disofenin (iminodiacetic acid derivative); HAM, human albumin microspheres; MIBI, methoxyisobutyl isonitrile; MDP, methylene diphosphonate; PYP, pyrophosphate; RBC, red blood cells; WBC, white blood cells; OIH, orthoiodohippurate; MIGB, metaiodobenzylguanidine; MAG3, mercaptoacetyltriglycine.

Source: Stabin MG, Breitz HB. Breast milk of radiopharmaceuticals: mechanisms, findings, and radiation dosimetry. *J Nucl Med* 2000; 41 (5): 863–873.

NARRATIVE AND EXAMPLE[1]

Recommended duration of interruption of breast-feeding following radiopharma-ceutical administration to a patient who is nursing an infant or child was provided in Chapter 21, Table 21-9. The interruption schedules for the nursing infant were derived using a dose criteria of 1 mSv effective dose to the infant. However, Stabin and Brietz recommend taking breast milk samples from subjects when possible to determine, on an individual basis, the best recommendation for the duration of inter-ruption. According to their recommendations in the article cited above, breast milk samples should be obtained: "(1) at about 3 h after administration (this is when the peak concentrations have most often been observed); (2) then, as many more samples as the patient is willing and able to give, over 2 to 3 effective half-times of the radiopharmaceutical in the body. If there is uncertainty about the biologic half-time, the radionuclide physical half-life may be used to estimate this overall time period. A minimum of two more samples (after the first sample at 3 h) should be obtained to calculate a good estimate of the retention half-time in the milk. Once the peak concentration and rate of decrease of the activity are determined, some approximate calculations can be performed by any physician or physicist to estimate the amount of activity that the infant will ingest starting at different points in time. One can set up a calculation in a simple spreadsheet that sums, for whatever sampling schedule the mother suggests that the infant is likely to follow, the amounts of activity likely to be ingested, using the observed concentrations and rate of elimination." Then, the dose conversion factors in Appendix F-4B can be used to calculate the infant dose.

This technique is illustrated in the following example from the Stabin and Breitz article: assume that for an administration of Tc-99m pertechnetate the breast-milk concentration reported at 3 h after administration to the mother is 2×10^{-2} MBq/ mL. Three more samples, taken over the next 8 h, show a clearance biologic half-time of 20 h. The effective half-time is

$$(6 \text{ h} \times 20 \text{ h})/(6 \text{ h} + 20 \text{ h}) = 4.6 \text{ h}$$

The mother wants to feed the baby (a newborn) approximately every 4 h. The volume ingested per feeding is assumed to be in feedings of 142 mL every 4 h (i.e., ~850 mL/d). Thus for the following times, starting at 12 h after administration (we are already at 11 h after administration), the baby's intakes for the next seven feedings would be

T (H)	A_T (MBq)
12	0.735
16	0.403
20	0.221
24	0.121
28	0.067
32	0.036
36	0.02
40	0.011
Total activity = 1.62 MBq	

---

[1]Source: Stalin MG, Breitz HB. Breast milk excretion of radiopharmaceuticals: mechanisms, findings and radiation dosimetry. *J Nucl Med* 2000;41(5):863–873.

Each value of A_t is given by the expression:

$$A_t = (142 \text{ mL} \times 0.02 \text{ MBq/mL}) \times e{-}0.693 \times (T{-}3)/(4.6)$$

A_t (MBq) is the activity ingested by the infant at the feeding at time T (h). We are assuming that the peak concentration (0.02 MBq/mL) occurred at 3 h and then decreased with the effective half-time (4.6 h) thereafter. We took the calculations out to 40 h, when the concentration seemed to have diminished to the point that further contributions would be negligible. The sum of the activity values listed previously is 1.62 MBq." In Appendix F-4B, we find a dose value for Tc-99m pertechnetate of 0.14 mSv/MBq for a newborn. The cumulative dose, assuming that feeding started at 12 h, would be 1.62 MBq × 0. 14 mSv/MBq = 0.23 mSv.

This dose is within the 1 mSv guideline used here, and one would conclude that breast-feeding could resume safely at 12 h after administration. If the dose had turned out to be too high, the calculation could be repeated easily, simply excluding some of the values in the table shown above from the sum, starting at 16 h, then at 20 h, and so on, until an acceptable dose value was obtained. The time at which this value was obtained would represent the time at which breast-feeding could be resumed.

APPENDIX F-4C BREAST DOSE FROM RADIOPHARMACEUTICALS EXCRETED IN BREAST MILK

RADIOPHARMACEUTICAL	ADMINISTERED ACTIVITY IN MBq (mCi)	BREAST DOSE (Gy)	
		[a]BEST CASE	[a]WORST CASE
[67]Ga-citrate	185 (5.0)	2.18E-04	1.10E-02
^{99m}Tc-DTPA	740 (20)	6.09E-06	1.20E-04
^{99m}Tc-MAA	148 (4)	1.55E-05	1.21E-03
[99m]Tc-pertechnetate	1110 (30)	1.86E-05	2.52E-03
[131]I-NaI	5550 (150)	–	1.96E+00
[51]Cr-EDTA	1.85 (0.05)	4.21E-09	2.52E-08
^{99m}Tc-DISIDA	300 (8)	1.94E-05	5.98E-05
[99m]Tc-glucoheptonate	740 (20)	3.58E-05	7.40E-05
^{99m}Tc-HAM	300 (8)	8.48E-06	2.33E-04
^{99m}Tc-MIBI	1110 (30)	5.54E-06	5.09E-05
^{99m}Tc-MDP	740 (20)	2.69E-05	3.76E-05
^{99m}Tc-PYP	740 (20)	4.16E-05	2.26E-04
^{99m}Tc-RBC *in vivo*	740 (20)	2.46E-06	1.14E-03
^{99m}Tc-RBC *in vitro*	740 (20)	9.25E-06	1.61E-05
[99m]Tc-sulfur colloid	444 (12)	3.17E-05	4.64E-04
^{111}In-WBCs	18.5 (0.5)	5.03E-06	2.52E-05
[123]I-NaI	14.8 (0.4)		4.74E-04
^{123}I-OIH	74 (2)	7.50E-05	5.84E-04
^{123}I-MIBG	370 (10)		2.71E-04
^{125}I-OIH	0.37 (0.01)		8.46E-07
^{131}I-OIH	11.1 (0.3)	4.97E-05	3.22E-04
^{99m}Tc-DTPA aerosol	37 (1)	1.22E-07	2.49E-06
^{99m}Tc-MAG3	185 (5)	3.04E-06	6.01E-05
^{99m}Tc-WBCs	370 (10)	1.11E-04	1.51E-02
[201]Tl-chloride	111 (3)	2.35E-05	4.14E-05

[a]Best and worst case as observed from the literature.
DTPA, diethylenetriamine pentaacetic acid; MAA, macroaggregated albumin; EDTA, ethylenediaminetetraacetic acid; DISIDA, disofenin (iminodiacetic acid derivative); HAM, human albumin microspheres; MIBI, methoxyisobutyl isonitrile; MDP, methylene diphosphonate; PYP, pyrophosphate; RBC, red blood cells; WBC, white blood cells; OIH, orthoiodohippurate; MIGB, metaiodobenzylguanidine; MAG3, mercaptoacetyltriglycine.
From Stabin MG, Breitz HB. Breast milk excretion of radiopharmaceuticals: mechanisms, findings, and radiation dosimetry. *J Nucl Med.* 2000;41(5):863–873.

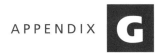

Convolution and Fourier Transforms

G.1 Convolution

Convolution is the mathematical property that describes the blurring process in medical imaging, among other physical phenomenon. It is the basis of optical physics and imaging physics. For a function $f(x)$ and a convolution kernel $h(x)$, convolution is performed as below resulting in the function $g(x)$:

$$g(x) = \int_{-\infty}^{\infty} f(x')\, h(x - x')\, dx' \qquad \text{[G-1a]}$$

where x' is a *dummy* variable used for integration. Convolution is also the basis of many image processing procedures. The shorthand symbol for convolution is described in Equation G-1b:

$$g(x) = f(x) \otimes h(x) \qquad \text{[G-1b]}$$

where $\otimes$ is the mathematical symbol for convolution. The convolution process can be extended to two dimensions:

$$g(x, y) = \int_{y'=-\infty}^{\infty} \int_{x'=-\infty}^{\infty} f(x', y')\, h(x - x', y - y')\, dx'dy' \qquad \text{[G-1c]}$$

Figure G-1A shows a one-dimensional convolution, and it is straightforward to extend convolution to a three-dimensional function as well. With the advent of near-isotropic three-dimensional image data sets, three-dimensional convolution techniques are used with increasing utility for many imaging applications.

Figure G-1 illustrates the effect of a five element rectangular (RECT) convolution kernel, $h(x)$, on an input signal $f(x)$ with some considerable noise. The output function $g(x)$ is much *smoother* than the input signal, but the edges are not as sharp. The RECT kernel is illustrated in the inset. A RECT kernel used in convolution is also known as a boxcar average. If the kernel is normalized to unit area as in this case ($5 \times 0.2 = 1$), the total amplitude of the convolved function will be equal to that of the input function. Convolution kernels that have all positive values (as in Fig. G-1) will always result in some degree of smoothing of the input function. Let [0.2, 0.2, 0.2, 0.2, 0.2] represent the RECT kernel (with highlighted color being the center element). Other kernels with all positive elements such as [0.1, 0.25, 0.4, 0.25, 0.1] will also result in smoothing, for example.

Convolution can be used to enhance edges as well, and Figure G-2 illustrates this with a kernel designated as [0.0, –0.5, 2.0, –0.5, 0.0] (see inset). In this case, the noise in the input function $f(x)$ is made worse by the convolution procedure resulting in the output function $g(x)$. Although the noise in the signal is amplified, the edges are enhanced as well. Edge enhancement (also known as high pass filtering) is a key part of filtered backprojection reconstruction in tomographic imaging applications.

The convolution operation can perform a number of interesting mathematical procedures on an input signal. Figure G-3 shows a convolution procedure with a

987

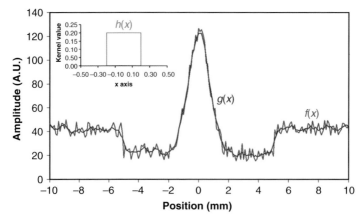

■ **FIGURE G-1** This figure illustrates the impact of convolution with a noise-suppressing kernel. The original signal *f(x)* was convolved with the five element RECT kernel *h(x)* shown in the inset, resulting in the smoothed function *g(x)*.

kernel [0.0, 0.0, –1.0, 1.0, 0.0]. In this case, the output function *g(x)* is the discrete derivative of the input function *f(x)*. Notice that in this example the sum of the kernel is zero, and the average value of the output function *g(x)* also becomes zero.

The convolution operation has a number of shifting and scaling properties. Figure G-4 illustrates a convolution kernel with eleven elements, all zeros with the tenth element set to –0.5: [0, 0, 0, 0, 0, 0, 0, 0, 0, –0.5, 0]. By placing the only non-zero element away from the center of the kernel, the output function *g(x)* is shifted laterally relative to the input function. By having only a negative element, the entire output function *g(x)* has its polarity flipped relative to the input function *f(x)*. Finally, because the amplitude of the kernel has a magnitude of 0.5, the output function is scaled to be 50% of the amplitude of the input function (albeit in the negative direction due to the negative value of the kernel).

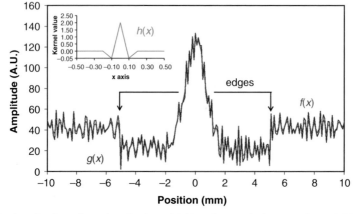

■ **FIGURE G-2** The role of an edge-enhancing kernel, *h(x)*, is illustrated. The original signal *f(x)* was convolved with *h(x)*, resulting in the noisier function *g(x)*. While *g(x)* is noisier than the original function, the two edges (*arrows*) have also been enhanced.

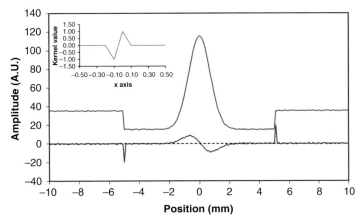

■ **FIGURE G-3** This figure illustrates the original signal (*blue*) with only a small amount of noise, and the kernel (**inset**) was used to compute the derivative signal (*red*). The numerical derivative was computed using convolution.

G.2 The Fourier Transform

In the analysis of time-based signals, the Fourier transform converts from the time domain (x-axis labeled in seconds) to the temporal frequency domain (x-axis labeled in sec^{-1}). While time-series analysis has applications in radiological imaging in ultrasound Doppler and magnetic resonance imaging, here we focus on input signals that are in the spatial domain (x-axis labeled typically in mm), which is pertinent to any anatomical medical image. The Fourier transform of a spatial domain signal converts it to the *spatial frequency* domain (x-axis labeled in mm^{-1}).

The one-dimensional Fourier transform of a spatial domain signal input function $f(x)$ is given by

$$F(v) = \int_{-\infty}^{\infty} f(x)\, e^{-2\pi i v x}\, dx \qquad \text{[G-2a]}$$

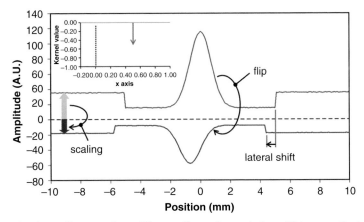

■ **FIGURE G-4** This figure illustrates three different effects of convolution—(1) because the total amplitude of the kernel was negative, the convolved function is flipped downward relative to the input signal (i.e., it has become negative); (2) because the amplitude of the kernel was 0.5, the convolved function has half of the (negative) amplitude as the original; and (3) because the δ-*function* used (see kernel—**inset**) was shifted from zero, the convolved function is shifted laterally compared to the original function.

where $F(v)$ is the Fourier transform of $f(x)$ and is in the units of amplitude versus spatial frequency $v(\text{mm}^{-1})$, and where i is equal to $\sqrt{-1}$. As with convolution, the Fourier transform can be performed in two dimensions as described by

$$F(v, \upsilon) = \int_{y=-\infty}^{\infty} \int_{x=-\infty}^{\infty} f(x, y)\, e^{-2\pi i (vx + \upsilon y)} \, dx \, dy \qquad \text{[G-2b]}$$

Three-dimensional Fourier transforms can also be performed. For simplicity, only one-dimensional Fourier transforms are described below. The shorthand notation for the Fourier transform in Equation G-2a is given by

$$F(v) = FT[f(x)] \qquad \text{[G-3a]}$$

Of course, other functions such as $h(x)$ can be transformed as well:

$$H(v) = FT[h(x)] \qquad \text{[G-3b]}$$

Multiplication of the two frequency domain functions $F(v)$ and $H(v)$ is the equivalent of convolution in the spatial domain,

$$G(v) = F(v) \times H(v) \qquad \text{[G-4]}$$

except that the product $G(v)$ then needs to be converted back to the spatial domain using the inverse Fourier transform (shorthand $FT^{-1}[]$):

$$g(x) = \int_{-\infty}^{\infty} G(v)\, e^{2\pi i x v} \, dv \qquad \text{[G-5]}$$

Notice that the use of the Fourier transform and its inverse in Equations G-3a, G-3b, G-4, and G-5 provides the same result as the convolution function described in Equation G-1a. Explicitly:

$$g(x) = f(x) \otimes h(x) = FT^{-1}\left\{ FT[f(x)] \times FT[h(x)] \right\} \qquad \text{[G-6]}$$

For most applications, the implementation of these equations in a computer is faster using Fourier transforms* than using convolution, and this has led to the widespread use of the Fourier transform in image processing, image reconstruction, and other image analysis operations.

G.3 The Fourier Transform in Filtered Backprojection

The purpose of this section is to tie the discussion of convolution and Fourier transforms into previous discussions on filtered backprojection in tomographic reconstruction (Chapters 10 and 19). The backprojection procedure results in a characteristic $1/r$ blurring phenomenon, and the filtering procedure in filtered backprojection is the mathematical operation described in Equation G-6 that corrects for this $1/r$ blurring. In the case of filtered backprojection, $h(x)$ is a convolution kernel that corrects for the $1/r$ blurring—and hence it can be called a deconvolution kernel. Deconvolution simply refers to convolution when it is used to correct for a specific effect (such as blurring). In the image reconstruction literature, it is common to talk about the filtering function $h(x)$ in the frequency domain, that is, $FT(h(x))$ or $H(v)$. As was seen in Chapter 10, $h(x)$ is an edge-enhancing kernel, more complicated (and wider in terms

---

*The Fast Fourier Transform is the principal tool used for computer implementation of the Fourier Transform, as it achieves computational efficiency over a general Discrete Fourier Transform.

of number of elements) but similar conceptually to that shown here in Figure G-2. In the frequency domain, $H(v)$ is a ramp filter that in clinical CT imaging always has an additional high-frequency roll-off term as well. Thus, $H(v) = R(v) A(v)$, where $R(v)$ is the RAMP filter (thus $R(v) = \alpha v$, where α is a scalar) and $A(v)$ is an apodization filter that approaches zero as v approaches the Nyquist frequency.

G.4 The Fourier Transform and the Modulation Transfer Function

The rigorous assessment of spatial resolution as discussed in Chapter 4 involves the measurement of the modulation transfer function (MTF) of an imaging system. There are several approaches to this, but the most widely used method is to measure the line spread function $l(x)$, and from it, the $MTF(f)$ is computed. In this section, more details about this process are provided. The line spread function (LSF) $l(x)$ is measured or synthesized as discussed in Chapter 4. Here we show the analytic description of MTF calculation, but in most practical situations, computer programs are used that perform the mathematics in a discrete manner—using a computer.

The first step of MTF assessment is to normalize the area of $l(x)$ to unity:

$$1 = \int_{-\infty}^{\infty} l(x)\, dx \qquad \text{[G-7]}$$

The Fourier transform of the line spread function is then computed, resulting in the optical spread function, $OTF(f)$.

$$OTF(f) = \int_{-\infty}^{\infty} l(x)\, e^{-2\pi i f x}\, dx \qquad \text{[G-8]}$$

The line spread function is a real function, whereas the $OTF(f)$ is a complex function; that is, it has real and imaginary components. As a reminder, a complex number c has a real component a and an imaginary component b, where $c = a + bi$, and as mentioned earlier, $i = \sqrt{-1}$. The $MTF(f)$ is computed as the modulus of the OTF(f):

$$MTF(f) = \sqrt{\Re\{OTF(f)\}^2 + \Im\{OTF(f)\}^2} \qquad \text{[G-9]}$$

where $\Re\{OTF(f)\}$ is the real component of the OTF and $\Im\{OTF(f)\}$ is the imaginary component. With this transformation, the MTF(f) represents the modulus of the OTF and as such is a real function. Another way to write Equation F-9 is

$$MTF(f) = \|OTF(f)\| \qquad \text{[G-10]}$$

Because of the properties of the Fourier transform, since $l(x)$ is normalized to 1.0, the $MTF(f)$ value at $f = 0$ is also unity, that is, $MTF(0) = 1$.

Fourier Transform Pairs

A set of three line spread functions is shown in Figure G-5. These $l(x)$ plots corresponding loosely to those for three imaging modalities—analog screen film radiography (curve A), computed tomography (curve B), and single photon emission computed tomography (SPECT, curve C). The full width at half maximum of these curves is approximately 0.14, 0.6, and 6 mm, respectively. The MTFs of these three $l(x)$ curves are shown in Figure G-6. It can be seen that the widest $l(x)$ (curve C) in Figure G-5 has the worst MTF in Figure G-6. Note that the limiting resolution for the three MTFs shown in Figure G-6 (at the 5% dashed line) corresponds approximately to 0.2, 1.4, and 6.6 mm^{-1}.

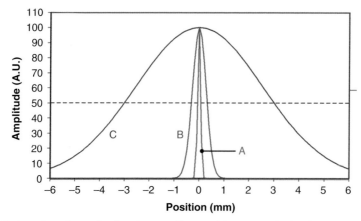

■ **FIGURE G-5** A number of gaussian functions are illustrated (A, B, and C). This figure shows the gaussian functions in the spatial domain, and these functions could represent line spread functions.

Gaussian

The Fourier transform of a gaussian is also a gaussian. Because the line spread function in many settings is well approximated by a gaussian function, that example will be used here to illustrate the utility of Fourier transform pairs.

Let the spatial domain function $l(x)$ be given by

$$l(x) = e^{-(\pi x^2)/a^2} \qquad \text{[G-11a]}$$

where a is a constant that affects the width of the line spread function. The analytical Fourier transform of Equation G-11a is given by

$$MTF(v) = a\,e^{-\pi v^2 a^2} \qquad \text{[G-11b]}$$

where the value of a in Equation G-11b is the same as that in Equation G-11a for the Fourier transform pair. The LSF/MTF curves shown in Figures G-5 and G-6 (respectively) were produced with values of a corresponding to 0.15, 0.68, and 6.0 (for curves A, B, and C as labeled in these figures).

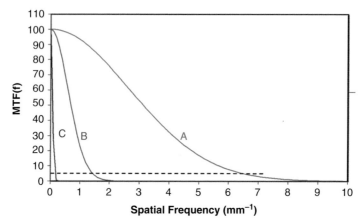

■ **FIGURE G-6** These gaussian functions are the Fourier transforms of the gaussian functions seen in Figure G-5. Notice that the widest gaussian in Figure G-5 results in the narrowest function on this plot. While the relationship between the gaussian functions shown in Figure G-5 and their FT counterparts in this figure is general and illustrates Fourier transform pairs, if the functions in Figure G-5 were line spread functions, then the functions illustrated here in Figure G-6 are the corresponding MTFs.

The LSF/MTFs shown in Figures G-5 and G-6 were meant to illustrate the use of the Fourier transform in image science, but they also illustrate gaussian Fourier transform pairs. It should be noted that gaussian FT pairs are not limited to LSFs and MTFs, but rather this is a general relationship. In addition, there are many LSFs and MTFs that do not fit a gaussian function.

RECT

The rectangle function, or $RECT\left(\dfrac{x}{a}\right)$, is a commonly used function in image science—in the absence of other sources of blur, the $RECT\left(\dfrac{x}{a}\right)$ function describes how a detector element (dexel) of width a integrates a signal incident upon it. $RECT\left(\dfrac{x}{a}\right)$ is defined by

$$RECT\left(\frac{x}{a}\right) = 1,\ |x| < \frac{a}{2} \qquad\qquad \text{[G-12]}$$
$$= 0,\ elsewhere$$

With this definition, the limits of integration of the Fourier transform can be modified resulting in the following analytical derivation:

$$F(v) = \int_{-\infty}^{\infty} RECT\left(\frac{x}{a}\right) e^{-2\pi i v x}\, dx = \int_{-a/2}^{a/2} e^{-2\pi i v x}\, dx = \frac{\sin(\pi a v)}{\pi v} \qquad \text{[G-13]}$$

The *SINC* function is defined as

$$SINC(x) = \frac{\sin(\pi x)}{\pi x} \qquad\qquad \text{[G-14]}$$

And thus Equation G-13 can be written as

$$F(v) = a\ SINC(av) \qquad\qquad \text{[G-15]}$$

The above derivation illustrates that $RECT\left(\dfrac{x}{a}\right)$ and $SINC(v)$ are Fourier transform pairs.

The SINC function is shown in Figure G-7, for different RECT apertures. As the aperture (a) gets smaller, the RECT function (detector element in this example) gets narrower, and

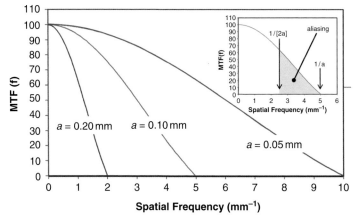

■ **FIGURE G-7** The analytical Fourier transform of a RECT function is SINC, and three SINC functions are illustrated in this figure. The SINC is the theoretically best physical MTF that can be achieved with a rectangular-shaped detector element with a given width a.

the spatial resolution (MTF) improves. Figure G-7 illustrates the MTF curves for rectangular detector element apertures corresponding to 0.05, 0.10, and 0.20 mm in width (value of a). Indirect detector systems that use an x-ray phosphor have other significant sources of resolution loss (optical blur), but for direct x-ray detectors, the RECT function characterizes the detector's response to the incident x-ray beam and thus the SINC function approximates the MTF of indirect detector systems. An MTF described by SINC reaches MTF(f) = 0 at $1/a$, whereas the Nyquist frequency (see Chapter 4) is given by $F_n = 1/(2a)$. This is shown in the inset in Figure G-7. For direct detector x-ray systems, the near SINC MTF results in potential signal intensity up to $1/a$, whereas all frequencies above $1/(2a)$ will be aliased.

Digital Sampling and Aliasing

A linear detector array with center-to-center spacing between dexels of Δ can be thought of as an array of delta functions (δ-functions) separated by a distance Δ (Fig. G-8). Mathematically, a "comb" of δ-functions describes this:

$$s(x) = \sum_{j=0}^{n} \delta(x - j\Delta) \qquad [\text{G-16}]$$

It is noted that $\delta(0) = 1$, and $\delta(x) = 0$ when $x \neq 0$. Using (for example) a rectangular sampling aperture of width a, $RECT\left(\dfrac{x}{a}\right)$, the digital sampling function, $g(x)$, is the convolution between these terms:

$$g(x) = s(x) \otimes RECT\left(\frac{x}{a}\right) \qquad [\text{G-16}]$$

Figure G-8A illustrates the comb of δ-functions with sampling interval Δ. Figure G-8B shows two different RECT functions, of width $a = \Delta$ and $b = 2\Delta$. Figure G-8C illustrates the combined effects of the aperture a and sampling interval Δ, as described

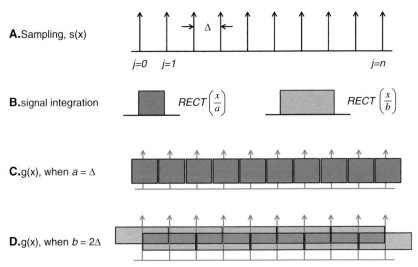

■ **FIGURE G-8 A** Illustrates the sampling of a detector system with a center-to-center spacing of Δ, represented as a *comb* of δ-functions. **B** shows the RECT aperture detector elements of width a (where a = Δ, and widith b, where b = 2 Δ). A contiguous detector array is shown in (**C**) where $\Delta = a$, and there are real examples of this in direct detection x-ray imaging. The function shown in (**D**) shows a nonphysical detector where the aperture width b = 2Δ. The consequences of this situation are shown in Figure G-9B.

by Equation G-16. Figure G-8D illustrates the shape of $g(x)$ when the sampling comb is convolved with the aperture function given by $RECT\left(\dfrac{x}{b}\right)$.

Figure G-9A shows the frequency domain interpretation of Figure G-8C, the Fourier transform of $g(x)$ in Equation G-16. The comb of δ-functions in the spatial domain separated by a sampling interval of Δ becomes a comb of δ-functions separated by $1/\Delta$ in the frequency domain. As seen in Figure G-7, the SINC function has nonzero amplitude to $1/a$, and so when $a = \Delta$ as in Figure G-9A, the MTF values overlap between samples and this means that aliasing can occur. Although the sampling scenario illustrated in Figure G-8D is not practical physically (except as proposed by Rowlands), it represents an optimal approach to the management of aliasing. Because the wider detector element results in more blurring of the detected signal, the magnitude of the MTF is degraded at higher spatial frequencies such that it reaches zero at the Nyquist frequency, and this is shown in Figure G-9B. In this situation, aliasing cannot occur because signal amplitude becomes zero above the Nyquist frequency. While aliasing is eliminated, the MTF is reduced and therefore the spatial resolution of the imaging system is degraded relative to that shown in Figure G-9A. Aliasing is most problematic in terms of a radiological signal when that signal is periodic in nature, such as the x-ray shadow of an antiscatter grid. It is recognized that Figure G-9A also allows periodic components of image noise to be aliased, meaning that high frequency image noise will wrap around the Nyquist frequency and increase noise levels in the image.

It is noted that in the case of indirect x-ray imaging systems that use an x-ray scintillator, the optical blurring that occurs in the system degrades the MTF at high spatial frequencies such that little if any signal amplitude exists above the Nyquist frequency. The influence of the optical blurring is to increase the effective aperture width, similar to that illustrated in Figure G-8D, although the blurring function is not RECT in shape.

G.5 Fourier Analysis of Noise: The Noise Power Spectrum

Image noise is measured in the absence of an object, so typically a constant image is produced by the imaging modality. Examples in radiography, mammography, or fluoroscopy would be air scans (no object), and in CT, a homogeneous cylinder of plastic

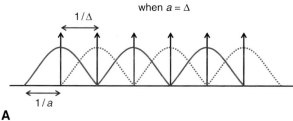

when $a = \Delta$

$1/\Delta$

$1/a$

A

■ **FIGURE G-9 A.** This figure shows the frequency domain consequences of the detector defined in Figure G-8C—a RECT aperture a sampled with a pitch of Δ where $a = \Delta$ **B.** This shows the frequency domain construct of function $g(x)$ shown in Figure G-8D, where $b = 2\Delta$. With this situation, the MTF approaches zero amplitude at the Nyquist frequency, eliminating the potential for aliasing.

when $b = 2\Delta$

$1/\Delta$

$1/b$

B

can be scanned. Every effort is made to make these images as "flat" as possible—one approach to "flatten" the image is to subtract two independently acquired images, and this reduces spatial bias due to the heel effect, inverse square law, or pincushion distortion effects. The variance of the noise on the subtracted image is divided by a factor of two in order to compensate for the noise propagation when two images

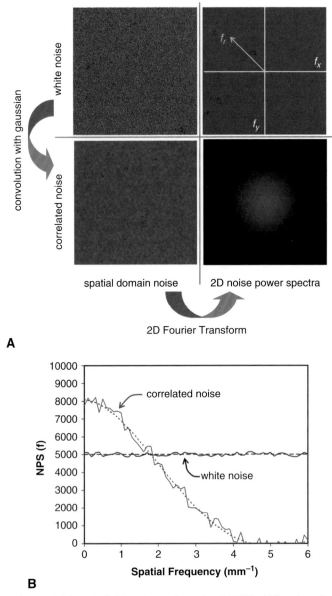

A

B

■ **FIGURE G-10 A.**The spatial domain (**left**) and two-dimensional $NPS(f_x, f_y)$ functions for two examples of noise are shown, white noise on the top row and correlated noise on the bottom row. Most imaging systems demonstrate correlated noise. The correlation was produced in this example by convolving the white noise example with a two-dimensional gaussian function. **B.** The two-dimensional NPS shown on the right side of (**A**) is radially symmetric, and this allows it to be integrated radially. Radial integration converts the function to a one-dimensional function, which is a function of frequency, as shown in (**B**). Here, two one-dimensional $NPS(f)$ functions are shown for the two-dimensional $NPS(f_x, f_y)$ shown in (**A**) (**top and bottom right side**). The $NPS(f)$ functions shown in this figure characterize the noise texture on an image.

are subtracted. In most settings, however, the NPS is measured on unsubtracted but sometimes detrended images. The NPS is computed as

$$NPS(f) \int_{-\infty}^{\infty} \left(I(x) - \bar{I} \right)^2 e^{-2\pi i f x} \, dx \qquad \text{[G-17]}$$

The integral of the NPS over all frequencies is the noise variance:

$$\sigma^2 = \int_{-\infty}^{\infty} NPS(f) \, df \qquad \text{[G-17]}$$

The variance describes the overall magnitude of the noise in an image, while the $NPS(f)$ is a measure of the noise texture, that is, the frequency-dependent character of the noise. Figure G-10 illustrates differences in noise texture. Figure G-10A illustrates white noise in the spatial domain, and the accompanying $NPS(f)$ is white as well. Figure G-10B illustrates noise that has a correlation structure in it, both in the spatial and the frequency domains. The spatial noise pattern in Figure G-10B was produced by convolving the noise pattern in Figure G-10A with an 11×11 gaussian. The $NPS(f)$ in Figure G-10B shows a bell shape, and indeed when radially averaged (Fig. G-10C), the $NPS(f)$ appears gaussian-like.

SUGGESTED READING

Barrett HH, Sindell W. *Radiological imaging: the theory of image formation, detection, and processing*, vol. 1, New York, NY: Academic Press, 1981.

Dainty JC, Shaw R. *Image science*. London: Academic Press, 1974.

Ji WG, Zhao W, Rowlands JA. Digital x-ray imaging using amorphous selenium: reduction of aliasing. *Med Phys* 1998;25(11):2148–2162.

Radiation Dose: Perspectives and Comparisons

Table H-1 provides the ICRP tissues and tissue weighting factors (w_T) that were used in the calculation of effective dose equivalent (H_E) in ICRP report 26 (ICRP 1977) and effective dose (E) in ICRP report 60 (ICRP 1990) and ICRP report 103 (ICRP 2007). Note that many of the effective dose estimates provided in Appendix E refer to references where the effective dose cited was that calculated using the previous (i.e., ICRP 60) system for effective dose and their associated tissue weighting factors. In some cases, the application of the ICRP 103 system to examinations provided in those tables will result in different (higher or lower) effective dose estimates.

Figure H-1 shows the relationships between the emission of radiation and the various quantities described in previous chapters to express radiation exposure; kerma; absorbed dose; equivalent dose (from which the dose to tissues and organs can be used along with other risk-modifying variables such as age at time of exposure and gender to estimate cancer incidence and mortality risk to an individual); and effective dose to the body, which can be used to estimate the stochastic health risk for a group that has the same general age and gender distribution as the general population.

Figure H-2 provides an example of estimated effective doses and weighted organ equivalent doses from some standard cardiac radionuclide and CT diagnostic studies using ICRP report 103 (2007) and ICRP report 60 tissue weighting factors.

Figure H-3 provides a comparison of estimated effective doses (mSv) for standard myocardial perfusion imaging protocols, determined with the use of ICRP and manufacturers' package insert dose coefficients.

Tables H-2 to H-4 and Figures H-4 and H-5 are presented to help put radiation exposure into perspective by providing examples of other sources of radiation, the doses from those sources as well as other public health risks, and their relative magnitude. Table H-2 provides information on doses from several sources of public and occupational radiation exposure. Table H-3 presents the estimated loss of life expectancy from several health risks including an estimate for the risk from background radiation. It is important to be aware of the assumptions incorporated into the values presented and limitations inherent in making risk comparisons (see table footnotes). Table H-4 provides some examples of the amount of radioactivity in various natural and artificially produced sources. Figure H-4 illustrates the variation in the annual effective dose from cosmic radiation in North America. Figure H-5 compares the average annual effective dose from natural background radiation sources in the United States to that of a number of European countries.

TABLE H-1   ICRP TISSUE WEIGHTING FACTORS w$_T$ (ICRP 1977; ICRP 1990; ICRP 2007)

ICRP REPORT	ICRP 26	ICRP 60	ICRP 103	ICRP 26	ICRP 60	ICRP 103
YEAR	1977	1990	2007	**Tissues Included in Remainder Tissues**		
Quantity	EDE	ED	ED	—	—	Adipose tissue
Tissue	Tissue Weighting Factors, w$_T$			—	Adrenals	Adrenals
Gonads	0.25	0.2	0.08	—	Brain	STWF
Breast	0.15	0.05	0.12	—	—	Connective tissue
Red bone marrow	0.12	0.12	0.12	—	—	Extrathoracic airways
Lung	0.12	0.12	0.12	—	—	Gall bladder
Thyroid	0.03	0.05	0.04	—	Brain	IMT
Bone surfaces	0.03	0.01	0.01	—	—	Heart wall
Colon	—	0.12	0.12	—	Kidney	Kidney
Stomach	—	0.12	0.12	—	—	Lymphatic nodes
Bladder	—	0.05	0.04	—	Muscle	Muscle
Esophagus	—	0.05	0.04	Liver	STWF	STWF
Liver	—	0.05	0.04	LLI	STWF	STWF
Brain	—	—	0.01	—	—	Pancreas
Salivary Glands	—	—	0.01	—	—	Prostate
Skin	—	0.01	0.01	SG	—	IMT
^{a}Remainder tissues	0.3	0.05	0.12	SI	SI	SI wall
Total	**1.0**	**1.0**	**1.0**	Stomach	STWF	STWF
				—	Spleen	Spleen
				—		Thymus
				ULI	ULI	STWF

^{a}Tissues selected to represent the remainder in ICRP reports 26, 60 and 103 are shown on the right side of the table.
EDE, Effective Dose Equivalent (H$_E$); ED, Effective Dose (E); STWF, See Tissue Weighting Factor Table; LLI, lower large intestine; SG, salivary glands; SI, small intestine; ULI, upper large intestine.
ICRP 26: ICRP Publication 26, Recommendations of the International Commission on Radiological Protection, Pergamon Press, Oxford, England (1977).
ICRP 60: International Commission on Radiological Protection. 1990 Recommendations of the International Commission on Radiological Protection, ICRP Publication 60, Ann.ICRP 21(1-3) (Elsevier, New York), (1991).
ICRP 103: The 2007 Recommendations of the International Commission on Radiological Protection. ICRP Publication 103. Ann ICRP 37, 1–332 (2007).

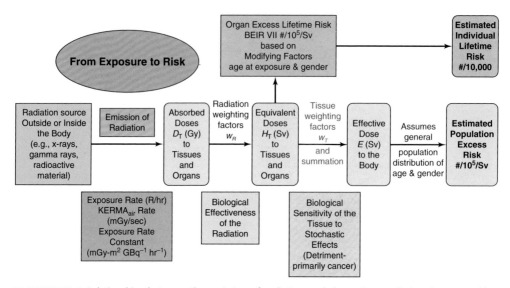

■ **FIGURE H-1** Relationships between the emission of radiation and the various radiation dose quantities described in Chapter 3 and discussed throughout the text. (Adapted from ICRP. The 2007 Recommendations of the International Commission on Radiological Protection, ICRP Publication 103. *Ann ICRP* 2007;37:1–332.)

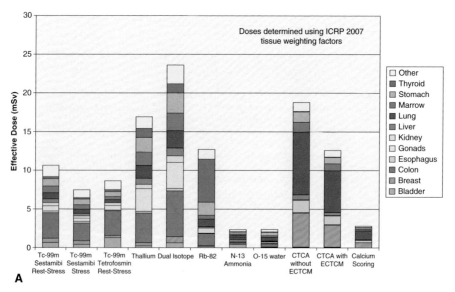

■ **FIGURE H-2** Estimated effective doses and weighted organ equivalent doses from cardiac radionuclide and CT studies. **A.** Doses determined using ICRP Publication 103 (2007) tissue weighting factors.

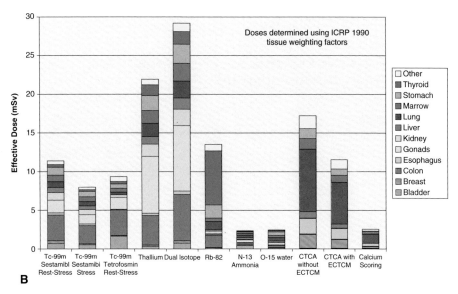

B

■ **FIGURE H-2** (*Continued*) **B.** Doses determined using ICRP Publication 60 (1990) tissue weighting factors. CTCA indicates 64-slice computed tomography coronary angiogram; CaSc, calcium scoring; and ECTCM, ECG-controlled tube current modulation. Calculations were performed with ImpactDose (VAMP GmbH, Erlangen, Germany); for Siemens Sensation 64 scanner with retrospective gating, voltage was 120 kVp, pitch 0.2, and scan length 15 cm. For CTCA, slice thickness was 0.6 mm and tube current-time product was 165 mAs; ECTCM was simulated by reducing tube current by a third, to 110 mAs. For CaSc, collimation was 20 × 1.2 mm, and tube current-time product was 27 mAs. Doses shown are arithmetic means of doses to standardized male and female phantoms. (From Einstein AJ, Moser KW, Thompson RC, et al. Radiation dose to patients from cardiac diagnostic imaging. *Circulation* 2007;116:1290–1305.)

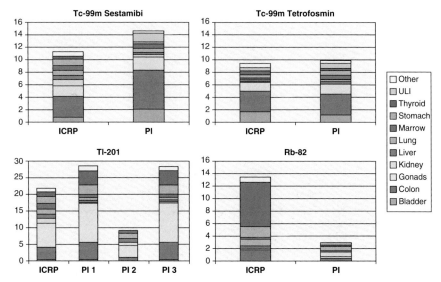

■ **FIGURE H-3** Comparison of estimated effective doses (mSv) for standard myocardial perfusion imaging protocols, determined with the use of ICRP and manufacturers' package insert dose coefficients. Weighted equivalent doses were determined with the use of ICRP Publication 60 tissue weighting factors. ULI indicates upper large intestine. Some notable differences exist between effective doses estimated with the use of ICRP dose coefficients and those estimated with the use of dose coefficients provided in package inserts (PI), as illustrated above. Most PIs were initially issued at the time of approval of a radiopharmaceutical, and dosimetry information included in subsequent revisions has not been updated to reflect new biokinetic data or changes in the ICRP dosimetry system. Note that in some cases there can also be substantial discordance in dose estimates between different manufactures' PIs (e.g., Tl-201). In general, the most recent ICRP data should be used for dosimetry estimates. PI should only be used as the source of dose information for new radiopharmaceuticals for which ICRP dosimetry data have not yet been published. (From Einstein AJ, Moser KW, Thompson RC, et al. Radiation dose to patients from cardiac diagnostic imaging. *Circulation* 2007;116:1290–1305.)

TABLE H-2 DOSES FROM SEVERAL SOURCES OF PUBLIC AND OCCUPATIONAL RADIATION EXPOSURE

RADIATION EXPOSURE	TYPICAL EFFECTIVE DOSE (mSv)
US annual average *per capita* dose from natural background radiation	3.1
US annual average *per capita* dose from medical radiation exposure	3
Total US annual average *per capita* dose from all sources	6.2
Commercial aviation aircrew average annual dose from cosmic radiation	3
Radiation workers annual average occupational dose	2–5
Whole body x-ray airport scanner (1 scan)	0.00003–0.0001
Flying on airplane at 35,000 ft (per minute)	0.00004

1. NCRP. National Council on Radiation Protection and Measurements. Ionizing Radiation Exposure of the Population of the United States, NCRP Report No. 160 National Council on Radiation Protection and Measurements, Bethesda, Maryland, 2009.
2. Commentary No. 16—Screening of Humans for Security Purposes Using Ionizing Radiation Scanning Systems. National Council on Radiation Protection & Measurements. Retrieved November 12, 2010.

TABLE H-3 ESTIMATED LOSS OF LIFE EXPECTANCY FROM HEALTH RISKS

[a]HEALTH RISK	ESTIMATES OF AVERAGE DAYS (YEARS) OF LIFE EXPECTANCY LOST
Smoking 20 cigarettes/d	2,250 (6.2 years)
All accidents combined	366 (1 year)
Auto accidents	207
Alcohol consumption	125
Home accidents	74
Drowning	24
Natural background radiation	30
Medical diagnostic x-rays	30

[a]With the exception of smoking, all risks are expressed as the loss of life expectancy averaged over the U.S. population.
Data from Cohen BL. Catalog of risks extended and updated. *Health Phys* 1991;61(3):317–335. It is important to note that there are a lot of assumptions that are incorporated into the numerical values presented in this table. The original text should be consulted for the details and caution should be exercised when comparing a risk from one source or activity to another (see: Covello, VT. Risk comparisons and risk communication: Issues and problems in comparing health and environmental risks. In Kasperson RE & Stallen PJM. (eds.), *Communicating risks to the public: International perspectives.* London, UK: Kluwer Academic. 1991:79–124. and Risk Communication, Risk Statistics, and Risk Comparisons: A Manual for Plant Managers by Vincent T. Covello, Peter M. Sandman, and Paul Slovic Washington, DC: Chemical Manufacturers Association, 1988 Appendix B Risk Comparison Tables and Figuresby Vincent T. Covello, Peter M. Sandman, and Paul Slovic accessed at http://www.psandman.com/articles/cma-appb.htm# on August 1, 2011.

TABLE H-4   RADIOACTIVITY OF SOME NATURAL AND OTHER MATERIALS

1 kg of granite	1,000 Bq	0.027 μCi
1 kg of coffee	1,000 Bq	0.03 μCi
1 kg of coal ash	2,000 Bq	0.054 μCi
The air in a 100 m² Australian home (radon)	3,000 Bq	0.08 μCi
1 kg superphosphate fertilizer	5,000 Bq	0.14 μCi
1 adult human (100 Bq/kg)	7,000 Bq	0.19 μCi
The air in many 100 m² European homes (radon)	up to 30,000 Bq	0.81 μCi
1 household smoke detector (with americium)	37 000 Bq	1.0 μCi
1 kg uranium	25 million Bq	676 μCi
Radioisotope for medical diagnosis	370 MBq	10 μCi
1 luminous exit sign (1970s)	1,000,000 million Bq (1 TBq)	27 Ci
Radioisotope source for medical radiotherapy (Gamma Knife)	222,222,222 million Bq (222 TBq)	6,000 Ci

Adapted from Hall E. *Radiation and Life*. 2nd ed. Pergamon Press, New York, 1984.

The annual outdoor effective dose (μSv) from cosmic radiation for Canada and the U.S.

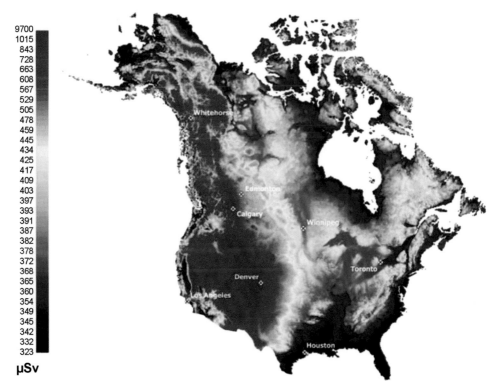

■ FIGURE H-4 Color plot of the annual outdoor effective dose from cosmic radiation (in microsievert) in North America. (Source: Grasty RL, Lamarre JR. The annual effective dose from natural sources of ionizing radiation in Canada. *Radiat Protect Dosim* 2004;108(3):215–226.)

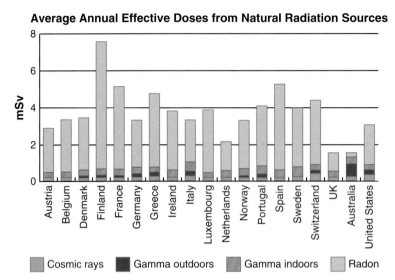

Average Annual Effective Doses from Natural Radiation Sources

■ FIGURE H-5 Examples of variation in natural background and the sources of the variation. (Adapted from Green BMR, Hughes JS, Lomas PR, et al. Natural radiation atlas of Europe. *Radiat Protect Dosim* 1992;45:491–493.)

APPENDIX

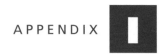

Radionuclide Therapy Home Care Guidelines

I.1 General Safety Guide for Outpatients Receiving Radioiodine Therapy: Less Than 10 mCi

The radioactive iodine that you have been treated with is for your benefit. You need to take some precautions so that others do not receive unnecessary radiation exposure.

A. Please follow the instructions below:
1. Breast feeding your infant must be discontinued.
2. Drink plenty of liquids.
3. Women of child bearing potential must have a negative pregnancy test prior to therapy. Results _____.

B. Please follow the steps below during the first 2 days after your treatment.
1. Most of the remaining radioiodine in your body will come out through the urine. A small portion of radioactivity will be found in your saliva and sweat. To decrease the spread of radioactivity:
   a. Use paper drinking cups, plates and plastic utensils. Put these items in the trash when you are done with them.
   b. Use towels and washcloth that only you will touch.
   c. You should sleep in a separate bed.
   d. At the end of 2 days wash your laundry separately. This need only be done once.
   e. Avoid touching and hugging babies and pregnant women.
2. Most of the radioactivity is in the urine during these first 2 days. If urine should be spilled or splashed, wash and rinse the affected area three times, using paper towels or tissue. Be sure to carefully wash your hands after using the bathroom.
3. Breast-Feeding: Breast-feeding must be discontinued. Your physician will advise you when you may resume.

C. During the rest of the week
Your body will still contain some radioactivity. Avoid sitting close to others for hours at a time. This will reduce their radiation exposure. Do not be concerned about being close to people for a few minutes. Avoid holding babies or young children for a long time each day.
If you have problems or questions about the above, please call: _____, M.D.

Nuclear Medicine Division — Ph. No._____

1005

I.2 **General Safety Guide for Outpatients Receiving Radioiodine Therapy: More Than 10 mCi**

The radioactive iodine that you have been treated with is for your benefit. You need to take some precautions so that others do not receive unnecessary radiation exposure.

A. Please follow the instructions below:

Young people are more sensitive to radiation. To minimize possible effects from radiation, do not hold children or spend time near pregnant women during the next week.

1. Go directly home. Do not stay at a hotel.
2. Sit as far from anyone as practical during your ride home from the hospital. Let us know if your trip is longer than 3 hours.
3. Breast feeding your infant must be discontinued.
4. Drink plenty of liquids.
5. Women of child bearing potential must have a negative pregnancy test prior to therapy. Results _____.

B. Please follow the steps below during the first 4 days after your treatment.

1. Most of the radioiodine in your body will come out in the urine and stool. A small portion of radioactivity will be found in your saliva and sweat. To decrease the spread of radioactivity:
   a. If possible, use a separate bath room.
   b. Flush the toilet two times after each use.
   c. Men should sit down when urinating.
   d. If urine is spilled/splashed, wash and rinse the spill area three times, using paper towels or tissue.
   e. Menstruating women should use tampons that can be flushed down the toilet.
   f. Be sure to carefully wash your hands after using the bathroom.
   g. Do not share utensils or food with others. (For example do not drink from the same glass or share a sandwich.)
   h. Use towels and washcloths that only you will touch.
   i. Run water in the sink while brushing your teeth or shaving and rinse the sink well after use.
   j. Nausea following therapy is very rare. However, if you feel sick to your stomach, try to vomit into the toilet. If necessary, wash and rinse any spill areas three times, using paper towel/tissue.
   k. At the end of 4 days wash your laundry, including the pillow cases, separately from others. This need only be done once.
2. To decrease the radiation exposure to others:
   a. You should sleep in a separate bed. Cover the pillow with two pillow cases or a water resistant cover if possible.
   b. Remain in your home for the first 4 days.
   c. Young people are more sensitive to radiation so do not hold children or spend time near pregnant women.
   d. Family members should stay six feet or more from you. After the first 2 days, they may be closer for brief periods such as a few minutes.
   e. Avoid sexual relations.

C. **Please follow the steps below until the end of the first week after your treatment.**
Your body will still contain some radioactivity. To minimize radiation exposure to other people, you should:
1. Avoid sitting close (within a foot) to others for hours at a time.
2. Minimize use of public transportation (bus, airplane, etc.) and going to public gatherings such as movies, plays, etc. Do not be concerned about being close to people for short times (less than an hour).
3. To minimize possible effects from radiation, avoid holding babies or children.

D. **Please follow the steps below for the next 6 to 12 months**
1. Avoid becoming pregnant for the next 12 months or fathering a child for the next 6 months.
2. If you are hospitalized or require emergency medical treatment within the next 2 weeks, please inform the doctor or nurse that you have been treated with _____ mCi of radioactive iodine on _____. Please contact the Nuclear Medicine Department at _____ as soon as possible. After hours, call the hospital operator at _____ and ask for the Nuclear Medicine on-call physician.

_____, M.D.   _____, M.D.

Nuclear Medicine Physician Signature   Nuclear Medicine Physician Printed Name

Date: _____

I understand the above instructions which have been discussed with me and I agree to follow them.

_____   _____

        Patient's Signature   Date

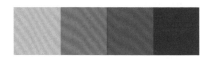

Index

(Note: Page numbers followed by *f* indicate figures; page numbers followed by *t* indicate tables)

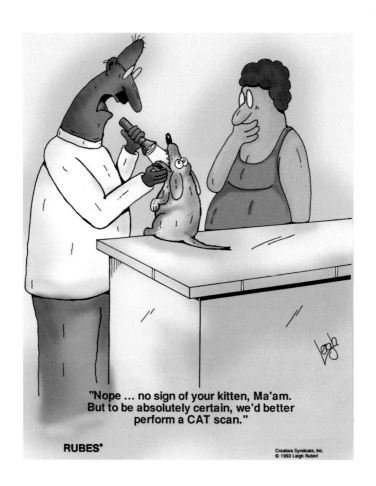

"Nope ... no sign of your kitten, Ma'am.
But to be absolutely certain, we'd better
perform a CAT scan."

RUBES®